CONTENTS

UNIT I INTRODUCTION TO PHARMACOLOGY

UNIT II A NURSE'S PERSPECTIVE OF PHARMACOLOGY

UNIT III DRUG CALCULATIONS

UNIT IV NUTRITION AND ELECTROLYTES

UNIT V AUTONOMIC NERVOUS SYSTEM AGENTS

UNIT VI NEUROLOGIC AND NEUROMUSCULAR AGENTS

UNIT VII PAIN AND INFLAMMATION MANAGEMENT AGENTS

UNIT VIII PSYCHIATRIC AGENTS

UNIT IX ANTIBACTERIAL AND ANTIINFECTIVE AGENTS

UNIT X ADDITIONAL ANTIINFECTIVE AGENTS

PHARMACOLOGY

A Patient-Centered Nursing Process Approach

8e

Joyce LeFever Kee, MS, RN
Associate Professor Emerita
School of Nursing
College of Health Sciences
University of Delaware
Newark, Delaware

Evelyn R. Hayes, PhD, MPH, FNP-BC
Professor
School of Nursing
College of Health Sciences
University of Delaware
Newark, Delaware

Linda E. McCuistion, PhD, RN, CNS
Professor
South University
Richmond Campus
Richmond, Virginia

ELSEVIER

ELSEVIER
SAUNDERS

3251 Riverport Lane
St. Louis, Missouri 63043

PHARMACOLOGY: A PATIENT-CENTERED NURSING PROCESS APPROACH
ISBN: 978-1-4557-5148-8

Library of Congress Cataloging-in-Publication Data

Kee, Joyce LeFever, author.
Pharmacology : a patient-centered nursing process approach / Joyce LeFever Kee, Evelyn R. Hayes, Linda E. McCuistion ; section editor, Marilyn Herbert-Ashton.—8th edition.
p. ; cm.
Previous edition has subtitle: "a nursing process approach."
Includes bibliographical references and index.
ISBN 978-1-4557-5148-8 (pbk. : alk. paper)
I. Hayes, Evelyn R., author. II. McCuistion, Linda E., author. III. Title.
[DNLM: 1. Pharmacological Phenomena—Nurses' Instruction. 2. Drug Therapy—Nurses' Instruction. 3. Patient-Centered Care—Nurses' Instruction. 4. Pharmaceutical Preparations—Nurses' Instruction. QV 4]
RM301
615.5′8—dc23

2013038375

Executive Content Strategist: Lee Henderson
Content Manager: Jennifer Ehlers
Publishing Services Manager: Jeff Patterson
Project Manager: Clay S. Broeker
Design Direction: Amy Buxton

Printed in Canada

Last digit is the print number: 9 8 7 6 5 4 3 2 1

In loving memory of my parents, Esther B. and Samuel H. LeFever
Joyce LeFever Kee

In loving memory of my parents, Margaret and Justin Hayes,
and in gratitude for the support of my family
Evelyn R. Hayes

To Dr. Gerald DeLuca for expert guidance,
and in memory of my parents, Otto and Pauline Schmidt
Linda E. McCuistion

MEET THE AUTHORS

JOYCE LEFEVER KEE

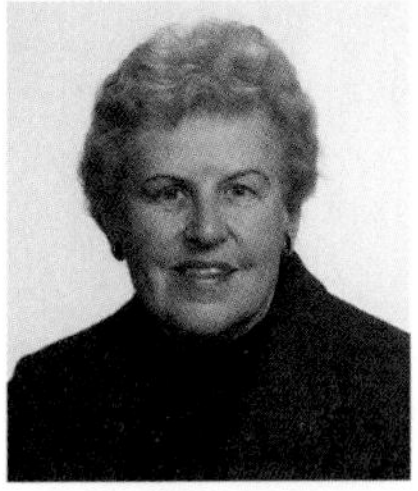

Joyce LeFever Kee received her Bachelor of Science and Master of Science degrees in Nursing from the University of Maryland and earned 36 postgraduate credits from the University of Delaware. She was a distinguished faculty educator at the University of Maryland for 4 years and at the University of Delaware for 27 years.

Joyce is a member of the Sigma Theta Tau Nursing Honor Society and Phi Kappa Phi Honor Society. She received the Excellence in Teaching Award from and was inducted into the Mentor's Circle at the University of Delaware.

Joyce gave numerous lectures and presentations throughout the United States from 1970 to 1990. She has written various articles, particularly on fluids and electrolytes, laboratory and diagnostic tests, and research projects, in the *American Journal of Nursing, Nursing Clinics of North America, Nursing Journal,* and *Critical Care Quarterly.* She has participated in several research studies on "Identification of Hypertensive Young Adults."

Joyce has authored and coauthored several text and reference books, including *Fluids and Electrolytes with Clinical Applications*, eighth edition; *Handbook of Fluid, Electrolyte, and Acid-Base Imbalances,* third edition; *Clinical Calculations in General and Specialty Areas,* seventh edition; *Laboratory and Diagnostic Tests with Nursing Implications,* ninth edition; and *Handbook of Laboratory and Diagnostic Tests with Nursing Implications,* seventh edition.

Joyce and her husband enjoy traveling all over the world.

EVELYN R. HAYES

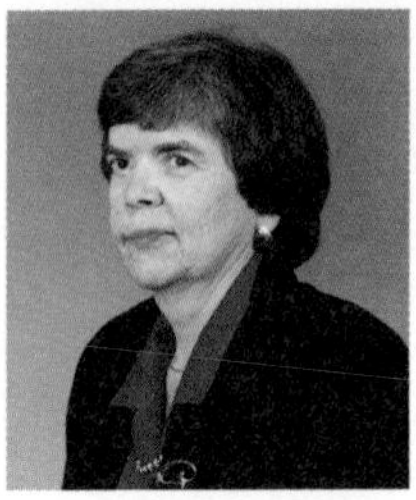

Evelyn (Lyn) R. Hayes received her Bachelor of Science in Nursing from Cornell University—New York Hospital School of Nursing; an MPH in Public Health Nursing from the University of North Carolina, School of Public Health, in Chapel Hill, North Carolina; and a PhD in Higher Education from Boston College. In addition, she completed a Post Master's Certificate as Family Nurse Practitioner at the University of Massachusetts at Amherst and is a certified family nurse practitioner. Her professional practice experience includes both acute care institutions and the community setting. Currently she is a Professor in the School of Nursing, College of Health Sciences, at the University of Delaware. In this role, she has vast experience with a variety of teaching modalities at both the undergraduate and graduate levels and experience with distance learning. Reflective of a global focus, Lyn has provided consultation to university faculty in Taiwan and Panama.

A strong advocate of health promotion, Lyn served as Project Director and co-investigator of a U.S. Public Health Service grant promoting healthy lifestyles in Delaware. She was a finalist for the Excellence in Community Based Nursing Practice Award sponsored by the Delaware Nurses Association and Delaware Organization of Nurse Executives.

As author, coauthor, and collaborative team member, she has published in multiple journals. Research interests include smoking cessation in teens and young adults, online caregiver support groups, and the meaning of storytelling of military experience by veterans at end of life. In addition, Lyn has made multiple presentations at regional, national, and international professional meetings.

Throughout her career, Lyn has assumed member and leadership positions at various levels within the University of Delaware as well as professional and community organizations. She ably provides long-term service and leadership to Sigma Theta Tau International, the American Nurses Association, the National League for Nursing Accrediting Commission (NLNAC), and the Delaware Nurses Association.

Now a retired colonel in the United States Army Reserve, Lyn's last assignment was as Principal Reservist to Deputy Commander for Nursing, Walter Reed Army Medical Center, Washington, DC. When at her home base, she enjoys being creative with crafts and spending time with family and friends.

LINDA E. MCCUISTION

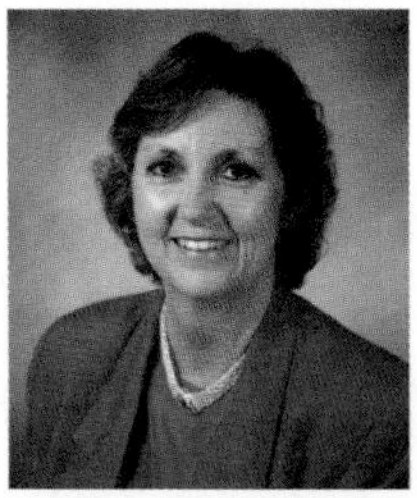

Dr. Linda E. McCuistion received a Diploma of Nursing from the Lutheran Hospital School of Nursing in Fort Wayne, Indiana; Bachelor of Science in Nursing from William Carey College in Hattiesburg, Mississippi; Masters in Nursing from Louisiana State University Medical Center; and PhD in Curriculum and Instruction from the University of New Orleans. She was licensed as an Advanced Practice Nurse in Louisiana and has many years of nursing experience, including acute care and home health nursing. For 20 years, Linda was a Nursing Professor at Our Lady of Holy Cross College in New Orleans, Louisiana. She received an Endowed Professorship Award in 2000 and 2003. Linda is currently a Nursing Professor at South University, Richmond, Virginia.

Linda has served as a past president, vice president, and faculty advisor of the Sigma Theta Tau International Honor Society in Nursing, Xi Psi chapter-at-large. She is a past associate editor of the *NODNA Times,* a New Orleans District Nurses' Association newsletter. She has been a member of Phi Delta Kappa and The American Society of Hypertension.

Linda was coordinator for the Graduate Plus Internship Program, a preceptorship program for new nursing graduates in the state of Louisiana. She has served as a legal nurse consultant; a member of a medical review panel; advisory board member, consultant, and reviewer of a software preparation company focused on the state licensure examination; advisory board member for a school for surgical technicians; and consultant to a local hospital to improve the quality of nursing care and assist acute care facilities in preparation for accreditation.

Linda was chosen as a "Great One Hundred Nurse" by the New Orleans District Nurses' Association in 1993. She is also listed in the 2005/2006 edition of the Empire Who's Who Executive and Professional Registry.

Linda has given numerous lectures and presentations regionally and nationally on a variety of nursing topics. She has published articles in nursing journals and authored many chapters in several nursing textbooks, including *Pharmacotherapeutics: Clinical Decision-Making in Nursing* (1999), *Saunders Manual of Medical-Surgical Nursing: A Guide for Clinical Decision-Making* (2002), and the *Saunders Nursing Survival Guide: Pathophysiology* (2007). She is author and coauthor of many chapters and co-editor of the *Saunders Nursing Survival Guide: Pharmacology* (2007).

Linda enjoys cruises and other travel. When at home, she enjoys family, friends, crafts, golf, and writing.

CONTRIBUTORS

Section Editor

Marilyn Herbert-Ashton, MS, RN, BC
Associate Professor
Director of Grants Development and Special Projects
Virginia Western Community College
Roanoke, Virginia

Contributors to the Textbook

Joseph Boullata, PharmD, RPh, BCNSP
Professor of Pharmacology and Therapeutics
School of Nursing
University of Pennsylvania
Pharmacy Specialist in Clinical Nutrition Support
Hospital of the University of Pennsylvania
Philadelphia, Pennsylvania
Tables 6–2 and 6–3

Jacqueline Rosenjack Burchum, DNSc, FNP-BC, CNE
Associate Professor, College of Nursing
Department of Advanced Practice and Doctoral Studies
University of Tennessee Health Science Center
Memphis Tennessee
Chapter 49

Karen Carmody, MSN, RN, FNP-BC
Family Nurse Practitioner
Limestone Medical Aid Unit
Wilmington, Delaware
Chapter 57

Robin Webb Corbett, PhD, RNC
Associate Professor
East Carolina University
Greenville, North Carolina
Chapters 53, 54, and 55

Janice Heinssen, MSN, FNP-BC, AAHIVS
Nurse Practitioner/Clinical Coordinator
Christiana Care Health Services HIV Early Intervention Services
Wilmington, Delaware
Chapter 35

Marilyn Herbert-Ashton, MS, RN, BC
Associate Professor
Director of Grants Development and Special Projects
Virginia Western Community College
Roanoke, Virginia
Chapters 1 and 24

Judith W. Herrman, PhD, RN
Professor
School of Nursing
University of Delaware
Newark, Delaware
Chapter 8

Bettyrae Jordan, MA, MEd, RN
Professor of Nursing
Instructor of Anthropology
Delgado Community College
New Orleans, Louisiana
Chapter 3

Robert J. Kizior, BS, RPh
Educational Coordinator
Alexian Brothers Medical Center
Elk Grove Village, Illinois
Chapter 35

Linda Laskowski-Jones, MS, RN, ACNS-BC, CEN, FAWN
Vice President
Emergency and Trauma Services
Christiana Care Health System
Newark, Delaware
Chapter 59

Ronald J. Lefever, RPh
Lead Pharmacist
VCU Medical Center
Ashland, Virginia
Appendix B

Patricia Lincoln, RN, BSN, ACRN
Site Director
Delaware Local Performance Site of the Pennsylvania/Mid-Atlantic AIDS Education and Training Center
Christiana Care Health Services
Wilmington, Delaware
Chapter 35

Jane F. Marek, MSN, DNP, RN
Instructor of Nursing
Frances Payne Bolton School of Nursing
Case Western Reserve University
Cleveland, Ohio
Chapter 16

Laura K. Williford Owens, PharmD, AAHIVP
Chief of Pharmacy Services
Carolina Family Health Centers, Inc.
Wilson, North Carolina
Chapters 53, 54, and 55

Carolee A. Polek, RN, PhD, AOCNS
Associate Professor
University of Delaware
Newark, Delaware
Chapters 37, 38, and 39

Patricia Smart, RN-BC, MN, CNE
Professor of Nursing
Delgado Community College
New Orleans, Louisiana
Selected NCLEX® Study Questions

Donald L. Taylor, MS, RN, PMHNP-BC
Instructor
Advanced Practice Nursing
School of Nursing
Department of Psychiatry
School of Medicine
Oregon Health and Science University
Portland, Oregon
Chapter 5

Lynette M. Wachholz, MN, PNP-C
Clinical Instructor
University of Washington
Department of Family and Child Nursing
Seattle, Washington
Pediatric Nurse Practitioner and Quality Program Manager
The Everett Clinic
Everett, Washington
Chapter 36

Marcia Welsh, CNM, MSN, DL
Assistant Professor
School of Nursing
University of Delaware
Newark, Delaware
Chapters 56 and 58

Contributors to the Teaching and Learning Resources

Valerie O'Toole Baker, ACNS, BC
Assistant Professor
Villa Maria School of Nursing
Morosky College of Health Professions and Sciences
Gannon University
Erie, Pennsylvania
PowerPoint Collection

Tim J. Bristol, PhD, RN, CNE, ANEF
Faculty Development, Owner
NurseTim, Inc.
TEACH® for Nurses *Lesson Plans*

Nancy Haugen, PhD, RN
Associate Professor and ABSN Program Chair
School of Nursing
Samuel Merritt University
Oakland, California
Pharmacology Online

Kathryn Schartz, BSN, MSN, RN, APRN, PNP-BC
Advanced Practice Registered Nurse
Assistant Professor of Nursing
Baker University School of Nursing
Topeka, Kansas
Test Bank

Allison Terry, PhD, MSN, RN
Associate Professor of Nursing
Auburn University at Montgomery
Montgomery, Alabama
Review Questions for the NCLEX® Examination

Jennifer J. Yeager, PhD-c, RN
Assistant Professor
Department of Nursing
Tarleton State University
Stephenville, Texas
Downloadable Key Points

REVIEWERS

Marilyn L. Adair, MSN, RN
Professor of Nursing
South Puget Sound Community College
Olympia, Washington

Zenesha R. Barkley, DNP, MSN
Instructor
Bethune-Cookman University
Daytona Beach, Florida

Katherine L. Byar, MSN, ANP, BC
Hematological Nurse Practitioner
University of Nebraska Medical Center
Omaha, Nebraska

Cheryl Cassis, MSN, RN
Professor of Nursing
Belmont College
St. Clairsville, Ohio

Sandra Fleischmann, MSN, RN
Nursing Instructor
Southern Vermont College
Bennington, Vermont

Margie L. Francisco, MSN, RN
Nursing Professor
Illinois Valley Community College
Oglesby, Illinois

Kathy L. Ham, RN, EdD
Associate Professor
Southeast Missouri State University
Cape Girardeau, Missouri

Jacqulene Pick Harris, MSN, APRN
Instructor
Benedictine College
Atchison, Kansas

Pamela M. Hendricks, RN, MS
Instructor
Blackhawk Technical College
Janesville, Wisconsin

Marilyn Herbert-Ashton, MS, RN, BC
Associate Professor
Director of Grants Development and Special Projects
Virginia Western Community College
Roanoke, Virginia

Lisa Hollett, RN, BSN, CFN
Trauma Program Manager
St. John Medical Center
Tulsa, Oklahoma

Abbie Lovatt, RN, BN
Nursing Instructor
Bow Valley College
Calgary, Alberta
Canada

Joshua J. Neumiller, PharmD, CDE, FASCP
Assistant Professor
Pharmacotherapy Department
Washington State University
Spokane, Washington

Diana Rangaves, PharmD
Director Pharmacy Technology Program
Santa Rosa Junior College
Santa Rosa, California

Harsha Sharma, PhD
Associate Professor
Nebraska Methodist College
Omaha, Nebraska

Rebecca L. Tyree, BSN, RN
Resource Nurse
Centra Health
Lynchburg, Virginia

Lisa Van Cleave, MSN, RN, CCRN
Assistant Professor
Patty Hanks Shelton School of Nursing
Abilene, Texas

PREFACE

The eighth edition of *Pharmacology: A Patient-Centered Nursing Process Approach* is written for students in a variety of nursing programs who can benefit from its presentation of the principles of pharmacology in a straightforward, student-friendly manner. It focuses on need-to-know content and helps students learn to administer drugs safely and eliminate medication errors through extensive practice of dosage calculations and careful application of the nursing process.

ORGANIZATION

Pharmacology: A Patient-Centered Nursing Process Approach is organized into 19 units and 59 chapters. **Unit I** is an introduction to pharmacology and includes thoroughly updated chapters on drug action, the drug approval process, cultural and pharmacogenetic considerations, drug interactions, over-the-counter drugs, drugs of abuse, herbal therapies, lifespan issues, patient collaboration in community settings, and the role of the nurse in drug research.

Unit II focuses on patient care and safety, with completely revised and updated chapters on the nursing process in patient-centered pharmacotherapy, safety and quality in pharmacotherapy, and medication administration. Unit II features an introduction to the QSEN (Quality and Safety Education for Nurses) initiative, with special emphasis on patient-centered care and on the QSEN competencies of safety and quality.

Unit III, a comprehensive review of drug dosage calculations for adults and children, is a unique strength of this book. This unit, tabbed for quick reference, consists of six sections: Systems of Measurement with Conversion, Methods for Calculation, Calculations of Oral Dosages, Calculations of Injectable Dosages, Calculations of Intravenous Fluids, and Pediatric Drug Calculations. Six methods of dosage calculation are presented, with color coding for easy identification: basic formula, ratio and proportion, fractional equation, dimensional analysis, body weight, and body surface area. Integral to Unit III are its clinical practice problems (featuring actual drug labels in full color), which provide extensive practice in real-world dosage calculations. With this wide array of practice problems in a variety of health care settings, the unit eliminates the need to purchase a separate dosage calculations book.

Unit IV addresses nutrition and fluids and electrolytes, with separate chapters covering vitamin and mineral replacement, fluid and electrolyte replacement, and nutritional support.

Units V through XIX make up the core of *Pharmacology: A Patient-Centered Nursing Process Approach* and cover the drug families that students must understand to practice effectively. Each drug family chapter includes a chapter outline, learning objectives, key terms, at least one Prototype Drug Chart, a drug table, and an extensive Nursing Process section.

- The **Prototype Drug Charts** are a unique tool that students can use to view the many facets of a prototype drug through the lens of the nursing process. Each prototype drug is one of the common drugs in its drug class. The charts include Drug Class, Trade Names, Contraindications, Dosage, Drug-Lab-Food Interactions, Pharmacokinetics, Pharmacodynamics, Therapeutic Effects/Uses, Side Effects, and Adverse Reactions. With these charts, students can see how the steps of the Nursing Process correlate with these key aspects of drug information and therapy.
- The **drug tables** provide a quick reference to routes, dosages, uses, and key considerations for the most commonly prescribed medications for a given class. They list drug names (generic, brand, and Canadian), dosages, uses and considerations, pregnancy categories, and specific information on half-life and protein-binding.
- The **Nursing Process sections** provide a convenient summary of how to assess a patient, develop nursing diagnoses, determine and follow through with the plan of care, and evaluate the outcomes of your efforts. These sections also include cultural content, nursing interventions, suggestions for patient teaching, and relevant herbal information.

ADDITIONAL FEATURES

Throughout this edition, we have retained, enhanced, and added a variety of features that teach students the fundamental principles of pharmacology and the role of the nurse in drug therapy:

- **NCLEX Study Questions** at the end of each chapter help prepare students for the NCLEX examination with its increasing emphasis on pharmacology; answers are listed upside down below the questions for quick feedback.
- **Safety: Preventing Medication Errors boxes** have been updated and include information on packaging, dosages, look-alike and sound-alike drugs, and other causes of medication errors.
- **Key Terms** include page numbers and are defined in the text to enhance this "built-in glossary" feature for students.
- **Canadian drug names** are identified with **a special maple-leaf icon (🍁)**.
- **Critical Thinking Case Studies** conclude many chapters. These clinical scenarios are followed by a series of questions, challenging students to carefully consider the scenario and apply their knowledge and analytical skills to respond to the situations.

- **Herbal Alerts** appear throughout the text, providing students with a quick reference to information on popular herbs and their side effects, drug interactions, and more.
- **Anatomy and physiology.** Unit openers for all drug therapy chapters include illustrated overviews of normal anatomy and physiology. These introductions give students the foundation for understanding how drugs work in various body systems.
- **High-alert drugs** (denoted with the symbol ▶), **evidence-based practice** (denoted with the symbol 🔍), and **safety concerns** (denoted with the symbol ⚡) are identified within the text with distinctive icons that make it easy to find crucial information.

TEACHING AND LEARNING RESOURCES

The eighth edition of *Pharmacology: A Patient-Centered Nursing Process Approach* is the core of a complete teaching and learning package for nursing pharmacology. Additional components of this package include resources for students, resources for faculty members, and resources for both students and faculty.

For Students

A comprehensive *Study Guide,* available for purchase separately, provides thousands of study questions and answers, including clinically based situational practice problems, drug calculation problems and questions (many with actual drug labels), and case studies to help students master textbook content. Answers are provided at the end of the *Study Guide.*

A completely updated Evolve website (http://evolve.elsevier.com/KeeHayes/pharmacology/) provides additional resources for students, including the following:

- **Review Questions for the NCLEX® Examination** organized by chapter
- **Downloadable Key Points** for content review on-the-go
- **Pharmacology animations** and **videos**
- **Unfolding Case Studies** with review questions
- **References** from the textbook

For Faculty Members

The updated faculty Evolve website (http://evolve.elsevier.com/KeeHayes/pharmacology/) includes all of the student resources mentioned previously, plus the following instructor-only resources:

- ***TEACH for Nurses*** **Lesson Plans (NEW for this edition!)** focus on the most important content from each chapter and provide innovative strategies for student engagement and learning. The Lesson Plans include strategies for integrating nursing curriculum standards (QSEN, concept-based learning, and BSN essentials), links to all relevant student and instructor resources, and an original instructor-only case study in each chapter.
- **ExamView Test Bank** features more than 1000 NCLEX® Examination–format questions, including alternate-item questions, as well as rationales and page references for each question.
- **PowerPoint Collection** features customizable slides with images, integrated Audience Response System Questions, and new unfolding case studies with questions.
- **Image Collection** provides approximately 125 full-color images from the book.

This textbook may be supplemented with the drug content found on government agency websites, which supply the latest information regarding changes to drug brand names. It is our hope that *Pharmacology: A Patient-Centered Nursing Process Approach* and its comprehensive ancillary package will serve as a dynamic resource for teaching students the basic principles of pharmacology and their vital role in drug therapy.

Joyce LeFever Kee
Evelyn R. Hayes
Linda E. McCuistion

ACKNOWLEDGMENTS

We wish to extend our sincere appreciation to the many professionals who assisted in the preparation of the eighth edition of *Pharmacology: A Patient-Centered Nursing Process Approach* by reviewing chapters and offering suggestions.

We wish to especially thank the original authors and those who updated the established chapters: Margaret Barton-Burke, Joseph Boullata, Jacqueline Rosenjack Burchum, Katherine L. Byar, Michelle M. Byrne, Karen Carmody, Robin Webb Corbett, Sandy Elliott, Linda Goodwin, Janice Heinssen, Marilyn Herbert-Ashton, Judith W. Herrman, Kathleen J. Jones, Bettyrae Jordan, Robert J. Kizior, Paula R. Klemm, Anne E. Lara, Linda Laskowski-Jones, Ronald J. Lefever, Patricia S. Lincoln, Patricia O'Brien, Laura K. Williford Owens, Byron Peters, Lisa Ann Plowfield, Larry D. Purnell, Nancy C. Sharts-Hopko, Jane Purnell Taylor, Donald L. Taylor, Lynette M. Wachholz, Marcia Welsh, Gail Wilkes, and M. Linda Workman.

Of course, we are deeply indebted to the many patients and students we have had throughout our many years of professional nursing practice. From them we have learned many fine points about the role of therapeutic pharmacology in nursing practice.

Our deepest appreciation goes to pharmaceutical companies for use of their drug labels. Pharmaceutical companies that extended their courtesy to this book include the following:

Abbott Laboratories
AstraZeneca Pharmaceuticals
Aventis
Bayer Corporation
Bristol-Myers Squibb (including Apothecon Laboratories and Mead Johnson Pharmaceuticals)
DuPont/Merck Pharmaceuticals
Eli Lilly and Company
Elkins-Sinn, Inc.
Glaxo-Wellcome
Marion Merrell Dow, Inc.
McNeill Laboratory, Inc.
Merck and Co., Inc.
Parke-Davis Co.
Pfizer Inc.
Rhone-Poulenc Rorer
SmithKline Beecham Pharmaceutical
Wyeth-Ayerst Laboratories

Thanks to Becton, Dickinson and Company for the syringe displays. Thanks to CareFusion Corporation for the photos of the infusion pumps.

Our sincere thanks to Elsevier, especially Lee Henderson, Executive Content Strategist; Jennifer Ehlers, Content Manager; Clay Broeker, Senior Project Manager; and Jeff Patterson, Publishing Services Manager, for their suggestions and assistance.

Joyce LeFever Kee
Evelyn R. Hayes
Linda E. McCuistion

UNIT I

Introduction to Pharmacology

Assessing a patient's response to drug therapy is an ongoing nursing responsibility. To adequately assess, plan, intervene, and evaluate drug effects, the nurse must have knowledge of the pharmaceutic, pharmacokinetic, and pharmacodynamic phases of drug action, all of which are described in Chapter 1, Drug Action: Pharmaceutic, Pharmacokinetic, and Pharmacodynamic Phases.

The rest of the unit is composed of nine chapters that cover a range of important issues affecting drug therapy and nursing. Chapter 2, The Drug Approval Process, discusses drug standards and federal legislation for American and Canadian drugs that establish safety guidelines for drug use, drug names, and drug resources.

Chapter 3, Cultural and Pharmacogenetic Considerations, helps the nurse understand and respond to unique cultural and genetic factors that may influence drug therapy for a particular patient. Factors such as heritage, communication styles, family organization, spirituality and religion, health beliefs and practices, biocultural ecology, and traditional medicine are discussed.

Chapter 4, Drug Interactions and Over-the-Counter Drugs, and Chapter 5, Drugs of Abuse, cover two areas of special interest to nurses. Assessing drug interaction has always been and remains an ongoing function of the nurse. Because drug abuse is a national problem from which no portion of the population is immune—including health professionals—it is a topic of great concern to nurses.

Chapter 6, Herbal Therapies, explores herbal-based preparations that are available over the counter. It covers the most commonly used herbs and discusses their indications, preparation, dosages, potential hazards, and tips for safe and effective use.

Chapter 7, Pediatric Pharmacology, and Chapter 8, Geriatric Pharmacology, cover pharmacokinetic and pharmacodynamic effects specific to these age groups. They also discuss the special attention required when administering drugs to these age groups.

With the increasing movement of health care into the community, nurses are gaining more responsibilities and opportunities to collaborate with patients in safe medication administration and use. Chapter 9, Collaboration in Community Settings, focuses on aspects of drug therapy unique to the home, school, workplace, and other alternative care settings.

Chapter 10, The Role of the Nurse in Drug Research, discusses the nurse's challenges regarding drug research. In general practice, the nurse identifies specific needs that may be met by medications. When part of clinical drug trials, the nurse must be aware of informed consent issues and patient responses to drugs.

CHAPTER

1

Drug Action: Pharmaceutic, Pharmacokinetic, and Pharmacodynamic Phases

evolve WEBSITE

http://evolve.elsevier.com/KeeHayes/pharmacology/

- Animations
- Content Updates
- Key Points
- Review Questions for the NCLEX® Examination
- References from the Textbook
- Unfolding Case Studies

OBJECTIVES

- Differentiate the three phases of drug action.
- Discuss the two processes that occur before tablets are absorbed into the body.
- Describe the four processes of pharmacokinetics.
- Explain the meaning of pharmacodynamics, dose response, maximal efficacy, receptors, and nonreceptors in drug action.
- Define the terms *protein-bound drugs, half-life, therapeutic index, therapeutic drug range, side effects, adverse reaction,* and *drug toxicity.*
- Check drugs for half-life, percentage of protein-binding effect, therapeutic range, and side effects in a drug reference book.
- Describe the nursing implications of pharmacokinetics and pharmacodynamics.

OUTLINE

KEY TERMS

The authors gratefully acknowledge the work of Marilyn Herbert-Ashton, who updated this chapter for the eighth edition.

metabolism, p. 6
nonselective drugs, p. 8
nonspecific drugs, p. 8
onset of action, p. 7
passive absorption, p. 3
peak action, p. 7
peak drug level, p. 10
pharmaceutic phase, p. 3
pharmacodynamics, p. 7
pharmacogenetics, p. 11
pharmacokinetics, p. 3
pinocytosis, p. 4
placebo effect, p. 11
protein-binding effect, p. 4
receptor families, p. 8
side effects, p. 10
tachyphylaxis, p. 11
therapeutic index, p. 9
therapeutic range (therapeutic window), p. 9
time-response curve, p. 7
tolerance, p. 11
toxic effects, p. 11
toxicity, p. 11
trough drug level, p. 10

A tablet or capsule taken by mouth goes through three phases—pharmaceutic, pharmacokinetic, and pharmacodynamic—as drug actions occur. In the **pharmaceutic phase,** the drug becomes a solution so that it can cross the biologic membrane. When the drug is administered parenterally by subcutaneous (subQ), intramuscular (IM), or intravenous (IV) routes, there is no pharmaceutic phase. The second phase, the pharmacokinetic phase, is composed of four processes: absorption, distribution, metabolism (or biotransformation), and excretion (or elimination). In the pharmacodynamic phase, a biologic or physiologic response results.

PHARMACEUTIC PHASE

Approximately 80% of drugs are taken by mouth. The pharmaceutic phase (dissolution) is the first phase of drug action. In the gastrointestinal (GI) tract, drugs need to be in solution so they can be absorbed. A drug in solid form (tablet or capsule) must disintegrate into small particles to dissolve into a liquid, a process known as *dissolution*. Drugs in liquid form are already in solution. Figure 1-1 displays the pharmaceutic phase of a tablet.

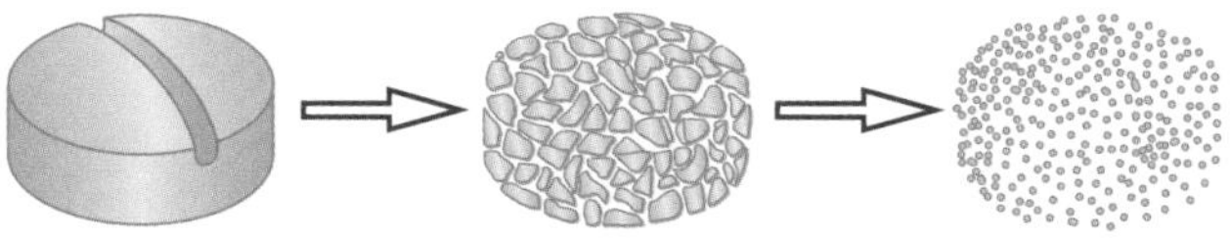

FIGURE 1–1 The two pharmaceutic phases are disintegration and dissolution.

Tablets are not 100% drug. Fillers and inert substances, generally called **excipients,** are used in drug preparation to allow the drug to take on a particular size and shape and to enhance drug dissolution. Some additives in drugs, such as the ions potassium (K) and sodium (Na) in penicillin potassium and penicillin sodium, increase the absorbability of the drug. Penicillin is poorly absorbed by the GI tract because of gastric acid. However, by making the drug a potassium or sodium salt, penicillin can then be absorbed. **Disintegration** is the breakdown of a tablet into smaller particles. **Dissolution** is the dissolving of the smaller particles in the GI fluid before absorption. Rate of dissolution is the time it takes the drug to disintegrate and dissolve to become available for the body to absorb it. Drugs in liquid form are more rapidly available for GI absorption than are solids. Generally, drugs are both disintegrated and absorbed faster in acidic fluids with a pH of 1 or 2 rather than in alkaline fluids. Alkaline drugs would become ionized and have difficulty crossing cell membrane barriers. Both the very young and older adults have less gastric acidity; therefore, drug absorption is generally slower for those drugs absorbed primarily in the stomach.

Enteric-coated drugs resist disintegration in the gastric acid of the stomach, so disintegration does not occur until the drug reaches the alkaline environment of the small intestine. Enteric-coated tablets can remain in the stomach for a long time; therefore, their effect may be delayed in onset. Enteric-coated tablets or capsules and sustained-release (beaded) capsules should not be crushed. Crushing would alter the place and time of absorption of the drug. Food in the GI tract may interfere with the dissolution of certain drugs. Some drugs irritate the gastric mucosa, so fluids or food may be necessary to dilute the drug concentration and to act as protectants.

PHARMACOKINETIC PHASE

Pharmacokinetics is the process of drug movement to achieve drug action. The four processes are absorption, distribution, metabolism (or biotransformation), and excretion (or elimination). The nurse applies knowledge of pharmacokinetics when assessing the patient for possible adverse drug effects. The nurse communicates assessment findings to members of the health care team in a timely manner to promote safe and effective drug therapy for the patient.

Absorption

Absorption is the movement of drug particles from the GI tract to body fluids by passive absorption, active absorption, or pinocytosis. Most oral drugs are absorbed into the surface area of the small intestine through the action of the extensive mucosal villi. Absorption is reduced if the villi are decreased in number because of disease, drug effect, or the removal of small intestine. Protein-based drugs such as insulin and growth hormones are destroyed in the small intestine by digestive enzymes. **Passive absorption** occurs mostly by diffusion (movement from higher concentration to lower concentration). With the process of diffusion, the drug does not

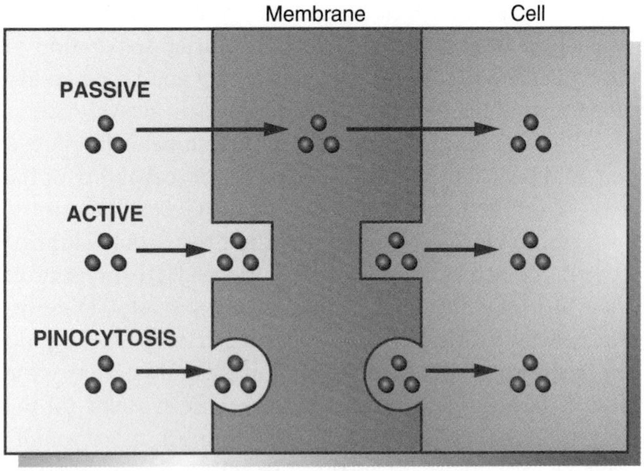

FIGURE 1–2 The three major processes for drug absorption through the gastrointestinal membrane are passive absorption, active absorption, and pinocytosis.

require energy to move across the membrane. **Active absorption** requires a carrier such as an enzyme or protein to move the drug against a concentration gradient. Energy is required for active absorption. **Pinocytosis** is a process by which cells carry a drug across their membrane by engulfing the drug particles (Figure 1-2).

The GI membrane is composed mostly of lipid (fat) and protein, so drugs that are lipid soluble pass rapidly through the GI membrane. Water-soluble drugs need a carrier, either enzyme or protein, to pass through the membrane. Large particles pass through the cell membrane if they are nonionized (have no positive or negative charge). Weak acid drugs such as aspirin are less ionized in the stomach, and they pass through the stomach lining easily and rapidly. An infant's gastric secretions have a higher pH (alkaline) than those of adults; therefore, infants can absorb more penicillin. Certain drugs such as calcium carbonate and many of the antifungals need an acidic environment to achieve greater drug absorption; thus food can stimulate the production of gastric acid. Hydrochloric acid destroys some drugs such as penicillin G; therefore a large oral dosage of penicillin is needed to offset the partial dose loss. Drugs administered by many routes do not pass through the GI tract or liver. These include parenteral drugs, eyedrops, eardrops, nasal sprays, respiratory inhalants, transdermal drugs, and sublingual drugs. **Remember**, drugs that are lipid soluble and nonionized are absorbed faster than water-soluble and ionized drugs.

Blood flow, pain, stress, hunger, fasting, food, and pH affect drug absorption. Poor circulation to the stomach as a result of shock, vasoconstrictor drugs, or disease hampers absorption. Pain, stress, and foods that are solid, hot, or high in fat can slow gastric emptying time, so the drug remains in the stomach longer. Exercise can decrease blood flow by causing more blood to flow to the peripheral muscle, thereby decreasing blood circulation to the GI tract.

Drugs given IM are absorbed faster in muscles that have more blood vessels (e.g., deltoids) than in those that have fewer blood vessels (e.g., gluteals). Subcutaneous tissue has fewer blood vessels, so absorption is slower in such tissue.

Some drugs do not go directly into the systemic circulation following oral absorption but pass from the intestinal lumen to the liver via the portal vein. In the liver, some drugs may be metabolized to an inactive form that may then be excreted, thus reducing the amount of active drug. Some drugs do not undergo metabolism at all in the liver, and others may be metabolized to drug metabolite, which may be equally or more active than the original drug. The process in which the drug passes to the liver first is called the **first-pass effect,** or hepatic first pass.

Most drugs given orally are affected by first-pass metabolism. Lidocaine and some nitroglycerins are not given orally because they have extensive first-pass metabolism and therefore most of the dose would be destroyed.

Bioavailability is a subcategory of absorption. It is the percentage of the administered drug dose that reaches the systemic circulation. For the oral route of drug administration, bioavailability occurs after absorption and first-pass metabolism. The percentage of bioavailability for the oral route is always less than 100%, but for the IV route it is 100%. Oral drugs that have a high first-pass hepatic metabolism may have a bioavailability of only 20% to 40% on entering systemic circulation. To obtain the desired drug effect, the oral dose could be higher than the drug dose for IV use.

Factors that alter bioavailability include (1) the drug form (e.g., tablet, capsule, sustained-release, liquid, transdermal patch, rectal suppository, inhalation), (2) route of administration (e.g., oral, rectal, topical, parenteral), (3) GI mucosa and motility, (4) food and other drugs, and (5) changes in liver metabolism caused by liver dysfunction or inadequate hepatic blood flow. A decrease in liver function or a decrease in hepatic blood flow can increase the bioavailability of a drug, but only if the drug is metabolized by the liver. Less drug is destroyed by hepatic metabolism in the presence of liver disorder.

With some oral drugs, rapid absorption increases the bioavailability of the drug and can cause an increase in drug concentration. Drug toxicity may result. Slow absorption can limit the bioavailability of the drug, thus causing a decrease in drug serum concentration.

Distribution

Distribution is the process by which the drug becomes available to body fluids and body tissues. Drug distribution is influenced by blood flow, the drug's affinity to the tissue, and the **protein-binding effect** (Figure 1-3). In addition, volume of drug distribution (Vd) is dependent on drug dose and its concentration in the body. Drugs with a larger volume of drug distribution have a longer half-life and stay in the body longer. See the section on metabolism, or biotransformation, later in this chapter.

Protein Binding

As drugs are distributed in the plasma, many are bound to varying degrees (percentages) with protein (primarily albumin). Drugs that are greater than 89% bound to protein are known as *highly protein-bound drugs*; drugs that are 61%

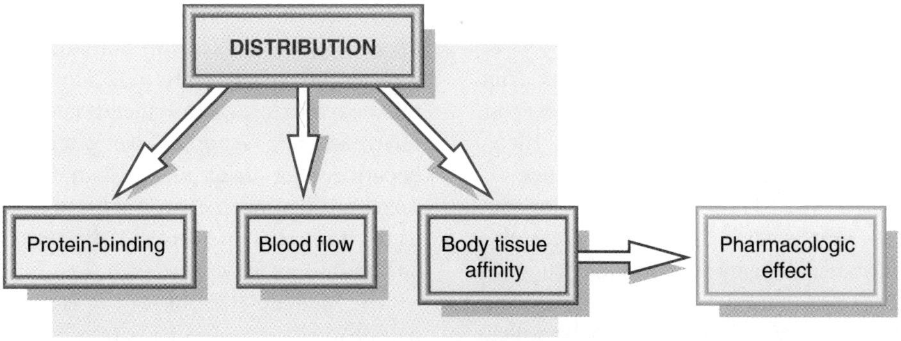

FIGURE 1–3 Drug distribution.

to 89% bound to protein are moderately highly protein-bound; drugs that are 30% to 60% bound to protein are moderately protein-bound; and drugs that are less than 30% bound to protein are low protein-bound drugs. Table 1-1 lists selected highly protein-bound drugs and moderately highly protein-bound drugs. The portion of the drug that is bound is inactive because it is not available to receptors, and the portion that remains unbound is free, active drug. Only **free drugs** (drugs not bound to protein) are active and can cause a pharmacologic response. As the free drug in the circulation decreases, more bound drug is released from the protein to maintain the balance of free drug. Drugs bound to proteins cannot leave the systemic circulation to get to the site of action. This is why only free drug is active.

When two highly protein-bound drugs are given concurrently, they compete for protein-binding sites, thus causing more free drug to be released into the circulation. In this situation, drug accumulation and possible drug toxicity can result. Also, a low serum protein level decreases the number of protein-binding sites and can cause an increase in the amount of free drug in the plasma. Drug toxicity may then result. Drug dose is prescribed according to the percentage in which the drug binds to protein.

Patients with liver or kidney disease or those who are malnourished may have an abnormally low serum albumin level. This results in fewer protein-binding sites, which in turn leads to excess free drug and eventually to drug toxicity. Older adults are more likely to have hypoalbuminemia. With some health conditions that result in a low serum protein level, excess free or unbound drug goes to nonspecific tissue binding sites until needed and excess free drug in the circulation does not occur. Consequently, a decreased drug dose is needed as there is not as much protein circulated for the drug to bind to.

Some drugs bind with a specific protein component such as albumin or globulin. Most anticonvulsants bind primarily to albumin. Some basic drugs such as antidysrhythmics (e.g., lidocaine, quinidine) bind mostly to globulins.

To avoid possible drug toxicity, checking the protein-binding percentage of all drugs administered to a patient is important. The nurse should also check the patient's plasma protein and albumin levels, because a decrease in plasma protein (albumin) decreases protein-binding sites, permitting

TABLE 1-1 PROTEIN-BINDING AND HALF-LIFE OF DRUGS

DRUG	PROTEIN-BOUND (%)	HALF-LIFE $(t_{1/2})$ (h)
Highly Protein-Bound Drugs (89%)		
amitriptyline	97	40
chlorpromazine	95	30
diazepam	98	30-80
dicloxacillin	95	0.5-1
furosemide	95	1.5
ibuprofen	98	2-4
lorazepam	92	15
piroxicam	99	30-86
propranolol	92	4
rifampin	89	2
sulfisoxazole	85-95	4.5-7.5
valproic acid	92	15
warfarin	97	20-60
Moderately High Protein-Bound Drugs (61% to 89%)		
erythromycin	70	3
nafcillin	86	2-20
phenytoin	88	10-40
quinidine	70	6
trimethoprim	70	11
Moderately Protein-Bound Drugs (30% to 60%)		
aspirin	49	0.25-2
lidocaine	50	2
meperidine	56	3
pindolol	40	3-4
theophylline	60	9
ticarcillin	45-65	1-1.5
Low Protein-Bound Drugs (30%)		
amikacin	4-11	2-3
amoxicillin	20	1-1.5
atenolol	6-16	6-7
cephalexin	10-15	0.5-1.2
digoxin	25	36
neostigmine bromide	15-25	1-1.5
terbutaline sulfate	25	3-11
timolol maleate	<10	3-4
tobramycin sulfate	10	2-3

h, Hour; >, greater than; <, less than.

more free drug in the circulation. Depending on the drug, the result could be life-threatening.

Abscesses, exudates, body glands, and tumors hinder drug distribution. Antibiotics do not distribute well at abscess and exudate sites. In addition, some drugs accumulate in particular tissues such as fat, bone, liver, muscle, and eye tissues.

The blood-brain barrier (BBB) is a semipermeable membrane in the central nervous system (CNS) that protects the brain from foreign substances. Highly lipid-soluble drugs are able to cross the BBB. Drugs that are not bound to proteins and are not lipid soluble are not able to cross the BBB, which makes it difficult to distribute the drug (Figure 1-4).

During pregnancy, both lipid-soluble and lipid-insoluble drugs are able to cross the placental barrier, which can affect the fetus and the mother. The risk-benefit ratio should be considered before drugs are given during pregnancy (Figure 1-5; see also Chapter 53). During lactation, drugs can be secreted into breast milk, which could affect the nursing infant. The nurse needs to check which drugs may cross into breast milk before administering to a lactating patient.

Metabolism, or Biotransformation

Metabolism is the process by which the body inactivates or biotransforms drugs. Drugs can be metabolized in several organs; however, the liver is the primary site of metabolism. Most drugs are inactivated by liver enzymes and are then converted or transformed by hepatic enzymes to inactive metabolites or water-soluble substances for excretion. A large percentage of drugs are lipid soluble; thus the liver metabolizes the lipid-soluble drug substance to a water-soluble substance for renal excretion. However, some drugs are transformed into active metabolites, causing an increased pharmacologic response. Liver diseases such as cirrhosis and hepatitis alter drug metabolism by inhibiting the drug-metabolizing enzymes in the liver. When the drug metabolism rate is decreased, excess drug accumulation can occur and lead to toxicity.

The **half-life** ($t\frac{1}{2}$) of a drug is the time it takes for one half of the drug concentration to be eliminated. Metabolism and elimination affect the half-life of a drug. For example, with liver or kidney dysfunction, the half-life of the drug is prolonged and less drug is metabolized and eliminated. When a drug is taken continually, drug accumulation may occur. Table 1-1 shows the half-life of selected drugs.

A drug goes through several half-lives before more than 90% of the drug is eliminated. If the patient takes 650 mg of aspirin and the half-life is 3 hours, it takes 3 hours for the first half-life to eliminate 325 mg, 6 hours for the second half-life to eliminate an additional 162 mg, and so on until the sixth half-life (or 18 hours), when 10 mg of aspirin is left in the body (Table 1-2). A short half-life is considered to be 4 to 8 hours, and a long one is 24 hours or longer. If the drug has a long half-life (such as digoxin at 36 hours), it takes several days for the body to completely eliminate the drug.

By knowing the half-life, the time it takes for a drug to reach a steady state of serum concentration can be computed. Administration of the drug for three to five half-lives

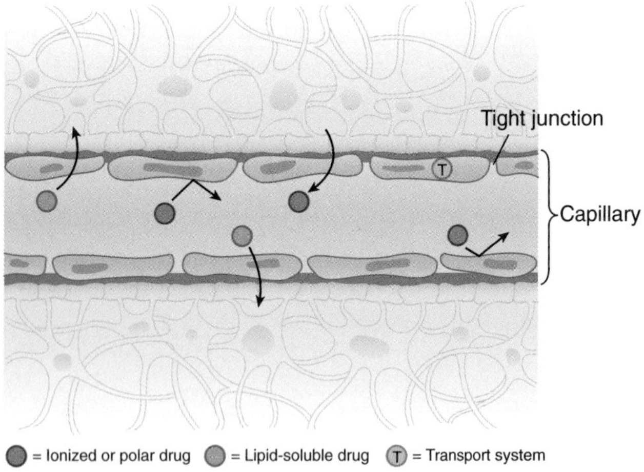

FIGURE 1–4 Drug movement across the blood-brain barrier.

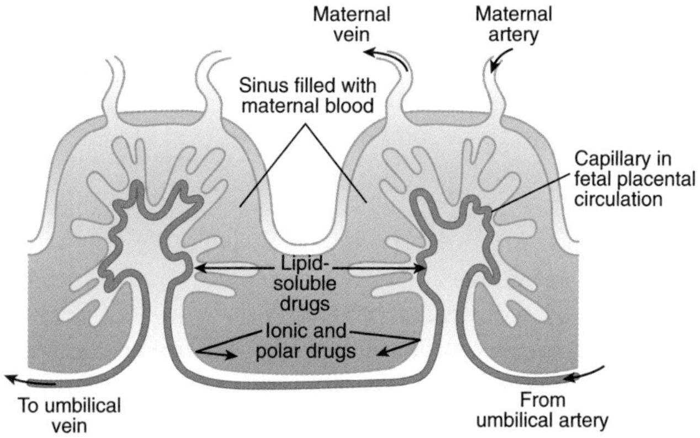

FIGURE 1–5 Drug crossing the placenta.

TABLE 1-2 HALF-LIFE OF 650 mg OF ASPIRIN

NUMBER ($t\frac{1}{2}$)	TIME OF ELIMINATION (h)	DOSAGE REMAINING (mg)	PERCENTAGE LEFT
1	3	325	50
2	6	162	25
3	9	81	12.5
4	12	40	6.25
5	15	20	3.1
6	18	10	1.55

h, Hour; $t\frac{1}{2}$, half-life.

saturates the biologic system to the extent that the intake of drug equals the amount metabolized and excreted. An example is digoxin, which has a half-life of 36 hours with normal renal function. It would take approximately 5 days to 1 week (three to five half-lives) to reach a steady state for digoxin concentration.

Excretion, or Elimination

The main route of drug **elimination** is through the kidneys (urine). Other routes include bile, feces, lungs, saliva, sweat, and breast milk. The kidneys filter free unbound drugs, water-soluble drugs, and drugs that are unchanged. The lungs eliminate volatile drug substances and products metabolized to carbon dioxide (CO_2) and water (H_2O).

The urine pH influences drug excretion. Urine pH varies from 4.5 to 8. Acidic urine promotes elimination of weak base drugs, and alkaline urine promotes elimination of weak acid drugs. Aspirin, a weak acid, is excreted rapidly in alkaline urine. If a person takes an overdose of aspirin, sodium bicarbonate may be given to change the urine pH to alkaline to promote excretion of the drug. Large quantities of cranberry juice can decrease urine pH, causing acidic urine and thus inhibiting the elimination of aspirin.

With a kidney disease that results in decreased glomerular filtration rate (GFR) or decreased renal tubular secretion, drug excretion is slowed or impaired. Drug accumulation with possible severe adverse drug reactions can result. A decrease in blood flow to the kidneys can also alter drug excretion.

Common tests used to determine renal function are **creatinine clearance (CLcr)** and blood urea nitrogen (BUN). Creatinine is a metabolic by-product of muscle that is excreted by the kidneys. The creatinine clearance test compares the level of creatinine in the urine with the level of creatinine in the blood. Creatinine clearance varies with age and gender. Lower values are expected in older adult and female patients because of their decreased muscle mass. GFR may be the best test, but it is expensive and not so commonly used. A decrease in GFR results in an increase in serum creatinine level and a decrease in urine creatinine clearance.

With renal dysfunction either in older adults or as a result of kidney disorders, drug dosage usually needs to be decreased. In these cases, the creatinine clearance needs to be determined to establish appropriate drug dosage. When the creatinine clearance is decreased, drug dosage likewise may need to be decreased. Continuous drug dosing according to a prescribed dosing regimen without evaluating creatinine clearance could result in drug toxicity.

PHARMACODYNAMIC PHASE

Pharmacodynamics is the study of the way drugs affect the body. Drug response can cause a primary or secondary physiologic effect or both. The primary effect is desirable, and the secondary effect may be desirable or undesirable. An example of a drug with a primary and secondary effect is diphenhydramine (Benadryl), an antihistamine. The primary effect of diphenhydramine is to treat the symptoms of allergy, and the secondary effect is a central nervous system depression that causes drowsiness. The secondary effect is undesirable when the patient drives a car, but at bedtime it could be desirable because it causes mild sedation.

Dose Response and Maximal Efficacy

Dose response is the relationship between the minimal versus the maximal amount of drug dose needed to produce the desired drug response. Some patients respond to a lower drug dose, whereas others need a high drug dose to elicit the desired response. The drug dose is usually adjusted to achieve the desired drug response.

All drugs have a maximum drug effect (maximal efficacy). For example, morphine and tramadol hydrochloride (Ultram) are prescribed to relieve pain. The maximum efficacy of morphine is greater than tramadol hydrochloride, regardless of how much tramadol hydrochloride is given. The pain relief with the use of tramadol hydrochloride is not as great as it is with morphine.

Onset, Peak, and Duration of Action

One important aspect of pharmacodynamics is knowing the drug's onset, peak, and duration of action. **Onset of action** is the time it takes to reach the minimum effective concentration (MEC) after a drug is administered. **Peak action** occurs when the drug reaches its highest blood or plasma concentration. **Duration of action** is the length of time the drug has a pharmacologic effect. Figure 1-6 illustrates the areas in which onset, peak, and duration of action occur.

Some drugs produce effects in minutes, but others may take hours or days. A **time-response curve** evaluates three parameters of drug action: the onset of drug action, peak action, and duration of action. Figure 1-6 indicates these parameters by using T (time) with subscripts (e.g., T_0, T_1, T_2, T_3).

It is necessary to understand the time response in relationship to drug administration. If the drug plasma or serum level decreases below threshold or MEC, adequate drug dosing is

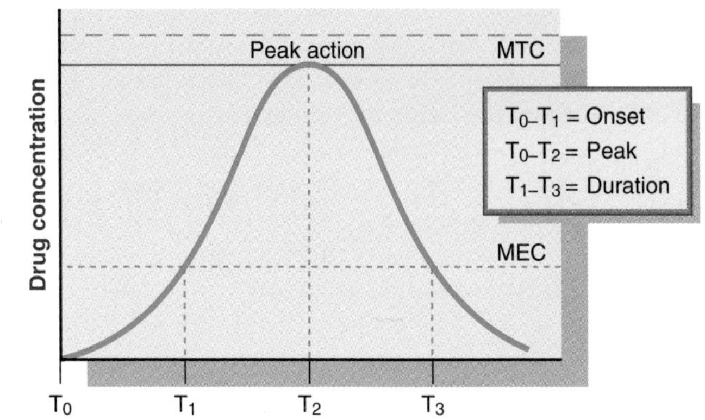

FIGURE 1–6 The time-response curve evaluates three parameters of drug action: (1) onset, (2) peak, and (3) duration. *MEC,* Minimum effective concentration; *MTC,* minimum toxic concentration.

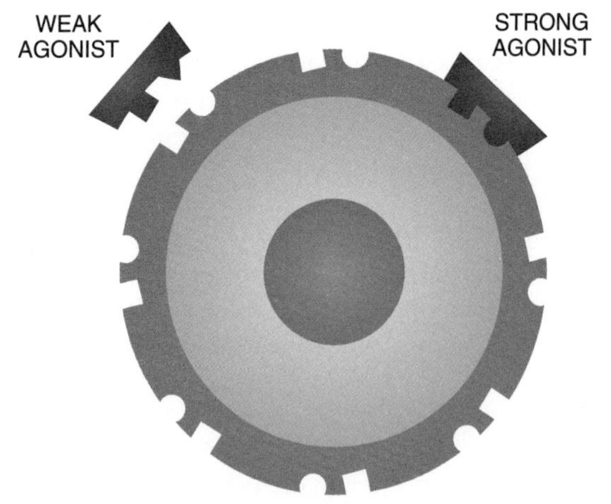

FIGURE 1–7 Two drug agonists attach to the receptor site. The drug agonist that has an exact fit is a strong agonist and is more biologically active than the weak agonist.

not achieved; too high a drug level above the minimum toxic concentration (MTC) can result in toxicity.

Receptor Theory

Drugs act through receptors by binding to the receptor to produce (initiate) a response or to block (prevent) a response. The activity of many drugs is determined by the ability of the drug to bind to a specific receptor. The better the drug fits at the receptor site, the more biologically active the drug is. It is similar to the fit of the right key in a lock. Figure 1-7 illustrates a drug binding to a receptor.

Most receptors, which are protein in nature, are found in cell membranes. Drug-binding sites are primarily on proteins, glycoproteins, proteolipids, and enzymes. There are four **receptor families:** (1) kinase-linked receptors, (2) ligand-gated ion channels, (3) G protein–coupled receptor systems, and (4) nuclear receptors. The **ligand-binding domain** is the site on the receptor at which drugs bind.

- *Kinase-linked receptors.* The ligand-binding domain for drug binding is on the cell surface. The drug activates the enzyme (inside the cell), and a response is initiated.
- *Ligand-gated ion channels.* The channel spans the cell membrane and, with this type of receptor, the channel opens, allowing for the flow of ions into and out of the cells. The ions are primarily sodium and calcium.
- *G protein–coupled receptor systems.* There are three components to this receptor response: (1) the receptor, (2) the G protein that binds with guanosine triphosphate (GTP), and (3) the effector that is either an enzyme or an ion channel. The system works as follows:

$$\text{drug} \xrightarrow{\text{activates}} \text{receptors} \xrightarrow{\text{activates}} \text{G protein} \xrightarrow{\text{activates}} \text{effect}$$

- *Nuclear receptors.* Found in the cell nucleus (not on the surface) of the cell membrane. Activation of receptors through the transcription factors is prolonged. With the first three receptor groups, activation of the receptors is rapid.

Agonists and Antagonists

Drugs that produce a response are called **agonists,** and drugs that block a response are called **antagonists.** Epinephrine (Adrenalin) stimulates $beta_1$ and $beta_2$ receptors, so it is an agonist. Atropine, an antagonist, blocks the histamine (H_2) receptor, thus preventing excessive gastric acid secretion. The effects of an antagonist can be determined by the inhibitory (I) action of the drug concentration on the receptor site. IC_{50} is the antagonist drug concentration required to inhibit 50% of the maximum biological response.

Nonspecific and Nonselective Drug Effects

Many agonists and antagonists lack specific and selective effects. A receptor produces a variety of physiologic responses, depending on where in the body the receptor is located. Cholinergic receptors are located in the bladder, heart, blood vessels, stomach, bronchi, and eyes. A drug that stimulates or blocks the cholinergic receptors affects all anatomic sites of location. Drugs that affect various sites are **nonspecific drugs** and have properties of nonspecificity. Bethanechol (Urecholine) may be prescribed for postoperative urinary retention to increase bladder contraction. This drug stimulates the cholinergic receptor located in the bladder, and urination occurs by strengthening bladder contraction. Because bethanechol affects the cholinergic receptor, other cholinergic sites are also affected. The heart rate decreases, blood pressure decreases, gastric acid secretion increases, the bronchioles constrict, and the pupils of the eye constrict (Figure 1-8). These other effects may be either desirable or harmful. Drugs that evoke a variety of responses throughout the body have a nonspecific response.

Drugs may act at different receptors. Drugs that affect various receptors are **nonselective drugs** or have properties of nonselectivity. Chlorpromazine (Thorazine) acts on the norepinephrine, dopamine, acetylcholine, and histamine receptors, and a variety of responses result from action at these receptor sites. Epinephrine acts on the $alpha_1$, $beta_1$, and $beta_2$ receptors (Figure 1-9). Drugs that produce a response but do not act on a receptor may act by stimulating or inhibiting enzyme activity or hormone production.

Categories of Drug Action

The four categories of drug action include (1) stimulation or depression, (2) replacement, (3) inhibition or killing of organisms, and (4) irritation. In drug action that stimulates, the rate of cell activity or the secretion from a gland increases. In drug action that depresses, cell activity and function of a specific organ are reduced. Replacement drugs such as insulin replace essential body compounds. Drugs that inhibit or kill organisms interfere with bacterial cell growth (e.g., penicillin exerts its bactericidal effects by blocking the synthesis of the bacterial cell wall). Drugs also can act by the mechanism of irritation (e.g., laxatives irritate the inner wall of the colon, thus increasing peristalsis and defecation).

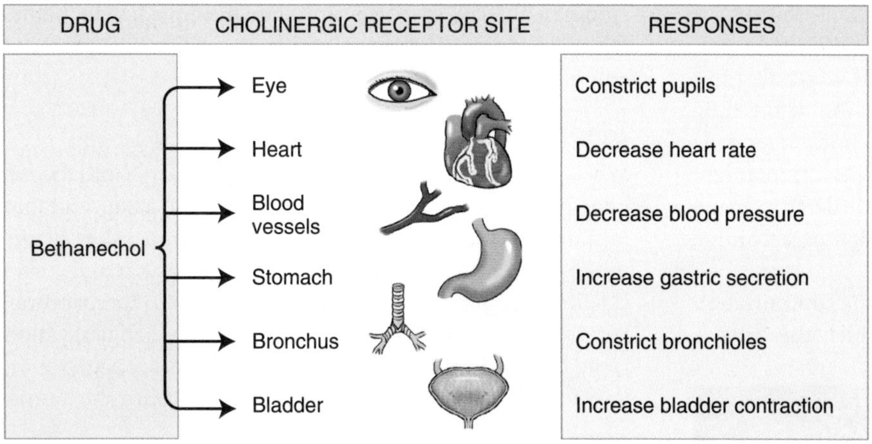

FIGURE 1–8 Cholinergic receptors are located in the bladder, heart, blood vessels, stomach, bronchi, and eyes.

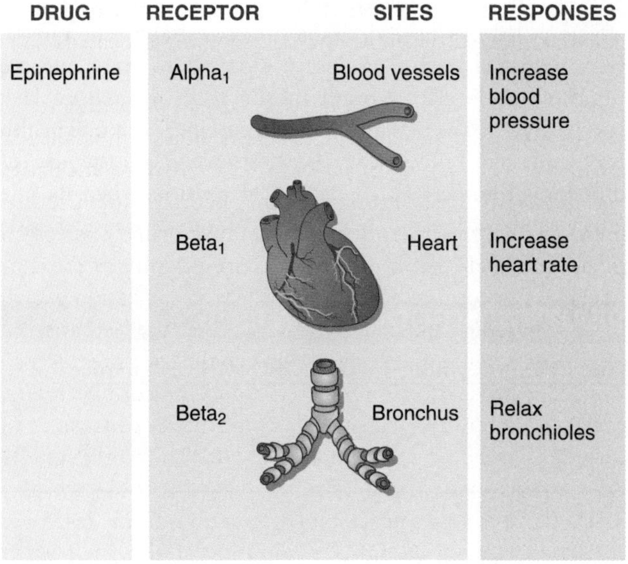

FIGURE 1–9 Epinephrine affects three different receptors: alpha$_1$, beta$_1$, and beta$_2$.

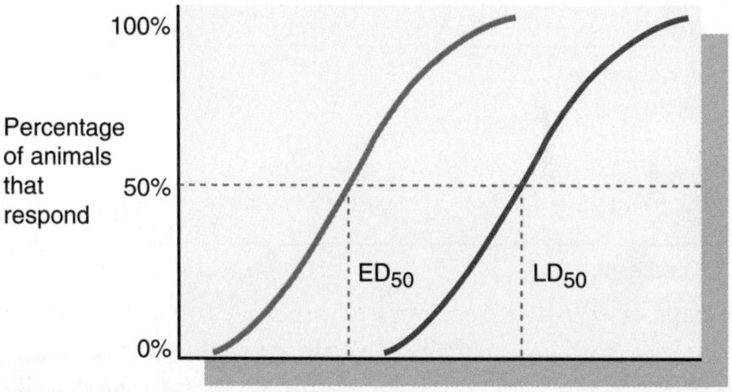

FIGURE 1–10 The therapeutic index measures the margin of safety of a drug. It is a ratio that measures the effective therapeutic dose and the lethal dose.

Therapeutic Index and Therapeutic Range (Therapeutic Window)

The safety of drugs is a major concern. The **therapeutic index (TI)** estimates the margin of safety of a drug through the use of a ratio that measures the effective (therapeutic) dose (ED) in 50% of people (ED_{50}) and the lethal dose (LD) in 50% of people (LD_{50}) (Figure 1-10). The closer the ratio is to 1, the greater the danger of toxicity.

$$TI = \frac{LD_{50}}{ED_{50}}$$

In some cases, the ED may be 25% (ED_{25}) or 75% (ED_{75}).

Drugs with a low therapeutic index have a narrow margin of safety (Figure 1-11, *A*). Drug dosage might need adjustment, and plasma (serum) drug levels need to be monitored because of the small safety range between the ED and LD. Drugs with a high therapeutic index have a wide margin of safety and less danger of producing toxic effects (Figure 1-11, *B*). Plasma (serum) drug levels do not need to be monitored routinely for drugs with a high TI.

The **therapeutic range (therapeutic window)** of a drug concentration in plasma is the level of drug between the minimum effective concentration in the plasma for obtaining desired drug action and the minimum toxic concentration (the toxic effect). When the therapeutic range is given, it includes both protein-bound and unbound portions of the drug. If the therapeutic range is narrow, such as for digoxin (0.5 to 1 ng/mL), the plasma drug level should be monitored periodically to avoid drug toxicity. Monitoring the therapeutic range is not necessary if the drug is not considered highly toxic. When the therapeutic range is given, it includes both protein-bound and unbound portions of the drug. Table 1-3 lists the therapeutic ranges and toxic levels for anticonvulsants.

Peak and Trough Drug Levels

Peak drug levels indicate the rate of absorption of the drug, and trough drug levels indicate the rate of elimination of the drug. Peak and trough levels are requested for drugs that have a narrow therapeutic index and are considered toxic, such as the aminoglycoside antibiotics (Table 1-4). If either the peak or trough level is too high, toxicity can occur. If the peak is too low, no therapeutic effect is achieved. **Peak drug level** is the highest plasma concentration of drug at a specific time. Peak drug levels indicate the rate of absorption. If the drug is given orally, the peak time might be 1 to 3 hours after drug administration. If the drug is given IV, the peak time might occur in 10 minutes. If a peak drug level is ordered, a blood sample should be drawn at the proposed peak time, according to the route of administration.

The **trough drug level** is the lowest plasma concentration of a drug, and it measures the rate at which the drug is eliminated. Trough levels are drawn immediately before the next dose of drug is given, regardless of route of administration.

TABLE 1-3 ANTICONVULSANTS: THERAPEUTIC RANGES AND TOXIC LEVELS

DRUG	THERAPEUTIC RANGE (mcg/mL)	TOXIC LEVEL (mcg/mL)
carbamazepine	6-12	>12-15
ethosuximide	40-80	>80-100
phenytoin	10-20	>30
primidone	5-10	>12-15
valproic acid	50-150	>150

>, Greater than.

Loading Dose

When immediate drug response is desired, a large initial dose, known as the **loading dose,** of drug is given to achieve a rapid minimum effective concentration in the plasma. After a large initial dose, a prescribed dosage per day is ordered. Digoxin (Digitek, Lanoxicaps, Lanoxin), a digitalis preparation, requires a loading dose when first prescribed. Digitalization is the process by which the minimum effective concentration level for digoxin is achieved in the plasma within a short time.

Side Effects, Adverse Reactions, and Toxic Effects

Side effects are physiologic effects not related to desired drug effects. All drugs have desirable or undesirable side effects. Even with a correct drug dosage, side effects occur and are predicted. Side effects result mostly from drugs that lack specificity, such as bethanechol (Urecholine). In some health problems, side effects may be desirable (e.g., the use of diphenhydramine HCl [Benadryl] at bedtime when its side effect of drowsiness is beneficial). At times, however, side

TABLE 1-4 AMINOGLYCOSIDE ANTIBIOTICS: PEAK AND TROUGH LEVELS

DRUG	PEAK (mcg/mL)	TROUGH (mcg/mL)	TOXIC PEAK LEVEL (mcg/mL)	TOXIC TROUGH LEVEL (mcg/mL)
amikacin	15-30	5-10	>35	>10
gentamicin	5-10	<2	>12	>2
tobramycin	5-10	<2	>12	>2

>, Greater than; <, less than.

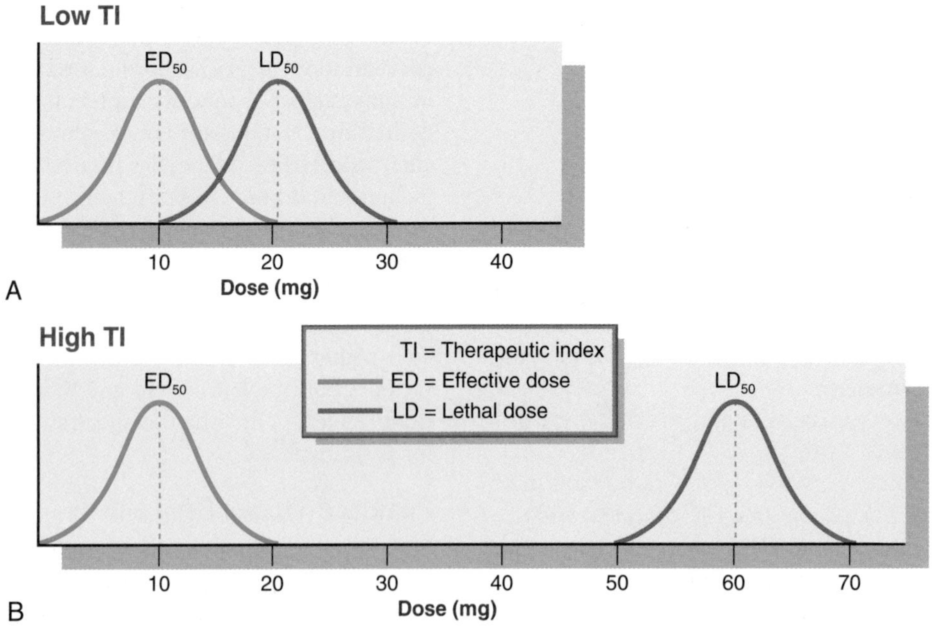

FIGURE 1–11 A, Low therapeutic index drug has a narrow margin of safety, and the drug effect should be closely monitored. **B,** High therapeutic index drug has a wide margin of safety and carries less risk of drug toxicity.

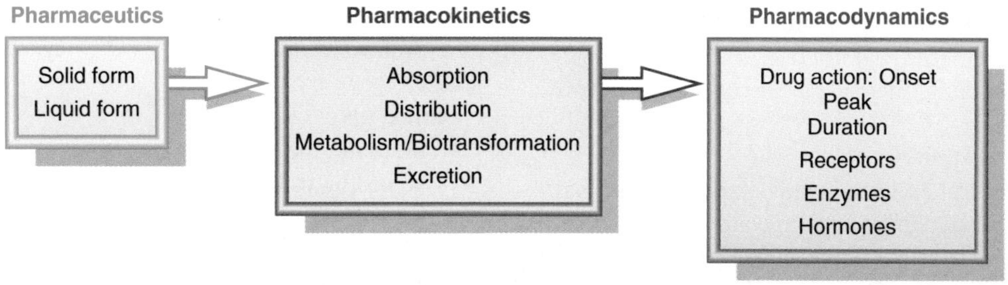

FIGURE 1–12 The three phases of drug action.

effects are called *adverse reactions.* The terms *side effects* and *adverse reactions* are sometimes used interchangeably in the literature and in speaking, but they are different. Some side effects are expected as part of drug therapy. The occurrence of these expected but undesirable side effects is not a reason to discontinue therapy. The nurse's role includes teaching patients to report any side effects. Many can be managed with dosage adjustments, changing to a different drug in the same class of drugs, or implementing other interventions. It is important to know that the occurrence of side effects is one of the primary reasons patients stop taking the prescribed medication. **Adverse reactions** are more severe than side effects. They are a range of untoward effects (unintended and occurring at normal doses) of drugs that cause mild to severe side effects, including anaphylaxis (cardiovascular collapse). Adverse reactions are always undesirable. Adverse effects must always be reported and documented because they represent variances from planned therapy.

Toxic effects, or **toxicity,** of a drug can be identified by monitoring the plasma (serum) therapeutic range of the drug. However, for drugs that have a wide therapeutic index, the therapeutic ranges are seldom given. For drugs with a narrow therapeutic index, such as aminoglycoside antibiotics and anticonvulsants, the therapeutic ranges are closely monitored. When the drug level exceeds the therapeutic range, toxic effects are likely to occur from overdosing or drug accumulation.

Pharmacogenetics

Pharmacogenetics is the scientific discipline studying how the effect of a drug action varies from a predicted drug response because of genetic factors or hereditary influence. Because people have different genetic makeup, they do not always respond identically to a drug dosage or planned drug therapy. Genetic factors can alter the metabolism of the drug in converting its chemical form to an inert metabolite; thus, the drug action can be enhanced or diminished. Some persons are less or more sensitive to drugs and their drug actions because of genetic factors. For example, African Americans do not respond as well as Caucasians to some classes of antihypertensive medications such as ACE inhibitors. (See Chapter 3 for a discussion of pharmacogenetics.)

Tolerance and Tachyphylaxis

Tolerance refers to a decreased responsiveness over the course of therapy. In contrast, **tachyphylaxis** refers to a rapid decrease in response to the drug. In essence, tachyphylaxis is an "acute tolerance." Drug categories that can cause tachyphylaxis include narcotics, barbiturates, laxatives, and psychotropic agents. For example, drug tolerance to narcotics can result in decreased pain relief for the patient. If the nurse does not recognize the development of drug tolerance, the patient's request for more pain medication might be interpreted as drug-seeking behavior associated with addiction. Prevention of tachyphylaxis should always be part of the therapeutic regimen (see Chapter 42).

Placebo Effect

A **placebo effect** is a psychological benefit from a compound that may not have the chemical structure of a drug effect. The placebo is effective in approximately one third of persons who take a placebo compound. Many clinical drug studies involve a group of subjects who receive a placebo. The nurse can increase the therapeutic effect of the drug (e.g., narcotics for pain management) but violate the truth-telling ethical principle if a nontherapeutic drug is presented as a therapeutic agent. Hence, it is required that participants in drug trials be told from the start that they might receive a placebo.

To review, the phases of drug action are pharmaceutic, pharmacokinetic, and pharmacodynamic. Figure 1-12 illustrates these three phases for drugs given orally, but drugs given by injection are involved only in the pharmacokinetic and pharmacodynamic phases. Nurses should be aware that tablets must disintegrate and go into solution (the pharmaceutic phase) to be absorbed.

To avoid toxic effects, the nurse must know the half-life, protein-binding percentage, normal side effects, and therapeutic ranges of the drug. This information can be obtained from drug reference books.

Nursing Process
Patient-Centered Collaborative Care

Assessment

- Take patient history to identify factors that may affect drug pharmacokinetics (e.g., gastric surgery will affect absorption; low serum albumin will affect protein binding; peripheral vascular disease may affect drug distribution to extremities).

- Examine the patient's history to identify factors that may affect pharmacodynamics (e.g., a G6PD deficiency may cause hemolytic anemia if some common drugs are given)
- Collect a medication history.
- Perform a physical exam to identify problems that may affect pharmacodynamics (e.g., elevated BP, dysrhythmias, or other abnormal findings may be an indication for drug therapy).
- Identify side effects of drugs that are nonspecific (same receptor at different tissue and organ sites). For example, when atropine is the drug to be administered, assess for tachycardia, dry mouth and throat, constipation, urinary retention, and blurred vision. If nonspecific drugs are given in large doses or at frequent intervals, many side effects are likely to occur.
- Check peak levels and trough levels of drugs such as aminoglycosides that have a narrow therapeutic range. If the trough level is high, toxic effects can result.
- Check the drug literature for the protein-binding percentage of the drug. Drugs with a high protein-binding effect have a large portion of drug bound to protein. This causes the drug to become inactive until it is released from the protein. The portion not bound to protein is a free and active drug.

Nursing Interventions
- Advise patient not to eat high-fat food before ingesting an enteric-coated tablet, because high-fat foods decrease absorption rate.
- Report to the health care provider if drugs with a long half-life (i.e., greater than 24 hours) are given more than once a day. Some drugs with a long half-life (e.g., the anticoagulant warfarin [Coumadin]) can be more dangerous than others and must be monitored frequently.
- Monitor the therapeutic range of drugs that are more toxic or have a narrow therapeutic range (e.g., digoxin).

Cultural Considerations
- Be aware that individuals of some ethnic or racial heritage metabolize drugs differently than the general population.
- Assess for adverse effects that may result from this variation in metabolism.

Evaluation
- Evaluate the determinants that affect drug therapy according to Figure 1-13.
- Assess for signs and symptoms of drug toxicity when giving two drugs that are highly protein-bound. The drugs compete for protein-binding sites, and displacement of drugs occurs. More free drug is in circulation because there are not enough protein-binding sites. Too much of a free drug can result in drug toxicity.

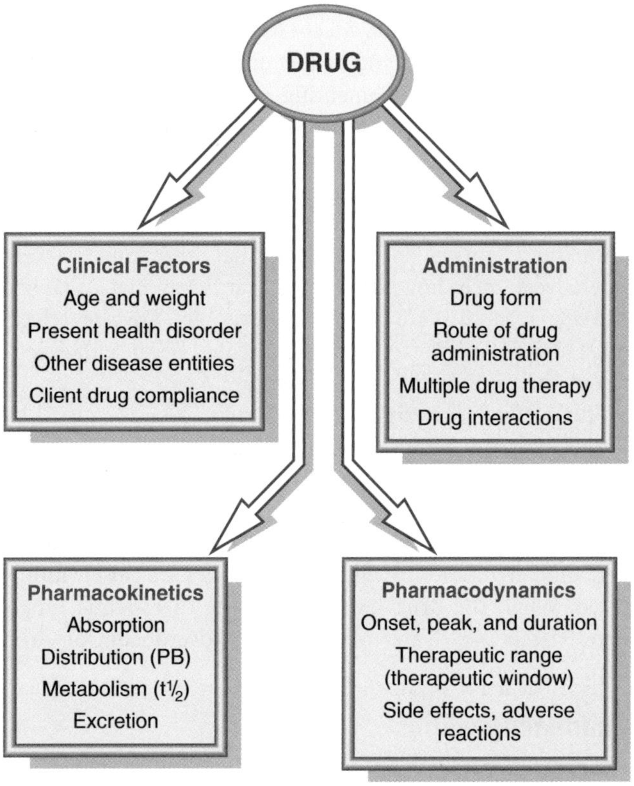

FIGURE 1–13 Determinants that affect drug therapy.

KEY WEBSITES

American Pharmaceutical Association: *www.aphanet.org*
Drug Topics: *www.drugtopics.com*
Pharm Web: *www.pharmweb.net*

CRITICAL THINKING CASE STUDY

The nurse is caring for JM, a patient who was admitted to the hospital with new onset of seizures. JM has been taking warfarin (Coumadin), a highly protein-bound drug that decreases blood clotting. The neurologist has ordered valproic acid (Depakote), an antiseizure medication. Valproic acid is also highly protein bound.

1. What information needs to be included in the interdisciplinary health/teaching plan for this patient?

NCLEX STUDY QUESTIONS

1. Which components of pharmacokinetics does the nurse need to understand before administering a drug? (Select all that apply.)
   a. Drugs with a smaller volume of drug distribution have a longer half-life.
   b. Oral drugs are dissolved through the process of pinocytosis.
   c. Patients with kidney disease may have fewer protein-binding sites and are at risk for drug toxicity.
   d. Rapid absorption decreases the bioavailability of the drug.
   e. When the drug metabolism rate is decreased, excess drug accumulation can occur, which can cause toxicity.
2. The nurse will question the health care provider if a drug with a half-life ($t\frac{1}{2}$) of more than 24 hours is ordered to be given more than how often?
   a. Once daily
   b. Every other day
   c. Twice weekly
   d. Once weekly
3. The nurse is explaining drug action to a nursing student. Which statement made by the nurse is correct?
   a. "Water-soluble and ionized drugs are quickly absorbed."
   b. "A drug not bound to protein is an active drug."
   c. "Most receptors are found under the cell membrane."
   d. "Toxic effects can result if the trough level is low."
4. The nurse is caring for a patient with congestive heart failure who is receiving digoxin (Digitek, Lanoxicaps, Lanoxin). The nurse plans to take which action when administering digoxin?
   a. Check the peak levels of digoxin.
   b. Check the trough levels digoxin.
   c. Monitor for tachyphylaxis.
   d. Monitor the therapeutic range of digoxin.
5. The nurse anticipates that the health care provider will order which laboratory test for an older adult with renal dysfunction?
   a. Creatinine clearance
   b. Glomerular filtration rate
   c. Urine specific gravity
   d. Urine pH
6. When reviewing the patient's medication regimen, the nurse understands that the interval of drug dosage is related to what?
   a. Half-life
   b. Stimulation of receptors
   c. Therapeutic index
   d. Trough level
7. Which nursing assessment(s) will the nurse include when developing a patient medication plan? (Select all that apply.)
   a. Check peak and trough levels of drugs.
   b. Check the drug literature for the protein-binding percentage of a drug.
   c. Identify side effects of drugs that are nonspecific.
   d. Evaluate the patient's reaction to a drug.
   e. To enhance absorption, advise the patient to crush an enteric-coated tablet before taking.
8. A student nurse is studying the phases of drug action. Which statement by the student indicates to the nursing instructor that the student understands the pharmaceutic phase?
   a. "To achieve drug action, drugs are moved by four processes."
   b. "For the drug to cross the biologic membrane, the drug becomes a solution."
   c. "In this phase, drugs are concentrated and a biologic or physiologic response occurs."
   d. "The pharmaceutic phase is the process by which the drug becomes available to body fluids and tissue."
9. The nurse plans to advise the patient to avoid which food(s) before ingesting an enteric-coated medication? (Select all that apply.)
   a. Bananas
   b. Baked lamb chops
   c. Broiled fish
   d. Ice cream
   e. Fried chicken

Answers: 1, c, e; 2, a; 3, b; 4, d; 5, a; 6, a; 7, a, b, c; 8, b; 9, d, e.

CHAPTER

2

The Drug Approval Process

evolve WEBSITE

http://evolve.elsevier.com/KeeHayes/pharmacology/

- Animations
- Content Updates
- Key Points
- Review Questions for the NCLEX® Examination
- References from the Textbook
- Unfolding Case Studies

OBJECTIVES

- Discuss the federal legislation acts related to U.S. Food and Drug Administration drug approvals.
- Explain the Canadian schedules for drugs sold in Canada.
- Describe the function of nurse practice acts.
- Differentiate between chemical, generic, and brand names of drugs.
- Describe useful drug references.

OUTLINE

KEY TERMS

Approval of new drugs by the **U.S. Food and Drug Administration** (FDA) has been steady since the early 2000s; the FDA's Center for Drug Evaluation and Research (CDER) has averaged 23 approvals per year. In 2004, the FDA established its Critical Path Initiative, a national strategy "to drive innovation in the scientific processes through which medical products are developed, evaluated, and manufactured." One focus is on "improving the prevention, diagnosis, and treatment of rare and neglected disorders." Successes of the initiative include developing biomarkers and other scientific tools, streamlining clinical trials, and ensuring product safety.

DRUG STANDARDS AND LEGISLATION

The combination of drug discovery and manufacturing takes 12 to 20 years, with a cost of more than $1 billion. Only a small percentage of drugs are approved. The steps of the process are shown in Figure 2-1.

Drug Standards

The set of drug standards used in the United States is the *United States Pharmacopeia* of 1820. The ***United States Pharmacopeia National Formulary (USP-NF),*** the current three-volume authoritative source for drug standards, is an annual

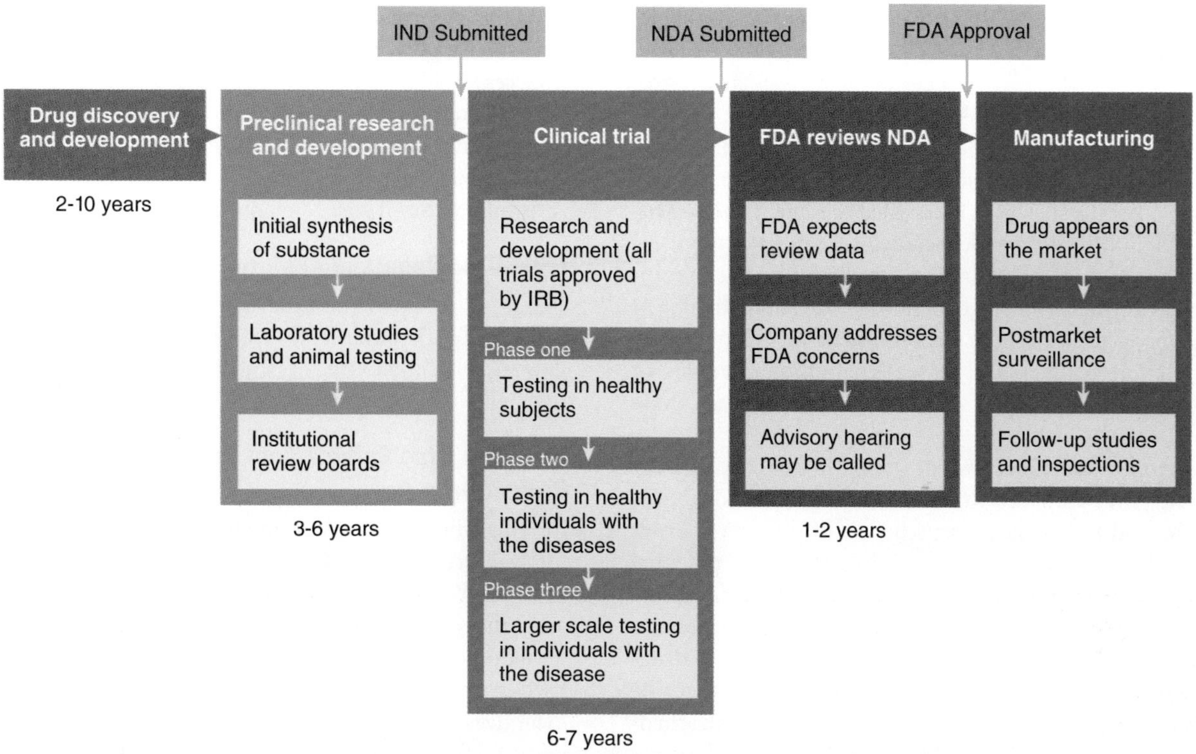

FIGURE 2–1 The drug approval process. *FDA,* U.S. Food and Drug Administration; *IND,* Investigation of New Drug; *NDA,* New Drug Application.

publication with two supplements. Experts in nursing, pharmaceutics, pharmacology, chemistry, and microbiology all contribute. Drugs included in the *USP-NF* have met high standards for therapeutic use, patient safety, quality, purity, strength, packaging safety, and dosage form. Drugs that meet these standards have the initials "USP" following their official name, denoting global recognition of high quality. The *USP-NF* is the official publication for drugs marketed in the United States, so designated by the U.S. Federal Food, Drug, and Cosmetic Act.

The *International Pharmacopeia,* first published in 1951 by the World Health Organization (WHO), provides a basis for standards in strength and composition of drugs for use throughout the world. The book is published in English, Spanish, and French. The fourth edition (Volumes I and II) was published in 2006, with the first supplement in 2008.

Federal Legislation

Through federal legislation, the public is protected from drugs that are impure, toxic, ineffective, or not tested before public sale. The primary purpose of the legislation is to ensure safety. America's first law to regulate drugs was the Federal Pure Food and Drug Act of 1906, which did not include drug effectiveness and drug safety.

1938: Food, Drug, and Cosmetic Act

The Food, Drug, and Cosmetic Act of 1938 empowered the FDA to ensure drug safety by monitoring and regulating the manufacture and marketing of drugs. It is the FDA's responsibility to ensure that all drugs are tested for harmful effects, have labels with accurate information, and enclose detailed literature in the drug packaging that explains adverse effects. The FDA can prevent the marketing of any drug it judges to be incompletely tested or dangerous. Only drugs considered safe by the FDA are approved for marketing.

1952: Durham-Humphrey Amendment to the 1938 Act

The Durham-Humphrey Amendment to the Food, Drug, and Cosmetic Act of 1938 distinguished between drugs that can be sold with or without prescription and those that should not be refilled without a new prescription. Those drugs that should not be refilled without a new prescription, such as narcotics, hypnotics, or tranquilizers, must be so labeled.

1962: Kefauver-Harris Amendment to the 1938 Act

The Kefauver-Harris Amendment to the Food, Drug, and Cosmetic Act of 1938 resulted from the widely publicized thalidomide tragedy of the 1950s in which European patients who took the sedative-hypnotic thalidomide during the first trimester of pregnancy gave birth to infants with extreme limb deformities. The Kefauver-Harris amendment tightened controls on drug safety, especially experimental drugs, and required that adverse reactions and contraindications must be labeled and included in the literature. The amendment also included provisions for the evaluation of testing methods used by manufacturers, the process for withdrawal of approved drugs when safety and effectiveness were in doubt, and the establishment of effectiveness of new drugs before marketing.

1970: The Controlled Substances Act

In 1970, Congress passed the Controlled Substances Act (CSA) of the Comprehensive Drug Abuse Prevention and Control Act, Title II. This act, designed to remedy the escalating problem of drug abuse, included several provisions: (1) promotion of drug education and research into the prevention and treatment of drug dependence; (2) strengthening of enforcement authority; (3) establishment of treatment and rehabilitation facilities; and (4) designation of schedules, or categories, for controlled substances according to abuse liability.

Controlled substances are described in five schedules, or categories, and are listed in Table 2-1. Schedule I drugs are not approved for medical use; schedule II through V drugs have accepted medical use. In addition, the abuse potential and extent of physical and psychological dependence are greatest with schedule I drugs. This dependency decreases as one moves through the schedule, with schedule V drugs having only limited abuse potential. Some drugs might be listed in more than one schedule category. Codeine is a schedule II drug, but when it is added to acetaminophen, it becomes a schedule III drug, and when it is used in combination as a cough preparation, it becomes a schedule V drug.

Nursing interventions for controlled substances are as follows:

- Account for all controlled drugs.
- Keep a special controlled-substance record for required information.
- Countersign all discarded or wasted medication; wastage must be witnessed.
- Ensure that documentation and drugs on hand match.
- Keep all controlled drugs in a locked storage area; keep narcotics under double lock. Be certain that only authorized persons have access to the keys, including keys for patient-controlled analgesia and epidural pumps. Medication may also be administered via an automated dispensing cabinet, with bioidentical identifiers used for access.
- The American Nurses Association (ANA) recognizes nurse drug diversion and recommends that all states have a peer-to-peer assistance program for addicted nurses. Reporting is mandatory if suspected or known diversion occurs.

1978: Drug Regulation Reform Act

This act shortened the time in which new drugs could be developed and marketed. It protects patients' rights and at the same time facilitates the investigational process and promotes research.

1983: The Drug Enforcement Administration and the Orphan Drug Act

In 1983, the **Drug Enforcement Administration** (DEA) of the Department of Justice was charged with the role of being the nation's sole legal drug enforcement agency. In the same year, the Orphan Drug Act was designed to promote the development and manufacture of orphan drugs, those drugs used in the treatment of rare diseases. The act's three primary incentives are (1) federal funding of grants and contracts to perform clinical trials of orphan products; (2) 50% tax credit for costs of clinical testing; and (3) exclusive right to market the drug for 7 years from the marketing approval date.

1997: The Food and Drug Administration Modernization Act

The five provisions in this act are (1) review and use of new drugs is accelerated; (2) drugs can be tested in children before marketing; (3) clinical trial data are necessary for experimental drug use for serious or life-threatening health conditions; (4) drug companies are required to give information on "off-label" drugs (non–FDA-approved drugs) and their uses and costs; and (5) drug companies that plan to discontinue drugs must inform health professionals and patients at least 6 months before stopping drug production.

TABLE 2-1 SCHEDULE CATEGORIES OF CONTROLLED SUBSTANCES

SCHEDULE	EXAMPLES OF SUBSTANCES	DESCRIPTION
I	Heroin, hallucinogens (LSD, marijuana [except when prescribed with cancer treatment], mescaline, peyote, psilocybin)	High potential for drug abuse. No accepted medical use. Labeled C-I.
II	Meperidine (Demerol), morphine, hydrocodone (Hycodan), hydromorphone (Dilaudid), methadone (Dolophine), oxycodone (Oxy-Contin), codeine, amphetamines, secobarbital, pentobarbital (Nembutal)	High potential for drug abuse. Accepted medical use. Can lead to strong physical and psychological dependency. Labeled C-II.
III	Codeine preparations, paregoric, nonnarcotic drugs (e.g., pentazocine [Talwin])	Medically accepted drugs. Potential abuse is less than that for schedules I and II. May cause dependence. Labeled C-III.
IV	Phenobarbital (Luminal), benzodiazepines (e.g., diazepam [Valium], oxazepam [Serax], lorazepam [Ativan], chlordiazepoxide [Librium]), chloral hydrate (Aquachloral), meprobamate	Medically accepted drugs. May cause dependence. Labeled C-IV.
V	Opioid-controlled substances for diarrhea and cough (e.g., codeine in cough preparations)	Medically accepted drugs. Very limited potential for dependence. Labeled C-V.

C, Control; *LSD*, lysergic acid diethylamide.

2002: Best Pharmaceuticals for Children Act

This act gives manufacturers extension of patents to evaluate drugs on the market for their safety and efficacy in children.

2003: Health Insurance Portability and Accountability Act

The Health Insurance Portability and Accountability Act (HIPAA) of 2003 set the standards for the privacy of individually identifiable health information. This rule gives patients more control over their health information, including boundaries on the use and release of health records. Implications of HIPAA related to the individual's therapeutic regimen include limitation on access to information from the pharmacy. For example, patient history can be released only to the patient, and the pharmacist must provide a private area for consultation and have all patients sign a statement that they have received a copy of the privacy statement.

2003: Pediatric Research Equity Act

This act authorizes the FDA to require that drug manufacturers test drugs and biologic products for their safety and effectiveness in children, noting that "children are not small adults."

2007: Food and Drug Administration Amendments Act

This act allows the FDA to mandate postmarketing safety studies and to affect the distribution of drugs that are found to be not as safe as premarket studies indicated.

2009: Family Smoking Prevention and Tobacco Control Act

This act allows the FDA to regulate cigarettes by various measures such as requiring prominent warning labels and complete ingredient lists and prohibiting youth marketing.

2010: Patient Protection and Affordable Care Act

This act was signed into law in 2010 but will not be fully executed until 2014. Essential components of the reform include (1) quality, affordable health care for all Americans; (2) improved quality and efficiency of health care; (3) prevention of chronic disease and improved public health; (4) improved access to innovative medical therapies; and (5) community living services and supports.

NURSE PRACTICE ACTS

Every state has its own laws regarding drug administration by nurses. Generally, nurses cannot prescribe or administer drugs without a health care provider's order. Practicing nurses should be knowledgeable about the nurse practice act in the state where they are licensed. (Nurse practice acts are available online.) Nurses are responsible for knowing their state's law and administrative code. Nurses who administer a drug without a licensed health care provider's order are in violation of the nurse practice act and can have their licenses revoked.

In a civil court, the nurse can be prosecuted for giving the wrong drug or dosage, omitting a drug dose, or giving the drug by the wrong route. The legal terms for these offenses are as follows:

- ***Misfeasance.*** Negligence; giving the wrong drug or drug dose that results in the patient's death
- ***Nonfeasance.*** Omission; omitting a drug dose that results in the patient's death
- ***Malfeasance.*** Giving the correct drug but by the wrong route that results in the patient's death

CANADIAN DRUG REGULATION

In Canada, the Health Protection Branch, Department of National Health and Welfare, is responsible for the administration of the two acts that are the foundation of national drug laws. The manufacture, distribution, and sale of drugs (except narcotics) are controlled by the Canadian Food and Drug Act, which was amended in 1953. The manufacture, distribution, and sale of narcotic drugs are controlled by the 1996 Controlled Drugs and Substances Act (CDSA). Like the U.S. Controlled Substances Act, the Canadian act requires prescriptions and strict recordkeeping for all narcotics.

Drugs sold in Canada are assigned to one of the following schedules:

1. *Schedule F Prescription Drugs.* All prescription drugs, except narcotics and controlled substances, are available only by prescription (written or verbal); thus, these drugs have essentially no potential for abuse. Manufacturing labels are required to include [Pr].
2. The CDSA regulates the control and sale of narcotics and controlled substances through identification of eight schedules based on potential for abuse. Recordkeeping and degree of control are specified for each. Labels must include a ⟨C⟩ for controlled agents and an ⟨N⟩ for narcotic agents. Benzodiazepines are "targeted substances," with *t/c* on all labels. The schedules are as follows:
    1. *Schedule I*: Opium poppy and its derivatives (e.g., morphine, heroin); methadone; coca and its derivates (e.g., cocaine)
    2. *Schedule II*: Cannabis and its derivatives (e.g., marijuana, hashish)
    3. *Schedule III*: Amphetamines, methylphenidate, lysergic acid diethylamide (LSD), methaqualone, psilocybin, mescaline
    4. *Schedule IV*: Sedative-hypnotic agents (e.g., barbiturates, benzodiazepines); anabolic steroids
    5. Schedules V through VIII are in development.

The CDSA covers select codeine preparations. Low-dose codeine (20 mg/30 mL and 8-mg tablets) is an exception and can be sold only by a pharmacist. Two additional medicinal ingredients (usually caffeine and acetylsalicylic acid) must be part of this codeine preparation.

Nonprescription drugs are administered by the pharmacy acts of the respective Canadian provinces that identify the place and conditions of sale. These drugs are assigned to one of three categories:

1. *Nonprescription drugs sold at any retailer.* There is no requirement for professional supervision. Labeling provides information for the patient to make an informed choice for safe use. An example of this category is antiulcer medications.
2. *Pharmacy-only nonprescription drugs.* A pharmacist must be available for advice. The patient self-selects a medication that may have risks for certain populations. An example of this category is antihistamines.
3. *Restricted access nonprescription drugs.* These are available only from the pharmacist. Consultation with a pharmacist is required, and referral to a health care provider is supplied if necessary. An example of this category is insulin.

To address the proliferation of a variety of provincial schedules and regulations, the National Association of Pharmacy Regulatory Authorities (NAPRA) has proposed to "harmonize" regulations nationwide by creating three national drug schedules using the same nomenclature and numbering as the controlled substances schedule system. The NAPRA website at *www.napra.ca* provides detailed information on this system. The schedules are as follows:

1. *Schedule I:* All prescription drugs, including narcotics and controlled substances
2. *Schedule II:* Restricted access of pharmacist-only nonprescription drugs
3. *Schedule III:* Pharmacy-only nonprescription drugs
4. *Unscheduled Drugs:* Drugs that are available at retail outlets and not placed in the above categories

In Canada, therapeutic and toxic levels are monitored according to the International System of Units (SI); this is also true in many European countries. The mole (mol) was adopted to express drug concentration in body fluid in molar units, such as millimoles per liter (mmol/L), instead of the traditional expression of mass units, milligrams per liter (mg/L). Some institutions in the United States use SI units, but the traditional use of mass units in the United States continues.

INITIATIVES TO COMBAT DRUG COUNTERFEITING

Use of counterfeit and adulterated prescription drugs is on the rise. Contributing reasons are that reporting of counterfeit incidents is not mandatory and that counterfeiting has features of a "perfect crime" (medicine is taken; evidence is gone). (See Chapter 12.) The FDA and consumer groups are working on strategies to combat this problem, including tougher oversight of distributors, a rapid alert system, and better-informed consumers. The role of the nurse is critical in consumer education. The nurse must advise patients to report any differences in taste or appearance of a drug or in its packaging. Patients should be alert to slight variations in packaging or labeling (e.g., color, package seal); should note any unexpected side effects; and should buy drugs from reputable sources. Reputable online pharmacies have the designation of Verified Internet Pharmacy Practice Site (VIPPS) and display an approval seal. If any suspicion of counterfeit arises, the patient, family, or nurse should contact the FDA at *www.fda.gov/Safety/MedWatch/HowToReport/.*

DRUG NAMES

Drugs have several names. The **chemical name** describes the drug's chemical structure. The **generic name** is the official, nonproprietary name for the drug. This name is not owned by any drug company and is universally accepted. Most drugs are ordered by generic name. The **brand (trade) name,** also known as the *proprietary name,* is chosen by the drug company and is usually a registered trademark owned by that specific company. Drug companies market a compound using its brand name. For example, Narcan is the brand (proprietary) name of a drug whose generic name is naloxone HCl.

Throughout this text, both generic and brand names are given for each drug at its first mention. Because many brand names may exist for a single generic name, the generic name is given first in lowercase letters, followed by the most commonly used brand name in parentheses. Brand names always begin with a capital letter. An example of a generic and brand-name drug listing is "furosemide (Lasix)."

Generic drugs must be approved by the FDA before they can be marketed. If the generic drug is found to be bioequivalent to the brand-name drug, then the generic drug is considered therapeutically equivalent and is given an "A" rating. If the peak serum concentration and the plasma-concentration curve of the generic drug fall within 80% to 125% of the brand-name drug, then the generic drug is considered equivalent to the brand-name drug.

Approved generic drugs can be checked at *www.accessdata.fda.gov/scripts/cder/drugsatfda/.* The FDA also publishes a list of approved generic drugs that are bioequivalent to brand-name drugs. Generic drugs have the same active ingredients as brand-name drugs but are usually less expensive because manufacturers do not have to do extensive testing; these drugs were clinically tested for safety and efficacy by the pharmaceutic company that first formulated the drug. However, some generic drugs have inert fillers and binders that may result in variations of drug effectiveness.

The health care provider and the patient must exercise care in choosing generic drugs because of possible variation in their action or the response to them. Brand-name drugs are preferred when ordering anticonvulsants for seizures; anticoagulants (e.g., Coumadin); medication for heart failure (e.g., Lanoxin); and aspirin in large doses for rheumatoid arthritis. The nurse should check with the health care provider or the pharmacist when generic drugs are prescribed. The health care provider must note on the prescription whether the pharmacist may substitute the generic drug when the brand name is prescribed.

DRUG RESOURCES

Many drug references are available, including nursing texts that identify related nursing interventions and areas for health teaching. Some recommended resources follow.

American Hospital Formulary Service (AHFS) Drug Information is published by the American Society of Health-System Pharmacists in Bethesda, Maryland. It provides accurate and complete drug information on nearly all prescription drugs marketed in the United States. This text contains drugs listed according to therapeutic drug classification. The information given for each drug includes chemistry and stability, pharmacologic actions, pharmacokinetics, uses, cautions per body system, precautions, contraindications, acute toxicity, drug interactions, dosage and administration, and preparations.

This reference is updated yearly with monthly supplements. The supplements contain information on new drugs such as dosage forms and strengths, uses, and cautions. The text is unbiased; it does not contain information about the drug only from the drug company.

United States Pharmacopeia—Drug Information (USP-DI) is a three-volume set that is available in most hospitals and pharmacies and supplies monthly supplements. The first two volumes, Volumes IA and IB, provide drug information for the health care provider. They include pharmacology, precautions to consider, side effects and adverse effects, patient consultation, general dosing information, and dosage forms. Volume II offers drug information for the patient. It explains the information in a way the patient can understand. The topics include administration of drugs, drug effects, indications, adverse reactions, dosage guidelines, and what to do for missed doses.

The *Medical Letter* on drugs and therapeutics is a non-profit publication for physicians, nurse practitioners, and other health professionals. Biweekly issues cover one of two themes, such as (1) drugs for the treatment of disease entities (e.g., human immunodeficiency virus, peptic ulcers) and (2) two to four new drugs that have been recently approved by the FDA. Information for each new drug includes pharmacokinetics, clinical studies, dosage, adverse effects, and interactions.

Prescriber's Letter is a newsletter published monthly by the Therapeutic Research Center in Stockton, California. It addresses new FDA-approved drugs, various uses of older drugs, and FDA warnings.

Handbook on Injectable Drugs by Lawrence A. Trissel is published by the American Society of Hospital Pharmacists. It is an excellent reference for injectable medications and lists drug compatibility with other drugs, base fluids, and drugs available in large-volume parenterals. Also, it includes the pH of each drug and offers some dosing administration guidelines.

MedlinePlus is a service of the U.S. National Library of Medicine. Available at *www.nlm.nih.gov/medlineplus/druginformation*, it offers extensive information on prescribed drugs as well as herbs and supplements, indexed by generic and brand names. Other key websites are listed at the end of each chapter of this text.

U.S. FOOD AND DRUG ADMINISTRATION PREGNANCY CATEGORIES

The FDA has developed a classification system related to the effects of drugs on the fetus. These categories are described in Chapter 12.

KEY WEBSITES

Critical Path Initiative: *www.fda.gov/ScienceResearch/SpecialTopics/CriticalPathInitiative/default.htm*

Health Insurance Portability and Accountability Act: *www.hhs.gov/ocr/hipaa*

U.S. Food and Drug Administration: *www.fda.gov/medwatch*

NCLEX STUDY QUESTIONS

1. The nurse is having a health teaching session with a patient who has many questions about the history of drug labels. What is the nurse's best legislation reference for drug labels and increased control on drug safety?
   a. Kefauver-Harris Amendment to the 1938 Act
   b. Controlled Substances Act
   c. Food, Drug, and Cosmetic Act
   d. Durham-Humphrey Amendment to the 1938 Act
2. The nurse is reviewing a patient's list of medications and notes that several have the highest abuse potential. According to U.S. standards, the highest potential for abuse of drugs with accepted medical use is found in drugs included in which schedule?
   a. II
   b. III
   c. IV
   d. V
3. The nurse is reviewing the drug-approval process in the United States and learns that the Food and Drug Administration Modernization Act of 1997 contains which provisions? (Select all that apply.)
   a. Review of new drugs is accelerated.
   b. Drug companies must provide information on "off-label" drugs.
   c. Privacy of individually identifiable health information must be protected.
   d. Drug companies must offer advanced notice of plans to discontinue drugs.
   e. Drug labels must describe side effects and adverse effects.

4. The patient has questions about counterfeit drugs. Which factors alert the patient or nurse that a drug is counterfeit or adulterated? (Select all that apply.)
   a. Variations in packaging
   b. Unexpected side effects
   c. Different taste
   d. Different chemical components
   e. Different odor
5. The nurse must be knowledgeable about the Nurse Practice Act. In the event the nurse gives the correct drug via the wrong route, resulting in the death of the patient, what may the nurse be charged with in a civil court?
   a. Misfeasance
   b. Nonfeasance
   c. Malfeasance
   d. Negligence
6. The nurse knows the importance of administering the right medication to the patient and that drugs have many names. It is therefore most important that drugs be ordered by which name?
   a. Generic
   b. Brand
   c. Trade
   d. Chemical
7. A drug label has "t/c" on it. The nurse knows that which statement is true about this designation? (Select all that apply.)
   a. It is on all schedule F prescription drugs.
   b. It is on targeted substances, such as benzodiazepines.
   c. It is a designation of the Canadian Controlled Drugs and Substances Act.
   d. It is on all narcotics.
   e. It is on over-the-counter drugs.
8. What provisions from the Controlled Substances Act of 1970 were designed to remedy drug abuse?
   a. The act established treatment and rehabilitation facilities.
   b. The act tightened controls on experimental drugs.
   c. The act required clinical trial data on drugs.
   d. The act required drug companies to give information on off-label drugs.

Answers: 1, a; 2, a; 3, a, b, d; 4, a, b, c; 5, c; 6, a; 7, b, c; 8, a.

CHAPTER

3

Cultural and Pharmacogenetic Considerations

Bettyrae Jordan

evolve WEBSITE

http://evolve.elsevier.com/KeeHayes/pharmacology/

- Animations
- Content Updates
- Key Points
- Review Questions for the NCLEX® Examination
- References from the Textbook
- Unfolding Case Studies

OBJECTIVES

- Recognize verbal and nonverbal communication practices of various social and cultural groups.
- Explain appropriate spatial configurations for patients when delivering nursing care.
- Discuss the importance of including significant members of the social group in planning and implementation of patient care.
- Compare patients' perception of time based on cultural constructs.
- Describe patients' need to exercise control in their environment.
- Anticipate potential unique responses to drugs based on social, cultural, and biologic influences.
- Safeguard patients' rights to confidentiality during inclusion of significant others in the plan of care.

OUTLINE

KEY TERMS

alternative health practices, p. 22
acculturation, p. 22
assimilation, p. 22
community, p. 22
complementary health practices, p. 22
culture, p. 22
cultural universals, p. 22
ethnopharmacology, p. 21
genomes, p. 24
healers, p. 22
pharmacogenetics, p. 21
pharmacogenomics, p. 24
polymorphisms, p. 24
traditional health practices, p. 22

ETHNOPHARMACOLOGY

Ethnopharmacology is the study of drug responses that may be unique to an individual owing to social, cultural, and biologic phenomena. The emergence of ethnopharmacology highlights the need for nurses to use knowledge and research from the social sciences as well as the biologic and physical sciences to provide holistic nursing care.

Pharmacogenetics integrates the study of pharmacokinetics, pharmacodynamics, and variations of the predicted response to a drug due to genetic factors. The nurse must integrate knowledge of pharmacogenetics within patients' cultural contexts. **Culture** is defined as sets of learned behavior and ideas that human beings acquire as members of a community. A **community** is a cluster of individuals who function as a group to attain cultural universals. **Cultural universals** are designed to meet the community's survival needs and common goals such as the obtainment of food and other practices that maintain the group. Providing culturally competent care complements the Quality and Safety Education for Nurses (QSEN) initiative (see Chapters 11 and 12 for more information on QSEN).

TRANSCULTURAL NURSING

The concept of transcultural nursing was formalized by Madeleine Leininger, a nurse anthropologist. She founded the Transcultural Nursing Society in 1974. A challenge for nurses worldwide is the degree of cultural diversity owing to migration and global movement. Numerous cultural groups engage in the use of **traditional health practices**, which may include use of teas, herbs, spices, and special foods as well as homeopathic remedies, poultices, and ointments. These practices can have neutral, beneficial, or deleterious effects on a patient's health. The nurse must obtain a thorough health history to determine all the pharmacotherapeutic agents the patient is using. Obtaining a thorough history is more difficult than it seems; patients may not reveal all information, assuming that because herbs, teas, and spices are natural substances, they are therefore not drugs. They may also be reluctant to share this information with a conventional health care practitioner.

Healers play a role in traditional health practices in about 80% of the population worldwide. Traditional healers usually have some practical knowledge of human anatomy and physiology, pharmacology, and pharmaceutical substances. Healers may combine practical knowledge with rituals that seek to control otherworldly forces such as deities or spirits. Every cultural group has its own traditions, superstitions, and belief systems. Throughout history, healing practices, religious ideology, and spirituality have been tightly intertwined.

Owing to varying degrees of assimilation and acculturation within and among cultural groups, it is essential for the nurse to not make generalizations about an individual's beliefs or behaviors. **Assimilation** occurs when a less powerful group changes its ways to blend in with the dominant cultural group. Adults who immigrate to a new region usually take longer to assimilate than do younger people. **Acculturation** is the process by which a group adjusts to living within a dominant culture while at the same time maintaining its original identity. This sets the stage for **complementary health practices** that combine traditional beliefs and mainstream health practices.

Adding to the challenges faced by nurses in countries with numerous cultural groups is the phenomenon of the dominant group borrowing traditional health practices from other groups. When a dominant group adopts health practices from a nondominant group, they are called **alternative health practices.**

Use of complementary and alternative health practices is growing in the United States. A major impetus for this movement is that many individuals experience difficulty accessing or paying for mainstream health care. Even individuals who have access to mainstream health care may perceive that it is not personalized or effective, so they may opt for complementary health care (using a new therapy along with a mainstream therapy already in use) or alternative health care (using a new therapy in place of a mainstream therapy). This is evidenced by the vast amounts of teas and herbs available in most supermarkets (see Chapter 6) and by the increase in the use of acupuncture, acupressure, and massage as therapies.

HERBAL ALERT 3-1

Gender-Specific Herb Protocols

Women have traditionally sought substitutes for hormonal replacement therapy. More women are now using phytoestrogens like those found in flaxseed, licorice, black cohosh, and soybeans. Health care providers should ask patients about the use of these naturally occurring phytoestrogens because they are contraindicated in women with a history of or risk for hormonally mediated cancers and benign tumors.

THE GIGER AND DAVIDHIZAR TRANSCULTURAL ASSESSMENT MODEL

The Transcultural Assessment Model, developed by Giger and Davidhizar in 1998, suggests that all cultures have six cultural phenomena. These cultural phenomena flow from a culturally unique individual (Figure 3-1). The model has been frequently reviewed for relevancy and has been clinically useful for nurses and other members of the health care team.

Communication

Communication occurs verbally and nonverbally. Nurses must be alert to different types of communication styles among patients to provide culturally competent care.

Language

Patients' use of languages other than English may pose a challenge to nurses working in the United States. Professional translators should be used whenever possible to safeguard a patient's confidentiality. If a professional translator is not available, the nurse must select an alternative person carefully. (For example, asking the teenage son of a patient with gynecological health issues to translate may create an uncomfortable situation that is better avoided.) Even with the use of a translator, nuances in languages are unique and may not lend themselves to accurate translation in another language. There can be miscommunication between the patient, the translator, and the nurse.

Nurses should not confuse politeness with meaningful communication. Many patients will nod in agreement to

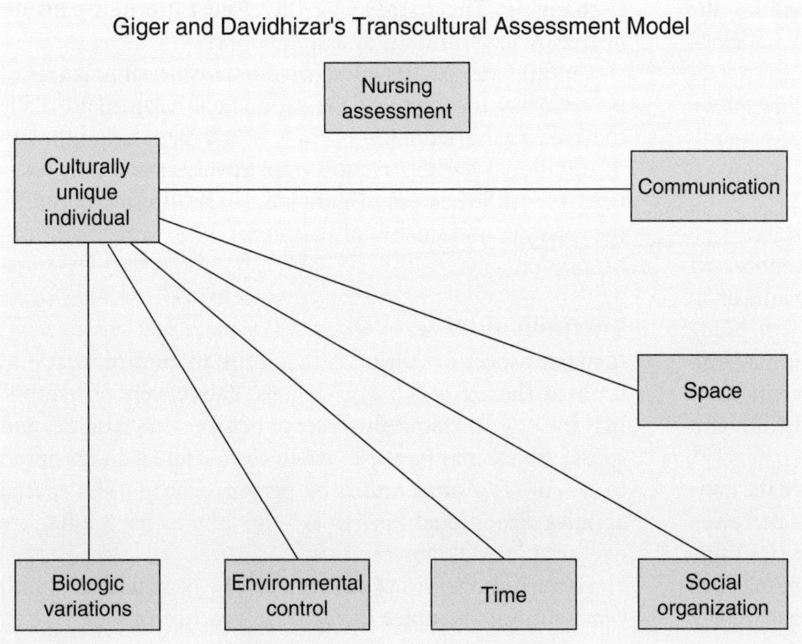

FIGURE 3–1 The Giger and Davidhizar Transcultural Assessment Model. (From Giger J, Davidhizar R: *Transcultural nursing: assessment and intervention,* ed. 6, St Louis, 2013, Elsevier.)

statements made by the nurse even if the statements are not well understood because of language differences.

Vernacular English

Adding to the challenge of communication is the pervasive use of words and phrases that are popular in particular social or cultural groups. For example, the term "African-American Vernacular English" has been used to describe a style of English speaking that is used among some African Americans. It is thought to have its roots in the myriad of West African languages spoken by slaves brought to America. More generally, vernacular English is any style of English that varies from standard English. Its use by patients can lead to misunderstanding by the nurse or to other communication difficulties.

Greetings and Communication Styles

All cultures have prescribed norms for greeting and addressing others. Americans of European descent may be more informal when greeting and addressing others than descendants of non-European cultures. Nurses must keep in mind that patient-nurse interactions in health care settings are considered formal and that informal styles of communication should be used only after careful consideration.

For example, a communication style that might hinder culturally competent nursing care may be found in some patients of Asian descent, who might speak in a soft tone of voice and avoid direct eye contact. The nurse who is unaware of this may miss cues that care is needed. Asian Americans and Native Americans may be comfortable with periods of silence, while persons of Latin American, African, or European descent may be uneasy during periods of silence. Being cognizant of these preferences will help the nurse provide a comfortable environment for the patient.

Space

The amount of space around a person's body is an important psychological consideration. Americans may desire a great deal of personal space. In some other cultures, population density may dictate limited personal space. Patients who are used to dense living quarters may feel insecure in a hospital room. It is important that the nurse have frequent contact with these patients and allow significant members of the social group to remain with the patient as much as possible.

A major challenge in caring for patients is the use of touch and the protection of modesty. Although nurses must touch patients to administer care, all cultures have taboos regarding touch. There are added considerations when the patient is of a different gender than the nurse. This is a particularly sensitive issue for groups within the Muslim, Orthodox Jewish, Amish, and Roma communities. For example, a Muslim woman may prefer to be cared for by a female nurse rather than a male nurse. Nurses should consider inquiring about patients' preferences regarding touch before implementing nursing care. It may be best to have a family member of the same gender as the patient present during procedures, if possible. There may also be apparent paradoxes within cultures; for example, persons of Hispanic descent may value human contact but also value modesty.

Social Organization

Families are basic social units. The definition of family and the criteria for inclusion varies among individuals and among cultures. Americans of western European descent may have small, nuclear families, whereas other cultural groups living in the United States may have larger, extended families. Delivery of nursing care can be enhanced by including family whenever appropriate; nurses are in a position to advocate for inclusion of family in health care settings. Limiting the amount of time a patient can visit with members of the social group is a long-standing practice in American health care settings, but in some other countries, such as the Philippines, it is expected that family members will stay by the patient's bedside and participate in his or her care.

Time

Nurses and their patients may have different perceptions of time. Time moves slowly for a patient who is anxious or in pain but moves quickly for a nurse who has a demanding workload. The use of vague terms to denote time may also cause a disparity between nurses' and patients' perceptions of time. Words like *now, soon,* or *later* may have vastly different nuances among individuals and groups.

Adding to the complexity of time perception are the concepts of *linear* time and *circular* time. When time is perceived as linear, the present flows into the future and is irretrievably lost. Viewing time as linear is likely to prompt thinking such as "I must do this now." When time is perceived as circular, the present has more stability and the need to do things at the moment has less urgency. Viewing time as circular is likely to prompt thinking such as, "I will have the opportunity to do this later."

The cultural aspect of time perception has a profound effect on pharmacotherapeutic adherence. All cultures have a concept of time as it is related to the past, present, and future. All humans are acutely aware that the present is here and now and in real time; it is the *relative importance* placed on the past, present, and future that directs the use of time.

People of western European descent may exhibit a great deal of future orientation. This can lead to health practices perceived to prevent illness, such as adhering to a low-fat diet to prevent higher cholesterol or wearing a condom during sex to prevent disease. Concern for the future also serves as motivation to take steps to control chronic illness, which is likely to lead to greater adherence to long-term pharmacotherapy. Explanations for these phenomena are that people of western European descent have historically experienced longevity and expect to have a lengthy future, and that their economic and social lives have revolved around calendars and clocks for centuries.

Non-European cultural groups such as those of African, Asian, Native American, or Latin American descent have exhibited less dependence on strict time schedules for economic and social activities. These groups' perception of time may be rooted in agrarian cultures that use daily and seasonal rhythms of the earth and the sun to direct activities. This could result in emphasis being placed on the present; measures to ease the discomfort of a current illness may take precedence over measures to promote long-term wellness or treat a chronic illness. Patients with a present-oriented perception of time are more likely to discontinue mainstream prescriptive therapies when they feel well. It must be noted, however, that with the shrinking of agrarian cultures and the spreading of European-style practices, this treatment of time is changing. The nurse must therefore assess the patient's degree of acculturation or assimilation.

Cultural groups that are steeped in traditional practices or perceive that their cultural identities are threatened are likely to have a past orientation of time, which may lead to the use of traditional health practices over mainstream health practices. Health behaviors of individuals are also influenced by the quantity and quality of past experiences with the health care system.

Environmental Control

A major aspect of culture is the desire to control nature to facilitate the needs of human beings. The concept of "nature" may include otherworldly forces or beings, such as deities and spirits. Illness may be attributed to cosmic forces and believed to be cured or ameliorated by persons who possess special abilities. Traditional healers are thought to have influence over otherworldly forces.

Healers and spiritual advisors can be beneficial in health care settings; examples include the practice of clergy (e.g., minister, priest, rabbi) visiting ill members of a congregation or the inclusion of a traditional healer in the plan of care.

The Indian Health Service is a federal agency within the U.S. Department of Health and Human Services that oversees the health care of approximately 2 million Native Americans who belong to federally recognized tribes. Similarly, the Canadian health care system has developed many initiatives to improve the health care of its indigenous peoples, known as *First Nation, Inuit,* and *Metis.* In both systems, the use of traditional healers and spiritual guides is incorporated into mainstream prescriptive therapies.

Biologic Variations

Through the work of the *Human Genome Project,* an international collaborative research program, the field of pharmacogenomics is rapidly expanding. In the United States, the project is managed by the National Human Genome Research Institute, which is part of the National Institutes of Health (NIH). **Pharmacogenomics** refers to the general study of all the different genes that determine drug behavior. An example of a significant finding of pharmacogenomics is the effect of the Cytochrome P-450 (CYP) enzymes on drug response, drug-drug interactions, and adverse drug events, which are described later in the chapter.

The Genographic Project has performed DNA testing on populations all over the world. Findings reveal that human beings are 99.9% genetically identical; this implies that there are not multiple races but multiple genotypes (an individual's genetic identity).

To illustrate the significance of these findings to the patient care setting, it is necessary to review additional terms used in the fields of pharmacogenomics and pharmacogenetics. **Genomes** are a complete set of chromosomes and make up a cell's DNA. **Polymorphisms** are DNA variants that occur within a specific population at a frequency greater than 1%. A **substrate** is a substance that binds to and is metabolized by one or more enzymes. Drugs are chemical substances and a type of substrate. The Cytochrome P-450 enzyme system either induces or inhibits the action of substrates. Induction or inhibition of a substrate accounts for the variations in drug metabolism in individuals and groups. The Division of Clinical Pharmacology at Indiana University Department of Medicine continually updates a clinically relevant table of drug interactions caused by the Cytochrome P-450 system.

Human migration around the world has been so vast over such a long period that most people have a variety of genetic markers. The study of pharmacogenetics can pave the way for pharmacotherapy that yields greater therapeutic benefits and causes fewer adverse reactions. The application of pharmacogenetics should be approached with caution. A person who is dark-skinned and appears to be of African descent is likely to have some European genetic markers.

Certain classifications of medications have different effects in individuals whose genetic markers are predominantly characteristic of a certain biologic group. For example, in the United States, Caucasian people are more likely than people of Asian or African heritage to have abnormally low levels of the CYP2D6 enzyme that metabolizes drugs belonging to a variety of therapeutic areas, such as antidepressants, antipsychotics, and beta blockers.

African Americans respond poorly to several classes of antihypertensive agents (beta blockers and angiotensin-converting enzyme inhibitors). Differences in skin structure and physiology can affect response to dermatologic and topically applied products. Clinical trials have demonstrated lower responses to interferon-alpha used in the treatment of hepatitis C among African Americans compared with other racial subgroups.

As another example, the U.S. Food and Drug Administration has entered into an agreement with the manufacturers of drugs containing carbamazepine (Tegretol) to include product labeling recommending that patients of Asian ancestry be genetically tested before starting on this agent. There is a strong association between serious skin reactions and an inherited variant of the *H 1502LA-B* gene found in Asians.

These intrinsic biologic factors must be considered along with extrinsic factors such as diet and environmental and sociocultural issues to prescribe effective therapies and provide holistic health care.

Researchers conducting clinical trials for development of new drugs are now required to obtain genetic testing of the participants in the study. Issues to be resolved before widespread testing are the cost-versus-benefit ratio and ethical considerations. Genetic testing is expensive and generally not covered by third-party payers. Genetic information can affect employment, insurability, and family relationships.

Table 3-1 applies the Giger and Davidhizar Transcultural Assessment model to four broad cultural categories of peoples of European descent, African descent, Latin and Native American descent, and Asian descent. It is important to keep in mind that there is no generic prototype for any of these categories. Italian Americans are likely to have different customs than German Americans. There may be a perception in the United States that most Asians are Chinese and most Hispanics are Mexican, but in fact there is great variation among these broad groups regarding geography of origin, language, customs, and spiritual systems. Another misperception in the United States is that people of African descent are from one country, but Africa comprises 54 countries over a large geographical area; language, customs, and spiritual systems vary extensively.

Box 11-1 in Chapter 11 supplies additional information on culturally sensitive care.

Nursing Process
Patient-Centered Collaborative Care

Cultural and Pharmacogenetic Considerations

Assessment
- Assess patient's ability to communicate using standard English.
- Determine if patient participates in traditional health practices and/or complementary or alternative medical practices.
- List patient's use of pharmacotherapeutic agents, including prescription medications, over-the-counter medications, herbs, and teas.
- Ascertain if including a traditional healer would facilitate compliance with prescriptive therapies.
- Inquire about patient's preferences regarding touch, modesty, and personal space.
- Gauge patient's perception of time.

Nursing Diagnoses
- Anxiety related to inability to communicate and understand diagnosis
- Impaired verbal communication related to not understanding primary language
- Ineffective community coping related to lack of relationships with members of the community
- Ineffective self–health management related to not accessing or understanding health care resources

Planning
- Patient's health care needs will be met within a culturally competent framework.
- Patient will effectively manage health care.

Nursing Interventions
- Use appropriate persons as translators when patient's use of standard English is limited.
- Anticipate that therapeutic communication with patient and significant others who use limited standard English will require additional time with each encounter.

TABLE 3-1 SELECTED ETHNIC/CULTURAL GROUPS AND COMPONENTS OF THE GIGER AND DAVIDHIZAR TRANSCULTURAL ASSESSMENT MODEL*

CULTURAL PHENOMENA	COMMUNICATION STYLES	SPATIAL PREFERENCES	SOCIAL ORGANIZATION	PERCEPTION OF TIME	ENVIRONMENTAL CONTROL	BIOLOGIC VARIATIONS
People of European descent	Prefer direct eye contact. Use moderate to loud vocal volume. Use many words to describe symptoms. Uncomfortable with periods of silence.	Prefer a large amount of personal space. Value privacy. Exhibit a low to moderate amount of touching among group members.	Small, nuclear families. Extended family members often live a far distance away. High degree of individualism.	High level of importance placed on the future. Expect that the present level of comfort be addressed. Little focus on the past.	Primarily believe that healthy behaviors prevent illness. Secondarily believe that illness is caused by cosmic forces. Believe in being united with a deity in the afterlife.	Poor metabolizers of antidepressants, antipsychotics, cardiovascular agents, and isoniazid (INH), which can lead to toxicity.
People of African descent	Prefer direct eye contact. Use moderate to loud vocal volume. Uncomfortable with periods of silence.	Comfortable with a smaller amount of personal space. Exhibit moderate amount of touching among group members.	Small, nuclear families in America but might classify nonrelated persons as family. Important to recognize these members of the social group.	High level of importance placed on the present. Connected with the past as evidenced by the use of home remedies passed through generations. Become more concerned with the future as longevity increases.	Spiritually oriented. Important to include clergy in care. Believe in being united with a deity in the afterlife.	May have diminished therapeutic effects from beta blockers, ACE inhibitors, and warfarin sodium (Coumadin).
People of Latin American descent and Native Americans	Not likely to make direct eye contact with persons perceived to be in authoritative positions. Varying degrees of comfort with silence.	Comfortable with a small amount of personal space. Latin Americans value touching. Native Americans use touch lightly.	Large, extended families. Important to include family members in care.	High level of importance placed on the present. Connected with the past as evidenced by the use of traditional healers. Become more concerned with the future as longevity increases.	Spiritually oriented. Followers of Christian religions derive comfort from religious artifacts such as rosary beads. There may be multiple deities in indigenous religions.	Native Americans have a high incidence of lactose intolerance resulting in low-calcium diets. Also exhibit enhanced vasomotor responses to alcohol.

*This table is limited in scope and does not necessarily reflect an individual's beliefs, behaviors, or biologic functioning.

- Provide appropriate spatial configurations for individual patients and members of their social groups when delivering nursing care.
- Include significant members of the social group in planning and implementation of patient care.
- Allow patient adequate time with significant members of the social group.
- Recognize the need for patients to exercise control in their environment.
- Anticipate unique responses to drugs based on social, cultural, and biologic influences.
- Consult with persons who are knowledgeable about the patient's culture and mainstream culture.
- Incorporate nonharmful traditional health practices with mainstream prescriptive therapies when appropriate.
- Facilitate adherence to mainstream prescriptive therapies within patient's social and cultural contexts.

Patient Teaching

- Include significant members of the social group, when appropriate, while teaching about prescriptive therapies.
- Provide health information written in the patient's primary language. Medline, an online service of the National Institutes of Health, offers a variety of patient education materials in a number of languages available at *www.nlm.nih.gov/medlineplus/languages/languages.html.*
- Use illustrations to explain prescriptive therapies.

Evaluation

- Monitor for patient adherence to prescriptive therapies.
- Evaluate physical, social, and psychological outcomes of prescriptive therapies.

KEY WEBSITES

EthnoMed: *www.ethnomed.org/patient-education*
Indian Health Service: *www.ihs.gov*
New York University School of Medicine Center for Immigrant Health: *www.med.nyu.edu/cih*
The Office of Minority Health: *www.minorityhealth.hhs.gov*
Transcultural Nursing Society: *www.tcns.org*

CRITICAL THINKING CASE STUDY

1. NS is a 72-year-old woman who immigrated to the United States from Egypt 5 years ago. She is a widow, has five grown children, and follows Islamic doctrine. She lives with her oldest daughter. A younger daughter and three sons live near her home. NS is currently hospitalized owing to a recent cerebral vascular accident. She has left-sided paralysis. The attending physician tells the patient she should go to a rehabilitation unit for 3 weeks for physical therapy. The oldest daughter is present for the physician's visit. Both the patient and her daughter appear anxious but do not ask the physician any questions.
   1. What cultural factors could explain the apparent anxiety?
   2. Which nursing interventions would help decrease the anxiety?
   3. How may the patient view the idea of physical therapy?
   4. What should the nurse consider before applying an ointment?

NCLEX STUDY QUESTIONS

1. The nurse is performing a health assessment on a newly admitted patient of Asian descent. The patient looks at the floor whenever the nurse asks a question. Communication is enhanced when the nurse does which action?
   a. Frequently touches the patient
   b. Asks questions that require only "yes" or "no" for answers
   c. Discontinues the health assessment
   d. Uses eye contact sparingly
2. The nurse has been measuring the blood pressure of an African-American patient every 4 hours for the past 3 days in a hospital setting. The blood pressure is consistently above 140/90. The patient has been compliant with the antihypertensive drug therapy while hospitalized. The nurse will initially perform which action?
   a. Question the patient about the types of food consumed in the last 3 to 4 days.
   b. Inform the prescriber that the antihypertensive drug therapy is not working.
   c. Increase blood pressure measurements to every 2 hours.
   d. Place the patient on a restricted fluid intake.
3. A nurse who is male is caring for a young, married woman who is an observant Muslim. It is important that the nurse perform which action?
   a. Touch no part of the patient's body.
   b. Identify the patient's preference regarding touch.
   c. Touch the patient only when her spouse is present.
   d. Tell the nurse manager he cannot care for female patients who practice Islam.

4. A nurse is teaching a 16-year-old female patient about a newly prescribed medication. The patient is bilingual in Spanish and English. Which behavior best indicates the patient's understanding of the instructions?
   a. The patient frequently nods her head while listening to the nurse's instructions.
   b. The patient states that she understands the instructions.
   c. The patient repeats the nurse's instructions to her parents.
   d. The patient does not ask the nurse for clarification of the instructions.
5. A Native American patient is newly diagnosed with diabetes mellitus type 2 and is prescribed the antidiabetic drug metformin (Glucophage) 500 mg PO with morning and evening meals. Which statement best indicates to the nurse that the patient will adhere to the pharmacotherapy?
   a. "I will no longer put sugar on my cereal because that will help me be healthier."
   b. "If I take this medicine, I will feel better soon and won't have to take it anymore."
   c. "To reduce the possibility of damage to my body, I must take the medicine as scheduled."
   d. "I have diabetes because of my ancestry, so there's not much I can do about it."

Answers: 1, d; 2, b; 3, b; 4, c; 5, c.

CHAPTER

4

Drug Interactions and Over-the-Counter Drugs

evolve WEBSITE

http://evolve.elsevier.com/KeeHayes/pharmacology/

- Animations
- Content Updates
- Key Points
- Review Questions for the NCLEX® Examination
- References from the Textbook
- Unfolding Case Studies

OBJECTIVES

- Differentiate the four pharmacokinetic processes related to drug interaction.
- Explain the three effects associated with pharmacodynamic interactions.
- Discuss drug interaction, and give examples
- Describe the effects of drug-food interactions.
- Explain the meaning of drug-induced photosensitivity.
- Discuss the nursing implications related to patients' use of over-the-counter drugs.

OUTLINE

KEY TERMS

additive effect, p. 32
adverse drug reaction, p. 30
antagonistic effects, p. 33
drug incompatibility, p. 30
drug interaction, p. 29
over-the-counter drugs, p. 29
photosensitivity, p. 34
synergistic effects, p. 33

Drug therapy is complex because of the great number of drugs available. Drug-drug, drug-food, and drug-laboratory interactions are an increasing problem. Because of the possibility of numerous interactions, the nurse should be knowledgeable about drug interactions and should closely monitor patient responses. Thorough and timely communication among members of the health team is essential. Patients at high risk for interactions include those who have chronic health conditions, take multiple medications, see more than one health care provider, and use multiple pharmacies. Older adults are at especially high risk for drug interactions; 75% take prescription drugs, and 82% take **over-the-counter (OTC) drugs**—drugs that are obtainable without a prescription.

DRUG INTERACTIONS

A **drug interaction** is defined as an altered or modified action or effect of a drug as a result of interaction with one or multiple drugs. It should not be confused with adverse drug reaction or drug incompatibility. An **adverse drug reaction** is an undesirable drug effect that ranges from mild untoward effects to severe toxic effects, including hypersensitivity reaction and anaphylaxis. **Drug incompatibility** is a chemical or physical reaction that occurs among two or more drugs in vitro. In other words, the reaction occurs between two or more drugs within a syringe, IV bag, or other artificial environment outside of the body.

Drug interactions can be divided into two categories: (1) pharmacokinetic interactions and (2) pharmacodynamic interactions.

Pharmacokinetic Interactions

Pharmacokinetic interactions are changes that occur in the absorption, distribution, metabolism or biotransformation, and excretion of one or more drugs.

Absorption

When a person takes two drugs at the same time, the rate of absorption of one or both drugs can change. One drug can block, decrease, or increase the absorption of another drug. It can do this in one of the following ways:

1. By decreasing or increasing gastric emptying time
2. By changing the gastric pH
3. By forming drug complexes

Drugs that increase the speed of gastric emptying (e.g., laxatives, metoclopramide [Reglan]) may cause an increase in gastric and intestinal motility and a decrease in drug absorption. Most drugs are absorbed primarily in the small intestine; exceptions include barbiturates, salicylates, and theophylline (Theo-24), which undergo gastric absorption. Opioids and anticholinergic drugs (e.g., atropine) decrease gastric emptying time and gastrointestinal (GI) motility, causing an increase in absorption rate. For drugs that undergo gastric absorption, the amount or extent of absorption increases the longer the drug remains in the stomach.

When the gastric pH is decreased, a weakly acidic drug like aspirin is less ionized and more rapidly absorbed. Drugs that increase the gastric pH decrease absorption of weak-acid drugs. Antacids such as magnesium hydroxide (Maalox) and aluminum hydroxide (Amphojel) raise the gastric pH and block or slow absorption. Some drugs may react chemically. For example, tetracycline and the heavy-metal ions (calcium, magnesium, aluminum, and iron) found in antacids or iron supplements may lead to the formation of a drug complex and thus prevent the absorption of tetracycline. This phenomenon may also be observed when products that contain divalent cations are ingested with fluoroquinolone antibiotics such as ciprofloxacin (Cipro). Consequently, dairy products, multivitamins, and antacids should be avoided 1 hour before and 2 hours after tetracycline or ciprofloxacin consumption.

Certain cholesterol-lowering drugs, such as cholestyramine and colestipol, also form complexes with drugs like carbamazepine (Tegretol) and furosemide (Lasix). The drugs are then less soluble, resulting in reduced drug absorption. Drug complexation may be desired; for example, activated charcoal may be administered after toxic ingestion of a medication to decrease its absorption and, consequently, diminish or eliminate any untoward effects associated with the overdose.

Alteration of bacteria normally found in the GI tract may affect the pharmacokinetics of a medication. For example, intestinal microflora have the ability to metabolize digoxin (Lanoxin). Digoxin is a digitalis preparation that is used to treat heart failure and arrhythmias. Metabolism of this drug by gut bacteria decreases its bioavailability. Erythromycin, a macrolide antibiotic, and tetracycline are broad-spectrum antibiotics (effective against both gram-positive and gram-negative organisms) that destroy or inhibit the growth of these GI microflora. Consequently, the administration of one of these drugs to a patient on digoxin therapy may lead to an increase in the absorption of digoxin and, ultimately, to toxicity. Another example of this phenomenon occurs with oral contraceptives. Gut bacteria are necessary to hydrolyze estrogen conjugates into free estrogens so they may be optimally absorbed to exert their contraceptive effect. Concurrent antibiotic administration may alter these intestinal bacteria, impairing this process and preventing the optimal absorption and effectiveness of the oral contraceptive. A patient who takes oral birth control to prevent pregnancy should use a barrier form of protection during sex when she takes a course of antibiotics.

Distribution

A drug's distribution to tissues can be affected by its binding to plasma/serum protein. Only drugs unbound to protein are free active agents and can enter body tissues. Two drugs that are highly protein bound and administered simultaneously can result in drug displacements. Factors that influence displacement of drugs are (1) drug concentration in the blood, (2) protein-binding power of the drugs, and (3) volume of distribution (Vd).

Two drugs that are highly bound to protein or albumin will compete for binding sites in the plasma. The result is a decrease in protein binding of one or both drugs; therefore, more free drug circulates in the plasma and is available for drug action. This effect can lead to drug toxicity. When two highly protein-bound drugs must be taken concurrently, the drug dosage of one or both drugs may need to be decreased to avoid drug toxicity.

Drugs that are highly protein bound include the anticoagulant warfarin, anticonvulsants such as phenytoin and valproic acid, gemfibrozil (antihyperlipidemic), most nonsteroidal antiinflammatory drugs (NSAIDs), sulfisoxazole (sulfonamide), glyburide (antidiabetic), and quinidine (antidysrhythmic). Warfarin (Coumadin) is 99% protein-bound, allowing only 1% to be free drug. If 2% to 3% of warfarin is displaced from albumin binding sites, the amount of free warfarin would be 3% to 4% instead of 1%. This action has the potential to increase the anticoagulant effect of warfarin; excess bleeding may result.

A significant decrease in serum albumin level because of liver disease or poor nutritional status can increase the free amount of highly protein-bound drugs such as phenytoin and warfarin, making more drug available to exert its pharmacologic effect.

Metabolism or Biotransformation

Many drug interactions of metabolism occur with the induction or inhibition of the hepatic microsomal system. A drug can increase the metabolism of another drug by stimulating liver enzymes. These enzymes produce a cascade effect in drug function. Drugs that promote induction of enzymes are called *enzyme inducers.* Barbiturates like phenobarbital are enzyme inducers. Phenobarbital increases the metabolism of most antipsychotics and methylxanthine (theophylline). Increased metabolism promotes drug elimination and decreases plasma concentration of the drug. The result is a decrease in drug action. Sometimes liver enzymes convert drugs to active or passive metabolites. The drug metabolites may be excreted or may produce an active pharmacologic response.

The anticonvulsant drugs phenytoin and carbamazepine and the antimicrobial medication rifampin are hepatic enzyme inducers that can increase drug metabolism—for example, for the anticoagulant drug warfarin. A larger dose of warfarin is usually needed while the patient takes a hepatic inducer, because metabolism aids in decreasing the amount of drug. If the drug inducer is withdrawn, warfarin dosages must be decreased, because less drug is eliminated by hepatic metabolism. Usually interaction occurs after 1 week of drug therapy and can continue for 1 week after the drug inducer is discontinued. Drugs with narrow therapeutic ranges should be closely monitored.

Some drugs are enzyme inhibitors. The antiulcer drug cimetidine (Tagamet) is an enzyme inhibitor that decreases metabolism of certain drugs such as theophylline, causing an increase in the plasma concentration of theophylline. The theophylline dose must be decreased to avoid toxicity. If cimetidine or any enzyme drug inhibitor is discontinued, the theophylline dosage should be adjusted. Other well-known hepatic enzyme inhibitors are erythromycin (an antibacterial) and itraconazole (an antifungal).

The use of tobacco and alcohol may have variable effects on drug biotransformation. Polycyclic aromatic hydrocarbons found in cigarette smoke induce production of the specific family of enzymes responsible for theophylline metabolism. Chronic cigarette smoking leads to an increase in hepatic enzyme activity and can increase theophylline clearance. Asthmatics who smoke and take theophylline to manage their disease may require an increase in theophylline dosage. The ingestion of alcohol may have variable effects on biotransformation. With chronic alcohol use, hepatic enzyme activities are increased; with acute alcohol use, metabolism is inhibited.

Natural or herbal products may also have an impact on metabolism. St. John's wort, an OTC herbal product used to manage symptoms of depression, induces the metabolism of certain drugs such as warfarin, digoxin, and theophylline. This action potentially decreases the effectiveness of these medications, possibly necessitating a dose increase to sustain efficacy. Flavonoids, a group of naturally occurring compounds found in the juice and pulp of citrus fruits, are potent inhibitors of the metabolism of certain drugs. Patients who are stabilized on therapeutic doses of carbamazepine, diazepam, statins, calcium channel blockers, or erectile dysfunction drugs may subject themselves to adverse effects from greater-than-expected drug levels if they eat or drink grapefruit products concurrently with the drug.

Certain drugs alter hepatic blood flow, causing a decrease in liver metabolism. Table 4-1 describes the effects of drug enzyme inducers and inhibitors.

TABLE 4-1 DRUGS: ENZYME INDUCERS AND ENZYME INHIBITORS

DRUG CATEGORY	DRUG EFFECT
Drug enzyme inducer	Onset and termination of drug effect is slow, approximately 1 week.
	Drug dosage may need to be increased with use of drug inducer.
	Drug dosage should be adjusted after termination of drug inducer.
	Monitor serum drug levels, especially if the drug has a narrow therapeutic drug range.
Drug enzyme inhibitor	Onset of drug effect usually occurs rapidly.
	Half-life ($t\frac{1}{2}$) of the second drug may be increased, causing a prolonged drug effect.
	Interaction may occur related to the dosage prescribed.
	Disease entities affect drug dosing.
	Monitor serum drug levels, especially if the drug has a narrow therapeutic range.

Excretion

Most drugs are filtered through the glomeruli and excreted in the urine. With some drugs, excretion occurs in the bile, which passes into the intestinal tract. Drugs can increase or decrease renal excretion and have an effect on the excretion of other drugs. Drugs that decrease cardiac output, decrease blood flow to the kidneys, and decrease glomerular filtration rate can also decrease or delay drug excretion. The antiarrhythmic drug quinidine decreases the excretion of digoxin; therefore, the plasma concentration of digoxin is increased, and digitalis toxicity can occur.

Diuretics promote water and sodium excretion from the renal tubules. Furosemide (Lasix) acts on the loop of Henle, and hydrochlorothiazide (HydroDIURIL) acts on the distal tubules. Both diuretics decrease reabsorption of water, sodium, and potassium. A renal loss of potassium, which may lead to a condition known as *hypokalemia*, can enhance the action of digoxin, and digitalis toxicity could occur (see "Drug-Laboratory Interactions" later in the chapter).

Two or more drugs that undergo the same route of excretion may compete with one another for elimination from the body. Probenecid, a drug for gout, decreases penicillin excretion by inhibiting the secretion of penicillin in the renal tubules of the kidneys. In some cases, this effect may be desirable to increase or maintain the plasma concentration of penicillin (which has a short half-life) for a prolonged period of time.

Changing urine pH affects drug excretion. The antacid sodium bicarbonate causes the urine to be alkaline. Alkaline urine promotes the excretion of drugs that are weak acids (e.g., aspirin, barbiturates). Alkaline urine also promotes reabsorption of weak base drugs. Acid urine promotes the excretion of weak base drugs such as quinidine.

With decreased renal or hepatic function, there is usually an increase in free drug concentration. It is essential to closely monitor these patients for drug toxicity when they take multiple drugs. Checking serum drug levels, a practice also known as *therapeutic drug monitoring (TDM)*, is especially important for drugs that have a narrow therapeutic range and are highly protein bound. Digoxin and phenytoin are two drugs that require TDM. Table 4-2 summarizes the drug interactions that affect pharmacokinetics.

Pharmacodynamic Interactions

Pharmacodynamic interactions are those that result in additive, synergistic, or antagonistic drug effects.

Additive Drug Effect

When two drugs with similar action are administered, the drug interaction is called an **additive effect** and is the sum of the effects of the two drugs. Additive effects can be desirable or undesirable. For example, a desirable additive drug effect occurs when a diuretic and a beta blocker are administered for the treatment of hypertension. In combination, these two drugs use different mechanisms to have a more pronounced blood pressure–lowering effect. As another example, aspirin and codeine are two analgesics that work by different mechanisms but can be given together for increased pain relief.

An example of an undesirable additive effect is that from two vasodilators: hydralazine (Apresoline) prescribed for hypertension and nitroglycerin prescribed for angina. The result could be a severe hypotensive response. Another example is the interaction of aspirin and alcohol. Aspirin is directly irritating to the stomach, causes platelet dysfunction, and inhibits prostaglandin-mediated mucus production of

TABLE 4-2 PHARMACOKINETIC INTERACTIONS OF DRUGS

PROCESS	DRUG	EFFECT
Absorption	Laxatives	Speeds gastric emptying time Increases gastric motility Decreases drug absorption
	Opioids Anticholinergics	Slows gastric emptying time Decreases gastric motility Increases or decreases drug absorption, depending on where the drug is delayed (gastric vs. intestinal)
	Aspirin	Decreases gastric pH Increases drug absorption
	Antacids	Increases gastric pH Slows absorption of acid drugs
	Antacids and tetracycline	Forms drug complexes Blocks drug absorption
Distribution	Anticoagulant and antiinflammatory (sulindac)	Competes for protein-binding sites Increases free drug (e.g., increases anticoagulant)
Metabolism or biotransformation	Barbiturates	Promotes induction of liver enzymes Increases drug metabolism Decreases plasma concentration of second drug
	Antiulcer cimetidine (Tagamet)	Inhibits liver enzyme release Decreases metabolism of diazepam (Valium), phenytoin (Dilantin), morphine, and so on Increases plasma concentration of second drug
Excretion	Antiarrhythmic (quinidine)	Decreases renal excretion of second drug (e.g., digoxin) Increases digoxin concentration
	Antigout (probenecid)	Decreases penicillin excretion by competing for renal tubular secretion Increases penicillin concentration
	Antacid (sodium bicarbonate)	Promotes excretion of weak acid drugs (e.g., aspirin, barbiturates, sulfonamides)
	Aspirin, ammonium chloride	Promotes excretion of weak base drugs (e.g., quinidine, theophylline)
Other: Decrease in cardiac output and renal blood flow	Most drug categories	Decreases drug excretion Increases drug plasma concentration

the gastric mucosa, which protects the underlying tissues of the stomach. Alcohol disrupts the gastric mucosal barrier and suppresses platelet production. Both aspirin and alcohol can prolong bleeding time and, when taken together, may result in gastric bleeding.

Synergistic Drug Effect or Potentiation

When two or more drugs are given together, one drug can potentiate or have a **synergistic effect** on another. In other words, the clinical effect is substantially greater than the combined effect of the two. An example of this is the combination of meperidine (Demerol, synthetic opioid analgesic) and promethazine (Phenergan, antihistamine). One of the major side effects of promethazine is sedation. When used with meperidine in postsurgery patients, promethazine enhances or potentiates the drowsiness effect of meperidine. Less meperidine is required when it is combined with promethazine, which can be desirable. An example of an undesirable effect occurs when alcohol and a sedative-hypnotic drug, such as chlordiazepoxide (Librium) or diazepam (Valium), are combined. The resultant effect of this example is increased central nervous system (CNS) depression.

Some antibacterials (antibiotics) have an enzyme inhibitor added to the drug to potentiate the therapeutic effect. Examples are ampicillin with sulbactam (Unasyn) and amoxicillin with clavulanate (Augmentin), in which sulbactam and clavulanate potassium are bacterial enzyme inhibitors. Ampicillin and amoxicillin can be given without these inhibitors; however, the desired therapeutic effect may not occur because of the bacterial beta-lactamase, which inactivates the drugs and causes bacterial resistance. The combination of the antibiotic with either sulbactam or clavulanate inhibits bacterial enzyme activity and enhances the effect or broadens the spectrum of activity of the antibacterial agent. Not all bacteria secrete beta-lactamase enzyme; only those that do will inhibit these antibiotics and result in bacterial resistance. (Refer to Unit IX for information on antibacterial agents.)

Antagonistic Drug Effect

When two drugs that have opposite effects, or **antagonistic effects,** are administered together, each drug cancels the effect of the other. In other words, the actions of both drugs are nullified. An example of an antagonistic effect occurs when the adrenergic beta stimulant isoproterenol (Isuprel) and the adrenergic beta blocker propranolol (Inderal) are given together. Isoproterenol is a drug that is used in emergency situations to treat bradycardia, which is defined as a heart rate of less than 60 beats per minute. If given to a patient receiving a drug that decreases blood pressure and heart rate, the action of each drug is canceled. Neither drug delivers the expected therapeutic effect.

There are some situations in which the antagonistic effect is desirable. In morphine overdose, naloxone is given as an antagonist (antidote) to block the narcotic response. This is a beneficial drug interaction of an antagonist.

The use of two prescription drugs can have additive, synergistic, antagonistic, or no effect. This is especially true of warfarin; when taken with another drug, the effects of the second drug can increase, decrease, or have no effect on the anticoagulant. Table 4-3 lists the drugs that may be taken with an anticoagulant and the effects that the second drug has on the anticoagulant.

Table 4-4 summarizes the drug responses associated with pharmacodynamic interactions, and Table 4-5 lists selected drug-drug interactions.

TABLE 4-3 DRUG INTERACTIONS WITH ANTICOAGULANTS AND PRESCRIPTION DRUGS

PRESCRIPTION DRUGS	ANTICOAGULANT EFFECTS
Selected Antilipidemics	
Fibrate Group	Increased effect; may cause increased bleeding
Statin Group	
Lovastatin	Increased effect
Pravastatin	No known effects
Angiotensin-Converting Enzyme Inhibitors	No known effects
Aminoglycosides	No known effects
Aspirin	Strong effects; can cause bleeding
Antineoplastic Drugs	
Cytoxan, 5-fluorouracil, methotrexate, doxorubicin, vincristine	Increased effects; can cause bleeding
Cytoxan, mercaptopurine, mitotane	Decreased effects; Cytoxan may cause increased or decreased effects
Barbiturates	Reduced effect of anticoagulants
Benzodiazepines	No known effects
Beta Blockers	No known effects
Selected Cephalosporins	
Cefamandole	Increased effects; may cause bleeding
Nonsteroidal Antiinflammatory Drugs (NSAIDs)	
Ibuprofen	Normal doses; no effects
Diclofenac, ketoprofen, tolmetin	May increase effects
Quinolone Antibiotics	Usually no effects
Ciprofloxacin, norfloxacin, ofloxacin	Increased effects in isolated cases
Sulfonamides	
Bactrim-cotrimoxazole	Increased effects in 35% of persons
Tricyclic Antidepressants	No known effects
Vitamin K	Decreased effects of anticoagulants
Food	
Aspartame (artificial sweetener)	Increased effects
Green vegetables (spinach, broccoli, brussels sprouts)	Decreased effects; vegetables are rich in vitamin K
Alcohol	
Mild to moderate drinking	No effects unless heavy drinking
Heavy drinking	Increased effects if liver function is impaired

TABLE 4-4 PHARMACODYNAMIC INTERACTIONS OF DRUGS

INTERACTION	EFFECT
Additive	In the same drug category, the drug effect is the sum of both drug effects.
Synergistic or potentiation	One drug potentiates or enhances the effect of the other drug (greater than the effect of each drug alone).
Antagonistic	Two drugs in opposing drug categories cancel the effects of both drugs.

Common symptoms of drug-drug interactions include nausea, GI upset, headache, and dizziness. The patient should contact the pharmacist or health care provider if he or she experiences any unusual reaction. The most feared interactions are those that result in a dramatic drop in blood pressure or cause a rapid or irregular heart rate. Also of concern are drug interactions that produce toxins that may damage vital organs such as the heart or liver. Fortunately, most interactions are not severe or life threatening. Patients should be aware that prescription and OTC drugs and herbal products can interact with each other. It is a myth that interactions occur only with prescription medications. Severe adverse reactions are highlighted with a boxed warning in the product literature.

DRUG-FOOD INTERACTIONS

Food is known to increase, decrease, or delay drug absorption. Food can bind with drugs, causing less or slower drug absorption. An example of food binding with a drug is the interaction of tetracycline and dairy products. The result is a decrease in the plasma concentration of tetracycline. Because of the binding effect, tetracycline should be taken 1 hour before or 2 hours after meals and should not be taken with dairy products. Another example is levothyroxine, an antithyroid used to treat hypothyroidism. The absorption of this drug is erratic in the presence of food.

Food may also have an impact on the absorption of different dosage forms of the same drug. Antifungal itraconazole solution (Sporanox) is best absorbed on an empty stomach. However, itraconazole capsules, which require an acidic environment for absorption, have a higher availability when administered with food. Other examples in which food increases drug absorption include the antibiotic nitrofurantoin (Macrodantin), the beta blocker metoprolol (Lopressor), and the cholesterol-lowering drug lovastatin (Mevacor). These drugs should be taken with food. The composition of a meal may also influence drug absorption. For example, the absorption of levodopa, one of the components of the antiparkinsonism drug Sinemet, is significantly reduced when it is taken with high-protein meals.

The classic drug-food interaction occurs when an antidepressant of the monoamine oxidase inhibitor (MAOI) type (e.g., phenelzine) is taken with tyramine-rich foods such as cheese, wine, organ meats, beer, yogurt, sour cream, or bananas. These foods have sympathomimetic-like effects; more norepinephrine is released, and the result could be a hypertensive crisis. These foods must be avoided when taking MAOIs.

DRUG-LABORATORY INTERACTIONS

Abnormal plasma or serum electrolyte concentrations can affect certain drug therapies. If the patient takes digoxin and serum potassium and serum magnesium levels are decreased or serum calcium level is increased, digitalis toxicity may result. Drugs from the thiazide diuretic group can cause abnormal electrolyte concentrations. An example is hydrochlorothiazide, which can decrease serum potassium, magnesium, and sodium levels and can increase serum calcium levels. Hydrochlorothiazide promotes potassium loss, and low serum potassium results in an increase in the uptake of digoxin by myocardial tissue. This sensitization of the myocardium to digoxin increases the risk of digitalis-induced arrhythmias. When digoxin and hydrochlorothiazide are taken together, the nurse should observe the patient for digitalis toxicity. Symptoms are nausea, vomiting, bradycardia, and stated visual problems. Patients on long-term therapy should have regular digoxin levels drawn to detect early toxicity.

DRUG-INDUCED PHOTOSENSITIVITY

A drug-induced **photosensitivity** reaction is a skin reaction caused by exposure to sunlight. It is caused by the interaction of a drug and exposure to ultraviolet A (UVA) light, which can cause cellular damage. Usually the skin area that is exposed is affected.

There are two types of photosensitivity reactions: photoallergy and phototoxicity. Photoallergy occurs when a drug (e.g., sulfonamide) undergoes activation in the skin by ultraviolet light to a compound that is more allergenic than the parent compound. Because it takes time to develop antibodies, photoallergenic reactions are a type of delayed hypersensitivity reaction. With phototoxicity, a photosensitive drug undergoes photochemical reactions within the skin to cause damage. This type of reaction is different from photoallergy in that it is not immune-mediated. The onset of phototoxicity with erythema can be rapid, occurring within 2 to 6 hours of sunlight exposure.

Both types of reactions are the result of light exposure, but they differ according to the wavelength of light and the photosensitive drug. Phototoxicity may be the result of the drug dose, whereas photoallergenic reactions are not and only require previous exposure, or sensitization, to the offending agent. Examples of drugs that can induce photosensitivity are listed in Table 4-6.

Most photosensitive reactions can be avoided by using sunscreen with a sun protection factor (SPF) greater than 15; avoiding excessive sunlight, especially at the height of the daylight hours; and wearing protective clothing. Decreasing

TABLE 4-5 SELECTED DRUG-DRUG INTERACTIONS

DRUGS AND DRUG CATEGORIES	INTERACTING EFFECTS WITH DRUGS
Acyclovir	IV incompatible with dobutamine, dopamine, and morphine.
Alteplase	IV incompatible with dobutamine, dopamine, heparin, morphine, and nitroglycerin.
Aminoglycosides	Cephalosporins, ethacrynic acid, furosemide, polymyxin, and vancomycin can increase the risk of nephrotoxicity and ototoxicity. This is especially true in young and older adults.
Aminophylline	IV incompatible with dobutamine, dopamine, meperidine, and ondansetron.
Angiotensin-converting enzyme (ACE) inhibitors (e.g., captopril)	Antacids decrease absorption of ACE inhibitors. Potassium-sparing diuretics decrease potassium excretion, and lithium use decreases lithium excretion. Antihypertensives, nitrates, and diuretics enhance hypotensive effects.
Anticoagulants (e.g., warfarin [Coumadin])	Drugs that may enhance anticoagulant effects include acetaminophen (high doses), alcohol, antiplatelet drugs, aspirin, aminoglycosides, cephalosporins, erythromycins, furosemide, fluoroquinolones, isoniazid, NSAIDs, sulfonamides, thiazides, tricyclic antidepressants, and vitamin E.
Anticonvulsants (e.g., phenytoin [Dilantin])	Alcohol decreases phenytoin effect. Warfarin absorption may be decreased. May decrease effectiveness of oral contraceptives and corticosteroids. Isoniazid increases phenytoin levels.
Antipsychotic agents (e.g., phenothiazides)	Alcohol increases CNS depression. Antacids and antidiarrheals decrease drug absorption. Tricyclic antidepressants may increase the risk of hypotension. Anticonvulsant dose may need to be increased because phenothiazides can decrease seizure threshold.
Antitubercular agents (e.g., isoniazid)	Alcohol increases the risk of hepatotoxicity. Antacids decrease absorption of isoniazid. Phenytoin levels can increase, resulting in phenytoin toxicity.
Aspirin (salicylates)	Anticoagulants can increase the risk of bleeding when taken with aspirin. Oral antidiabetic agents may increase the risk of hypoglycemia.
Benzodiazepines (e.g., diazepam, lorazepam)	Alcohol, narcotics, and anticonvulsants can increase CNS depression. Cimetidine can increase diazepam and lorazepam toxicity. May decrease levodopa effects. May increase phenytoin serum levels.
Beta (adrenergic) blockers (e.g., propranolol [Inderal])	Diuretics, antihypertensives, and phenothiazines can increase the state of hypotension. Atropine can correct bradycardia. Antacids decrease propranolol absorption. Cimetidine decreases drug clearance and increases beta blocker effects.
Calcium channel blockers (e.g., nifedipine [Procardia])	May increase digoxin levels. Beta blockers have an additive effect and can cause bradycardia. H_2 blockers decrease drug clearance, resulting in elevated calcium blocker levels.
Cardiac glycosides (e.g., digoxin [Lanoxin])	Thiazide and loop diuretics, corticosteroids, laxatives, and amphotericin B can cause hypokalemia, which may cause digitalis toxicity. Antacids, antidiarrheals, and colestipol decrease absorption of digoxin. Quinidine, verapamil, and erythromycin increase digoxin levels.
Diazepam	IV incompatible with dobutamine, heparin, meperidine, and potassium in D_5W.
Diuretics (potassium-wasting) (thiazide and loop)	Digoxin toxicity may result from hypokalemia because of loop or thiazide diuretics. Corticosteroids increase potassium loss. May increase lithium levels.
Fluoroquinolones (e.g., ciprofloxacin [Cipro])	May increase theophylline and warfarin (Coumadin) levels. Antacids and iron products can decrease ciprofloxacin absorption.
Furosemide	IV incompatible with dobutamine, meperidine, morphine, and ondansetron.
Lithium carbonate	Diuretics, NSAIDs, tetracyclines, and methyldopa can increase lithium toxicity. Theophylline, sodium bicarbonate, and potassium or sodium citrate can promote lithium excretion.
Narcotics (e.g., morphine and meperidine [Demerol])	Alcohol, sedatives, benzodiazepines, barbiturates, and tricyclic antidepressants can increase CNS depression. Monoamine oxidase inhibitors (MAOIs) may cause hypertensive crisis.
Nonsteroidal antiinflammatory drugs (NSAIDs) (e.g., ibuprofen [Motrin])	Warfarin, heparin, and alcohol may prolong bleeding time. May increase lithium and methotrexate levels, resulting in lithium toxicity. Corticosteroids may cause peptic ulcer.
Penicillins	May decrease warfarin effects. NSAIDs prolong the effects of penicillin. Diuretics with penicillin G-K may cause hyperkalemia. May decrease effectiveness of oral contraceptives. Rifampin inhibits the action of penicillin.
Phenytoin	IV incompatible with dobutamine, heparin, meperidine, morphine, nitroglycerin, and potassium in D_5W.
Sulfonylureas	Alcohol, aspirin, anticoagulants, some NSAIDs, anticonvulsants, sulfonamides, and oral contraceptives may increase the risk of hypoglycemia. Corticosteroids, thiazide diuretics, estrogen, calcium channel blockers, phenytoin, and thyroid drugs may increase the blood sugar level.
Tetracyclines	Milk, antacids, and iron supplements decrease tetracycline absorption. May decrease effectiveness of oral contraceptives.
Theophylline	Erythromycins, fluoroquinolones, and tacrine can increase theophylline levels. May increase lithium excretion. Cigarette smoking decreases theophylline levels.
Tricyclic antidepressants (e.g., amitriptyline)	Can increase anticoagulant effects of warfarin. Alcohol, narcotics, and sedatives increase CNS depression. MAOIs must not be taken with tricyclic antidepressants. May reduce antihypertensive drug effects. Cimetidine may increase tricyclic serum levels.

TABLE 4-6 DRUG-INDUCED PHOTOSENSITIVITY

DRUG-INDUCED	OCCURRENCE
Amantadine	Confirmed by positive photopatch testing.
Amiodarone	Frequency may be 10% to 75%. Sunscreen lotion with UVA can help reduce incidence.
Benzodiazepines	Reported cases with alprazolam and chlordiazepoxide.
Carbamazepine	Frequency is less than 1%; however, photocopy machines can trigger photosensitivity.
Corticosteroids	Reported cases with positive photopatch testing and with use of hydrocortisone.
Fluorouracil	Avoid sunlight with topical or intravenous use; erythema and hyperpigmentation may occur.
NSAIDs	Aspirin, ibuprofen, and indomethacin have been reported to have a low phototoxic effect; however, there is a possibility for a dose-related photosensitive effect with ibuprofen.
Methotrexate	Avoid sunlight to prevent severe photosensitive reaction (sunburn).
Calcium blockers	Diltiazem: possible phototoxic reaction nifedipine: may cause phototoxicity with high doses.
Phenothiazines	Reported cases of phototoxic reaction with chlorpromazine and other phenothiazines at high drug doses.
Piroxicam	Was confirmed with positive photopatch testing; photosensitive reaction occurs after a few days of piroxicam and exposure to sunlight.
Pyrazinamide	Skin color may change to reddish brown; usually occurrence is dose-related.
Quinolones (fluoroquinolones)	Phototoxicity occurs with lomefloxacin, enoxacin, ofloxacin, and nalidixic acid; ciprofloxacin causes less photosensitivity.
Sulfonamides	Reported cases of photosensitive reaction.
Sulfonylureas	Reported cases of photosensitive reaction.
Tetracyclines	Highly photosensitive; demeclocycline and doxycycline have a higher degree of photosensitive reaction than minocycline.
Thiazides	Thiazide-induced photosensitivity has been reported; hydrochlorothiazide has a greater photosensitivity than bendroflumethiazide.
Trimethoprim	Reported cases of photosensitive reaction.
Vinblastine	Reported cases of photosensitive reaction.

NSAID, Nonsteroidal antiinflammatory drug; *UVA,* ultraviolet A.

the drug dose may decrease the risk of photosensitivity if treatment is required. It may be necessary, however, to discontinue use of the offending drug.

OVER-THE-COUNTER DRUGS

OTC drugs are found in most households. According to the U.S. Food and Drug Administration (FDA), OTC drugs have been found to be safe and appropriate for use without the supervision of a health care provider, and individuals can access them without a prescription. More than 90% of illnesses are initially treated with OTC drugs, and their use is unknown to many health care providers. A study of 7 resident physicians and 414 adult patients revealed that more than 50% of the patients reported OTC use, and physicians questioned OTC use in 33% of the visits. Almost 60% of those reporting OTC use did not tell the physician; at the same time, only 14% of the patients indicated it was not important to report OTC use to the physician.

Many drugs that were previously available only by prescription are available OTC. Examples include proton pump inhibitors (e.g., Prilosec-OTC) and Plan B® emergency contraception. Knowing all of the medications a patient is taking is an important part of the nursing history. For example, aspirin can increase the risk of bleeding if the patient is taking anticoagulants such as warfarin. The nurse needs to reconcile medications as part of the patient safety standards on admission to the hospital; this includes both prescription medications and OTC drugs (e.g., baby aspirin 81 mg for patients with coronary artery disease). (Refer to Chapter 12 for discussion of medication reconciliation.)

Many factors contribute to the increase in the number and use of OTC products. Mass-media marketing of drugs surrounds us. Many people turn to "self-treatment" because they lack the time, money, or health insurance for regular doctor visits. It is one of the nurse's responsibilities to advocate for the patient making educated choices.

OTC drugs include vitamin supplements, cold and cough remedies, analgesics for pain, antacids, laxatives, antihistamines, sleep aids, nasal sprays, weight-control drugs, and herbal products. Some patients do not consider herbal products to be OTC drugs. More than $4 billion is spent annually on herbal products, nutraceuticals, and dietary supplements; most of these products are minimally regulated by the FDA. (Refer to Chapter 6 for a discussion of herbal therapies.)

The FDA has been working to standardize OTC labeling. OTC labeling is designed to provide consumers with better information and to describe the benefits and risks associated with taking OTC medications. Multiple OTC drugs may have the same active ingredients; patients should avoid taking an excess amount of an ingredient.

Nurses must be aware of OTC products and the implications of their use for their patients' drug therapy. OTC drugs provide both advantages and potential serious complications for the consumer. The nurse needs to emphasize that many of these drugs are potent medications and can cause moderate to severe side effects, especially when taken with other drugs. Self-diagnosis and self-prescribing OTC drugs may mask the seriousness of a clinical condition. Based on an increase in serious adverse reactions and deaths of infants and toddlers, the FDA recalled all OTC medications with directions/dosages for children 2 years of age and younger in 2007. Refer to Chapter 2 for detailed information on drug regulation.

The FDA has the responsibility for monitoring the safety of drug therapy and is charged with identifying standards for known active ingredients and establishing mandatory

BOX 4-1 FDA OVER-THE-COUNTER DRUG CATEGORIES

- Allergy treatment products (internal)
- Analgesics—antipyretics (internal)
- Antacids and antiflatulents
- Antidiarrheal products
- Antimicrobials
- Antiperspirants
- Antirheumatic products
- Antitussives
- Bronchodilators and antiasthmatic products
- Cold remedies and decongestants
- Contraceptive products
- Dandruff products
- Dentifrices and other dental products
- Dermatologic products
- Emetics and antiemetics
- Hematinics
- Hemorrhoidal products
- Herbal products
- Laxatives and cathartics
- Nicotine gum or transdermal patches
- Ophthalmic products
- Oral-hygiene drug products
- Sedatives and sleep aids
- Stimulants
- Sunburn prevention and treatment products
- Vitamin-mineral supplements
- Weight-control aids
- Miscellaneous products (not covered in above categories)

FDA, U.S. Food and Drug Administration.

labeling to assist consumers in the proper use of drugs. The FDA OTC drug categories are listed in Box 4-1.

As a result of review by the FDA, drugs are placed in one of three categories:

- Category I: Drugs judged to be both safe and effective
- Category II: Drugs judged to be either unsafe or ineffective; these drugs should not be included in nonprescription products
- Category III: Drugs for which there are insufficient data to judge safety or efficacy

The FDA has recommended that drugs in category II be reformulated to be included in category I or removed from the market. (Manufacturers can maintain the brand name after changing the components of an OTC product.)

The FDA has also recommended that selected prescription drugs be reclassified so they can be sold OTC. For example, the prescription drug Motrin became available as the OTC drug ibuprofen in 1984; Tagamet, another prescription drug, was made available as the OTC drug cimetidine. Because of this process, hundreds of thousands of OTC products have ingredients or dose strengths that were once available only by prescription. As a result, it is vitally important that nurses be aware of current drug information, any changes in FDA recommendations, and the implications of this information for an informed patient population. The following cautions may be of assistance when OTC preparations are considered:

- Delay in professional diagnosis and treatment of serious or potentially serious conditions may occur if the patient self-prescribes OTC drugs.
- Symptoms may be masked, making diagnosis more complicated.
- Labels and instructions should be followed carefully.
- The patient's health care provider or pharmacist must be consulted before OTC preparations are taken.
- Ingredients in OTC products may interact with medications prescribed by the health care provider or self-prescribed by the patient.
- Inactive ingredients (e.g., alcohol, dyes, preservatives) may result in adverse reactions.
- Potential for overdose exists because of the use of several preparations with similar active ingredients. A double dose does not translate into a quicker recovery.
- The risk for adverse drug reactions and drug-drug interactions will increase as more medications, whether prescription or OTC, are added to drug therapy regimens.

Interactions of selected prescription medications and OTC preparations are potentially dangerous. Many individuals routinely reach for aspirin, acetaminophen, and ibuprofen to relieve discomfort or pain without being aware of these interactions. For example, ibuprofen increases fluid retention, which could worsen the condition of a patient with heart failure; use of ibuprofen on a long-term basis may decrease the effectiveness of antihypertensive drugs.

Several OTC drugs, such as cough and cold preparations, are composed of two to four compounds. For patients who are already taking maintenance medicine, it is conceivable that there could be a drug-drug interaction with a cough medicine and one of the medications prescribed by the patient's health care provider.

Patients with asthma should be aware that aspirin can trigger an acute asthma episode. Patients may be allergic to aspirin, or aspirin may act as a deregulator of leukotrienes. Aspirin is also not recommended for children with influenza symptoms or chickenpox, because it has been associated with Reye syndrome. Patients with impaired renal function should avoid aspirin, acetaminophen, and ibuprofen because each can further decrease renal function, especially with long-term use. Also, patients taking moderate to high doses of aspirin, ibuprofen, or naproxen concurrently with an oral anticoagulant may be at increased risk for bleeding.

The previous examples are not all-inclusive. Caution is advised before using any OTC preparation, including antacids, decongestants, and laxatives. Patients should check with their health care providers and read drug labels before taking OTC medications so they are aware of possible contraindications and adverse reactions. They should look for product name, active ingredients, purpose, uses, warnings, directions, storage information, and inactive ingredients (e.g., color, flavors). The acronym SAFER is a mnemonic for the instructions that the FDA recommends before taking any medicine: **S**peak up, **A**sk questions, **F**ind the facts, **E**valuate your choices, and **R**ead the labels. (Refer to Chapter 12 for a comprehensive discussion of medication safety.)

Polypharmacy is a problem in the United States, and older adults are especially at risk. (Refer to Chapter 8 for more information on geriatric pharmacology.)

A good source for OTC drug information is *The Handbook of Nonprescription Drugs*, published by the American Pharmacists Association in Washington, DC. The Internet can be another great resource if only credible sites are used. Key websites are listed at the end of this chapter.

Cough and Cold Remedies

Most OTC cough and cold remedies are used to relieve coughs and nasal and sinus congestion. These products contain ingredients such as guaifenesin, dextromethorphan, pseudoephedrine, an analgesic, and an antihistamine.

The majority of ingredients to treat nasal congestion are sympathomimetic (i.e., they stimulate the sympathetic nervous system). Examples include phenylephrine and pseudoephedrine. The FDA has ordered removal of phenylpropanolamine from OTC cold remedies because of the increased risk of hemorrhagic stroke in young women who take the drug. It has been reported that phenylpropanolamine may also cause psychosis, hypertension, renal failure, and cardiac dysrhythmias.

OTC cough and cold remedies are primarily safe for children older than 6 years. For children ages 2 to 6 years, consult with a health care provider. The use of these medications in children younger than 2 years is not recommended. In fact, the Centers for Disease Control and Prevention (CDC) has reported that cough and cold medications can be harmful and should be used with caution in children younger than 2 years. This statement was issued in response to the discovery of three infant deaths in 2005 from the toxic effects of these medications. The report stated that more than 1500 emergency department visits in 2004 and 2005 were due to adverse effects associated with cough and cold medication use in children younger than 2 years.

Patients with heart disease, hypertension, or thyroid disease should not take these OTC preparations without approval from their health care provider. Side effects of cough and cold OTC drugs that contain a sympathomimetic include headache, nervousness, increased blood pressure, and insomnia. The most common side effect of the antihistamine is drowsiness.

Health professionals should discuss the pros and cons of taking cough and cold remedies with their patients and read labels carefully. The recommended dose should not be exceeded for either adults or children. Iatrogenic conditions (treatment-induced disorders) are another concern. In situations with limited choices in pharmacotherapy, the patient and the health care provider at times have to deal with a second condition resulting from the treatment with a particular drug. An example of an iatrogenic condition is when a person medicated with antiinflammatory steroids develops a Cushing's appearance. People on long-term acetylsalicylic acid (ASA) therapy are prone to developing ulcers.

Sleep Aids

The FDA restricts the number of OTC sleep aids available. Before 1979, most OTC sleep aids contained bromides, scopolamine, or a combination of antihistamines. Now, most OTC sleep aids contain an antihistamine with or without an analgesic such as aspirin or acetaminophen (e.g., Tylenol PM). The side effect of an antihistamine is drowsiness, which is useful as a sleep aid. If the patient has night pain that causes sleeplessness, an analgesic with antihistamine is helpful. In young children or older adults, these sleep aids may cause CNS stimulation instead of sedation. These drugs should not be taken with a depressant because they can have an additive depressive effect on the CNS.

Weight-Control Drugs

For years, most weight-control drugs contained amphetamines. They were prescription drugs prescribed to suppress the appetite. The effectiveness of the amphetamines was short-term because they were effective only as long as the therapeutic blood level of the drug was maintained. Side effects included nervousness, heart palpitations, increased blood pressure, and insomnia. Drug dependence was a problem associated with amphetamines. They are no longer used in weight-control preparations.

Currently, many OTC weight-control products are on the market. They are contraindicated for patients with heart disease, hypertension, diabetes mellitus, and thyroid disease, and their effectiveness is not proven.

In February 2007, the FDA approved the marketing of orlistat (Alli) as an OTC weight-control medication. Alli was the first FDA-approved weight-control medication to be sold in the United States without a prescription; it inhibits lipase enzymes within the GI tract and blocks the dietary absorption of fat by about 30%. For use in adults age 18 years and older, it is to be used as part of a weight-control program that includes a reduced-calorie, low-fat diet and an exercise program. A daily multivitamin should be taken when orlistat is used. The most common side effects of orlistat are oily spotting on underwear, flatulence, urgent bowel movements, and fatty or oily stools. Additionally, in May 2010, the FDA announced that rare cases of serious liver injury have been reported with use of prescription and OTC orlistat. Symptoms of possible liver failure include weakness or fatigue, fever, jaundice, brown urine, abdominal pain, nausea, vomiting, light-colored stools, itching, and loss of appetite.

Nursing Process
Patient-Centered Collaborative Care

Drug Interactions

Assessment

- Obtain a medication history on your patient. Include questions regarding OTC drug and herbal product use.

There could be a drug interaction with the prescribed drug.
- Review all literature provided by drug companies and pharmacy.
- Assess for drug reaction when two highly protein-bound drugs are taken together daily. For example, the anticoagulant warfarin (Coumadin) and the anticonvulsant phenytoin have a high affinity to protein. When warfarin is displaced from the plasma protein binding sites, this leads to more free warfarin and a possible increase in bleeding risk.
- Determine the potential for drug interaction problems related to an increased or decreased absorption rate of two drugs. Drug enzyme inducers that increase the metabolism of an affected drug may result in a decrease in effect of that drug.
- Assess the patient for drug toxicity when a drug enzyme inducer has been discontinued or when a drug enzyme inhibitor is taken concurrently with other drugs.
- Determine whether or not the patient is a cigarette smoker. Tobacco is an enzyme inducer and can increase the metabolic rate of drugs. If patient is a smoker and is taking a drug such as theophylline to control asthma, the drug dosage may need to be increased. For nonsmokers, the theophylline dosage should be within the suggested drug dosing range.
- Determine renal function by checking for adequate urine output; it should be greater than 600 mL daily. The guideline is 30 mL/hr for adults.

Nursing Diagnoses
- Readiness for enhanced knowledge related to therapeutic regimen
- Deficient knowledge related to lack of information about drug interactions and OTC drugs
- Risk for injury related to adverse reaction to drug interaction

Planning
- Patient will be aware of drug interactions, will avoid drugs that may cause a severe reaction, and will know what to report immediately to the health care provider.
- Patient will not take any OTC drugs without consultation with the health care provider.

Nursing Interventions
- Contact the health care provider to assess the need for a drug dose adjustment if one has not been ordered after a drug enzyme inducer has been discontinued.
- Recognize drugs of the same category that might have an additive effect. The additive drug effect might be undesirable and could cause a severe physiologic response.
- Notify the health care provider of drugs ordered that have antagonistic or opposite effects, such as beta stimulants and beta blockers.
- Consult a pharmacist about the use of a drug interaction computer program.
- Encourage the patient to use one pharmacy; drug reconciliation is to be done for hospitalized patients and patients on community-based visits to the health care provider.

Patient Teaching
- Advise patients not to take OTC drugs with prescribed drugs without first notifying the health care provider.
- Remind patients to be cautious about taking herbal products, especially if taking OTC or prescription medications; check with health care provider first.

Evaluation
- Evaluate the effectiveness of the drugs, and determine that patient is free from side effects.

KEY WEBSITES

Facts and Comparisons' Guide to Popular Natural Products: *www.drugfacts.com*

National Library of Medicine: *www.nlm.nih.gov*

PubMed: *www.ncbi.nlm.nih.gov/pubmed*

CRITICAL THINKING CASE STUDY

A patient is taking phenytoin, warfarin (Coumadin), promethazine, (Phenergan), meperidine (Demerol), and diazepam (Valium).

1. What general teaching is appropriate for this patient? Be certain to include specifics about probable drug interactions.
2. During a teaching session, the patient shares that he plans to start taking OTC products to boost his energy. What is the nurse's best response to the patient's comment? Explain your answer.

NCLEX STUDY QUESTIONS

1. The rate of absorption of drugs can change when two drugs are taken at the same time. The nurse is aware that the rate of absorption can be changed by which actions? (Select all that apply.)
   a. Modifying gastric emptying time
   b. Changing gastric pH
   c. Decreasing inflammation
   d. Forming drug complexes
   e. Eating too slowly
2. The nurse is reviewing a patient's medications as part of patient teaching. The nurse is aware that which drug is least likely to cause photosensitivity?
   a. Penicillins
   b. Sulfonamides
   c. Sulfonylureas
   d. Thiazides
3. A patient asks the nurse about the drug qualities that determine the category in which a drug is placed. What is the nurse's best response? (Select all that apply.)
   a. "Drugs that are in clinical trials"
   b. "Drugs judged to be both safe and effective"
   c. "Drugs judged to be either unsafe or ineffective"
   d. "Drugs with insufficient data to judge safety or efficacy"
   e. "Herbal products"
4. The nurse is meeting with a community group about medication safety. The nurse must emphasize that patients at high risk for drug interactions include which groups? (Select all that apply.)
   a. Older patients
   b. Patients with chronic health conditions
   c. Patients taking three or more drugs
   d. Patients dealing with only one pharmacy
   e. Patients covered by Medicare or Medicaid
5. The nurse recognizes that when a patient takes a hepatic enzyme inducer, the dose of the warfarin (Coumadin) is usually modified in which way?
   a. It is increased.
   b. It is decreased.
   c. It remains the same.
   d. It is unpredictable.
6. The nurse is conducting a patient assessment and notes that the patient has alkaline urine, which promotes excretion of drugs that are weak acids. Which drug is a weak acid?
   a. phenytoin (Dilantin)
   b. acetylsalicylic acid (aspirin)
   c. quinidine (Apo-Quinidine)
   d. warfarin (Coumadin)
7. The nurse is describing to a patient the synergistic effects of two of his medications. Which statement by the nurse is correct about synergistic drug effects?
   a. "Two drugs have antagonistic effects on each other."
   b. "The action of a drug is nullified by another drug."
   c. "One drug acts as an antidote to the side effects of another drug."
   d. "A greater effect is achieved when two drugs are combined."
8. A patient asks the nurse about cautions related to use of OTC medications. What is the nurse's best response? (Select all that apply.)
   a. "Over-the-counter drugs may delay professional diagnosis."
   b. "They may mask symptoms."
   c. "They may make diagnosis easier."
   d. "Their inactive ingredients may cause adverse reactions."
   e. "They may be more expensive."
9. Patients on long-term digoxin (Lanoxin) therapy need regular digoxin-level monitoring to detect early toxicity manifested by which symptoms? (Select all that apply.)
   a. Visual problems
   b. Nausea and vomiting
   c. Skin eruptions
   d. Urinary retention
   e. Dizziness
10. The nurse is reviewing a teaching plan with a patient who was recently diagnosed with asthma. What cautions about the use of aspirin are important for the nurse to advise the patient? (Select all that apply.)
    a. It may trigger an acute asthma attack.
    b. It may trigger a heart attack.
    c. There is an increased risk for bleeding if also taking an anticoagulant.
    d. It may decrease renal function.
    e. It may decrease hepatic function.
11. A patient asks the nurse about drug interactions with OTC preparations. What is the nurse's best response?
    a. "Discuss this with the health care provider."
    b. "There are not many interactions, so don't worry about it."
    c. "Read the labels carefully, and check with your health care provider."
    d. "Avoid over-the-counter preparations."

Answers: 1, a, b, d; 2, a; 3, b, c, d; 4, a, b, c; 5, a; 6, b; 7, d; 8, a, b, d; 9 a, b, d; 10 a, c, d; 11, c.

CHAPTER

5

Drugs of Abuse

Donald L. Taylor

evolve WEBSITE

http://evolve.elsevier.com/KeeHayes/pharmacology/

- Animations
- Content Updates
- Key Points
- Review Questions for the NCLEX® Examination
- References from the Textbook
- Unfolding Case Studies

OBJECTIVES

- Define and differentiate among drug abuse, drug misuse, addiction, dependence, tolerance, detoxification, withdrawal, and abstinence.
- Describe the short-term and long-term effects of the relationships among brain structures and neurotransmitters involved in the neurobiology of addictive drugs.
- Identify the physical and psychological assessment findings associated with the use of commonly abused central nervous system stimulants and depressants, cannabis, psychedelic agents, and inhalants.
- Explain the rationale for the use of pharmacologic treatments during toxicity, withdrawal, and maintenance of abstinence of commonly abused drugs.
- Prioritize appropriate nursing interventions to use during treatment of patients with substance toxicity and withdrawal.
- Identify nursing interventions appropriate during management of surgical experiences and pain in patients who abuse drugs.
- Describe the nurse's role in recognizing and promoting treatment of chemical impairment among nurses.
- Implement the nursing process in the care of patients who abuse drugs.

OUTLINE

KEY TERMS

abstinence, p. 43
addiction, p. 42
brain reward system, p. 42
chemical impairment, p. 58
craving, p. 43
cross-tolerance, p. 52
cue-induced craving, p. 43
dependence, p. 42
detoxification, p. 43
drug abuse, p. 42
drug addiction, p. 42
drug misuse, p. 42
intoxication, p. 43
Korsakoff's psychosis, p. 52
opioids, p. 54
physical dependence, p. 42
potentiation, p. 52
psychological dependence, p. 44
relapse, p. 43
tolerance, p. 43
Wernicke's encephalopathy, p. 52
withdrawal syndrome, p. 43

Most drugs are used safely and within prescribed guidelines, but it is possible for all drugs to be misused or abused. Drug abuse and addiction are serious and complex social and health problems that nurses address in all areas of practice. However, this chapter focuses primarily on the physiologic effects of abused drugs and the pharmacologic treatment of abuse.

CONTEXT OF DRUG ABUSE

Cultural Considerations

Cultural and social expectations influence the definitions and perception of drug abuse versus acceptable usage. In Moslem Middle Eastern populations, any use of alcohol or mind-altering drugs may be considered abuse. The same might be true in the United States among conservative religious groups. Yet in many European cultures, alcohol use is expected and present at all family and social gatherings. For many people in the United States, occasional use of marijuana and alcohol is not considered abuse, nor is the use of psychedelic agents in some Native American religious rites. Cigarette smoking, which was glamorized in the past, is now less socially acceptable than moderate alcohol use in the United States.

Sociocultural factors arising from unemployment, poverty, or adverse social conditions affect the incidence of substance abuse. Individual factors, such as age, educational status, and geographic region, also affect rates of use. Metropolitan and urban areas have higher rates of substance abuse than rural areas in the United States. Additionally, the West Coast has a higher rate of use (11.0%) than the Northeast, Midwest, or South (9.4%, 8.2%, and 7.8%, respectively). A major responsibility of nurses in addressing drug abuse in ethnic and cultural groups is to assess and treat patients within their cultural perspectives, as described in Chapter 3.

Definitions

Although small differences exist in their definitions, the terms *drug, substance,* and *chemical* are often used interchangeably within the context of drug abuse. **Drug misuse** generally refers to indiscriminate or recreational use of a chemical substance or its use for purposes other than those for which it is intended. **Drug abuse** is culturally defined and may be considered drug use inconsistent with medical or social norms. It generally refers to an overindulgence of a chemical substance that results in a negative impact on the psychological, physical, or social functioning of an individual. Chronic abuse of a drug may lead to addiction. **Drug addiction** should be considered a complex disease of the central nervous system (CNS) characterized by a compulsive, uncontrolled craving for and **dependence** on a substance to such a degree that cessation causes severe emotional, mental, and/or physiologic reactions. **Physical dependence** is not necessary or sufficient for addiction to occur. Terms used in describing drug abuse are presented in Table 5-1.

Drugs abused most often are psychoactive agents that result in pleasure or modify thinking and perception. They include legal substances such as alcohol, tobacco, and prescription drugs such as analgesics, sedative-hypnotics, tranquilizers, and amphetamines. Common illegal substances that are abused include marijuana and hashish, cocaine, MDMA, and heroin.

NEUROBIOLOGY OF ADDICTIVE DRUGS

Most addictive drugs increase the availability of dopamine and other neurotransmitters in the mesolimbic system of the brain. This area has been identified as the "pleasure center" or **brain reward system**, an ancient system that creates the sensation of pleasure for certain behaviors necessary for survival, such as eating and sexual behavior.

Normally dopamine is released at a stable rate in the mesolimbic system, maintaining a normative mood. Certain drugs such as opioids and cocaine increase the release of dopamine or decrease its reuptake at the synapse. Nicotine, alcohol, marijuana, amphetamines, and caffeine are also believed to increase dopamine activity at the synapse. The resulting increase in dopamine in the system leads to mood elevation or euphoria, factors that provide strong motivation to repeat the experience. Many addictive drugs also increase the availability of other neurotransmitters such as serotonin and gamma-aminobutyric acid (GABA), but dopamine's effect on the reward system appears to be pivotal to the addictive process.

Addiction (a compulsive, uncontrollable craving for and dependence on a substance to such a degree that cessation causes severe reactions) results from the prolonged effects of addictive drugs on the brain. Repeated use of drugs remodels the neural circuitry of the brain cells and reduces the responsiveness of receptors. This decreased responsiveness leads to

TABLE 5-1 TERMINOLOGY OF DRUG ABUSE

TERM	DEFINITION
Abstinence	Sustained avoidance of substance use.
Addiction	A compulsive, uncontrollable craving for and dependence on a substance to such a degree that cessation causes severe emotional, mental, or physiologic reactions.
Chemical impairment	A term used by health professionals to describe behaviors related to the effects of drugs or substances on performance.
Craving	Subjective need for a substance, usually experienced after decreased use or abstinence. Cue-induced craving is stimulated in the presence of situations previously associated with drug taking.
Dependence	Reliance on a substance that has reached the level that its absence will cause impairment in function.
Psychological	Compulsive need to experience pleasurable response from the substance.
Physical	Altered physiologic state from prolonged substance use; regular use is necessary to prevent withdrawal syndrome.
Drug abuse	Overindulgence in and dependence on a substance that has a negative impact on psychological, physiologic, and social functioning of an individual; synonymous with chemical dependence.
Drug misuse	Indiscriminate use of a drug for purposes other than those for which it is intended.
Relapse	Return to substance use during abstinence.
Substance	Drug, chemical, or biologic entity.
Tolerance	Decreased effect of a substance that results from repeated exposure. It is possible to develop cross-tolerance to other substances in the same category.
Withdrawal syndrome	Constellation of physiologic and psychological responses that occur when there is abrupt cessation or reduced intake of a substance on which an individual is dependent or when the effect is counteracted by a specific antagonist.

tolerance—the need for a larger dose of a drug to obtain the original euphoria. As drugs of abuse result in levels of dopamine that do not naturally occur, tolerance also reduces the sense of pleasure from experiences that previously resulted in positive feelings, such as food, sex, or relationships. Without the drug, the individual may experience depression, anxiety, and/or irritability. **Craving** is another characteristic of addiction; one type of craving is **cue-induced craving**, which occurs in the presence of people, places, or things patients have previously associated with drug use. These encounters produce surges in dopamine levels, and these surges push the individual toward active drug seeking and drug taking. Cue-induced craving may occur after long periods of **abstinence** and is a common cause of **relapse.**

Continued research into the biologic and genetic basis of addiction is crucial to the development of drugs to treat addiction. Increasing evidence shows that genetics play a significant role in alcoholism and nicotine use and that there are significant gender differences in drug abuse risk. A natural genetic mutation that inhibits nicotine metabolism in the brain has been identified. Men with the mutation are less likely to become addicted to nicotine and find it easier to quit smoking. However, the presence or absence of the defective gene does not affect women's smoking. Women also have less stomach metabolism of alcohol, resulting in higher blood alcohol levels than men after the same amount of alcohol intake. A genetic difference in the activity of a liver enzyme in African Americans results in slower metabolism of nicotine, potentially resulting in the consumption of fewer cigarettes per day than Caucasian people may consume.

Biologic and genetic research has led to the development of drugs to treat opioid, nicotine, and alcohol addiction. However, currently no medications are approved by the U.S Food and Drug Administration (FDA) for treating addiction to cocaine, lysergic acid diethylamide (LSD), phencyclidine hydrochloride (PCP), marijuana, methamphetamine and other stimulants, or inhalants.

OVERVIEW OF ADDICTIVE STATES

Intoxication

Intoxication is a state of being influenced, or affected by a drug or other toxic substance. This may be a very small amount of drug in the drug-naïve person, or a potentially lethal amount in the chronic user. The signs and symptoms seen for either are the toxic effects of the drug when taken in excessive amounts.

Detoxification

Detoxification involves treating an intoxicated patient to diminish or remove drugs or their effects from the body. Treatments may involve administration of antagonistic drugs, promotion of metabolism and elimination of the drug, or intensive supportive care until the drug is naturally eliminated.

Withdrawal Syndrome

Withdrawal syndrome is a group of signs and symptoms that occurs in physically dependent persons when drug use is stopped. The symptoms are often opposite the effects the drug produced before it was withdrawn. Opioids, alcohol, barbiturates, and anxiolytics cause relatively strong physical dependence and withdrawal syndrome. Cannabinoids and amphetamines cause weaker physical dependence. Hallucinogens such as LSD do not cause physical dependence or abstinence signs. Withdrawal syndrome is treated by slow weaning of the drugs, or use of "cross-tolerant" drugs to control symptoms, and supportive care.

Cessation and Maintenance of Abstinence

To promote cessation and abstinence of the abused drug, treatment with other drugs may be used to decrease craving and prevent withdrawal syndrome. Specific receptor blockers, less potent drugs of the same class, or nonaddicting substitutes are treatment options. In addition to the use of drugs to maintain abstinence, cognitive-behavioral therapies enhance the effectiveness of medications and are recommended for treatment of all drug abuse and addiction.

STIMULANTS

Nicotine

Nicotine is the alkaloid in tobacco that causes dependence and is the most rapidly addicting of the drugs of abuse. Smoking cigarettes is the most damaging method of nicotine use. Cigarette smoke contains more than 4000 chemicals and gases, including at least 45 cancer-causing or tumor-promoting agents and a number of hydrocarbons or solvents. Although nicotine is not believed to be carcinogenic, it is the addictive substance and has no therapeutic value.

Pharmacokinetics Nicotine is rapidly absorbed into the blood through the lungs in smoking and more slowly through the buccal mucosa in chewing and the nasal mucosa in snuffing. It crosses membranes easily and is widely distributed throughout the body. Nicotine passes freely into breast milk and may be toxic to the nursing infant. Plasma protein binding of nicotine is less than 5%. The liver is the major site of nicotine metabolism. Nicotine and its more than 20 metabolites are eliminated in the urine. The elimination half-life of nicotine is 1 to 2 hours.

Pharmacodynamics In low doses, such as those obtained through cigarettes, nicotine activates nicotinic receptors. Most effects occur from activated receptors in autonomic ganglia and the adrenal medulla. In the CNS, nicotine rapidly acts on the mesolimbic reward system of the brain, promoting the release of dopamine and mimicking the effects of cocaine and other highly addictive substances.

Side Effects and Adverse Reactions

Stimulation of nicotinic receptors in the sympathetic ganglia and the adrenal medulla result in marked cardiovascular stimulation and increased myocardial oxygen consumption. In the brain, the action of nicotine causes general CNS stimulation. Physical effects include increased respiratory rate and tremors. Psychological effects include increased alertness and arousal. In the gastrointestinal (GI) tract, nicotine increases GI secretions and smooth-muscle tone. Many abusers of nicotine report that nicotine has a depressant effect, promoting relaxation and relief of anxiety. However, it is thought that these effects actually occur when periodic nicotine withdrawal is relieved by further nicotine.

Nicotine causes a very strong **psychological dependence**. In addition, physiologic dependence occurs with regular heavy use. Withdrawal symptoms may occur within the first few hours after stopping smoking, peak in 24 to 48 hours, and last from a few weeks to several months. After withdrawal subsides, cue-induced craving may cause smoking relapse. The effects of nicotine and symptoms of withdrawal are presented in Table 5-2.

Treatment

Treatment of nicotine addiction has received considerable attention in the past few years because of its association with preventable illness and death. Chronic smoking can affect nearly every organ of the body. In addition to cardiovascular disease, chronic lung disease, and cancers of the larynx, lung, esophagus, oral cavity, and bladder, smoking is now associated with leukemia, cataracts, abdominal aortic aneurysm, and cancers of the cervix, kidney, pancreas, and stomach. To help end thousands of these unnecessary health problems, nurses must be proactive in identifying and talking with tobacco users and providing them with information on ways to stop the use of tobacco.

Several drug products are available to aid smoking cessation. Except in special circumstances, nicotine replacement therapy (NRT) or other smoking cessation agents are recommended for all tobacco users in addition to behavioral and support therapies. Five NRTs in the form of gum, lozenges, transdermal patches, nasal spray, and inhalers have been approved by the FDA to reduce the craving and withdrawal symptoms associated with tobacco cessation. These agents enable a smoker to reduce nicotine previously obtained from cigarettes with a system that provides slower delivery of the drug and eliminates the carcinogens and gases associated with tobacco smoke. Table 5-3 describes various nicotine replacement products.

Bupropion is an atypical (heterocyclic) antidepressant unrelated to nicotine that has been approved by the FDA for smoking cessation. The exact mechanism of action of bupropion is unknown. It is thought to inhibit neuronal reuptake of dopamine, and to a lesser degree norepinephrine, and this reduces the urge to smoke and minimizes some symptoms of nicotine withdrawal. Bupropion may be combined with NRT to provide additional benefit. Bupropion is marketed as Zyban for smoking cessation. Serious negative effects of bupropion use include agitation, hostility, increased depression or other psychiatric symptoms, and suicidality.

Varenicline (Chantix) is a novel drug approved for smoking cessation that is an alternative to NRT and bupropion. It is a nicotinic receptor partial agonist that reduces cravings for nicotine and decreases the pleasurable effects of cigarettes and other tobacco products if tobacco is used. The approved course of varenicline treatment is 12 weeks, and those who successfully quit smoking during treatment may continue with an additional 12 weeks to increase long-term cessation. In clinical trials, the most common adverse effects were nausea, headache, vomiting, flatulence, insomnia, abnormal dreams, and a change in taste perception; serious negative effects are similar to those for bupropion.

Nortriptyline (Aventyl, Pamelor) and clonidine (Catapres) are used as second-line drugs to reduce nicotine withdrawal symptoms and promote cessation. These drugs are not approved by the FDA for this purpose, and their action in nicotine addiction is not clearly understood. Nortriptyline is a tricyclic antidepressant (see Chapter 28). Clonidine is a centrally acting $alpha_2$ agonist used to treat hypertension (see Chapter 44).

Research related to the development of new agents and new uses of approved drugs in smoking cessation is a priority of the National Institute for Drug Abuse. Clinical trials are currently in progress to examine the effects of various combinations of nicotine-replacement agents, combinations of nicotine-replacement agents with antidepressants, neurotransmitter modulators, nicotine vaccines that produce antibodies that bind in the blood with nicotine, and nicotine receptor–blocking agents. More information on nicotine

TABLE 5-2 EFFECTS OF FREQUENTLY ABUSED DRUGS

SUBSTANCE	PHYSIOLOGIC AND PSYCHOLOGICAL EFFECTS	TOXICITY	WITHDRAWAL SYNDROME
Stimulants			
Nicotine	Increased arousal and alertness; performance enhancement; increased heart rate, cardiac output, and blood pressure; cutaneous vasoconstriction; fine tremor, decreased appetite; antidiuretic effect; increased gastric motility	Rare: Nausea, abdominal pain, diarrhea, vomiting, dizziness, weakness, confusion, decreased respirations, seizures, death from respiratory failure	Craving, restlessness, depression, hyperirritability, headache, insomnia, decreased blood pressure and heart rate, increased appetite
Cocaine/Amphetamines amphetamine (Benzedrine) bath salts/khat/cathinone benzphetamine (Didrex) dextroamphetamine (Dexedrine) methamphetamine (Desoxyn) methylphenidate (Ritalin) pemoline (Cylert) phenmetrazine (Preludin)	Euphoria, grandiosity, mood swings, hyperactivity, hyperalertness, restlessness, anorexia, insomnia, hypertension, tachycardia, marked vasoconstriction, tremor, dysrhythmias, seizures, sexual arousal, dilated pupils, diaphoresis	Agitation; increased temperature, pulse, respiratory rate, blood pressure; cardiac dysrhythmias; myocardial infarction; hallucinations; seizures; possible death	Severe craving, severely depressed mood, exhaustion, prolonged sleep, apathy, irritability, disorientation
Caffeine	Mood elevation, increased alertness, nervousness, jitteriness, irritability, insomnia, increased respirations, increased heart rate and force of myocardial contraction, relaxation of smooth muscle, diuresis	Rare: Nervousness, confusion, psychomotor agitation, anxiety, dizziness, tinnitus, muscle twitching, elevated blood pressure, tachycardia, extrasystole, increased respiratory rate	Headache, irritability, drowsiness, fatigue
Depressants ***Alcohol*** ***Sedative Hypnotics*** *Barbiturates* secobarbital (Seconal) pentobarbital (Nembutal) amobarbital (Amytal) *Benzodiazepines* diazepam (Valium) chlordiazepoxide (Librium) alprazolam (Xanax) *Nonbarbiturates/ Nonbenzodiazepines* methaqualone (Quaalude) chloral hydrate (Noctec)	Initial relaxation, emotional lability, decreased inhibitions, drowsiness, lack of coordination, impaired judgment, slurred speech, hypotension, bradycardia, bradypnea, constricted pupils	Shallow respirations; cold, clammy skin; weak, rapid pulse; hyporeflexia; coma; possible death	Anxiety, agitation, insomnia, diaphoresis, tremors, delirium, seizures, possible death
Opioids heroin morphine opium codeine fentanyl (Sublimaze) meperidine (Demerol) hydromorphone (Dilaudid) oxycodone (OxyContin, Percocet) methadone (Dolophine)	Analgesia, euphoria, drowsiness, detachment from environment, relaxation, constricted pupils, constipation, nausea, decreased respiratory rate, slurred speech, impaired judgment, decreased sexual and aggressive drives	Slow, shallow respirations; clammy skin; constricted pupils; coma; possible death	Watery eyes, dilated pupils, runny nose, yawning, tremors, pain, chills, fever, diaphoresis, nausea, vomiting, diarrhea, abdominal cramps

Continued

TABLE 5-2 EFFECTS OF FREQUENTLY ABUSED DRUGS—cont'd

SUBSTANCE	PHYSIOLOGIC AND PSYCHOLOGICAL EFFECTS	TOXICITY	WITHDRAWAL SYNDROME
Cannabis			
Marijuana ***Hashish*** ***Synthetic Marijuana***	Relaxation, euphoria, amotivation, slowed time sensation, sexual arousal, abrupt mood changes, impaired memory and attention, impaired judgment, reddened eyes, dry mouth, lack of coordination, tachycardia, increased appetite	Fatigue, paranoia, panic reactions, hallucinogen-like psychotic states	With heavy use: insomnia, restlessness, irritability, tremor, weight loss, hyperthermia, chills
Psychedelics lysergic acid diethylamide (LSD) psilocybin (mushrooms) dimethyltryptamine (DMT) diethyltryptamine (DET) 3,4-methylendioxyamphetamine (MDMA, Ecstasy) herbal ecstasy (contains herbs and ephedrine) mescaline (peyote) phencyclidine (PCP)	Perceptual distortions, hallucinations, delusions (PCP), depersonalization, heightened sensory perception, euphoria, mood swings, suspiciousness, panic, impaired judgment, increased body temperature, hypertension, flushed face, tremor, dilated pupils, constricted pupils (PCP), nystagmus (PCP), violence (PCP)	Prolonged effects and episodes, anxiety, panic, confusion, blurred vision, increases in blood pressure and temperature	No physical withdrawal, but psychological desire may occur
Inhalants			
Aerosol Propellants fluorinated hydrocarbons nitrous oxide (in deodorants, hair spray, pesticide, whipped cream spray, spray paint, cookware coating products) ***Solvents*** gasoline, kerosene, nail polish remover, typewriter correction fluid, cleaning solutions, lighter fluid, paint, paint thinner, glue ***Anesthetic Agents*** nitrous oxide, chloroform ***Nitrites*** amyl nitrite, butyl nitrite	Euphoria; decreased inhibitions; giddiness; slurred speech; illusions; drowsiness; clouded sensorium; tinnitus; nystagmus; dysrhythmias; cough; nausea; vomiting; diarrhea; irritation to eyes, nose, and mouth	Anxiety, respiratory depression, cardiac dysrhythmias, loss of consciousness, sudden death	None

abuse and its effects can be found in the discussion of lower respiratory disorders in Chapter 41.

Cocaine

Cocaine is a naturally occurring potent stimulant, an alkaloid that was originally obtained from the leaves of the coca plant but today can be prepared synthetically. Historically, cocaine was used as a local anesthetic, but it has been largely replaced by synthetic agents with no abuse potential. Cocaine is a Schedule II drug under the Controlled Substances Act. Illicit cocaine is available as white powder (cocaine hydrochloride) and as cocaine base (alkaloidal cocaine, freebase), a crystalline substance. "Crack," a cocaine base that gets its name from the popping sound the crystals make when heated, is popular because it is less expensive, readily available, and easy to use, and has increased purity over cocaine hydrochloride.

Pharmacokinetics Absorption rates of cocaine depend on the route of administration. Cocaine hydrochloride is usually "snorted" intranasally. Cocaine can also be smoked as crack cocaine or in "freebase" form, injected intravenously (IV), taken orally, or absorbed through the mucous membranes. Smoking and IV methods result in the fastest absorption and the highest "rush." Peak blood levels develop within 5 to 30 minutes with most methods of administration. The longest effects occur following intranasal use because absorption is delayed by vasoconstriction of the nasal vessels. Cocaine is rapidly metabolized by the liver. Elimination half-lives by oral, intranasal, and IV routes are 50, 80, and 60 minutes, respectively. Tolerance appears to occur with long-term use, but users can also become more sensitive to

TABLE 5-3 NICOTINE-REPLACEMENT AGENTS

GENERAL CONSIDERATIONS FOR NICOTINE REPLACEMENT THERAPY (NRT)

NRT should not be used by pregnant or nursing patients.
Smoking while using NRT may cause nicotine overdose.
Tapering of all agents except transdermal patches is required.
Replacement agents used are usually a matter of personal preference.
The stronger doses of agents should be used by heavy smokers.
Using more than one agent at the same time should be discussed with the health care provider.
Generic preparations are available for some agents.

AGENTS	ABSORPTION	SIDE EFFECTS	CONSIDERATIONS
Gum (OTC)			
Nicorette 2 mg, 4 mg	Buccal mucosa	Hiccups, mouth ulcers, indigestion, jaw pain	Specific 30-minute chewing regimen with periods of holding the gum between cheek and teeth; food and drink should be avoided 15 minutes before or during use.
Lozenge (OTC)			
Commit 2 mg, 4 mg	Buccal mucosa	Nausea and indigestion, hiccups, headache, cough, mouth soreness, flatulence	Dissolves in the mouth in 20 to 30 minutes; chewing and swallowing the lozenge increases GI side effects.
Patch (OTC)			
NicoDerm CQ Nicotine transdermal system 18-hour, 24-hour doses	Skin	Skin rash at patch site, headache, dizziness, weakness, indigestion, diarrhea, sleep disturbances with 24-hour patch	Differs from other agents in that it helps prevent craving; cannot be used by those with adhesive allergies.
Nasal Spray			
Nicotrol NS	Nasal mucosa	Nose and throat irritation, sneezing, rhinitis, watery eyes, cough	Requires a prescription; nasal irritation may limit use; affects airways and not a good choice for those with asthma, allergies, or sinus problems.
Inhaler			
Nicotrol nicotine inhalation system, delivers 4 mg	Oral mucosa	Cough; nose, mouth, and throat irritation; heartburn and nausea	Requires a prescription; simulates smoking with mouthpiece and nicotine cartridge; may not be advisable for those with asthma or pulmonary disease.

GI, Gastrointestinal; *OTC,* over-the-counter.

the drug's anesthetic and convulsant effects. Cocaine readily crosses the placenta in pregnant patients and accumulates in the fetal circulation. Conflicting research exists about the effect of prenatal cocaine exposure on the development of the child.

Pharmacodynamics Cocaine inhibits the neuronal uptake of dopamine in the brain and increases the activation of dopamine receptors in the brain reward system. This action magnifies pleasures and leads to rapid dependence. Cocaine also increases norepinephrine at postsynaptic receptor sites, producing intense vasoconstriction and cardiovascular stimulation. Drug interactions with cocaine are identified in Table 5-4.

Side Effects and Adverse Reactions

At usual doses, cocaine produces euphoria and increased energy and alertness. In addition to CNS stimulation, effects include peripheral adrenaline-like actions (see Table 5-2). Chronic use may lead to impairment of concentration and memory, irritability and mood swings, paranoia, and depression.

A stimulant psychosis may occur with the chronic use of any stimulant. A cocaine psychosis usually progresses from paranoid delusions to visual hallucinations of "snow lights" (colored lights when cocaine is administered) and tactile hallucinations of bugs crawling under the skin. Skin excoriations from scratching; needle marks; and elevated blood pressure, heart rate, and temperature are findings that help differentiate a stimulant psychosis from schizophrenia.

Acute cocaine toxicity may be manifested by cardiac palpitations, tachycardia, increased respiratory rate, and fever. At high levels of overdose, grand mal seizures, hypertension, and dysrhythmias or myocardial ischemia can occur. The patient experiences restlessness, paranoia, agitated delirium, and confusion. Bizarre, erratic, and violent behavior may occur. Death is often related to a cerebrovascular accident, fatal dysrhythmias, or myocardial infarction.

The degree of physical dependence produced by cocaine appears to vary among individuals. Some users report little or no evidence of physical withdrawal with abstinence, but others report symptoms similar to those associated with amphetamine withdrawal: dysphoria, fatigue, depression, and a need to sleep. In the first 9 hours to 14 days of abstinence, many users experience an intense psychological response

TABLE 5-4 DRUG INTERACTIONS: DRUGS OF ABUSE

DRUG OF ABUSE	INTERACTING DRUGS/DRUG CATEGORIES	EFFECTS
Nicotine/Smoking*	isoproterenol (Isuprel) phenylephrine (Neo-Synephrine)	Increased effects with use of nicotine/smoking (After smoking cessation, dosages may need to be increased.)
	pentazocine (Talwin NX) propoxyphene (Darvon) Benzodiazepines (diazepam [Valium]) Tricyclic antidepressants propranolol (Inderal) theophylline (Theo-Dur, others) heparin insulin	Decreased effects with use of nicotine/smoking (After smoking cessation, dosages may need to be reduced.)
Cocaine	Sympathomimetics/adrenomimetics Central nervous system (CNS) stimulants Cholinesterase inhibitors (neostigmine)	May increase CNS and cardiac effects of cocaine
	Tricyclic antidepressants, digoxin, methyldopa (Aldomet)	May increase cocaine-induced dysrhythmias
	Beta-adrenergic blockers	Cocaine may decrease effects
Amphetamines	Tricyclic antidepressants Sympathomimetics/adrenomimetics CNS stimulants	Increased effect of tricyclic antidepressants and sympathomimetics; increased effect of amphetamines
	GI antacids/urinary alkalinizing agents Monoamine oxidase inhibitors (MAOIs)	Increased effect of amphetamine
	meperidine (Demerol)	Amphetamines increase analgesic effect; meperidine increases risk of seizures and vascular collapse.
	Thyroid hormone	Reciprocal increase in effects
	Adrenergic blockers Antihistamines Antihypertensives	Amphetamines may decrease effects.
Alcohol	Other CNS depressants: Sedative-hypnotics Opioids General anesthetics	Increased CNS depression with increased risk of death from respiratory depression
	Nonsteroidal antiinflammatory drugs	Combined effect increases risk of gastric bleeding
	acetaminophen (Tylenol)	Increased risk for liver injury
	Antihypertensives	Decreased effect of antihypertensives
Barbiturates	Other CNS depressants: Alcohol Opioids General anesthetics Other sedative/hypnotics MAOIs valproic acid (Depakene)	Increased CNS depression
	Oral anticoagulants Corticosteroids and other steroid hormones griseofulvin (Fluvicin) doxycycline	Effect decreased by barbiturates
Benzodiazepines	Other CNS depressants: Alcohol Opioids General anesthetics Other sedative/hypnotics Herbs: Kava kava, valerian	Increased CNS depression

TABLE 5-4 DRUG INTERACTIONS: DRUGS OF ABUSE—cont'd

DRUG OF ABUSE	INTERACTING DRUGS/DRUG CATEGORIES	EFFECTS
Opioids	Other CNS depressants: Alcohol, General anesthetics, Sedative/hypnotics, Phenothiazines, Antiemetics	Increased CNS depression
	Mixed agonist/antagonist opioids	Reduces the effect of pure opioid agonists and may precipitate withdrawal syndrome
	MAOIs	May cause severe fatal reaction
	Diuretics	Opioids may decrease effect
Marijuana/Hashish	CNS stimulants/sympathomimetics Anticholinergic agents Tricyclic antidepressants	Additive hypertension, tachycardia, drowsiness
	CNS depressants	Additive drowsiness and CNS depression
	theophylline	Decreased effect of theophylline

CNS, Central nervous system; *GI,* gastrointestinal; *MAOIs,* monoamine oxidase inhibitors.
*Interactions may be due to nicotine or the effect on the liver by hydrocarbons found in cigarette smoke.

characterized by intense craving and cocaine-seeking behavior (see Table 5-2). Eventually, mood becomes more normal, but a desire to return to the drug, especially prompted by cue-induced craving, remains for an indefinite period. In rare instances, withdrawal can be prolonged and difficult.

Treatment

Emergency management of cocaine toxicity depends on the patient findings at the time of treatment. Treatment may be complicated by the possibility that the patient has combined the use of cocaine with heroin, alcohol, or PCP. There is no specific antidote for cocaine toxicity, but during an overdose most symptoms can be controlled with a variety of drugs. Emergency interventions for assessment findings in cocaine toxicity are presented in Table 5-5.

Cognitive-behavioral therapies are often the only effective approach to cocaine addiction, but maintenance of cocaine abstinence with behavioral therapies has been difficult to achieve in most users. No drugs are currently approved to promote cocaine abstinence; however, disulfiram (Antabuse), a well-established medication for treatment of alcoholism, has helped nonalcoholic people addicted to cocaine reduce drug use from 2.5 days per week to 0.5 days per week on average. It has also been found that when modafinil (Provigil), a CNS stimulant used for treatment of narcolepsy, is combined with behavioral therapy, the likelihood of cocaine abstinence increases. The anticonvulsant topiramate (Topamax) and the antiemetic ondansetron (Zofran) have shown some efficacy for treating cocaine addiction and may benefit some individuals, but they are not approved for this use by the FDA. Additionally, research shows promise for a vaccine that works by stimulating the production of

TABLE 5-5 DRUG THERAPY FOR COCAINE AND AMPHETAMINE TOXICITY

ASSESSMENT FINDINGS	DRUG THERAPY
Cardiovascular	
Palpitations Tachycardia Hypertension Dysrhythmias Myocardial ischemia or infarction	Establish IV access, and initiate fluid replacement as appropriate. Anticipate the need for propranolol (Inderal) or labetalol (Normodyne) for hypertension and tachycardia. Severe hypertension may require administration of nitroprusside (Nipride) or phentolamine (Regitine). Treat ventricular dysrhythmias as appropriate with lidocaine, bretylium (Bretylol), or procainamide (Pronestyl). Aspirin may be administered to lower the risk of myocardial infarction.
Central Nervous System (CNS)	
Feeling of impending doom Euphoria Agitation Combativeness Seizures Hallucinations Confusion Paranoia Fever	Naloxone (Narcan) IV should be given if CNS depression is present and concurrent opiate use is suspected. Administer diazepam (Valium) or lorazepam (Ativan) IV for agitation and seizures. Administer chlorpromazine (Thorazine) or haloperidol (Haldol) IV for psychosis and hallucinations.

IV, intravenous.

cocaine-specific antibodies that bind to cocaine molecules, rendering them ineffective.

Amphetamines

Amphetamine is a synthetic drug and, with its derivatives and similar stimulants, is strictly regulated today as a Schedule II drug of the Controlled Substances Act. Specific drugs classified as amphetamines are identified in Table 5-2 and Chapter 20. Because amphetamines may be used therapeutically as CNS stimulants, abuse may rise out of slow escalation of a prescribed dose. However, they are more often initially used a cheaper alternative to cocaine.

Methamphetamine (crank) and methamphetamine crystals (crystal meth) are very potent stimulants and can be easily made in clandestine settings with relatively inexpensive over-the-counter (OTC) ingredients. Methamphetamine abuse is a growing problem in all segments of the population and geographic regions.

Pharmacokinetics Amphetamines are prescribed for oral use, with peak effects occurring within 60 to 90 minutes and lasting 2 to 4 hours. More rapid effects are obtained by smoking, snorting, or IV injection; and they are therefore more frequently used illicitly in these manners. Amphetamines have a longer half-life than cocaine and a longer, more intense effect. Additional information regarding the pharmacodynamics and pharmacokinetics of amphetamines can be found in Chapter 20.

Pharmacodynamics Amphetamines act similarly to cocaine, stimulating the release of dopamine and norepinephrine in the brain and the sympathetic nervous system. The dopamine release in the brain reward system produces euphoria and an increase in self-confidence. Drug interactions with amphetamines are identified in Table 5-4.

Side Effects and Adverse Reactions

Initial use of amphetamines results in increased alertness, improved performance, relief of fatigue, and anorexia. Stimulation of the sympathetic nervous system leads to cardiovascular stimulation with increased heart rate and blood pressure. Amphetamine use over time can lead to irritability, anxiety, paranoia, and hostile and violent behaviors. The physical effects of extended methamphetamine abuse are notable in tooth decay and dermatologic deterioration (Figure 5-1).

Toxic reactions to amphetamines are similar to those to cocaine. Increased levels of stimulation, sometimes described as "overamping," may result in amphetamine psychosis, paranoia, seizures, and death (see Table 5-2). Without medical intervention, death may occur as a result of dysrhythmias, myocardial infarction, hyperthermia, and cerebral hemorrhage.

Withdrawal symptoms of amphetamine use are similar to those of cocaine use and are presented in Table 5-2. Amphetamines usually cause only mild physical dependence, but craving can be intense during abstinence. IV use will cause the onset of withdrawal symptoms in approximately 2 hours, whereas oral use results in withdrawal symptoms in 8 to 10 hours.

"Bath salts" is the name for a group of synthetic stimulants that mimic many effects of amphetamines. These drugs contain synthetic versions of cathinone, a compound found in the khat plant that causes amphetamine-like stimulant

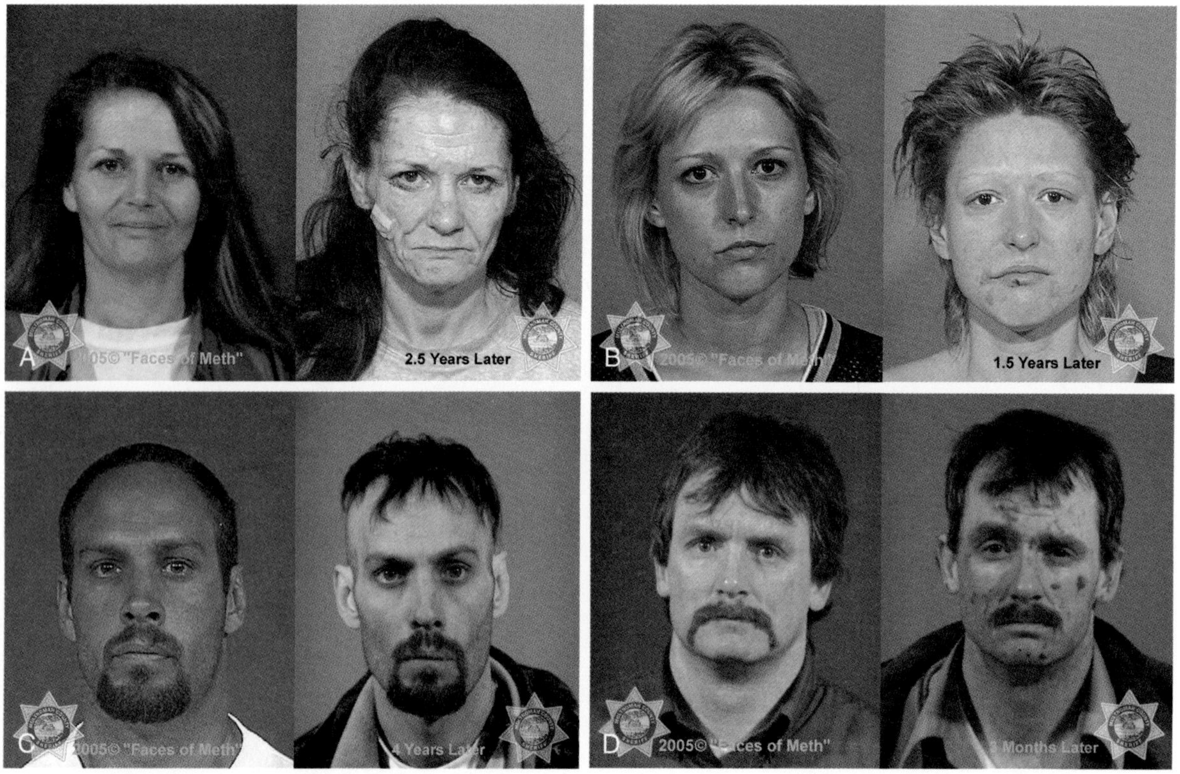

FIGURE 5–1 Methamphetamine abuse can cause significant physical deterioration. (Copyright 2014 by Faces of Meth™. Used with permission.)

effects. These are not for use in bathing; the name "bath salts" has been used to evade authorities and sell the intoxicant in retail settings. It has also been sold as jewelry cleaner or plant food, often labeled "Not for human consumption," with brand names like "White Lightning," "Cloud Nine," or "Vanilla Sky." Negative effects of these drugs are tachycardia; hypertension; psychiatric symptoms of hallucinations, paranoia, and panic attacks; kidney failure; and death.

Treatment

Patients often seek treatment for complications of amphetamine abuse such as panic reactions, psychosis, or depression. Emergency management of amphetamine toxicity is the same as that for cocaine. Elevated blood pressure and tachycardia can be controlled with vasodilators and beta-adrenergic blockers. Drug elimination can be enhanced by administering agents such as ammonium chloride that acidify the urine. Emergency treatment of amphetamine toxicity is shown in Table 5-5.

Cessation and maintenance of abstinence are difficult in amphetamine abuse. Like cocaine, withdrawal causes more psychological symptoms than physical symptoms. Depression can last for months and is a common cause of relapse. No specific drug therapy is indicated to help maintain abstinence. It is possible that agents being tested to promote cocaine abstinence may also be effective for amphetamine abuse.

Caffeine

Caffeine is the most widely used psychoactive substance in the world. Its use to promote alertness and to alleviate fatigue is safe in most people. However, of concern to health professionals is the marketing of caffeine-laden "energy" drinks directed specifically to teenagers and young adults. Used by about 30% of 18- to 24-year-olds in the United States, these products provide a "buzz" to fight fatigue, brighten mood, and increase physical and mental performance. Caffeine is also added to some brands of alcoholic drinks, and energy drinks may be used as mixers with alcohol.

Caffeine combined with alcohol appears to improve response time but does not reduce the errors in judgment caused by alcohol. Although weaker than other stimulant drugs, caffeine shares characteristics of intoxication, tolerance, and withdrawal symptoms in some individuals, especially when high doses are used.

Pharmacokinetics Caffeine is readily absorbed from the GI tract and reaches peak plasma levels in about 1 hour. Additional information regarding the pharmacodynamics and pharmacokinetics of caffeine is presented in Chapter 20.

Pharmacodynamics Caffeine is a methylxanthine that stimulates the CNS, especially the medullary respiratory center. It also is a diuretic and myocardial stimulant. It can worsen peripheral vasoconstriction in those with hypertension and causes cerebral vasodilation, making it an effective treatment for migraines and headaches.

Side Effects and Adverse Reactions

Oral doses of 200 mg of caffeine (two cups of coffee) can elevate mood and offset fatigue, but can also produce insomnia, increase irritability, and cause anxiety. Intake of 500 mg or more per day is known to cause intoxication with symptoms of nervousness, insomnia, gastric hyperacidity, muscle twitching, confusion, chest pain, tachycardia, and cardiac dysrhythmias. In toxic doses, caffeine influences behavior patterns and may precipitate states of panic. Until the advent of caffeine pills and highly caffeinated energy drinks, caffeine overdoses were very rare because people developed undesirable symptoms before they could ingest enough. Now toxicity can result from several cans of energy drinks or from caffeine supplements. Also of concern is caffeine toxicity in young children, who may show symptoms with much smaller doses. Although the government does not require food and drink manufacturers to list caffeine content, public concern about children's access to energy drinks has induced soft drink manufacturers to start labeling caffeine content on drinks.

Physical and psychological dependence on caffeine have been found with chronic use of more than 500 mg/day. However, dependence may occur in some individuals at lower doses. The most commonly reported withdrawal symptoms are headache, irritability, drowsiness, and fatigue occurring within 12 to 24 hours after abstinence. Caffeine withdrawal may be responsible for some cases of headache that occur after general anesthesia. It is thought that weekend headaches may also be related to caffeine withdrawal, because caffeine consumption may be different during the workweek than on the weekend. Effects of caffeine are shown in Table 5-2.

Treatment

Toxic reactions to caffeine and lethal doses of caffeine are managed symptomatically. Attention is given to controlling hypertension, dysrhythmias, and seizures, as with other CNS stimulants. Management of the patient with symptoms of caffeine dependence includes assisting the patient to reduce or stop caffeine intake gradually. Supplying a list of caffeinated products with their dosages may help the patient avoid caffeine intake. Substituting decaffeinated beverages may also help (decaffeinated coffee and tea contain 2 to 4 mg of caffeine per cup).

DEPRESSANTS

Drugs classified as depressants have common physiologic and psychological effects of sedation, decreased respiratory and cardiac rates, and depressed CNS function. Drugs in this category include alcohol, sedative-hypnotics, anxiolytics, and opioid narcotics. With the exception of alcohol and some federally regulated drugs, most CNS depressants are medically useful. These drugs are also widely recognized for their abuse potential, which leads to rapid tolerance, dependence, and medical emergencies involving overdose and withdrawal.

Alcohol

Alcohol is the most widely consumed substance of abuse in the United States. Most people use alcohol in moderation, with some positive cardiovascular and cognitive benefits. Abuse of alcohol, however, can lead to dependence and significant health, social, legal, and interpersonal problems. Alcoholism (alcohol dependency) is a chronic, progressive, potentially fatal disease if left untreated.

Pharmacokinetics Alcohol is absorbed directly from the stomach and small intestine. Absorption from the stomach is slower in the presence of water or food, especially proteins and fats. Faster absorption occurs when alcohol is mixed with carbonated liquids. Alcohol is distributed to all body tissues and fluids. It crosses the placenta and can affect fetal development. Alcohol is primarily metabolized in the liver, although a small amount is metabolized in the stomach. Unlike most other drugs in which the metabolic rate increases as plasma drug levels rise, alcohol is usually metabolized at a relatively constant rate. In an occasional or moderate drinker, that metabolic rate is approximately one drink (7 g of alcohol) per hour. One drink is equal to 12 ounces of beer, 5 ounces of wine, or 1 ounce of distilled spirits. However, regular or heavy use of alcohol increases the rate of liver metabolism of alcohol and other drugs. Because women have significantly lower rates of alcohol metabolism, they have higher blood alcohol levels than men after ingesting the same amount of alcohol.

Pharmacodynamics Alcohol affects almost all cells of the body and has complex effects on the neurons in the CNS. Alcohol is a general CNS depressant. Additionally, alcohol binds with receptors in the brain reward system, resulting in the release of dopamine and promoting the addictive process.

The concentration of alcohol in the body can be determined by assessing the blood alcohol concentration (BAC). For the nondependent drinker, the BAC is fairly predictable of alcohol's effects (Table 5-6). The relationship between BAC and behavior is different in a person who has developed tolerance to alcohol and its effects. This individual is commonly able to drink large amounts without obvious impairment at BAC levels several times higher than those that would produce obvious impairment in the nontolerant drinker. However, little tolerance develops to respiratory depression. Chronic heavy alcohol users reach the lethal BAC at almost the same level as nonusers.

Alcohol interacts with many commonly prescribed or OTC medications (see Table 5-4). **Potentiation** and cross-tolerance with other CNS depressants also may occur. Potentiation occurs when an additional CNS depressant is taken with alcohol, increasing the effect. **Cross-tolerance**, the need for an increased dose of other drugs, also develops to general anesthetics, barbiturates, and other general CNS depressants. No cross-tolerance develops to opioids.

TABLE 5-6 BLOOD ALCOHOL CONCENTRATION AND RELATED EFFECTS

BAC* (MG%)	PHYSICAL AND PSYCHOLOGICAL EFFECTS
20 (0.02)	Light and moderate drinkers begin to feel some effects after one drink.
40 (0.04)	Most people begin to feel relaxed.
60 (0.06)	Judgment is mildly impaired. People are less able to make rational decisions about their capabilities (e.g., driving skills).
80 (0.08)	Definite impairment of muscle coordination and driving skills occurs. Person is legally intoxicated in some states.
100 (0.10)	Clear deterioration of reaction time and control is observed. Person is legally intoxicated in most states.
120 (0.12)	Vomiting occurs unless this level is reached slowly.
150 (0.15)	Balance and movement are impaired. Equivalent of one half pint of whiskey is circulating in the bloodstream.
300 (0.30)	Many people lose consciousness.
400 (0.40)	Most people lose consciousness, and some die.
450 (0.45)	Breathing stops; person eventually dies.

*Blood alcohol concentration (BAC) is generally recorded in milligrams of alcohol per deciliter (mg/dL) of blood or milligrams percent (mg%). Percentage is used for legal definitions of intoxication. BAC is dependent on how much alcohol is consumed, how fast it is consumed, and the individual's weight.

Side Effects and Adverse Reactions

Alcohol intoxication is evidenced with an increasing BAC and results in behavioral and physical changes (see Tables 5-2 and 5-6). Acute overdose produces vomiting, coma, and respiratory depression. Alcohol-induced hypotension may lead to renal failure and cardiogenic shock, common causes of alcohol-related death.

The effects of chronic alcohol use are numerous. One condition that can be prevented is **Wernicke's encephalopathy**, an inflammatory, hemorrhagic, degenerative condition of the brain resulting from a deficiency of thiamine owing to malnutrition associated with chronic alcohol use. Untreated or progressive Wernicke's encephalopathy may lead to **Korsakoff's psychosis**, a form of amnesia characterized by loss of short-term memory and an inability to learn.

After excessive drinking, nondependent individuals experience malaise, nausea, headache, thirst, and a general feeling of fatigue. In those with an alcohol addiction, sudden withdrawal from alcohol may have life-threatening effects. Withdrawal syndrome should be anticipated if the patient reports consumption of more than 10 drinks every day for a period of 2 weeks. Characteristic signs of withdrawal are gross tremors, seizures, hallucinations, and alcohol withdrawal delirium; they develop because the brain has adapted to the consistent presence of alcohol, a depressant. The brain is accustomed to functioning in the presence of a substance inhibiting its activity; thus, symptoms of withdrawal develop when alcohol is removed.

The onset of withdrawal symptoms is variable, depending on the person's drinking pattern. Symptoms (see Table 5-2) may occur the first 4 to 6 hours after the last drink, peak at 24 to 36 hours, and last up to 5 days. Anticipation of withdrawal syndrome should always include assessment of the time of the last alcohol intake. Seizures are most likely to occur 7 to 48 hours after the last drink. Alcohol withdrawal delirium is a serious complication that may occur from 30 to 120 hours after the last drink. Delirium components include disorientation, visual or auditory hallucinations, and increased hyperactivity without seizures. Death may be caused by hyperthermia, peripheral vascular collapse, or cardiac failure.

Treatment

Initial treatment of acute alcohol intoxication or overdose requires implementation of the basic principles of airway, breathing, and circulation (ABCs). No antidote for alcohol is available, and stimulants should not be given. Alcohol-induced hypotension cannot be corrected with vasoconstrictors. Alcohol may be removed from the body by gastric lavage and dialysis. Because symptoms of Wernicke's encephalopathy may be difficult to distinguish from those of intoxication, and because Wernicke's encephalopathy is potentially reversible, IV thiamine at a dose of 100 mg/day is often administered to intoxicated patients. Patients with alcohol intoxication may also be hypoglycemic because of lack of food intake. Treatment with IV glucose solutions may precipitate Wernicke's encephalopathy in a previously unaffected patient. For this reason, thiamine should be started before treatment with IV glucose solution in all patients with alcoholism and continued until the patient resumes regular eating.

Although specific drugs are not indicated for acute alcohol toxicity, drugs are available to facilitate alcohol withdrawal and help maintain abstinence. Management of alcohol withdrawal frequently includes the use of a variety of drugs. Anticipating withdrawal syndrome in patients is important because alcohol withdrawal delirium can usually be prevented by administration of benzodiazepines such as chlordiazepoxide (Librium) or lorazepam (Ativan) if the patient has liver dysfunction. Benzodiazepines with long half-lives are the most effective drugs in alcohol withdrawal to stabilize vital signs, reduce symptoms, and decrease the risk of seizures and delirium. Benzodiazepines are discussed further in Chapter 21. Additional drugs used as adjuncts to benzodiazepines are included in Table 5-7.

Rehabilitation and sustained abstinence are the primary long-term goals of alcohol treatment. Drugs approved to maintain abstinence may be used in addition to cognitive-behavioral therapy for long-term treatment. These include disulfiram (Antabuse), which prevents drinking by causing an unpleasant reaction if alcohol is consumed, and naltrexone, which blocks the desired effects of alcohol. Disulfiram disrupts alcohol metabolism, causing accumulation of acetaldehyde when alcohol is ingested. An adverse reaction to the accumulated acetaldehyde begins with flushing in the face and develops into intense vasodilation of the face, neck, and upper part of the body. Hyperventilation and palpitations may occur. Nausea occurs in 30 to 60 minutes with copious vomiting. Headache, sweating, thirst, chest pain, weakness, blurred vision, and hypotension follow. Blood pressure may decline to shock levels. The reaction lasts from 30 minutes to several hours and can be brought on by ingesting as little as 7 mL of alcohol. In its most severe form, it can be life threatening. In the absence of alcohol, disulfiram may cause drowsiness and skin eruptions that diminish over time. Disulfiram is metabolized by the liver, and excretion of metabolites occurs through the kidneys and lungs. Up to 20% of the drug is excreted unchanged in the feces. Effects may persist for up to 2 weeks after the last dose is taken. Patient education regarding disulfiram therapy is extremely important. Patients must be made aware that consumption of any alcohol, even use of alcohol-based mouthwash, while taking disulfiram can cause a severe, potentially fatal reaction. All food and liquid medication labels must be checked for the presence of alcohol, and alcohol must not be used on the skin. Because disulfiram is self-administered, patients must be highly motivated to abstain from alcohol for it to be effective. Additionally, using a family or other strong support system improves adherence to daily dosing of disulfiram.

TABLE 5-7 DRUG THERAPY FOR ALCOHOL WITHDRAWAL

CLINICAL MANIFESTATIONS	MEDICATIONS
Minor Withdrawal Syndrome	
Tremulousness, anxiety Insomnia Increased heart rate Increased blood pressure Sweating Nausea Hyperreflexia	Long-acting benzodiazepines (e.g., lorazepam [Ativan], chlordiazepoxide [Librium]) to stabilize vital signs, reduce anxiety, and prevent seizures and delirium Thiamine to prevent Wernicke's encephalopathy Multivitamins (folic acid, B vitamins) for nutritional support Magnesium sulfate if serum magnesium is low Glucose solutions IV if hypoglycemia is present (after thiamine)
Major Withdrawal Syndrome	
Disorientation Visual/auditory hallucinations Increased hyperactivity without seizures Gross tremors Seizures Alcohol withdrawal delirium	Continue use of benzodiazepines and add: Antipsychotic drugs (e.g., haloperidol [Haldol]) for hallucinations and delirium Carbamazepine (Tegretol) or phenytoin (Dilantin) to prevent or treat seizures

IV, Intravenous.

HERBAL ALERT 5-1

St. John's Wort

St. John's wort, if taken with disulfiram (Antabuse), may cause a reaction similar to alcohol.

Naltrexone is a pure opioid antagonist that decreases craving for alcohol and blocks the "high" of alcohol use. It was originally approved for treatment of opioid addiction but was also approved for alcohol dependency when clinical trials found that it reduced alcohol relapse rates by 50% when combined with extensive counseling. Naltrexone (ReVia, Depade) 50 mg once a day by mouth is the usual dose for alcohol dependency. Naltrexone is also available in an injectable extended-release form (Vivitrol) that is given intramuscularly once a month. This drug is indicated for alcohol-dependent patients who are able to abstain from drinking in an outpatient setting and are not actively drinking when starting treatment. Naltrexone is discussed further with opioid abuse later in this chapter and in Chapter 26.

Acamprosate (Campral) is used to decrease unpleasant feelings such as tension, dysphoria, anxiety, and cravings brought about by abstinence from alcohol. It is thought to act on the brain pathways related to alcohol abuse. Dosing should start immediately after detoxification and continue even if relapse occurs. Acamprosate is not addicting but is somewhat less effective than naltrexone. Combining acamprosate with naltrexone is more effective than acamprosate alone but no better than naltrexone alone. The most common adverse effects reported include headache, diarrhea, flatulence, and nausea.

Two marketed drugs are currently being studied for their use in long-term alcohol abstinence. Ondansetron (Zofran), an antagonist of receptors in the brain reward system, decreases motivation for drinking in early onset alcoholism; and topiramate (Topamax), an anticonvulsant, may be helpful in decreasing craving for alcohol as well as cocaine.

Sedative-Hypnotics

Commonly abused sedative-hypnotic agents include barbiturates, benzodiazepines, and barbiturate-like drugs. Benzodiazepines have largely replaced barbiturates as therapeutic agents for anxiety and insomnia, because they have less risk of toxicity, tolerance, and dependence. The short-acting barbiturates are preferred as recreational drugs because they more frequently produce euphoric effects. Chapter 21 covers the topic of CNS depressants in greater detail.

Pharmacokinetics and Pharmacodynamics Sedative-hypnotic drugs act primarily on the CNS. Benzodiazepines enhance the effects of gamma-aminobutyric acid (GABA), an inhibitory neurotransmitter in the brain. Barbiturates not only enhance the inhibitory effect of GABA, but they can directly mimic the actions of GABA. Barbiturates are powerful respiratory depressants and can readily cause death by overdose. For more on the pharmacodynamics and pharmacokinetics of these drugs, see Chapter 21.

Side Effects and Adverse Reactions

The abuse potential is much greater for barbiturates than benzodiazepines. The drugs are usually taken orally, but both may be injected intravenously. Excessive doses produce an initial euphoria and intoxication similar to that of alcohol. Effects of sedative-hypnotics are presented in Table 5-2.

Tolerance develops rapidly to the sedative effects of barbiturates, requiring higher doses to achieve euphoria. Little tolerance develops to respiratory depression, however, and increasing doses may trigger hypotension and respiratory depression, resulting in death. Cross-tolerance also develops between barbiturates and other CNS depressants such as alcohol, benzodiazepines, and general anesthetics. Little cross-tolerance occurs with opioids, however. In addition, many drug interactions are associated with barbiturates and benzodiazepines (see Table 5-4). An overdose of a sedative-hypnotic produces respiratory depression and coma. Other symptoms of overdose are listed in Table 5-2.

Withdrawal from sedative-hypnotics can be very serious. In the first 12 to 16 hours after the last dose, the patient may develop anxiety, tremors, weakness, nausea, vomiting, muscle cramps, and increased reflexes. After 24 hours, the patient craves the drug and may experience delirium, grand mal seizures, and respiratory and cardiac arrest (see Table 5-2). Symptoms of withdrawal peak on the second or third day for short-acting (shorter half-life) drugs (e.g., alprazolam, secobarbital, pentobarbital) and on the seventh or eighth day for long-acting (longer half-life) drugs (e.g., diazepam, chlordiazepoxide).

Treatment

Overdoses of benzodiazepines are treated with flumazenil (Romazicon), a specific benzodiazepine antagonist. No antagonists are known to counteract the effects of barbiturates or other sedative-hypnotic drugs. Emergency life support measures must be taken in cases of overdose. Gastric lavage may be used in extremely toxic cases if the drug was taken orally within the last hour. Dialysis may be required to decrease the drug level. Gradual withdrawal of the drug is required during withdrawal syndrome. Phenobarbital, a long-acting barbiturate, may be used to control withdrawal symptoms in a patient dependent on barbiturates. Phenobarbital is gradually withdrawn when the patient is stable. To manage symptoms safely, hospitalization is recommended during drug withdrawal for patients who have been abusing large amounts of barbiturates.

Opioids

Opioids include the naturally occurring opiates derived from opium and the many semisynthetic and synthetic narcotic agents used as analgesics. Individuals who abuse opioids include those who use illegal drugs sold on the street and individuals who misuse prescription opioids. Those who begin drug use illegally constitute the largest group of abusers. Street use is usually of heroin. In the medical setting, some people misuse prescribed analgesics, including health care professionals, who may have the highest rate of opioid abuse and dependence of any middle-class population. Ready access to drugs, stresses of the workplace environment, and long hours that interfere with family life are considered contributing factors in health care professionals. Drug abuse and chemical dependency in nurses are discussed later in this chapter.

Pharmacokinetics and Pharmacodynamics Pharmacokinetics and pharmacodynamics of opioids are presented in Chapter 26. Important to the abuse potential of opioids is their ability to activate the brain reward system, reinforcing an addictive effect. As drugs of abuse, opioids are taken orally, sniffed, smoked, or injected subcutaneously ("skin-popping") or intravenously ("mainlining"). IV use will produce effects in seconds. Smoking or sniffing produces a longer onset and effect. Drug interactions with opioids are identified in Table 5-4.

Side Effects and Adverse Reactions

The primary effects of opioids include analgesia, drowsiness, slurred speech, and detachment from the environment. IV use usually causes a "rush" of feelings in the lower abdomen, along with warm skin flushing and a strong sense of euphoria. Opioid use leads to rapid tolerance and physical dependence after short-term use. Cross-tolerance among opioids is common, but cross-tolerance to other CNS depressants does not occur. However, additive effects of other CNS depressants may lead to increased CNS depression.

Signs of overdose of opioids include pinpoint pupils, clammy skin, depressed respiration, coma, and death, if not treated (see Table 5-2). Unintentional overdose frequently occurs with recreational use of the drugs because of the unpredictability in potency and purity. Withdrawal symptoms occur with decreased amounts or cessation of the drug after prolonged moderate to heavy use. The administration of a narcotic antagonist such as naloxone (Narcan) will cause withdrawal symptoms in dependent individuals. Symptoms may include craving, abdominal cramps, diarrhea, nausea, and vomiting (see Table 5-2). Symptoms appear about 8 to 10 hours after the last dose, peak within 36 to 48 hours, and usually subside in 96 hours. Although opioid withdrawal is acutely uncomfortable, it is not usually life threatening.

Treatment

Overdose of opioids can precipitate a medical emergency. A narcotic antagonist such as naloxone should be given as soon as life support is instituted. (The use of naloxone and other narcotic antagonists is discussed in Chapter 26.) Treatment of withdrawal syndrome is symptom-based and does not always require the use of medication. Methadone (Dolophine) in decreasing doses over 10 to 14 days is most often used to decrease symptoms during opioid detoxification. Some patients obtain relief from withdrawal symptoms with the use of clonidine (Catapres), a centrally acting alpha$_2$-adrenergic agonist that may also be used for nicotine addiction (see Chapter 44). It is most effective against GI hyperactivity but does not decrease craving. The action of clonidine in nicotine and opioid addiction is not fully understood.

Long-term management of opioid addiction involves the use of opioid agonists, opioid antagonists, and mixed opioid agonist-antagonists (Table 5-8; see also Chapter 26). Methadone is the most commonly used opioid agonist. By substituting oral methadone for the abused opioid, withdrawal syndrome can be avoided, and the euphoria that leads to craving can be prevented. Methadone is an addictive drug, but its use in maintenance programs alters the drug-using lifestyle, reduces exposure to infectious disease, and controls drug use. To prevent methadone abuse, it is available for addiction treatment only through agencies approved by the FDA and state authorities.

Buprenorphine (Buprenex) is an agonist-antagonist opioid that may be used for detoxification and maintenance therapy. Because of its action on specific opiate receptors, it

TABLE 5-8 DRUGS USED IN OPIOID ADDICTION

STATE WITH SIGNS AND SYMPTOMS	DRUGS
Toxicity Respiratory depression Coma	**Opioid Antagonists** naloxone (Narcan): Short-acting and may need to be repeated until opioid levels decrease; too much will cause withdrawal symptoms. nalmefene (Revex): Long-acting; may cause prolonged withdrawal if dose is excessive
Detoxification/withdrawal Nausea, vomiting, diarrhea Abdominal cramping Bone and muscle pain Muscle spasms Tremor, chills, diaphoresis	**Opioid Substitution** methadone (Dolophine): An opioid agonist that may be used to prevent withdrawal syndrome; when used for withdrawal, it is given in decreasing oral doses over 10 to 14 days after the patient is stabilized. buprenorphine (Subutex): an opioid agonist-antagonist that can be substituted for abused opioids to prevent withdrawal syndrome but can cause withdrawal if an opioid agonist is in the bloodstream; for treatment of withdrawal, it must be given after withdrawal symptoms begin. **Centrally Acting Alpha$_2$-adrenergic agonist** clonidine (Catapres): effective in decreasing GI hyperactivity and some other symptoms of withdrawal; does not reduce craving for the drug.
Maintenance of abstinence Craving, cue-induced craving	**Opioid Agonists** methadone (Dolophine): substitution for abused opioids may be used for long-term treatment of dependency. Addiction is maintained with this method and withdrawal occurs if methadone is stopped, but drug use can be controlled and drug-using lifestyles changed with methadone maintenance. **Opioid Antagonists** naltrexone (ReVia, Depade): blocks opioid receptors, preventing the desired effects if opioids are used; long-acting oral preparation that must be used voluntarily. **Mixed Opioid Agonist/Antagonists** buprenorphine (Subutex), a sublingual tablet, can be used instead of methadone for maintenance therapy. To prevent abuse of buprenorphine itself, it is also marketed in combination with naltrexone as Suboxone. If this preparation is crushed and injected, opioid withdrawal will occur in an opioid-addicted individual. When Suboxone is used sublingually, the opioid agonist effect predominates.

can decrease the symptoms of withdrawal and suppress drug craving, yet it has low potential for abuse. For treatment of withdrawal symptoms, it is available in a sublingual tablet marketed as Subutex. For long-term maintenance, it is combined with naloxone in a sublingual tablet marketed as Suboxone. In this preparation, naloxone is added to the buprenorphine to prevent injection use of the tablets. Because it contains naloxone, Suboxone can produce intense withdrawal symptoms if it is used intravenously. However, the potential for withdrawal is minimal when Suboxone is taken as prescribed because little naloxone is absorbed with sublingual administration in comparison to buprenorphine, which has a significantly higher bioavailability with sublingual administration. Buprenorphine in other forms (e.g., Buprenex) is not approved for treatment of opioid addiction and is used only as a Schedule III analgesic.

SAFETY: Preventing Medication Errors

Do not confuse ...
Buprenorphine/naloxone (Suboxone) with

- **Buprenorphine** (Subutex/Buprenex), the same active drug, but without the combination of naloxone
- **Bupropion** (Wellbutrin), an antidepressant
- **Buspirone** (BuSpar), an anxiolytic

Naltrexone (oral ReVia, injectable Vivitrol) is an opioid antagonist that blocks euphoria and all other opioid effects. Like naloxone, it will precipitate withdrawal symptoms when administered to opioid-dependent individuals. When naltrexone is used, administration of an opioid produces no effect, eliminating the reinforcing properties of drug use. It does not prevent craving, however. Naltrexone is used rather than naloxone for maintenance treatment, because it is longer acting and can be taken orally. Usual dosing is orally once a day or alternate days, or intramuscularly once a month.

OTHER DRUGS OF ABUSE

Cannabis

In North America, cannabis is usually sold as marijuana or hashish. Tetrahydrocannabinol (THC) is the active ingredient in cannabis responsible for most of the psychoactive effects. Although a number of potential benefits of THC have been reported, the only approved THC preparation is dronabinol (Marinol), which is used to control nausea and vomiting resulting from cancer chemotherapy. Dronabinol is also used to stimulate appetite in patients with acquired immunodeficiency syndrome (AIDS).

Pharmacokinetics When marijuana is smoked, effects usually occur in 20 to 30 minutes and may last up to 7 hours. Because THC is stored in body fat, it is eliminated slowly, resulting in a half-life of 2 to 7 days. When taken orally, it is almost completely absorbed but undergoes extensive first-pass metabolism.

Pharmacodynamics At low to moderate doses, THC produces fewer physiologic and psychological alterations than do other classes of psychoactive drugs, including alcohol. Although its mechanism of action is uncertain, THC affects cannabinoid receptors in the brain and may act in part through the same reward system as opioids and cocaine.

Side Effects and Adverse Reactions

Marijuana and hashish are usually smoked with the usual effects of euphoria, sedation, and hallucinations. Responses are varied and depend on dose, expectations of the user, and the setting of drug use. Low to moderate doses result in euphoria and relaxation, enhanced sensory perception, and distortion of time perception. Undesirable responses include short-term memory loss, decreased ability to perform multistep tasks, and temporal disintegration. High doses may cause serious psychological effects; intense anxiety, delusions, paranoia, and a state of toxic psychosis can occur. Effects vary among individuals (see Table 5-2). Some individuals experience ill effects only at extremely high doses, while others routinely experience adverse effects at moderate doses. Physiologic effects are seen most commonly in the cardiovascular and respiratory systems. Decreased sperm production, and decreased reproductive hormones in both men and women may occur. Problems of chronic heavy use include decreased motor coordination, tremors, and increased heart and respiratory rates. A condition known as *amotivational syndrome*, characterized by apathy, dullness, and disinterest, may also occur.

Acute reactions, including intoxication and withdrawal, are usually mild and time-limited. Marijuana has low toxicity and no known level of lethal dose. Complications may result when marijuana is used with other drugs, such as heroin and cocaine (see Table 5-4). When taken in extremely high doses, marijuana can produce tolerance and physical dependence. Abrupt cessation of high-dose marijuana may cause irritability, restlessness, nervousness, insomnia, and tremor. In rare instances, withdrawal can be prolonged and difficult.

Synthetic marijuana has been growing in availability. Referred to as "Spice" or "K2," synthetic marijuana is purported to be a combination of various natural, plant-based, materials; chemical analysis, however, has shown that synthetic cannabinoids are the active ingredient. These products were legal in the United States because none of the identified ingredients were explicitly banned by controlled substances acts; however, many states have moved to make the sale or possession of synthetic marijuana illegal. It is usually smoked and causes intoxication with similar effects to marijuana. It is known to cause nausea, vomiting, hypertension, and myocardial ischemia and has been associated in some cases with myocardial infarction.

Treatment

Individuals using marijuana may seek treatment for anxiety or mood symptoms or may be treated for toxic reactions to a combination of drugs that includes marijuana. Treatment is directed toward relief of symptoms, and administration of drugs is avoided if possible. There is no antidote or substitution therapy for cannabis.

Psychedelic Agents

Psychedelic drugs are often referred to as *hallucinogens*. These drugs produce a change in level of consciousness and induce hallucinations and mental states that resemble psychosis. Primarily, they bring about alterations in thoughts, perceptions, and feelings that normally only occur in dreams. Common agents and their effects are identified in Table 5-2. Although LSD originally was thought to provide a model for the study of psychosis, this idea was found to be incorrect. As a result, the drugs have no recognized medical use. Currently ecstasy (3,4-methylenedioxymethamphetamine or MDMA) is the most commonly used psychedelic. It is popular among adolescents and young adults and may also be abused as a "rape drug."

The effects of psychedelic drug use are primarily psychological, but cardiovascular and neurologic toxicity may occur. Little or no physical dependence develops, but acute panic reactions are common with toxicity. Panic attacks may be treated with an antianxiety agent such as diazepam (Valium) and by providing a nonthreatening environment. Although a toxic reaction may mimic psychosis, the use of antipsychotic agents such as phenothiazines (e.g., haloperidol, chlorpromazine) can intensify rather than ameliorate the experience.

Inhalants

Inhalation is the major route of ingestion for a number of common household and industrial volatile substances. Forms of use include sniffing, huffing, bagging, or spraying. Because inhalants are readily accessible, inexpensive, and produce a rapid high, they are more often used by preadolescents and adolescents.

The four main classes of inhalants are volatile solvents, aerosols, anesthetic agents, and nitrites. They act as CNS depressants but are also extremely damaging to the cardiovascular and respiratory systems. Common agents and their effects are presented in Table 5-2. Users may develop peripheral neuropathies and exhibit tremors and weakness. Sudden death may occur from direct toxic effects, aspiration of gastric contents, trauma, and suffocation. No antidotes are available for these substances, and treatment of toxicity is symptomatic.

Prescription Drugs

The growing popularity of prescription medication abuse is due in part to ease of access as well as to misplaced belief that these drugs always are safe. The types of prescription medications most frequently misused are pain medications and sedative-hypnotics. Individuals may obtain these medications as valid prescriptions for legitimate health issues but use the drug in a nonprescribed manner; others may use someone else's prescription with or without their knowledge or permission. Nurses must be active in addressing this health concern. One way this can be done is by thorough patient education on safe storage and disposal of medications (see Chapter 12).

BOX 5-1 SURGICAL CONSIDERATIONS: PATIENTS WITH DRUG ABUSE

- Standard amounts of anesthetic and analgesic medication may not be sufficient because of cross-tolerance.
- Anesthetic agents may have a prolonged sedative effect if the patient has liver dysfunction.
- Increased doses of pain medication may be required if the patient is dependent on opioids.
- Dosage of pain medications must be reduced gradually.
- Patients have an increased susceptibility to cardiac and respiratory depression.
- Patients have an increased risk for bleeding, postoperative complications, and infection.
- Withdrawal symptoms from central nervous system depressants may be delayed for up to 5 days because of effects of anesthetics and pain medications.

SPECIAL NEEDS OF DRUG-ABUSING PATIENTS

Surgical Patients

An individual who abuses drugs is at high risk for drug interactions, complications, and death when surgery is required (Box 5-1). Preoperative assessment of all patients must include an assessment of drug use. Respiratory changes in smokers make introduction of endotracheal and suction tubes more difficult and increase the risk for postoperative respiratory problems. Postoperative headaches may be caused by caffeine withdrawal in heavy users. During the patient's postoperative period, the nurse should be alert for signs and symptoms of drug interactions with pain medications or anesthesia and for signs of drug withdrawal.

Special precautions must be taken for the patient who is intoxicated or alcohol dependent and requires surgery. Alcohol use may be overlooked in an accident victim if there are injuries that cause CNS depression. In addition, many persons are undiagnosed as alcoholics at the time of admission for elective surgery. The patient who is alcohol dependent but is not currently drinking usually requires an increased level of anesthesia because of cross-tolerance. The intoxicated individual needs a decreased level of anesthesia because of the synergistic effect of alcohol. Whenever possible, surgery is postponed in alcohol-intoxicated individuals until the BAC is less than 200 mg%. Synergistic effects occur with anesthesia when the BAC is >150 mg%, and a patient with a BAC >250 mg% has a significantly increased surgical risk and mortality rate. Alcohol withdrawal delirium may be triggered by surgery and the cessation of alcohol consumption. Anesthetics and pain medications used in the acute period can delay withdrawal syndrome for up to 5 days postoperatively.

Pain Management

Although nurses and physicians may be reluctant to administer opioids to drug-dependent patients for fear of promoting or enhancing addictions, there is no evidence that providing opioid analgesia to these patients in any way worsens their addictive disease. When addicted patients experience any type of acute pain, the goal is to treat the pain. Addiction treatment is not the priority while the patient is in pain.

If the patient acknowledges opioid use, it is important to determine the types and amounts of drugs used. It is best to avoid exposing the patient to the drug of abuse, and effective equianalgesic doses of other opioids can be determined if daily drug doses are known. If a history of drug abuse is unknown or if the patient denies drug abuse, the nurse should consider the potential of drug abuse when normal doses of analgesics do not relieve the patient's pain or when signs of withdrawal occur. Withdrawal symptoms can exacerbate pain and lead to drug-seeking behavior or illicit drug use. Toxicology screens may be helpful in determining recently used drugs.

Severe pain should be treated with opioids, but at much higher doses than those used with drug-naïve patients. The use of one opioid is preferred. Mixed opioid agonist-antagonists such as butorphanol (Stadol), buprenorphine (Buprenex), or nubain (Nalbuphine) should be avoided because they may precipitate withdrawal symptoms. Nonopioid and adjuvant analgesics and nonpharmacologic pain relief measures may also be used. To maintain opioid blood levels and prevent withdrawal symptoms, analgesics should be provided around the clock. Supplemental doses should be used to treat breakthrough pain. Although patient-controlled analgesia (PCA) is controversial for treating addicted patients, its use may improve pain control and reduce drug-seeking behavior.

A written agreement or treatment plan that describes the pain management should be developed with the patient. The plan should ensure that pain will be treated based on the patient's perception and report of pain but also clearly outline the gradual tapering of the analgesic dose and eventual substitution of long-acting oral preparations for parenteral analgesics.

CHEMICAL IMPAIRMENT IN HEALTH PROFESSIONALS

Chemical impairment is a term used by health professionals to indicate impaired performance as a result of drug use. Drug use and abuse is a serious concern in health care professions. Alcohol is the most commonly abused drug. Others include opiates and benzodiazepines, abuse of which occurs at higher rates than in the general population, likely due to ease of access. It is estimated that 10% to 20% of nurses have substance-abuse problems and that 3% to 6% demonstrate impaired practice resulting from the use of drugs (chemicals).

Contributing Factors

Factors contributing to drug abuse among nurses have been identified as chronic fatigue, illness, responsibility for patients' responses to illness and dying, professional dissatisfaction, access to drugs, marital and child care problems, and downsizing. Other factors include nurses' false belief that knowledge of drugs provides immunity to drug problems. The issue has become less of a priority within the nursing community over the past several years, partly because the nursing shortage and workplace hazards have received more attention. Yet these issues lead to increasing stressful working conditions that put nurses at even greater risk for substance-related disorders.

Characteristics

Evidence of chemical dependence may be seen by changes in personality and behavior, job performance, and attendance. Behaviors related to influence of the drug or signs of withdrawal may also be present. Poor judgment, errors, inappropriate behavior, and illogical documentation are common in the chemically impaired nurse. Discrepancies in controlled-drug handling and records may indicate *drug diversion,* the deliberate redirecting of a drug from a patient or facility to the employee for personal use. Nurses often enable substance abuse among coworkers by covering up their mistakes or tardiness, excusing their behavior, or simply ignoring obvious signs and symptoms. When it is recognized that a nurse is impaired, help for the nurse requires sharing observations and concerns with the nurse and supervisor to provide the means for rehabilitation.

Management

Management of drug abuse in nurses largely depends on the state in which the nurse practices and the policies of the employing facility. Sometimes employment is simply terminated, allowing the nurse to work elsewhere with no resolution of the problem. Some states or facilities require that management report the nurse to regulatory agencies that may revoke licensure to practice or refer the case to the criminal justice system. These approaches are disciplinary and contribute to the reluctance by nurses to report impaired coworkers.

The tragedy of allowing a treatable disease to go untreated is costly in both human and economic terms. In an effort to help impaired nurses, the American Nurses Association, the National Student Nurse Organization, and other nursing organizations and nurse substance-abuse experts strongly advocate rehabilitation for nurses who are chemically dependent. Alternatives to discipline have been developed in most states. Alternatives include diversion programs associated with the state board of nursing that allow nurses to maintain their licenses while being monitored through recovery; state nurses' association peer assistance programs; and employee assistance programs. The goals of these programs are to protect the safety of the public, to maintain the integrity of the profession, and to ensure that the nurse is offered the possibility of treatment and rehabilitation before the license to practice is revoked or the job is terminated. Other efforts are under way to prevent chemical dependency in nurses through substance abuse educational programs, for both nursing students and nurse employees.

All nurses care for patients who are dependent on drugs, whether they are identified as dependent or not, simply because of the prevalence of drug abuse. It is important for nurses to identify and intervene with patients who are abusing drugs. Knowledge of the commonly abused drugs and treatment during intoxication, overdose, withdrawal, and cessation are critical to maintaining life and promoting healthy lifestyles.

Nursing Process
Patient-Centered Collaborative Care

Smoking (Nicotine) Cessation

Assessment
- Assess current smoking status and smoking history.
- Identify the cultural context of patient's smoking pattern.
- Determine the willingness of patient to attempt to quit.
- Have patient identify negative consequences of smoking and the potential benefits of quitting.
- Ask patient to identify any barriers or impediments to quitting.
- Identify what rewards for quitting are most important to patient.

Nursing Diagnoses
- Readiness for enhanced knowledge related to smoking cessation as manifested by a stated desire to quit smoking and a request for professional assistance

Planning
- Patient will eliminate tobacco use.

Nursing Interventions
- Set a quit date with patient, ideally within 2 weeks.
- Teach patient about the nicotine-replacement systems and other agents available to assist in smoking cessation.
- Help patient choose the best method to quit smoking based on patient preferences and anticipated benefits.
- Refer patient to support groups or programs available in the community.
- Teach patient to anticipate withdrawal symptoms and challenges of quitting.
- Advise patient to keep a list of "slips" and "near-slips" to learn to avoid their causes.
- Encourage patient to avoid environments and activities previously associated with smoking.
- Schedule frequent follow-up contacts with patient to offer encouragement; help patient deal with lapses.

Evaluation
- Evaluate effectiveness of the cessation plan, including use of drugs and support systems, to avoid relapse.
- Determine the smoking status of patient.

KEY WEBSITES

National Institute on Drug Abuse: *www.nida.nih.gov*

Substance Abuse and Mental Health Services Administration: *www.samhsa.gov*

Substance Abuse Treatment Facility Locator: *www.findtreatment.samhsa.gov*

CRITICAL THINKING CASE STUDY

LM, a 57-year-old man, is admitted to the surgical unit in preparation for back surgery, after conservative treatment for a recent back injury has not relieved his pain. His wife tells the nurse she hopes the surgery will be successful. She confides that her husband has just been sitting around the house drinking more beer than usual, because he has not been able to work. LM appears relaxed and unconcerned about his anticipated surgery. He jokes with the nurse, telling her that his back would be cured if "a cute young thing" like her "would only rub his back."

1. What assessments of LM's alcohol use should the nurse make and communicate to the surgeon and anesthesiologist before he is further prepared for surgery?
2. How would the nurse's approximation of LM's BAC affect his surgical experience?
3. During LM's postoperative period, when will the nurse expect signs of withdrawal syndrome to occur? Explain your answer.
4. What early signs and symptoms would alert the nurse to the development of withdrawal syndrome?
5. What drug regimens might be used during LM's postoperative period to manage problems associated with his alcohol use?

NCLEX STUDY QUESTIONS

1. When caring for a patient recovering from an episode of opioid toxicity, the nurse determines that the patient has an addiction to the drug based on which finding?
   a. Physical withdrawal signs
   b. A history of daily use
   c. Craving that results in drug-seeking behaviors
   d. Intravenous rather than oral use of the drug

2. While teaching the parents of an adolescent who has been using marijuana, the nurse explains that the euphoria that results from the use of abused psychoactive substances is believed to be caused by which factor?
   a. Blockade of opioid receptors in the mesolimbic system of the brain
   b. Stimulation of the dopamine pathways in the pleasure areas of the brain
   c. Increased release of serotonin in all areas of the brain
   d. Reduction in the responsiveness of brain receptors
3. A patient hospitalized with a fractured femur following an automobile accident develops diarrhea and vomiting with abdominal cramps, chills with goose bumps, and dilated pupils. The nurse suspects that the patient is experiencing which reaction?
   a. Opioid withdrawal
   b. Alcohol toxicity
   c. Flashbacks from psychedelic abuse
   d. Barbiturate withdrawal
4. Which agent(s) will the nurse anticipate administering to a patient who has been admitted with acute alcohol intoxication? (Select all that apply.)
   a. naloxone (Narcan)
   b. thiamine
   c. lorazepam (Ativan)
   d. naltrexone (ReVia)
   e. intravenous glucose solution
   f. flumazenil (Romazicon)
5. A patient is admitted to the emergency department with acute cocaine toxicity. Which is the most important intervention by the nurse?
   a. Institute cardiac monitoring, and obtain frequent blood pressures.
   b. Monitor the patient for decreasing respiratory function and level of consciousness.
   c. Provide reality orientation with a calm, quiet approach.
   d. Administer oral fluids with caffeine to prevent withdrawal symptoms.
6. A nurse observes another nurse taking oral opioids from the medication room at the hospital. Which is the best action by the nurse?
   a. Report the finding to the nursing supervisor to enable the nurse's participation in a diversion program.
   b. Ignore the situation to protect the nurse from dismissal and possible loss of licensure.
   c. Confront the nurse and demand that the drugs be returned before someone notices their absence.
   d. Ask the nurse to request pain medications from a physician rather than stealing them from the hospital.
7. A patient is to start disulfiram (Antabuse) to help with alcohol abuse. The nurse providing medication education about the drug will include which topics in the education plan? (Select all that apply.)
   a. Importance of taking this medication every day
   b. That better results are experienced when a support group helps with adhering to treatment
   c. Common food and hygiene products containing alcohol
   d. That disulfiram treatment should be stopped 1 day before alcohol consumption
   e. That disulfiram works by disrupting the metabolism of alcohol
   f. That use of alcohol with disulfiram may cause nausea and vomiting and may even be fatal
8. A patient in the hospital is experiencing methamphetamine withdrawal. What does the nurse expect the symptoms and treatment to be?
   a. Hypertension, tachycardia, and autonomic overactivity; treated by benzodiazepines
   b. Hypersomnia, irritability; treated by supportive care including pushing food and fluids
   c. Minimal notable symptoms; no treatment needed
   d. Anxiety, insomnia, hyperactivity, and rapid, pressured speech; treated by symptom management

Answers: 1, c; 2, b; 3, a; 4, b, c, e; 5, a; 6, a; 7, a, b, c, e, f; 8, b.

CHAPTER

6

Herbal Therapies

evolve WEBSITE

http://evolve.elsevier.com/KeeHayes/pharmacology/

- Animations
- Content Updates
- Key Points
- Review Questions for the NCLEX® Examination
- References from the Textbook
- Unfolding Case Studies

OBJECTIVES

- Discuss at least six important points associated with herbal therapy for consumer and health care provider education.
- Compare at least six common herbs and their associated toxicity.
- Differentiate at least eight of the most common herbal therapies and the potential use for each.
- Describe the recommendations for labels on herbal products.
- Discuss the nursing implications, including patient teaching, related to herbal products.

OUTLINE

KEY TERMS

It is critical for nurses to know about herbal therapy and to include herbal preparations as part of their assessment. Herbal products can have both positive and negative effects and important interactions with prescription and over-the-counter (OTC) medications. Nurses are in an excellent position to educate patients about these interactions.

An **herb**, according to MedlinePlus, is "a plant or plant part used for its scent, flavor or therapeutic properties. Herbal medicine products ... are sold as tablets, capsules, powders, teas, extracts, and fresh or dried plants. However, some can cause health problems, some are not effective and some may interact with other drugs."

Herbs have long been and continue to be sources of old and new drugs: foxglove (source of digitalis), snakeroot (source of reserpine), willow bark (source of aspirin), and Pacific yew tree (source of Taxol), to name just a few. The therapeutic value of **phytomedicine** (medicine derived from plants) relates to several factors, including dosage, potency, and purity. Research into the effects of herbal medicine is increasing.

Many Americans use herbal products for therapeutic or preventive reasons. Herbal therapy has surged in popularity; marketing and media have fueled the demand, with advertisements and promotions on television, in magazines, and on the Internet. It is estimated that herbal products are used by almost one third of Americans, many of whom do not share the use of these products with their health care providers. Worldwide annual sales of herbal products represent greater than $60 billion, and the strong market is expected to continue.

Few pharmacy schools in the United States offer courses in botanical remedies, but herbal therapy is being addressed in the professional literature with increasing frequency and seriousness. Health care providers and consumers are asking questions about herbal therapy's effectiveness, potential toxicity, and reactions with conventional medications. Consumers are right to question advertisements that imply that herbs will cure anything. Herbs can be useful, but they can also be ineffectual or even dangerous (Herbal Alert 6-1).

HERBAL ALERT 6-1

Patient Responsibility

To optimize the therapeutic regimen, the patient has the responsibility to (1) consult with the health care provider before taking any herbal preparation, (2) report all herbal preparations taken to all health care providers, (3) inform health care providers of any allergy or sensitivity to any herbal products, (4) use caution if pregnant or lactating, and (5) not take a greater dose than recommended.

In 1992, Congress instructed the National Institutes of Health (NIH) to develop an Office of Alternative Medicine to support studies of alternative therapies. This office is now called the National Center for Complementary and Alternative Medicine (NCCAM). NCCAM lists current clinical trials with herbal products on their website *(www.nccam.nih.gov/research/clinicaltrials)*. The Natural Standard Research Collaboration also reviews global literature on herbal studies by clinicians and researchers. These studies are important because botanical remedies cannot be patented, so their manufacturers generally cannot justify the expenses associated with safety and efficacy testing in an already booming conventional medicine economy.

This chapter describes selected aspects of herbal therapy, including (1) herbal monographs, (2) the Dietary Supplement Health and Education Act of 1994, (3) varieties of herbal preparations, (4) the most commonly used herbs, (5) herbs used to treat selected common ailments, (6) potential hazards of herbs, (7) tips for consumers and health care providers, and (8) herbal resources.

HERBAL MONOGRAPHS

The two primary types of **herbal monographs** are therapeutic and qualitative. Therapeutic monographs contain information on use, dosage, side effects, and contraindications. Qualitative monographs have information on areas such as compliance with compounding guidelines and standards of purity. Integrating herbs into the American health care system requires both types of monographs, which the United States currently does not have.

Work to develop these monographs is in progress by several organizations, including the United States Pharmacopeia (USP), the World Health Organization (WHO), the American Herbal Pharmacopeia (AHP), the European Scientific Cooperative of Phytomedicines (ESCOP), and the German Commission E.

The German Commission E, an oversight commission in Germany, works to determine the safety of an herbal product with "reasonable certainty." The American Botanical Council has translated the German Commission E monographs into English in an effort to bring more information to the American public. Much work remains to be done related to the effects of preparations and the improvement of manufacturing and marketing processes.

Standardization is movement toward consistency and comparison of herbal preparations. A standardized herbal extract has one or multiple ingredients whose levels are guaranteed in the sold product. Examples of standardized herbal products are presented in Table 6-1.

DIETARY SUPPLEMENT HEALTH AND EDUCATION ACT OF 1994

The **Dietary Supplement Health and Education Act of 1994 (DSHEA)** clarified marketing regulations for herbal remedies. DSHEA reclassified herbals as "dietary supplements" distinct from food or drugs. Herbal supplements can be marketed with suggested dosages. Consumers are reminded that premarket testing for safety and efficacy is not required, and manufacturing is not standardized. The physiologic effects of the product can be noted, but no claims can be made about preventing or curing specific conditions. For example, a

TABLE 6-1 SELECTED HERBAL PRODUCTS WITH STANDARDIZED CONCENTRATIONS

HERB	STANDARDIZED CONCENTRATION OF ACTIVE INGREDIENT
Bilberry	25% anthanocyanosides
Feverfew	0.2% parthenolide
Ginkgo biloba	24% flavone glycosides; 6% terpene lactones
Goldenseal	8% to 12% alkaloid
Hawthorn	20% procyanidins
St. John's wort	0.13% to 0.30% hypericin
Saw palmetto	85% to 95% fatty acids

product label cannot claim that the agent "prevents heart disease," but it can say that the agent "helps increase blood flow to the heart." In addition, a disclaimer is required that indicates that the herb is not approved by the U.S. Food and Drug Administration (FDA) and that it is not meant to be used as a drug.

In January 2000, the FDA finalized rules for claims on dietary supplements, noting that supplements may make structure and function claims without FDA approval. However, it may not be claimed that the supplement can prevent, treat, cure, mitigate, or diagnose diseases. This ruling caused label changes on products but did not affect product availability or consumer access. Health maintenance claims (e.g., "maintains a healthy immune system") and claims for relief of minor symptoms related to life stages (e.g., "alleviates hot flashes") are acceptable because they do not relate to disease. Herbal products using a "may be beneficial" disclaimer rather than claims of definite benefit are appropriate legally. Dietary supplement manufacturers are still required to substantiate any claims they make.

CURRENT GOOD MANUFACTURING PRACTICES

The FDA proposed standards for marketing and labeling for dietary supplements in 2003. Known as the **Current Good Manufacturing Practices (CGMPs)**, these standards are multifaceted and require that package labels give quality and strength of all contents and products be free of contaminants and impurities. Manufacturing quality control procedures are part of the CGMPs.

Additionally, a "seal of approval" is awarded to products meeting criteria similar to the CGMPs by four organizations (the USP, ConsumerLab, National Products Association, and NSF International). The fee-based tests provide information on herbal products' identity, potency, dissolution, purity, and labeling accuracy.

HERBAL PREPARATIONS

Herbal remedies are available in a variety of preparations and forms. Following is a description of selected preparations and forms of herbs, including dried herbs, fresh oils, salves, teas, tinctures, syrups, capsules, and tablets. The consumer and health care provider must be knowledgeable about the differences in dosages between extracts and powders as well as the issues associated with standardization.

Dried herbs are fresh herbs that have had the moisture removed by sun or heat. They can be stored for about 6 months. **Extracts** are made by isolating certain components, resulting in more reliable dosing. Dissolving the herb in a solvent such as alcohol or water is a common way to prepare an extract, which may or may not be standardized. **Fresh herbs** may decay after a few days because of enzyme activity; hence they have a short life.

Oils are made by soaking dried herb in olive or vegetable oil and heating it for an extended time. The oil promotes concentration of some of the herb's active components, and it may last for months if stored correctly. These infused oils are not "essential oils" (volatile oils extracted from plants that produce an odor and stimulate taste sensations). **Salves**, semisolid fatty preparations, are made by melting a wax in oil (or crushing the herb and mixing it in a petroleum jelly base) and allowing it to cool and harden. If stored correctly, they last for several months as balms, creams, and ointments. **Teas** are made by steeping fresh or dried herbs in boiling water. Tea made from bark and roots is often simmered. It is recommended that only a 2- to 3-day supply be prepared at one time and that it be stored in the refrigerator. Teas may be used as a drink, added to baths, and applied topically in a compress. **Tinctures** are commonly made by soaking fresh or dried herbs in a solvent such as water or alcohol. Both water- and fat-soluble components are concentrated in the final form. Alcohol promotes preservation, yielding a shelf life of 1 year. Alcohol-free, glycerin-based tinctures are available for people who do not consume alcohol. **Syrups** are made by adding a sweetener, usually honey or sugar, to the herb and then cooking it. Syrups are used to treat colds, coughs, and sore throats.

Capsules commonly contain a powdered form of dried supplement, but they may hold juices or oils. They have a slower effect than liquids because of decreased absorption. They store and travel well. Tablets are similar to capsules; they are a powder compressed with stabilizers and binders.

COMMONLY USED HERBAL REMEDIES

Most herbal therapies are used for chronic conditions, are unlikely to cause harm, and may provide some relief in selected situations. This section discusses some of the more commonly used herbs.

Aloe Vera *(Aloe barbadensis)*

The juice is used externally for treatment of minor burns, insect bites, and sunburn. Fresh aloe leaves are most effective. There has been some success with the treatment of dandruff, oily skin, and psoriasis. Taken internally, aloe vera is a powerful laxative. Menstrual flow is increased with small doses.

Black Cohosh *(Cimicifuga racemosa)*

This is a popular supplement used to treat hot flashes, palpitations, and irritability (short-term menopausal symptoms; short-term use is recommended). It potentiates the effects of insulin, oral hypoglycemics, and antihypertensive drugs (Herbal Alert 6-2).

HERBAL ALERT 6-2

Black Cohosh

Do not confuse black cohosh with blue cohosh, an herbal preparation said to induce labor in pregnant patients.

Chamomile *(Matricaria recutita)*

Dried flower heads of *Matricaria recutita* are the ingredients of a popular tea for relief of digestive and gastrointestinal (GI) complaints. Chamomile tea's antispasmodic and anti-inflammatory effects on the GI tract make it useful for relief of irritable bowel syndrome and infant colic. In addition, chamomile may have sedative effects.

Chamomile tea is prepared by steeping 1 teaspoon of flower heads for 10 to 15 minutes in boiling water; suggested use is three to four times per day. An extremely rare reaction of urticaria and bronchoconstriction may occur in an individual who is allergic to daisy or ragweed-type plants. Pharmacokinetics and pharmacodynamics are not known.

Dong Quai *(Angelica sinensis)*

Dong quai, an all-purpose woman's tonic herb, has long been popular in China and Japan for the treatment of menstrual cramps and to regulate the menstrual cycle. This herb has not been well studied, and preparations are frequently mixed with fillers. Dong quai contains vitamin B_{12}, which may promote manufacture of blood cells. Rare side effects include fever and excessive menstrual bleeding. Pharmacokinetics and pharmacodynamics are not known. The recommendation is to avoid the use of this herb.

Echinacea *(Echinacea angustifolia)*

Echinacea, a popular oral and topical supplement, is used as an immune enhancer; it acts by furthering phagocytosis by means of increasing leukocytes and spleen cells and activating granulocytes. In addition, echinacea inhibits hyaluronidase activity and increases the release of tumor necrosis factor. The leaf preparation is given for respiratory and urinary tract infections. The root extract is used to treat flulike symptoms. German Commission E recommends that echinacea preparations be avoided by persons with autoimmune diseases and those with abnormal T-cell functioning (e.g., human immunodeficiency virus [HIV], acquired immunodeficiency syndrome [AIDS], tuberculosis).

Echinacea should be purchased only from reliable sources. There are many reports of fraudulent substitution with other plants and varying potency. Recommendations for duration of treatment are inconsistent. However, treatment should begin immediately with the onset of symptoms to "catch it early." German Commission E recommends the use of echinacea for up to 8 weeks; others recommend a week-long "drug holiday" (i.e., not taking the preparation for a specific time period) before continuing therapy. Pharmacokinetics is not known. Immunosuppression may occur after extended therapy.

Evening Primrose *(Oenothera biennis)*

Evening primrose is a native North American biennial plant. Oil in its seeds contains gamma-linolenic acid (GLA), a fatty acid believed to help prevent cirrhosis, eczema, premenstrual syndrome, hypertension, hardening of the arteries, and heart disease. It aids in lowering cholesterol and relieving pain and inflammation. The bark and leaves have astringent qualities, and the oil affects uterine muscles, metabolism, and the nervous system. It should not be used during pregnancy and lactation. It may lower the seizure threshold if taken with anticonvulsants; the anticonvulsant dose may need modification, or it should not be used concurrently. Pharmacokinetics and pharmacodynamics are not known.

Feverfew *(Tanacetum/Chrysanthemum parthenium)*

The plant compound parthenolide is believed to inhibit platelet aggregation and act as a serotonin antagonist in mediating vascular headaches. Feverfew is popular for prophylaxis and for relief of migraine headaches and their accompanying nausea and vomiting. Postfeverfew syndrome (fatigue, headache, joint pain, nervousness) is experienced by some. Local ulceration and irritation may result from chewing feverfew leaves. Only standardized extracts should be used. Wide variation in the amount of active compound in plants and commercial capsules is a potential dosing problem. Pharmacokinetics and pharmacodynamics are not known.

Garlic *(Allium sativum)*

Garlic is reported to lower cholesterol and triglyceride levels, decrease blood pressure, and reduce the clotting capability of blood (increases precursor of nitric oxide). It also acts as an antibiotic to treat infections and wounds both internally and externally. Warm garlic oil is used in the ear for treatment of earache. Garlic may be used for some types of heavy-metal poisoning. Pharmacokinetics and pharmacodynamics are not known.

Ginger *(Zingiber officinale)*

Ginger boosts the immune system. It is used to treat migraine headache, stomach problems, and digestive disorders, including motion sickness. Long-time use for relief from nausea is validated by modern research. In addition, it may provide relief from pain, swelling, and stiffness of both osteoarthritis and rheumatoid arthritis (dosage 500 to 4000 mg/day). Information on pharmacokinetics and pharmacodynamics is limited. Metabolites are excreted via urine within 24 hours, and it is 90% protein-bound.

Ginkgo *(Ginkgo biloba)*

Ginkgo biloba, an extract of one of the oldest plant species, is the most commonly prescribed herbal remedy worldwide. When it crosses the blood-brain barrier, ginkgo has central nervous system (CNS) effects, increasing both cerebral arterial dilation and uptake of oxygen and glucose. It assists cells during periods of hypoxia (e.g., during transient ischemic attacks) and decreases free-radical damage to neurons. In addition, there is inhibition of platelet adhesion and degranulation. German Commission E Monograph #55 lists the use of ginkgo for dementia syndromes, intermittent claudication, vertigo, and tinnitus when these symptoms are secondary to diminished blood flow. There is some evidence that ginkgo improves cognition and may be helpful in Alzheimer's disease, early stroke, and Raynaud's phenomenon. Some men take ginkgo to treat erectile dysfunction.

Ginkgo biloba is generally given as 120 to 240 mg/day in two to three divided doses for up to 90 days. Rare side effects include headache and GI disturbances. Limited information is available on pharmacokinetics and pharmacodynamics. Bioavailability is not affected by food; urinary excretion is less than 30% metabolites.

Ginseng *(Panax ginseng)*

Preparations of ginseng are taken for short-term relief of stress, to boost energy, and to give digestive support. Ginseng tends to support the immune system and assist in the prevention of chronic infections. Red Korean or Chinese ginseng may be overstimulating in chronic inflammatory conditions such as arthritis. Pharmacokinetics and pharmacodynamics are not known.

Goldenseal *(Hydrastis canadensis)*

Goldenseal is frequently used with echinacea to ward off infection and promote wound healing. Common uses include treatment of GI ulcers, mouth ulcers, bladder infection, eye and skin irritation, and postpartum hemorrhage. It is used to treat congestion associated with the common cold. In addition, it is used as a tonic and astringent. Active ingredients are deactivated in the stomach. Goldenseal is expensive and scarce; thus it is frequently adulterated with fillers. Its ability to stimulate the immune system has been questioned, and it can be toxic if overused. Goldenseal is contraindicated during pregnancy (stimulates uterus). Pharmacokinetics and pharmacodynamics are not known.

Kava *(Piper methysticum)*

Kava promotes sleep and muscle relaxation and is an antiepileptic, antidepressant, and antipsychotic. Kava also promotes wound healing. Tea can help with urinary tract infections. Kava may be used in combination with other herbs, such as valerian and St. John's wort, for relaxation. Kava may cross the placenta and be present in breast milk. In 2002, the FDA issued a consumer advisory about the potential for liver damage with kava use. Long-term use may result in a pellagra-like skin disorder that disappears when kava is discontinued. Little is known about its pharmacokinetics and pharmacodynamics.

Licorice *(Glycyrrhiza glabra)*

Licorice may have physiologic effects similar to aldosterone and corticosteroids related to glycyrrhizin, a major ingredient. Licorice may help with chronic fatigue syndrome. The deglycyrrhizinated form is used to treat ulcers. It relieves heartburn and indigestion by decreasing stomach acid; it also has a laxative effect. Side effects from excessive licorice include increased blood pressure, headache, lethargy, water retention, increased potassium excretion, and, rarely, heart failure. Licorice root is considered safe in dosages of 5 to 15 mg when taken as tea. Its recommended use is limited to 6 weeks. Pharmacokinetics and pharmacodynamics are not known (Herbal Alert 6-3).

HERBAL ALERT 6-3

Black Licorice

Consuming 2 ounces of black licorice daily for 14 days may cause arrhythmia in people age 40 years and older.

Milk Thistle *(Silybum marianum)*

This herbal extract has the remarkable ability to prevent damage to liver cells and stimulate regeneration of liver cells. Milk thistle is widely used in Europe to treat hepatitis, cirrhosis, and fatty liver associated with drug and alcohol abuse. Pharmacokinetics and pharmacodynamics are not known.

Peppermint *(Mentha piperita)*

Peppermint stimulates appetite and aids in digestion when taken internally. The digestive tract is protected by the tannins, and peppermint is used in the treatment of bowel disorders. Hot peppermint tea stimulates circulation, reduces fever, clears congestion, and helps restore energy. Peppermint oil is an effective treatment for tension headache when rubbed on the forehead. In research in Germany, peppermint has been shown to be comparable with acetaminophen (extra-strength Tylenol) in relieving headache. Pharmacokinetics and pharmacodynamics are not known.

Sage

Sage has a long history of use for medicinal and culinary purposes. Sage tea is used as an aid for sore throat and cough; it may also be used as a gargle to decrease inflammation of mouth, gums, and throat. According to clinical studies, antibacterial, antifungal, and antiviral effects are found in sage and result in its medicinal effects. Its recommended use is limited to 2 weeks to avoid the toxic effects of tannins.

St. John's Wort *(Hypericum perforatum)*

Current research suggests that St. John's wort is not effective when used by individuals with moderate to severe depression. Botanical experts indicate that it is to be used for mild depression. St. John's wort has at least 10 pharmacologically active components. The compound used for standardization is hypericin. Researchers recommend that prospective trials be conducted to compare St. John's wort with standard antidepressant medication and to identify dosages, effectiveness in different stages of depression, and implications of long-term use. St. John's wort has been nicknamed "herbal Prozac" because of its great popularity in the United States and its use as a "tonic" for the nervous system. St. John's wort is used in combination with yarrow to treat enuresis. When taken concomitantly with a prescription antidepressant, an adverse effect of St. John's wort may be suicidal ideation. This herbal remedy is considered a dietary supplement in the United States and has not been FDA approved. In Germany, it is licensed for relief of anxiety, depression, and insomnia. The 1984 German Commission E monograph on hypericin indicated that the agent was an experimental monoamine oxidase inhibitor (MAOI) for use in depression, anxiety, and psychogenic disturbances. The mechanism of action is unknown.

The usual dose of St. John's wort is 300 mg of extract three times a day (standardized to 0.3% hypericin). A tea can be prepared from 1 to 2 teaspoons of herb steeped for 10 minutes. One to two cups of tea per day for 4 to 6 weeks is recommended. Users should apply sunscreen freely when outdoors, although phototoxicity has not been reported in humans. St. John's wort crosses the blood-brain and placental barriers and may enter breast milk. Minimal information is known about the pharmacokinetics and pharmacodynamics.

Saw Palmetto *(Serenoa repens)*

Double-blind studies indicate that saw palmetto relieves symptoms of benign prostatic hypertrophy and urinary conditions. Saw palmetto has earned the nickname "plant catheter." Individuals who use saw palmetto can get false-negative test results for PSA. Other indications for this herb include use as an expectorant and a treatment for colds, asthma, bronchitis, and thyroid deficiency. The recommended dose is 160 mg of standardized extract twice a day. Pharmacokinetics and pharmacodynamics are not known.

Valerian *(Valeriana officinalis)*

Valerian, a mild sedative and sleep-inducing agent, has an effect similar to benzodiazepines. It is popularly known as "herbal Valium." Most researchers report no hangover effect. A "dirty socks" odor is related to the dried plant, resulting in low risk of overdose. Preparations from fresh root are reported to be better relaxants and have a sweet aroma. There have been no reports of habituation and addiction. Drowsiness may occur, as with any relaxant. The dosage depends on the symptoms, such as insomnia and anxiety. To treat insomnia, 400 mg of tincture extract or 2.5 to 5 mg of solid extract is recommended at bedtime. For anxiety, a tea steeped with 1 teaspoon of dried herb is taken several times a day. About 5% to 10% of users report a stimulant effect. Pharmacokinetics and pharmacodynamics are not known.

Table 6-2 describes aspects of selected herbs. Vitamins and elements commonly used in conjunction with herbal therapy are vitamins B_6, A, C, and E; selenium; and zinc. The American Herbal Products Association has categorized herbal products based on "reasonable use" into four classes. See the note at the end of Table 6-2 for a description of the classes.

POTENTIAL HAZARDS OF HERBS

Both consumers and health care providers should remember that although herbs are natural substances, they are not necessarily safe. No preparations are safe in all situations, and herbs are no exception. Consumers and health care providers must be alert to potential hazards with herbal therapy. It is essential that the health care provider get a complete list of all of the herbal preparations the patient takes, the reason they are taken, and their perceived effectiveness. This assessment should be updated regularly along with information on the patient's prescription and OTC drug use.

Patients may not disclose use of herbal products to health care providers for a variety of reasons, including the sense that the health care provider is biased against or not knowledgeable about herbal products or the belief that these products are not considered medications. Herbal use should be encouraged as an "integrative" modality rather than as a replacement for a medical therapy. The patient must inform the health care provider of any use of herbal products to ensure that they do not interfere with the use and actions of prescribed medication. When taking a health history, it is important for the nurse collecting data to ask about these remedies and to specifically mention homeopathic remedies as well as teas (infusions), tinctures, tablets, and herbs in dried forms.

Without regulations, manufacturers of herbal products may make unsubstantiated claims on their labels. Companies manufacturing for drugstores and grocery stores are suspect. Their supplements may contain many fillers not mentioned on the labels. However, several companies (e.g., Nature's Way, Nature's Sunshine, Gaia) do label their products accurately and include in the bottle only what the ingredient list indicates.

Contamination is another area of concern, most likely resulting from lack of standards in the manufacture and regulation of herbs. It is the responsibility of consumers to educate themselves about herbs before use and to purchase products only from reputable dealers. Determination of the purity and concentration of a particular product can be done only through assays, a costly process; thus, most products have not had appropriate human toxicological analysis.

Interaction with conventional drugs is another area in which health care providers should be alert. For example, an additive effect of digoxin can result from the use of the laxative herbs cascara and senna. Also, elevation of the blood level of lithium may result from juniper, dandelion, and other herbs with diuretic properties. Patients at high risk for interactions include older adults and those taking three or more drugs for chronic conditions. See Table 6-3 for selected herbal ingredients and drug interactions.

Text continued on p. 75

TABLE 6-2 SUMMARY OF SELECTED HERBS*

HERB	ACTIONS AND USES	DOSAGE	INTERACTIONS/PRECAUTIONS	SIDE/ADVERSE EFFECTS
Common and *Botanical* Names ***Class and Part Used***				
aloe/aloe vera *Aloe barbadensis* Class 1 Leaf gel Class 2b/2d Dried, juice Class 2d Topical bladelike leaf	Uses: Internal for constipation; externally to relieve pain and promote healing of burns, wounds, sunburn, psoriasis	Internal: Tincture/extract: 50-300 mg External: t.i.d. or PRN	Internal use contraindicated if pregnant or lactating, and in children <12 y Consult with HCP before taking if have ulcerative colitis or Crohn's disease or if taking cardiac glycosides, antiarrhythmics, thiazide diuretics, licorice, or corticosteroids Monitor electrolytes	Internal: Overdose/long-term use: arrhythmias, neuropathies, edemas, albuminuria, hematuria (side effects are rare)
bilberry *Vaccinium myrtillus L.* Class 4 Extract of dried fruit and leaf	Uses: Fruit may promote healthy vision, increase visual pigment regeneration; decrease diarrhea in children Leaf used for diabetes, arthritis, dermatitis, gout	Fruit extract: 80-160 mg t.i.d. (St: 25% anthocyanosides) Leaf: no information	Avoid use if pregnant or lactating, and in children No reported significant interaction with fruit Leaf: May decrease blood sugar and triglyceride levels; may increase action of anticoagulants and NSAIDs; monitor for dose adjustments	Leaf: Long-term higher doses (in animals): anemia, icterus, excitation, death
black cohosh (bugwort, snakeroot, squaw root) *Cimicifuga racemosa* Class 2b/2c Root	Suppresses luteinizing hormone, optimizes estrogen levels Uses: Antispasmodic, astringent, diuretic, vasodilator, PMS, dysmenorrhea, infertility, menopausal symptoms	Cap/tab: 20 mg b.i.d. Tincture: 2-5 mg b.i.d.	Avoid use if pregnant or lactating, and in children Limit use to 6 mo; no data on long-term use Under supervision of qualified herbalist, increases action of antihypertensives; may alter effects of HRT May decrease iron absorption	Higher doses: dizziness, headache, nausea, change in heart rate
chamomile (green chamomile) *Matricaria recutita* Class 2b Dried flower tops	Stimulates normal digestion, antiinflammatory, antispasmodic, mild sedative, mild diuretic, mild antibacterial with topical use Uses: Anxiety, insomnia, indigestion, inflammatory skin conditions	*Between meals:* Cap/tab: 2-3 g t.i.d., Tea: 1-4 c/d Tincture: max: 1 tsp t.i.d.	Avoid use if allergic to daisy family (e.g., ragweed, asters, chrysanthemums) May increase effects of sedatives and interfere with action of anticoagulants H/F, H/H: None known	None known
cranberry *Vaccinium macrocarpon Ait.* Class 4 Berries	Prophylaxis (not treatment) of urinary tract infections; to treat kidney stones	Extract: 300-400 mg concentrated juice b.i.d. Cocktail: 300 mL/d commercial cranberry juice	Caution: Avoid use with oliguria and anuria. Patients with DM should use sugar-free cranberry juice; lactating patients, children <12 y, and patients with history of oxalate kidney stones limit to 1 L/day. H/D, H/F, H/H: None known	Doses of >3 L/day may produce diarrhea

Continued

TABLE 6-2 SUMMARY OF SELECTED HERBS—cont'd

HERB	ACTIONS AND USES	DOSAGE	INTERACTIONS/PRECAUTIONS	SIDE/ADVERSE EFFECTS
dong quai *Angelica Sinensis* Class 2b (root) Roots, rhizomes	Phytoestrogen activity; vasodilation, small muscle relaxation Decreased IgE antibody production Uses: PMS, menopausal symptoms, cardiovascular support	Tea: 1-4 c/d (equivalent 1-2 g dried herb) Tincture: 0.5-4 mL, Max: 6 times a day	Caution: Avoid use with prescription anticoagulants, history of bleeding disorders, or if pregnant or at risk for breast cancer H/D: additive bleeding effect with anticoagulants, aspirin, NSAIDs	Rash and photosensitivity; fever, bleeding
echinacea (purple coneflower) *E. purpura; E. angustifolia, E. pallida* Class 1 (root/seed) Aerial parts of *E. pallida;* root of *E. pallida* and *E. angustifolia*	Stimulates immune system; antibacterial, antiviral, antipyretic Antifungal as topical Uses: Prevention and early treatment of colds and flu; recurrent respiratory, ear, and urinary tract infections Topical: Canker sores, fungal infections Investigational use: Stimulate immune system of HIV/AIDS patients.	Tab: 500 mg-1 g t.i.d. Tea: 1-5 c/d Tincture: max: 2 tsp t.i.d.	Short-term use: 2 wk; 8 wk if low dose; may be hepatotoxic if taken continuously Avoid use with immunosuppressants such as corticosteroids (may counteract) and with chronic systemic disease of immune system (e.g., SLE, HIV, TB, MS) Safety not determined in pregnancy, lactation, and children <2 y	Lozenge/tincture: Temporary numbness or tingling of tongue Cross-sensitivity in patients allergic to daisy family, GI upset, diarrhea
evening primrose *Oenothera biennis* Class 4 Oil of seed	Natural estrogen promoter Uses: PMS, problems with synthesis of fatty acids, abnormal prostaglandin production, diabetic neuropathies, chronic inflammatory conditions (eczema), overactive immune systems	Take with meals (increases absorption): Oil: PMS: 3-6 g/d for 6 mo, 14 days before menses Inflammatory conditions: 4-8 g/d for 3-4 mo MS: 500 mg/d for 3 wk with exacerbation	Avoid use if pregnant or lactating May lower seizure threshold if taken with anticonvulsants; anticonvulsant dose may need modification, or do not use concurrently H/F, H/H: None known	GI upset, nausea, headache, rash Immunosuppression with long-term use
feverfew *Tanacetum parthenium; chrysanthemum parthenium* Class 2b (whole herb) Leaves, flowering tops	Interferes with platelet aggregation, inhibits release of serotonin from platelets, blocks proinflammatory mediators, digestive relaxant Uses: Prevention and long-term management of migraine headaches; rheumatoid arthritis; menstrual problems; allergies	Cap/tab (at least 2% parthenolide) 125 mg/d; increase to 1-2 g with acute attack	May be 4-6 wk before effect; use continuously for best outcome Cross-sensitivity to plants in daisy family Avoid use if pregnant or lactating, with prescription anticoagulants, and in children <2 y Consult HCP before use if taking prescription NSAIDs (decreases effectiveness) May interfere with SSRI antidepressants (e.g., Prozac)	Possible gastric distress or mouth sores if using raw leaves; muscle stiffness; may have rebound headache if discontinued abruptly
garlic *Allium sativum* Class 2c Bulb	Detoxifies body and increases immune function; decreases platelet aggregation; increases HDL and decreases cholesterol and triglycerides, broad antimicrobial activity, mild antihypertensive; hypoglycemia Uses: Hypercholesterolemia, mild HTN, colds and flu	Caps (enteric coated): (ED of 5000 mcg/d of allicin in divided doses) Raw garlic clove is best source; minimum: 1/d	Avoid use if pregnant or lactating (may stimulate labor or cause infant colic) and in hypothyroidism Blood pressure may decrease in 30 min and return to baseline in about 2 hr Caution: Use with caution with prescription anticoagulants because of increased fibrinolysis and decreased platelet aggregation; modify antidiabetic doses H/F: None; H/H: Acidophilus decreases absorption of garlic	Heartburn, flatulence, gastric irritation, decreased RBCs; dizziness, diaphoresis

ginger *Zingiber officinale* Class 1 (fresh root) Class 2b/2d Dried root, rhizome	Stimulates digestion, increases bile and motility; antispasmodic; decreased platelet aggregation; decreases absorption and increases excretion of cholesterol; antioxidant Uses: Nausea, pregnancy morning sickness (short term, low dose ONLY); motion sickness; gastric protection with NSAIDs	Take with food Cap/tab/tea: 2-4 g in 2-3 divided doses For motion sickness, start 2 d to 2 hr before travel Inflammatory joint disease: 4 g in 2-3 divided doses Nausea (pregnancy related): 1 g in divided doses for 1-4 d Tincture: 1.5-3 mL in 8 oz juice q.i.d., PRN	Avoid long-term use with pregnancy, thrombocytopenia (abortifacient in large amounts) Caution: Use with caution with prescription anticoagulants (additive effect) Consult with HCP before use if have gallstones May increase absorption of all PO medications H/F, H/H: None known	May cause gastric discomfort if not taken with food; anorexia
Ginkgo biloba *Gingko folium* Class 1 (leaf) Leaves	Antioxidant; peripheral vasodilation and increased blood flow to CNS, reduces platelet aggregation Uses: Allergic rhinitis, Alzheimer's disease, anxiety/stress, dementia, Raynaud's disease, tinnitus, vertigo, impotence, poor circulation; altitude sickness	Cap/tab: 120-240 mg/d in 2-3 divided doses (standardized to at least 24% ginkgo flavone glycosides and 6% Terpene lactones) Tincture: 5-10 mL b.i.d., t.i.d. Circulation/memory: 120 mg/d in 2-3 divided doses Alzheimer's dementia, tinnitus: up to 240 mg/d in 2-3 divided doses	Effects seen in 2-3 wk; 12-wk course recommended Avoid use if pregnant or lactating, in children, and with MAOIs Caution: Use with caution with prescription anticoagulants; monitor bleeding and prothrombin times. Use with extra caution if using ginger, garlic, or feverfew May increase BP if used with thiazide diuretics Discontinue use 2 wk before surgery Ginkgo fruit may result in severe rash; seeds are toxic H/F, H/H: None known	Initially, mild transient headache that usually stops in 2 d; mild gastric distress Toxicity: vomiting, diarrhea, dermatitis, irritability
ginseng, eleuthera, or Siberian *Eleutherococcus senticosus, Acanthopanax senticosus* Class 2b/2c/2d Root	Supports adrenal glands, enhances energy levels by inhibiting alarm phase SNS response, stimulates RBC production, decreases blood sugar levels, protects from cellular mutation from carcinogens Uses: Cold and flu prevention, adaptation to stress, chronic fatigue syndrome, SLE, HIV, mental fatigue and physical exhaustion, following chemotherapy or radiation treatments, recovery from chronic or long-term illness	Cap/tab: 2-3 g/d in 3-4 divided doses Tea: 1-4 c/d Tincture: 5-20 mL/d in 3-4 divided doses	Take for 6-8 wk; then 1 wk drug holiday, and resume for total of 3 mo Avoid use with BP >170/90, if pregnant or lactating, in children, and with bipolar or psychic disorders, DM, and anticoagulants (may increase or decrease anticoagulants, dependent on species) May increase effects of caffeine and HRT, falsely elevate digoxin levels, and interact with antipsychotic drugs H/F: Overstimulation may occur with caffeinated coffee, cola, and tea; H/H: None	Hypertension, palpitations, occasional diarrhea, possible insomnia if taken at bedtime Ginseng abuse syndrome: Edema, insomnia, hypertonia; may be life threatening

Continued

TABLE 6-2 SUMMARY OF SELECTED HERBS—cont'd

HERB	ACTIONS AND USES	DOSAGE	INTERACTIONS/PRECAUTIONS	SIDE/ADVERSE EFFECTS
goldenseal *Hydrastis canadensis* Class 2b Root, rhizome	Stimulates immune system and bile secretion, antipyretic, broad-spectrum antibiotic activity Uses: For infection: respiratory, digestive, urinary tract, mucous membranes, cholecystitis, cirrhosis	Cap/tab: 2-4 g/d in divided doses (standardized to 8%-12% alkaloid content)	Avoid use if pregnant or lactating, with HTN, and in children Higher dosing >5-7 d may increase liver enzymes or malabsorption of B vitamins May decrease effect of heparin, anticoagulants, cardiac glycosides; increased effect of antiarrhythmics, antihypertensives, beta blockers, and CNS depressants Caution: Use with caution in patients with cardiovascular disease, DM, or glaucoma	High doses may be hepatotoxic Toxicity: CNS depression, restlessness, seizures, cardiovascular collapse Endangered plant species
hawthorn *Crataegus laevigata, C. oxycantha, C. monogyna* Class 1 Ripe fruit, leaves, flowers	Peripheral dilation and increased coronary circulation, improves cardiac oxygenation, antioxidants, mild diuretic, decreases proinflammatory substances Uses: Mild HTN, early HF, stable angina	Cap/tab: 100-900 mg/d in divided doses (standardized to 20% procyanidins) Average dose: 100-250 mg t.i.d. Tea: 2.5-5 mL t.i.d. Tea: 1 c t.i.d. (4-5 g dried/day)	May need to modify doses of beta blockers, digitalis, and ACE inhibitors Increased effects of digitalis, beta blockers, ACE inhibitors, and CNS depressants High doses contraindicated with chronic atrial fibrillation and hypotension from dysfunction of valve H/F: None known; H/H: increases action of Lily of the Valley	Hypotension, fatigue Sedation, nausea, vomiting, anorexia
kava *Piper methysticum* Class 2b/2c/2d Dried rhizome, roots	CNS sedation without loss of mental acuity or memory Uses: Anxiety, insomnia, skeletal muscle spasm Good with psychotic disorders, no risk of tolerance	Cap/tab: Anxiety: 50-100 mg up to t.i.d. Insomnia: 180-210 mg at bedtime (standardized to 70% kavalactones) Max: 300 g/wk	Avoid use if pregnant or lactating, with parkinsonism, and if taking levodopa; not for young children Avoid alcohol use and if patient needs to be alert or will operate machinery Increases CNS-sedating drugs, especially benzodiazepines Fat soluble, so may have delayed effects H/F: increased absorption when taken with food; H/H: None known Unstable gait, numb tongue, mild GI upset	Leaf: Long-term higher doses (in animals): anemia, icterus, excitation, death High doses: may cause loss of balance, pulmonary hypertension May cause liver toxicity Banned in several European countries Use >3 mo may turn skin yellow: discontinue drug if HTN, headache, weakness
licorice *Glycyrrhiza glabra* Class 2b/2c/2d (root) Root, leaf	Antiinflammatory, antibacterial, antiviral, hepato- and gastric-protective, antidepressant, estrogenic, laxative Uses: Viral infection, upper respiratory infection, inflammation, Addison's disease, depression, ulcers Topically: Herpes, psoriasis, eczema DCL: IBS, mouth ulcers	Cap/tab: 200-600 mg glycyrrhizin in 3 divided doses; max: 4-6 wk Tea: 3 c/d (equivalent to 1-2 g/d) Tincture: 2.5-5 mL t.i.d. DGL: 300-380 mg; max: 1200 mg/d in chewable form 20 min before meals for 8-16 wk	Avoid use if pregnant or lactating, with HTN, with kidney or liver disorders, or if at risk for hypokalemia; avoid in children Caution with DM Increased aldosterone effect with increasing dose and duration Antagonizes antihypertensive drugs and spirolactone Potentiates corticosteroids and digitalis H/F: none known; H/H: may cause hypokalemia if used with aloe vera	Doses >5000 mg/d result in aldosterone-like syndrome that reverses when herb is discontinued

milk thistle (Mary thistle, wild artichoke) *Silybum marianum* Class 1 Seeds of dried flowers	Increased regeneration of liver cells; increases antioxidant activity Uses: Liver disease (hepatitis), cholecystitis, psoriasis	Cap/tab: Initially: 500 mg/d in 3 divided doses for 6-8 wk With improvement: 120-240 mg/d in divided doses; may take 7-10 d for effect; 4-8 wk if liver is diseased with alcohol Tincture: 1 mL t.i.d. (avoid ETOH-based tinctures)	Avoid use if pregnant or lactating, in children, and with drugs metabolized by P-450 enzyme Does not reverse cirrhotic liver changes, but may slow the disease and increase quality of life H/F, H/H: None known	Diarrhea first days of therapy, nausea, vomiting, menstrual changes
peppermint *Mentha piperita, var. officinalis* or *vulgaris* Class 4 Aerial parts	Antispasmodic, increase bile flow, carminative, external analgesic Uses: IBS, indigestion, cholecystitis, infant colic, nasal decongestant Topically: Musculoskeletal pain, itching, colds	Cap/tab: enteric coated: 1-2 t.i.d. between meals Tea: 2-3 c/d (equivalent 3-6 g dried herb) Tincture/oil: 6-12 gtts/d diluted in divided doses	Consult HCP before taking if have cholecystitis or obstructed bile duct No known drug interactions; may interfere with iron absorption	None known
psyllium *Plantago psyllium* Class 4	Uses: Laxative, treatment of hemorrhoids, colitis, Crohn's disease, IBS Herb of longevity, poultice: wound healing effects	½ tsp soaked in water for 15-60 min at bedtime with at least 8 oz water PO extract: 1-4 mL t.i.d.	Major ingredient in Metamucil May decrease lithium absorption Avoid use if pregnant or lactating, and in children	None known
sage *Salvia officinalis* Class 2b/2d (leaf) Whole plant	Gargle tea for sore throat, dries up mother's milk, decreases hot flashes Antidepressant and antiviral activity	Take with food Cap/tab: (standardized to at least 0.1% hypericin) 300 mg t.i.d.	Limit use to 2 wk to avoid toxic effects of tannins Caution patients with DM and seizure disorders	Nausea, vomiting, anorexia, oral irritation
St. John's wort *Hypericum perforatum* Class 2d Flowers	Uses: Mood swings, mild to moderate depression, anxiety, sleep disorders Topically: Burns/wounds	Tea: 1-2 c/d for 4-6 wk Tincture: 1-2 mL t.i.d.	Long-term use recommended; effects seen in 4-8 wk Avoid use if pregnant or lactating; with prescription antidepressants, MAOIs, and indinavir; and in children <2 y May decrease effect of digoxin related to bioavailability Monitor serum digoxin levels Use with amphetamines, trazodone, or tricyclic antidepressants may cause serotonin syndrome Interferes with absorption of iron and other minerals; high doses may increase liver enzymes	Skin photosensitivity, headache, occasional GI upset, dry mouth, dizziness, confusion

Continued

TABLE 6-2 SUMMARY OF SELECTED HERBS—cont'd

HERB	ACTIONS AND USES	DOSAGE	INTERACTIONS/PRECAUTIONS	SIDE/ADVERSE EFFECTS
saw palmetto *Serenoa repens, Sabal serrulata* Class 4 Berries	Decreases size of prostate; increases breakdown of estrogen, progesterone, and prolactin: antiandrogenic Diuretic Uses: BPH, chronic cystitis; sexual potency	Cap/tab: 230 mg/d in 1-2 doses (standardized to 85%-95% fatty acids) Tea: 1 c t.i.d. (equivalent dose 1-2 g/d) Liquid extract: 5-6 mL daily	Recommend 45-90 d of treatment; effects seen after 30 d. If effective, may take long term Avoid use if pregnant or lactating, in children, and in patients with breast cancer Effectiveness of prophylactic treatment not shown May interfere with PSA test; discontinue use 1-2 wk before test May increase or decrease effects of antiinflammatories and immunostimulants; may antagonize hormone therapy	Headache, dysuria, back pain Gastric disturbance (rare)
valerian *Valeriana officinalis* Class 1 Root	Sedative/hypnotic, antispasmodic, increases deep sleep Uses: Insomnia, stress headaches, mild anxiety, muscle cramps and spasms	Cap/tab: (standardized to 0.5% essential oils, equivalent to 2-3 g up to b.i.d.) Tea: 1-3 c/d or at bedtime Tincture: 1-3 mL; may repeat 2-3 times over 6 h	Effects may take several doses For long-term use; monitor liver function, and discontinue use if elevated Avoid if pregnant or lactating, in children, and with prescription sedative/hypnotics, MAOIs, and anticoagulants Increased sedative effect with barbiturates; negates effects of phenytoin Foul smell; no dependence or tolerance	Anxiety, headache, occasional GI upset and hangover effect with high doses, CNS depression

ACE, Angiotensin-converting enzyme; *AIDS,* acquired immunodeficiency syndrome; *b.i.d.,* twice a day; *BP,* blood pressure; *BPH,* benign prostatic hypertrophy; *c,* cup; *cap,* capsule; *CNS,* central nervous system; *d,* day; *DCL,* deglycyrrhizinated licorice; *DM,* diabetes mellitus; *ED,* effective dose; *Eq,* equivalent to; *ETOH,* alcohol; *GI,* gastrointestinal; *HCP,* health care provider; *H/D,* herb-drug interaction; *HDL,*high-density lipoprotein; *H/F,* herb-food interaction; *HF,* heart failure; *H/H,* herb-herb interaction; *HIV,* human immunodeficiency virus; *HRT,* hormone replacement therapy; *HTN,* hypertension; *IBS,* irritable bowel syndrome; *MAOI,* monoamine oxidase inhibitor; *max,* maximum; *mo,* month; *MS,* multiple sclerosis; *NSAIDs,* nonsteroidal antiinflammatory drugs; *PMS,* premenstrual syndrome; *PO,* orally; *PRN,* as needed; *RBCs,* red blood cells; *SLE,* systemic lupus erythematosus; *SNS,* sympathetic nervous system; *SSRI,* selective serotonin reuptake inhibitor; *St,* standardized to; *tab,* tablet; *TB,* tuberculosis; *t.i.d.,* three times a day; *wk,* week; *y,* year; >, greater than; <, less than.

Table revised by Joseph I. Boullata, Pharm D, BCNSP.

*The American Herbal Products Association (described in the *Botanical Safety Handbook*) has categorized herbal products based on "reasonable use" of the herb into the following four classes: **Class 1,** herbs that can be safely consumed when used appropriately; **Class 2,** herbs for which the following use restrictions apply unless otherwise directed by an expert qualified in the use of the herbal substance: for external use only, not to be used during pregnancy, not to be used while nursing, and other specific use restrictions as noted; **Class 3,** herbs for which significant data exist to recommend the following labeling: "To be used only under the supervision of an expert qualified in the appropriate use of this substance." Labeling must include proper use information as follows: Dosage, contraindications, potential adverse effects and drug interactions, and any other relevant information related to safe use of the substance; **Class 4,** herbs for which insufficient data are available for classification.

TABLE 6-3 SELECTED HERB-DRUG INTERACTIONS*

HERBAL INGREDIENT: COMMON AND BOTANICAL NAMES	DOCUMENTED DRUG INTERACTION	COMMENT	POTENTIAL DRUG INTERACTION	COMMENT
alfalfa *(Medicago sativa)*	—	—	anticoagulants	⇓ Drug effect
			oral contraceptives	⇓ Drug effect
aloe *(Aloe vera)*	—	—	antidiabetics	⇑ Drug effect
			antiplatelets	⇑ Drug effect
			digoxin	⇑ Drug effect
			diuretics	⇑ Hypokalemia
angelica root *(Angelica sp.)*	—	—	warfarin	⇑ Drug effect
arnica flower *(Arnica montana)*	—	—	warfarin	⇑ Drug effect
astragalus *(Astragalus membranaceus)*	—	—	cyclophosphamide	⇓ Drug effect
betel nut *(Areca catechu)*	fluphenazine	⇑ Drug toxicity	—	—
bilberry *(Vaccinium myrtillus)*	—	—	anticoagulants	⇑ Drug effect
			antidiabetics	⇑ Drug effect
black cohosh *(Actaea racemosa* or *Cimicifuga racemosa)*	—	—	antihypertensives	⇑ Drug effect
			digoxin	⇑ Drug absorption
			estrogen	⇓ Drug absorption
			iron salts	⇓ Drug absorption
bladderwrack *(Fucus vesiculosus)*	—	—	lithium	⇑ Drug effect
			thyroxine	⇑ Drug effect
boldo *(Peumus boldus)*	warfarin	⇑ Drug effect	—	—
cascara *(Rhamnus purshiana)*	—	—	corticosteroids	⇑ Hypokalemia
			digoxin	⇑ Drug effect
cat's claw *(Uncaria tomentosa)*	—	—	cyclosporine	⇑ Drug effect
			protease inhibitors	⇑ Drug effect
cayenne *(Capsicum annuum)*	theophylline	⇑ Drug absorption	antiplatelets	⇑ Drug effect
chamomile *(Matricaria chamomilla)*	simvastatin	—	sedatives	⇑ Drug effect
	warfarin			⇑ Drug effect
				⇑ Drug effect
chasteberry *(Vitex agnuscastus)*	—	—	prolactin inhibitors	⇑ Drug effect
cocoa *(Theobroma cacao)*	—	—	antidiabetics	⇓ Drug effect
cranberry *(Vaccinium macrocarpon)*	—	—	warfarin	⇑ Drug effect
dandelion *(Taraxacum officinale)*	—	—	antidiabetics	⇑ Drug effect
			diuretics	⇑ Drug effect
			lithium	⇑ Drug levels
danshen *(Salvia bowelyana; Saliva miltorrhiza)*	warfarin	⇑ Drug effect	antiplatelets	⇑ Drug effect
devil's claw *(Harpagophytum procumbens)*	warfarin	⇑ Drug effect	antiplatelets	⇑ Drug effect
dong quai *(Angelica sinensis)*	warfarin	⇑ Drug effect	antiplatelets	⇑ Drug effect
echinacea *(Echinacea spp.)*	—	—	immunomodulators	Altered drug effect
			protease inhibitors	⇑ Drug effect
elder *(Sambucus nigra)*	—	—	antidiabetics	⇑ Drug effect
evening primrose *(Oenothera biennis)*	—	—	anticoagulants	⇑ Drug effect
			antiplatelets	⇑ Drug effect
			phenothiazines	⇑ Seizure risk
fennel *(Foeniculum vulgare)*	—	—	fluoroquinolones	⇓ Drug absorption
fenugreek *(Trigonella sp.)*	warfarin	⇑ Drug effect	iron	⇓ Drug absorption
feverfew *(Tanacetum parthenium)*	—	—	antiplatelets	⇑ Drug effect
flaxseed *(Linum usitatissium)*	—	—	warfarin	⇑ Drug effect
garcinia *(Garcinia cambogia)*	—	—	warfarin	⇓ Drug effect
garlic *(Allium sativum)*	protease inhibitors	⇓ Drug levels	anticoagulants	⇑ Drug effect
	warfarin	⇑ Drug effect	antidiabetics	⇑ Drug effect
			antiplatelets	⇑ Drug effect
			cyclosporine	⇑ Drug effect
			non-nucleoside RTIs	⇑ Drug effect

Continued

TABLE 6-3 SELECTED HERB-DRUG INTERACTIONS—cont'd

HERBAL INGREDIENT: COMMON AND BOTANICAL NAMES	DOCUMENTED DRUG INTERACTION	COMMENT	POTENTIAL DRUG INTERACTION	COMMENT
ginger *(Zingiber officinale)*	phenprocoumon	⇑ Bleeding risk	anticoagulants	⇑ Drug effect
			antiplatelets	⇑ Drug effect
ginkgo *(Ginkgo biloba)*	trazodone	⇑ Drug effect	anticoagulants	⇑ Drug effect
	antiplatelet agents	⇑ Bleeding risk	antiepileptics	⇓ Drug effect
	nifedipine	⇑ Drug effect	cyclosporine	⇓ Drug absorption
	omeprazole	⇑ Drug effect	Ca^{++} channel blockers	⇓ Drug effect
			MAOIs	⇑ Drug effect
ginseng (Panax ginseng, *Panax quinquefolia*)	warfarin	⇓ Drug effect	anticoagulants	Altered drug effect
	phenelzine	⇑ Drug effect	antidiabetics	⇑ Drug effect
			antiplatelets	Altered drug effect
			immunomodulators	Altered drug effect
			MAOIs	⇑ Drug effect
goldenseal (*Hydrastis canadensis*)	midazolam	⇑ Drug effect	anticoagulants	⇓ Drug effect
			antihypertensives	⇓ Drug effect
			immunomodulators	Altered drug effect
			CYP3A substrate	⇑ Drug effect
green tea *(Camellia sinensis)*	warfarin	⇓ Drug effect	—	—
guggul *(Commiphora mukul)*	—	—	anticoagulants	⇑ Drug effect
			antiplatelets	⇑ Drug effect
			diltiazem	⇓ Drug effect
hawthorn *(Crataegus laevigata)*	—	—	CNS depressants	⇑ Drug effect
			antiarrhythmics	Altered drug effect
			digoxin	⇑ Drug effect
hibiscus *(Hibiscus sabdarifa)*	—	—	chloroquine	⇓ Drug absorption
juniper *(Juniperus communis)*	—	—	antidiabetics	⇓ Drug effect
			diuretics	⇑ Drug effect
			lithium	⇑ Drug levels
kava *(Piper methysticum)*	alprazolam	⇑ Drug effect	antiepileptics	⇑ Drug effect
	levodopa	⇓ Drug effect	CNS depressants	⇑ Drug effect
lemon balm *(Melissa officinalis)*	—	—	CNS depressants	⇑ Drug effect
licorice *(Glycyrrhiza glabra)*	spironolactone	⇓ Drug effect	antihypertensives	⇓ Drug effect
			antiplatelets	⇑ Drug effect
			corticosteroids	⇑ Drug effect
			digoxin	⇑ Drug effect
			diuretics	⇑ Hypokalemia
meadowsweet *(Filipendula ulmaria)*	—	—	warfarin	⇑ Drug effect
milk thistle *(Silybum marianum)*	indinavir	⇓ Drug concentration	CYP3A substrate	Altered drug effect
oleander *(Nerium oleander)*	—	—	digoxin	⇑ Drug effect
papaya *(Carica papaya)*	warfarin	⇑ Drug effect	—	—
passionflower *(Passiflora incarnate)*	—	—	antiepileptics	⇑ Drug effect
			CNS depressants	⇑ Drug effect
			warfarin	⇑ Drug effect
peppermint *(Mentha piperita)*	—	—	iron salts	⇓ Drug absorption
piperine or black pepper *(Piper nigrum)*	phenytoin	⇑ Drug absorption	P-glycoprotein substrate	⇑ Drug absorption
	propranolol	⇑ Drug absorption		
	rifampin	⇑ Drug absorption		
	theophylline	⇑ Drug absorption		
psyllium *(Plantago spp.)*	lithium	⇓ Drug absorption	digoxin	⇓ Drug effect
red clover *(Trifolium pretense)*	—	—	warfarin	⇑ Drug effect
rosemary *(Rosmarinus officinalis)*	—	—	antidiabetics	⇓ Drug effect
St. John's wort *(Hypericum perforatum)*	alprazolam	⇓ Drug effect	amiodarone	⇓ Drug level and effect
	amitriptyline	⇓ Drug level and effect	amsacrine	⇓ Drug effect
	cyclosporine	⇓ Drug level and effect	carbamazepine	⇓ Drug level and effect
	digoxin	⇓ Drug level and effect	diltiazem	⇓ Drug level and effect
	fexofenadine	⇓ Drug level	etoposide	⇓ Drug effect

TABLE 6-3 SELECTED HERB-DRUG INTERACTIONS—cont'd

HERBAL INGREDIENT: COMMON AND BOTANICAL NAMES	DOCUMENTED DRUG INTERACTION	COMMENT	POTENTIAL DRUG INTERACTION	COMMENT
	imatinib	⇓ Drug level	protease inhibitors	⇓ Drug level and effect
	indinavir	⇓ Drug level and effect	triptans	Serotonin syndrome
	irinotecan	⇓ Drug level	verapamil	⇓ Drug level and effect
	ivabridine	⇓ Drug level	CYP3A4 substrate	⇓ Drug level and effect
	midazolam	⇓ Drug level	P-glycoprotein substrate	⇓ Drug level and effect
	nifedipine	⇓ Drug level		
	omeprazole	⇓ Drug level		
	oral contraceptives	⇓ Drug effect		
	SSRIs	Serotonin syndrome		
	simvastatin	⇓ Drug level		
	tacrolimus	⇓ Drug level and effect		
	talinolol	⇓ Drug level		
	theophylline	⇓ Drug level		
	voriconazole	⇓ Drug level		
	warfarin	⇓ Drug effect		
saw palmetto *(Serenoa repens)*	—	—	hormone therapy	⇓ Drug effect
			warfarin	⇑ Drug effect
schisandra *(Schisandra chinensis, S. sphenanthera)*	midazolam	⇑ Drug effect	CYP3A substrate	⇑ Drug effect
	tacrolimus	⇑ Drug effect	P-glycoprotein substrate	⇑ Drug effect
	talinolol	⇑ Drug effect		
senna *(Cassia senna)*	—	—	corticosteroids	⇑ Hypokalemia
			digoxin	⇑ Drug effect
soy (Glycine max)	warfarin	⇓ Drug effect	—	—
uva ursi *(Arctostaphylos uva ursi)*	—	—	iron	⇓ Drug absorption
valerian *(Valeriana officinalis)*	barbiturates	⇑ Drug effect	antiepileptics	⇑ Drug effect
			CNS depressants	⇑ Drug effect
willow bark *(Salix spp.)*	—	—	warfarin	⇑ Drug effect
yohimbe *(Pausinystalia yohimbe)*	—	—	antihypertensives	⇓ Drug effect
			MAOIs	⇑ Hypertension

MAOI, Monoamine oxidase inhibitor; *RTI,* reverse transcriptase inhibitor.

*Interaction risk will depend on patient age, sex, genotype, and comorbid conditions as well as herb or drug dosage form, composition, quality, and duration of use.

Table revised by Joseph I. Boullata, PharmD, BCNSP.

Herbal products can also affect laboratory test results. One significant interaction is the effect of herbal products on blood coagulation as measured by the International Normalized Ratio (INR) system. Examples of herbs that that may decrease INR include St. John's wort, yarrow, and green tea (dose dependent). Herbs that may increase INR and put the patient at increased risk for bleeding include bilberry, black cohosh, chamomile, dong quai, feverfew, garlic, kava kava, and milk thistle.

Not all compounds are safe via all routes. For example, comfrey *(Symphytum officinale)* has both internal and external preparations. Internal use is discouraged because hepatic damage may be fatal. For external use, comfrey is used as an ointment for relief of swelling associated with abrasions and sprains.

Many products have significance for patients facing surgery because they may interfere with the absorption, breakdown, and excretion of anesthetics, anticoagulants, and other surgery-related medications (Herbal Alert 6-4). For example, valerian may increase or prolong the sedative effects of anesthetic agents. Echinacea and St. John's wort have the potential of immunosuppression required for transplant surgeries. Consult the health care provider about the length of herb-free "washout" before surgery. Guidelines reflective of the complexities of surgery related to herbal products are needed.

HERBAL ALERT 6-4

Anticoagulants

The following commonly used herbal products have been reported to interfere with anticoagulants: bilberry, cat's claw, chamomile (German), dong quai, feverfew, garlic, ginseng, ginger, ginkgo, and licorice.

Herbal product advocates have petitioned the FDA to reconsider herbal dietary supplement classification and change to a drug model consistent with European herbal regulations. The FDA is formulating rules that set standards for preparing and labeling dietary supplements to enable the consumer to make more informed choices, for example, the appropriate dosage. For dietary supplement alerts and safety information, visit *www.fda.gov/Food/Dietary/Supplements/Alerts/default.htm.*

TIPS FOR CONSUMERS AND HEALTH CARE PROVIDERS

The following are guidelines for prudent use of herbs:

- Do not take herbs if pregnant or attempting to become pregnant.
- Do not take herbs if nursing.
- Do not give herbs to infants or young children.
- Do not take a large quantity of any one herbal preparation.
- Do not delay in seeking care from the health care provider for persistent or severe symptoms.
- Buy only preparations that have the plant and its quantity listed on the packet.
- Use only herbs that have been bought currently and are fresh.
- Contact the health care provider before stopping use of a prescription medication.
- Store herbal remedies in a cool, dry, dark place; dark containers are preferred.
- Be wary of unsubstantiated claims of "miracle cures."

It is essential that both consumers and health care providers become aware of several crucial factors before trying herbal therapy:

- Consumers must regard herbs as medicines; more is not necessarily better.
- Herbs are not placebos.
- Most herbal remedies are less potent than conventional drugs. However, when prescription or OTC drugs and herbs with similar actions are combined, there is an increased risk of adverse reactions.
- Results may come faster with conventional medicine.
- Safety, efficacy, and dosage are important; multiple reliable sources should be consulted.

Labeling of herbal products is an important safety aspect. The following information should be on the label of herbal products:

- Scientific name of the product and parts of the plant used in preparation
- Manufacturer's name and address
- Batch and lot number
- Dates of manufacture and expiration; many products have a short shelf life

HERBAL RESOURCES

Many herbal resources are available on the Internet. The reader must evaluate each website and decide if the information is credible and appropriate. Following are a few examples of the many Internet resources that provide herbal information.

- American Botanical Council: *www.herbalgram.org*
- NCCAM Clearinghouse: *www.nccam.nih.gov*

The NCCAM Clearinghouse provides information on complementary and alternative medicine (CAM) and NCCAM, including publications and searches of federal databases of scientific and medical literature. The Clearinghouse does not provide medical advice, treatment recommendations, or referrals to practitioners.

- U.S. Food and Drug Administration (FDA): *www.fda.gov*
- Office of Dietary Supplements (ODS), NIH: *www.ods.nih.gov*
- CAM on PubMed: *www.nccam.nih.gov/camonpubmed*

CAM on PubMed is a service of the National Library of Medicine (NLM). PubMed contains publication information and (in most cases) brief summaries of articles from scientific and medical journals.

- U.S. Library of Medicine's MedlinePlus: *www.nlm.nih.gov/medlineplus/herbalmedicine.html*
- The Cochrane Database of Systematic Reviews: *www.cochrane.org/reviews/*

The Cochrane Database of Systematic Reviews is a collection of evidence-based reviews produced by the Cochrane Library, an international nonprofit organization. Reviews summarize the results of clinical trials on health care interventions.

- United States Pharmacopeia: *www.usp.org*
- Herbnet: *www.herbnet.com*
- Herb Research Foundation: *www.herbs.org*

Nursing Process
Patient-Centered Collaborative Care

Herbal Preparations

Assessment

- Obtain baseline information about patient's use of nonconventional therapeutic agents and all prescription and OTC products used.
- Determine product name, brand, dosage, frequency, side effects, and patient's perception of effectiveness.
- Identify all prescription and OTC medications taken by patient; include dosage, frequency, side effects, and perceived effectiveness.

Nursing Diagnosis

- Enhanced readiness about therapeutic regimen related to use of herbal products

Planning

- Patient/family will verbalize understanding of herbal therapy, prescription and OTC medications, interaction between herbal therapy and prescription and OTC medications, and strategies for optimal participation in the therapeutic regimen

Nursing Interventions

- Check patient's response to herbal therapy.
- Monitor patient's response to prescription and OTC medications.
- Consult a dietitian and other specialists as necessary.
- Continue with the same brand of herbal therapy, and advise patient to notify health care provider if considering changing brands or preparations.

Patient Teaching

General

- Explain rationale for herbal therapy (see Herbal Alert 6-1).
- Advise patient to first notify health care provider before substituting any herbal product for prescription or OTC medication.
- Encourage patient to read labels and heed the recommended information displayed on the label.
- Advise patient of portion of plant used in preparation (e.g., flower or root).
- Advise patient about optimal storage conditions of the herbal remedy.

Diet

- Teach patient about foods that enhance or diminish the action of specific herbs.
- Advise patient about foods to avoid, if any, while taking herbs.

Side Effects

- Advise patient of potential side effects of herbal therapy.
- Counsel patient about symptoms that require prompt reporting to the health care provider.

Self-Administration

- Teach patient about preparation of special remedies (e.g., steeping of specific teas).

Cultural Considerations

- Assess personal beliefs of patients from different cultures.
- Modify communication to meet patient's/family's cultural needs.
- Communicate respect for patient's/family's culture.
- Evaluate effectiveness of cultural competence in interactions. If patients believe the health care provider is not sensitive to their beliefs regarding the use of herbs, they are less likely to disclose herbal regimens to future providers.
- Inquire about nutritional practices, and incorporate harmless or nonconflicting practices into the diet.
- Refrain from making prejudicial comments that may inhibit collaboration with healers.
- Do not criticize folk practices; it deters patients from seeking follow-up care and decreases trust and confidence.

Evaluation

- Evaluate the effectiveness of herbal remedies for alleviating symptoms.
- Evaluate patient's use of resources.

KEY WEBSITES

American Herbal Pharmacopoeia: *www.herbal-ahp.org*
The Mayo Clinic: *www.mayoclinic.com*
The Natural Medicines Comprehensive Database: *naturaldatabase.therapeuticresearch.com*

CRITICAL THINKING CASE STUDY

AB, a 49-year-old accountant, reports periods of feeling tired that are increasing in frequency and intensity. On her health history, she lists "no medications on a regular basis." During the nursing history, the nurse learns that AB has been taking ginseng 2 g, b.i.d., ginkgo biloba 300 mg b.i.d., and licorice root 2 mg b.i.d. for the past 6 months. Occasionally, she takes 300 mg t.i.d. of St. John's wort extract.

1. Is AB taking the recommended dose of ginseng and ginkgo biloba? If not, what modifications should the nurse suggest that she consider?
2. AB tells the nurse that she has arthritis. What modifications would be appropriate based on this new information?
3. What specific patient teaching is appropriate for AB at this time?

NCLEX STUDY QUESTIONS

1. What provisions of the Dietary Supplement Health and Education Act of 1994 are most important for the nurse to know related to patient health teaching? (Select all that apply.)
   a. Clarified marketing regulations
   b. Reclassified herbs as dietary supplements
   c. Stated that herbal products can be marketed with suggested dosages
   d. Required that package labels give quality and strength of all contents
   e. Stated that herbs can be used as drug
2. The nurse discovers that a patient has recently decided to take four herbal preparations. Which action will the nurse take first?
   a. Discuss the cost of herbal products.
   b. Instruct the patient to inform the health care provider of all products taken.
   c. Instruct the patient to stop taking all herbal products immediately.
   d. Suggest that the patient taper off use of herbal products over the next 2 weeks.
3. Labeling of herbal products is important. Which is an appropriate claim for an herbal product?
   a. "Prevents diabetes"
   b. "Helps increase blood flow to the extremities"
   c. "Cures Alzheimer's disease"
   d. "Is safe for all"
4. The nurse is reviewing a patient's current medications. Which herbal products interfere with the action of anticoagulants? (Select all that apply.)
   a. aloe
   b. feverfew
   c. ginger
   d. licorice
   e. cranberry
5. A patient has multiple prescription medications and is not able to recall which herbal product he uses for relief of migraine headaches. He notes that it is a serum antagonist and asks the nurse to assist him. What is the best response by the nurse?
   a. "Valerian"
   b. "Feverfew"
   c. "Milk thistle"
   d. "Ginkgo"
6. A patient is being followed by a cardiovascular clinic and takes garlic, which is reported to decrease cholesterol, triglycerides, blood pressure, and blood-clotting capability. Which patient statement indicates a need for further teaching? (Select all that apply.)
   a. "I can just take garlic for my heart problems."
   b. "Garlic may provide some decrease in blood pressure."
   c. "Garlic is very effective in preventing depression."
   d. "Garlic may promote healing of my incision."
   e. "Garlic will not cure impotence."
7. The nurse notes that many patients are taking herbal remedies for relief of depression and anxiety. Which herbal preparation has at least 10 pharmacologically active components for relief of depression and anxiety?
   a. St. John's wort
   b. licorice
   c. saw palmetto
   d. goldenseal
8. A patient who is pregnant asks the nurse, "What herbal products can I take?" What is the best response by the nurse?
   a. "What are you taking now?"
   b. "Taking a product at bedtime is usually not a problem."
   c. "How long have you been taking herbal products?"
   d. "Discuss this with your health care provider."
9. A patient reports taking aloe, ginkgo, and licorice on a regular basis. Which patient statement indicates a need for health teaching about potential drug interactions?
   a. "Aloe decreases the effect of my digoxin."
   b. "Ginkgo decreases the effects of my antiepileptics."
   c. "Licorice increases the effect of my digoxin."
   d. "Licorice decreases the effect of my antihypertensives."

Answers: 1, a, b, c; 2, b; 3, b; 4, b, c, d; 5, b; 6, a, c; 7, a; 8, d; 9, a.

CHAPTER

7

Pediatric Pharmacology

Judith Herrman

evolve WEBSITE

http://evolve.elsevier.com/KeeHayes/pharmacology/

- Animations
- Content Updates
- Key Points
- Review Questions for the NCLEX® Examination
- References from the Textbook
- Unfolding Case Studies

OBJECTIVES

- Apply principles of pharmacokinetics and pharmacodynamics to pediatric medication administration.
- Differentiate components of pharmacology unique to pediatric patients.
- Synthesize knowledge about pediatric medication safety and administration to current or potential nursing practice.

OUTLINE

Pharmacokinetics
- Absorption
- Distribution
- Metabolism
- Excretion

Pharmacodynamics

Nursing Implications
- Pediatric Medication Dosing and Monitoring
- Pediatric Medication Administration

Considerations for the Adolescent Patient

Nursing Process: Patient-Centered Collaborative Care
- Nursing Process: Patient-Centered Collaborative Care: Pediatrics

Key Websites

Critical Thinking Case Studies

NCLEX Study Questions

KEY TERMS

atraumatic care, p. 83
family-centered care, p. 82
first-pass effect, p. 81
pharmacodynamics, p. 82
pharmacokinetics, p. 80

A nurse who is providing care to children must make certain adaptations in assessments, treatments, and evaluations of nursing care because of the physiologic, psychological, and developmental differences inherent in this population. This is especially true in the science of pharmacology, in both the administration of medications to children and evaluation of the therapeutic and adverse effects of a medication. This chapter addresses pediatric nursing adaptations and discusses the impact of a child's growth and development on many aspects of pharmacology: pharmacokinetics, pharmacodynamics, dosing and monitoring, methods of medication administration, and nursing implications.

Pharmacology as it relates to the nursing care of infants, children, and adolescents is limited by the research available in providing protocols of recommended dosages, safe practices, key assessments, and important nursing implications. Most information available about medications is concluded from studies that use adult samples, small sample sizes, or samples with healthy children. Few studies have been conducted to determine the effectiveness of medication for target populations of children diagnosed as having applicable illnesses. Generalizing results of adult studies to pediatric populations (as in applying principles of adult pharmacology to dictate pediatric nursing practice) may result in serious errors

SAFETY: Preventing Medication Errors

Pediatric Pharmacology

- Owing to developmental factors and smaller body size, infants and young children may receive very small dosages of medications. Careful calculations, double-checking math, and checking with another registered nurse may prevent medication errors.
- Ensure that families understand the units of measurement for a medication. Confusion may occur with the discussion of metric, household, and other measurement systems.
- For safety when administering injectable medications to children, use the smallest syringe that ensures the most exact measurement of the medication.
- Use the correct medication and procedure to ensure safe dosing. Dilutions, different concentrations, and different solutions of a prescribed medication can complicate giving appropriate pediatric dosages.
- Infants and children may not be able to confirm identity, allergies, or medications. The nurse must be positive of such information before medication administration.
- Nurses must be vigilant for severe side effects or adverse reactions to medications, because information related to pediatric responses to medications is limited.
- Regulatory agencies caution that medication errors are more common in pediatric patients, warranting increased precautions in medication administration.

and ignore the impact of growth and development on pharmacology.

Research related to pediatric patients is limited because of several factors. Research risks and obtaining informed consent make it difficult to recruit a pediatric sample. Parents and guardians are reluctant to provide permission for children to participate in research studies because of the risk involved and the potentially invasive nature of data gathering. Pharmaceutical companies invest fewer resources in pediatric drug research because of the smaller market share afforded to pediatric medications. Many perceive pediatric pharmacologic research as unethical if it involves profit-margin factors. Others contend that lack of pediatric data reflects lack of due diligence, especially when medications are administered to pediatric patients without supporting research data on which to base safe practices. As a result, less is known about the effects, uses, and dosages of pediatric medications, and nurses must investigate pediatric medications carefully to provide knowledgeable nursing care for children.

Closely aligned with the conflicts that affect pediatric pharmacologic research are those associated with medication labeling and dosing instructions. Because many drugs have not undergone the clinical trials required for federal approval, they have not been approved for pediatric use. Safe use for children may be guided by small studies or the judgment of the clinician and may be based on anecdotal rather than scientific study. These conflicts have generated new legislation designed to protect pediatric patients and provide health care professionals with better information and resources.

In the United States, approximately 25% of all medications carry federally approved indications for use in children, but almost 75% of drugs marketed for adults are also prescribed for children. As a result of legislation presented in 1992 and 1994, the U.S. Food and Drug Administration (FDA) requires many medications to include known dosages, adverse effects, precautions, and effectiveness to provide health care professionals and the public some level of security when using medications. In 2003, a law known as the *Pediatric Research Equity Act* joined the Best Pharmaceuticals Act of 2002 to require drug manufacturers to study pediatric medication use and offer incentives for pediatric pharmacology research. Current research agendas reinforce the need for pediatric medication research and establishment of safe guidelines for pediatric medication dosing, administration, and evaluation. Even with increasing data, many drugs are prescribed based on off-label instructions, expert opinions, small clinical trials, or practitioners' personal experiences with the medication.

PHARMACOKINETICS

Significant differences exist in drug pharmacokinetics for pediatric patients versus adults. These distinctions stem from differences in body composition and organ maturity and appear to be more pronounced in neonates and infants but less significant in school-age and adolescent children. **Pharmacokinetics** may be defined as the study of the time course of drug absorption, distribution, metabolism, and excretion.

Absorption

The degree and rate of absorption are based on factors such as the child's age, health status, and weight, and the route of administration. As children grow and develop, the absorption of medications generally becomes more effective; therefore, less developed absorption in neonates and infants must be considered in dosage and administration. In contrast, during the adolescent years, poor nutritional habits, changes in physical maturity, and hormonal differences may cause slowing of medication absorption. Hydration status, presence of underlying disease, and gastrointestinal (GI) disorders in the child may be significant factors in the absorption of medications.

Drug absorption is initially influenced by the route of administration. For oral medication, conditions in the stomach and intestine, such as gastric acidity, gastric emptying, gastric motility, GI surface area, enzyme levels, and intestinal flora, all mediate drug absorption. Lack of maturation of the GI tract is most pronounced in infancy, making the neonatal and infancy periods those most affected by changes in absorption physiology. Gastric pH is alkaline at birth; acid production begins in the neonatal period. Gastric pH may not reach adult acidity until age 1 to 3 years. A low pH or acidic environment favors acidic drug absorption, whereas a high pH or alkaline environment favors basic drug formulations; therefore, differences in pH may hinder or enhance the absorption of medications. Gastric emptying is generally prolonged in neonates and infants but increases as the child grows. Nurses should be aware that delayed emptying in children reduces the peak serum concentrations of medications.

Varying transit times through the GI system may also hinder or enhance absorption of oral medications, depending on the usual site of chemical absorption. For this reason, feeding methods may affect infant absorption; for example, breastfed infants have faster gastric emptying than formula-fed infants. Frequent infant feedings also affect GI transit times. The more frequent the feedings, the less time the food is in contact with the gastric or intestinal lining.

Irregular peristalsis associated with immaturity or with symptoms of vomiting or diarrhea decreases the absorption time available for medications. In contrast, many pediatric medications actually cause diarrhea, which again bears on absorption rates. In younger infants and children, the GI surface area is greater than in adults, allowing for more absorptive area in the stomach and intestines. This difference in pediatric anatomy and physiology may affect the speed and effectiveness of absorption, especially in the small intestine. Immature enzyme function may also affect drug absorption; for example, low lipase levels deter the absorption of lipid-soluble medications. Microorganism colonization of the intestine, as it changes with pH and flora, creates different environments that may change medication absorption. All of these factors must be considered when assessing the effectiveness of medications administered by the oral route.

For medications administered via the subcutaneous (subQ) or intramuscular (IM) routes, absorption occurs at the tissue level. The level of peripheral perfusion and effectiveness of circulation affects the medication's ability to be absorbed. Conditions that alter perfusion (e.g., dehydration, cold temperatures, alterations in cardiac status) may impede absorption of medications in the tissues. Intravenous (IV) medications are administered directly into the bloodstream and are immediately absorbed and distributed.

Topical medications—those absorbed through the skin—may be altered by the condition of the skin tissue. Because children's skin is thinner and more porous, absorption may be enhanced. The skin surface area for children is proportionately higher than for adults such that many medications are more readily absorbed than in adults.

Distribution

The distribution of medication throughout the body of a child is affected by factors such as body fluid composition, body tissue composition, protein-binding capability, and effectiveness of various barriers to medication transport. In neonates and young infants, the human body is about 70% water. (As the child grows, this percentage decreases to 50% to 60%.) This increased body fluid proportion in the very young allows for a greater volume of fluid in which to distribute medication and a lower concentration of the drug. Until about age 2 years, the pediatric patient requires higher doses of water-soluble medications to achieve therapeutic levels. Younger patients also have higher levels of extracellular fluids, which increase the tendency for children to become dehydrated and change the distribution of water-soluble medications.

Neonates and young infants tend to have less body fat than older children. The difference means that this age group requires less fat-soluble medications than adults, because fat-soluble drugs saturate fat tissue before acting on body tissues. Less fat available for saturation creates a need for less medication.

Drugs become bound to circulating plasma proteins in the body. Only drugs that are free, or unbound, are available to cross the cell membrane and exert an effect. Infants and neonates have less albumin than older patients and fewer protein receptor sites available for binding with medication; this allows medication to be more available for use and dictates a decrease in the dosage needed in young patients to produce the same therapeutic effect. Greater quantities of circulating drugs caused by reduced plasma proteins increase the propensity for adverse or toxic reactions in infants younger than 1 year. In neonates, high bilirubin levels may pose a health risk related to the administration of medications. Bilirubin molecules may bind with plasma protein sites, making the sites unavailable to medications and allowing large amounts of drug to remain free and available for effect. If neonatal medications are prescribed, dosages must be decreased and closely monitored to both ensure therapeutic effectiveness and avoid adverse effects.

Anatomic barriers to medication distribution, such as the skin or the blood-brain barrier, must be considered when drugs are administered to pediatric patients. The skin is more absorptive in young children, as previously described, and allows rapid distribution of medication. Infants' blood-brain barriers are relatively immature, allowing medications to pass easily into nervous system tissue and increasing the likelihood for toxicity. As a child matures, both of these barriers become more impervious to medication, and dosages must be titrated accordingly.

Metabolism

The metabolism of medications depends greatly on the maturation level of the pediatric patient and varies from child to child. Metabolism is carried out primarily in the liver, with the kidneys and lungs playing a small part in the metabolic stage. For most children younger than 2 years, sustained decreases in levels of hepatic enzymes result in slower metabolism of medications. Hepatic metabolic activity is lower in neonates; infant hepatic function matures at age 1 to 2 months. This issue, as with other pharmacokinetic factors, reinforces the importance of the nurse evaluating therapeutic effects and monitoring adverse effects of medications.

Children inherently have higher metabolic rates than adults, causing metabolism to occur more rapidly. This may necessitate a higher medication requirement than for adults. For example, pain medication for children may require increased dosages or decreased durations between dosages. After oral medications are absorbed, they are metabolized in the liver. This phenomenon, called the **first-pass effect,** causes drugs administered by the oral route and absorbed via the GI tract to undergo some metabolism in the hepatocytes in the liver before they are made available to the body tissues. For select medications, when the oral route is ordered, the first-pass effect must be considered in the calculation of dosages. Some medications are administered by the rectal route to avoid the hepatic first-pass effect.

Excretion

The excretion of medications occurs in the kidneys, intestines, lungs, sweat glands, salivary glands, and mammary glands, with the kidneys providing the most elimination. Before about age 9 months, infants experience a reduction in the elimination capacity of the kidneys because of decreased renal blood flow, decreased glomerular filtration rate, and reduced renal tubular function. (At the onset of adolescence, renal tubular function is again decreased.) Because medications are excreted more slowly as a result of this decreased renal function, they can accumulate and may reach toxic levels. Water is needed for the effective excretion of medication, so patients must be evaluated for dehydration. Nurses need to carefully monitor renal function, urine flow, and medication effectiveness to evaluate the impact of medication excretion on patient status.

PHARMACODYNAMICS

Pharmacodynamics have also been used to describe differences in pediatric pharmacology. **Pharmacodynamics** refers to the mechanisms of action and effect of a drug on the body and includes the onset, peak, and duration of effect of a medication. It can also be described as the intensity and time course of therapeutic and adverse effects of medications. The variables of pharmacokinetics—absorption, distribution, metabolism, and excretion—all affect the parameters of pharmacodynamics. These processes determine the time a medication begins to function, reaches its peak, and sustains its length of action. The half-life of a medication may be different in children than in adults. Pediatric variables such as organ function, developmental factors, and administration issues affect drug pharmacodynamics and require nurses to knowledgeably evaluate the action and effectiveness of pediatric medications.

NURSING IMPLICATIONS

Pediatric Medication Dosing and Monitoring

Because of the changes in pharmacokinetics and pharmacodynamics inherent in pediatric patients, a key nursing role is to monitor the patient for therapeutic effect and adverse reactions. The processes described earlier in the chapter may be measured using plasma or serum drug levels, which indicate the amount of medication in a patient's body. Close monitoring of serum drug levels can assist in establishing appropriate dosages, schedules, and routes of administration. Monitoring can also assist in indicating when the dose is too high (toxic) or too low (not therapeutic). The therapeutic ranges established for many drug levels are based on adult studies, so it is important for the nurse to assess pediatric patients in conjunction with monitoring blood levels. Serum blood levels are not available for all medications, so patient clinical responses to medications are especially important when monitoring drug effects.

The calculation of pediatric dosages is based in part on FDA recommendations, approved protocols, research studies, and provider experience. Most medications are ordered based on the child's weight in kilograms; therefore, a "dose per unit of weight" calculation is required. In caring for children of higher weights, dosages are, at times, calculated on lean body mass to ensure an appropriate dose. Some medications, such as chemotherapies, are prescribed based on body surface area (BSA, or mg/m^2). Dosing must also consider the individual child's status, including age, organ function, health, and route of administration.

Pediatric Medication Administration

A key issue with pediatric medication administration is confirming the identification of the patient who is to receive the dose. Using the patient's identification wristband in inpatient settings is the most effective method to ensure patient identity; outpatient and other settings pose a greater challenge. Children may not be able to communicate or want to divulge their names. To ensure safe medication administration, a reliable method to identify patients for each setting must be created. Automated computerized and bar-coding systems are especially effective in ensuring safe medication administration in the pediatric population. It is the nurse's responsibility to check medication dosages and ensure that they are safe and effective.

Developmental and cognitive differences must always be considered when administering medication to children. It is important for the nurse to differentiate the child's developmental age from the chronologic age, because this difference has an impact on the child's response and responsiveness to medication. The pediatric patient's ability to understand the process, the reasons for medication, and the need to cooperate with the procedure must always figure prominently in the pediatric nurse's plan of care. The child's temperament may influence understanding and level of cooperation. Especially in pediatric nursing, the concept of **family-centered care** is essential to ensuring safe care during and after health care intervention. Teaching is directed toward family caregivers and patients commensurate with the cognitive level of the child. When possible, family members or caregivers should be solicited to assist in medication administration, taught how to administer the medications, and instructed on methods to evaluate effectiveness. These significant persons in the child's life, individuals who know the child on a day-to-day basis, are usually in the best position to evaluate the effectiveness of a medication and observe for adverse reactions. Some adverse reactions of medication in a child (e.g., ringing in ears, nausea) may be difficult to evaluate; those closest to the child may be in the best position to assess for these responses. However, parents or other family members may request not to participate in invasive procedures. This request should be respected, and parents or guardians should be encouraged to provide comfort to the child after medication is administered. Caregivers should always be supported in their caring function so that the child feels safe and secure.

Cognitive issues must be addressed such as the ability to understand (1) the reason for the medication, (2) the need for the medication despite unpleasant taste or method of administration, and (3) the need to complete all doses and courses of medication. When the family is taught about pediatric drug administration, education for the child—at a developmentally appropriate level—must also be included. Communication with the child and family must always consider level of knowledge, developmental age, cultural factors, and levels of anxiety. The nurse should use optimal interpersonal skills to ensure the best outcome in the administration of medications to pediatric patients.

The primary concerns in administering medications to infants are maintaining safety with the minimum restraint necessary, administering the correct dosage, and providing care with as much comforting as possible. Toddlers may react violently and negatively to medication administration. Simple explanations, a firm approach, and enlisting the imagination of a toddler through play may enhance success with medication administration. Preschoolers are fairly cooperative and respond well to age-appropriate explanations. Allowing some level of choice and control may facilitate success with preschool children. School-age children, although often cooperative, may fear bodily injury and should be permitted even more control, involvement in the process, and information. Age-appropriate fears related to pain, changes in body image, and injury are prevalent among older school-age and adolescent patients. The nurse should establish a positive rapport with the patient, contract with the adolescent related to the plan of care, and ensure privacy in all aspects of medication administration. Parents or guardians must be able to practice and repeat the psychomotor skills associated with medication administration.

Most pediatric medications are administered via the oral route. This route is the least invasive and easiest to use and can be used by family and home caregivers. Topical, rectal, and parenteral routes (i.e., subQ, IM, IV) are also used to deliver medications to pediatric patients for whom the oral route is contraindicated. Because of tissue differences among children, the IV route is more predictable than other routes.

Most oral medications are administered to children using an oral syringe. Oral syringes ensure more exact dosing and are relatively easy to use. Syringes may be marked to ensure correct dosages. The syringe is inserted into either side of the mouth and pointed toward the buccal mucosa. Depositing the medication too close to the front of the mouth increases the likelihood that the medication will be spit out. Pointing the syringe directly toward the back of the mouth may increase the risk for gagging or choking. Infants may suck medication from a bottle nipple into which the measured medication has been squirted from the oral syringe. Preschool and school-age children are usually able to inject oral medication into their own mouths, enhancing their sense of control over what can be an anxiety-provoking situation.

Nurses may need to crush pills or dissolve capsules in fluid for administration to pediatric patients. It is the nurse's responsibility to access information on the advisability of crushing or dissolving a medication before administration; some medications, such as time-released or enteric-coated medications, should *not* be crushed or dissolved. Some medications may be made more palatable by adding jelly, syrup, or honey (infants younger than 1 year should not be given honey because of the risk of botulism). Small volumes should be used to dilute medications so the patient is ensured the full dose. As pediatric medication research increases, more medications will be available in stable liquid pediatric forms. Until then, the nurse should work closely with pharmacy and hospital policies to ensure safe administration of oral medications to children. For children who refuse to take medication by mouth or children who require tube feeding, oral medications can be administered via nasogastric, orogastric, or gastrostomy tubes. Precautions required when giving medications via this route are similar to those implemented when administering feedings.

The administration of subQ, IM, and IV medications to children includes many of the same principles as adults, with additional considerations. Safe restraint and atraumatic care principles should be used when possible. Hockenberry defines **atraumatic care** as the delivery of therapeutic care through the implementation of interventions that "eliminate or minimize the psychological and physical distress experienced by children and their families in the health care system." Depending on developmental age, the child may have incorrect interpretations about the need for medication, believing that the medication is a punishment or a result of wrongdoing. The nurse should provide preparation for the procedure at the appropriate level for the child and involve caregivers in all aspects of care. One method to ensure atraumatic care is through the use of topical analgesics on the site before IM, subQ, or IV injections. Eutectic mixture of local anesthetics (EMLA), a topical cream, anesthetizes the site of injection if applied 1 to 2.5 hours before injection. After EMLA is applied to the injection site, the site is covered with a transparent dressing for containment. Also available are iontophoresis (Numby Stuff), a vasocoolant spray, and buffered lidocaine injections. Powdered lidocaine preparations are effective in reducing the pain and fear associated with invasive procedures in children, such as venipuncture. LET (lidocaine, epinephrine, and tetracaine) is another topical anesthetic agent used for children undergoing invasive procedures.

Based on the cognitive level of the child, distraction and other nonpharmacologic methods of pain and anxiety control can also be used to decrease the perception of pain. The use of creative imagery and hypnosis with toddlers and preschool children has been explored as a pain-management strategy. Wallace and colleagues describe the "cough trick," in which children are taught to initiate a cough during injections. This method is effective in reducing perceptions of pain in children during immunizations. Injections should *never* be given to a sleeping child with the intent to surprise the child with a quick procedure. The child may subsequently experience a lack of trust and be reluctant to sleep in the future.

IV infusion sites must be protected, especially in infants and toddlers, who do not understand the rationale or importance of maintaining the IV site. Commercial products are available to protect the IV site and maintain an intact IV infusion set. Stocking-like covers may hide the IV site from infants before they master the concept of object permanence. The patency of an IV site should be checked before each medication administration to avoid infiltration and extravasation. Any injection site on a preschooler should be covered with a bandage, preferably a decorated one, so that the child does not fear "leakage" from the area. Selection of injection and IV sites is made based on developmental variables, site of preference, and access to administration sites. The dorsogluteal site is no longer recommended for pediatric patients because of lack of development of the muscle and potential for sciatic nerve damage. The ventrogluteal or the vastus lateralis are preferred sites for pediatric IM injections. The length of the needle depends on the child's muscle mass and subQ tissue and the site of injection. The child may prefer subQ injections in the leg or upper arm rather than in the abdomen. IV sites may be difficult to find in children. Amount of fat tissue, hydration status of the child, and ability to isolate and immobilize veins are all mitigating factors.

When administering medications to children, follow these basic principles: honesty, respect, age-appropriate teaching and explanations, attention to safety, atraumatic care, using the least amount of restraint necessary, providing positive reinforcement for age-appropriate cooperation, refraining from use of negative messages or behaviors, and upholding family-centered principles. These standards may be used throughout the pediatric life span and highlight the need for nursing intervention that is sensitive, individualized, and caring.

CONSIDERATIONS FOR THE ADOLESCENT PATIENT

Adolescent patients need individualized nursing care specific to this developmental stage. Age-oriented developmental considerations include physical changes, cognitive level and abilities, emotional factors, and impact of chronic illness.

Physically, adolescence is a highly diverse period of growth and development. Growth rates during these years may be affected by nutrition, factors within the environment, genetics and heredity, and gender. A group of adolescents of similar ages may manifest very different sizes, height-to-weight proportions, timing of secondary sex characteristics, and other indicators of physical maturity. These differences may warrant individualization of dosages based on weight or body surface area, even when the adolescent meets or exceeds the size of standard adults. For example, an adjustment may be required in the dosage of a lipid-soluble medication, because of the changes in lean-to-fat body mass, especially in young adolescent males, that coincide with physical maturation. Hormonal changes and growth spurts may necessitate changes in medication dosages; many children with chronic illnesses require dosage adjustments in the early teen years as a result of these transitions. Sleep requirements and metabolic rates may greatly increase during the teen years, along with appetite and food consumption, which may affect their scheduling of and response to medications. Although adolescents' physical appearance and organ structure and function resemble those of adults, their bodies continue to grow and change, requiring increased vigilance in monitoring therapeutic and toxic drug levels.

The cognitive level and abilities of adolescents may pose additional considerations for the pediatric nurse. Cognitive theorists have posited that adolescents progress from concrete to abstract reasoning. Individuals who are still in the concrete operational stage may have difficulty comprehending how a medication exerts its effects on the body and the importance of meticulous dosing and administration. Teenagers may also have difficulty understanding such concepts as drug interactions, side effects, adverse reactions, and therapeutic levels. For example, the patient taking birth control pills may or may not be able to comprehend the potential implications and extra precautions needed when taking an antagonistic antibiotic during an acute infection. Patient teaching must consider the cognitive level of the individual; as adolescents learn to reason in an abstract manner, teaching may be based on more complex information. Potentially, teen perceptions of invulnerability and their difficulty in relating future consequences to current actions may dictate that the nurse adapt teaching to address specific adolescent thought processes. Newer research into the teenage brain and the ongoing development of decision-making, social, and reasoning skills may inform how nurses assess and intervene with the pediatric patient. An adolescent who is told that an insulin injection schedule must be adhered to in order to avoid long-term complications may not understand the rationales for treatment if he or she is only substantiated by abstract, future-oriented risks. The same patient may find the relationship between using insulin to maintain normoglycemia and the ability to participate in sports more immediate and relevant.

Emotional development of the teenager also occurs on an individual basis. The teen years are characterized by sensation seeking, risk taking, questioning, formation of identity, and increasing influences exerted by peer groups. The nurse should assess for high-risk behaviors, including use of alcohol, tobacco, and recreational drugs, to avoid potential drug interactions. Other issues, including sexual practices and stressful family and social situations, may affect the patient's response to medications. Nurses must be respectful of the emotional needs of adolescence while attending to the mental health issues that may surface during these years. A comprehensive history must be solicited from teenage patients to ensure appropriate medication administration.

The nurse is often positioned in a key role for establishing a productive working relationship with the patient and providing the patient with appropriate levels of privacy. Allowing the adolescent to verbalize concerns about the medication and its regimen may offer opportunities for clarifying misconceptions and teaching new concepts. The nurse must also be conscious of the need to exercise care in offering confidentiality in the event that information needs to be divulged to other health care providers, parents, or caregivers to ensure patient safety.

As adolescents attain greater levels of independence from their parents, self-care behaviors increase. The nurse should assess the patient's abilities to self-administer medication and self-monitor therapeutic and adverse reactions. Teenagers spending less time with parents and caregivers may need increased instruction about their medication regimen and the key observations that are needed. Although teenagers frequently display "breaking away" behaviors in response to parental bonds, they often continue to use parent or caregiver medication habits as models for their own medication behaviors.

For the child with a chronic illness, issues may change in the teen years. Engaging peers in the medication plan of care, allowing the teenager to make safe choices and have flexibility within that plan, setting up mutual medication contracts, and permitting the patient to design his or her own adult-monitored medication regimen may facilitate adherence. The family's key role in management of chronic illness changes during adolescence. Such issues as rebellion against rules, refusal to take medications, and participation in high-risk behaviors may need to be dealt with. The nurse can facilitate required adaptations and support both the patient and the family during these times.

Teenagers who need to receive medications may require assistance with decision making, organization of a medication schedule, and understanding of the key physical, cognitive, and emotional changes characteristic of this stage. Nurses' levels of knowledge and caring support may offer a great contribution to adolescent patients and their families.

NURSING PROCESS: PATIENT-CENTERED COLLABORATIVE CARE

In working with pediatric patients, key developmental differences must be considered when administering and monitoring medications. The nursing process provides the framework to guide nursing practice in administering medications, planning and evaluating nursing care, providing patient and family teaching, and incorporating the family into all aspects of treatment.

Family and patient teaching is a key role for the nurse. Issues such as indications for the medication, the side effects, the dose, how to measure the dose, how to administer the dose, the therapeutic effect, adverse effects to monitor for, the duration, and the frequency are all important information needed by the family or caregiver. Specifics such as the need for refrigeration, the need to shake the medicine, the difference between household and prescriptive measurements, and other issues should be addressed to ensure patient safety. Adherence to the medication regimen is of paramount importance with children and families; providing written instructions or a medication calendar may facilitate this through concrete reminders.

Nurses should also be aware of the tendency for parents to treat infants and children with over-the-counter (OTC) analgesics. Parents may provide frequent analgesia to their children and may be largely unaware of the potential for misuse and overuse in the pediatric population. Additional concern has arisen regarding the inappropriate use of OTC cough and cold remedies with children. Deaths and significant illness have been attributed to lack of label recommendations, misuse of adult medications, poor medication instructions, and overdose, warranting rigid restrictions on their use in the pediatric population.

HERBAL ALERT 7-1

Pediatric

Herbal preparations are generally not recommended for use in children.

Nursing Process
Patient-Centered Collaborative Care

Pediatrics

Assessment

- Record the age, weight, and height of the child. Drug calculations are based on these three factors.
- Assess the allergy history of the child, and determine family allergy history.
- Assess developmental age, health status, nutritional status, and hydration status.
- Assess history of drug use (prescriptions, OTC, herbal).
- Assess family's understanding and child's cognitive level.

Nursing Diagnoses

- Delayed growth and development related to physiologic, congenital, or environmental factors
- Risk for ineffective peripheral tissue perfusion related to decreased fluid volume, decreased cardiac output, or developmental physiologic differences
- Impaired urinary elimination related to decreased fluid volume, renal immaturity, congenital anomalies, or decreased renal perfusion
- Deficient knowledge related to new parenting role, lack of exposure to children and adolescents, language barrier, cognitive discrepancy, or new diagnosis
- Risk for injury related to developmental, cognitive, and environmental factors
- Ineffective health maintenance related to cognitive, experiential, environmental, and social factors
- Readiness for enhanced knowledge related to parenting and progression through child's developmental stages

Planning

- The child will receive drug dosage based on age, weight, and height. Most drug calculations for children are related to weight in kilograms or BSA.
- Consider developmental factors and elements of family-centered care in all medication administration.

Nursing Interventions

- Use appropriate drug references to obtain the drug parameters or ranges, side effects, and contraindications for use when administering drugs to children.
- Monitor infants and young children closely for side effects of drugs because of their developmental differences. Because infants and young children have limited communication skills, changes in their usual behavior pattern may indicate side effects.
- Communicate with the health care provider about drug dosages that are questionable for infants and young children because of developmental differences. Calculate the child's drug dose according to weight in kilograms or BSA.

Patient Teaching

- Teaching patients and families about medications, dosages, therapeutic effects, side effects, and precautions is key in the pediatric population, especially with nonverbal, young, or at-risk children.
- Advise the responsible family member not to give OTC drugs to children without first consulting the health care provider.
- Advise the family member to immediately report side effects of the medication to the health care provider.
- Advise mothers who are breastfeeding their newborn or infant to consult a health care provider when taking any medication, because a portion of most drugs is excreted in breast milk.
- Nurses must be aware that parents and families frequently believe that all pediatric infections are treated with an antibiotic. The nurse plays a key role in raising awareness about avoiding the overuse of antibiotics for viral infections and allergic responses to avoid the development of resistant organisms.
- Advise the family member to keep medications out of the reach of children.
- Suggest that the family member use child-resistant medication containers.

Cultural Considerations

- Consider cultural differences when providing care and teaching about medications to children and families. These may include areas such as eye contact, personal space, time orientation, parenting roles/beliefs, value of children, and communication styles.
- Some cultures may adhere to folk and other health practices, including using herbal preparations for children. Nurses should ensure that families understand the contraindications and precautions associated with use of herbal products in children.
- When soliciting adolescent health histories, consider issues related to sexual practices, risk behaviors, recreational drug use, and other issues that may affect medication administration and safety. Provide privacy when asking sensitive questions.

Evaluation

- Evaluate the family member's knowledge about the drug, the dosage, the schedule for administration, and the side effects.
- Evaluate the child's physiologic and psychological response to the drug regimen.
- Evaluate the therapeutic and adverse effects of the medication(s).

KEY WEBSITES

American Academy of Pediatrics: *www.aap.org*

General pediatric information: *www.keepkidshealthy.com* and *www.kidshealth.org*

CRITICAL THINKING CASE STUDY

A 6-month-old child enters the emergency department with a 3-day history of vomiting with diarrhea. The patient is started on IV hydration. A stool culture indicates a bacterial infection in the GI tract.

1. How might the diagnosis of dehydration affect the pharmacokinetics of IV antibiotic therapy?
2. What physiologic factors make young babies prone to dehydration?
3. What components of family-centered care are critical for infants and their families when ill or hospitalized?

NCLEX STUDY QUESTIONS

1. An 8-month-old patient is discharged from the hospital with a plan of care to receive IM injections each day. The parents have been taught how to administer IM injections. Which statement by the parents indicates a need for further teaching?
   a. "I should administer the injection in the upper, outer quadrant of her buttocks."
   b. "IM injections are safe for infants and children if administered correctly."
   c. "When I give my daughter this injection, the safest place for insertion is the thigh."
   d. "I need someone to assist me and hold my daughter while I give the injection."
2. A 4-year-old patient is discharged on an oral liquid drug suspension of 4 mL per dose. Which device will the nurse recommend to ensure the highest level of accuracy in home administration of the medication?
   a. Measuring spoon
   b. Graduated medicine cup
   c. Household teaspoon
   d. Oral syringe
3. A child is ordered to receive naloxone (Narcan) IV, STAT. The child's weight is 20 kg. The recommended child's dosage is 0.01 mg/kg. Naloxone is available in a 400 mcg/mL solution. How much medication will the nurse plan to administer?
4. A child is ordered to receive 3 mg/kg of medication. The child weighs 88 pounds. The medication is available in a 15 mg/mL elixir. How much medication will the patient receive?
5. The nurse understands the differences between drug excretion in children and that in adults. With this knowledge, what does the nurse consider when administering medications to children?
   a. Most children need a higher dose of medication, so the nurse will contact the physician for an increase in the ordered dose.
   b. Children excrete drugs rapidly, so the nurse must assess carefully for therapeutic effects of the medication.
   c. The most important assessment is to evaluate for drug accumulation, because the excretion of drugs in children is slower.
   d. Excretion of most drugs is the same in children as in adults, but assessments are important to avoid side effects.
6. A parent is learning to administer medication to a school-age child. Which strategy will the nurse teach the parent to achieve cooperation in a child of this age?
   a. Enlisting physical restraint
   b. Establishing medication contracts
   c. Providing age-appropriate explanations
   d. Tolerating violent reactions
7. The nurse is caring for a neonate with lower-than-normal albumin levels. The nurse is ordered to administer a medication that is highly protein bound. The nurse knows that what must occur in response to these factors?
   a. The dose must be doubled to compensate for low albumin levels.
   b. The dose must be decreased because of increased unbound, active medication.
   c. Highly protein-bound drugs must be contraindicated.
   d. The nurse must further clarify the medication order before administration.
8. A nurse caring for a child with developmental delay prepares to teach the patient about prescribed medications. Which actions are essential in ensuring patient safety? (Select all that apply.)
   a. Assess the child's developmental age.
   b. Assess for side effects the same as those experienced by adults.
   c. Consider the actions and uses of the medication.
   d. Focus on the child's chronological age.
   e. Involve the family in teaching sessions.
9. A 2-year-old patient is to receive a topical medication. The nurse considers which factor when administering this medication?
   a. Children's skin is less vascular, slowing absorption.
   b. Decreased hair follicles enhance absorption.
   c. Medications are absorbed slower due to less BSA than adults.
   d. Thinner skin in children allows for rapid absorption.

Answers: 1, a; 2, d; 3, 0.5 mL; 4, 8 mL; 5, c; 6, c; 7, b; 8, a, c, e; 9, d.

CHAPTER

8

Geriatric Pharmacology

evolve WEBSITE

http://evolve.elsevier.com/KeeHayes/pharmacology/

- Animations
- Content Updates
- Key Points
- Review Questions for the NCLEX® Examination
- References from the Textbook
- Unfolding Case Studies

OBJECTIVES

- Explain the physiologic changes of the aging process that have a major effect on drug therapy.
- Explain the pharmacokinetics and pharmacodynamics of the older adult that relate to drug dosing.
- Differentiate the effects of two drug categories on the older adult.
- Discuss reasons for noncompliance to drug regimen by the older adult.
- Describe nursing implications related to drug therapy in the older adult.

OUTLINE

KEY TERMS

In coming years, nurses will care for increasing numbers of older adults, who will represent the "core business" of health care. Geriatric pharmacology for the **older adult** requires special attention to the age-related factors of drug absorption, distribution, metabolism, and excretion. Drug dosages are adjusted according to the older adult's weight, adipose tissue, laboratory results (e.g., serum protein, electrolytes, liver enzymes, blood urea nitrogen [BUN], creatinine clearance), and current health problems. Modifications in drug therapy for the older adult are frequently required. Because of declining organ functioning in older adults, the effects of drug therapy must be closely monitored to prevent adverse reactions to drugs and possible drug toxicity.

Approximately 85% of adults older than 65 years take medications. By 2030, it is expected that the number of older adults will be nearly twice the number in 2000. Women 65 years old presently outnumber men of that age by 134 to 100; in the 75-year-old age group, there are 100 women to 55 men. A fast-growing population is those age 85 years and older, and their use of drug therapy will likely continue to grow.

Older adults take pain, sleep, and laxative over-the-counter (OTC) drugs more frequently than younger populations. At the time of hospital admission, only about 15% of patients older than 65 years are not taking any medications (prescribed or self-medicated). During hospitalization, older adults take an average of three to five drugs. In nursing homes, 33% of patients receive 6 to 12 drugs daily.

The adverse reactions and drug interactions that occur in the older adult are three to seven times greater than those for middle-aged and young adults. Older adults consume numerous drugs because of chronic and multiple illnesses; therefore, they are susceptible to adverse reactions and interactions. Additional problems that can cause adverse reactions from drugs include self-medicating with OTC drugs, taking drugs prescribed for other health problems, taking drugs ordered by several different health care providers, overdosing when symptoms do not subside, taking new drugs to treat the side effects of other drugs, using drugs that were prescribed for another person, and, of course, the ongoing physiologic aging process. Intentional noncompliance (possibly related to drug costs or side effects) and unintentional noncompliance (possibly related to complicated, confusing drug regimens or impaired mental status) must be assessed, as should alcohol use or abuse and its interactions with medications.

Drug toxicity may develop in the older adult for drug doses that are within the therapeutic range for the younger adult. These therapeutic drug ranges are usually safe for young and middle-aged adults but are not always within safe range for older adults. It has been suggested that the drug dose for older adults should initially be prescribed at a low to low-average therapeutic range and then gradually increased according to tolerance and lack of adverse reactions; *start low and go slow* is an important concept. This approach prevents a toxic reaction to the drug in older adults. Older adults who are at risk for problems with medication administration frequently have common characteristics such as lack of coordinated care, recent discharge from the hospital, self-treatment, multiple diagnoses, sensory and physical changes associated with aging, multiple health care providers, and cognitive impairment.

PHYSIOLOGIC CHANGES

The physiologic changes associated with the aging process have a major effect on drug therapy. Table 8-1 describes the physiologic changes that occur in the gastrointestinal (GI), cardiac and circulatory, hepatic, and renal systems of the older adult and how these changes can affect pharmacologic response to drug therapy.

POLYPHARMACY

Polypharmacy (administration of many drugs together) is more common in older adults because of the use of (1) multiple health care providers, (2) herbal therapy, (3) OTC drugs, and (4) discontinued prescription drugs. Polypharmacy can cause confusion, falls, malnutrition, renal and liver dysfunction, and nonadherence. The nurse should coordinate the health care of older adults, including drug therapy, to avoid

TABLE 8-1 PHYSIOLOGIC CHANGES IN THE OLDER ADULT

SYSTEM	PHYSIOLOGIC CHANGE	EFFECT ON DRUG ADMINISTRATION
Gastrointestinal	↑ pH (alkaline) gastric secretions ↓ peristalsis with delayed intestinal emptying time ↓ motility ↓ first-pass effect	Slower absorption of oral drugs
Cardiac and circulatory	↓ cardiac output ↓ blood flow	Impaired circulation can delay transportation of drugs to the tissues
Hepatic	↓ enzyme function ↓ blood flow	Drugs metabolized more slowly and less completely
Renal	↓ blood flow ↓ functioning nephrons (kidney cells) ↓ glomerular filtration rate	Drugs excreted less completely

↓, decrease; ↑ increase.

duplication of drugs from various health care providers and misuse of OTC and herbal supplements. For example, an older patient may take a prescribed drug, ranitidine (Zantac), with an OTC drug, famotidine (Pepcid AC), for GI discomfort; this drug combination causes duplication to occur. Some older adults do not think herbal drugs are actually drugs that could cause adverse reactions when taken with other prescription or OTC drugs. Older adults should be encouraged to use one pharmacy and give the pharmacist a list of all drugs they take, both prescribed and OTC. Pharmacists conduct clinical reviews of medications that focus primarily on drug interactions.

PHARMACOKINETICS

Parameters of pharmacokinetics for the older adult are described in Table 8-2.

Absorption

Drug absorption from the GI tract is slowed in the older adult because of decreases in both blood flow and GI motility. In this age group, acidic drugs are poorly absorbed because of increased alkaline gastric secretions, but enteric-coated tablets dissolved in alkaline fluid can break down more rapidly. Drugs remain in the GI tract longer because there is a decrease in gastric motility, causing delayed onset. Iron and calcium tablets may not be absorbed as readily; generally, however, the amount of an oral dose that is absorbed is not affected by age.

Distribution

Older adults have a loss of protein-binding sites for drugs, which causes increased circulation of free drug and increased chance for adverse drug reaction. During the aging process,

TABLE 8-2 **PHARMACOKINETICS IN GERIATRIC PHARMACOLOGY**

PHASES	BODY EFFECTS AND POSSIBLE DRUG RESPONSES
Absorption	Decrease in gastric acidity (increased gastric pH) alters absorption of weak acid drugs such as aspirin. Decrease in blood flow to the GI tract (up to 40% to 50% less) may be caused by decrease in cardiac output. Because of reduced blood flow, absorption is slowed but not decreased. Reduction in GI motility rate (peristalsis) may delay onset of action. Reduction in gastric emptying time occurs.
Distribution	Because of a decrease in body water, water-soluble drugs are more concentrated. Increase in fat-to-water ratio in older adult; fat-soluble drugs are stored and likely to have decreased effect. Decrease in circulating serum protein. Acidic drugs (e.g., nonsteroidal antiinflammatory drugs [NSAIDs], aspirin, benzodiazepines, phenytoin, and warfarin) bind to albumin; basic drugs (e.g., beta-adrenergic blockers, tricyclic antidepressants, lidocaine) bind to alpha$_1$ acid glycoprotein. With fewer protein-binding sites, there is more free drug available to body tissue at receptor sites. Drugs with a high affinity for protein (>90%) compete for protein-binding sites with other drugs. Drug interactions result because of lack of protein sites and increase in free drugs.
Metabolism	Decrease in hepatic enzyme production, hepatic blood flow, and total liver function. These decreases cause a reduction in drug metabolism. With reduction in metabolic rate, t½ of drugs increases; drug accumulation can result and lead to toxicity.
Excretion	Decrease in renal blood flow and decrease in glomerular filtration rate. A decrease in renal function results in a decrease in drug excretion; thus drug accumulation results. Drug toxicity should be assessed continually while the patient takes the drug.

GI, Gastrointestinal; *t½,* half-life.

there is a loss of body water, and water-soluble drugs become more concentrated in the body. Because of an increase in body fat in the older adult, a greater amount of lipid-soluble drugs is absorbed into fat, causing a decrease in desired drug effects.

Metabolism or Biotransformation

Hepatic blood flow in the older adult may be decreased by 40% to 45%, and aging causes a decrease in liver size. Drug clearance by hepatic metabolism is affected more in older male adults than in older female adults.

Liver dysfunction, caused by the aging process, decreases enzyme function, which decreases the liver's ability to metabolize and detoxify drugs, thereby increasing the risk of drug toxicity.

The liver and kidneys are the major organs responsible for drug clearance from the body. *Biotransformation* refers to drug metabolism that occurs in the liver and contributes to drug clearance. Biotransformation during hepatic metabolism can occur either in phase I by oxidation reaction or in phase II by conjugation reaction. Hepatic microsomal enzymes are responsible for phase I, oxidation reaction. Hepatic microsomal oxidation can be impaired by the aging process, liver diseases (e.g., cirrhosis, hepatitis), and drugs that reduce oxidation capability. Drug clearance by the liver is then reduced. An example of a drug that undergoes a phase I biotransformation oxidation reaction is diazepam (Valium). Diazepam is biotransformed to its active metabolite, desmethyldiazepam. In the older adult, the plasma-serum diazepam level would remain high because of an impaired phase I oxidation reaction. Other drugs that are biotransformed by phase I include barbiturates, codeine, ibuprofen, phenytoin, meperidine, lidocaine, certain benzodiazepines (alprazolam [Xanax], midazolam [Versed]), and warfarin (Coumadin).

Phase II of biotransformation involves the conjugation or attachment of the drug to an inactive state. Hepatic conjugation is usually not influenced by older age, liver diseases, or drug interaction, so the drug is inactivated and excreted in the urine. Examples of drugs that are biotransformed or metabolized by phase II are aspirin, acetaminophen, certain benzodiazepines (lorazepam [Ativan], oxazepam [Serax], temazepam [Restoril]), procainamide, and sulfanilamide. The benzodiazepines lorazepam, oxazepam, and temazepam that undergo conjugation reaction do not have active metabolites. The drug metabolic process, phase I or II, for drug clearance for the older adult patient is an important consideration with drug selection.

To assess liver function, liver enzymes must be checked. Elevated levels indicate possible liver dysfunction. The older adult could have normal liver function test (LFT) results and still have impaired hepatic microsomal enzyme-drug oxidation reactions.

Excretion

Cardiac output and blood flow throughout the circulatory system are decreased in older adults, affecting blood flow to the liver and kidneys. After age 65 years, nephron function may be decreased by 35%; after age 70 years, blood flow to the kidneys may be decreased by 40%.

Kidney function is assessed by monitoring urine output, laboratory values of BUN and serum creatinine (Cr), and creatinine clearance (CLcr or CrCl) (estimated). Creatinine clearance is an indicator of glomerular filtration rate (GFR). To evaluate renal function based on serum creatinine alone may not be accurate for the older adult because of the decrease in muscle mass that can cause a decrease in serum creatinine. Creatinine, a by-product of muscle catabolism, is primarily excreted by the kidneys. With older adult patients, serum creatinine may be within normal values because of a lack of muscle mass, but there still could be a decrease in renal function.

The 24-hour creatinine clearance test and the serum creatinine level should be used to evaluate renal function. If a 24-hour creatinine clearance test is not feasible, the following formulas can be used to estimate creatinine clearance:

$$\text{CLcr (men)} = (140 - \text{age}) \times \text{kg}/72 \times \text{serum Cr level} = \text{mL/min}$$

$$\text{CLcr (women)} = \text{value of men} \times 0.85 = \text{mL/min}$$

The normal creatinine clearance value for an adult is 80 to 130 mL/min.

With liver and kidney dysfunction, the efficacy of a drug dose is usually increased. Multiple drug use may intensify drug effect in the older adult. When the efficiency of the hepatic and renal systems is reduced, the half-life of the drug is prolonged and drug toxicity is probable.

Adverse Reactions

Factors contributing to adverse reactions in the older adult include a loss of protein-binding sites, which increases the amount of free circulating drug; a decline in hepatic first-pass metabolism; and a prolonged half-life of the drug because of decreased liver and kidney function. Because of these factors, the time interval between doses of a drug may need to be increased, or the dose decreased, for the older adult patient.

PHARMACODYNAMICS

Because there is a lack of affinity to receptor sites throughout the body in the older adult, the pharmacodynamic response may be altered. The older adult could be more or less sensitive to drug action because of age-related changes in the central nervous system (CNS), changes in the number of drug receptors, and changes in the affinity of receptors to drugs. Frequently, the drug dose must be lowered. Consideration of changes in organ function is important in drug dosing.

In the older adult patient, the compensatory response to physiologic changes is decreased. When a drug with vasodilator properties is administered and the sympathetic feedback does not occur quickly, orthostatic hypotension (i.e., rapid decrease in blood pressure when changing position quickly) could result. In the younger adult, the sympathetic response of vasoconstriction works to avert a severe hypotensive effect.

EFFECTS OF SELECTED DRUG GROUPS ON OLDER ADULTS

Hypnotics, diuretics and antihypertensives, cardiac glycosides, anticoagulants, antibacterials (antibiotics), GI drugs (antiulcers, laxatives), antidepressants, and opioid analgesics are drug categories for which drug effects on the older adult are possible. The number of drugs taken, drug interactions (see Chapter 4), and physical health of the older adult (cardiac, renal, and hepatic function) are factors associated with drug effects in the older adult population. Drug selection is extremely important. Drugs with a shorter half-life are less likely to cause problems as a result of drug accumulation than drugs with a long half-life. If severe side effects occur, the drug with a shorter half-life is eliminated more quickly than the drug with a longer half-life.

Evaluation of hepatic and renal function is imperative, especially if the older adult takes multiple drugs. When side effects and adverse reactions occur, prescription and nonprescription drugs should be assessed (Herbal Alert 8-1).

HERBAL ALERT 8-1

Older Adults

Advise patients to consult with the health care provider before starting herbal products. Common herbal preparations (e.g., ginger, gingko, ginseng, garlic) interact with many drugs (e.g., anticoagulants) that older adult patients take to treat chronic health disorders.

Hypnotics

Insomnia (having difficulty in falling asleep, frequently awakening during the night, or awakening early in the morning with difficulty falling back to sleep) is a frequent problem in the older adult population. Sedatives and hypnotics are the second most common group of drugs prescribed or taken OTC. Types of hypnotics differ according to the cause of insomnia. Five benzodiazepine hypnotics (flurazepam, quazepam, temazepam, triazolam, and estazolam) have been approved by the U.S. Food and Drug Administration (FDA) as hypnotics to control insomnia. For the older patient, low doses of benzodiazepines with short or intermediate half-lives are usually prescribed. Short-term therapy is suggested. Usually benzodiazepines are prescribed at higher doses for sedative and hypnotic effects and at lower doses for antianxiety effects. About 35% of older adults take a hypnotic.

Flurazepam HCl (Dalmane), the first benzodiazepine hypnotic, was introduced in 1970. It has three metabolites and is considered to be both a short- and long-acting hypnotic. Its principal metabolite is desalkylflurazepam, which is long-acting, has a long half-life, and is slowly eliminated. This drug is not suggested for persons older than 65 years. Drug hangover is a problem. Quazepam (Doral) has effects similar to flurazepam. It is a precursor of desalkylflurazepam and has a prolonged half-life.

Temazepam (Restoril) was introduced in 1981. Because it is biotransformed in the liver by conjugation and not by oxidation, it is prescribed frequently for the older adult patient. Temazepam's principal metabolite, glucuronide, is conjugated with no pharmacologic effects and excreted in the urine. Temazepam is slowly absorbed, so it should be taken 1 to 2 hours before bedtime. It is classified as an intermediate-acting benzodiazepine. Food delays its action. Temazepam is more effective for frequent awakenings during the night than for problems falling asleep.

Triazolam (Halcion) is an intermediate-acting benzodiazepine. It has a short half-life and at low doses (0.0625 to 0.125 mg) is considered safe for the older adult. It is metabolized by hepatic microsomal oxidation, although the drug doses differ from oxidized benzodiazepines. Triazolam helps with problems falling asleep, and it also decreases frequent awakenings during the night. To avoid rebound insomnia when the drug is discontinued, doses should be tapered rather than abruptly stopped.

Estazolam is an intermediate- to long-acting drug. It is metabolized in the liver to two metabolites that are not highly potent.

The benzodiazepines lorazepam and oxazepam can be used for insomnia. These agents have an intermediate half-life and should be taken 1 hour before bedtime. Other benzodiazepines are more effective as anxiolytics (antianxiety drugs) than as hypnotics.

Diuretics and Antihypertensives

Diuretics are frequently prescribed for treatment of hypertension or heart failure. For the older adult, the dose is usually reduced because of dose-related side effects. Hydrochlorothiazide (HydroDIURIL) is generally prescribed in low doses of 12.5 mg/day. Higher doses of 25 to 50 mg/day with chronic use can cause electrolyte imbalances (e.g., hypokalemia, hyponatremia, hypomagnesemia, hypercalcemia), hyperglycemia, hyperuricemia, and hypercholesterolemia.

Many older adult patients are hypertensive (blood pressure >140/90 mm Hg). Nonpharmacologic methods to reduce blood pressure such as exercise, reduction of salt and alcohol intake, and adequate rest are suggested. These actions can reduce the systolic and diastolic pressure by 8 to 10 mm Hg. Diuretics, beta-adrenergic blockers or antagonists, calcium channel blockers, angiotensin-converting enzyme (ACE) inhibitors, angiotensin II receptor antagonists (A-II blockers), and centrally acting $alpha_2$ agonists are used as antihypertensive drugs. Calcium blockers, angiotensin-converting inhibitors, and A-II blockers are frequently the agents of choice because of their low incidence of electrolyte imbalance and CNS side effects (see Chapter 44). Usually antihypertensive dosing for older adults begins with reduced doses that are gradually increased according to need, tolerance, and adverse reactions. Because of adverse reactions such as orthostatic hypotension, $alpha_1$ blockers or antagonists (prazosin, terazosin) and centrally acting $alpha_2$ agonists (methyldopa, clonidine, guanabenz, guanfacine) are infrequently prescribed for older adults.

Cardiac Glycosides

Digoxin (Lanoxin) is commonly prescribed for older adults; however, long-term use of the drug should be carefully monitored because of its narrow therapeutic range (0.5 to 2 ng/mL) and the possibility of digitalis toxicity. Digoxin is given for left ventricular heart failure, chronic atrial fibrillation, and atrial tachycardia. Its half-life is doubled (70 hours) in patients older than 80 years. Most of the digoxin is eliminated by the kidneys, so a decline in kidney function (decreased GFR) could cause digoxin accumulation. With close monitoring of serum digoxin levels, creatinine clearance tests, and vital signs (pulse should be >60 beats per minute), digoxin is considered safe for the older adult.

Anticoagulants

Bleeding may occur with chronic use of anticoagulants in older adult patients. Warfarin (Coumadin) is 99% protein bound; with a decrease in serum albumin, which is common among older adults, there is an increase in free, unbound circulating warfarin and a potential risk for bleeding. Older adult patients should have their prothrombin time (PT) or international normalized ratio (INR) checked periodically, and the nurse should check for signs of bleeding. Older adults are more at risk for falls and injury that can cause bleeding complications from drug interactions affecting Coumadin levels.

Antibacterials

Penicillins, cephalosporins, tetracyclines, and sulfonamides are normally considered safe for the older adult. If renal drug clearance is decreased and the drug has a prolonged half-life, the drug dose should be reduced. Aminoglycosides, fluoroquinolones (quinolones), and vancomycin are excreted in the urine. These drug agents are not frequently prescribed for patients older than 75 years, and, if they are prescribed, the drug dose is usually reduced.

Gastrointestinal Drugs

Histamine (H_2) blockers and sucralfate are safer drugs than other antiulcer agents for the treatment of peptic ulcers. Cimetidine (Tagamet) was the first histamine blocker or antagonist and is not suggested for the older adult because of its side effects and multiple potential drug interactions. Ranitidine (Zantac), famotidine (Pepcid), and nizatidine (Axid) may be prescribed for older adult patients instead of cimetidine.

Laxatives are frequently taken by older adults. In long-term facilities such as nursing homes, 75% of residents take laxatives on a daily basis. Fluid and electrolyte imbalances may occur with excessive use. Increased GI motility with laxative use could decrease absorption of other drugs. Nonpharmacologic measures such as increasing fluid intake, consuming high-fiber foods, and exercising should be encouraged.

Antidepressants

An antidepressant drug dose for older adults is normally 30% to 50% of the dose for young and middle-aged adults. Drug dose should be gradually increased according to the patient's tolerance and the desired therapeutic effect. Close monitoring for possible adverse reactions is important.

Although tricyclic antidepressants are generally effective in the older adult population, their anticholinergic properties can cause side effects such as dry mouth, tachycardia, constipation, and urinary retention. Tricyclic antidepressants can also contribute to narrow-angle glaucoma. Fluoxetine (Prozac), a bicyclic antidepressant, has fewer side effects than the tricyclic antidepressants, and the side effects are mostly dose-related. Monoamine oxidase inhibitors (MAOIs) are not often prescribed for older adults because of adverse reactions such as drug-food interactions that could result in hypertensive crisis and severe orthostatic hypotension. (Refer to Chapter 28 for a discussion of antidepressants.)

Opioid Analgesics

Opioids can cause dose-related adverse reactions when taken by the older adult. Hypotension and respiratory depression may result from opioid use, so close monitoring of vital signs is essential when providing nursing care and support to the older adult patient on opioid analgesics. Constipation is another side effect; patients taking these medications must also take stool softeners.

Table 8-3 presents a list of drugs not generally recommended for use in older adult patients.

ADHERENCE AND NONADHERENCE

Nonadherence with a drug regimen can be a problem in all patient age groups, but it is especially troublesome in older adult patients. Frequently the older adult fails to ask questions during interactions with health care providers; therefore the drug regimen may not be fully understood or precisely followed. Nonadherence can cause underdosing or overdosing that could be harmful to the patient's health. Table 8-4 lists barriers to effective medication use by older adults.

> **SAFETY: Preventing Medication Errors**
>
> **Do not confuse ...**
> - **Celebrex**, a COX-2 inhibitor, with **Celexa**, an SSRI
> - **Ditropan**, an antispasmodic/anticholinergic, with **Diflucan**, an antifungal
> - **Digoxin** (Lanoxin), a cardiac glycoside used to treat heart failure, with **levothyroxine**, synthetic T_4 used to treat hypothyroidism
> - **Xanax**, a benzodiazepine used to treat panic disorder, with **Zantac**

TABLE 8-3 DRUGS NOT GENERALLY RECOMMENDED FOR USE IN OLDER ADULT PATIENTS

DRUGS	DRAWBACKS	ALTERNATIVES
Analgesics		
ketorolac (Toradol and others)	Serious GI toxicity	
meperidine (Demerol and others)	Confusion, convulsions	Morphine preferred
Antidepressants, Tricyclic		
amitriptyline (Elavil) doxepin (Sinequan)	Anticholinergic effects (constipation, urinary retention, blurred vision, confusion), orthostatic hypotension, sedation, and cardiac arrhythmias	Selective serotonin reuptake inhibitors (SSRIs) other than daily fluoxetine; other antidepressants preferred
Antihistamines, First-Generation		
chlorpheniramine (Chlor-Trimeton) diphenhydramine (Benadryl) hydroxyzine (Vistaril) promethazine (Phenergan)	Anticholinergic effects; some such as diphenhydramine and promethazine are highly sedating	Second-generation antihistamines such as fexofenadine (Allegra) or loratadine (Claritin) preferred
Antispasmodics		
belladonna alkaloids (Donnatal) dicyclomine (Bentyl) hyoscyamine (Levsin) propantheline (Pro-Banthine)	Anticholinergic effects	
Muscle Relaxants		
carisoprodol (Soma) cyclobenzaprine (Flexeril) methocarbamol (Robaxin) metaxalone (Skelaxin)	Anticholinergic effects, sedation, limited effectiveness at tolerated doses	
Sedatives		
Barbiturates	Sedation, addiction	
benzodiazepines, long-acting	Prolonged sedation	Low doses of shorter-acting benzodiazepines such as lorazepam (Ativan) preferred
chlordiazepoxide (Librium) diazepam (Valium)	Sedation, addiction	
Other		
cimetidine (Tagamet)	Confusion, many drug interactions	Other H_2 agonists preferred
nitrofurantoin (Macrobid)	Limited efficacy in renal impairment	Other antibiotics preferred
trimethobenzamide (Tigan)	Extrapyramidal side effects, limited effectiveness	

TABLE 8-4 BARRIERS TO EFFECTIVE MEDICATION USE BY OLDER ADULTS

CAUSES	NURSING ACTIONS
Taking too many medications at different times	Develop a chart indicating times to take drugs. Provide space to place a mark for each drug taken. Coordinate medication regimen with activities of daily living (e.g., meals) and events. Use an organizer container (daily or weekly). Have the patient bring all medications, including over-the-counter drugs and herbal, vitamin, and mineral supplements, to all health appointments.
Failure to understand purpose or reason for drug	Explain the purpose, drug action, and importance of the medication. Provide time for questions and reinforcement. Reinforce with written information.
Impaired memory	Encourage family members or friends to monitor the patient's drug regimen.
Decreased mobility and dexterity	Advise family members or friends to have drugs and water or other fluid accessible. Assist older adults as needed.
Visual and hearing disturbances	Suggest eye and ear examinations (glasses or hearing aids).
High cost of prescriptions	Contact the social services department of your institution; contact "compassionate care programs" as appropriate.
Childproof drug bottles	Suggest that the patient request non-childproof bottle caps.
Side effects or adverse reactions from the drug	Educate the patient and family about side effects to report to the health care provider.

Nonadherence can lead to adverse reactions, admission and/or readmission to health care institutions, and even death. Complex medication regimens promote nonadherence. Education is the cornerstone of adherence—education of the patient, family, and formal and informal caregivers.

Working with older adult patients is an ongoing nursing responsibility. The nurse should plan strategies with the patient and family or friends to encourage **adherence** with prescribed regimens. Daily contact may be necessary at first. Mere ordering of medication does not mean that the patient is able to get the drugs or is taking them correctly. Older adults should have their prescriptions filled at one pharmacy so possible drug interactions can be identified and monitored closely.

Older adults often do not have insurance that includes prescription drug coverage, so they choose to buy food and other necessities before medication. Some will delay purchasing or never purchase the drugs prescribed. The older adult is more apt to experience serious side effects from drug administration than the young or middle-aged adult. If a drug such as ibuprofen (Advil, Motrin) irritates the GI tract, the older adult may not take it because he or she is unaware that another drug such as magnesium hydroxide (Maalox) taken before the ibuprofen dose will decrease this side effect. He or she may not know that food can also decrease gastric irritation from ibuprofen.

Health care professionals (nurses, pharmacists, and health care providers) need to work collaboratively to enhance safety and adherence of older adult patients and to avoid errors and unwarranted concerns. Nurses are in a unique position to educate patients and monitor the effectiveness of the therapeutic regimens. (Refer to Chapter 12 for additional information on medication safety.) A handout of tips for patients on talking with their pharmacist can be found at *www.fda.gov/downloads/Drugs/ResourcesForYou/UCM163349.pdf.*

Cost of medications may be a factor in nonadherence. Potential patient strategies for cutting costs include telling the health care provider about concerns related to expense, asking for senior-citizen discounts, obtaining medication samples from health care providers, buying in bulk for chronic conditions, and buying OTC medications on sale.

HEALTH TEACHING WITH THE OLDER ADULT

A comprehensive discussion of health teaching in the nursing process is presented in Chapter 11. Specific factors that promote adherence in the older adult include the following:

- Ensure that the patient is wearing eyeglasses and has working hearing aids in place, if needed. Check sensory aids to be sure they are clean and working.
- Speak in a tone of voice that the patient can hear; sit facing the patient, and limit distractions.
- Treat the patient with respect; never infantilize; expect that he or she can learn.
- Use large print and bright colors in teaching aids if the patient is vision-impaired.
- Review all medications at each patient visit; ask the patient to bring all medications to each appointment; advise use of only one pharmacy.
- Advise the patient to complete the "vial of life" and keep it in the refrigerator where safety personnel know to look for it. Instruct the patient to keep a list of all medications taken, bring it to all health appointments, and carry it when out of the house.
- Encourage a simple dosing schedule when possible.
- Suspect recently prescribed medication(s) if new confusion or disorientation occurs.
- Encourage the patient to report if a drug is not improving the condition for which it was prescribed.
- Consider use of memory aids such as pill organizers or planners, alarms, blinking lights, or prerecorded messages.

The National Institutes of Health (NIH) websites on aging are excellent resources for both health care providers and older adults and their families. The website for health care providers is *www.nia.nih.gov*; it has sections on health information, research, grants, training, news, and events. The website for older adults is *www.nihseniorhealth.gov.*

Nursing Process
Patient-Centered Collaborative Care

Geriatrics

Assessment

- Assess the older adult's sensorium, mental awareness, and visual and auditory acuity. Assess the patient's use of eyeglasses, and check date of last eye examination.
- Is the patient confused or disoriented? If so, is this state transitory? Does the patient live alone, with or without social support, and need assistance with medications (including costs) or transportation?
- Obtain a history of cardiac, kidney, liver, or GI disorders. Kidney or liver disorders can cause a decrease in the function of these organs and increase the half-life of drugs.
- Assess lab rest results and monitor, as appropriate. Longer drug half-life and frequent drug dosing can result in drug toxicity.
- Assess laboratory test results, and follow up as appropriate.
- Determine whether or not patient takes OTC drugs or supplements (including herbal preparations), how often, and for what length of time. Specifically, ask about laxatives and antacids, which can affect gastric pH, electrolyte balance, and GI motility. Many people do not think of these agents as drugs. Remind patient and family to tell the pharmacist about prescribed drugs when contemplating the purchase of OTC preparations.
- Assess patient's and family's knowledge of the purpose of each medication, how it works, and its possible side effects.
- Assess for patient adherence with taking drugs correctly and reasons for noncompliance. Does the patient have difficulty opening drug containers, or with side effects or adverse effects?

Nursing Diagnoses

- Risk for constipation related to analgesics
- Urinary retention related to drug therapy
- Imbalanced nutrition, less than body requirements, related to metabolism of drugs
- Ineffective health maintenance related to lack of transportation
- Deficient knowledge related to lack of understanding about reason for taking medication
- Noncompliance related to lack of insurance with prescription drug coverage

Planning

- Patient will take prescribed medications as ordered.
- Drug therapy will be effective with no, few, or minimal side effects.

Nursing Interventions

- Monitor patient's laboratory results in relation to kidney and liver function. Are BUN, serum creatinine, and creatinine clearance levels within normal range? Are liver enzymes within normal range? Discuss findings with the health care provider.
- Check patient's serum drug level as ordered and report abnormal findings to nurse manager or health care provider. Remember: Older adults who take water-soluble drugs such as digoxin are likely to have higher blood levels because of reduced body water.
- Communicate with pharmacist or health care provider when drug dose is in question. Check drug references for recommended drug doses for older adults.
- Observe patient for adverse reactions when multiple drugs are being taken. An older adult with hypertension and heart failure might take a diuretic (e.g., hydrochlorothiazide [HydroDIURIL]) and digoxin. The diuretic may cause potassium loss, and if potassium replacement is not ordered, digitalis toxicity may occur. Hypokalemia (low serum potassium) enhances action of digoxin, causing toxicity. Symptoms of digitalis toxicity may be a slow (bradycardia is <60 beats/min) or irregular pulse rate, nausea and vomiting, and blurred vision.
- Recognize a change in usual behavior or an increase in confusion. One of the first signs of drug toxicity is confusion. Report changes to the health care provider.
- Ascertain whether financial problems are preventing patient from purchasing prescribed drugs. Assistance programs are available.

Patient Teaching

General

- Review medications with patient and family, including reason for medication, route of administration, frequency, common side effects, and when to notify health care provider.
- Explain to patient and family the importance of adherence to the drug regimen. Emphasize taking drug as prescribed, discarding unused or old drugs, and keeping a record of medication taken. Remember: Drugs are the property of the patient and may not be disposed of without his or her permission.
- Be available to answer patient's questions. Be supportive of the older adult and the family. Discuss problems related to the medications.
- Advise patient to use one pharmacy to fill prescriptions. Tell patient to inform pharmacist of all OTC and herbal drugs taken.
- Advise patient and family to request a non–childproof cap from the pharmacy if patient has arthritis in the hand joint or difficulty opening childproof bottle caps. Patient may need to sign for this at the pharmacy; safety of children or pets in the environment must be ensured.

- Counsel patient not to share prescribed medications with others or to take medications prescribed for another person.

Self-Administration
- Advise patient to keep a medication record of drugs and when they are to be taken. Consider offering patient a sample log for recording information. This removes barriers, increases drug adherence, and avoids drug errors.

Diet
- Encourage patients controlling hypertension with a potassium-wasting diuretic (e.g., hydrochlorothiazide) to eat foods rich in potassium (bran cereal, tomatoes, raisins, potatoes, bananas, avocados) and to take potassium supplements if recommended by the health care provider.
- Advise patient about how to maintain a generally well-balanced diet, and give examples.

Side Effects
- Advise patient and family to immediately report mental and physiologic changes (confusion, GI bleeding) to health care provider.

Cultural Considerations
- Recognize that language difficulties may interfere with older adults' understanding of the prescribed drug regimen if English is not their first language.
- Provide additional time for verbal and written explanation to ensure that the older adult will take drugs as prescribed.
- Do not assume that lack of eye contact means the patient is not listening or does not care; it might indicate respect. More traditional or older individuals in some cultures do not maintain eye contact.

Evaluation
- Evaluate compliance with the drug regimen, and answer any questions the older adult may have.
- Evaluate drug effect, and ascertain side effects or adverse reactions.

KEY WEBSITES

American Society of Consultant Pharmacists: *www.ascp.com*

Beers Criteria for Potentially Inappropriate Medication use in the Elderly: *www.omfire.org/links/files/beerscriteria.pdf*

National Council on Patient Information and Education: *www.talkaboutrx.org*

Senior Care Pharmacist: *www.seniorcarepharmacist.com*

CRITICAL THINKING CASE STUDY

An older adult patient has osteoarthritis. The patient had previously taken aspirin for the condition and later was prescribed naproxen (Naprosyn). Both drugs caused GI distress. The health care provider discontinued the naproxen and prescribed celecoxib (Celebrex) 100 mg twice a day. Celecoxib is a non-opioid, cyclooxygenase-2 (COX-2) inhibitor.

1. How does celecoxib differ from naproxen? (See Chapters 25 and 26.)
2. Describe the advantages and disadvantages of taking celecoxib for osteoarthritis.
3. What is the rationale for checking the patient's renal and liver function before prescribing celecoxib? Explain your answer.
4. What should be included in the nursing assessment in regard to the patient's physical and drug histories?

   The patient states that the arthritic pain is not relieved with the new drug. The patient wants to take naproxen with the celecoxib.
5. Explain the effects of these two medications when taken together.
6. What is the most appropriate response to the patient's request? Explain your answer.
7. Develop a teaching plan for the patient that includes medication use and nursing measures to relieve pain.

NCLEX STUDY QUESTIONS

1. A patient has nine medications prescribed to take daily. Which are common reasons for nonadherence to the drug regimen in the older adult? (Select all that apply.)
   a. Taking multiple drugs at one time
   b. Impaired memory
   c. Decreased dexterity
   d. Increased mobility
   e. Increased visual acuity

2. The nurse is reviewing a patient's list of medications with the patient. The nurse understands that the older adult's slower absorption of oral medications is primarily because of which phenomenon?
   a. Decreased cardiac output
   b. Increased blood flow
   c. Decreased enzyme function
   d. Increased pH of gastric secretions
3. The older adult patient has questions about oral drug metabolism. What is the most important information to include in this patient's teaching plan?
   a. First-pass effect
   b. Enzyme function
   c. Glomerular filtration rate
   d. Motility
4. A 97-year-old patient asks why a protein supplement has been prescribed. What is the nurse's best response?
   a. "You have increased circulation of free drug."
   b. "You have decreased hepatic size."
   c. "You have decreased calcium absorption."
   d. "You have increased motility."
5. An 80-year-old patient complains of recent onset of insomnia, saying, "If only I could get to sleep!" If a drug is prescribed, which drug characteristics would be best for this situation? (Select all that apply.)
   a. Short-intermediate acting
   b. Rapidly eliminated
   c. Slowly eliminated
   d. Multiple metabolites
   e. Few metabolites
6. An older patient has just started on hydrochlorothiazide (HydroDiuril) and is advised by the health care provider to eat foods rich in potassium. What is the nurse's best recommendation of foods?
   a. Cabbage and corn
   b. Pineapple and orange juice
   c. Bran cereal and raisins
   d. Brown rice and fish
7. Insomnia is a frequent complaint voiced by the patient. What are the most important elements for the nurse to include in the teaching plan? (Select all that apply.)
   a. There are a limited number of FDA-approved medications to treat insomnia.
   b. Benzodiazepines with long half-lives are preferred.
   c. 17% of the older adult population take hypnotics.
   d. Temazepam is to be taken 1 to 2 hours before bedtime.
   e. Triazolam should be tapered rather than abruptly stopped.

Answers: 1, a, b, c; 2, d; 3, a; 4, a; 5, a, b, e; 6, c; 7, a, d, e.

CHAPTER

9

Collaboration in Community Settings

evolve WEBSITE

http://evolve.elsevier.com/KeeHayes/pharmacology/

- Animations
- Content Updates
- Key Points
- Review Questions for the NCLEX® Examination
- References from the Textbook
- Unfolding Case Studies

OBJECTIVES

- Describe common elements of patient teaching about medication administration in community settings.
- Explain specific points related to administration of medications in the home.
- Discuss specific points related to administration of medications in the school.
- Describe specific points related to administration of medications in the work site.
- Explain the application of the nursing process to medication administration in community settings.

OUTLINE

Health and illness care has shifted from traditional institutions to community settings. The faces of a community are many, varied, and ever-changing. With the movement of health care into the community, nurses—more than any other health care provider—have the opportunity to shape the health care of society. This chapter describes selected aspects of medication administration of prescription, over-the-counter (OTC), and herbal preparations within each of the major community settings: home, school, and work. In all settings, patient safety is the primary concern. (Refer to Chapter 13 for a detailed discussion of medication administration.)

This chapter discusses a small, but significant, portion of the nurse's role in a variety of community settings. Specifically, the focus is on selected concerns associated with the administration of medications and the need to practice in accordance with the Nurse Practice Act of a specific state. The role of the nurse in drug administration is growing in complexity. Most medications are taken by community-dwelling residents (not hospitalized patients), which clearly shows the importance of patient education in all settings. The nurse in the twenty-first century must have a strong knowledge base.

The process of medication administration in the home, school, and work site must be consistent with professional, legal, and regulatory requirements. In each setting, it must first be determined what the nursing personnel will teach patients about medications and then the routes by which the medications can be administered. Once these decisions have been made, criteria for administration, instruction and patient teaching, and ongoing supervision must be developed, implemented, and evaluated. Mechanisms for communication and electronic or paper tracking must be in place to promote efficacy of the medication and avoidance of untoward responses and medication errors.

With the escalating costs of medications, the nurse in any community setting is likely to meet patients who need assistance paying for their prescriptions. A possible resource for the nurse and patient are pharmaceutical companies' patient-assistance programs (PAPs). Some PAPs provide medications for free or at a reduced cost, but often patients must demonstrate that they do not qualify for private or public health insurance and that their income is below a certain level. An application process is required; the health care provider, nurse, or social worker may need to apply for the patient. Online resources that assist in finding PAPs or other programs include rxassit.org (sponsored by Volunteers in Health Care), RxHope.com (supported by the Pharmaceutical Research and Manufacturers of America), and PPARx.org (Partnership for Prescription Assistance).

The backbone of health promotion and disease prevention is the patient knowledge base. The role of the nurse in establishing this base is critical. (A comprehensive discussion of patient teaching is offered in Chapter 11.) Assessment of learning needs and styles is another essential component to achieving the identified teaching goal.

PATIENT TEACHING

Regardless of the state and agency regulations related to medication administration in community settings, the following format for patient teaching associated with medication administration is recommended. Hints are grouped into five categories: (1) general, (2) diet, (3) self-administration, (4) side effects, and (5) cultural considerations.

General

Patient safety is of primary concern, so a patient's physical abilities require ongoing assessment. Capabilities of the patient may be temporarily impaired with the use of certain drugs (e.g., narcotics, selected eye medications, psychotropics). It is essential that patients be advised not to drive a vehicle or operate hazardous machinery during such times and to use caution at all other times. It is appropriate to discuss with patients and families what situations in the daily routine require full alertness and cannot be influenced by medication for the sake of safety.

Numerous safety concerns are associated with the storage of medications. Medications should be kept in their original labeled containers, with childproof caps when needed, and stored away from light and moisture.

Advise the patient and family about any necessary laboratory tests to monitor the blood level of the medication and any possible drug-laboratory test interactions. Also educate the patient and family about assessments—such as heart rate, blood pressure, or blood sugar levels—that should be done before taking the medication. This information, and all other information about the drug regimen, should be provided as written instructions (or audio instructions if the patient is sight impaired or unable to read). Large print may be helpful or necessary.

Important yet frequently misunderstood components of the instructions are the expected therapeutic effect and the length of time required to achieve a therapeutic response from the medication. These vary widely among different medications (e.g., most opioids act within 30 minutes; many antibiotics act within 24 hours; some psychotropics act within 6 weeks). Patient understanding of the expected time frame for results can markedly diminish concerns and promote adherence to the therapeutic plan.

The patient and family must also be aware of the need to have an adequate supply of necessary medications available at all times: at home, school, work, and while traveling. It is best to order prescription refills in advance. If the pharmacy is local, at least 1 week should be allowed; several weeks should be allowed if drugs are ordered through the mail. It is a good idea to pack extra medication when going on trips, both short and extended. This is preferred at all times and is essential for foreign travel.

Advise the patient and family to contact the health care provider before using OTC preparations. Common OTC preparations that may cause problems are laxatives, diet aids, cold and cough preparations, nonsteroidal anti-inflammatory drugs (NSAIDs), antacids, and medications for sleep. Reinforce with the patient and family the importance of follow-up appointments with health care providers. Encourage wellness checkups, including preventive and restorative dental care, because the presence of other conditions may affect the current therapeutic regimen. In addition, advise patients of the need to complete laboratory studies in a timely manner. Encourage patients to wear medical alert bands that indicate the patient's condition or disease (e.g., diabetes, parkinsonism), medications, and allergies (Herbal Alert 9-1). See Chapter 12 for guidelines on the safe disposal of drugs.

Reinforcement of the availability of community resources is important. Availability does not always equate with accessibility, so the patient or family needs to know how to mobilize resources according to individual needs. Matching community resources and patient needs is a prerequisite. While acknowledging the variability of each patient, family, and setting need, the following are offered as examples:

- The Internet, medical libraries with medical librarians, and telephone listings can direct patients and families to contact information for associations of relevant health conditions (e.g., American Heart Association, American Cancer Society). Most agencies and associations have or can direct the caller to a wealth of health education resources available in a variety of media (e.g., print, audio, video, Braille). In addition, many organizations have "Ask a Nurse" programs.
- Houses of worship may have volunteer outreach groups to pick up prescriptions and deliver them to homebound patients.

HERBAL ALERT 9-1

Community

Encourage the patient to consult the health care provider before taking herbal preparations or vitamin and mineral supplements; some products may interact with prescription or over-the-counter medications.

- Pharmacists can frequently clarify a patient's or family's concern over the telephone.
- Meals on Wheels enables patients to remain at home and adhere to taking medications with food.
- In a college town, students of the health professions may be motivated caregivers to assist patients or families in the community.

Patients or families need to be encouraged to have a contact person for their concerns and questions, frequently a nurse. Use of appropriate resources is likely to increase compliance with and effectiveness of the therapeutic regimen.

Diet

Nurses should advise patients or families about possible drug-food interactions, detailing which foods are to be avoided and which foods are encouraged for specific nutrient value. For example, tyramine-rich foods are contraindicated with monoamine oxidase inhibitors (MAOIs), and potassium-rich foods are recommended for patients taking potassium-wasting diuretics. Alcohol may be contraindicated with selected medications. Lists of foods, with pictures when appropriate, may be helpful to patients and their families.

Self-Administration

Based on the level of the patient's or family's knowledge, instructions should be given on all skills related to the drug regimen, how to take the pulse for patients who take digitalis preparations, how to use and clean inhalers, how to administer parenteral medications, and how to decrease the risk for infection in patients taking immunosuppressants. The nurse should allow time for instruction and questions, including demonstration of the skill and return demonstration. Patients should be given graphic illustrations for future reference as appropriate. It is essential that the nurse provide the patient or family with the name and telephone number of a contact person for questions and concerns. It is not uncommon for a patient or family member to return-demonstrate a skill (e.g., administration of insulin, use of inhaler) with relative ease and then forget information or become confused when attempting self-administration of the drug while alone. Resources must be provided to the patient and family if this occurs.

Side Effects

The patient or family should be advised about general side effects of medications. This is not done to scare patients but rather to let them know what they might expect. Patients should know when and how to notify their health care provider if they experience an adverse reaction; this information should be kept in an easily accessible location for ready access if needed.

Cultural Considerations

Initially, the nurse assesses the patient's personal beliefs. Based on these beliefs, the nurse then modifies communication to meet patient and family cultural practices. The nurse should communicate respect for the patient or family culture at all times. It is important for the nurse to assess his or her own beliefs and biases related to cultural competence and diversity, and then evaluate the effectiveness of interactions and their acceptability within the cultural realm. Culturally sensitive and competent health care promotes patient and family adherence to the therapeutic regimen. Respect for cultural diversity may be demonstrated by inclusion of traditional practices into the plans for improved communication, health promotion, and disease prevention. Refer to Chapter 3 for a discussion of cultural differences.

COMMUNITY-BASED SETTINGS

Home Setting

The home setting provides nurses with opportunities and challenges related to medication administration. The patient and family are generally more comfortable in their home; the nurse is a guest. The nurse has a comprehensive view of the patient and family during a home visit (e.g., support system, resources, adherence). A question that may quickly arise is, "Who can administer medications in the home setting?" The response does not develop so quickly.

In general, medications are administered by licensed nurses in the home setting according to the health care provider's order. Drugs that are administered by nursing personnel in the home must be approved by the U.S. Food and Drug Administration (FDA). The nurse must provide instructions about the medication to the patient and family. The licensed nurse may also administer the medication on a short-term basis for a disease-related condition if the patient or a caregiver with an order from the health care provider is unable to do so.

The order from the health care provider must be current and complete (drug, dosage, frequency, route of administration, and signature). The medication must be labeled by the pharmacist or health care provider; the nurse should not administer any medication that is not properly labeled. It is the nurse's responsibility to contact the health care provider, pharmacist, or other contact identified by the agency with any concerns about the medication for a specific patient. The expiration date must be checked at the time of each administration. Storage and deterioration of the medication are also evaluated. Significant side effects, allergies, and adverse reactions are reported promptly to the health care provider. Each patient is assessed for allergies before administering the drug.

The establishment of policy and procedures for medication administration promotes safety and consistency; however, errors do occur. When a medication error occurs, it is reported to the health care provider and nursing supervisor. The patient and family are instructed when to notify the nurse or health care provider if an adverse drug reaction is suspected. Ultimately, the health care provider should be notified of all adverse drug reactions.

SAFETY: Preventing Medication Errors

Community Settings

- Do not give or take medications in the dark; proper lighting is important to avoid errors.
- Apply the rights of medication administration (see Chapter 13).
- Dispose of unused medications in a safe manner (see Chapter 12).

An agency policy for medication administration generally addresses guidelines for specific medications, such as allergy vaccines, chemotherapy, gamma globulin, gold therapy, experimental drugs, and narcotics. The guidelines are agency-specific and may include that the first dose of allergy vaccine be given by the health care provider in a controlled environment or that family members be taught how to administer narcotics to the patient by the parenteral route if the order is so written by the health care provider. When the order is discontinued, the health care provider should be notified if any unused narcotics are in the home. Licensed practical nurses may not administer gamma globulin intravenously, and family members may not be taught to administer selected drugs (e.g., iron dextran [Imferon]). Chemotherapy for cancer commonly presents a special challenge. The patient's blood work must be current before the administration of chemotherapeutic drugs, the patient must be under regular and ongoing care of a health care provider, and safety requirements may be identified (e.g., gloves and goggles may be used).

Certified home health aides work under the supervision of a registered nurse. Home health aides are commonly asked to administer medications to a patient by the patient, family, or friends. The home health aide may receive pressure to administer medications, but legally home health aides may only *assist* with medications the patient customarily self-administers.

Additional challenges related to medication administration in the home setting include adherence to the therapeutic regimen, especially the right drug, right dose, and right time. Some patients need, but do not have, a primary caregiver to oversee follow-up with medications and other aspects of care. The quality and preparation of meals may also be a factor related to medication administration, such as what foods to avoid with certain medications and what foods complement a medication. In addition, it may be difficult for patients to get their medications and to get them in a timely manner. Coordinated skill may be required by the patient or family—for example, with use of an inhaler or administration of insulin. In all of these situations, the nurse is frequently the person who coordinates the resources.

School Setting

Administration of medications in the school setting is of special concern. One study reports that in any given 2-week period, about 13 million children in grades kindergarten through senior year take medications. The most frequently taken medications are OTC preparations and prescription medications for attention deficit hyperactivity disorder (ADHD) or asthma. In addition, there has been a dramatic increase in the kinds of medications taken at school: from 58 different types in the late 1980s to more than 200 currently.

School health services are not immune to the phenomenon of downsizing personnel, and many school systems are dealing with questions like "Where are the nurses?" and "Who is responsible for the administration of medication?" In the absence of federal and state law, some school districts have elected not to employ school nurses. The average national caseload for a school nurse is more than 3,100 students, despite the long-standing recommendation of having one registered nurse for every 750 students. Coupled with this is the impact of a federal law that entitles children with disabilities to attend public schools in their residential areas. It is not unreasonable to assume that these children have special needs that may require professional nursing services.

Massachusetts has developed a model with the goal "to develop regulations that provide minimum standards for the safe and proper administration of prescription medications in the Commonwealth schools." This model has many strengths including representation of professional associations, community groups, and regulatory bodies. Consistent consent forms have been designed and adopted, and orientation and training programs have been instituted for all personnel in school health positions. The established regulations apply to both public and nonpublic schools. The Massachusetts model appears to have applicability to other states that are grappling with the important child health issue of medication administration in schools.

It is essential that nurses be aware of the policies and procedures for medication administration in their own state, county, and school system. Standardized policies for medication administration are necessary for safe practice and promote self-management programs for students with chronic conditions such as asthma and diabetes. Nurses must be actively involved in developing these policies and in ensuring that the needs of individual students are met.

In some states or school systems, people who are not nurses may be responsible for medication administration. This presents additional concerns that must be addressed, such as adherence to instructions and to the principle that medication administration is a process, more than merely "giving the student a pill." A major component of medication administration is assessment of the need for the medication and its effectiveness of action. The effectiveness of action includes being alert to side effects and adverse reactions that the patient may experience.

The National Association of School Nurses (NASN) released their Summary of Position Statement on the Administration of Medications in 2012. This document contains helpful information, including delegation, alternative medications, controlled substances, emergency medications, and research medications. The full position statement is available at *www.nasn.org*.

Child care and adult day care services have similar rules for the administration of medications. In general, these facilities administer medications or supervise self-administration within the Nurse Practice Act of the specific state. In addition, most facilities require labeling of medications in accordance with the Pharmacy Rules and Regulations of the specific state. Guidelines for safe storage of medications must be followed, including the rule that medications be accessible only to personnel responsible for their administration or for distribution of self-administered medications. Some states require that internal and external medications be stored separately. Care must be taken to ensure that prescription medications be used only by those for whom the medication was prescribed.

Work Setting

Healthy employees are more productive than unhealthy employees. This fact, coupled with the escalating costs of health care and insurance, has inspired many businesses to offer some type of health care at the work site. This care may range from emergency first aid and work-related safety initiatives to the provision of primary care and referral services.

Occupational and environmental health nursing is a specialty practice that provides for and delivers health care services to workers and worker populations. The practice is autonomous and focuses on the promotion, protection, and restoration of workers' health within the context of a safe and healthy work environment. According to the American Association of Occupational Health Nurses (AAOHN), occupational and environmental health nurses may function in a variety of roles, including but not limited to solo practitioner, manager, educator, consultant, nurse practitioner, case manager, and corporate director, and these nurses often work with the other members of an occupational health and safety team (e.g., medicine, safety, industrial hygiene).

The nurse needs to be aware of the policies and procedures for administration of medication at the specific work site. There is great diversity in policy and procedure among settings. Following are two examples of the many current practices at work sites:

- At one setting, the registered nurse follows protocols for selected employee complaints (e.g., back injuries: acute and chronic; burns: thermal, chemical, and electrical; eye emergencies; herpes; adult immunizations). Each protocol includes the following areas with relevant information for the specific complaint: assessment, treatment/medications, patient education, referral, and follow-up. Medications are identified as appropriate and noted under the treatment/medications section with the stated drug, dosage, frequency, and route.
- Another work site has established self-care stations for minor illnesses and injuries. Each station has designated criteria for use. Examples include stations for colds, superficial cuts, and menstrual cramps. Employees are familiarized with this service as part of the orientation process. Upon arrival at the stations, employees note date, time, and signature on the sign-in sheet posted at each station. They indicate their chief complaint or reason for seeking medication and the specific medication they have taken from the OTC preparations supplied at each station.

An excellent resource for care of patients in the work setting is the AAOHN website at *www.aaohn.org*.

Nursing Process
Patient-Centered Collaborative Care

Overview of Medication Administration

Assessment

- Obtain appropriate vital signs and relevant laboratory test results for future comparisons and evaluation of the therapeutic response.
- Obtain drug history (prescription, OTC, and herbal preparations), including drug, food, latex, and environmental allergies.
- Identify patients/students/employees at high risk for reactions.
- Assess patient's/student's/employee's capability to follow therapeutic regimen.
- Determine patient/student/employee learning needs.

Nursing Diagnoses

- Risk for injury related to possible adverse reaction
- Deficient knowledge related to therapeutic regimen
- Risk-prone health behavior (taking medications not as prescribed or without first contacting health care provider)

Planning

- Identify goals.
- Promote therapeutic response, and prevent or minimize adverse reactions.
- Identify strategies to promote adherence.
- Identify interventions.

Nursing Interventions

- Prepare equipment and environment; wash hands.
- Verify patient/student/employee identification.
- Determine allergies and other assessment data.
- Check drug label three times; check expiration date.
- Be certain of drug calculation; verify dose with another registered nurse as necessary.
- Pour liquids at eye level on flat surface.
- Avoid contact with topical and inhalation preparations.
- Administer only drugs you have prepared.
- Assist patient to desired position.
- Discard needles and syringes in "sharps" container.
- Keep all drugs stored properly, especially related to temperature, light, and moisture.
- Follow policy related to discarding drugs and controlled substances.
- Report drug errors immediately.
- Document all appropriate information in a timely manner.
- Record effectiveness of drugs administered and reason for any drugs refused.

Cultural Considerations

- When language barriers are present, use literature and videos in the patient's preferred language and with pictures of the patient's cultural group to promote adherence with health interventions.
- Obtain an interpreter when necessary; do not rely on family members, who may not fully disclose because of honor or guilt. Provide interpreter with the same ethnic background and gender if possible, especially with sensitive topics.
- When offering a prescription, instructions, or pamphlets to Asians and Pacific Islanders, use both hands to show respect.
- Include grandparents when providing support and health teaching for African Americans.
- Encourage patients to disclose the use of folk healers and treatments prescribed. Incorporate harmless and nonconflicting practices into the therapeutic plan.

Evaluation

- Evaluate effectiveness of medication(s) administered.
- Identify expected time frame of desired drug response; consider need for modification of therapy.
- Determine patient/student/employee satisfaction with regimen.
- Determine patient/student/employee knowledge of medication regimen.

KEY WEBSITES

Directory of Prescription Drug Patient Assistance Programs: *www.phrma.org*

IMS Institute for Healthcare Informatics: *www.imshealth.com*

2013 National Patient Safety Goals: *www.jointcommission.org/standards_information/npsgs.aspx*

CRITICAL THINKING CASE STUDY

The junior high school nurse is reflecting on the activities and events at the school during the last several weeks. Several students have chronic conditions and require medications during the school day for optimum effectiveness.

1. What is key information for medication administration in the school setting?
2. A student reports to the nurse's office and states that he needs his medicine for his chronic condition. What must be in place before the nurse can administer medication to the student?
3. A student asks the school nurse about starting herbal products "to feel stronger." What is the best response by the nurse?
4. The school has a culturally diverse student population. What cultural resources are recommended to provide the students with the optimal level of care?

NCLEX STUDY QUESTIONS

1. The nurse is preparing a health teaching session for a patient. Which topic is the most important for the nurse to include in health teaching?
   a. Foods to avoid
   b. Patient safety
   c. Storage of medication
   d. Laboratory test results
2. Community-dwelling individuals may take over-the-counter (OTC) preparations. The nurse includes in health teaching related to OTC preparations the importance of contacting the health care provider in which situations? (Select all that apply.)
   a. When planning to use OTC products
   b. When symptoms persist
   c. When prescriptions are filled
   d. When adding an herbal product
   e. When quick relief is not achieved
3. Patients in the community often have questions about how long it takes for various types of medications to "work." The nurse correctly reports which general guidelines? (Select all that apply.)
   a. Psychotropics—6 weeks
   b. Antibiotics—24 hours
   c. Opioids—many within 30 minutes
   d. Antiinflammatories—within 1 week
   e. Glucocorticoids—immediately
4. An adult Hispanic patient comes to the mobile health unit for evaluation of his cardiac condition. An interpreter will be present during the visit. Which qualities are most important for the nurse to consider when matching an interpreter with a patient? (Select all that apply.)
   a. About same age as patient
   b. Same ethnicity as patient
   c. Same gender as patient
   d. Member of patient's family
   e. Similar likes and hobbies as patient

5. The role of the nurse in the community setting is multifaceted and commonly includes which actions? (Select all that apply.)
   a. Assist patient to identify community resources.
   b. Take patient to health appointments.
   c. Emphasize importance of follow-up health appointments.
   d. Educate on safe disposal of medications.
   e. Administer daily oral medications.
6. The nurse makes a home visit to a patient who was discharged from the hospital the previous day. Which are regulations for the nurse administering medications in the home setting to follow? (Select all that apply.)
   a. May administer medication on a long-term basis
   b. Must be an FDA-approved drug
   c. Drug is ordered by the health care provider
   d. May administer drug on a short-term basis if caregiver is unable
   e. May compound medications in the home
7. The school nurse is updating the policy and procedure manual for medication administration. Which are examples of content? (Select all that apply.)
   a. The nurse is accountable for state law and regulations.
   b. Medication can be given with parents' verbal permission.
   c. Policy to address how OTC medications are received, stored, and labeled
   d. Medications must be stored in a secure, locked, and clean area.
   e. Electronic health record must be maintained on a daily basis.

Answers: 1, b; 2, a, d; 3, a, b, c; 4, a, b, c; 5, a, c, d; 6, b, c, d; 7, a, c, d.

CHAPTER 10

The Role of the Nurse in Drug Research

evolve WEBSITE

http://evolve.elsevier.com/KeeHayes/pharmacology/

- Animations
- Content Updates
- Key Points
- Review Questions for the NCLEX® Examination
- References from the Textbook
- Unfolding Case Studies

OBJECTIVES

- Discuss basic ethical principles.
- Relate the basic ethical principles governing informed consent and risk-to-benefit ratio.
- Describe the objectives of each phase of human clinical experimentation.
- Discuss the role of the nurse in clinical drug trials using the nursing process.

OUTLINE

KEY TERMS

active control, p. 109
autonomy, p. 106
beneficence, p. 106
control group, p. 107
Declaration of Helsinki, p. 107
double-blind, p. 109
experimental group, p. 107
FDA Modernization Act of 1997, p. 108
Good Clinical Practice: Consolidated Guideline, p. 107
informed consent, p. 106
open-label study, p. 109
placebo, p. 109
Prescription Drug User Fee Act, p. 108
single-blind, p. 109
triple-blind, p. 109
veracity, p. 106

In the United States, all prescription drugs must be approved by the U.S. Food and Drug Administration (FDA) before they are made available on the market. Drug studies take place in a variety of inpatient and outpatient settings. Drug research involves risk and is a "high-cost item," with the estimated average cost to develop each new drug being more than $1 billion.

Drug research and development are complex processes that are of particular interest and importance to professional nursing practice. The nursing process facilitates the integration of cutting-edge research.

This chapter is devoted to a description of basic ethical principles governing informed consent and risk-to-benefit ratio, preclinical testing and human clinical experimentation, and the nurse's role and nursing process in clinical drug trials.

BASIC ETHICAL PRINCIPLES

Four basic ethical principles are relevant to research involving human subjects: respect for persons, beneficence, justice, and veracity. These are integral to the issues of informed consent and risk-to-benefit ratio in research involving human beings.

Respect for Persons

Individuals undergoing treatment in any health care system should be treated as independent persons who are capable of making decisions in their own best interests. Individuals whose decision-making capability is diminished are entitled to protection. The nurse can determine this with consistent reassessment of the patient's cognitive state. Patients should be made aware of the alternatives available to them in their health care, as well as the consequences that stem from those alternatives. The patient's choice should be honored whenever possible. It is imperative that the nurse recognize when the patient is not capable of rational decision making and therefore entitled to protection.

Autonomy is an integral component of respect for persons. **Autonomy** is the right to self-determination. In health care settings, health care personnel must respect the patient's right to make decisions about themselves, even if the decision is not what the personnel want or think is best for the patient. Generally, patients can refuse any and all treatments (right of autonomy) except when the decision poses a threat to others—such as with tuberculosis, when taking medications is legally mandated. Patients have the right to refuse to participate in a research study and may withdraw from studies at any time without penalty of any kind.

Beneficence

Beneficence is the duty to do good and to not harm others, to maximize possible benefits, and to minimize possible harm that might occur in research. It is often not possible to know whether something is beneficial unless it is tested and individuals have been exposed to the risks. A question central to this issue is: Who makes this decision—the patient, or those caring for the patient?

Justice

Justice requires that all people be treated fairly. Expansion of justice includes equal access to health care for all. Justice can be limited when it interferes with the rights of others. The principle of justice, in the context of clinical drug trials, means that social benefits and burdens can be allocated objectively and that those with equivalent circumstances should be treated equally. A challenge to the nurse is the allocation of scarce resources.

Veracity

Veracity requires health care personnel to tell the truth and the whole truth. When there is "bad news" to tell the patient, the health care provider may be reluctant to tell the truth and answer questions honestly. The patient has the right to know the truth, including the bad news.

INFORMED CONSENT

Informed consent has its roots in the 1947 Nuremberg Code. The two most relevant aspects of this Code are the participant's right to be informed and the fact that participation is voluntary, without coercion. If the nurse suspects that a patient is being coerced to participate in a study, the nurse is obligated to report this promptly to the party named on the informed consent (the patient should have a copy of the consent for reference). **Informed consent** has dimensions beyond protection of the individual patient's choice and includes the following:

1. Promotion of individual autonomy
2. Protection of patients and subjects from harm
3. Avoidance of fraud and duress in health care
4. Encouragement for professionals to be thorough and clear in communicating information
5. Promotion of educated decision making among patients
6. Promotion of self-determination of the patient

It is the role of the health care provider, *not* the nurse, to explain the study to the patient (including what is expected of the patient) and to respond to questions. While giving written consent, the patient must be alert and able to comprehend.

It is the nurse's role to protect patients from any anticipated harm. The nurse, in collaboration with the health care provider and pharmacist, must be knowledgeable about all aspects of a drug study, including all inclusion and exclusion criteria for participants (Box 10-1).

BOX 10-1 INCLUSION AND EXCLUSION CRITERIA FOR A HYPOTHETIC PROTOCOL FOR AN EXPERIMENTAL DIURETIC MEDICATION

Inclusion

- Persons between 18 and 65 years of age
- Persons with weight between 50 and 100 kg
- Persons who receive cardiac medications only if dose has been stable for past 3 months
- Persons on sodium-restricted diet

Exclusion

- Pregnant or nursing women
- All women of childbearing age who do not use oral contraceptives
- Persons with severe damage or disease of cardiac, hepatic, renal, neurologic, or musculoskeletal system
- Persons with clinically significant laboratory values

Memorial Hospital

PERMISSION FOR CLINICAL INVESTIGATION

Completed by Client:

1. I hereby authorize Dr. ____________ and/or such assistants as may be selected by him/her to conduct studies upon ____________ for the following: ____________
2. I further authorize Dr. ____________ and/or such assistants as may be selected by him/her, to prescribe drugs or to perform certain procedures in connection with the diagnosis and treatment of my condition including the following drugs and/or extraordinary procedures: ____________
3. I have (have not) been made aware of certain risks, possible consequences and discomfort associated with these drugs or extraordinary procedures which are: ____________
4. I understand that no guarantee or assurance has been made as to the results that may be obtained although I have (have not) been advised of the possibility that certain benefits may be expected such as: ____________
5. I have (have not) had explained to me alternative procedures/treatments/drugs that may be advantageous and they include the following: ____________
6. I have (have not) received an offer to answer any inquiries concerning the procedures involved ____________
7. I have (have not) had explained to me all medical terminology in connection with this study ____________
8. I understand that it is in the intent of the principal investigator to maintain the confidentiality of records identifying subjects in this study. The Food and Drug Administration, however, may possibly inspect the records to monitor compliance with published federal regulations.
9. I understand that I may withdraw this consent and discontinue participation in this study at any time, without prejudice to my care, by informing Dr. ____________ of my desire to withdraw. ______ Yes, I understand ______ No, I do not understand
10. I understand that Department of Health and Human Services regulations require the Memorial Hospital to inform me of any provisions to provide for medical treatment for any physical injury which may occur as a result of this study. In this connection, I understand that the Memorial Hospital does not have a formal plan or program to provide for the cost of medical treatment or compensation for any physical injury which occurs as a result of this study and for which they do not have legal liability. However, in the unlikely event that I am injured as a result of my participation, I understand that I should promptly inform Dr. ____________

SIGNED ____________

RELATIONSHIP ____________

ADDRESS ____________

DATED ____________

Completed by witness:

I, the undersigned, hereby acknowledge that I was present during the explanation of the above consent for clinical investigation given by Dr. ____________ to ____________ during which the nature, purpose, risks, complications and consequences thereof were fully set forth and all questions answered and I was present while ____________ signed the above consent.

Dated ____________

____________ (witness)

____________ (address)

FIGURE 10–1 An example of informed consent.

Figure 10-1 shows an example of Permission for Clinical Investigation, and Box 10-2 shows an Informed Consent Checklist.

RISK-TO-BENEFIT RATIO

The risk-to-benefit ratio is one of the most complex problems faced by the researcher. All possible consequences of a clinical study must be analyzed and balanced with the inherent risks and the anticipated benefits. Physical, psychological, and social risks must be identified and weighed against the benefits. A requirement of the Department of Health and Human Services (DHHS) is that institutional review boards (IRBs) determine that risks to subjects be reasonable in relation to the anticipated benefits, if any, for subjects. No matter how noble the intentions, the calculation of risks and benefits by the researcher cannot be totally accurate or comprehensive.

BOX 10-2 INFORMED CONSENT CHECKLIST

- Participates voluntarily
- Identifies related drugs, treatments, and techniques
- Describes benefits and risks
- Describes other forms of treatment available
- Describes laboratory tests to monitor patient's reactions
- Identifies extent of confidentiality of results
- Describes availability of emergency treatment for illness/injury, if any
- States compensation for study-related injury, if any
- States compensation for participation, if any
- Writes consent clearly and understands easily at tenth-grade reading level
- Provides name and telephone number of contact person for patient questions and concerns

Varying amounts of time are required for the process of identifying a potentially useful chemical and having it become available to the general population; in many cases, 15 years may elapse. Only 1 in 10,000 potential drugs endures the research and development process and is used in a clinical situation.

OBJECTIVES AND PHASES OF HUMAN CLINICAL EXPERIMENTATION

Good Clinical Practice (GCP): Consolidated Guideline, an international ethical and scientific standard for design, conduct, performance, monitoring, auditing, recording, analysis, and reporting, is the foundation of clinical trials. Guidance and information sheets are available from the FDA on multiple topics related to clinical trials. Examples include information sheets for IRBs and Clinical Investigators and Choice of Control Groups and Related Issues in Clinical Trials. Websites with this and expanded information are the U.S. National Institutes of Health at http://clinicaltrials.gov and TrialsCentral at http://trialscentral.org. In addition, the World Medical Association **Declaration of Helsinki** has crafted ethical principles for medical research involving human subjects. This and other relevant websites are listed at the end of the chapter.

Preclinical Testing

Preclinical testing consists of in vitro and in vivo systems. In vitro experimentation is generally conducted in a test tube or other laboratory equipment, and in vivo testing is conducted with living organisms. This testing is followed by toxicity screening to identify (1) abnormal changes in animal organs related to drug administration and (2) the parameters of the safe therapeutic dose. Control and experimental groups of animals are compared. Participants in the **experimental group** receive the experimental intervention or treatment. Those in the **control group** do not receive the experimental intervention or treatment and provide a baseline against which to measure the effects of the treatment. Before initiating human studies, an assessment is made of the seriousness of the disease to be treated using this drug in relation to the drug's toxicity.

Human Clinical Experimentation

For every 5,000 to 10,000 compounds screened as potential new medications, only 5 are entered into clinical trials. To bring a new drug to market takes an average of 6 to 15 years, and costs continue to rise. The **FDA Modernization Act of 1997** increased the minimum age for subjects of human clinical experimentation. The Act has five provisions, one of which requires pediatric evaluation of new products intended for use by children. The Act advocates for children and appropriate testing for drugs to be used by the pediatric population. The automatic universal exclusion of children from clinical trials is not justified. Refer to Chapter 2 for a listing of the provisions of this act.

Drug research was historically done only with white males, causing uncertainty as to the validity of research results for people of other ethnicities and for white women. In 1993, Congress passed the NIH Revitalization Act to include white women and minorities.

Clinical experimentation in drug research and development encompasses four phases, each with its own objectives (Figure 10-2). A multidisciplinary team approach (nurses, physicians, pharmacologists, statisticians, and research associates) is required to ensure throughout the phases that the data collected will answer the clinical questions. A brief description of each phase follows.

Phase I

Phase I trials are primarily designed to assess safety. Their objectives are to determine the human dosage range based on response in healthy human beings and to identify the pharmacokinetics (i.e., absorption, distribution, metabolism/biotransformation, and excretion/elimination) of the drug. Progression to the next phase occurs if no serious adverse effects are demonstrated, the drug is eliminated in a reasonable amount of time, and the dose range is below that known to induce pathology in animals.

Phase II

The objective of phase II is to demonstrate the safety and efficacy of the drug in subjects who have the disease the drug is designed to treat. Phase III is initiated only when acceptable efficacy and safety data are generated and clearly documented in Phase II.

Phases III and IV

Phase III studies involve large numbers of subjects who have the disease intended for treatment. The objectives of Phases III and IV are to demonstrate the safety and efficacy of the drug for a wide patient population and to include long-term data if a chronic regimen is under consideration. Phase IV studies may also examine potential new indications for approved drugs. The sponsor submits all relevant and analyzed data in a new drug application (NDA) to the FDA. The FDA decides to approve, reject, or recommend withdrawal or resubmission. After the NDA research has been approved, Phase IV addresses the long-term use of the drug.

The pharmaceutic industry is eager to get new drugs to market. Delays in the FDA approval process were decreasing the valuable life of a drug's patent; therefore, in 1992 Congress passed the **Prescription Drug User Fee Act,** which provided the FDA with funds to expedite the review process. As a result, the average drug approval time has decreased from 30 to 12 months.

Challenges and new directions await clinical trial programs of the future. Specifically, future trials are needed for certain populations at risk, such as profiling patient and tumor for cancer-related trials. In addition, research is needed on drugs to treat orphan disease conditions.

Study Designs

An appropriate experimental design is important in being able to answer questions about drug safety and efficacy. The experimental design uses different groups of subjects (i.e., some groups who receive treatment and control groups who receive no treatment, an alternative treatment, or a combination of both) and assigns subjects randomly to treatment or control groups. Treatment groups and control groups do not differ in terms of baseline characteristics or demographics. If the subjects are different, variability is introduced and it becomes more difficult to determine a treatment effect. The examples in the following paragraphs illustrate selected research designs.

A *quasi-experimental* design would be a comparison of intermittent intravenous (IV) device patency of those hospitalized patients who received heparin flushes and those who

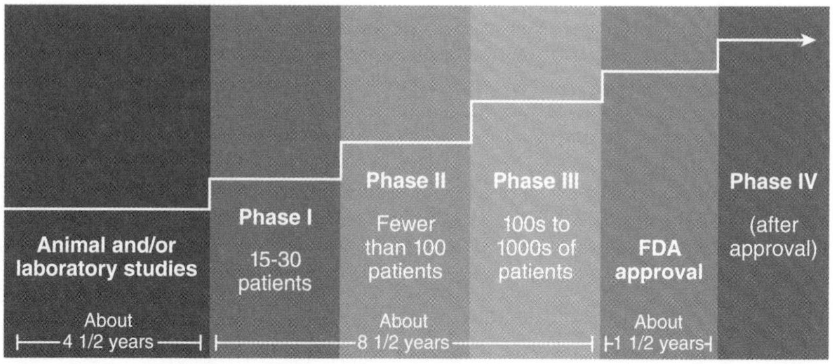

FIGURE 10–2 Clinical trials process.

received saline flushes. This study would have a nonmatched comparison group but no random assignment to a treatment group. Such quasi-experimental designs may contribute valuable information but ultimately lack the power to ascribe *cause*, because the variables are uncontrolled and potentially influential. Ethical decisions do not permit the use of this experimental design in all situations. For example, an experimental study to determine whether nicotine causes cancer would be unethical because individuals would have to be exposed to a carcinogenic substance. However, it might be possible to use an already-exposed group (smokers) as a comparator.

A researcher designs a study to show the effect of the independent variable (the drug) on the dependent variables (clinical responses or reactions). Intervening variables are specific to the research question and may include age, sex, weight, disease and its state of severity, diet, and the subject's social environment. It is important to control for as many of the intervening variables as possible to make it easier to determine whether there is a drug effect. Controlled treatment groups in drug research trials can receive no drug; a different drug; a **placebo** (pharmacologically inert substance); or the same drug with a different dose, route, or frequency of administration. A control group receiving a different drug is called an **active control.** In some cases, such as cancer treatment, it would not be ethical to use a placebo as a control.

A *crossover* design uses each subject in several different situations. In the first instance, the experimental group receives the drug and the control group receives an alternative form of treatment or no treatment. Then both groups receive no therapy. Finally, the experimental group receives the control form of therapy and the control group receives the drug. In this design, the subject serves as his or her own control.

The researcher wants to generalize the findings from the sample of subjects to the larger target population, such as all women with breast cancer. A statistical method called *probability sampling* (subjects are randomly selected from the entire population) is typically used to provide relative confidence in the generalization of findings.

In a *matched-pair* design, the researcher identifies several variables that may influence the outcome such as age, weight, or family history; the subjects are matched for these variables. One of the pair is randomly assigned to the experimental group and the other to the control group. A less effective technique is nonrandom assignment to treatment group.

The **double-blind** technique is a powerful tool wherein neither the health care provider nor the subject knows whether the subject is receiving the experimental or control form of therapy. In **triple-blind** studies, a researcher other than the prescribing health care provider collects data and is also unaware of the subject's treatment group. In a **single-blind** study, only the subjects are unaware of which group to which they are assigned. An **open-label study** indicates that all parties (data collectors, prescribing health care provider, and subject) know the treatment group assignment. The double-blind and triple-blind techniques are preferred for drug research, because those involved in the study are not aware of the subject's treatment group, thereby removing a source of bias.

Nurse's Role

The nurse has a pivotal role in drug clinical trials. The research and development process for drug research requires the multifaceted roles of professional nursing practice. Nurses must first consider their own thoughts, feelings, and beliefs about clinical trials. The nurse is both the patient and family advocate and the liaison between the patient, the health care provider, and the research nurse responsible for the specific protocol. Thorough and timely communication is essential in all aspects of the nurse's role. Nursing involvement is pivotal to the successful completion of clinical trials.

Asking relevant questions about informed consent and risk-to-benefit ratio is a major role of the nurse. Refer to the website for the Health Insurance Portability and Accountability Act (HIPAA) for implications for clinical trials (e.g., consent and privacy issues). Awareness of initial indicators of change in the patient and prediction of increased risk for adverse drug reaction are also dimensions of professional nursing practice.

Nursing responsibilities related to the specific research or clinical trial span the nursing process. Critical to the assessment phase are the recruitment and assessment of study subjects; a thorough understanding of the protocol, including inclusion and exclusion criteria for subjects; validity and reliability of measurement instruments; ongoing teamwork; and communication with the health care providers and sponsors.

Nursing input is important in the budget negotiations of the clinical trial as well as staff education on protocol requirements. Protocol guidelines are an essential component of staff education with special attention to ensuring that the subject's consent is "informed consent" obtained by the health care provider. The nurse is an ongoing resource when subject and family questions arise.

Protocol-based nursing implementations include comprehensive screening of subjects and monitoring parameters per protocol with relevant and timely communication with the entire health care team. Documentation on all predetermined components throughout the clinical trial is mandatory, including input from study subjects.

During the evaluation phase, the nurse's role involves examining the research statement or question. In addition, it considers elements such as: Are the conclusions valid and data-based? Are the findings clinically significant?

Nursing Process
Patient-Centered Collaborative Care

Clinical Drug Trials

Assessment

- Explore own beliefs about clinical trials.
- Recruit subjects.

- Assess protocol.
- Demonstrate thorough knowledge of all inclusion/exclusion criteria for subjects (see Box 10-1).
- Articulate observations and concerns to health care providers and sponsors/pharmaceutical company.
- Communicate need for drug to address a specific need with the appropriate individuals.

Planning

- Develop fact sheet of protocol guidelines.
- Educate involved staff about protocol requirements.
- Provide input into budget negotiations.
- Coordinate personnel and budget, including office visits, special tests, and laboratory work.
- Ensure that subject consent is informed (see Box 10-2 and Figure 10-1).
- Respond to subject's questions.

Nursing Interventions

- Screen subjects accurately and thoroughly based on established protocol.
- Adhere to protocol guidelines, including administration of drug.
- Monitor selected parameters. Observe and report toxicities promptly.
- Collect all data required by the sponsor (e.g., drug company).
- Communicate information in a complete, concise, accurate, and timely manner to the principal investigator and sponsor.
- Document data in a clear and timely manner.
- Record subjects' own evaluation; seemingly unrelated responses may be significant. At times, a drug is actually marketed for a different indication than the original testing.
- Report all adverse effects, including deaths, to physician, sponsor, Institutional Review Board, and FDA, whether or not the cause of death is drug related.

Cultural Considerations

- Be alert to specific side effects in selected drug groups from patients of different ethnic backgrounds (e.g., African Americans and their side effects from tricyclic antidepressants).
- Use an interpreter when necessary, preferably from the same ethnicity and gender, especially for sensitive and anxiety-raising topics.
- Depending on patient's background, include the extended family in the teaching and support system.

Evaluation

- Was the research design appropriate and maintained?
- Are the conclusions valid and based on data?
- Are the clinical findings significant?

KEY WEBSITES

Declaration of Helsinki: Recommendation for Conduct of Clinical Research: *www.wma.net/en/30publications/10policies/b3/index.html*

Good Clinical Practice: *www.fda.gov/oc/gcp/default.htm*

Health Insurance Portability and Accountability Act (HIPAA): *www.hhs.gov/ocr/privacy/*

Human Genome project: *www.genome.gov/27549135*

NCLEX STUDY QUESTIONS

1. The nurse in the clinical research setting is knowledgeable about ethical principles and protection of human subjects. What principle is demonstrated when ensuring the patient's right to self-determination?
   a. Beneficence
   b. Autonomy
   c. Justice
   d. Informed consent
2. The research nurse is meeting with a patient and, based on the assessment, determines that the patient meets the criteria. The patient agrees to participate in the clinical trial. The nurse advises the patient that which member of the health care team has the responsibility to explain the study and respond to questions?
   a. Registered nurse
   b. Pharmacist
   c. Research associate
   d. Health care provider
3. The clinical research nurse knows that only a small proportion of drugs survives the research and development process. An appreciation of the process and associated costs grows when the nurse is aware that approximately one in how many potential drugs is actually used in clinical situations?
   a. 100
   b. 1000
   c. 10,000
   d. 100,000
4. The nurse is interviewing a patient in a Phase I clinical trial. Which patient statement indicates an understanding of this trial phase?
   a. "I am doing this to be sure this drug is safe."
   b. "I am doing this to be sure this drug is efficacious."
   c. "I hope this drug has no side effects."
   d. "I can be part of demonstrating a cure."

5. The nurse is reviewing the protocols associated with a triple-blind study. The nurse understands that this technique is preferred in clinical trials because it removes which factor?
   a. Knowledge
   b. Conflicts
   c. Prejudice
   d. Bias
6. The foundation of clinical trials, Good Clinical Practice (GCP) is a helpful resource for nurses. The nurse is correct in choosing GPC as a reference for standards in which areas? (Select all that apply.)
   a. Design and performance
   b. Monitoring and auditing
   c. Analyses
   d. Reporting
   e. Outcomes evaluation
7. The nurse has an important role in working with patients on aspects of care that require informed consent. The patient and the nurse must be aware of the dimensions of informed consent. Which dimensions are included? (Select all that apply.)
   a. Protection of subjects from harm
   b. Promotion of finding cure of disease
   c. Protection of patient's self-determination
   d. Promotion of patient's educated decision making
   e. Promotion of individual autonomy
8. The nurse researcher reviews the proposed informed consent form for a future clinical trial. The nurse expects to find which in the document? (Select all that apply.)
   a. Description of benefits and risks
   b. Identification of related drugs, treatments, and techniques
   c. Description of outcomes
   d. Statement of compensation for participants, if any
   e. Description of serious risks
9. The nurse knows that the patient should be informed about available alternatives and consequences. What ethical principle does this describe?
   a. Respect for persons
   b. Veracity
   c. Justice
   d. Beneficence

Answers: 1, b; 2, d; 3, c; 4, a; 5, d; 6, a, b, c, d; 7, a, c, d, e; 8, a, b, d, e; 9, a.

UNIT II

A Nurse's Perspective of Pharmacology

The steps of the nursing process are described in Chapter 11, The Nursing Process in Patient-Centered Pharmacotherapy. Patient collaboration, also discussed in Chapter 11, is essential to promoting patient and family understanding of and adherence to drug therapy.

Chapter 12, Safety and Quality in Pharmacotherapy, provides information related to the medication culture of safety, including the rights of drug administration and the Quality and Safety Education for Nurses (QSEN) initiative. Chapter 13, Medication Administration, contains basic learning material for the administration of medications. It describes drug orders, drug distribution, drug charts, drug administration guidelines, and drug administration routes (with illustrated parenteral sites).

Chapter 13 and Unit III are recommended for drug administration and calculation in place of a nursing fundamentals text or a drug calculation text.

CHAPTER

11

The Nursing Process in Patient-Centered Pharmacotherapy

evolve WEBSITE

http://evolve.elsevier.com/KeeHayes/pharmacology/

- Animations
- Content Updates
- Key Points
- Review Questions for the NCLEX® Examination
- References from the Textbook
- Unfolding Case Studies

OBJECTIVES

- Discuss QSEN and the Guiding Principles for Patient Engagement in relation to medication safety.
- Differentiate the steps of the nursing process and their purpose in relation to drug therapy.
- Develop patient-centered goals.
- Discuss at least eight principles for health teaching related to drug therapy plans.
- Describe at least six culturally sensitive health teaching tips.
- Analyze the nurse's role related to drug therapy plans.

OUTLINE

KEY TERMS

Nurses have a significant role in the management and delivery of safe drug therapy. Influences on this role include technology, increased longevity of populations in general, and survival of persons with multiple and varied biopsychosocial needs. Variables in drug therapy are numerous and, at times, unknown. The nurse is most often the one person who follows the patient most closely and the one who is first to assess the patient's response to drugs. The nurse applies knowledge of pharmacology to anticipate drug responses in the individual patient.

This chapter explores the use of the nursing process as it relates to drug therapy and patient education about pharmacotherapy. Careful attention to each phase of the process fosters the patient's success with the prescribed medication regimen. Initiatives such as Quality and Safety Education for Nurses (QSEN) and the Guiding Principles for Patient Engagement are resources to help nurses ensure and advocate for patient-centered collaborative care.

The overall goal through all phases of QSEN is to prepare future nurses with the knowledge, skills, and attitudes necessary to improve the quality and safety of the health care systems in which they work.

The QSEN competencies are as follows:

1. Patient- and family-centered care: Recognize the patient as the source of control and full partner in providing compassionate and coordinated care based on respect for patient preferences, values, and needs.

2. Collaboration and teamwork: Function effectively in nursing and interprofessional teams, fostering open communication, mutual respect, and shared decision making to achieve quality patient care.
3. Evidence-based practice: Integrate best current evidence with clinical expertise and patient/family preferences and values for delivery of optimal health care.
4. Quality improvement: Continuously improve the quality and safety of health care systems by using data to monitor outcomes of care processes and improvement methods to design and test changes.
5. Safety: Minimize risk of harm to patients and providers through both system effectiveness and individual performance.
6. Informatics: Use information and technology to communicate, manage knowledge, mitigate error, and support decision making.

This chapter focuses on patient- and family-centered care, and Chapter 12 offers additional information on safety in pharmacotherapy. QSEN competencies are also integrated throughout the book and are highlighted in special features such as Safety: Preventing Medication Errors boxes and High-Alert Drug icons. Patient-centered collaborative care is demonstrated in each nursing process.

Guiding Principles for Patient Engagement are core principles to support health care providers in their practice of patient-centered, quality care. These principles were developed by the Alliance for Quality Care (NAQC) and supported by the Robert Wood Johnson Foundation with the aim of "patient relationship as the cornerstone of patient safety and quality."

The core principles address the dynamic partnership among patients, their families, and the providers of their health care, confidentiality, mutual responsibilities and accountabilities, levels of engagement, advocacy, respecting boundaries, appreciation of patient's rights, mutuality, and health care literacy, and acknowledgment and appreciation of diverse backgrounds.

Both QSEN and the Guiding Principles for Patient Engagement assert principles that are foundational to patient-centered practice and safety in pharmacotherapy.

NURSING PROCESS: PATIENT-CENTERED COLLABORATIVE CARE

The phases of the nursing process are assessment, nursing diagnosis, planning, implementation (nursing interventions), and evaluation. Each phase is dependent on the preceding phase; sometimes revisiting a preceding phase is required. The phases are discussed as each relates to health teaching in drug therapy.

Assessment

The **assessment** phase of the nursing process is characterized by the systematic validation and documentation of information. Assessments are made throughout the nursing process. Assessment is particularly important because the data provided by the assessment form the basis on which nursing diagnoses are made and care is planned, implemented, and evaluated. Data collection must include both subjective and objective information.

Subjective Data

Subjective data are symptoms described by and apparent to the patient. The following components are reflective of subjective data related to the medication regimen:

- Current health history, including any problems with swallowing
- Patient symptoms
- Current medications, including over-the-counter (OTC) drugs, herbal remedies, and nutritional supplements
  - Dosage, frequency, and route of all drugs, and prescribing health care provider, if any
  - Patient knowledge about drug, its side effects, and reason drug is taken
  - Patient adherence with regimen and reasons for deviations (Were prescriptions filled and finished? Are deviations based on valid data/rationale and clinically sound?)
  - Patient expectation and perception of drug effectiveness
  - Patient knowledge about what effects or drug reactions to report to health care provider
  - Drug allergies or reactions both past and present; also reactions to food and dye
  - Use of tobacco products, alcohol, caffeine, and recreational drugs, including frequency and duration of use
- Past health history
  - Past illnesses, major injuries, drug therapy
  - Mental status
  - Medications saved from previous use, reason for saving them, and expiration date
- Patient's environment
  - Home safety (stairs, lighting, rugs, smoke detectors, supplies) and neighborhood safety (lighting, sidewalks) to meet patient's and family's specific needs.
  - Patient's language and communication needs (including language of origin)
  - Patient's ability and readiness to read and follow instructions from the health care provider and the pharmacy
  - Patient knowledge of specific drug storage requirements, if any
  - Availability, willingness, and psychomotor ability to administer or assist in the administration of medications; capability for activities of daily living (This information is essential for third-party payment for continued home visits or for admission to an extended care facility.)
  - Household members (neighbors and friends and their roles, if possible); ages of household members
  - Learning style preferences
  - Readiness to learn

- Dietary patterns, cultural and economic influences, safety
- Financial resources or limitations (drugs can be expensive)

Remember: Patients, even those who do not intend to withhold information, do not always share everything about their medications. Therefore, in addition to asking about prescription drugs, ask specifically about vitamin and mineral supplements, herbal supplements, all contraceptives, and OTC drugs. Identify caffeine and nicotine use, and include questions about use of skin patches; laypersons often fail to see patches as a mechanism of drug administration. Home health nurses should ask to see the contents of the medicine chest at home (or other storage area for medications) and should ask if the patient practices pill-splitting as a cost-saving measure and whether a pharmacist is consulted. Based on the response, appropriate teaching can be initiated.

Objective Data

Objective data are signs that are measured and detected by another person. The following components are reflective of objective data related to the medication regimen:

- Physical health assessment: Limitations in gross- and fine-motor control; hand and joint range of motion; hand and finger muscle strength; visual impairment; and ability to read labels and correctly measure dosages.
- Laboratory test results and diagnostic studies: Baseline data are essential for future comparisons.

Data collection should provide additional information about the patient's symptoms and should also target those organs most likely to be affected by drug therapy. For example, if a drug is nephrotoxic, the patient's creatinine clearance should be assessed. Assess major body systems for any signs of reaction to or interaction of drugs or ineffectiveness of therapy.

Based on assessment data, the nurse must identify high-risk patients (those likely to have adverse reactions). The patient's health history, physical assessment, and laboratory test results are sources of these data.

Enhancing patient adherence with the drug therapy regimen is an essential component of health teaching. The patient and family response to the following three questions provides the nurse with critical information unique to each patient's teaching situation:

1. What things help you take your medicine as prescribed?
2. What things prevent you from taking your medicine as prescribed?
3. What would you do if you forgot to take a dose of medication?

Frequently cited factors for nonadherence include forgetfulness, knowledge deficit, side effects, low self-esteem, depression, lack of trust in the health care system, family problems, language barriers, high cost of medications, anxiety, value systems (e.g., religion), and lack of motivation. Drug shortages create additional concerns because patients may be dissatisfied with the effectiveness, cost, and side effects of alternative drug choices.

The patient's attitudes and values about taking medication are very important considerations when determining the patient's and family's readiness to learn. These attitudes and values should be considered when planning interventions to support the patient's decision to adopt healthy behaviors related to taking medications. The patient's social support system is emphasized. This special support system, unique to the individual, may be composed of persons who assist in preparing medications, organizing pills, and ordering medications, and can be alert to side effects—all actions that promote taking medication as prescribed and notifying the health care provider if a problem arises.

Nursing Diagnosis

A **nursing diagnosis** is made based on the analysis of the assessment data. Abnormal data collected during the assessment serve as the defining characteristics (for an actual problem) or risk factors (for a high risk for a problem) to support the appropriate nursing diagnosis. More than one applicable nursing diagnosis may be generated. The registered nurse formulates nursing diagnoses and uses them to guide the development of a care plan.

Common nursing diagnoses related to drug therapy include the following:

- Pain (acute or chronic) related to hesitancy in taking prescribed pain medications because of fear of addiction
- Acute confusion related to adverse reaction to medication
- Ineffective health maintenance related to not receiving recommended preventive care
- Deficient knowledge related to effects of anticoagulant medication on clotting mechanism
- Noncompliance related to forgetfulness
- Risk for injury related to side effects of drug (e.g., dizziness, drowsiness)
- Ineffective self-health management related to lack of finances or health care coverage to purchase medications
- Readiness for enhanced knowledge related to medication schedule and medication side effects

Use of these nursing diagnoses is beneficial to the patient because it facilitates the development of an individualized care plan for each patient. Note: To strengthen comprehensiveness of nursing diagnoses, consider using well/health promotion diagnoses.

Planning

The **planning** phase of the nursing process is characterized by **goal setting** or expected outcomes. Goals are patient centered, describe the specific activity, and include a time frame for achievement/reevaluation. Planning also includes development of nursing interventions that will be used to assist the patient to meet the goals. Effective goal setting has the following qualities:

- Is patient centered (accomplished through collaboration with the patient and/or family to develop goals that focus on patient outcomes)

- Clearly states the expected change: realistic, measurable, with reasonable deadlines
- Is acceptable to both patient and nurse (dependent on patient's decision-making ability)
- Is shared with other health care providers and with patient's family or caregiver
- Identifies components for evaluation

Examples of well-written comprehensive goals are (1) patient will independently administer prescribed dose of insulin by end of the fourth session of instruction; (2) patient will prepare a medication recording sheet that correctly reflects prescribed medication schedule within 3 days.

Implementation and Nursing Interventions

The **implementation** phase is the part of the nursing process in which the nurse provides education, medication administration, patient care, and other interventions necessary to assist the patient in accomplishing the established goals. In most practice settings, administration of drugs and assessment of drug effectiveness are also important nursing responsibilities. (See Chapters 12 and 13 for more information.)

Patient Teaching

Readiness to learn is paramount. Patient education is an ongoing, complex, multifaceted process and a dynamic interaction between nurse and patient in which both communicate information and emotions. Teaching is focused on health promotion and/or a specific skill to optimize patient health status. Teaching is more effective in an environment free of distractions, and the information should be tailored to the patient's interests and level of understanding. Assessment data suggest the complexity, number, and length of teaching sessions that may be required. Be sensitive to the patient's motivation to learn, attention span, and level of frustration. Readiness to learn is paramount. Readiness should be assessed first, before information is presented to the patient. Use a positive approach—for example, "This narcotic is usually effective for the relief of the type of pain you have." Be an active listener and observer.

Assessment data guide the nurse to the appropriate persons to be included. The inclusion of a family member or friend in the teaching plan is an excellent idea. This person may (1) act as a psychological support, (2) actually administer all or part of the drug therapy, (3) observe the effectiveness and side effects of the drug therapy, and (4) implement other changes such as food shopping or instituting new methods of food preparation. Provide simple written materials appropriate for individual patient needs. The patient and family must have the appropriate information (e.g., telephone number, email address) to reach the health care provider for questions and concerns. Health care providers should be available to provide timely responses.

With patient teaching being critical to the success of pharmacotherapy, it might be helpful for the nurse to use an outline format for patient education. Suggested topics related to pharmacotherapeutics include the following:

- *General.* Instruct the patient to take the drug as prescribed. Adherence is of utmost importance because discontinuing the drug before the course is completed may result in relapse or future ineffectiveness of the drug. Do not adjust dose, frequency, or time of day taken unless directed by the health care provider. Advise women contemplating pregnancy to check first with their health care provider before taking prescription or OTC medications and herbal products. Advise patients to consult with their health care provider about laboratory tests such as liver enzymes, blood urea nitrogen (BUN), creatinine, and electrolytes, which should be monitored when taking selected drugs.
- *Self-administration.* The patient's psychomotor skills and abilities are critical. Based on assessment of these, consider recommendations for modifications as appropriate. Reassess psychomotor skills on an ongoing basis. Instruct the patient on the administration of the drug according to the prescribed route: eyedrops or nose drops, subcutaneous insulin injections, suppositories, swish-and-swallow suspensions, and metered-dose inhalers with and without spacers. Include demonstration and return demonstration in the instructions when appropriate. Give written instructions for the sighted patient and audio instructions for the visually impaired. Teach more than one person when possible, because this aids in reinforcement and retention of information. It also provides a "backup" if the patient is unable to self-administer the drug.
- *Diet.* Advise patients about foods to include in their diet and foods to avoid. Many foods interact with certain drugs. Depending on the nature of the interaction, certain foods have the ability to decrease drug absorption, increase the risk of drug toxicity, or create other problems that make them an important safety concern.
- *Side effects.* Instruct the patient to report unusual symptoms immediately to the designated health care provider—usually a nurse, physician, or pharmacist. Give the patient instructions that help minimize any side effects (e.g., avoiding direct sunlight when there is risk of photosensitivity or sunburn). Advise the patient of any expected changes in the color of urine or stool. Advise the patient who has dizziness caused by orthostatic hypotension to rise slowly from a sitting to a standing position.
- *Cultural considerations.* A **culturally sensitive** nurse is one who has an awareness of the implications of culture for the patient and family. Be alert to patient and family cultural expectations. For example, the patient may not view time as important, which may affect the patient's adherence to taking medications at specific times during the day. The nurse applies knowledge of cultural considerations to individualize a teaching plan (Box 11-1). Refer to Chapter 3 for more information; cultural content is also found in the Nursing Process boxes in each chapter.

A teaching plan with interventions that involves stimulation of several senses and active participation by the patient enhances learning. Inclusion of return demonstrations by the

BOX 11-1 CULTURALLY SENSITIVE HEALTH TEACHING TIPS

- Flexibility in timing appointments may be necessary for those who have a circular sense of time rather than a linear sense of time.
- The nurse should consider whether appointments are something deemed culturally relevant.
- Discuss the ethnicity of the interpreter as well as the language desired when translation is needed. Provide an interpreter with the same ethnic background and gender if possible, especially with sensitive topics. Speak clearly and slowly, giving time for translation. Ask family members to assist with translation only if an interpreter is not available.
- Use videos and literature in the patient's preferred language to enhance adherence to health interventions when language and cultural barriers exist.
- Use simple and clear instructions that employ user-friendly terminology at the fourth-grade level. Avoid use of acronyms and abbreviations. Allow adequate time for information processing; failure to do this may result in an inaccurate response or no response. Allow time response to questions, especially for patients who have language barriers.
- Ask open-ended questions, and have patients demonstrate, rather than verbalize, their understanding of treatments. Because politeness and "saving face" may be important, do not assume that a positive response means a definite yes.

patient and others, when applicable, gives the nurse important feedback about the patient's learning and gives the patient confidence in carrying out the regimen or selected aspects of the regimen. Additional teaching tips include the following:

- Establish a trusting relationship.
- Teach patient and family the importance of bringing a medication list (including OTC, herbal, and vitamin products) or medications to all health care provider appointments in all settings.
- Provide written instructions in addition to other teaching aids.
- Use colorful charts and graphs.
- Consider using a variety of media, including audio and video.
- Encourage questions from patient and family; provide time for this. Do not rush.
- Use materials and language appropriate to patient's level of understanding; supply patient medication information sheets in different languages and appropriate reading levels.
- Space instruction over several sessions, if appropriate.
- Review community resources related to patient's nursing and medical diagnoses.
- Collaborate with patient and family and other health care staff and agencies to mobilize resources to meet patient's needs.
- Identify patients at risk for noncompliance with regimen. Alert health care provider and pharmacist so they can develop a plan to minimize the number of drugs and times administered.

BOX 11-2 POINTS FOR PATIENTS AND FAMILIES TO REMEMBER

Take medication as prescribed by your health care provider. If you have questions, call.

Keep medication in the original labeled container, and store as instructed.

Keep all medicines out of the reach of children. Remind grandparents and visitors to monitor their purses and luggage when visiting.

Before using any over-the-counter (OTC) drugs, check with your health care provider. This includes use of aspirin and laxatives. Consider asking the pharmacist before buying or using a product.

Bring all medications with you when you visit the health care provider.

Know the purpose of each medication and under what circumstances to notify the health care provider.

Do not drink alcoholic beverages around the time you take your medications. Alcohol is absolutely contraindicated with certain medications. Alcohol may alter the action and absorption of medications.

Be aware that smoking tobacco also alters the absorption of some medications (e.g., theophylline-type drugs, antidepressants, pain medications). Consult your health care provider or pharmacist for specific information.

- Evaluate patient's understanding of medication regimen on a regular basis.
- Empower patient to take responsibility for managing medications.

The use of teaching drug cards is helpful. These cards provide information about a specific drug or drug group. They may be developed by the health care provider or obtained from drug manufacturers. Helpful components for the teaching drug cards include name of the drug; reason for taking the drug; dosage; specific times to take the drug; possible side effects; possible adverse effects and when to notify health care provider; and specific things that should or should not be done while taking the medication (e.g., do not crush, take with food)

Group classes are useful for patients with certain diagnoses or who require certain drugs. A variety of formats can be developed. Be creative!

General points to remember and tips for successful patient education are presented in Box 11-2.

Many people take multiple medications simultaneously several times each day, which presents a challenge to the patient, his or her family, and the nurse. This complex activity of taking medications can be segmented into several simple tasks, including the following:

- Preparation of 1 day's or 1 week's supply of medication. The day's medication can be put into one container. Sorting of a day's supply allows the patient and the nurse to see at a glance what medications have and have not been taken. Keep in mind that a missing pill may have been dropped and not actually taken. A variation in accomplishing this task is to take a day's medication and sort or package the pills according to the time each is to be taken. Multi-compartment dispensers (available at drugstores) or an egg carton may help some patients sort their drugs.

- A recording sheet may be helpful. The patient or a family member marks when each medication is taken. The sheet is designed to meet the patient's individual needs; for example, the time can be noted by the patient or can be entered beforehand, with the patient marking when each dose is taken. A generic format follows.

	DOSAGE	DAY OF WEEK						
MEDICATION	(mg DAILY)	S	M	T	W	TH	F	S
captopril (Capoten)	12.5							
digoxin	0.25							
furosemide (Lasix)	40							

Alternatives to recording sheets are also available. Alarm reminder devices may be helpful to some patients. A combination of daily supply and recording may be helpful. Consider color-coding. Visual acuity, manual dexterity, and mental processes have a major effect on which system works best for each patient.

Throughout the teaching plan, the nurse promotes patient independence (e.g., self-administering medications, safely storing medications, ordering medications). The nurse should not lose sight of the goals or outcomes and become immersed in the intervention process (e.g., teaching a patient with short-term memory loss). Box 11-3 presents items for a checklist for health teaching in drug therapy.

BOX 11-3 CHECKLIST FOR HEALTH TEACHING IN DRUG THERAPY

- Comprehensive drug use and health history
- Reason for medication therapy
- Expected results
- Side effects and adverse reactions
- When to notify health care provider or pharmacist
- Drug-drug, drug-food, drug-laboratory, and drug-environment interactions
- Required changes in activities of daily living (ADLs)
- Demonstration of learning; may take several forms, such as listening, discussing, or return demonstration of psychomotor skills (insulin administration)
- Medication schedule, associated with ADLs and drug level of action as appropriate
- Recording system
- Discussion and monitoring of access to financial resources, medication, and associated equipment
- Development and support of backup system
- Community resources available

Evaluation

In the **evaluation** phase of the nursing process, the nurse determines how well goals are obtained. Nursing interventions are revised and teaching is focused to improve goal attainment if goals are not met.

The specific outcomes must be articulated with the patient and significant others to determine if they have been met. Additional data may be needed to assess if adherence to the drug regimen is not done. For example, patients may be denying or minimizing their diagnosis, financial problems may prevent timely prescription refill, or vision or physical limitations may inhibit administration of the drug. When the evaluation of a goal will occur depends on the time frame specified in the statement of the goal. Evaluation should be ongoing and related to progress as well as to attainment of the final goal.

If goals are not met, the nurse, in collaboration with the patient or family, must determine the reasons and revise the plan accordingly. This includes additional assessment data and the setting of new goals.

To complete the care for any current patient, review with the patient and family the need for follow-up care, if required, and refer the patient to community resources as necessary.

KEY WEBSITES

National Quality Forum: *www.qualityforum.org*
Patient Advocate Foundation: *www.patientadvocate.org*
QSEN: *www.qsen.org*
The Nursing Alliance for Quality Care: *www.gwumc.edu/healthsci/departments/nursing/naqc/index.cfm*

CRITICAL THINKING CASE STUDY

MZ, a 66-year-old man, lives in a two-story home in rural Vermont. He complains of shortness of breath, wheezing, and cough, primarily at night. MZ takes multiple asthma medications, and one of them (albuterol) is administered via nebulizer. He is 5 feet 11 inches tall and weighs 118 pounds. He admits to loss of appetite and reports, "I eat enough to keep going."

1. What are the most relevant nursing diagnoses for this patient?

NCLEX STUDY QUESTIONS

1. During a medication review session, a patient says, "I just do not know why I am taking all of these pills." Based on this piece of subjective data, which diagnosis will the nurse identify?
   a. Risk for injury
   b. Deficient knowledge
   c. Risk for aspiration
   d. Anxiety
2. The nurse is developing goals in collaboration with a patient. Which is the best goal statement?
   a. The patient will self-administer albuterol by tomorrow.
   b. The patient will self-administer the prescribed dose of albuterol by the end of the second teaching session.
   c. The patient will independently self-administer the prescribed dose of albuterol by the end of the second teaching session.
   d. The patient will organize her medications by tomorrow.
3. When developing an effective medication teaching plan, which component will the nurse identify as most essential?
   a. Provide written instructions.
   b. Establish a trust relationship.
   c. Use colorful charts.
   d. Review community resources.
4. When developing an individualized medication teaching plan, which topics will the nurse include? (Select all that apply.)
   a. Importance of adherence to the prescribed regimen
   b. How to administer medication(s)
   c. What side/adverse effects to report to the health care provider
   d. Foods that must be eaten
   e. Follow-up laboratory tests, if needed
5. The Guiding Principles for Patient Engagement are most important for health care providers as they strive for which goal?
   a. Nurses to focus care on quality and safety
   b. Confidentiality as determined by the patient
   c. All health care providers to have patient relationship for cornerstone of safety and quality
   d. Patient advocacy
6. The QSEN focus on safety is best exemplified by which competency?
   a. Patient advocacy
   b. Technology-enhanced medication administration
   c. Quality improvement
   d. Patient-centered collaborative care
7. Which teaching strategy is most likely to succeed in health teaching with the patient and family?
   a. Have patient verbalize understanding
   b. Have patient answer closed-ended questions
   c. Have patient demonstrate information
   d. Have patient identify pill by color

Answers: 1, b; 2, c; 3, b; 4, a, b, c, e; 5, c; 6, d; 7, c.

CHAPTER

12

Safety and Quality in Pharmacotherapy

evolve WEBSITE

http://evolve.elsevier.com/KeeHayes/pharmacology/

- Animations
- Content Updates
- Key Points
- Review Questions for the NCLEX® Examination
- References from the Textbook
- Unfolding Case Studies

OBJECTIVES

- Discuss the QSEN initiative related to safe administration of medications.
- Describe the "five-plus-five" rights of medication administration.
- Analyze safety risks for medication administration.
- Discuss safe disposal of medications.
- Discuss high-alert drugs and strategies for safe administration.
- Describe application of safe practices when ordering medications on the Internet.
- Discuss safety bases of pregnancy categories.
- Apply the nursing process to safe administration of medications.

OUTLINE

KEY TERMS

Nearly 4 billion prescriptions were written in the United States in 2010, according to the IMS Institute for Healthcare Informatics. Prescription medicines, over-the-counter (OTC) drugs, or dietary supplements are used by 80% of adults. The Institute for Safe Medication Practices reports that 33% of adults take at least five medications daily.

Medication errors are the most frequent malpractice claims against hospitals and nurses, costing about $5000 per error. More than $3 million is awarded (on average) by the courts for serious errors. The cost of the patient and family suffering is not calculable.

The focus of this chapter is the Quality and Safety Education for Nurses (QSEN) initiative as it relates to safe medication administration and prevention of medication-related errors. The six QSEN competencies focus on patient/family–centered care, collaboration and teamwork, evidence-based practice, quality improvement, safety, and informatics. (Refer to Chapter 11 and the QSEN website, *www.qsen.org.*)

"FIVE-PLUS-FIVE" RIGHTS OF MEDICATION ADMINISTRATION

The rights of medication administration are the foundation for medication safety. The nurse following the original five rights of medication administration will give (1) the *right patient* the (2) *right drug* (3) in the *right dose* via (4) the *right route* at the (5) *right time.* Experience shows that five additional rights are essential to professional nursing practice: (1) *right assessment,* (2) *right documentation,* (3) *patient's right to education,* (4) *right evaluation,* and (5) *patient's right to refuse.*

The **right patient** determination is essential. The Joint Commission (TJC) requires two forms of identification before administration of the medication. Some patients are unable to respond or answer to any name, so the nurse must verify patient identification each time he or she administers a medication.

Nursing implications include the following:

- Verify the patient by checking the patient's identification bracelet. Some facilities put the patient's photo on the health record.
- Distinguish between two patients with the same first or last name; have warnings highlighted in a bright color on identification (ID) tools such as a med card, bracelet, or Kardex.
- Some institutions have ID bracelets coded for allergy status. Be aware of whether such a policy exists at your institution.
- When patients do not wear ID bracelets (e.g., in schools, occupational health departments, outpatient departments, or health care provider offices), the nurse must accurately identify the individual by other means when administering a medication.

The nurse must be sure that the **right drug** is administered. Medication orders may be prescribed by any licensed health care provider (HCP) having authority from the state to prescribe drugs. These include a physician (MD), dentist (DDS), podiatrist (DPM), advanced practice registered nurse (APRN), or physician assistant (PA). In some health care settings, medical students write drug orders; these orders must be countersigned by an attending or staff physician or other prescribing health care provider before they are considered official. The law requires that handwritten prescriptions be written on a tamperproof prescription pad and filled by a pharmacist at a drugstore or hospital pharmacy. Depending on agency policy, drug orders may be written on order sheets and signed by the duly authorized person. A telephone order (TO) or verbal order (VO) for medication must be "read back" to the HCP as an accuracy check and cosigned by the prescribing health care provider within 24 hours. The nurse must comply with the institution's policy regarding a TO, which sometimes requires that two licensed nurses listen to and sign the order.

As part of the electronic health record (EHR), prescriptions may also be entered directly into the patient's record, electronically signed by the HCP, sent directly to the pharmacy, and recorded as part of the patient record. A strong safety feature of the EHR is the ability to identify untoward drug interactions with the patient's current drugs and the newly prescribed/ordered medications. The EHR has decreased medication errors by eliminating some opportunities for errors such as transcription errors.

The use of computerized order systems has added speed and a safety feature to the order process. Orders can be written from virtually any location and sent electronically. The computer will not process the order unless all necessary information is included. Because the order is computerized, illegible orders or signatures are prevented.

The components of a drug order are as follows:

- Date and time the order is written
- Drug name (generic preferred)
- Drug dosage
- Route of administration
- Frequency and duration of administration (e.g., × 7 days, × 3 doses)
- Any special instructions for withholding or adjusting dosage based on nursing assessment, drug effectiveness, or laboratory results
- Physician or other health care provider's signature or name if TO or VO
- Signatures of licensed staff taking TO or VO

Although the nurse's responsibility is to administer drugs as ordered, the drug order is incomplete and the drug should not be administered if any one of the components is missing. Clarification of a questionable order must be done in a timely manner. The health care provider is usually contacted, and the conversation content is documented. Nurses must know all of the components of a drug order and question any orders that are incomplete or unclear, give a dosage outside of the recommended range, or are contraindicated by patient allergy or laboratory test results. Nurses are legally liable if they give a prescribed drug and the dosage is incorrect or the drug is contraindicated for the patient's health status. Once the drug has been administered, the nurse becomes liable for the predicted effects of that drug.

The following is an example of a drug order and its interpretation:

1/1/14, 1010 Lasix 40 mg, PO, daily [signature]. (Give 40 mg of Lasix by mouth daily.)

To avoid drug error, the drug label should be read three times: (1) at the time of contact with the drug bottle/container or the prepackaged drug unit, (2) before measuring the drug, and (3) after measuring the drug. First dose, one-time, and "as needed" (PRN) medication orders should be checked against the original orders. Nursing interventions related to a drug order include the following:

- The nurse should be well versed in the patient's health history and previously performed assessments.
- Check that the medication order is complete and legible. If the order is not complete or legible, notify the nurse manager and health care provider.
- Know the patient's allergies.
- Know the reason the patient is to receive the medication.
- Check the drug label three times before administration of the medication.
- Know the date the medication was ordered and any ending date (e.g., for controlled substances and antibiotics and for limited or a specific number of doses). Some agencies have "automatic stop orders" that are generally facility specific. Examples of such orders include controlled drugs that need to be renewed every 48 hours, antibiotics to be renewed every 7 to 14 days, and cancellations of all medications when the patient goes to surgery.

The **right dose** refers to verification by the nurse that the dose administered is the amount ordered and that it is safe for the patient for whom it is prescribed. The right dose is based on the patient's physical status, including renal and hepatic function. Renal and hepatic function are important considerations because many drugs are cleared through the kidneys and metabolized by the liver. Patient weight is another important consideration in multiple contexts, such as pediatrics and many medical, surgical, and critical care situations. In most cases, the right dose for a specific patient is within the recommended range for the particular drug. Nurses must calculate each drug dose accurately (see Chapter 14).

Before calculating a drug dose, the nurse should have a general idea of the answer based on knowledge of the basic formula or ratios and proportions. Recheck the calculation of drug doses if a fraction of a dose or an extremely large dose is calculated. Consult a peer or a pharmacist whenever doubt exists.

The stock drug method and unit dose method are the two most frequently used methods to dispense drugs (Table 12-1). In the traditional **stock drug method,** the drugs are dispensed to all patients from the same containers. In the **unit dose method,** drugs are individually wrapped and labeled for single doses for each patient. The unit dose method, which is popular in many institutions and community settings, has reduced dosage errors because no calculations are required.

Automated dispensing cabinets assist the nurse in correctly and quickly administering medications. This technology improves patient care by promoting accurate and quick access to medications, locked storage for all medications, and electronic tracking for controlled substances. Pharmacists can review orders using a link to the pharmacy information system and current clinical patient data, interface with other databases (e.g., the laboratory), and bar-code doses. Automation of medication administration saves time, decreases costs associated with the administration of medications, and allows the ability to automatically collect documentation information. An activity report menu is a useful feature. Flexible dose modes are available, including single-dose, multi-dose, and multiple medications.

TABLE 12-1 DRUG DISTRIBUTION METHODS

STOCK DRUG METHOD	UNIT DOSE METHOD
Description	
Drugs are stored on unit and dispensed to all patients from the same container	Drugs are packaged in doses for 24 h by the pharmacy
Advantages	
Always available	Saves time for nurse; no dose calculation required
Cost-efficiency of large quantities	Billed for specific doses
	More accountability
	Less chance for contamination and error
Disadvantages	
Drug errors are more prevalent with multiple "pourers"	Potential delay in receiving drug
More risk of abuse by health care workers	Not immediately replaceable if contaminated
Less accountability for amount used; unable to track usage	More expensive
Increased opportunity for contamination (multiple pourers challenge aseptic/sterile status)	

Nursing interventions related to the right dose include the following:

- Calculate the drug dose correctly. When in doubt, recalculate the drug dose and check with another nurse. In many settings, the first nurse to administer the particular drug to the patient must calculate the dose according to the stated formulary doses and sign in the nurse's signature space once the safety parameter has been established. In some settings, two registered nurses (RNs) are required to check dosage for specific medications such as insulin and heparin.
- Check the American Hospital Formulary, the drug package insert, or other drug references for the recommended range of specific drug doses.

The **right time** is the time the prescribed dose is ordered to be administered. Daily drug dosages are given at specified times during a day, such as twice a day (b.i.d.), three times a day (t.i.d.), four times a day (q.i.d.), or every 6 hours (q6h), so that the plasma level of the drug is maintained at a

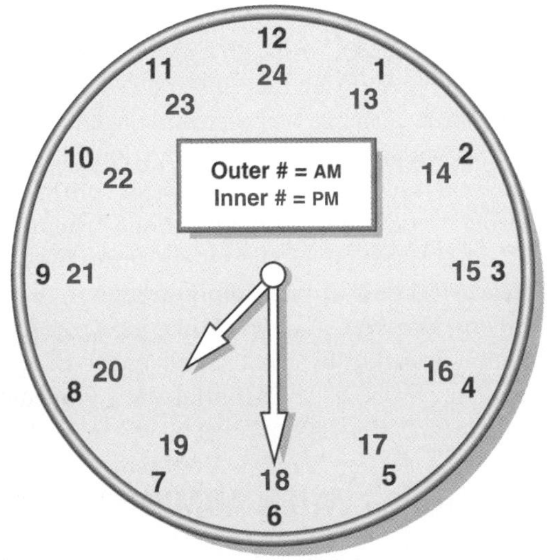

FIGURE 12–1 Military time.

therapeutic level. Every drug cannot be given exactly when ordered; therefore, health care agencies have policies that specify a range of times within which drugs can be administered before or after the appointed time. When a drug has a long half-life ($t\frac{1}{2}$), it is usually given once a day, although many depot preparations have a $t\frac{1}{2}$ of days. Drugs with a short $t\frac{1}{2}$ are given several times a day at specified intervals. Some drugs are given before meals, and others are given with meals or other food depending on the effect of the gastrointestinal (GI) environment on absorption of the drug.

Use of military time reduces administration errors and decreases documentation. Many nursing settings use military time, which is a 24-hour clock. See Figure 12-1 for military time in comparison with standard time. Nursing interventions related to the right time include the following:

- Administer drugs at the specified times (refer to agency policy).
- Administer drugs that are affected by food (e.g., tetracycline) 1 hour before or 2 hours after meals.
- Administer drugs that can irritate the stomach (gastric mucosa)—for example, potassium and aspirin—with food. Some medications are absorbed better after eating.
- Adjust the medication schedule to fit the patient's lifestyle, activities, **tolerances**, or preferences, as appropriate and if possible.
- Check whether or not the patient is scheduled for any diagnostic procedures such as endoscopy or fasting blood tests that contraindicate the administration of medications. Determine per policy if the medication should be given before or after the test is completed.
- Check the expiration date. Discard the medication or return it to the pharmacy (depending on policy) if the date has passed.
- Administer antibiotics at even intervals (e.g., q8h rather than t.i.d.) throughout a 24-hour period so therapeutic blood levels are maintained.

The **right route** is necessary for adequate or appropriate absorption. The right route is ordered by the health care provider and indicates the mechanism by which the medication enters the body. The more common routes of absorption include *oral* (by mouth): liquid, elixir, suspension, pill, tablet, or capsule; *sublingual* (under the tongue for venous absorption); *buccal* (between the gum and cheek); via feeding tube; *topical* (applied to the skin); *inhalation* (aerosol sprays); *instillation* (in nose, eye, or ear); *suppository* (rectal or vaginal); and five *parenteral* routes: intradermal, subcutaneous (subQ), intramuscular (IM), intravenous (IV), or intraosseous (IO).

Nursing interventions related to the right route include the following:

- Assess the patient's ability to swallow before administering oral medications; make sure that the patient is not NPO.
- Do not crush or mix medications in other substances without consulting a pharmacist or a reliable drug reference. Do not mix medications with sweet substances to trick children into taking them. Do not mix medications in an infant's formula feeding.
- If the medication is or must be mixed with another substance, explain this to the patient. For example, many children's medicines have flavor added (e.g., bubble gum– or banana-flavored antibiotics) to make them palatable.
- Use aseptic technique when administering drugs. Sterile technique is required with the parenteral routes.
- Administer drugs at the appropriate sites for the route.
- Stay with the patient until oral drugs have been swallowed.

The **right assessment** requires collection of appropriate data before administration of the drug. Examples of assessment data include apical heart rate before the administration of digitalis preparations or serum blood sugar levels before the administration of insulin.

The **right documentation** requires the nurse to immediately record the appropriate information about the drug administered. This includes (1) the name of the drug, (2) the dose, (3) the route (injection site if applicable), (4) the time and date, and (5) the nurse's initials or signature. Documentation of the patient's response to the medication is required with a variety of medications: (1) opioids (How effective was pain relief?); (2) non-opioid analgesics (How effective was pain relief?); (3) sedatives (How effective was relaxation?); and (4) antiemetics (Was nausea/vomiting decreased or eliminated?). Unexpected reactions to the medication (Was there any GI irritation or signs of skin sensitivity?) should also be documented. Patient responses are not necessarily verbal; they could be physiologic (e.g., Did blood pressure go down in response to an antihypertensive? Did LDL cholesterol go down in response to a statin?). Delay in charting could result in forgetting to chart the medication, and another nurse could administer the drug, assuming that the drug was not administered because it was not charted. Do not sign off medications before administration because the medication may not be administered to the patient for some reason. Graphic formats or computerized systems (Figure 12-2) assist in accurate and timely recording of drugs administered.

The **right to education** requires that patients receive accurate and thorough information about the medication and

```
6SB  -7530-01      W J M C   DEVELOPMENT   HOSP #6
     09:00 AM  SCHEDULED MEDICATIONS DUE   6SB    (QJB$$N)      PAGE 001
                                                  ISSUED:  07:47 AM 02/12/05

  6116A  MARILYN, MARILYN          0001393300      0215500019   GIV NGIV

  U   (ADVIL, MOTRIN, NUPRIN, RUFEN) IBUPROFEN TAB 400MG
        DOSE: #1, PO
      BID-PC (08/06/02 06PM-..)

  U   (DELTASONE, METICORTEN, ORASONE) PREDNISONE TAB 5MG
        DOSE: #1, PO
      QD-AM/Q24H (08/07/02 09AM-..)

  U   (FERGON) FERROUS GLUC TAB 320MG
        DOSE: #1, PO
      (URINE AND STOOL MAY DARKEN) BID/Q12H (12/06/02 09PM-..)

  U   (LANOXIN) DIGOXIN TAB 0.25MG
        DOSE: #1, PO
      QD-AM/Q24H HOLD FOR HR < 50 (01/15/04 09AM-..)

           ALLERGIES: CEPHALORSPORINS, PENICILLIN,
          MORPHINE, GENTAMICIN SULFATE, IODINE,
          PENICILLIN, SHELLFISH, POISON IVY/OAK,
          ANIMAL DANDER/HAIR, BEE STINGS

* * * * * * * * * * * * * * * * * * * * * * * * * * * * * * * * * * * * *
```

A

UNIVERSITY HOSPITAL

Nurse's Signature/Title		Initials
Evelyn Hayes	RN	EH
Joyce Kee	RN	JK
Rodney Brown	LPN	RB
Jody Smith	LPN	JS

Allergies: Codeine

Continuing Medical Record

				Date	Initials		
				8/14	8/15	8/16	8/17
8/14		Digoxin 0.125 mg po qd	0900	EH	EH	JK	
EH				AR=74	AR=70	AR=70	
8/14		Capoten 12.5 mg po bid	0900	EH	EH	JK	
EH			2100	RB	RB	RB	
8/15	8/22	Amoxicillin 250 mg po q6h	0600	X	X	JS	
EH	LD 0600	x7d	1200		EH	JK	
1100			1800		RB	RB	
			2400		JS	JS	

One-Time/PRN/STAT Medications

Date	Medication/Dosage/Route/Frequency	Time/Initials	Reason	Result
8/14	Nitroglycerin 1/150 gr sublingual PRN	1600 EH	Chest pain	Relief of pain
	Chest pain			

B

FIGURE 12–2 Medication record. **A,** Computerized format. **B,** Written format.

how it relates to their particular condition. Patient teaching also includes therapeutic purpose, expected result of the drug, possible side effects of the drug, any dietary restrictions or requirements, skill of administration, and laboratory test result monitoring. This right is a principle of **informed consent,** which is the individual having the knowledge necessary to make a decision. An informed patient and family is critical to preventing medication errors.

The **right evaluation** refers to an appraisal of a drug's therapeutic and adverse effects. Evaluation in this context asks, "Did the medication do for the patient what it was supposed to do?" It is essential for the nurse's practice to evaluate the therapeutic effect of the medication as well as any side effects and adverse reactions. This evaluation is an important aspect of patient safety.

The patient has the **right to refuse** the medication. Patients can and do refuse to take a medication. It is the nurse's responsibility to determine, when possible, the reason for the refusal and, if the reasoning is not sound, to take reasonable measures to facilitate the patient's taking the medication. Explain to the patient the risk of refusing to take the medication, and reinforce the reason for the medication. When a medication is refused, the refusal must be documented immediately, and follow-up is always required. The nurse manager, primary nurse, or health care provider should be informed when the omission may pose a specific threat to the patient, and when a change is expected in the laboratory test values, such as with insulin and warfarin (Coumadin).

Consider all medication errors serious or potentially serious. A medication error may involve one or more of the following: administration of the wrong medication or IV fluid; the incorrect dose or rate; administration to the wrong patient, by the incorrect route, or at the incorrect schedule interval; administration of a known allergenic drug or IV fluid; omission of a dose; or discontinuation of medication or IV fluid that was not discontinued.

NURSES' RIGHTS WHEN ADMINISTERING MEDICATIONS

In addition to the rights of medication administration, there are six rights for nurses who administer medications. These rights provide an additional layer of safety by ensuring that the nurse has what is needed to provide safe medication administration.

The nurses' six rights are (1) the right to a complete and clear order; (2) the right to have the correct drug, route (form), and dose dispensed; (3) the right to have access to information; (4) the right to have policies to guide safe medication administration; (5) the right to administer medications safely and to identify problems in the system; and (6) the right to stop, think, and be vigilant when administering medications. Discussion of these rights can assist in increasing the safety of medication administration.

The *right to a complete and clear order* requires that the drug, dose, route, and frequency be ordered by the health care provider. Prescription orders entered directly into a computer ensure that the prescription is legible. However, the nurse must question the health care provider if the order is not complete or is unclear.

The nurse has the *right to have the correct drug, route (form), and drug dispensed.* Dispensing medications correctly is the role of the pharmacist. Automated medication administration systems may be programmed to allow nurses access to many kinds of medications, rather than the safer unit dose access.

The *right to have access to information* includes the right to expect current and readily accessible drug information (e.g., hospital formulary, nursing drug reference). This right is a must. Nurses are only to administer drugs with which they are knowledgeable.

Nurses have the *right to have policies to guide safe medication administration.* Health care administration's role is to provide the structure on which nurses administer drugs safely. In each facility, policies guide nursing practice. Not following policy or administering medication without policies is not acceptable and places nurses at risk for losing their nursing license.

The *right to administer medications safely and to identify problems in the system* encompasses nurses' right and responsibility to speak up when they are first aware of situations that impinge negatively on safe administration of medications. Nurses should be an advocate for safety in the health care setting.

Nurses have the *right to stop, think, and be vigilant when administering medications.* When unsure, nurses have the right and responsibility to stop and think, consult with other health professionals, and check their institution's policies. Safety is the basis for these actions.

CULTURE OF SAFETY

The Institute of Medicine (IOM) classic report of 1999, *To Err Is Human: Building a Safer Health Care System,* spurred work on identifying health care system changes to decrease errors. A medication error may be defined as "any preventable event that may cause or lead to inappropriate medication use or harm to a patient."

Possible causes of medication errors include dramatic increase in the number of drugs available; violation of the rights of nursing medication administration; lack of drug knowledge; memory lapses; transcription, dispensing, or delivery problems; inadequate monitoring; distractions; overworked staff; lack of standardization; equipment failures; inadequate patient history; and poor interdepartmental communication.

In response to the escalating number of medication errors causing human deaths and costing billions of dollars, in 2002 the FDA proposed a rule titled *Bar Code Label Requirements for Human Drug Products and Blood,* which has increased the prominence of this coding. At a minimum, the bar code contains the drug's national drug code that "uniquely identifies the drug, its strength, and its dosage form." A revision to this rule eliminates blood and blood products because they have had bar codes since 1985. Most staff embrace bar coding once they are proficient with its use. They note, however, that bar coding is a tool but not a substitute for critical thinking.

Computerized prescriber order entry systems interact with laboratory, pharmacy, and patient data. This integrated system of patient data is the basis for the success of bar coding. With bar coding, the patient's medication administration record (MAR), a part of the database that is encoded in the patient's wristband, is accessible to the nurse using a handheld device. After scanning the patient's wristband, the nurse sees the individual's MAR on the device. To administer a medication, nurses first scan the drug's bar code, then the number of the patient's medical record, and finally the nurse's own ID badge code. The patient's MAR is then updated accordingly. (Figure 12-3 shows a nurse scanning a patient's wristband.) The nurse receives verification on the handheld device of the five rights, warnings, and clinical alerts (e.g., drug is discontinued, drug is not ordered for patient).

Additionally, TJC has taken steps to prevent drug errors. As part of their National Patient Safety Goals, TJC announced in 2004 that all accredited organizations may no longer use selected abbreviations, acronyms, and symbols because they can be misinterpreted or misread. See Table 12-2 for this "Do Not Use" list, and see Table 12-3 for a list of acceptable abbreviations. Visit TJC's website at *www.jointcommission.org* and the Institute for Safe Medication Practices at *www.ismp.org* for current detailed safety information.

Another safety feature is the *black box,* or *boxed,* warning, the FDA's strongest labeling requirement, which warns health care providers of risks associated with certain drugs.

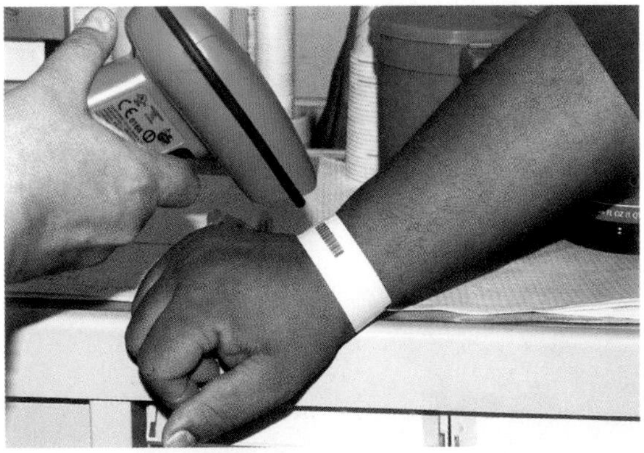

FIGURE 12–3 Bar code reader used to scan the patient's wristband. (From Kee JL, Marshall SM: *Clinical calculations: with applications to general and specialty areas,* ed. 7, St. Louis, 2013, Elsevier.)

TABLE 12-2 "DO NOT USE" ABBREVIATIONS

In 2005, The Joint Commission issued a new list of abbreviations that should not be used, but instead should be written out to avoid misinterpretation. Below is the list of "Do Not Use" abbreviations followed by a list of abbreviations that could possibly be included in future "Do Not Use" lists.

Abbreviation	Preferred
q.d., Q.D.	Write "daily" or "every day."
q.o.d., Q.O.D.	Write "every other day."
U	Write "unit."
IU	Write "International Unit."
MS, MSO_4	Write "morphine sulfate."
$MgSO_4$	Write "magnesium sulfate."
.5 mg	Use zero before a decimal point when the dose is less than a whole (write 0.X mg).
1.0 mg	Do not use a decimal point or zero after a whole number (write X mg).

The following abbreviations could **possibly be included** in future TJC "Do Not Use" lists.

Abbreviation	Preferred
c.c.	Use "mL" (milliliter).
Mg	Use "mcg" (microgram).
>	Write "greater than."
<	Write "less than."
Drug name abbreviations	Write out the full name of the drug.
Apothecary units	Use metric units instead.
@	Write "at."

Please visit *www.jointcommission.org* and *www.ismp.org* for more detailed safety information.

TABLE 12-3 ACCEPTABLE ABBREVIATIONS

TJC lists acceptable abbreviations in three categories: drug measurements and drug forms, routes of medication administration, and times of administration. Selected abbreviations are listed here. These are frequently used in drug therapy and must be known by the nurse.

Drug Measurements and Drug Forms

Abbreviation	*Meaning*
Cap	Capsule
Dr	Dram
Elix	Elixir
g, gm, G, GM	Gram
Gr	Grain
Gtt	Drops
Kg	Kilogram
l, L	Liter
m^2	Square meter
mcg, µg	Microgram
mEq	Milliequivalent
Mg	Milligram
mL, ml	Milliliter
m, min	Minim
Oz	Ounce
Pt	Pint
Qt	Quart
SR	Sustained release
ss., $\overline{ss}$	One half
Supp	Suppository
Susp	Suspension
T.O.	Telephone order
T, tbsp.	Tablespoon
t, tsp	Teaspoon
V.O.	Verbal order

Routes of Medication Administration

Abbreviation	*Meaning*
A.D., ad	Right ear
A.S., as	Left ear
A.U., au	Both ears
ID	Intradermal
IM	Intramuscular
IV	Intravenous
IVPB	Intravenous piggyback
KVO	Keep vein open
L	Left
NGT	Nasogastric tube
O.D., od	Right eye
O.S., os	Left eye
O.U., ou	Both eyes
PO, po, os	By mouth
®	Right
SC, subc, sc, SQ, subQ	Subcutaneous
SL, sl, subl	Sublingual
TKO	To keep open
Vag	Vaginal

Times of Administration

Abbreviation	*Meaning*
AC, ac	Before meals
ad lib	As desired
B.i.d., b.i.d.	Twice a day
$\bar{c}$	With
Hs	Hour of sleep
NPO	Nothing by mouth
PC, pc	After meals
PRN, p.r.n.	Whenever necessary, as needed
Q	Every
Qam	Every morning
Qh	Every hour
q2h	Every 2 hours
q4h	Every 4 hours
q6h	Every 6 hours
q8h	Every 8 hours
$\bar{s}$	Without
SOS	Once if necessary: if there is a need
Stat	Immediately
T.i.d., t.i.d.	Three times a day

Please visit *www.jointcommission.org* and *www.ismp.org* for more detailed safety information.

Joint Commission 2013 National Patient Safety Goals

TJC 2013 National Patient Safety Goals focus on problems in health care safety and how to solve them. National Patient Safety Goals program links for ambulatory health care, behavioral health care, critical access hospital, home care, hospitals, laboratory services, long-term care, long-term care (Medicare/Medicaid), and office-based surgery are found at *www.jointcommission.org/standards_information/npsgs.aspx*. As an example, the first three National Patient Safety Goals for hospitals have relevance for medication safety. They are as follows: Goal 1. Identify patients correctly; Goal 2. Improve staff communication; and Goal 3. Use medicines safely. The full text of the goals is available on TJC's website.

Medication Reconciliation

Medication reconciliation is an important component of the culture of safety. Medication discrepancies are not new in the literature. There are three transition points where many discrepancies occur: hospital admission, intrahospital transfer, and discharge. Medication reconciliation was created to provide medication continuity during care transitions, thereby promoting patient safety.

Medication reconciliation is the process of comparing a patient's medication orders to all of the medications that the patient has been taking. The purpose is to avoid errors (e.g., omissions, duplications, dosing errors, drug interactions). Reconciliation must be conducted at every transition of care when the patient is taking any medications. Transitions include changes in care setting, service, health care provider, or level of care.

The medication reconciliation process comprises five steps:

1. Develop a list of current medications.
2. Develop a list of medications to be prescribed.
3. Compare the medications on the two lists.
4. Make clinical decisions based on the comparison.
5. Communicate the new list to appropriate caregivers and to the patient.

Tips for Medication Reconciliation

- Conduct a thorough medication interview with patient and/or caregivers to obtain and verify current medication status and regimens.
- Teach patient/caregiver the key role of managing medication information at all transitions.
- Advise patient to give a list to his or her primary care provider; update own list when change in dose, deletion/addition of medication, including OTCs; and carry medication information at all times in case of an emergency.
- Enlist support of primary care physicians (all health care providers) and community pharmacists to encourage patients to carry and update their medication list at every encounter.
- The Agency for Healthcare Research and Quality (AHQR) has created a patient handout that can help patients play an active role in their own safety. Nurses can distribute the handout, found at *www.ahrq.gov/consumer/20tips.pdf*, during patient teaching.

Since 2005, TJC has required hospitals to perform medication reconciliation for all patients. The revised NSPG 03.06.01 requires facilities to "maintain and communicate accurate patient medication information." In addition, the Centers for Medicare and Medicaid Services Process of Care (Core) Measures require incorporating a reconciled medication list in the discharge instructions of all heart failure patients. In December 2011, the AHQR published *Medications at Transitions and Clinical Handoffs (MATCH) Toolkit for Medication Reconciliation;* it can be found at *www.ahrq.gov/qual/match/match1.htm*.

BOX 12-1 MEDICATIONS RECOMMENDED FOR DISPOSAL BY FLUSHING

MEDICINE	ACTIVE INGREDIENT
Abstral, tablets (sublingual)	Fentanyl
Actiq, oral transmucosal lozenge	Fentanyl citrate
Avinza, capsules (extended release)	Morphine sulfate
Daytrana, transdermal patch system	Methylphenidate
Demerol, tablets	Meperidine hydrochloride
Demerol, oral solution	Meperidine hydrochloride
Diastat/Diastat AcuDial, rectal gel	Diazepam
Dilaudid, tablets	Hydromorphone hydrochloride
Dilaudid, oral liquid	Hydromorphone hydrochloride
Dolophine hydrochloride, tablets	Methadone hydrochloride
Duragesic, patch (extended release)	Fentanyl
Embeda, capsules (extended release)	Morphine sulfate; naltrexone hydrochloride
Exalgo, tablets (extended release)	Hydromorphone hydrochloride
Fentora, tablets (buccal)	Fentanyl citrate
Kadian, capsules (extended release)	Morphine sulfate
Methadone hydrochloride, oral solution	Methadone hydrochloride
Methadose, tablets	Methadone hydrochloride
Morphine sulfate, tablets (immediate release)	Morphine sulfate
Morphine sulfate, oral solution	Morphine sulfate
MS Contin, tablets (extended release)	Morphine sulfate
Nucynta ER, tablets (extended release)	Tapentadol
Onsolis, soluble film (buccal)	Fentanyl citrate
Opana, tablets (immediate release)	Oxymorphone hydrochloride
Opana ER, tablets (extended release)	Oxymorphone hydrochloride
Oramorph SR, tablets (sustained release)	Morphine sulfate
Oxecta, tablets (immediate release)	Oxycodone hydrochloride
Oxycodone hydrochloride, capsules	Oxycodone hydrochloride
Oxycodone hydrochloride, oral solution	Oxycodone hydrochloride
Oxycontin, tablets (extended release)	Oxycodone hydrochloride
Percocet, tablets	Acetaminophen; oxycodone hydrochloride
Percodan, tablets	Aspirin; oxycodone hydrochloride
Xyrem, oral solution	Sodium oxybate

Disposal of Medications

The FDA collaborated with the White House Office of National Drug Control Policy (ONDCP) and in 2009 issued guidelines for appropriate disposal of prescription drugs. General guidelines include the following: Follow specific information on the drug label or drug insert. Unless specifically instructed, do not flush medications down the toilet, where they will pollute the environment and may be a danger to humans and animals. (Exceptions to this rule are listed in Box 12-1.) It is recommended that you remove the drug from its original container and dispose of it in a sealed bag with an undesirable substance such as used cat litter or used coffee grounds. This method is intended to make medications less attractive to people and animals. As needed, patients may take advantage of local community "drug take-back" programs that provide an opportunity for consumers to dispose of unwanted, unneeded, and/or expired medications in a safe manner. Some pharmacies will also take unused medications; this varies by state.

Before disposing of medication containers, all identifying information should be removed or obscured. Nurses and patients can consult a pharmacist with questions related to medication disposal.

Sharps Safety

The Occupational Safety and Health Administration (OSHA) Needlestick Safety and Prevention Act of 2000 resulted from the American Nurses Association's (ANA) campaign, *Safe*

Needles Save Lives. The Needlestick Safety and Prevention Act requires that employers do the following:

- Identify, evaluate, and implement safer medical devices.
- Maintain a sharps injury log.
- Involve health care workers in deciding which devices are used.
- Implement engineering controls for sharps disposal containers, self-sheathing needles, and safer medical devices like sharps with engineered injury protection and needleless systems. These engineering controls must be used to eliminate or lessen employee exposure to blood borne pathogens.
- Train employees in the proper usage of the engineering and work practice controls to help keep them safe.

Employers must ensure that no preventable sharps injuries occur. The Consensus Statement and Call to Action (2012), a collaboration of the ANA, the International Healthcare Worker Safety Center at the University of Virginia, and many health care colleagues, focuses on five areas: (1) improving sharps safety in surgical settings; (2) understanding and reducing exposure risks in nonhospital settings (e.g., offices, clinics, and home settings); (3) involving front-line workers in the selection of safety devices; (4) addressing gaps in available safety devices and encouraging innovative designs and technology; and (5) enhancing worker education and training.

SAFETY RISKS FOR MEDICATION ADMINISTRATION

It is estimated that for every 100 medication administrations, there are 5 medication errors. Several reports indicate that the majority of medication errors occur when administering the drug (41%), followed by documenting (21%), dispensing (17%), prescribing (11%), monitoring (1%), and other (9%).

Examples of risks to safety include the following:

- *Pill splitting.* In an effort to counteract steeply rising drug costs, some patients are cutting their pills in half. In the Half Tablet Program, with physician approval, patient costs are cut in half. However, splits can be dangerous. A minor dose change from uneven splitting can have a major effect on the patient. Patient attributes such as diminished vision, cognitive problems, and hand coordination problems can all contribute to the risk.
- *Buying drugs over the Internet.* This may be easy, but the buyer must be sure it is safe. Some websites are not state licensed or affiliated with pharmacies. They may not protect personal information; may not label, store, or ship medications correctly; and may sell expired medications. The FDA reports that consumers do not always get what they order and may not have someone available to verify if the drug is correct. Some sites may also sell counterfeit drugs (see the following paragraph). Patients should look for websites that require a prescription from a health care provider, have a licensed pharmacist to answer questions and a contact person if problems arise, are located in the United States, and are licensed by the state board of pharmacy.

Counterfeit Drugs

Counterfeit drugs look like the desired drug but may have no active ingredient, the wrong active ingredient, or the wrong amount of active ingredient. Improper packaging or contamination can also be problems. Counterfeit drugs may look remarkably like the real thing! To report suspect counterfeit products, call the FDA Office of Counterfeit Issues at 1-800-551-3989 or email *DrugSupplyChainIntegrity@fda.hhs.gov*.

To reduce the risk of exposure to counterfeit drugs, patients should do the following:

1. Purchase drugs only from licensed pharmacies. Refer to the National Association of Boards of Pharmacy (NABP) at *www.nabp.net* for information. The NABP reviews Internet pharmacies; after review, the NABP grants the Verified Internet Pharmacy Practice Sites (VIPPS) Accreditation Program seal. Visit *www.nabp.net/programs/accreditation/vipps/*.
2. Check the color, texture, shape, and taste (if applicable) of the drug when refilling a prescription. Patients should check with the pharmacist if they notice any changes.
3. Follow legislation in process to promote safe handling of drugs after they leave the authorized wholesaler by introducing "pedigree" requirements at federal and state levels.

Dosage Forms: To Crush or Not to Crush

Some medications can be crushed; consult with the health care provider or pharmacist. Do not crush any medication that has the suffix ER, SR, XR, SA, CR, MR, or XL; these are extended-release or sustained-release drugs, and crushing will change the location and speed of absorption. For a current complete listing of drugs that should not be crushed, see *www.ismp.org/Tools/Donotcrush.pdf*.

HIGH-ALERT MEDICATIONS

When high-alert drugs are involved in medication errors, the consequences to patients are more serious. Classes/categories of high-alert medications include IV adrenergic agents, IV adrenergic antagonists, IV antiarrhythmics; IV inotropic agents, IV moderate sedation agents, anesthetic agents, antithrombotic agents, cardioplegic solutions, chemotherapeutic agents, dextrose (hypertonic >20%), dialysis solutions, epidural or intrathecal agents, hypoglycemics, liposomal forms of drugs, moderate sedation agents, narcotics/opiates, neuromuscular blocking agents, IV radiocontrast agents, total parenteral nutrition solutions, sterile water for injection, inhalation and irrigation in containers of >100 mL, and sodium chloride for injection (hypertonic, >0.9% concentration). See *www.ismp.org/Tools/highalertmedications.pdf* for a complete list of classes/categories and specific medications. The ISMP recommends the following strategies to optimize safety when dealing with high-alert drugs: standardizing the ordering, storage, preparation, and administration of these products; improving access to information about these drugs; limiting access to high-alert medications; using auxiliary labels and automated alerts; and employing redundancies such as automated or independent double-checks when necessary.

LOOK-ALIKE AND SOUND-ALIKE DRUG NAMES

Nurses should be aware that certain drug names sound alike and are spelled similarly. Examples of drugs involved in medication errors and recognized as confused drug names include amaryl with reminyl; avinza with evista; cisplatin with carboplatin; Depakote with Depakote ER; ephedrine with epinephrine; and humalog mix 75/25 with Humulin 70/30. The FDA, ISMP, and TJC advocate the use of "tall man" letters as a safety strategy to reduce confusion between similar-sounding drugs. For example, rispiridone (Risperdal) is written as rispiriDONE, and ropinirole (Requip) is written as ropiniROLE to call attention to differences in spelling. Tall man letters should be used for computer listing and storage labeling.

OTHER FACTORS IN PREVENTION OF MEDICATION ERRORS

Creating a distraction- and interruption-free environment is critical to safe administration of medications. Effective strategies include creating a taped area on the floor surrounding the unit dose machine and hanging a sign stating, "Medication preparation/administration in progress. Please do not disturb"; hanging a card stating "Please do not interrupt during medication administration" on every computerized cart; designating a "quiet zone" for medication preparation; and wearing a vestlike garment that reads "Thank you for not interrupting" during medication preparation and administration.

Overall, the nurse's role is best achieved by the application of the nursing process. The nursing process related to medication safety follows.

Nursing Process
Patient-Centered Collaborative Care

Medication Safety

Assessment

- Assess vital signs and other patient parameters as appropriate. Report abnormal findings.
- Assess patient including patient history and ability to swallow (for PO medications).
- Assess medication order for completeness and with recommended parameters. Know purpose and expected effect of medication and interactions with other medications, including OTC and herbal preparations.
- Assess medication storage area (e.g., Does refrigerator storage meet requirements for medication storage?).

Planning

- Patient safety will be maintained/protected related to medication administration and use.

Nursing Interventions

- Calculate dose correctly.
- Use relevant resources appropriately.
- Avoid contamination of own skin or inhalation of substances to minimize exposure.
- Wash hands.
- Administer only medications you prepared.
- Determine patient's preferred language for communication, and mobilize resources to provide communication in this language.
- Identify patient by appropriate means (scanned name band, verbal confirmation).
- Remain with patient until medication has been taken.
- Administer medications according to the five-plus-five rights: right patient, right drug, right dose, right time, right route; plus right assessment, right documentation, right evaluation, right to education, right to refuse.
- Monitor subjective responses, physiologic alterations, and laboratory test results to identify therapeutic effects and adverse effects.
- Discard needles and syringes in appropriate container; be alert to sharps safety.
- Use aseptic/sterile technique appropriate for route of administration.
- Thoroughly document administration of medication(s) in the designated format in a timely manner.
- Document patient refusal to take medication, and notify health care provider.
- Follow up on effects of medication on patient.

Patient Teaching

- Counsel patient and family on anticipated effects of medications.
- Counsel patient on side effects and adverse reactions and what to report promptly to health care provider.
- Advise patient what foods to eat and/or avoid.
- Advise patient on taking medications before, with, or after meals, as appropriate, to promote optimal absorption.

Evaluation

- Evaluate patient's understanding of expected results from medication and what to report to health care provider.
- Evaluate effectiveness of medications administered to treat condition for which they were prescribed.

RESOURCES FOR PREVENTING ERRORS IN MEDICATION ADMINISTRATION

Several resources address medication errors and their prevention: (1) Pathways for Medication Safety was developed through the collaborative efforts of the American Hospital Association, the Health Research and Educational Trust, and the ISMP, with support from the Commonwealth Fund. Pathways for Medication Safety is a set of tools designed to assist hospitals through a system-based approach to reduce medication errors. (2) An FDA database of medication errors and "near misses" assists all health care personnel to identify, implement, and evaluate strategies to prevent medication errors. It is strongly suggested that health care workers report errors or near misses to the FDA. Reports are confidential. (3) The National Coordinating Council for Medication Error Reporting and Prevention (NCCMERP) specializes in medication errors from an interdisciplinary perspective. (4) The nurse must consult drug references (e.g., *United States Pharmacopeia, National Formulary,* and *American Hospital Formulary* drug reference handbook); human resources (e.g., pharmacists); and technology resources (Micromedix, Palm Pilot Epocrates) when unsure about the expected therapeutic effect, contraindications, dosage, potential side effects, or adverse reactions and interactions of a medication. (5) FDA MedWatch: Subscribe at *fda@service.govdelivery.com* for notifications on drug recalls, counterfeit products, and safety alerts.

PREGNANCY CATEGORIES

The FDA has developed a classification system related to the effects of drugs on the fetus. Table 12-4 lists the FDA's pregnancy categories and describes each category's effect on the fetus. Note: Prescription drug labeling revisions for health care providers are expected from the FDA. The purpose of the changes is to optimize informed decision making for pregnant patients and for patients of childbearing age who may wish to become pregnant. Both the pregnancy and lactation subsections will have three principal components: risk summary, clinical considerations, and a data section. The current pregnancy categories will be eliminated when the revisions have been completed.

FACTORS THAT MODIFY DRUG RESPONSE

Effects on the patient from drugs are complex owing to alterations in physiology. Nurses must complete thorough assessments of patients to accurately evaluate drug effects. Examples of factors that modify drug responses specifically related to safety include **absorption, distribution,** metabolism, excretion, **toxicity, pharmacogenetics,** pre-existing disease state, and drug-drug interaction. See discussions of factors that modify drug response in Chapters 1, 3, 4, 6, 7, and 8.

GUIDELINES FOR MEDICATION ADMINISTRATION

General guidelines for medication administration are listed in Boxes 12-2 and 12-3. Nurses should follow these guidelines to enhance safety when administering medications. Application of the nursing process to medication administration is presented in Chapter 13.

TABLE 12-4 FDA PREGNANCY CATEGORIES

PREGNANCY CATEGORY	DESCRIPTION
A	No risk to fetus. Studies have not shown evidence of fetal harm.
B	No risk in animal studies, and well-controlled studies in pregnant women are not available. It is assumed there is little to no risk in pregnant women.
C	Animal studies indicate a risk to the fetus. Controlled studies on pregnant women are not available. Risk versus benefit of the drug must be determined.
D	A risk to the human fetus has been proved. Risk versus benefit of the drug must be determined. It could be used in life-threatening conditions.
X	A risk to the human fetus has been proved. Risk outweighs the benefit, and drug should be avoided during pregnancy.

BOX 12-2 GUIDELINES FOR CORRECT ADMINISTRATION OF MEDICATIONS

Preparation

1. Wash hands before preparing medications.
2. Check for drug allergies; check the assessment history and Kardex.
3. Check medication order with health care provider's orders, Kardex, medicine sheet, or medicine card.
4. Check label on drug container three times.
5. Check expiration date on drug label, card, and Kardex; use only if date is current.
6. Recheck drug calculation of drug dose with another nurse as needed or by agency policy.
7. Verify doses of drugs that are potentially toxic with another nurse or pharmacist.
8. Pour tablet or capsule into the cap of the drug container. With unit dose, open packet at bedside after verifying patient identification.
9. Pour liquid at eye level. The meniscus (the lower curve of the liquid) should be at the line of desired dose (see Figure 13-2).

BOX 12-2 GUIDELINES FOR CORRECT ADMINISTRATION OF MEDICATIONS—cont'd

10. Dilute drugs that irritate the gastric mucosa (e.g., potassium, aspirin), or give with meals.

Administration

11. Administer only drugs that you have prepared. Do not prepare medications to be administered by another person.
12. Identify the patient by ID band or ID photo.
13. Offer ice chips to numb the patient's taste buds when giving bad-tasting drugs.
14. When possible, give bad-tasting medications first, followed by pleasant-tasting liquids.
15. Assist the patient to an appropriate position, depending on the route of administration.
16. Provide only amounts and kinds of liquids allowed on the diet.
17. Stay with the patient until the medications are taken.
18. Administer no more than 2.5 to 3 mL of solution intramuscularly at one site. Infants receive no more than 1 mL of solution intramuscularly at one site and no more than 1 mL subcutaneously. Never recap needles (Universal Precautions).
19. When administering drugs scheduled at the same time to a group of patients, give drugs last to patients who need extra assistance.
20. Discard needles and syringes in appropriate containers.
21. Drug disposal is dependent on agency policy and state law. For example, discard drugs in the sink or toilet, not in the trash can. Controlled substances must be returned to the pharmacy. Some disposals need signatures of witnesses; refer to agency policy.
22. Discard unused solutions from ampules.
23. Appropriately store (some require refrigeration) unused stable solutions from open vials.
24. Write date and time opened and your initials on the label.
25. Keep narcotics in a double-locked drawer or closet. Medication carts must be locked at all times when a nurse is not in attendance.
26. Keys to the opioids drawer must be kept by the nurse and not stored in a drawer or closet.
27. Keep opioids in a safe place, out of reach of children and others in the home.
28. Avoid contamination of one's own skin or inhalation to minimize chances of allergy or sensitivity development.

Recording

29. Report drug error immediately to the patient's health care provider and to the nurse manager.
30. Complete an incident report.
31. Charting: record drug given, dose, time, route, and your initials.
32. Record drugs promptly after given, especially STAT doses.
33. Record effectiveness and results of medication administered, especially PRN medications.
34. Report to the patient's health care provider and record drugs that were refused with the reason for refusal.
35. Record amount of fluid taken with medications on input and output chart.

ID, Identification; *PRN,* as needed; *STAT,* immediately.

BOX 12-3 BEHAVIORS TO AVOID DURING MEDICATION ADMINISTRATION

Do not be distracted when preparing medications.
Do not give drugs poured by others.
Do not pour drugs from containers with labels that are difficult to read or whose labels are partially removed or have fallen off.
Do not transfer drugs from their original, labeled container to another for storage.
Do not pour drugs into the hand.
Do not give medications for which the expiration date has passed.
Do not guess about drugs and drug doses. Ask when in doubt.
Do not use drugs that have sediment, are discolored, or are cloudy (and should not be).
Do not leave medications by the bedside or with visitors.
Do not leave prepared medications out of sight.
Do not give drugs if the patient says he or she has allergies to the drug or drug category.
Do not call the patient's name as the sole means of identification.
Do not give drug if patient states drug is different from drug he or she has been receiving. Check order.
Do not recap needles. Use Universal Precautions.
Do not mix drugs with large amount of food or beverages.

KEY WEBSITES

National Coordinating Council for Medication Error Reporting and Prevention (NCCMERP): *www.nccmerp.org*

Proper disposal of prescription drugs: *http://www.whitehouse.gov/sites/default/files/ondcp/issues-content/prescription-drugs/rx_abuse_plan.pdf*

U.S. Food and Drug Administration (FDA): *www.fda.gov*

NCLEX STUDY QUESTIONS

1. A patient asks about disposal of medications. What are the nurse's best responses?
(Select all that apply.)
   a. "Mix medications with coffee grounds before disposal."
   b. "Pour medications down the sink."
   c. "Remove identifying information on the original container."
   d. "Pulverize all tablets before disposal."
   e. "Dilute the medication with bleach before disposal."
2. The patient is taking duastride (Avodart). Which patient statement indicates the need for more education about the drug?
   a. "I'm glad I can take the medication with or without food."
   b. "It is good that no lab tests and monitoring are required."
   c. "This drug is expensive; I'm glad I have prescription coverage."
   d. "I prefer to chew the drug before swallowing it."
3. The nurse educator on the unit receives a list of high-alert drugs. Which strategy is recommended to decrease the risk of errors with these medications? (Select all that apply.)
   a. Store medications alphabetically on their usual shelf.
   b. Limit access to these drugs.
   c. Use special labels for these drugs.
   d. Provide increased information to staff.
   e. Standardize the ordering and preparation of these drugs.
4. The nurse is aware that, according to TJC, which abbreviation is on the "Do Not Use" list for ordering or documenting medications?
   a. QD
   b. h.s.
   c. T.I.W.
   d. b.i.d.
5. A patient refuses to take his prescribed medications. Which is the nurse's best response to this patient?
   a. Explain the benefits and side effects of the drug.
   b. Leave the medication at the patient's bedside to be taken later.
   c. Persuade the patient to take the medication.
   d. Explain the risks of not taking the medication.
6. What information is essential for the nurse to know related to right documentation? (Select all that apply.)
   a. Necessity to document all medications given at the end of shift
   b. Correct site of injectable medication
   c. Patient response to antiemetic
   d. Drug name, dose, route
   e. Date and time of dose and necessity for RN initial/signature
7. The nurse prepares to administer medications. Which are complete drug orders? (Select all that apply.)
   a. Aspirin 81 mg, PO, daily
   b. Multivitamin 1 daily
   c. Vitamin D, 2000 units, PO
   d. Ciprofloxacin HCl (Cipro) 500 mg PO q 12h × 7d
   e. Promethazine 50 mg IV q3-6h PRN for nausea

Answers: 1, a, c; 2, d; 3, b, c, d, e; 4, a; 5, d; 6, b, c, d, e; 7, a, d, e.

CHAPTER

13

Medication Administration

evolve WEBSITE

http://evolve.elsevier.com/KeeHayes/pharmacology/

- Animations
- Content Updates
- Key Points
- Review Questions for the NCLEX® Examination
- References from the Textbook
- Unfolding Case Studies

OBJECTIVES

- Differentiate routes of administration.
- Compare and contrast the various sites for parenteral therapy.
- Explain the equipment and technique used in parenteral therapy.
- Explain documenting medication administration.
- Analyze the nursing interventions related to administration of medications by various routes.
- Apply the nursing process to the administration of medication.

OUTLINE

KEY TERMS

Administration of medications is a basic activity in nursing practice. As a result of the transition from hospitals and institutions to community-based services, an increasing number of nurses are practicing in a variety of settings. Nurses therefore must be knowledgeable about specific drugs and their administration, patient response, drug interactions, patient allergies, and related resources. Safety and prevention of medication errors are essential (see Chapter 12).

SELF-ADMINISTRATION OF MEDICATION

Self-administration of medication (SAM) is common in the home and in many community-based settings like the workplace. However, SAM is relatively new to patients and staff in institutional settings. In practical terms, SAM means that the nurse gives the patient the appropriate medications and instructions that are kept at the bedside and then go home with the patient on discharge. Patients are responsible for taking their medication according to the instructions. Patients play a key role in and exercise control associated with taking selected medications. SAM allows patients to manage their medications during the hospital admission and prepares them to manage their medications at home for optimal benefits. Refer to Chapters 53 and 54 for a description of SAM for maternity patients and Chapter 12 for the "five-plus-five rights," the "do's and don'ts" of medication administration, factors that alter drug responses, high-alert medications, and pregnancy categories.

FORMS AND ROUTES FOR DRUG ADMINISTRATION

A variety of forms and routes are used for the administration of medications, including **sublingual, buccal,** oral (tablets, capsules, liquids, suspensions, elixirs), transdermal, topical, instillation (drops and sprays), **inhalation,** nasogastric and gastrostomy tubes, **suppositories,** and **parenteral** (Figure 13-1).

Tablets and Capsules

- Tablets and capsules are the most common drug forms; they are convenient and less expensive and do not require additional supplies for administration.

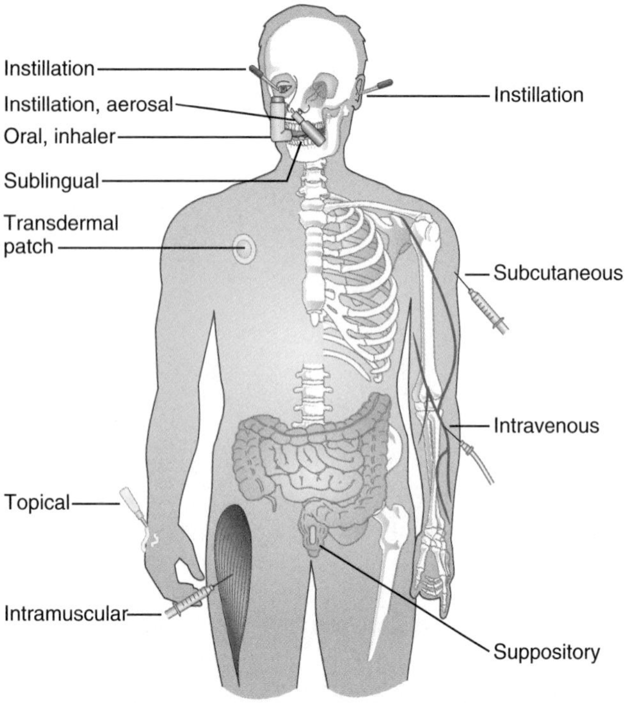

FIGURE 13–1 Some routes for medication administration.

- Oral medications are not given to patients who are vomiting, lack a gag reflex, or who are comatose. Patients who gag may need a brief rest before proceeding with further intake of medications.
- Do not mix medication with a large amount of food or beverage or with contraindicated food. Patients may not be able to eat all of the food and will not get a full dose of medication. Do not mix medication in infant formula.
- Enteric-coated and timed-release capsules must be swallowed whole to maintain a therapeutic drug level. If crushed, the initial excessive drug release poses a risk of toxicity. Because the drug is absorbed prematurely, the drug drops to a subtherapeutic level later in the cycle. To maintain a therapeutic drug level (not toxic and not subtherapeutic), the drug must be swallowed whole so it is released gradually. These medications should never be cut in half or crushed for administration. Follow agency policy for resources available for changing or altering such drugs if patients are unable to swallow them. At times, these medications can be given in liquid or IV form or in a non–extended-release form that may be given in more frequent doses—for example, Roprol XL (metaprolol succinate), which is long-acting, may be changed to Lopressor (metaprolol tartate), which is immediate-release and can be given more frequently.
- Be aware of medications without "extended-release" in the name that should never be cut in half or crushed (e.g., Mucinex tablets, which can be changed to liquid guaifenesin if needed).
- Administer irritating drugs with food to decrease GI discomfort.
- Administer drugs on an empty stomach if food interferes with medication absorption.
- Drugs given sublingually (placed under the tongue) or buccally (placed between the cheek and gum) remain in place until fully absorbed. No food or fluids should be taken while the medication is in place.
- Encourage the use of child-resistant caps. However, if patients have difficulty opening child-resistant caps, they might leave the caps off or not completely tightened, which is a safety hazard. Non–child-resistant caps are available for these patients on request.

Liquids

- Forms of liquid medication include elixirs, emulsions, and suspensions. Elixirs are sweetened hydroalcoholic liquids used in preparation of oral liquid medications. Emulsions are a mixture of two liquids that are not mutually soluble. Suspensions are liquids in which particles are mixed but not dissolved.
- Read the labels to determine whether dilution or shaking is required. As a general rule, suspensions and emulsions need to be shaken before administration; elixirs do not.
- The **meniscus** is the slightly concave curved line of a dose of liquid. The bottom of the meniscus should be used to measure the desired dose of medication (Figure 13-2).
- Many liquids require refrigeration once reconstituted.

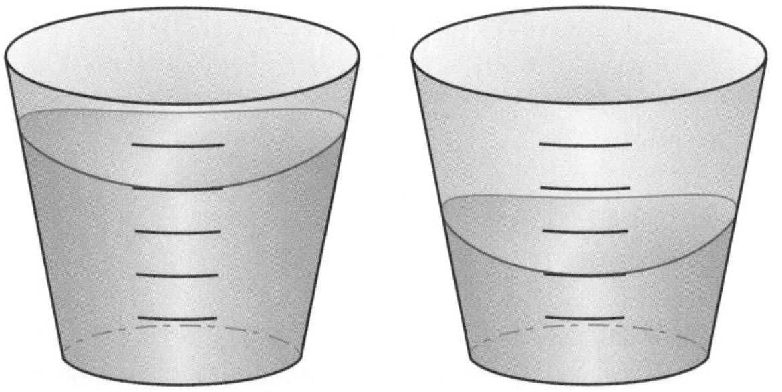

FIGURE 13–2 To read the meniscus, locate the lowest fluid mark.

Transdermal

- **Transdermal** medication is stored in a patch placed on the skin and absorbed through skin, having a systemic effect. Widespread use of such patches began in the 1980s. Patches for neoplastic drugs, drugs to treat allergic reactions, and insulin are in production or being developed. Transdermal drugs provide more consistent blood levels than oral and injection forms and avoid GI absorption problems associated with oral products. Transdermal patches should be rotated to different sites and not reapplied over the exact same area when changed. Additionally, the area should be thoroughly cleansed before administration of a new transdermal patch. This practice will prevent errors in overdosing the patient.
- Wash hands and wear gloves to administer medicated patches to prevent transfer of medication. Nurses should educate patients to wash hands after applying a patch to avoid transferring medicine to another part of body or to someone else.
- A common question is whether or not to cut the patches in half. A nurse might suggest using patches with a lower dosage rather than cutting patches and guessing the dose the patient will receive. There are two patch designs: (1) If the drug is embedded in a matrix patch and diffuses into the skin (e.g., Climara, Vivelle, Nicotrol, Testoderm), the drug is spread over the entire surface of the patch, which probably may be cut. Patients must be alert for underdosing or overdosing. (2) If the drug is pooled in a reservoir patch and is released via a semipermeable membrane (e.g., Catapres-TTS, Duragesic, Estraderm, Transderm-Nitro, Androderm), the patch should not be cut because too much drug may be released. Advise patients to secure the patch with tape, being careful not to apply it too tightly, which could alter the drug delivery.

Topical

- **Topical** medications are most frequently applied to the skin. They can be applied to the skin in several ways, such as with a glove, tongue blade, or cotton-tipped applicator. Nurses should never apply a topical medication without first protecting their own skin with gloves.
- Use appropriate technique to remove the medication from the container, and apply it to clean, dry skin, when possible. Do not contaminate the medication in a container; instead use gloves or an applicator.
- Gloves and applicators that come in contact with a patient should not be reinserted into the container. Estimate the amount needed and remove it from the container, or use a fresh sterile applicator each time the container is entered.

BOX 13-1 ADMINISTRATION OF EYEDROPS

1. Wash hands and wear gloves.
2. Instruct patient to lie down or sit down and look at ceiling.
3. Remove any discharge by gently wiping out from inner canthus. Use a separate cloth for each eye.
4. Gently draw skin down below affected eye to expose conjunctival sac.
5. Notify patient immediately before drops are administered so patient is prepared to avoid blinking when drops hit the conjunctiva.
6. Administer prescribed number of drops into center of sac. Medication placed directly on the cornea can cause discomfort or damage. Avoid touching eyelids or eyelashes with dropper. Self-administration of drops is enhanced with use of a Drop-eze, a cuplike device that holds the eyelids open.
   a. Gently press on lacrimal duct with a sterile cotton ball or tissue for 1 to 2 minutes after instillation to prevent systemic absorption through the lacrimal canal.
   b. Instruct patient to keep eyes closed for 1 to 2 minutes after application to promote absorption.

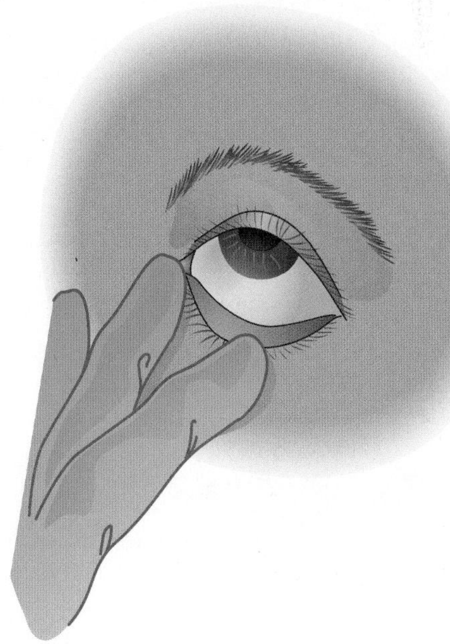

FIGURE 13–3 To administer eyedrops, gently pull down the skin below the eye to expose the conjunctival sac. Apply drops to the middle third of the sac, and apply gentle pressure over the lacrimal duct after administration.

Instillations

Instillations are liquid medications usually administered as drops, ointment, or sprays in the following forms:

- Eyedrops (Box 13-1 and Figure 13-3)
- Eye ointment (Box 13-2 and Figure 13-4)

BOX 13-2 ADMINISTRATION OF EYE OINTMENT

1. Wash hands and wear gloves.
2. Instruct patient to lie down or sit down and look at ceiling.
3. Remove any discharge by gently wiping out from inner canthus. Use a separate cloth for each eye.
4. Gently draw skin down below affected eye to expose conjunctival sac.
5. Prepare patient by explaining that ointment will be placed in the eye so patient can help by not blinking.
6. Squeeze a strip of ointment (about ¼ inch unless stated otherwise) onto conjunctival sac. Medication placed directly on the cornea can cause discomfort or damage. Avoid touching eyelids or eyelashes with tip of applicator.
7. Instruct patient to close eyes for 2 to 3 minutes.
8. Instruct patient to expect blurred vision for a short time. Apply at bedtime if possible.

BOX 13-3 ADMINISTRATION OF EARDROPS

1. Wash hands.
2. Have medication at room temperature.
3. Instruct patient to sit up with head tilted slightly toward unaffected side. This position straightens the external ear canal for better visualization. Maintain this position for 2 to 3 minutes to facilitate drops reaching the affected area (see Figure 13-5).
4. Pull down and back on the auricle for a child younger than 3 years of age. (For children 3 years of age and older, use the same procedure as for an adult.) For an adult, pull up and back on the auricle.
5. Instill prescribed number of drops. Take measures to avoid allowing drops to fall directly on tympanic membrane. Drops should be aimed at side of ear canal and allowed to run down into ear.
6. Do not contaminate dropper.

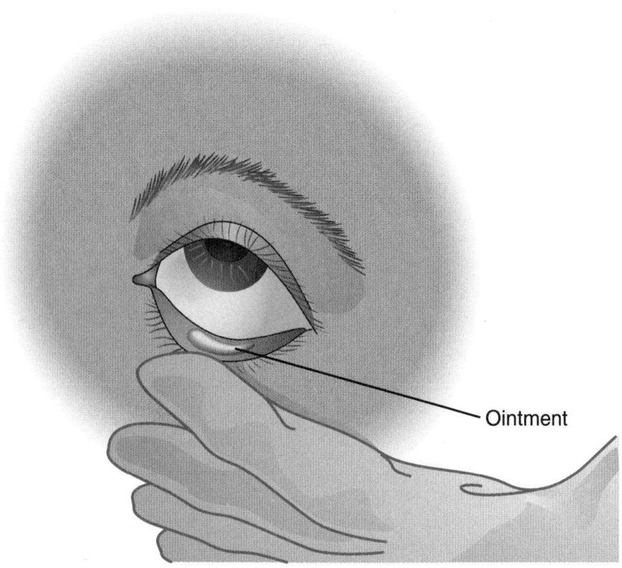

FIGURE 13–4 To administer eye ointment, squeeze a ¼-inch–wide strip of ointment onto the conjunctival sac.

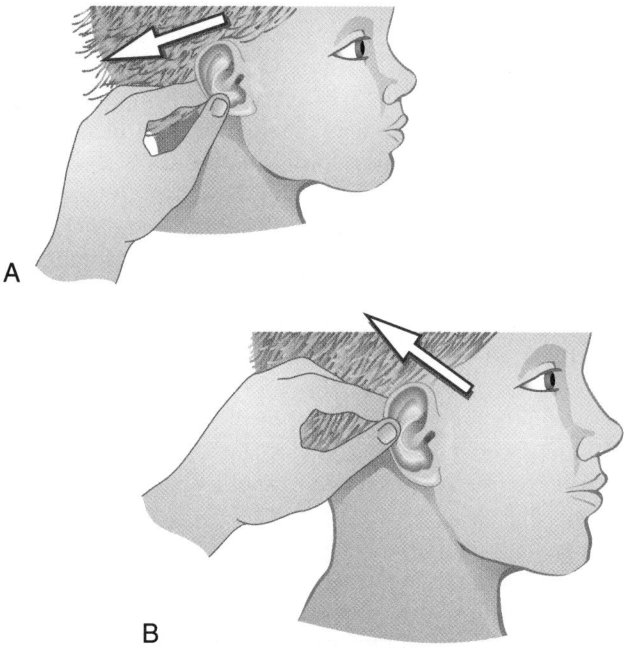

FIGURE 13–5 To administer eardrops, straighten the external ear canal by pulling down on the auricle in children younger than 3 years of age **(A)** or pulling back on the auricle in older children and adults **(B)**.

- Eardrops (Box 13-3 and Figure 13-5)
- Nose drops and sprays (Box 13-4 and Figures 13-6 and 13-7)

Inhalations

- **Metered-dose inhalers (MDIs)** are handheld devices that deliver medication to the lower respiratory tract (Box 13-5). Some MDIs have a counter to indicate the number of inhalations used. For those that do not, the most accurate way to determine this number is for the patient to count and record (e.g., on the box or a calendar) the number of inhalations used; however, this is often not practical. Inhalation counters are now on some inhalation products and are a most welcome addition. Every effort should be made to have the patient know how much medication is in the canister and to anticipate/obtain refills in a timely manner.

BOX 13-4 ADMINISTRATION OF NOSE DROPS AND SPRAYS

1. Wash hands and wear gloves.
2. Advise patient to blow nose.
3. Advise patient to tilt head back for drops to reach frontal sinus and tilt head to affected side to reach ethmoid sinus.
4. Administer prescribed number of drops or sprays without touching tip of medication applicator to nasal passages.
5. Some sprays have instructions to close one nostril, tilt head to closed side, and hold breath or breathe through the nose for 1 minute.
6. If patient is using a nasal spray to reach the sinuses, proper head position is with patient looking down at feet and spray tip aimed toward eye.
7. Advise patient to keep head tilted backward for 5 minutes after instillation of drops.

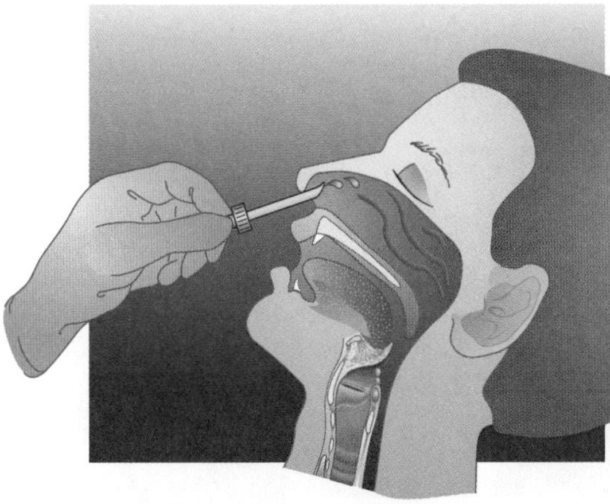

FIGURE 13–6 Administering nose drops.

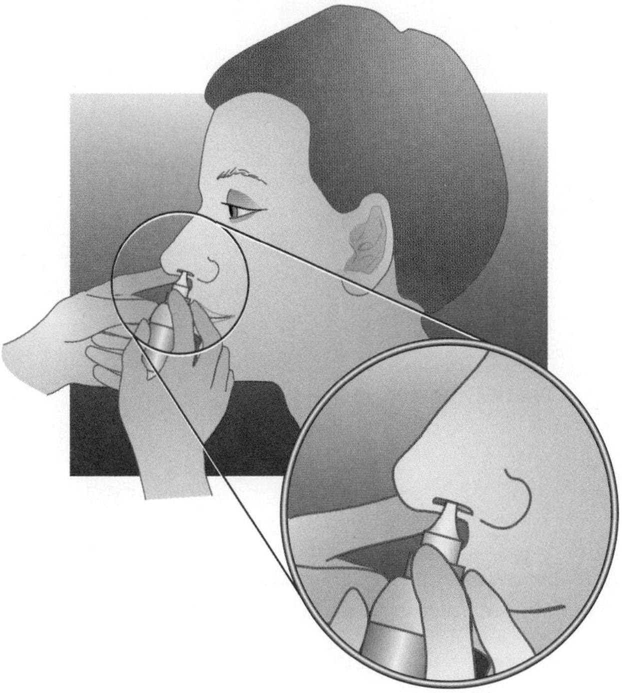

FIGURE 13–7 Administering nasal spray.

- Take special measures when handling the capsules used in some MDIs to prevent the transfer of medication (for example, with Spiriva, if the powder from the punctured capsule gets on the nurse's hands and transfers to the eyes, it will dilate the pupils).
- **Spacers** are devices used to enhance the delivery of medications from the MDI. Figure 13-8 illustrates the distribution of medication with and without a spacer. A nebulizer is a device that changes a liquid medication into a fine mist or aerosol that has the ability to reach the lower, smaller airways. Handheld nebulizers deliver a very-fine–sized particle spray of medication.
- When administering drugs via an MDI or nebulizer, the preferred patient position is the semi-Fowler's or high Fowler's position.

BOX 13-5 CORRECT USE OF METERED-DOSE INHALER

1. Discuss preferred techniques with health care provider.
2. Insert medication canister into plastic holder.
3. Shake inhaler well before using. Remove cap from mouthpiece.
4. Breathe out through mouth. Open mouth wide, and hold mouthpiece 1 to 2 inches from mouth. Do not put mouthpiece in mouth unless using a spacer.
5. Take slow, deep breath through mouth and, during inspiration, push top of medication canister once.
6. Autohalers do not require coordination of pushing down top of canister and taking deep breath. With autohaler in upright position, raise lever and shake. Inhale deeply through mouthpiece with steady, moderate force, which triggers the release of medicine, making a "click" sound and puffing out medicine. Continue to take deep breaths.
7. Hold breath for 10 seconds; exhale slowly through pursed lips.
8. Wait 1 to 2 minutes, and repeat procedure by first shaking canister in plastic holder with cap on, if a second dose is required.
9. "Test spray" before administering metered dose if inhaler has not been used recently or when it is first used.
10. Wait 5 minutes before using inhaler containing steroid, if a glucocorticoid inhalant is to be used with a bronchodilator.
11. Teach patient to monitor pulse rate.
12. Caution against overuse, because side effects and tolerance may result.
13. Teach patient to monitor amount of medication remaining in canister. Advise patient to ask health care provider or pharmacist to estimate when a new inhaler will be needed based on dosing schedule.
14. Teach patient to rinse mouth after using metered-dose inhaler. This is especially important when using a steroid drug. Rinsing mouth helps prevent irritation and secondary infection to oral mucosa.
15. Advise patient to avoid smoking.
16. Teach patient to do daily cleaning of equipment, including (1) wash hands; (2) take apart all washable parts of equipment and wash with warm water; (3) rinse; (4) place on clean towel, and cover with another clean towel to air-dry; and (5) store in clean plastic bag when completely dry. Recommendation: alternate two sets of washable equipment to make this process easier.

- Instruct the patient on the correct use and cleaning of MDIs or nebulizers.

Nasogastric and Gastrostomy Tubes

- Check for proper tube placement before administering medications. Replace any aspirated gastric fluid.
- Pour drug into syringe without plunger or bulb, release clamp, and allow medication to flow in properly, usually by gravity.
- Flush tubing with 50 mL of water, or the prescribed amount. (Refer to agency policy for exact amount.)
- Clamp tube and remove syringe.
- If the patient has a nasogastric tube to suction, clamp the tube for 30 minutes before placing the patient back on suction to allow medication to be absorbed.

Suppositories

Rectal Suppositories

- Medications administered as suppositories or enemas can be given rectally for local and systemic absorption. The

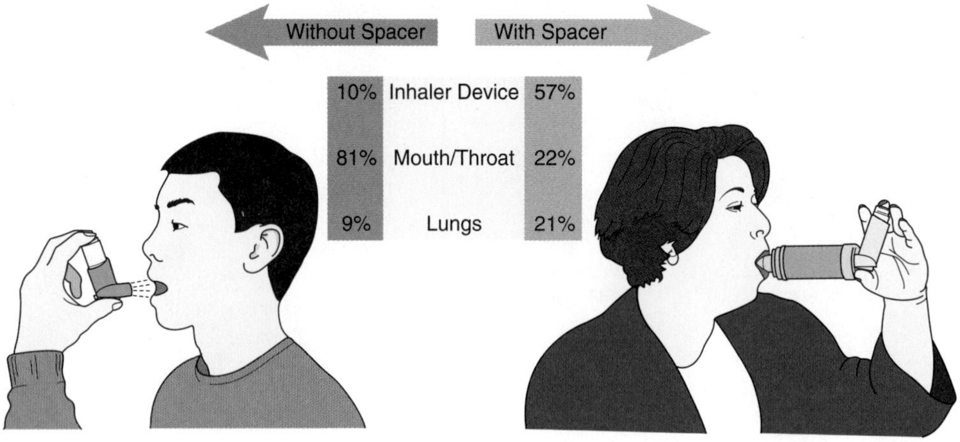

FIGURE 13–8 Distribution of medication with and without a spacer.

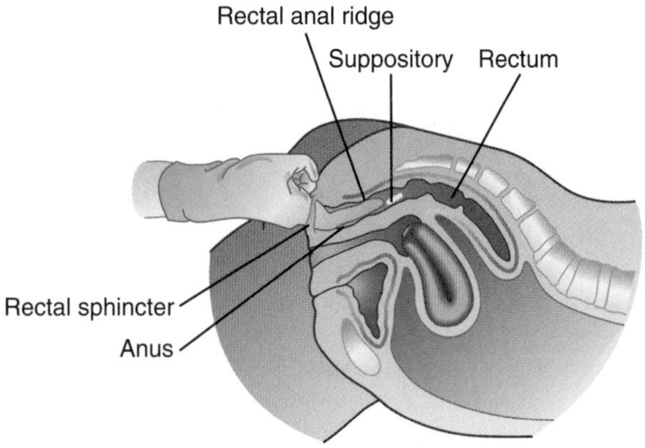

FIGURE 13–9 Inserting a rectal suppository.

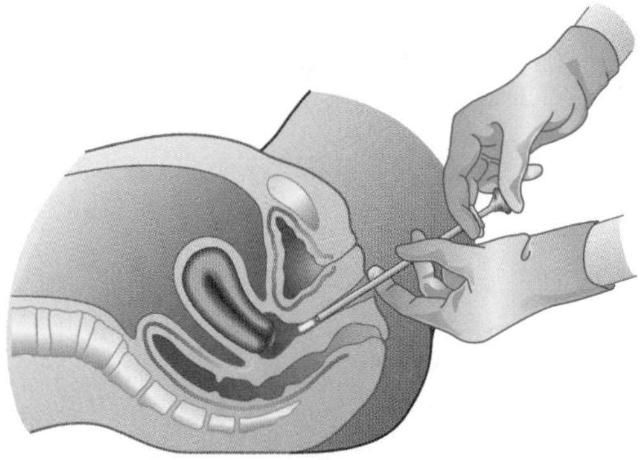

FIGURE 13–10 Inserting a vaginal suppository.

numerous small capillaries in the rectal area promote medication absorption.

- The foil around the suppository is removed, and the suppository may be lubricated before insertion. When medications such as antipyretics and bronchodilators are given, the patient must be reminded to retain the medication, not expel it.
- Suppositories tend to soften at room temperature and therefore must be refrigerated before use.
- Explain the procedure to the patient, and provide privacy.
- Use a glove for insertion.
- Instruct the patient to lie on the left side and breathe through the mouth to relax the anal sphincter.
- Apply a small amount of water-soluble lubricant to tip of unwrapped suppository, and gently insert suppository beyond the internal sphincter (Figure 13-9).
- Have patient lie on the side for 20 minutes after insertion.
- If indicated, teach patients how to self-administer suppositories, and observe a return demonstration for teaching effectiveness.

Vaginal Suppositories

Vaginal suppositories are similar to rectal suppositories. They are generally inserted into the vagina with an applicator supplied with the medication (Figure 13-10); gloves should be worn. The patient should be in the lithotomy position. Advise patient to remain lying for a period of time to allow medication absorption; times vary depending on medication. After insertion, provide the patient with a sanitary pad.

Parenteral

Safety is a special concern with parenteral medication (medication administered via injection to bypass the first-pass effect of the liver). Manufacturers have responded with safety features to help decrease or eliminate needlestick injuries and possible transfer of bloodborne diseases such as hepatitis and human immunodeficiency virus (HIV). (Figure 13-11 shows examples of safety needles.) Types of parenteral routes include **intradermal, subcutaneous, intramuscular, Z-track technique, intravenous,** and **intraosseous.** A description of each follows with special considerations noted for the pediatric patient.

Intradermal

Action

- Local effect
- Used for observation of an inflammatory (allergic) reaction to foreign proteins. Examples include tuberculin testing, testing for drug and other allergic sensitivities, and some immunotherapy for cancer.

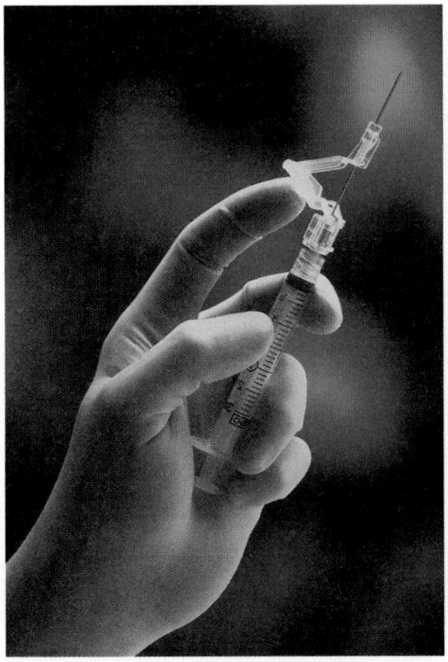

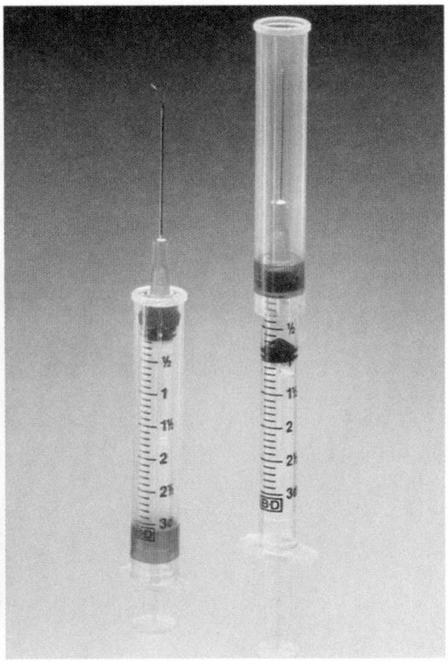

FIGURE 13–11 Safety needles. (Courtesy of Becton, Dickinson and Company, Franklin Lakes, New Jersey.)

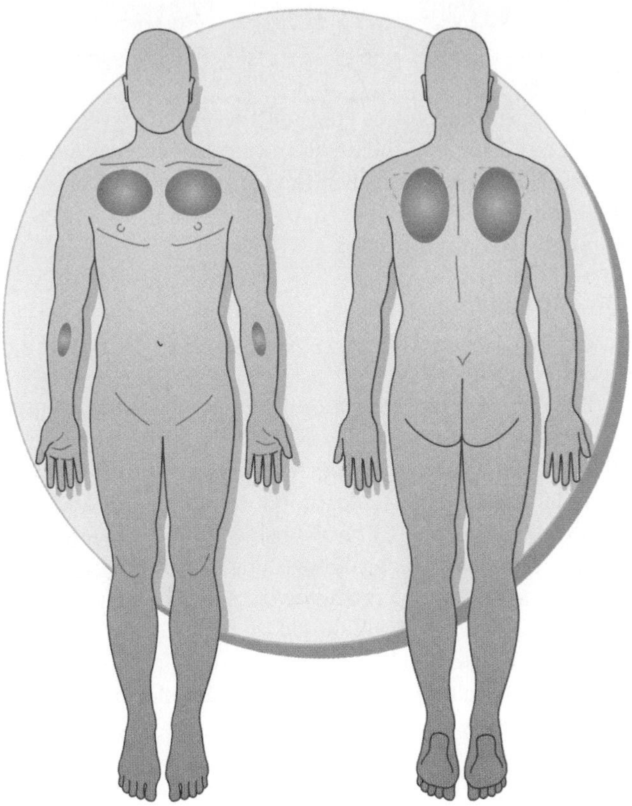

FIGURE 13–12 Common sites for intradermal injection.

Sites

- Locations are chosen so an inflammatory reaction can be observed. Preferred areas are lightly pigmented, thinly keratinized, and hairless, such as the ventral mid-forearm, clavicular area of the chest, or scapular area of the back (Figure 13-12).

Equipment

- Needle: 25- to 27-gauge; ⅜ to ⅝ inch long
- Syringe: 1 mL calibrated in 0.01-mL increments (usually 0.01 to 0.1 mL injected)

Technique

- Wash hands and wear gloves.
- Cleanse the area with a circular motion using aseptic technique.
- Hold the skin taut.
- Insert the needle, bevel up, at a 10- to 15-degree angle; the outline of the needle under the skin should be visible (Figure 13-13).
- Inject the medication slowly to form a wheal (blister or bleb). A small amount is injected so volume will not interfere with wheal formation or cause a systemic reaction. If the wheal does not appear, the needle is too deep; the medication may not be effective, and the injection will have to be given at another site.
- Remove the needle slowly; do not recap.
- Do not massage the area; instruct the patient not to do so.
- Mark the area with a pen, and ask the patient not to wash it off until read by a health care provider.
- Assess for allergic reaction in 24 to 72 hours; measure the diameter of local reaction. For tuberculin testing, measure only the indurated area; do not include the area of erythema in the measurement.

Subcutaneous

Action

- Systemic effect
- Sustained effect; absorbed mainly through capillaries; usually slower in onset than with IM route

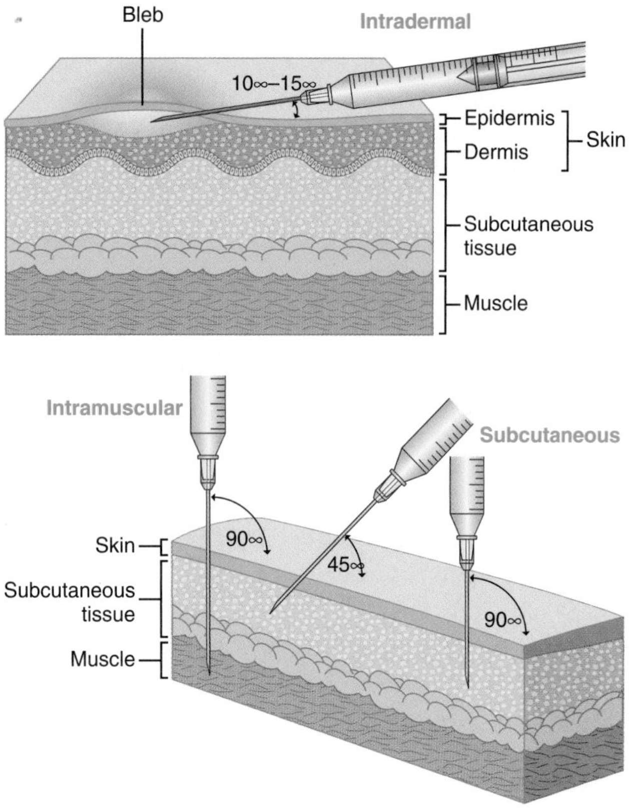

FIGURE 13–13 Needle-skin angle for intradermal, subcutaneous, and intramuscular injections.

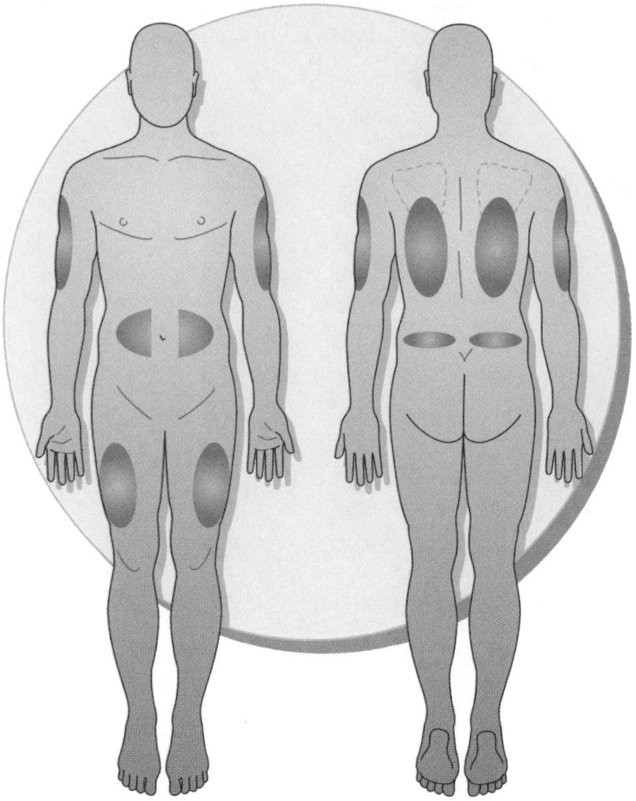

FIGURE 13–14 Common sites for subcutaneous injections.

Sites

- Locations for subQ injection are chosen for adequate fat-pad size (Figure 13-14). Sites should be rotated with subcutaneous injections, such as insulin and heparin, and documented on appropriate records to avoid overuse of an individual site.
- A larger amount of medication may have to be divided and administered at two sites, or else the medication route may be changed. Refer to agency policy for the maximum amount of medication to be administered via this route.

Equipment

- Needle: 25- to 27-gauge; ½ to ⅝ inch long
- Syringe: 1 to 3 mL (usually 0.5 to 1 mL injected)
- Insulin syringe measured in units for use with insulin only

Technique

- Wash hands and wear gloves.
- Cleanse the area with a circular motion using aseptic technique.
- Pinch the skin.
- Insert the needle at an angle appropriate to body size: 45 to 90 degrees (45 degrees for those with little subQ tissue) (see Figure 13-14).
- Release the skin.
- Do not aspirate.
- Inject the medication slowly.
- Remove the needle quickly; do not recap.
- Gently massage the area unless contraindicated.
- Apply gentle pressure to the injection site to prevent bleeding or oozing into the tissue and subsequent bruising and tissue damage, especially if the patient is on anticoagulant therapy.
- Apply bandage if needed.

Intramuscular

Action

- Systemic effect
- Usually more rapid effect of drug than with subQ route
- Used for solutions in oils and deep IM for irritating drugs

Sites. Locations are chosen for adequate muscle size and minimal major nerves and blood vessels in the area (see Figures 13-15 to 13-18). Other considerations include volume of drug administered, needle size, angle of injection, patient position, site location, and advantages and disadvantages of site. Underweight patients should be evaluated for sites with adequate muscle. The ventrogluteal is the preferred site for adults and toddlers with gluteal muscle development associated with firmly established walking.

Equipment

- Needle: 20- to 23-gauge; 18-gauge for blood products; 1 to 1½ inches long

Technique

- Wash hands and wear gloves.
- Same as for subQ injection, with two exceptions: Flatten the skin area using the thumb and index finger, and inject between them; insert the needle at a 90-degree angle into the muscle (see Figure 13-14).
- Syringe: 1 to 3 mL (usually 0.5 to 1.5 mL injected)

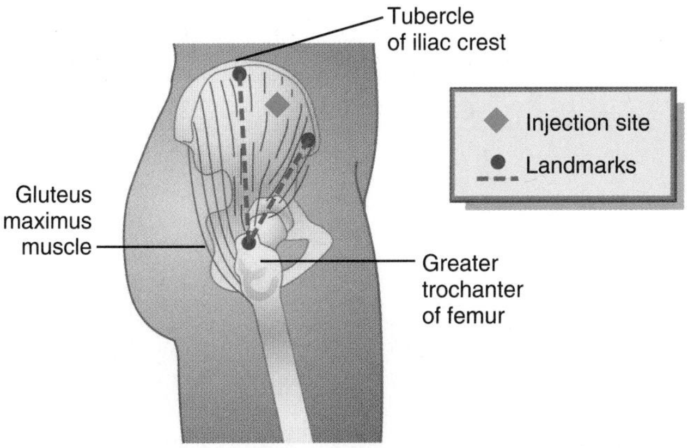

FIGURE 13–15 Ventrogluteal injection site.

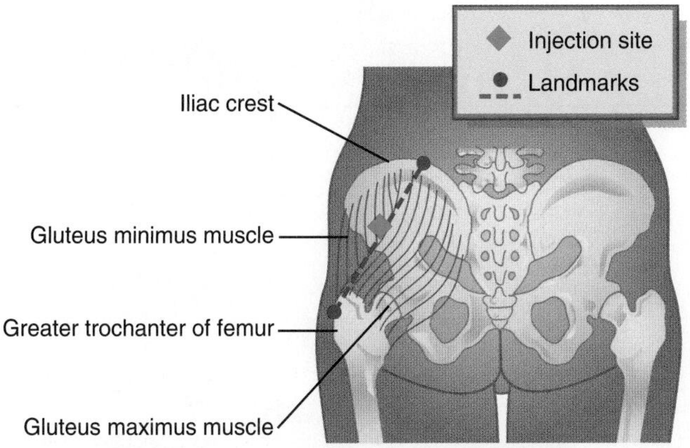

FIGURE 13–16 Dorsogluteal injection site.

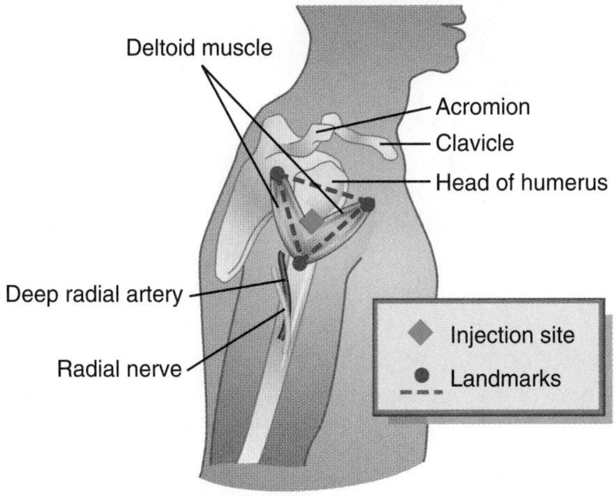

FIGURE 13–17 Deltoid injection site.

Preferred Intramuscular Injection Sites. Table 13-1 shows the four sites, patient position, advantages, and disadvantages of each injection site.

- *Ventrogluteal* (Figure 13-15). Volume of drug administered is 1 to 3 mL, with a 20- to 23-gauge, 1¼- to 2½-inch needle. Slightly angle the needle toward the iliac crest.
- *Dorsogluteal* (Figure 13-16). Volume of drug administered is 1 to 3 mL; 5 mL gamma globulin with 18- to 23-gauge, 1¼- to 3-inch needle. Place the needle at a 90-degree angle to the skin with the patient in the prone position.

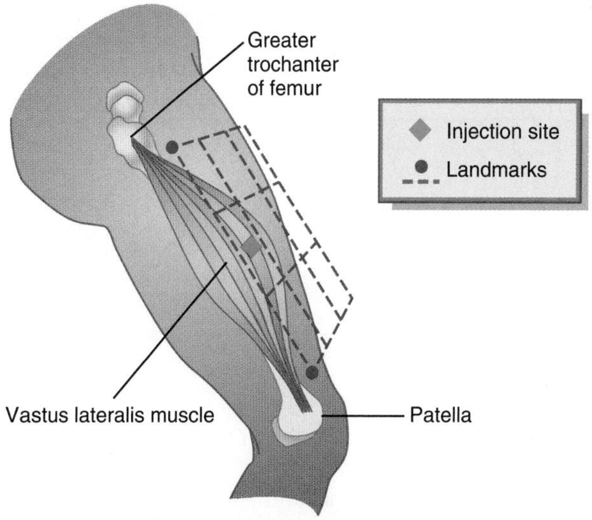

FIGURE 13–18 Vastus lateralis injection site in children.

- *Deltoid* (Figure 13-17). Volume of drug administered is 0.5 to 1 mL, with a 23- to 25-gauge, ⅝ to 1½-inch needle. Place the needle at a 90-degree angle to the skin or slightly toward the acromion.
- *Vastus lateralis* (Figure 13-18). Volume of drug administered is 0.5 mL in infants (max = 1 mL), 1 mL in pediatric patients, and 1 to 1.5 mL in adults (max = 2 mL). Direct the needle at the knee at a 45- to 60-degree angle to the frontal, sagittal, and horizontal planes of the thigh.

Z-Track Injection Technique

This technique (Figure 13-19) prevents medication from leaking back into the subQ tissue. It is frequently advised for medications that cause visible and permanent skin discolorations (e.g., iron dextran). The gluteal site is preferred. Using aseptic technique, draw up the medication. Replace the first needle with a second needle of appropriate gauge and length to penetrate muscle tissue and deliver the medication to the selected site. The first needle is removed to prevent the medication adhering to the needle shaft from being taken into the subQ tissue. Consider having the medication prepared in the pharmacy.

Intravenous

Action

- Systemic effect
- More rapid than IM or subQ routes

Sites. Accessible peripheral veins (e.g., cephalic or cubital vein of arm; dorsal vein of hand) are preferred (Figure 13-20). When possible, ask the patient about preference. Avoid needless body restriction. In newborns, the veins of the feet, lower legs, and head may also be used after the previous sites have been exhausted.

Equipment

- Needle
- Adults: 20- to 21-gauge, 1 to 1½ inches
- Infants: 24-gauge; 1 inch
- Children: 22-gauge; 1 inch

TABLE 13-1 INTRAMUSCULAR INJECTION SITES: PATIENT POSITION, ADVANTAGES, AND DISADVANTAGES

SITE	PATIENT POSITION	ADVANTAGES	DISADVANTAGES
Ventrogluteal	Supine, lateral	Anatomic landmarks well defined Muscle mass suited for deep IM or Z-track injections Free of major nerves	In the event of hypersensitivity reaction, medication absorption cannot be delayed by tourniquet
Dorsogluteal	Prone	Muscle mass suited for deep IM or Z-track injections	Requires correct/accurate site and technique to avoid injury to major nerves and vascular structures In the event of hypersensitivity reaction, medication absorption cannot be delayed by tourniquet
Deltoid	Lateral, prone, sitting, supine	Readily accessible In the event of hypersensitivity reaction, medication absorption can be delayed by tourniquet	Small muscle mass; limited to small volume doses Close to nerves; requires accurate technique
Vastus lateralis	Sitting, supine	Good site for infants Size acceptable for multiple injections Free of major nerves	Special attention required to avoid sciatic nerve or femoral structures if long needle is used

IM, Intramuscular.

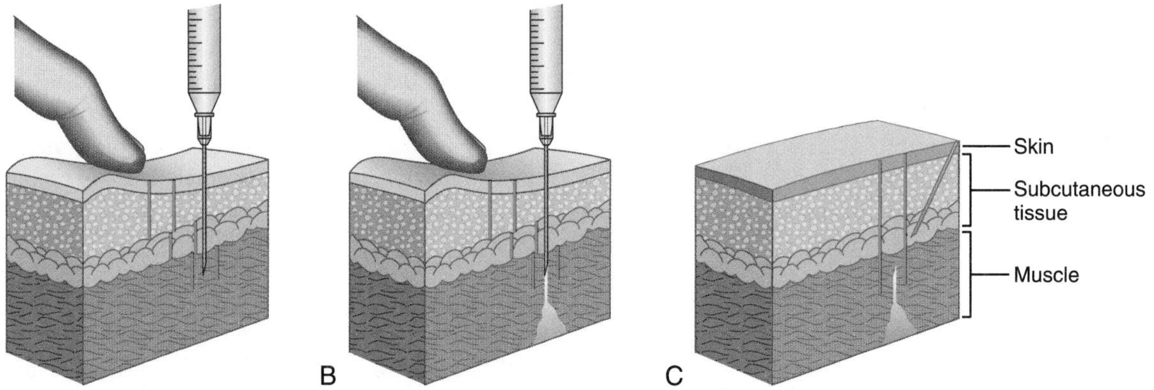

FIGURE 13–19 Z-track injection. **A,** Pull skin to one side and hold; insert needle. **B,** Holding skin to the side, inject medication. **C,** Wait 6 to 10 seconds before withdrawing needle and releasing skin. This technique prevents medication from entering subcutaneous tissue.

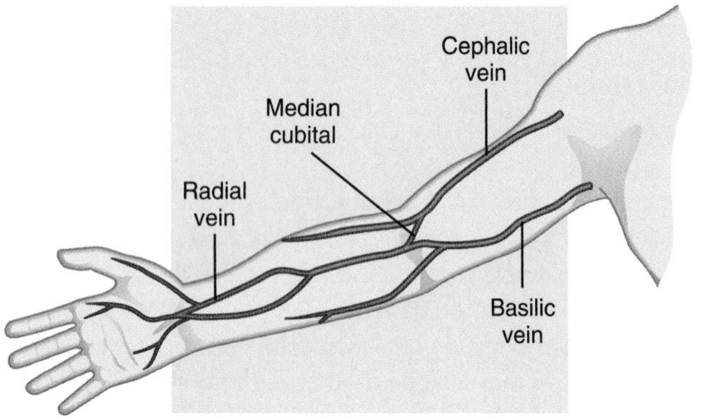

FIGURE 13–20 Common sites for intravenous administration.

- Larger bore for viscous drugs, whole blood or fractions; large volume for rapid infusion
- Electronic IV delivery device, an infusion controller, or pump
- Patient-controlled analgesia (PCA) system, if ordered
- Eutectic mixture of local anesthetics (EMLA), if appropriate

Technique

- Wash hands and wear gloves.
- Apply a tourniquet.
- Apply EMLA 1 hour before procedure on unbroken skin.
- Cleanse the area using aseptic technique with an appropriate solution.
- Insert butterfly or a catheter and feed up into the vein until blood returns. Remove tourniquet.
- Stabilize the needle or IV catheter, and apply dressing to site.

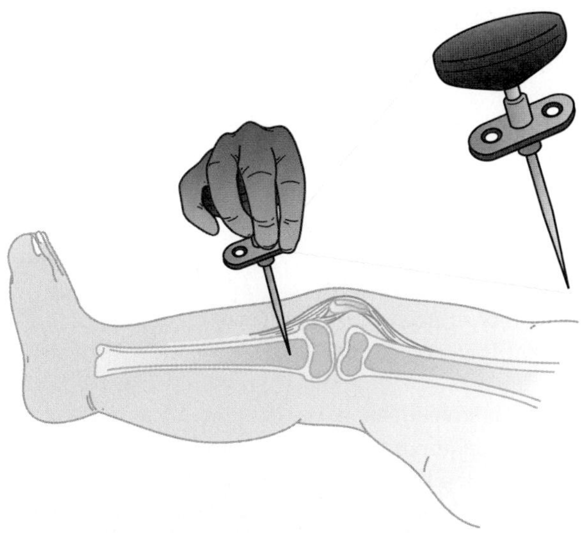

FIGURE 13–21 Intraosseous access.

- Monitor flow rate, distal pulses, skin color and temperature, and insertion site.
- Consult agency policy regarding addition of medications to bottle or bag, piggyback technique, and IV push. Be alert that all tubing is connected correctly.

Intraosseous

Action

- Fluids, crystalloids, blood products, and medications administered via intraosseous (IO) infusion into the bone marrow enter circulation through the network of venous sinusoids (Figure 13-21). IO is used when IV access is not possible; it is removed within 24 hours. Contraindications include fracture in insertion limb, infection at insertion site, severe osteoporosis and other bone abnormalities, and prosthetic joints in close proximity to insertion site.

Sites

- BIG: proximal tibia and humerus
- EZ-IO: proximal and distal tibia and humerus
- FAST1: sternum

Equipment

- Common intraosseous devices include BIG (blue cap for adults and red cap for children); EZ-IO; and First Access for Shock and Trauma I (FAST1)

Technique

- Wash hands and wear gloves.
- Palpate insertion site.
- Cleanse area using aseptic technique.
- Use insertion process appropriate to device (manual pressure, battery-operated power driver).
- Right after patency is confirmed, instill 1% lidocaine (usually 2 to 4 mL) if patient is awake.
- Stabilize the needle/device.
- Attach intravenous extension set; flush with isotonic saline (usually 5 to 10 mL), and attach IV tubing.

NURSING IMPLICATIONS FOR ADMINISTRATION OF PARENTERAL MEDICATIONS

Sites

- Ventrogluteal site is preferred for IM injections in adults and toddlers with gluteal muscle development associated with firmly established walking.
- For toddlers not walking alone for at least 1 year, the vastus lateralis is preferred.
- Do not use the dorsogluteal site for IM injections in children.

Equipment

- The syringe size should approximate the volume of medication to be administered.
- Use the tuberculin syringe for amounts <0.5 mL.
- Use the filter needle to draw up the medication from a glass vial or ampule. Change the needle before administration to prevent tissue irritation from any glass fragment or medication left on the needle.

Technique

- Wash hands and wear gloves.
- Correctly identify the patient.
- Explain to the patient what is going to be done. Gain the patient's cooperation. Allow the patient time to cooperate, if possible.
- Demonstrate empathy and concern for patient and family. Allay anxiety, and encourage expression of feelings.
- Position the patient.
- Follow the rights of medication administration (see Chapter 12).
- Inspect the skin before each injection.
- Inject medication slowly to minimize tissue damage.
- Stabilize skin during needle removal to reduce pain.
- Do not administer injections if sites are inflamed, edematous, or lesioned (e.g., moles, scars).
- Rotate the injection site to enhance absorption of the drug. Document the injection site.
- Observe patient for drug effectiveness. Report any untoward reactions immediately.
- Multiple products are available to reduce pain of parenteral medication administration, such as EMLA, lidocaine, and tetracaine in topical patch, and "shot buster"—a mechanical device based on the gate control theory of pain management.

DEVELOPMENTAL NEEDS OF PEDIATRIC PATIENTS

Anticipate developmental needs. Examples of needs associated with administration of medications include the following (refer to Chapter 7 for additional examples):

- Stranger anxiety (infant): Act to instill a sense of safety and security in the infant.

- Hospitalization, illness, or injury viewed as punishment (3 to 6 years of age): Allow control where appropriate; obtain child's view of situation; encourage positive relationships and expression of feelings in acceptable manner and activities. Include family or support person if appropriate.
- Fear of mutilation (3 to 6 years of age): Explain procedures carefully; use less intrusive routes, such as the oral route, whenever possible; allow children to give "play" injections to a doll or stuffed animal.

TECHNOLOGICAL ADVANCES

Advances in drug administration therapy continue to enhance safety, increase accessibility to sites, promote patient mobility, and improve patient adherence. Examples of these advances include the following:

- Pain-free delivery of insulin through patch
- Insulin pumps that deliver insulin based on monitoring of serum glucose levels
- Drugs implanted in contact lenses
- Intelligent infusion technology that programs IV infusions based on scanned information.
- Electronic order entry system
- Computerized unit dose dispensing cabinets
- Bar code technologies that scan medications and reconcile them with patient ID band
- Electronic medication administration records

SAFETY: Preventing Medication Errors

Medication Administration

- Remove foil-backed patches before magnetic resonance imaging (MRI) and in code situations when using AED equipment to prevent burns.
- Observe sterile technique when the skin is broken. Take precautions to avoid medication stains.
- Use firm strokes if the medication is to be rubbed in.

Nursing Process

Patient-Centered Collaborative Care

Overview of Medication Administration

Assessment

- Obtain appropriate vital signs and relevant laboratory test results for future comparisons and evaluation of therapeutic response.
- Determine patient's level of consciousness, risk for aspiration, and ability to take medications.
- Obtain drug history, including drug allergies.
- Identify high-risk patients for reactions.
- Assess patient's capability to follow therapeutic regimen.
- Assess possible contraindications in certain medication regimens.

Potential Nursing Diagnoses

- Risk for injury related to possible adverse reaction
- Readiness for enhanced management of medication regimen

Planning

- Identify goals.
- Promote therapeutic response, and prevent or minimize adverse reactions.
- Identify strategies to promote adherence.
- Identify interventions.

Nursing Interventions

- Prepare equipment and environment; wash hands.
- Check for allergies and other assessment data.
- Check drug label three times; check expiration date; apply rights of medication administration
- Be certain of drug calculation; verify dose with another RN or licensed personnel as necessary.
- Pour liquids at eye level on flat surface.
- Avoid contact with topical and inhalation preparations.
- Verify patient identification.
- Administer only drugs you have prepared.
- Assist the patient to appropriate position.
- Discard needles and syringes in "sharps" container. Do not recap needles.
- Keep all drugs stored properly, especially related to temperature, light, and moisture.
- Follow agency policy related to discarding drugs and controlled substances.
- Report drug errors immediately.
- Document all appropriate information in a timely manner.
- Record effectiveness of drugs administered, side effects or adverse effects, and reason for any drugs refused.

Patient Teaching

General

- Emphasize safety.
- Monitor patient's physical abilities regularly as needed.
- Keep or store medications in original labeled containers with child-resistant caps when needed.
- Provide patient and family with written instructions (or audio instructions if visually impaired or unable to read) about the drug regimen.
- Advise patient and family about expected therapeutic effect, anticipated onset of action, and expected duration of treatment.
- Educate patient and family on possible side effects or signs of an adverse reaction.
- Instruct patient and family about possible drug-laboratory test interaction.
- Advise patient of nonpharmacologic measures to promote therapeutic response.

- Encourage patient and family to have adequate supply of necessary medications available.
- Caution against use of OTC preparations, including herbal remedies without *first* contacting the health care provider.
- Reinforce importance of follow-up appointments with health care providers.
- Encourage patient to wear Medic-Alert band with medications or allergies indicated.
- Encourage lifestyle changes associated with medication administration, as needed (e.g., smoking cessation, exercising, limiting salt or fat in diet).
- Encourage use of community resources to assist with patient and family needs.

Diet
- Advise patient and family about possible drug-food interactions and contraindicated foods, if any.
- Advise patient and family about possible drug-alcohol interactions.

Self-Administration
- Advise patient and family regarding drug dose and dosing schedule.
- Teach patient and family about psychomotor skills related to drug regimen.
- Provide patient and family with contact information for questions and concerns.

Side Effects
- Counsel patient and family about general side effects and adverse reactions of the medications.
- Teach patient and family to monitor effects of drug, as appropriate (e.g., check blood pressure if drug is to treat hypertension).
- Advise patient and family when and how to notify health care provider.

Cultural Considerations
- Assess personal beliefs of patients and family.
- Modify communications to meet cultural needs of patient and family.
- Communicate respect for culture and cultural practices of patient and family.

Evaluation
- Evaluate effectiveness of medications administered.
- Identify expected time frame of desired drug response; consider modification of therapy as needed.
- Determine patient satisfaction with regimen.

KEY WEBSITES

The Institute for Safe Medication Practices: *www.ismp.org*
Medication Administration Safety: *www.ncbi.nlm.nih.gov/books/NBK2656/*
CDC's Medication Safety Program: *www.cdc.gov/medicationsafety/*

NCLEX STUDY QUESTIONS

1. The nurse is administering oral medications to a patient. Which are important considerations? (Select all that apply.)
   a. Administer irritating drugs with food.
   b. Avoid mixing medications in infant formula.
   c. Enteric-coated capsules may be chewed or crushed.
   d. Oral medications should be held if the patient is vomiting.
   e. Cut all transdermal patches to the correct dose.
2. The clinic nurse is preparing to administer an intradermal injection to the patient. Which supplies are most appropriate for this procedure?
   a. 21-gauge, ⅝-inch needle
   b. 27-gauge, ⅝-inch needle, 3-mL syringe
   c. 25-gauge needle, insulin syringe
   d. 25-gauge needle, tuberculin syringe
3. The nurse is administering iron dextran to a patient. What special considerations are associated with this?
   a. Gluteal site is preferred, best with different needle to draw up and to administer.
   b. Deltoid site is preferred; increased chance of "self sticks."
   c. Vastus lateralis site is preferred.
   d. Gluteal site is preferred with use of one needle.
4. The nurse administers a variety of medications to a patient. Which patient statement indicates a need for further teaching?
   a. "I do not drink or eat when I have sublingual nitroglycerin in place."
   b. "I mix all these meds in my dessert and hope I am not too full to finish."
   c. "I keep the meds in their original labeled containers."
   d. "I store medications away from children and pets."

5. The nurse is teaching a patient to use an inhaler. What common teaching point is essential for the nurse to include?
   a. Handheld nebulizers deliver a large molecule particle spray of medication.
   b. The semi- or high-Fowler's position is recommended.
   c. Spacers decrease delivery of medication.
   d. Nebulizers change medications to a fine powder mist.
6. A 3-year-old patient has an IM medication ordered. What is the most appropriate approach to gain the child's cooperation?
   a. Engage in fantasy play.
   b. Give a pretend injection to a toy animal.
   c. Restrain the patient's upper extremities.
   d. Ask family members to leave the room.
7. The nurse prepares to administer oral medications to a patient. What nursing intervention in addition to the "rights" is necessary to ensure safety?
   a. Assess the patient for risk for aspiration.
   b. Mix 2 of the 4 ordered medications into the meal.
   c. Administer drugs on a full stomach if food interferes with medication absorption.
   d. Administer irritating drugs without food to decrease gastrointestinal discomfort.
8. A patient is to start on a lidocaine transdermal patch. What is essential for the nurse to include in patient teaching? (Select all that apply.)
   a. Wear gloves when applying the patch.
   b. Cut the patch in half if a reduced dose is needed.
   c. Wear gloves when removing the patch.
   d. Remove the patch before an MRI.
   e. Remove the patch if the end becomes loose.

Answers: 1, a, b, d; 2, d; 3, a; 4, b; 5, b; 6, b; 7, a; 8, a, c, d.

UNIT III

Drug Calculations

Unit III (Chapter 14) provides practice in the calculation of drug dosages. The chapter is divided into six sections: (A) systems of measurement; (B) four general methods for calculating drug dosages, and two individualized methods; (C) calculations of oral dosages; (D) calculations of injectable dosages; (E) calculations of intravenous fluids; and (F) pediatric drug calculations. Although the sections in Chapter 14 are condensed, many practice problems are provided.

This unit may be used by students in place of a separate drug calculation text. It may also serve as a review of drug calculation when preparing for state boards or for nurses returning to practice settings.

CHAPTER

14

Medications and Calculations

OVERVIEW

This chapter on medications and calculations is subdivided into six sections: (A) systems of measurement with conversion, (B) methods for calculation, (C) calculations of oral dosages, (D) calculations of injectable dosages, (E) calculations of intravenous (IV) fluids, and (F) pediatric drug calculations. The nurse may proceed independently through Sections A to F to practice and master calculation of drug dosages during the fundamental nursing or pharmacology course. This chapter also serves as a review of drug calculation for nurses in practice settings.

Numerous drug labels are used in the drug calculation problems to familiarize the nurse with important information on a drug label. This information is then used in correctly calculating the drug dose.

Six calculation methods are explained. Four are general methods: (1) basic formula, (2) ratio and proportion, (3) fractional equation, and (4) dimensional analysis. The nurse should select one of these general methods for the calculation of drug dosages. The other two methods are used to individualize drug dosing by body weight and body surface area. Each calculation method has a color-coded icon that identifies the method used in the chapters.

The drug calculation chart in Table 14A-3 may be used in the clinical setting. The nurse might find it helpful to review Chapter 13 on medication administration.

Keeping in mind that the goal is to prepare and administer medications in a safe and correct manner, the following recommendations are offered:

- Think. Focus on each step of the problem. This applies to simple and difficult problems.
- Read accurately. Pay particular attention to the location of the decimal point and to the operation to be done, such as conversion from one system of measurement to another.
- Picture the problem.
- Identify an expected range for the answer.
- Seek to understand the problem. Do not merely master the mechanics of how to do it. Ask for help when unsure of the calculation.

Section 14A: Systems of Measurement with Conversion

OBJECTIVES

- Discuss the two systems of measurement.
- Convert measurement within the metric system, larger units to smaller units, and smaller units to larger units.
- Convert measurements within the household system, larger units to smaller units, and smaller units to larger units.
- Convert metric, apothecary, and household measurements among the three systems of measurement as appropriate. See Table 14A-3.

OUTLINE

KEY TERMS

apothecary system, p. 150
gram, p. 149
household measurement, p. 149
liter, p. 149
meter, p. 149
metric system, p. 149
minim, p. 150
ounce, p. 149

Two systems of measurement—metric and household—are used to measure drugs and solutions. The metric system, developed in the late eighteenth century, is the internationally accepted system of measure. It is replacing the apothecary system, which dates back to the Middle Ages and had been used in England since the seventeenth century. Household measurement is commonly used in community and home settings in the United States.

METRIC SYSTEM

The **metric system** is a decimal system based on the power of 10. The basic units of measure are **gram** (g, gm, G, Gm) for weight; **liter** (l, L) for volume; and **meter** (m, M) for linear measurement, or length. Prefixes indicate the size of the units in multiples of 10. Table 14A-1 gives the metric units of measurement in weight (gram), volume (liter), and length (meter) in larger and smaller units that are commonly used.

Kilo is the prefix used for larger units (e.g., kilometer), and *milli, centi, micro,* and *nano* are the prefixes used for smaller units (e.g., millimeter). The prefix stands for a specific degree of magnitude; for instance, *kilo* stands for thousands, *milli* for one thousandth, *centi* for one hundredth, and so on. Because the difference between degrees of magnitude is always a multiple of 10, converting from one magnitude to another is relatively easy.

Conversion within the Metric System

The metric units most frequently used in drug notation are the following:

$$1\,g = 1000\,mg$$

$$1\,L = 1000\,mL$$

$$1\,mg = 1000\,mcg$$

To be able to convert a quantity, one of the values must be known, such as gram or milligrams, liters or milliliters, and milligrams or micrograms. Gram, liter, and meter are larger units; milligram, milliliter, and millimeter are smaller units.

Metric Conversion

A. When converting larger units to smaller units in the metric system, move the decimal point one space to the right for each degree of magnitude change.

Note: This does *not* apply to micro and nano units.

EXAMPLE

Change 1 gram to milligrams.

Grams are three degrees of magnitude greater than milligrams (see Table 14A-1). Move the decimal point three spaces to the right.

$$1\,g = 1.000\,mg \quad \text{or} \quad 1\,g = 1000\,mg$$

B. When converting smaller units to larger units in the metric system, move the decimal point one space to the left for each degree of magnitude of change.

EXAMPLE

Change 1000 milligrams to grams.

Milligrams are three degrees of magnitude smaller than grams. Move the decimal point three spaces to the left.

$$1000\,mg = 1.000.\,g \quad \text{or} \quad 1000\,mg = 1\,g$$

REMEMBER: When changing larger units to smaller units, move the decimal point to the right, and when changing smaller units to larger units, move the decimal point to the left.

TABLE 14A-1 METRIC UNITS OF MEASUREMENT

UNIT	NAMES AND ABBREVIATIONS	MEASUREMENTS
Gram (weight)	1 kilogram (kg, Kg)	1000 g
	1 gram (g, gm, G, Gm)	1 g
	1 milligram (mg)	0.001 g
	1 microgram (mcg)	0.000001 g
	1 nanogram (ng)	0.000000001 g
Liter (volume)	1 kiloliter (kl, KL)	1000 L (l)
	1 liter (L, l)	1 L (l)
	1 milliliter (mL)	0.001 L (l)
Meter (length)	1 kilometer (km)	1000 m
	1 meter (m, M)	1 m
	1 centimeter (cm)	0.01 m
	1 millimeter (mm)	0.001 m

NOTE: 1 mL (milliliter) = 1 cc (cubic centimeter). Values are the same in drug and fluid therapy. 1 mg (milligram) = 1000 mcg (micrograms).

PRACTICE PROBLEM 1

Metric Conversion

Larger to Smaller Units	Smaller to Larger Units
1. Change 2 g to mg	4. Change 1500 mg to g
2. Change 0.5 (½) g to mg	5. Change 3 g to kg
3. Change 2.5 L to mL	6. Change 500 mL to L

HOUSEHOLD SYSTEM

Household measurement is not as accurate as the metric system because of the lack of standardization of spoons, cups, and glasses. The measurements are approximate. A teaspoon (t) is considered to be equivalent to 5 mL according to the official United States Pharmacopeia. Milliliters (mL) are the same as cubic centimeters (cc) in value. Three teaspoons equals 1 tablespoon (T). **Ounces** (oz) are fluid ounces in the household measurement system; the word *fluid* in front of

SECTION 14A

TABLE 14A-2 HOUSEHOLD EQUIVALENTS IN FLUID VOLUME

1 MEASURING CUP	=	8 OUNCES (oz)
1 medium-size glass (tumbler size)	=	8 ounces (oz)
1 coffee cup (c)	=	6 ounces (oz) (varies with cup size)
1 ounce (oz)	=	2 tablespoons (T)
1 tablespoon (T)	=	3 teaspoons (t)
1 teaspoon (t)	=	60 drops (gtt)*
1 drop (gt)*	=	1 **minim** (min, or m)

*Varies with viscosity of liquid and dropper opening.

ounce is usually not used. One milliliter of water fills a cubic centimeter exactly.

Table 14A-2 gives the household equivalents in fluid volume. The measurements with asterisks are frequently used in drug therapy and should be remembered.

Household Conversion

A. When converting larger units to smaller units within the household system, multiply the requested number by the basic equivalent value.

EXAMPLE

Change 2 glasses of water to ounces.

The equivalent value is 1 medium-sized glass = 8 oz (fl oz)

2 glasses × 8 oz = 16 oz (fl oz)

With discharge teaching for a patient who requires liquid medication(s) at home, the nurse may find it necessary to convert metric measurements to household measurements.

PRACTICE PROBLEM 2

Household Conversion

REMEMBER: To change larger units to smaller units, multiply the requested number of units by the basic equivalent value. To change smaller units to larger units, divide the requested number of units by the basic equivalent value. Refer to Table 14A-2 as needed.

Larger to Smaller Units

1. Change 3 oz to T ______
2. Change 5 T to t ______
3. Change 3 coffee cups to oz ______

Smaller to Larger Units

4. Change 3 T to oz ______
5. Change 16 oz to a measuring cup ______
6. Change 12 t to T ______

METRIC, APOTHECARY, AND HOUSEHOLD EQUIVALENTS

Although the **apothecary system** is no longer used, Table 14A-3 is included to show metric and apothecary equivalents by weight, and metric, apothecary, and household equivalents by volume.

PRACTICE PROBLEM 3

Summary: Metric and Household Measurements

Metric System: Refer to Table 14A-1 as needed.

1. 2 g = ________ mg
2. 1.2 kg = ________ g
3. 5 mg = ________ mcg
4. 2.5 L = ________ mL
5. 500 mg = ________ g
6. 10,000 mcg = ________ mg
7. 2400 mg = ________ g
8. 1500 mL = ________ L

Household System: Refer to Table 14A-2 as needed.

1. 5 glasses = ______ oz
2. 3 T = ________ t
3. 2 c = ________ oz
4. 4 oz = ________ T
5. 15 t = ________ T
6. 5 T = ________ oz

ANSWERS TO PRACTICE PROBLEMS

1 METRIC CONVERSION

1. 2.0 g = 2.000 mg or 2.0 g = 2000 mg

   The gram is three degrees of magnitude greater than the milligram, so the decimal point is moved three spaces to the right.
2. 0.5 g = 0.500 mg or 0.5 g = 500 mg

   The gram is three degrees of magnitude greater than the milligram, so the decimal point is moved three spaces to the right.
3. 2.5 L = 2.500 mL or 2.5 L = 2500 mL

   The liter is three degrees of magnitude greater than the milliliter, so the decimal point is moved three spaces to the right.
4. 1500 mg = 1.500. g or 1500 mg = 1.5 g

   The milligram is three degrees of magnitude smaller (less) than the gram, so the decimal point is moved three spaces to the left.
5. 3 g = 003. kg or 3 g = .003 mg

   The gram is three degrees of magnitude smaller than the kilogram, so the decimal point is moved three spaces to the left.
6. 500 mL = 500. L or 500 mL = 0.5 L

   The milliliter is three degrees of magnitude smaller than the liter, so the decimal point is moved three spaces to the left.

2 HOUSEHOLD CONVERSION

1. 3 oz = 6 T;

   the equivalent value is 3 oz × 2 = 6 T
2. 5 T = 15 t;

   the equivalent value is 1 T = 3 t
3. 3 c = 18 oz;

   the equivalent value is 1 c = 6 oz
4. 3 T = 1½ oz;

   the equivalent value is 3 T ÷ 2 or 1½ oz
5. 16 oz = 2 c;

   the equivalent value is 1 measuring cup = 8 oz
6. 12 t = 4 T;

   the equivalent value is 1 T = 3 t

TABLE 14A-3 APPROXIMATE METRIC, APOTHECARY, AND HOUSEHOLD EQUIVALENTS

	METRIC SYSTEM		APOTHECARY SYSTEM	HOUSEHOLD SYSTEM
Weight	1 kg	1000 g	2.2 lb	2.2 lb
	*1 g	1000 mg	15 (16) gr	
	0.5 g	500 mg	7½ gr	
	0.3 g	300 (325) mg	5 gr	
	0.1 g	100 mg	1½ gr	
	*0.06 g	60 (65) mg	1 gr	
	0.03 g	30 (32) mg	½ gr	
	0.01 g	10 mg	⅙ gr	
		0.6 mg	1/100 gr	
		0.4 mg	1/150 gr	
		0.3 mg	1/200 gr	
Volume	1 L; 1000 mL		1 qt; 32 oz (fl oz)	
	0.5 L; 500 mL		1 pt; 16 oz (fl oz)	
	0.24 L; 240 mL		8 fl oz	1 glass
	0.18 L; 180 mL		6 fl oz	1 c
	*30 mL		1 fl oz; 8 fl dr	2 T; 6 t
	15 mL		½ fl oz; 4 fl dr	1 T; 3 t
	†5 mL			1 t
	4 mL		1 fl oz; 60 ♏ (min)	1 t
	1 mL		15 (16) ♏	15-16 gtt
Height/distance	2.54 cm		1 in	1 in
	25.4 mm		1 in	1 in

*Equivalents commonly used for computing conversion problems by ratio.
†5 mL = 1 t (teaspoon); official United States Pharmacopeia measurement.
fl dr, Fluid dram; *fl oz*, fluid ounce; ♏ minim; *cm*, centimeter; *g*, gram; *gr*, grain; *gtt*, drops, *in*, inch; *kg*, kilogram; *L*, liter; *lb*, pound; *mg*, milligram; *mL*, milliliter; *mm*, millimeter; *pt*, pint; *qt*, quart; *T*, tablespoon; *t*, teaspoon; *c*, coffee cup.

3 SUMMARY: METRIC AND HOUSEHOLD MEASUREMENTS

Metric Conversion

1. 2000 mg (1 g = 1000 mg)
   2 × 1000 mg = 2000 mg
   or 2.000 mg
   (three spaces to the right)
2. 1200 g
3. 5000 mcg (1 mg = 1000 mcg)
4. 2500 mL
5. 0.5 g (1000 mg = 1 g)
   500 ÷ 1000 = 0.5
   or 500. g = 0.5 g
   (three spaces to the left)
6. 10 mg
7. 2.4 g
8. 1.5 L

Household Conversion

1. 40 oz
2. 9 t
3. 12 oz
4. 8 T
5. 5 T
6. 2½ oz

Section 14B: Methods for Calculation

OBJECTIVES

- Select a formula—the basic formula, the ratio-and-proportion method, fractional equation, or dimensional analysis—for calculating drug dosages.
- Convert all measures to the same system and same unit of measure within the system before calculating drug dosage.
- Calculate drug dosage using one of the general formulas.
- Calculate drug dosage according to body weight and body surface area.
- Discuss meanings for abbreviations used in drug therapy.

OUTLINE

Interpreting Oral and Injectable Drug Labels
- Method 1: Basic Formula (BF)
- Method 2: Ratio and Proportion (RP)
- Method 3: Fractional Equation (FE)
- Method 4: Dimensional Analysis (DA)
- Method 5: Body Weight (BW)
- Method 6: Body Surface Area (BSA)
- BSA with the Square Root

KEY TERMS

basic formula, p. 153
body surface area (BSA), p. 157
body weight (BW), p. 156
dimensional analysis (DA), p. 155
drug label, p. 152
fractional equation, p. 154
ratio and proportion, p. 153

The four general methods for the calculation of drug doses are (1) basic formula, (2) ratio and proportion, (3) fractional equation, (4) and dimensional analysis. These methods are used to calculate oral and injectable drug doses. The nurse should select one of the methods to calculate drug doses and use that method consistently.

For drugs that require individualized dosing, calculation by body weight (BW) or by body surface area (BSA) may be necessary. In the past, these two methods, (5) and (6), have been used for the calculation of pediatric dosages and for drugs used in the treatment of cancer (antineoplastic drugs). BW and BSA methods of calculation are especially useful for individuals whose BW is low, who are obese, or who are older adults.

Before calculating drug doses, all units of measure must be converted to a single system (see Section 14A). It is most helpful to convert to the system used on the **drug label**. If the drug is ordered in grams (g, G) and the drug label gives the dose in milligrams (mg), then convert grams to milligrams (the measurement on the drug label) and proceed with the drug calculation. Nursing programs prefer to use only the metric system for drug calculations.

INTERPRETING ORAL AND INJECTABLE DRUG LABELS

Pharmaceutic companies usually label their drugs with the brand name of the drug in large letters and the generic name in smaller letters. The dose per tablet, capsule, or liquid (for oral and injectable doses) is printed on the drug label. Two examples of drug labels are given below, the first for an oral drug and the second for an injectable drug.

EXAMPLE 1 Oral Drug

Tagamet is the brand (trade) name, cimetidine is the generic name, and the dose is 200 mg/tablet.

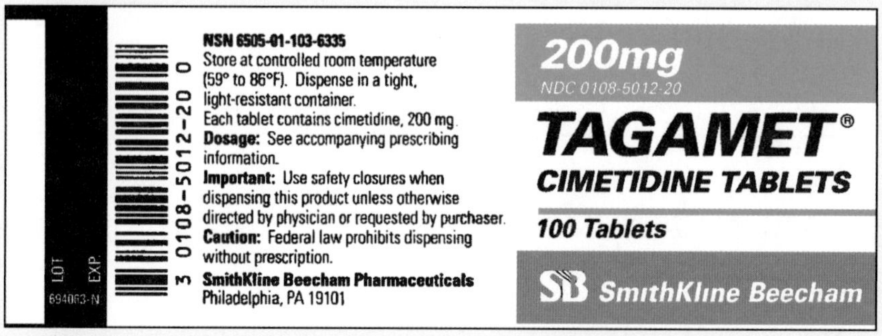

EXAMPLE 2 Injectable Drug

Compazine is the brand (trade) name, prochlorperazine is the generic name, and the dose is 5 mg/mL injectable.

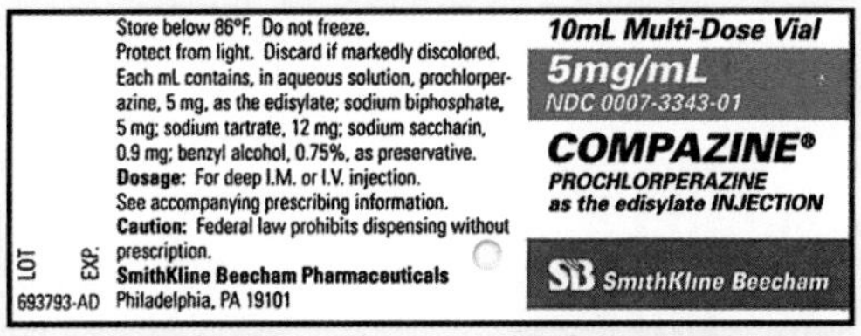

METHOD 1: BASIC FORMULA (BF)

The **basic formula** is easy to recall and is most frequently used in calculating drug dosages. The basic formula is the following:

$$\frac{D}{H} \times V = A$$

where D is the desired dose (i.e., drug dose ordered by the health care provider),

H is the on-hand dose (i.e., drug dose on label of container [bottle, vial]),

V is the vehicle (i.e., drug form in which the drug comes [tablet, capsule, liquid]), and

A is the amount calculated to be given to the patient.

Examples

1. Order: cefaclor (Ceclor) 0.5 g PO b.i.d.

   Available:

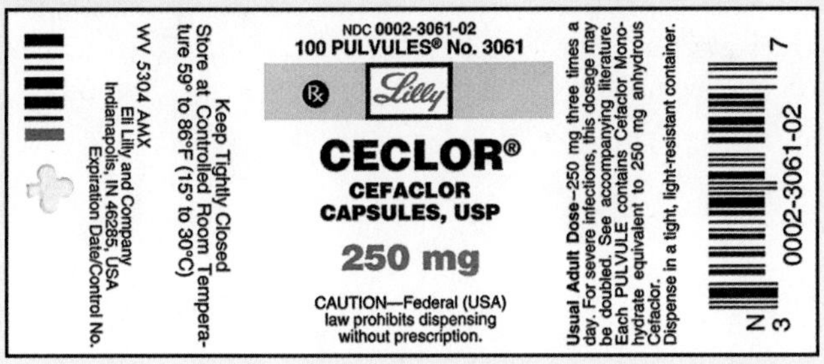

   a. The unit of measure that is ordered (grams) and the unit on the bottle (milligrams) are from the same system of measurement—the metric system. Conversion to the same unit is necessary to work the problem. Because the bottle is in milligrams, convert grams to milligrams.

To convert grams (large value) to milligrams (smaller value), move the decimal point three spaces to the right (see Section 14A: Systems of Measurement with Conversion).

$$0.5\text{ g} = 0.500\text{ mg or } 500\text{ mg}$$

   b. $\frac{D}{H} \times V = \frac{500}{250} \times 1\text{ capsule} = \frac{500}{250} = 2\text{ capsules}$

2. Order: codeine 60 mg PO STAT

   Available:

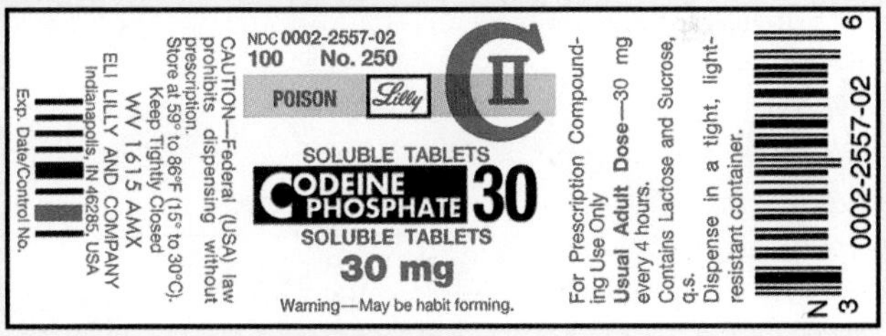

   a. $\frac{D}{H} \times V = \frac{60}{30} \times 1\text{ tablet} = \frac{60}{30} = 2\text{ tablets}$

METHOD 2: RATIO AND PROPORTION (RP)

The **ratio and proportion** method is the oldest method currently used in the calculation of drug dosages. The formula is as follows:

$$\overset{\text{Known}}{H : V} :: \overset{\text{Desired}}{D : x}$$

(means: V and D; extremes: H and x)

$x =$

where *H* is the drug on hand (available),

V is the vehicle or drug form (tablet, capsule, liquid),

D is the desired dose (as ordered),

x is the unknown amount to give,

and :: stands for "as" or "equal to."

Multiply the means and the extremes. Solve for *x*; *x* is the divisor.

Continued

Examples

1. Order: amoxicillin (Amoxil) 100 mg PO q.i.d.

   Available:

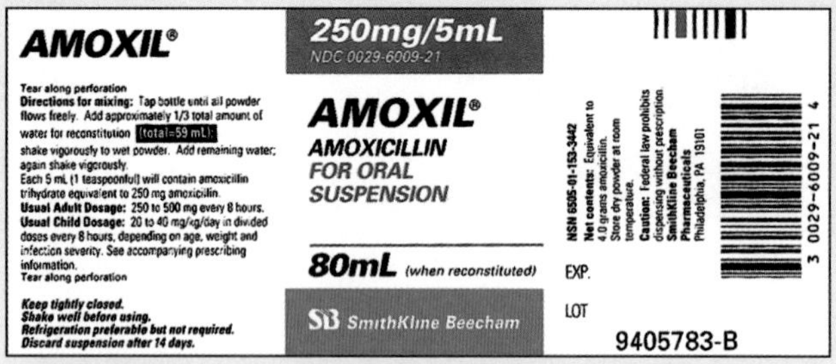

   a. Conversion is not needed because both are expressed in the same unit of measure.

   b.
$$\begin{array}{ccccccc} H & : & V & :: & D & : & x \\ 250\text{ mg} & : & 5\text{ ml} & :: & 100\text{ mg} & : & x\text{ mL} \end{array}$$

   means (5 ml × 100 mg); extremes (250 mg × x mL)

$$250x = 500$$
$$x = 2\text{ mL}$$

Answer: amoxicillin 100 mg = 2 mL

2. Order: aspirin/ASA 600 (650) mg q4h PRN

   Available: aspirin 325 mg/tablet

$$\begin{array}{ccccccc} H & : & V & :: & D & : & x \\ 325\text{ mg} & : & 1\text{ tab} & :: & 600\ (650)\text{ mg} & : & x \end{array}$$

$$325x = 600\ (650)$$
$$x = 1.8 \text{ tablets or 2 tablets}$$

(round off or use 650 instead of 600)

Answer: aspirin 650 mg = 2 tablets

METHOD 3: FRACTIONAL EQUATION (FE)

The **fractional equation** method is similar to ratio and proportion except it is written as a fraction.

$$\frac{H}{V} = \frac{D}{X} \qquad \frac{H \text{ dosage on hand}}{V \quad \text{Vehicle}} = \frac{D \text{ desired dosage}}{X \quad \text{unknown}}$$

Cross-multiply and solve for *x*.

Examples

Order: ciprofloxacin (Cipro) 500 mg PO q12h

Available:

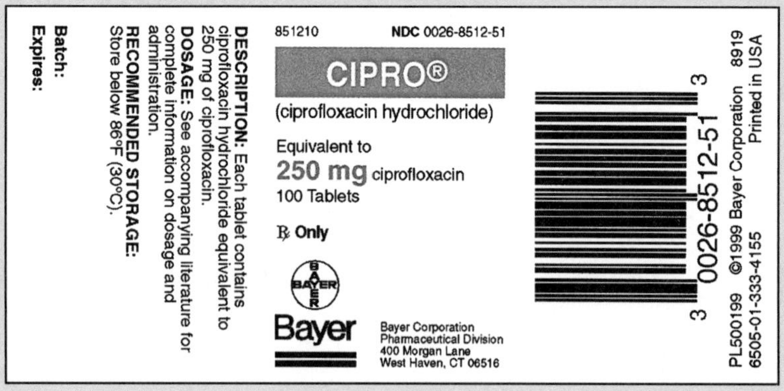

How many tablet(s) should the patient receive per dose?

Answer:

$$\frac{H}{V} = \frac{D}{X} \quad \frac{250\text{ mg}}{1\text{ tab}} = \frac{500\text{ mg}}{X\text{ tab}}$$

Cross-multiply and solve for x.

$250x = 500$

$x = 2$ tablets of Cipro per dose

METHOD 4: DIMENSIONAL ANALYSIS (DA)

Dimensional analysis (DA) is a calculation method known as units and conversions. The advantage of DA is that it decreases the number of steps required to calculate a drug dosage. It is set up as one equation.

Examples

1. Identify the unit/form (tablet, capsule, mL) of the drug to be calculated. If the drug comes in tablet, then tablet = (equal sign).
2. The known dose and unit/form from the drug label follows the equal sign.

   Order: amoxicillin 500 mg
   On the drug label: 250 mg per capsule

$$\text{capsule} = \frac{1\,\text{cap}}{250\,\text{mg}}$$

3. The mg (250 mg) is the denominator, and it must match the next numerator, which is 500 mg (desired dose or order). The NEXT denominator would be 1 (one) or blank.

$$\text{capsule} = \frac{1\,\text{cap} \times \overset{2}{\cancel{500}}\,\cancel{\text{mg}}}{\underset{1}{\cancel{250}}\,\cancel{\text{mg}} \times 1} =$$

4. Cancel out the mg, 250 and 500. What remains is the capsule and 2.

   Answer: 2 capsules When conversion is needed between milligrams (drug label) and grams (order), then a conversion factor is needed, which appears between the drug dose on hand (drug label) and the desired dose (order).

Metric Equivalent

$$1\,\text{g} = 1000\,\text{mg}$$

$$1\,\text{mg} = 1000\,\text{mcg}$$

Examples

Order: amoxicillin 0.5 g, PO, q8h

Available: 250 mg = 1 capsule (drug label). A conversion is needed between g and mg. Remember that 250 mg is the denominator; therefore 1000 mg (conversion factor, which is 1000 mg = 1 g) is the NEXT numerator, and 1 g becomes the NEXT denominator. The third numerator is 0.5 g, and the denominator is 1 (one) or blank.

$$\text{cap} = \frac{1\,\text{cap} \quad \times 1000\,\cancel{\text{mg}} \times 0.5\,\text{g}}{250\,\cancel{\text{mg}} \quad \times 1\,\text{g} \qquad \times 1} = \frac{500}{250} = 2 \text{ caps of amoxicillin}$$

If conversion from grams to milligrams is not needed, the middle step can be omitted.

The following are formulas for dimensional analysis (DA):

$$\text{V (form of drug)} = \frac{\text{V (drug form)} \quad \times \text{D (desired dose)}}{\underset{\text{(Drug label)}}{\text{H (on hand)}} \times \underset{\text{(Drug label)}}{\text{1 or blank}}}$$

$$\text{For conversion: v (form of drug)} = \frac{\text{V (drug form)} \quad \times \text{C (H)} \qquad \times \text{D (desired dose)}}{\underset{\text{(Drug label)}}{\text{H (on hand)}} \times \underset{\text{(Conversion factor)}}{\text{C (D)}} \times \underset{\text{(Drug order)}}{\text{1 or blank}}}$$

As with other methods for calculation, the three components are D, H, and V. With dimensional analysis, the conversion factor is built into the equation and is included when the units of measurement of the drug order and the drug container differ. If the two are of the same units of measurement, the conversion factor is eliminated from the equation.

Examples

Order: acetaminophen (Tylenol) 1 g, PO, PRN

Available:

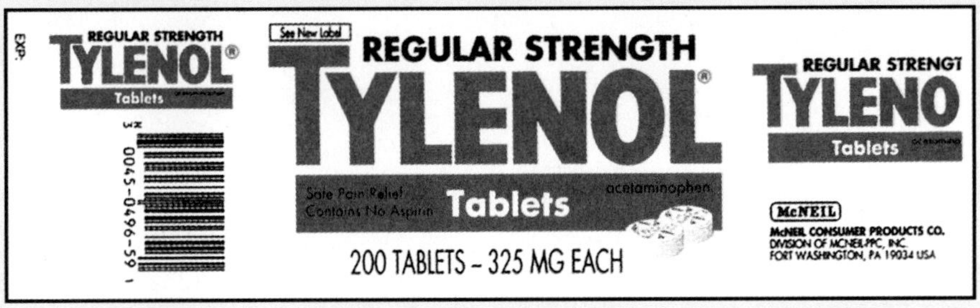

Factors: 325 mg = 1 tablet (from drug label)
1 g/1 (from drug order)
Conversion factor: 1000 mg = 1 g(G)
How many tablet(s) should be given? _____

$$\text{tab} = \frac{1\,\text{tab} \quad \times 1000\,\cancel{\text{mg}} \times \cancel{1}\,\text{g}}{325\,\cancel{\text{mg}} \times \cancel{1}\,\text{g} \qquad \times 1} = \frac{1000}{325} = 3.07 \text{ tab or } 3 \text{ tab}$$

METHOD 5: BODY WEIGHT (BW)

The **body weight** (BW) method of calculation allows for the individualization of the drug dose and involves the following three steps:

1. Convert pounds to kilograms if necessary (lb ÷ 2.2 = kg).
2. Determine drug dose per BW by multiplying as follows:

$$\text{Drug dose} \times \text{body weight} = \text{patient's dose per day}$$

3. Follow the basic formula, ratio and proportion, fractional equation, or dimensional analysis method to calculate the drug dosage.

Examples

1. Order: fluorouracil (5-FU), 12 mg/kg/day IV, not to exceed 800 mg/day. The adult weighs 132 lb.
   a. Convert pounds to kilograms by dividing the number of pounds by 2.2 (1 kg = 2.2 lb).

      $132 \div 2.2 = 60\,\text{kg}$

   b. mg × kg = patient's dose

      $12 \times 60 = 720\,\text{mg IV/day}$

   Answer: Fluorouracil 12 mg/kg/day = 720 mg

2. Order: cefaclor (Ceclor) 20 mg/kg/day in three divided doses. The patient weighs 31 lb.

   Available:

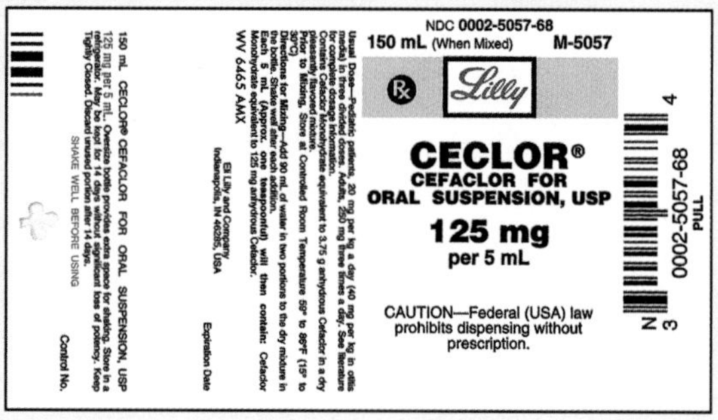

   a. Convert pounds to kilograms.

      $31 \div 2.2 = 14\,\text{kg}$

   b. 20 mg × 14 g = 280 mg/day

      $280\,\text{mg} \div 3\,\text{divided doses} = 93\,\text{mg/dose}$

   c. $\text{BF: } \frac{D}{H} \times V = \frac{93}{125} \times 5 = \frac{463}{125} = 3.7\,\text{mL}$

      or

      $\text{DA: ml} = \frac{5\,\text{mL} \times 93\,\text{mg}}{125\,\text{mg} \times 1} = \frac{465}{125} = 3.7\,\text{mL}$

      or

      $\text{RP: } H : V :: D : x$

      $125\,\text{mg} : 5\,\text{mL} :: 93\,\text{mg} : x\,\text{mL}$

      $125x = 465$

      $x = \frac{465}{125} = 3.7\,\text{mL}$

      or

      $\text{FE: } \frac{H}{V} = \frac{D}{x} \quad \frac{125}{5} = \frac{93}{x} =$

      cross-multiply $125x = 465$

      $x = 3.7\,\text{mL}$

Answer: cefaclor 20 mg/kg/day = 3.7 mL per dose

SECTION 14B

METHOD 6: BODY SURFACE AREA (BSA)

The **body surface area** (BSA) method is considered the most accurate way to calculate the drug dose for infants, children, older adults, and patients who are on antineoplastic agents or whose BW is low. The BSA, in square meters (m^2), is determined by where the person's height and weight intersect the nomogram scale (Figures 14B-1 [children] and 14B-2 [adults]). To calculate the drug dosage using the BSA method, multiply the drug dose ordered by the number of square meters.

$$100\,\text{mg} \times 1.8\,\text{m}^2\ (\text{BSA}) = 180\,\text{mg/day}$$

Examples

1. Order: cyclophosphamide (Cytoxan) 100 mg/m²/day, IV

   Available:

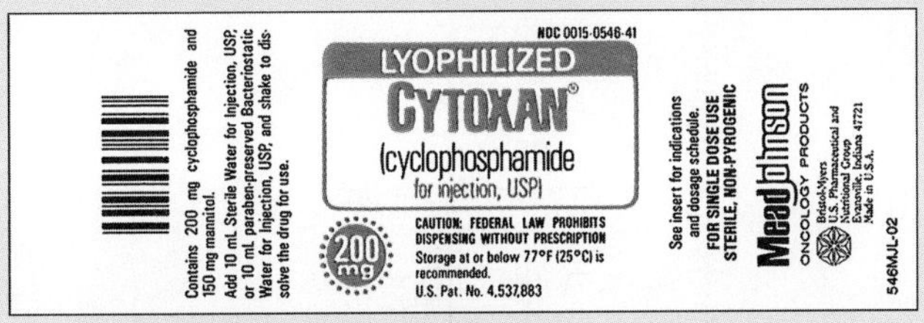

   Patient is 70 inches tall and weighs 160 lb.

   a. 70 inches and 160 lb intersect the nomogram scale at 1.97 m² (BSA)

   b. 100 mg × 1.97 = 197 mg.

Answer: Administer cyclophosphamide 197 mg or 200 mg/day.

2. Order: mephenytoin (Mesantoin) 200 mg/m² PO in three divided doses. Patient is 42 inches tall and weighs 44 lb.

   a. 42 inches and 44 lb intersect the nomogram scale at 0.8 m².

   b. 200 mg × 0.8 = 160 mg/day or 50 mg (53) t.i.d.

Answer: Administer mephenytoin 50 mg t.i.d.

BSA with the Square Root

BSA can be calculated by using the square root and a fractional formula of height and weight divided by a constant. Now that calculators are readily available, research has shown that this method results in fewer errors than drawing intersecting lines on a nomogram. The formula for BSA using the square root is as follows:

$$\text{BSA} = \sqrt{\frac{\text{height (inches)} \times \text{wt (lb)}}{3131\,(\text{constant})}}$$

Examples

Order: melphalan (Alkeran) 16 mg/m² q2wk. Patient is 68 inches tall and weighs 172 lb.

a. Use the BSA inches and pounds formula.

$$\text{BSA} = \sqrt{\frac{68\,\text{in} \times 172\,\text{lb}}{3131}}$$

$$\text{BSA} = \sqrt{\frac{11696}{3131}}$$

$$\text{BSA} = \sqrt{3.73}$$

$$\text{BSA} = 1.9\,\text{m}^2$$

b. 16 mg × 1.9 m² = 30.4 mg/m² or 30 mg/m². Patient should receive 30 mg every 2 weeks.

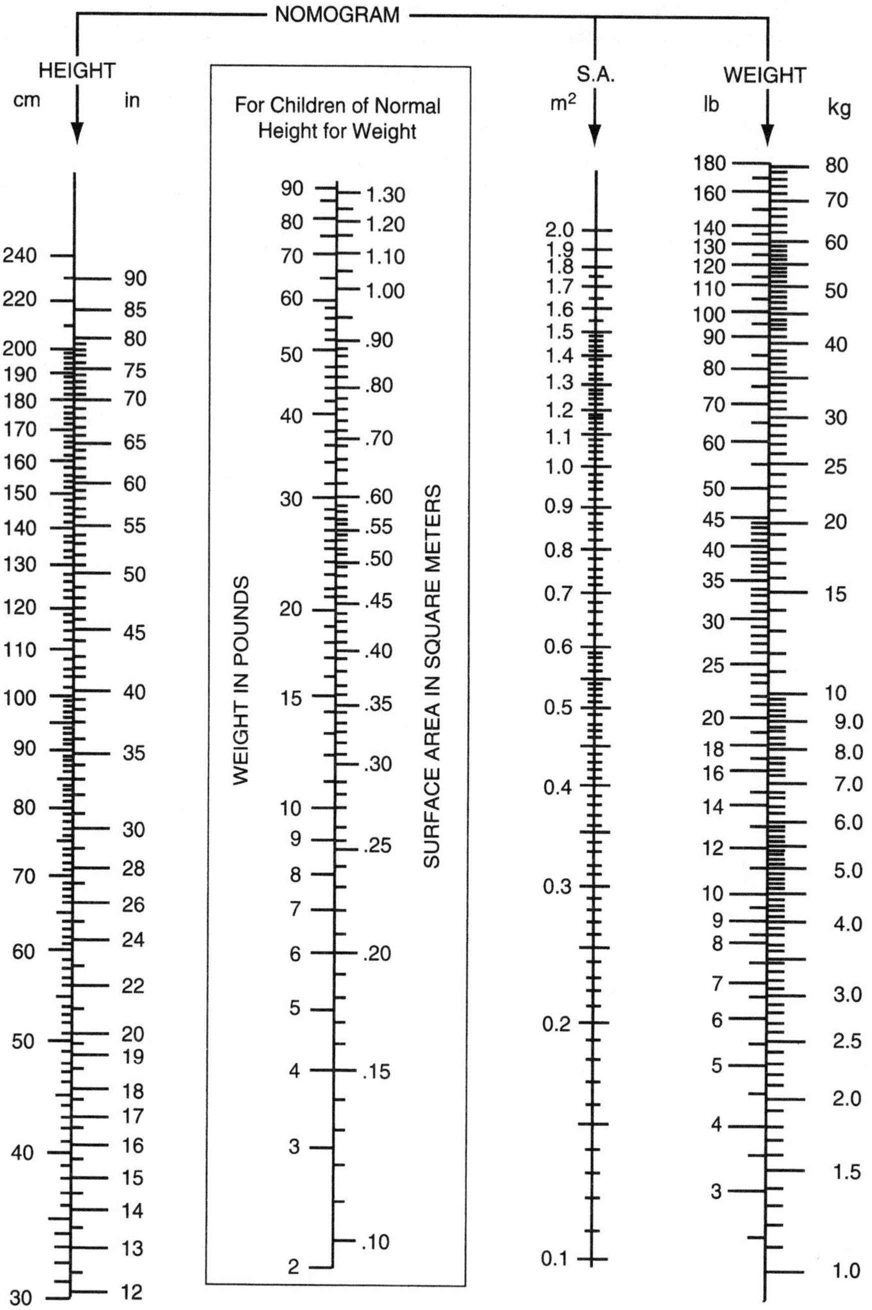

FIGURE 14B–1 West nomogram for infants and children. Directions: (1) Find height. (2) Find weight. (3) Draw a straight line that connects the height and weight. (4) Where the line intersects on the surface area column is the body surface area (m^2). (Modified from data by Boyd E, West CD. In Behrman RE, Kliegman RM, Jensen HB: *Nelson textbook of pediatrics,* ed. 18, Philadelphia, 2007, Saunders.)

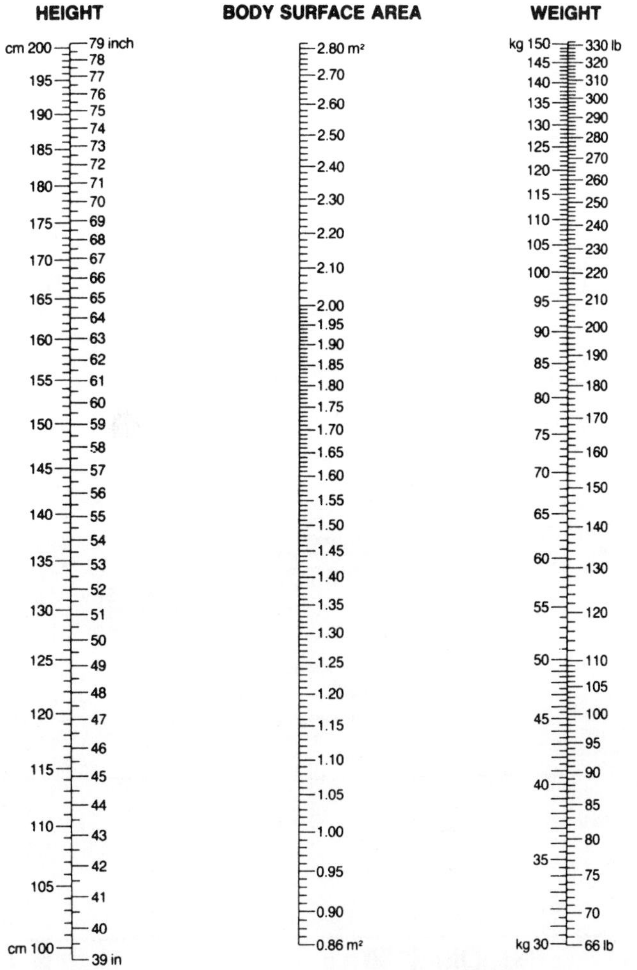

FIGURE 14B–2 Nomogram of body surface area for adults. Directions: (1) Find height. (2) Find weight. (3) Draw a straight line that connects the height and weight. (4) Where the line intersects on the body surface area column is the body surface area (m^2). (From Deglin JH, Vallerand AH, Russin A: *Davis's drug guide for nurses,* ed. 2, Philadelphia, 1991, FA Davis; Lentner C (ed). *Geigy scientific tables,* ed. 8, vol. 1, Basel, Switzerland, 1981, Ciba-Geigy, pp. 226-227. In RE Behrman, RM Kliegman, HB Jensen: *Nelson textbook of pediatrics,* ed. 18, Philadelphia, 2007, Saunders.)

PRACTICE PROBLEM 1

Drug Dosage Using Basic Formula, Ratio and Proportion, or Fractional Equation

Solve the problem and determine the drug dose given the following:

1. Order: cimetidine (Tagamet) 0.4 g PO, q6h

   Available:

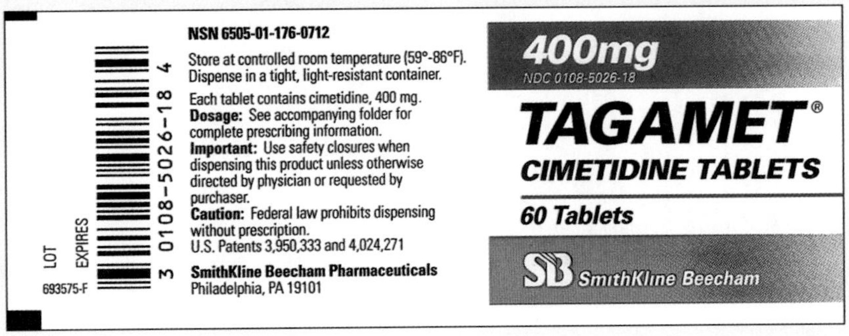

How many tablet(s) of Tagamet should the patient receive? _______

Continued

2. Order: doxycycline hyclate (Vibra-Tab), PO, initially 200 mg; then 50 mg PO, b.i.d.

   Available (scored tablets):

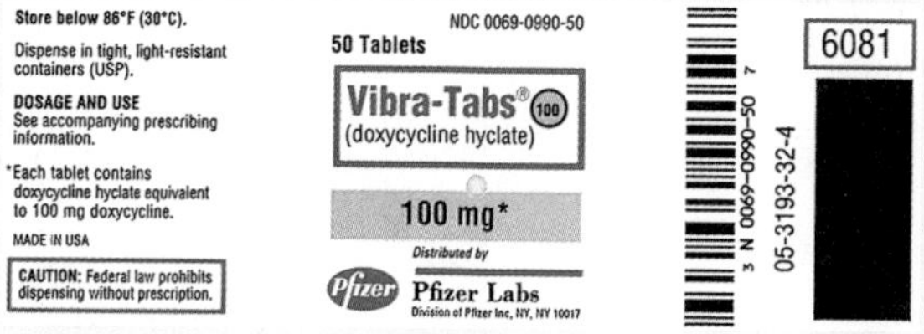

   a. How many scored tablets would you give as the initial dose? ______

   b. How many scored tablets would you give for each dose after the initial dose? ______

3. Order: azithromycin (Zithromax) 250 mg, PO, daily

   Available:

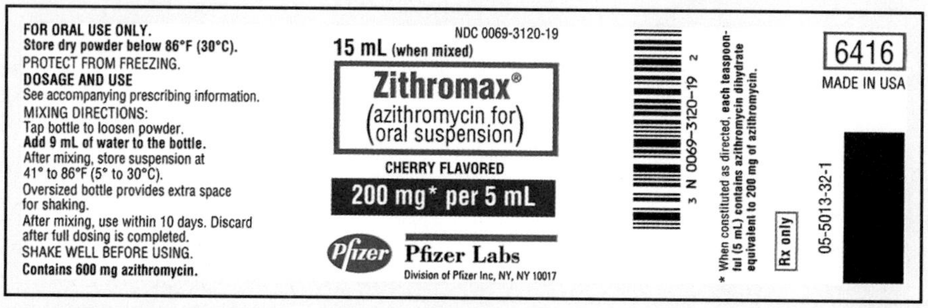

   How many milliliters should the patient receive per day? ______

4. Order: hydrochlorothiazide (HydroDIURIL) 25 mg PO, daily

   Available (scored tablets):

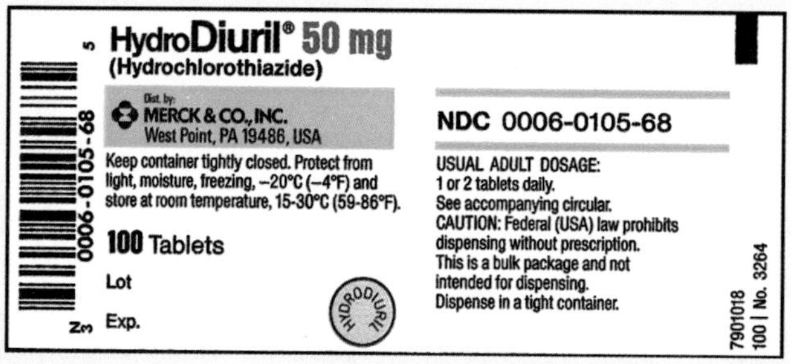

   How many scored tablets should the patient receive? ______

5. Order: cefadroxil (Duricef) 500 mg PO, b.i.d.

   Available:

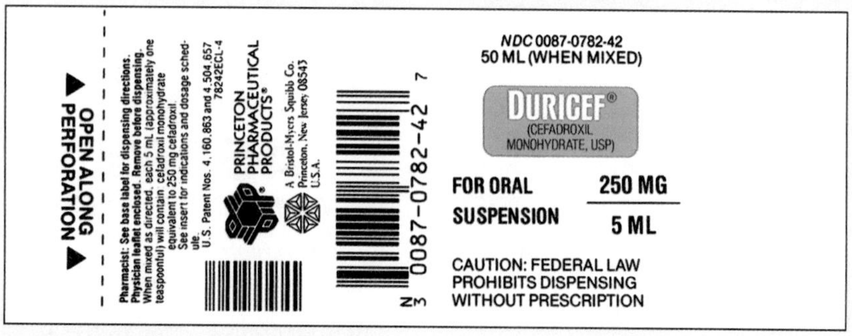

   How many milliliters should the patient receive? ______

SECTION 14B

6. Order: dicloxacillin 100 mg PO, q8h

   Available dicloxacillin 62.5 mg/5mL:

   How many milliliters should the patient receive? ______

7. Order: meperidine (Demerol) 35 mg IM STAT

   Available:

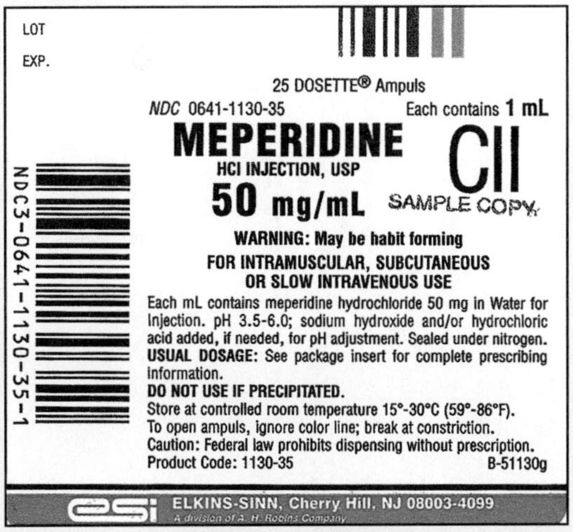

   How many milliliters should the patient receive? ______

8. Order: atropine sulfate 0.4 mg, SC on call

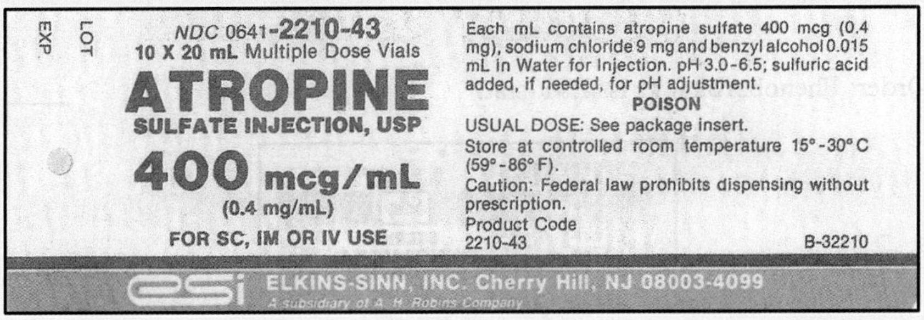

   Available:

   a. How many milliliters should the patient receive? ______

PRACTICE PROBLEM 2

Drug Dosage Using Dimensional Analysis

9. Order: erythromycin (ERY-TAB) 0.5 g, PO, q8h

   Available:

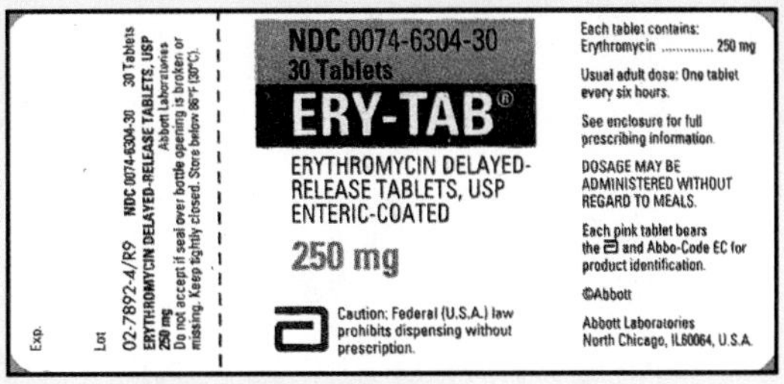

   Conversion factor: 1 g = 1000 mg

   a. How many milligrams (mg) should the patient receive per dose? ____________

   b. How many milligrams should the patient receive per day? ____________

   c. How many tablet(s) should the patient receive per dose? ____________

Continued

SECTION 14B

10. Order: loracarbef (Lorabid) oral suspension, 0.4 g, PO, q12h for 10 days

Available:

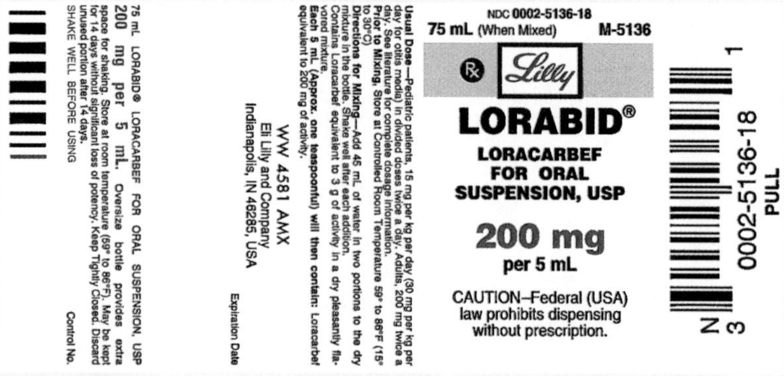

a. Factors: 200 mg = 5 mL (from drug label)

b. Conversion factor: 1000 mg = 1 g

c. How many milliliters should the patient receive? ____________

11. Order: ciprofloxacin (Cipro) 0.5 g PO, b.i.d.

Available:

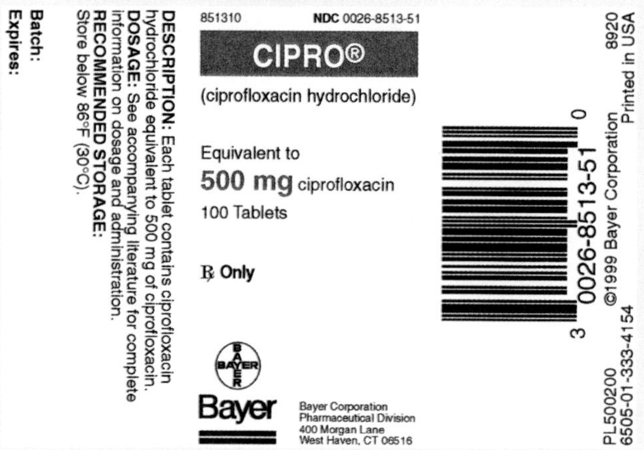

a. How many tablets should the patient receive per dose? ____________

PRACTICE PROBLEM 3

Drug Dosage Using Body Weight

12. Order: sulfisoxazole (Gantrisin) 50 mg/kg/day PO in four divided doses (q6h). Patient weighs 44 lb. How many mg should the patient receive per day? ______ Per dose? ______

13. Order: albuterol (Proventil) 0.1 mg/kg/day PO in four divided doses. Patient weighs 86 lb.

14. Order: cefprozil (Cefzil) 15 mg/kg/day PO in two divided doses. Patient weighs 33 lb.

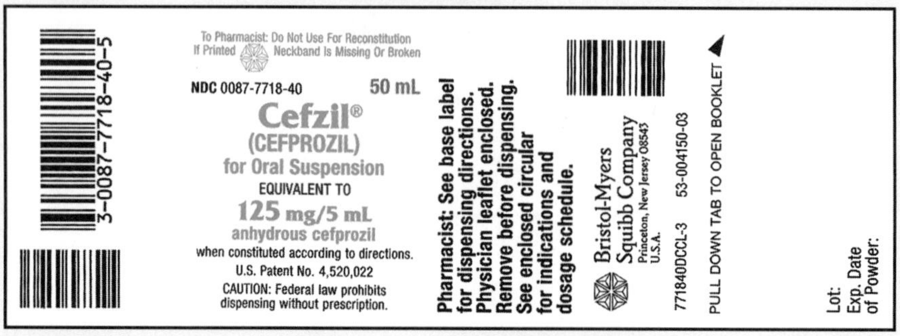

a. How many milligrams should be given per day? ______

b. How many milliliters should the patient receive per dose? ______

SECTION 14B

PRACTICE PROBLEM 4

Drug Dosage Using Body Surface Area

15. Patient is 62 inches tall and weighs 130 lb. What is the BSA? _____
16. Order: bleomycin sulfate 20 units/m^2 IV. Patient is 70 inches tall and weighs 160 lb.
    How many units should the patient receive?
17. Order: sulfisoxazole (Gantrisin) 2 g/m^2 in four divided doses. Patient is 50 inches tall and weighs 60 lb.
    Available: sulfisoxazole 500 mg/5 ml
    a. What is the BSA? _____
    b. How many gram(s) should the child receive per day? _____
    c. How many milliliters should the child receive per dose? _____

ANSWERS TO PRACTICE PROBLEMS

1 DRUG DOSAGE USING BASIC FORMULA, RATIO AND PROPORTION, OR FRACTIONAL EQUATION

1. a. Convert grams to milligrams by moving the decimal point three spaces to the right.

$$0.4\,g = 0.400\,mg$$

b. $BF: \frac{D}{H} \times V = \frac{400\,mg}{400\,mg} \times 1\,\text{tablet} = 1\,\text{tablet}$

2. a. Initially:

$$BF: \frac{D}{H} \times V = \frac{\overset{2}{\cancel{200}}}{\underset{1}{\cancel{100}}} \times 1 = 2\,\text{tablets}$$

or

$$\begin{aligned} &RP{:}H \;:\; V \;::\; D \;:\; x \\ &100\,mg \;:\; 1\,tab \;::\; 200\,mg \;:\; x \\ &100x = 200 \\ &x = 2\,\text{tablets} \end{aligned}$$

or

FE (cross-multiply):

$$\frac{100}{1} = \frac{200}{x} =$$

$$100x = 200$$

$$x = 2\,\text{tablets}$$

or

DA: No conversion factor

$$\text{Tablet(s)} = \frac{1 \times \overset{2}{\cancel{200}}}{\underset{1}{\cancel{100}} \times 1} = 2\,\text{tablets}$$

b. Daily:

$$\begin{aligned} &RP{:}H \;:\; V \;::\; D \;:\; x \\ &100\,mg \;:\; 1\,tab \;::\; 50\,mg \;:\; x \\ &100x = 50 \\ &x = \tfrac{1}{2}\,\text{tablet} \end{aligned}$$

DA: No conversion factor

$$\text{Tablet(s)} = \frac{1\,tab \times \overset{1}{\cancel{50\,mg}}}{\underset{2}{\cancel{100\,mg}} \times 1} = \tfrac{1}{2}\,\text{tablet}$$

3. a. $BF: \frac{D}{H} \times V = \frac{\overset{5}{\cancel{250\,mg}}}{\underset{4}{\cancel{200\,mg}}} \times 5\,mL =$

$$\frac{25}{4} = 6.25\,mL \text{ or } 6\,mL$$

4. ½ tablet
5. 10 mL
6. $FE: \frac{H}{V} = \frac{D}{x} \quad \frac{62.5\,mg}{5\,mL} = \frac{100\,mg}{x\,mL}$

   (cross-multiply $62.5x = 500$)

   $x = 8\,mL$
7. 0.7 mL
8. a. 400 mcg/ml = 0.4 mg/ml

$$\frac{D}{H} \times V = \frac{0.4\,mg}{0.4\,mg} \times 1 = 1\,mL \text{ of atropine}$$

SECTION 14B

2 DRUG DOSAGE USING DIMENSIONAL ANALYSIS

9. a. 0.5 = 500 mg (move the decimal point 3 spaces to the right for milligrams)

   answer: 500 mg

   b. q 8h = 3 times a day; 500 mg × 3 = 1500 mg per day (0.5 g × 3 = 1.5 g per day)

   c. DA: $\text{tab} = \dfrac{1\,\text{tab} \quad \times 1000\,\text{mg} \times 0.5\,\text{g}}{250\,\text{mg} \times 1 \quad\quad \times 1} = \dfrac{500}{250} = 2$ tablets of ERY-TAB

10. $\text{mL} = \dfrac{5\,\text{mL} \quad \times \overset{5}{\cancel{1000}}\,\cancel{\text{mg}} \times 0.4\,\cancel{\text{g}}}{\underset{1}{\cancel{200}}\,\cancel{\text{mg}} \times 1\,\cancel{\text{g}} \quad\quad \times 1} = 10\,\text{mL}$

11. $\text{tab} = \dfrac{1\,\text{tab} \quad \times \overset{2}{\cancel{1000}}\,\cancel{\text{mg}} \times 0.5\,\cancel{\text{g}}}{\underset{1}{\cancel{500}}\,\cancel{\text{mg}} \times 1\,\cancel{\text{g}} \quad\quad \times 1} = 1\,\text{tablet}$

3 DRUG DOSAGE USING BODY WEIGHT

12. a. 44 lb ÷ 2.2 kg = 20 kg

    b. 50 mg × 20 kg = 1000 mg/day

    1000 ÷ 4 times a day = 250 mg q.i.d. or q6h

13. a. 86 ÷ 2.2 = 39 kg

    b. 0.1 mg × 39 = 3.9 mg, or 4 mg (round to the whole number)

    4 ÷ 4 = 1 mg q6h

14. 33 ÷ 2.2 = 15 kg

    15 mg × 15 = 225 mg/day

    225 ÷ 2 times a day = 112.5 mg, q12h per dose

    $\dfrac{D}{H} \times V = \times \dfrac{112.5}{125} \times 5\,\text{mL} = \dfrac{562.5}{125} = 4.5\,\text{mL q12h}$

    a. Administer cefprozil 225 mg/day

    b. Administer 112.5 mg = 4.5 mL, q12h

4 DRUG DOSAGE USING BODY SURFACE AREA

15. 1.65 m^2

16. a. Patient's height and weight intersect the nomogram scale at 1.97 m^2.

    b. 20 Unit × 1.97 = 39.4, or 39 Unit (round to the whole number)

17. a. Height and weight intersect the nomogram scale at 0.98 m^2.

    b. 2 g × 0.98 = 1.96 g, or 2 g/day (round to the whole number)

    c. 5 mL (convert grams to milligrams)

    0.5 g = 0.500 mg or 500 mg

Section 14C: Calculations of Oral Dosages

OBJECTIVES

- Calculate oral dosages from tablets, capsules, and liquids with selected formula.
- Calculate oral medications according to body weight and body surface area.
- Calculate the amount of tube feeding solution needed for dilution according to the percentage ordered.

OUTLINE

KEY TERMS

body surface area (BSA), p. 157
capsules, p. 165
enteric-coated, p. 165
sustained-release, p. 165
tablets, p. 165
tube feeding, p. 173

Eighty percent of all drugs consumed are given orally. Oral drugs are available in tablet, capsule, powder, and liquid form. The written abbreviation for drugs given orally is P.O. or PO (*per os*, or *by mouth*). Oral medications are absorbed by the gastrointestinal (GI) tract, mainly from the small intestine.

Oral medications have the following advantages: (1) the patient frequently can take oral medications without assistance, (2) the cost of oral medications is usually less than when given via other routes (e.g., parenteral), and (3) oral medications are easy to store. The disadvantages include (1) variation in absorption as a result of food in the GI tract and pH variation of GI secretions, (2) irritation of the gastric mucosa by certain drugs (e.g., potassium chloride), and (3) destruction or partial inactivation of the drugs by liver enzymes. This section discusses oral dosages for adults; Section 14F discusses oral dosages for children.

TABLETS, CAPSULES, AND LIQUIDS

Tablets come in different forms and drug strengths. Most tablets are scored and thus can be readily broken when half of the drug amount is needed. **Capsules** are gelatin shells that contain powder or time-release pellets (beads). **Sustained-release** (pellet) capsules and controlled-release capsules *should not* be crushed and diluted, because the medication will be absorbed at a much faster rate than indicated by the manufacturer. Many medications that are in tablet form are also available in liquid form. When the patient has difficulty taking tablets, the liquid form of the medication is given. The liquid form can be in a suspension, syrup, elixir, or tincture. Some liquid medications that irritate the stomach, such as potassium chloride, are diluted. The tincture form is always diluted.

Enteric-coated (hard-shell) tablets must *not* be crushed, because the medication could irritate the gastric mucosa. Enteric-coated drugs pass through the stomach into the small intestine where the drug's coating dissolves and then absorption occurs. Oral drugs (tablets, capsules, liquids) that irritate the gastric mucosa should be taken with 6 to 8 ounces of fluids or taken with food. Figure 14C-1 shows the different forms of tablets and capsules.

Liquid medications are poured into a medicine cup that is calibrated in ounces, teaspoons, tablespoons, and milliliters. Figure 14C-2 shows the markings on a medicine cup.

INTERPRETING ORAL DRUG LABELS

Pharmaceutic companies usually label their drugs with the brand (trade) name of the drug in large letters and the generic name in smaller letters. The dose per tablet, capsule, or liquid is often printed under the drug name.

DRUG DIFFERENTIATION

Preventing Medication Errors

Some drugs' spellings look alike or sound alike but have different chemical drug structures and are prescribed for different health problems. When ordering drugs, make sure the spelling of the drug is correct, and be extremely careful when administering drugs whose names look alike. Caution: Physicians' handwriting of drug names.

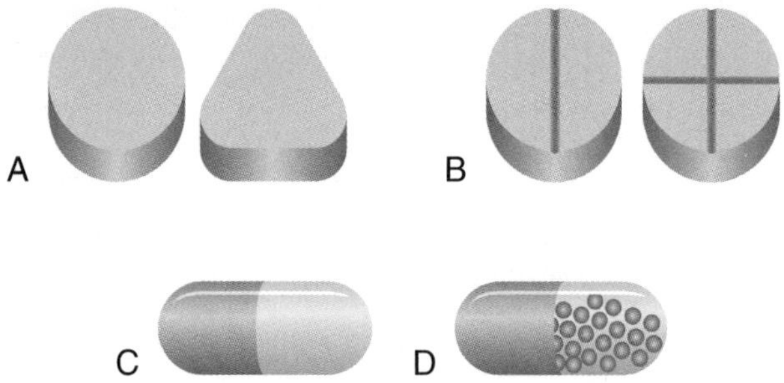

FIGURE 14C–1 Shapes of tablets and capsules. **A** and **B,** Tablets; **C** and **D,** capsules.

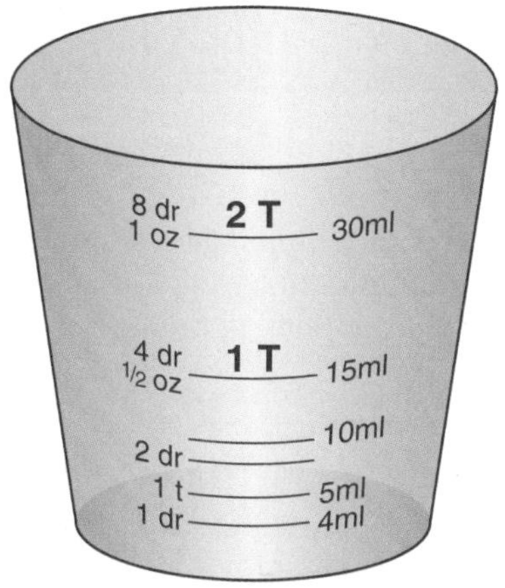

FIGURE 14C–2 Medicine cup for liquid measurement. (From Kee JL, Marshall SM: *Clinical calculations,* ed. 7, St. Louis, 2013, Elsevier.)

EXAMPLES

Ceftin is the brand (trade) name, and cefuroxime axetil is the generic name. The dose is 125 mg/5 mL (oral suspension).

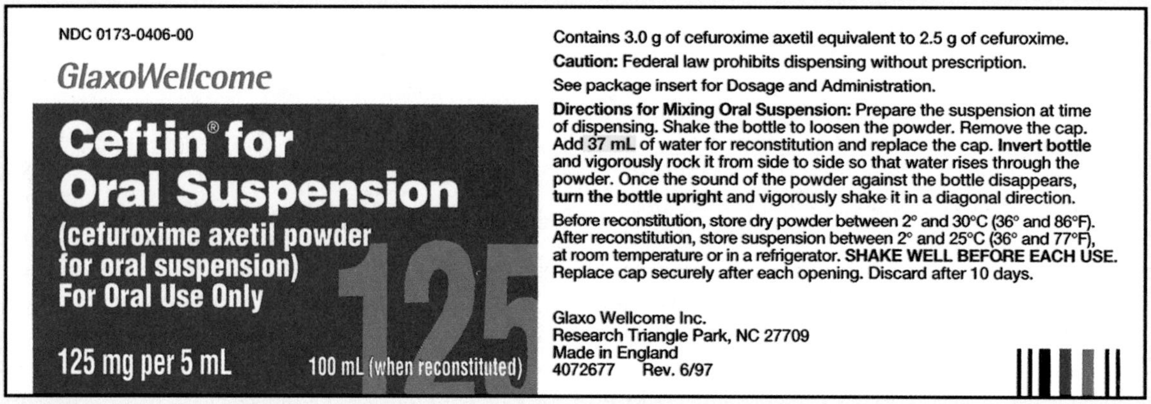

EXAMPLE 1 Quinidine and Quinine

Quinidine is an antiarrhythmic drug, and quinine is an antimalarial drug. Read the drug label three times before pouring the drug.

EXAMPLE 2 Celebrex, Celexa, and Cerebyx

All three drugs are brand name drugs and have a similar spelling. Celebrex (celecoxib) is an analgesic, a cyclo-oxygenase 2 (COX-2) inhibitor; Celexa (citalopram) is an antidepressant, a selective serotonin reuptake inhibitor (SSRI); and Cerebyx (fosphenytoin sodium) is an anticonvulsant.

EXAMPLE 3 Percodan and Percocet

Percodan contains oxycodone and aspirin, and Percocet contains oxycodone and acetaminophen. A patient may be allergic to aspirin or should not take aspirin because of a stomach ulcer; therefore it is important that the patient take Percocet. Read the drug labels carefully.

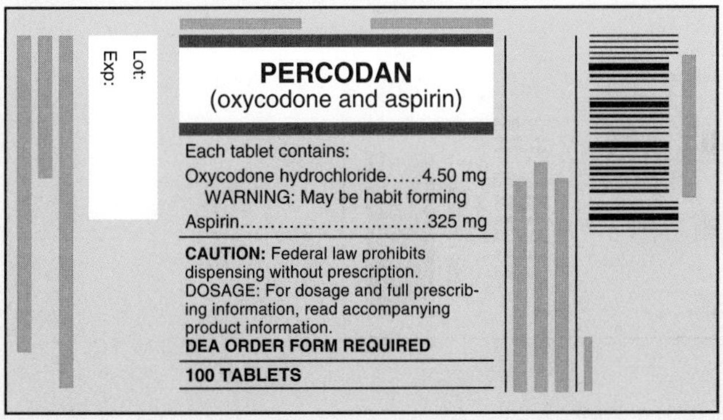

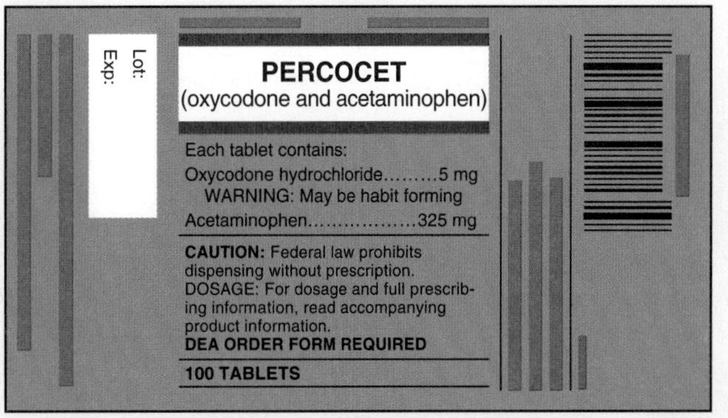

EXAMPLE 4 Hydroxyzine and Hydralazine

Hydroxyzine is an antianxiety drug, and hydralazine is an antihypertensive drug.

CALCULATION FOR TABLET, CAPSULE, AND LIQUID DOSES

When calculating oral dosages, choose one of the methods for calculation from Section 14B.

1. Order: diltiazem (Cardizem) 60 mg PO, b.i.d.

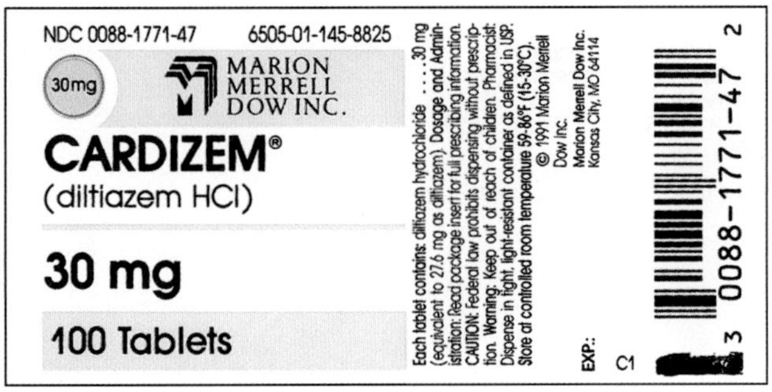

How many tablets would you give? ______

a. BF: $\frac{D}{H} \times V = \frac{60}{30} \times 1 = 2$ tablets

b. RF: $H : V :: D : x$

$30 \text{ mg} : 1 \text{ mg} :: 60 \text{ mg} : x \text{ tab}$

$30x = 60$

$x = 2$ tablets

Answer: diltiazem (cardizem) 60 mg = 2 tablets

c. FE: $\frac{H}{V} = \frac{D}{x}\quad \frac{30}{1} = \frac{60}{x}$ (cross-multiply) $= 30x = 60$

$x = 2$ tablets

d. DA: $\text{tab} = \frac{1 \text{ tab} \times \overset{2}{\cancel{60}} \cancel{\text{mg}}}{\underset{1}{\cancel{30}} \cancel{\text{mg}} \times 1} = 2$ tablets

Conversion is not needed.

2. Order: clarithromycin (Biaxin) 100 mg PO q6h
Available:

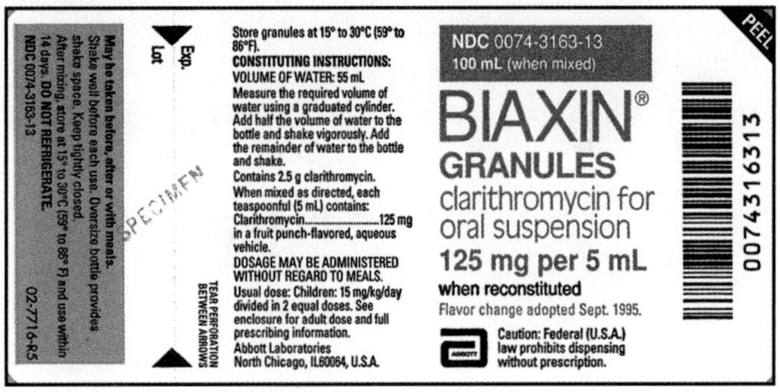

How many milliliters should the patient receive per dose? ______

a. BF: $\frac{D}{H} \times V = \frac{100}{\underset{25}{\cancel{125}}} = \overset{1}{\cancel{5}} = 4 \text{ mL}$

or

b. RP: $H : V :: D : V$

$125 : 5 :: 100 : x$

$125x = 500$

$x = 4 \text{ mL}$

or

c. DA: $\text{mL} \frac{5 \text{ mL} \times \overset{4}{\cancel{100}} \text{ mg}}{\underset{5}{\cancel{125}} \text{ mg} \times 1} = \frac{20}{5} = 4 \text{ mL}$

PRACTICE PROBLEM 1

Oral Medications

Solve the drug problems for *x*, the unknown amount of drug to be given.

1. Order: doxepin HCl (Sinequan) 30 mg PO at bedtime (h.s.)

   Available:

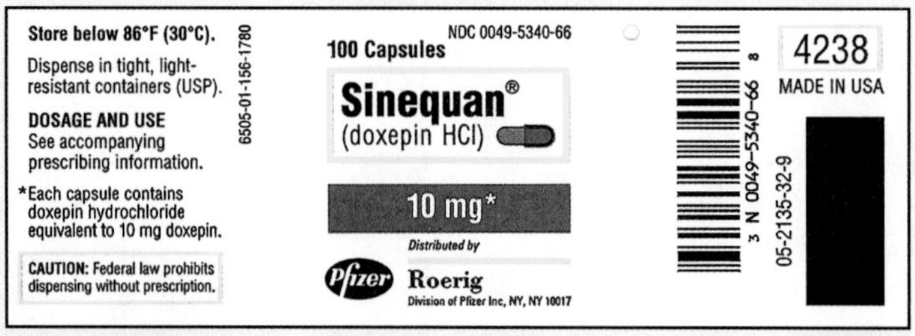

   How many capsule(s) should the patient receive?______

2. Order: lisinopril (Zestril) 5 mg PO, daily

   Available:

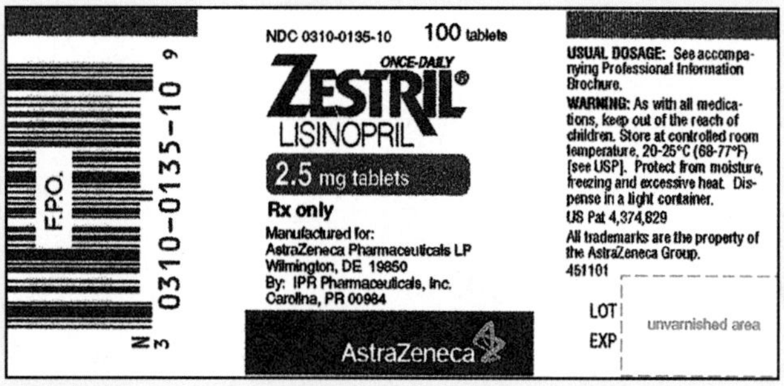

   How many tablets should the patient receive?______

3. Order: zidovudine (Retrovir) 300 mg PO, q12h

   Available:

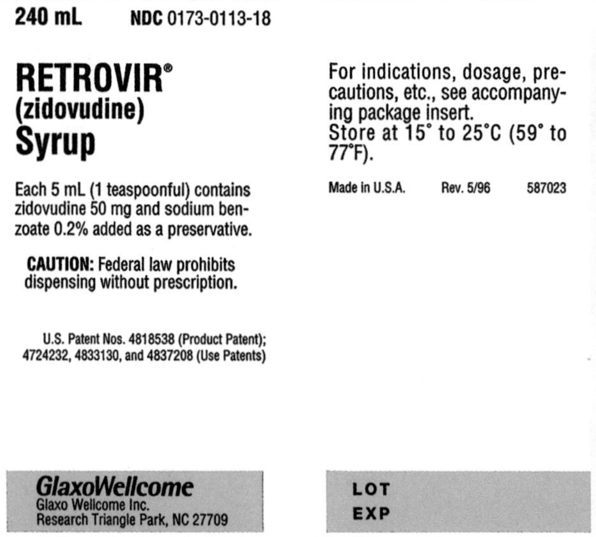

   a. How many milligrams should the patient receive per day?______

   b. How many milliliters should the patient receive per day?______

4. Order: digoxin (Lanoxin) 0.5 mg PO, daily

   Available:

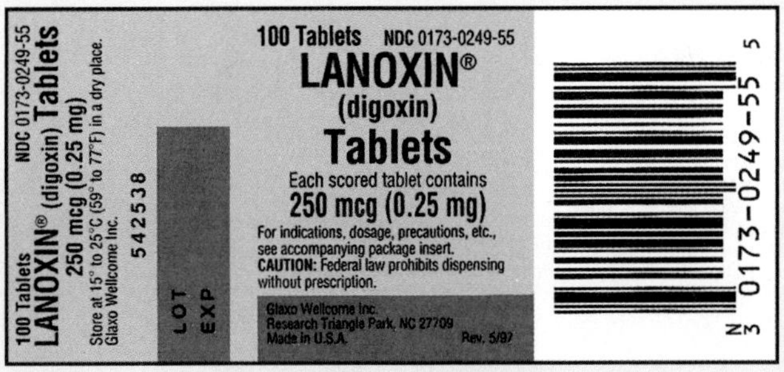

   How many tablet(s) should the nurse administer?______

5. Order: nitroglycerin (Nitrostat) $\frac{1}{150}$ gr sublingual STAT

   Available:

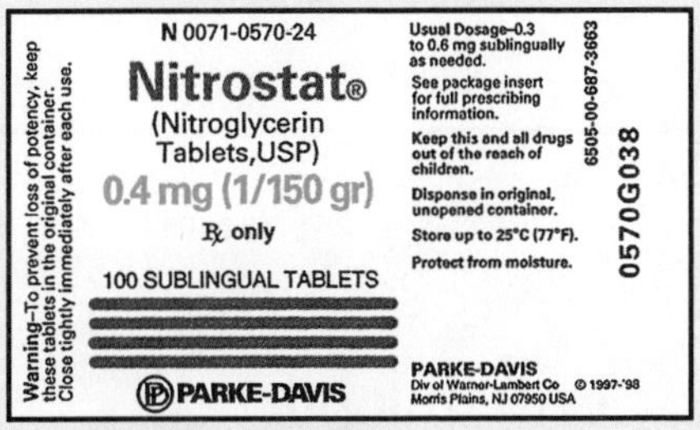

   How many sublingual tablet(s) should the patient take?______

6. Order: bethanechol Cl (Urecholine) 20 mg PO, t.i.d.

   Available:

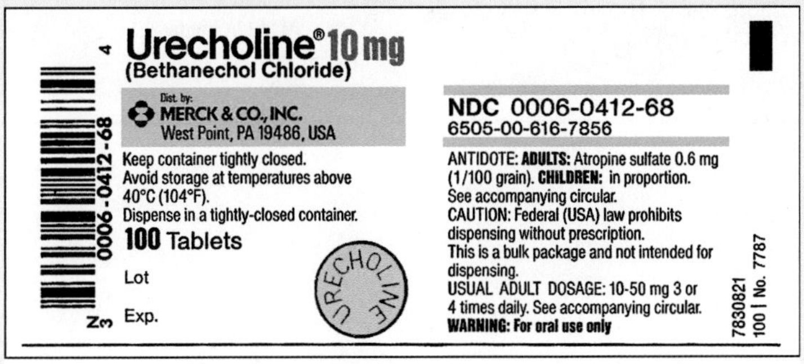

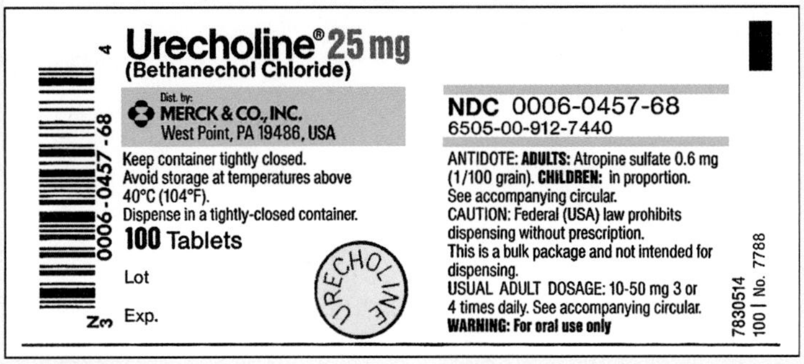

   a. Which Urecholine bottle should the nurse select?______

   b. How many tablet(s) should the patient receive per dose?______

Continued

SECTION 14C

7. Order: amoxicillin clavulanate (Augmentin) 500 mg PO, b.i.d.

   Available:

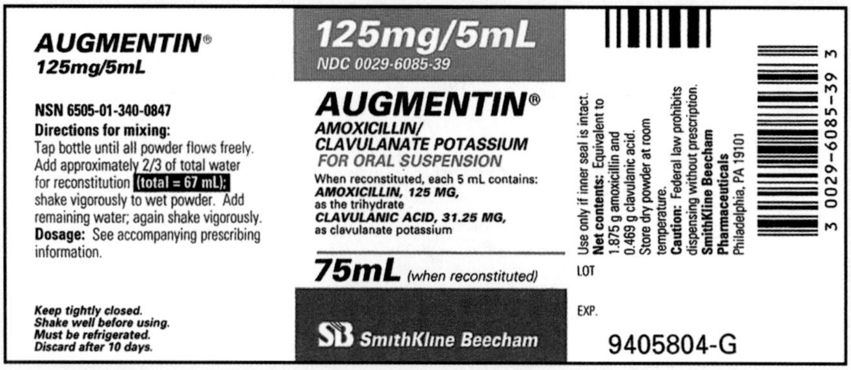

   How many milliliters should the patient receive per dose?______

8. Order: ondansetron HCl (Zofran) 6 mg PO, 30 minutes before chemotherapy, then q8h × 2 doses

   Available:

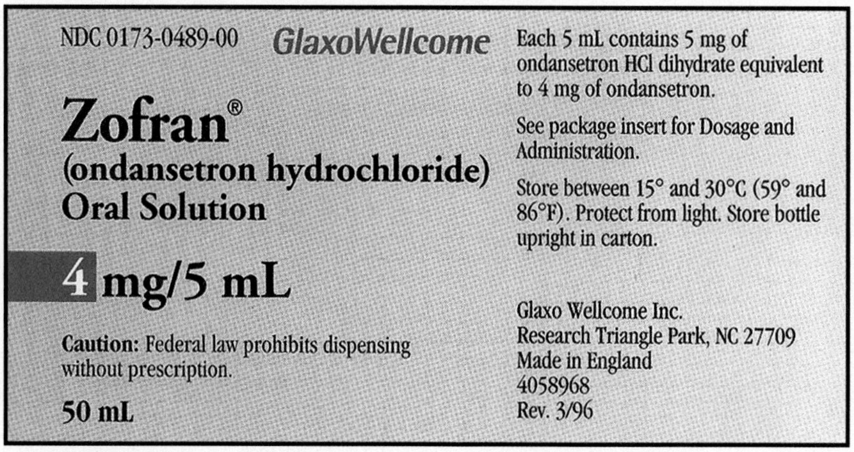

   How many milliliters would you give per dose? ______

9. Order: prazosin (Minipress) 10 mg PO, daily.

   Available: prazosin 1-mg, 2-mg, and 5-mg tablets

   a. Which tablet should be selected? ______

   b. How much should be given? ______

10. Order: capropril (Capoten) 25 mg, PO, b.i.d., for an older adult patient with heart failure.

    Available:

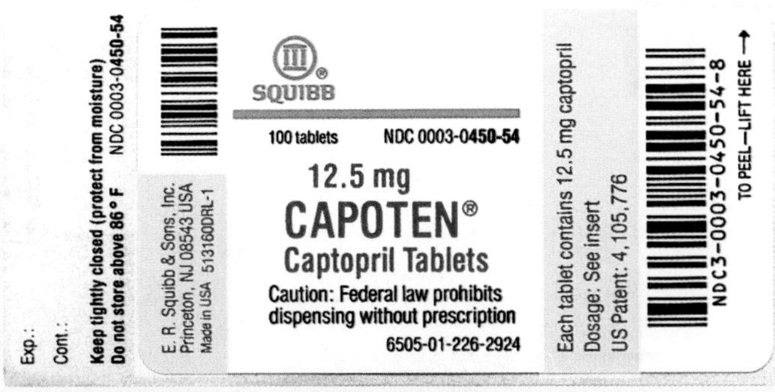

    a. How many milligrams should the patient receive per day? ______

    b. How many tablet(s) would you give per dose? ______

11. Order: carbidopa-levodopa (Sinemet) 12.5 to 125 mg PO, b.i.d.

    Available: Sinimet 25-100, 25-250, 10-100–mg tablets

    a. Which tablet should be selected? ______

    b. How much should the patient receive? ______

12. Order: cefuroxime axetil (Ceftin) 400 mg, PO, q 12 h.

    Available:

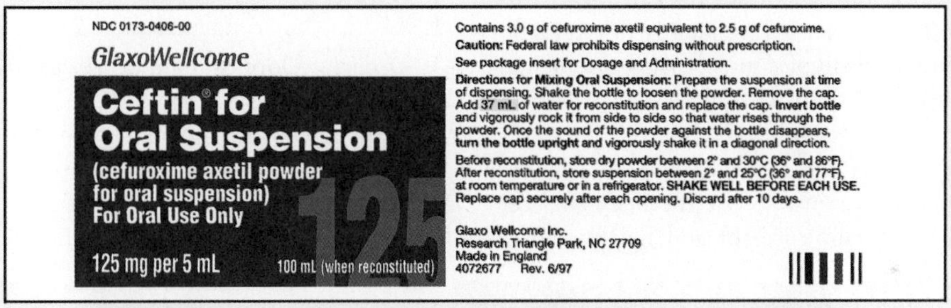

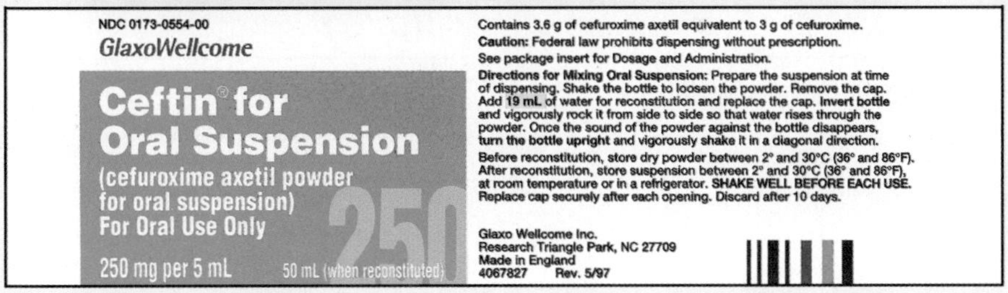

    a. How many milliliters should the patient receive per dose? ______

    b. Which drug bottle would use? Explain your answer. ______

Additional Dimensional Analysis

13. Order: omeprazole (Prilosec) 20 mg PO, daily.

    Available:

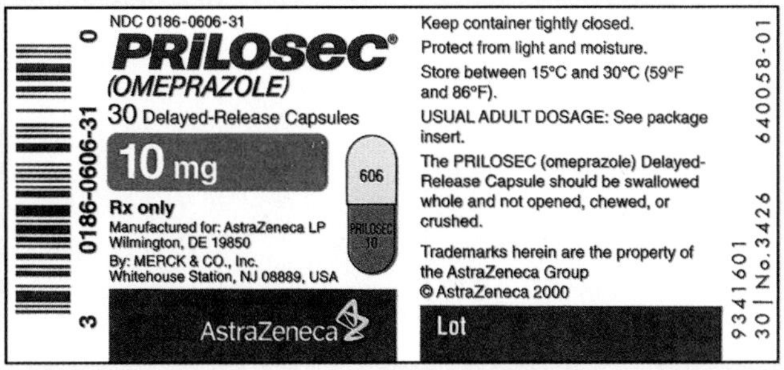

    Conversion factor: none (both are in milligrams)

    How many capsules should the patient receive? ______

Continued

14. Order: amoxicillin (Amoxil) 0.1 g PO, q8h

 Available:

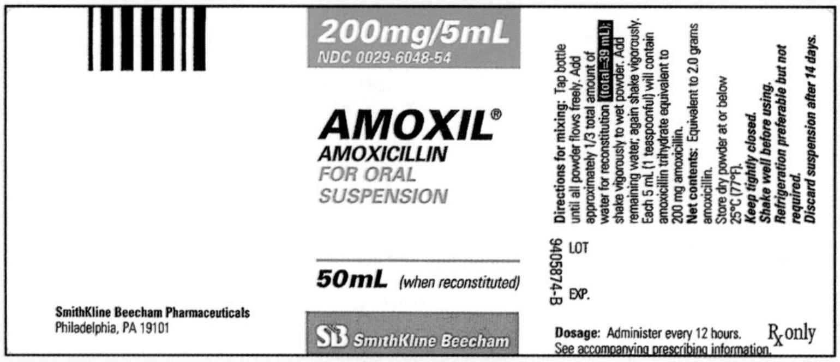

 Conversion factor: 1000 mg = 1 g

 How many milliliters should the patient receive per dose? ______

BODY WEIGHT AND BODY SURFACE AREA

Calculating the drug dosage for adults by body weight (BW) and **body surface area** (BSA) is used mostly when administering drugs to treat cancer (antineoplastic drugs). These two individualized methods are also used frequently to calculate drug dosages for children. Examples and practice problems for pediatrics are given in Section 14F.

To use the body weight method, convert the patient's weight in pounds to kilograms (kg). To convert, divide pounds by 2.2 to equal kilograms. To use the body surface area (BSA) method, the person's weight and height and a nomogram are needed (see Sections 14B and 14F). Daily requirements are usually divided into two to four doses per day.

EXAMPLE

1. Order: cyclophosphamide (Cytoxan) 2 mg/kg PO daily. Patient weighs 143 lb.
 How much does the patient weigh in kilograms? ______
 How many milligrams should the patient receive? ______
 Answer: 143 lb ÷ 2.2 = 65 kg
 2 mg × 65 = 130 mg of cyclophosphamide daily

PRACTICE PROBLEM 2

Body Weight

1. Order: valproic acid (Depakene) 8 mg/kg/day in four divided doses. Patient weighs 165 lb.
 How much Depakene should be administered per dose? ______
2. Order: cyclophosphamide (Cytoxan) 4 mg/kg/day. Patient weighs 176 lb.
 How much should the patient receive per day? ______

ANSWERS TO PRACTICE PROBLEMS

1 ORAL MEDICATIONS USING BASIC FORMULA, RATIO AND PROPORTION, FRACTIONAL EQUATION, OR DIMENSIONAL ANALYSIS

1. 3 capsules of Sinequan
2. 2 tablets of Zestril
3. a. 600 mg

 b. BF: $\frac{D}{H} \times V = \frac{\overset{6}{\cancel{300\text{ mg}}}}{\underset{1}{\cancel{50\text{ mg}}}} \times 5\text{ mL} = 30\text{ mL per dose}$
 (twice a day = 60 mL)

 or

 RP: H : V :: D : X
 50 mg : 5 mL :: 300 mg : X mL
 50 X = 1500
 X = 30 mL per dose
 (twice a day = 60 mL)

 or

 FE: $\frac{H}{V} = \frac{D}{x} = \frac{50\text{ mg}}{5\text{ mL}} = \frac{300\text{ mg}}{x} =$
 (cross-multiply) 50 X = 1500
 X = 30 mL per dose
 (twice a day = 60 mL)

 DA: $\text{mL} = \frac{5\text{ mL} \times \overset{6}{\cancel{300\text{ mg}}}}{\underset{1}{\cancel{50\text{ mg}}} \times 1} = 30\text{ mL per dose}$
 (twice a day = 60 mL)

4. 2 tablets

a. BF: $\frac{D}{H}\times V=\frac{0.5}{0.25}\times 1=0.25\overline{)0.500}=2.0=2$ tablets

or

b. RP: H : V :: D : x

0.25 mg : 1 tab :: 0.5 mg : x tab

$0.25x = 0.5 = 2$ tablets

c. DA: $\text{tab}=\frac{1 \quad \times 0.5\ \cancel{mg}}{0.25\ \cancel{mg}\times 1}=2$ tablets

5. 1 sublingual tablet

Convert grains to milligrams. $\frac{1}{150}$ gr = 0.4 mg

6. a. Select Urecholine 10-mg bottle.

b. BF: $\frac{D}{H}\times V=\frac{20\ \cancel{mg}}{10\ \cancel{mg}}\times 1\text{ tab}=\frac{20}{10}=2$ tablets

or

DA: $\text{tab}=\frac{1 \quad \times 20\ \cancel{mg}}{10\ \cancel{mg}\times 1}=2$ tablets

No conversion needed

7. 20 mL of Augmentin suspension

8. $\frac{D}{H}\times V=\frac{6\text{ mg}}{4\text{ mg}}\times 5=\frac{30}{4}=7.5$ mL of Zofran

9. Select 5-mg tablets. Give two tablets.

10. a. b.i.d. = 2 times a day; $25\times 2=50$ mg per day

b. RP: H : V :: D : V

12.5 mg : 1 tab :: 25 mg : X

12.5 X = 25

X = 2 tablets of Capoten

DA: $\text{tab}=\frac{1 \quad \times 25\text{ mg}}{12.5\text{ mg}\times 1}=2$ tablets of Capoten

11. a. Select 25- to 250-mg strength.

b. Give half a tablet.

2 capsules DA: $\text{capsules}=\frac{1\text{ cap} \times \overset{2}{\cancel{20}}\ \cancel{mg}}{\underset{1}{\cancel{10}}\ \cancel{mg}\times 1}=2$ capsules

12. a. BF: $\frac{D}{H}\times V=\frac{400\text{ mg}}{125\text{ mg}}\times 5\text{ mL}=\frac{2000}{125}=16$ mL using 125-mg Ceftin bottle

FE: $\frac{H}{V}=\frac{D}{X}=\frac{250\text{ mg}}{5\text{ mL}}=\frac{400\text{ mg}}{X}=$

(cross multiply) 250 X = 2000

X = 8 mL using 250 mg Ceflin bottle

b. Use the Ceftin bottle 250 mg/5 ml to give fewer milliliters Either bottle could be used.

13. DA: $\text{capsules}=\frac{1\text{ cap} \times \overset{2}{\cancel{20}}\ \cancel{mg}}{\underset{1}{\cancel{10}}\ \cancel{mg}\times 1}=2$ capsules

14. 2.5 mL per dose

$\text{mL}=\frac{5\text{ mL} \times \overset{5}{\cancel{1000}}\ \cancel{mg}\cdot 0.1\ \cancel{g}}{\underset{1}{\cancel{200}}\ \cancel{mg}\times \quad 1\ \cancel{g} \quad \cdot 1}$

= 2.5 mL per dose

2 BODY WEIGHT

1. 75 kg; 150 mg/dose; 600 mg/day
2. 80 kg; 320 mg/day

DRUGS ADMINISTERED VIA NASOGASTRIC TUBE

Oral medications can be administered through a nasogastric tube but should not be mixed with the entire **tube feeding solution.** Mixing the medications in a large volume of tube feeding solution decreases the amount of drug the patient receives for a specific time. The medication (NOT time-released or sustained-release capsules and psyllium hydrophilic mucilloid [Metamucil]) should be diluted in 1 ounce (30 mL) of warm water unless otherwise instructed, administered through the tube, and followed with extra water to ensure that the drug reaches the stomach and is not left in the tube. Check the policy at your institution.

Section 14D: Calculations of Injectable Dosages

OBJECTIVES

- Describe the difference between vials and ampules.
- Describe the types of syringes and needles and their uses.
- Explain how to administer intradermal, subcutaneous, and intramuscular injections.
- Calculate the dosage of drugs for subcutaneous and intramuscular injections.
- Identify the amount of insulin dosage with the use of an insulin syringe.
- Explain the methods for mixing two insulins in one insulin syringe and for mixing two injectable drugs in one syringe.
- Describe the procedure for the preparation and calculation of medications in powdered form for injectable use.

OUTLINE

KEY TERMS

When medications cannot be taken by mouth because of (1) an inability to swallow, (2) a decreased level of consciousness, (3) an inactivation of the drug by gastric juices, or (4) a desire to increase the effectiveness of the drug, the parenteral route may be the route of choice. **Parenteral** medications are administered intradermally (under the skin), subcutaneously (into the fatty tissue), intramuscularly (IM, within the muscle), and intravenously (IV, in the vein). IV injectables are discussed in Section 14E. The injectables in this section include intradermal, subQ (including insulin and heparin), and IM from prepared liquid and reconstituted powder in vials and ampules. Prefilled drug cartridges (syringes) are also discussed.

This section is divided into five parts: (1) injectable preparations, (2) intradermal injections, (3) subQ injections, (4) insulin injections, and (5) IM injections. Examples and practice problems to solve for the correct dosage are provided.

SECTION 14D

INJECTABLE PREPARATIONS

The appropriate drug container (vial or ampule) and the correct selection of needle and syringe are essential in the preparation of the prescribed drug dose. The route of administration is part of the medication order.

VIALS AND AMPULES

A **vial** is usually a small glass container with a self-sealing rubber top. Some are multiple-dose vials, and when properly stored, they can be used over time. An **ampule** is a glass container with a tapered neck for snapping open and using only once. Drugs that deteriorate readily in liquid form are packaged in powder form in vials and ampules for storage. Once the dry form of the drug is reconstituted (usually with sterile water, bacteriostatic water, or saline), the drug is used immediately or must be refrigerated. Check the accompanying drug circular for specific storage length and other instructions. The person reconstituting the drug should write on the label when the drug is to be discarded and include his or her initials. Usually a vial should be used within 96 hours.

Drug labels on vials and ampules provide the following information: (1) generic and brand name of the drug, (2) drug dose in weight (milligrams, grams, milliequivalents) and amount (milliliters), (3) expiration date, and (4) directions about administration. If the drug is in powdered form, mixing instructions and dose equivalents (e.g., milligrams equal milliliters) may be given. Figure 14D-1 shows a vial and an ampule.

SYRINGES

The syringe is composed of a barrel (outer shell), plunger (inner part), and the tip where the needle joins the syringe (Figure 14D-2). Syringes are available in various types and sizes, the most common of which are the 3-mL and 5-mL tuberculin, insulin, and metal and plastic syringes for prefilled cartridges. Glass syringes may be used in the operating room and on special instrument trays. The tip of the syringe and inside of the plunger should remain sterile.

The 3-mL syringe is calibrated in tenths (0.1 mL) and minims. The amount of fluid in the syringe is determined by the black rubber end of the plunger (the inner end of the plunger) that is closest to the tip (Figure 14D-3). REMEMBER: Milliliter (mL) and cubic centimeter (cc) may be used interchangeably, but milliliter (mL) is preferred. An advance in safety needle technology is the SafetyGlide shielding hypodermic needle (see Chapter 13). This type of needle reduces needlestick injuries.

The 5-mL syringe is calibrated in 0.2-mL marks. A 5-mL syringe is usually used when the fluid needed is more than 2.5 mL. It is frequently used when reconstituting the dry drug form with sterile bacteriostatic water or saline. The needleless syringes are used primarily for intermittent infusion therapy to irrigate the intermittent infusion device for maintaining patency and to administer IV medication through the IV tubing device. See intermittent infusion adapters/devices in Section 14E. Figure 14D-4 shows the 5-mL syringe and 5-mL needleless syringe. (See also Chapter 13.)

The **tuberculin syringe** is a 1-mL slender syringe with markings in tenths (0.1) and hundredths (0.01). It is also marked in minims (Figure 14D-5). This syringe is used when the amount of drug solution to be administered is less than 1 mL and for pediatric and heparin dosages. The tuberculin

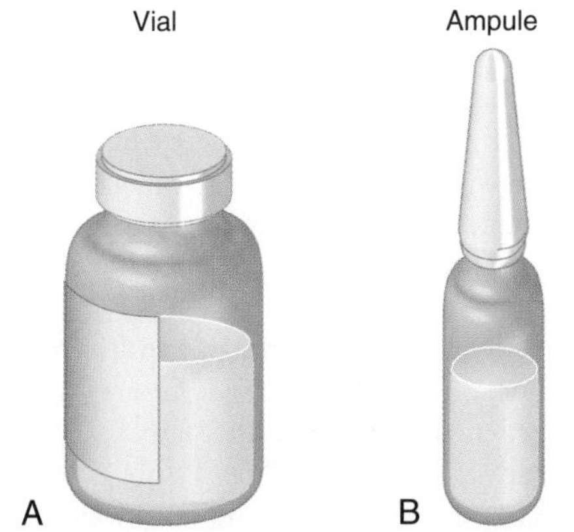

FIGURE 14D–1 **A,** Vial. **B,** Ampule. (From Kee JL, Marshall SM: *Clinical calculations,* ed. 7, St. Louis, 2013, Elsevier.)

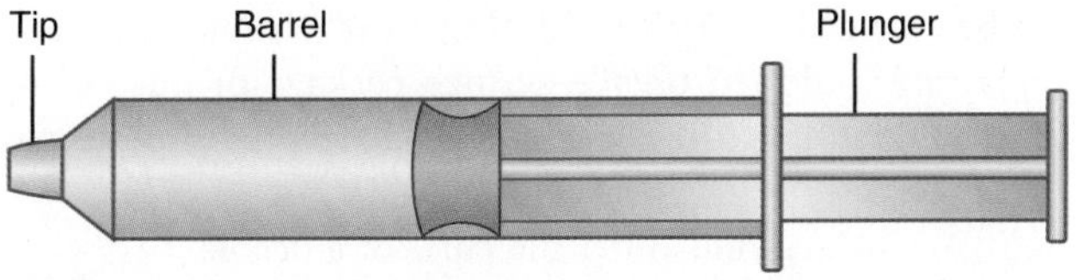

FIGURE 14D–2 Parts of a syringe. (From Kee JL, Marshall SM: *Clinical calculations,* ed. 7, St. Louis, 2013, Elsevier.)

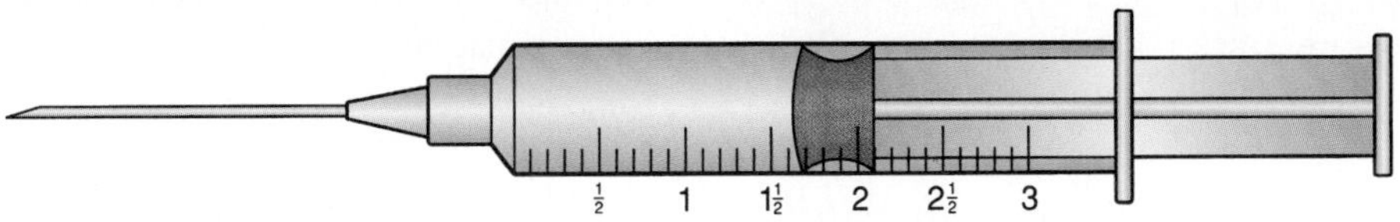

FIGURE 14D–3 A 3-mL syringe. (From Kee JL, Marshall SM: *Clinical calculations,* ed. 7, St. Louis, 2013, Elsevier.)

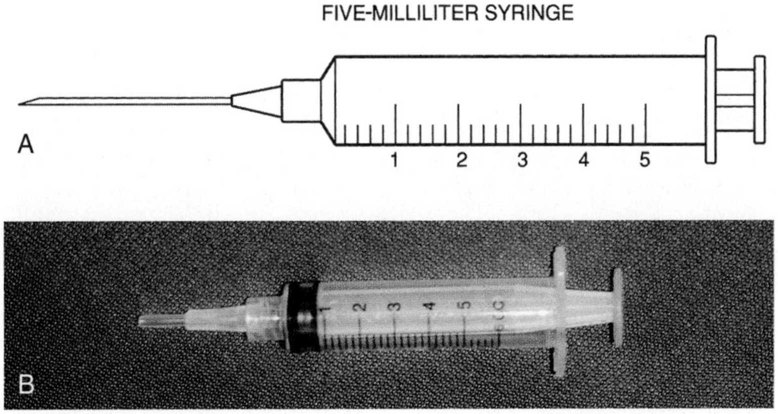

FIGURE 14D–4 5-mL syringes: **A,** 5-mL syringe with 0.2-mL markings. **B,** Needleless 5-mL BD syringe that can penetrate a rubber-top vial.

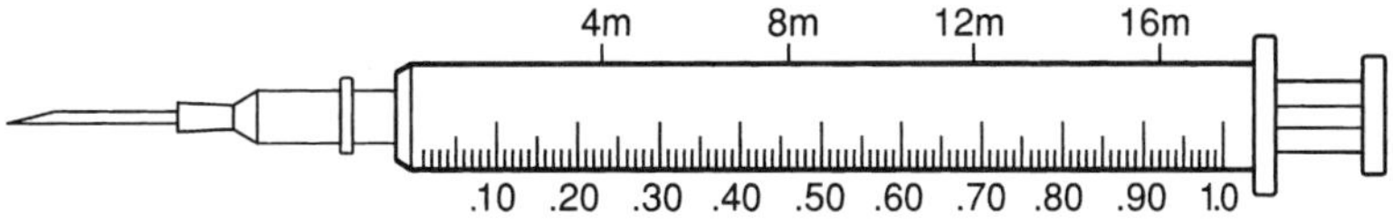

FIGURE 14D–5 Tuberculin syringe. (From Kee JL, Marshall SM: *Clinical calculations,* ed. 7, St. Louis, 2013, Elsevier.)

syringe is also available in a 0.5-mL syringe. Figure 14D-6 illustrates the 0.5-mL and 1-mL tuberculin syringes.

The **insulin syringe** has the capacity of 1 mL; however, insulin is measured in units, and insulin dosage must *not* be calculated in milliliters. Insulin syringes are calibrated as 2-unit marks, and 100 units equal 1 mL (Figure 14D-7). *Insulin syringes must be used for the administration of insulin.*

Insulin syringes are available as low-dose insulin syringes. The 1-mL insulin syringe may be purchased with a permanent attached needle or a detachable needle (Figure 14D-8).

Prefilled Drug Cartridges and Syringes

Many injectable drugs are packaged in prefilled, disposable cartridges. The disposable cartridge is placed into a Tubex injector or a reusable metal or plastic holder. Usually the prefilled cartridge contains 0.1 to 0.2 mL of excess drug solution. Based on the amount of drug to be administered, the excess solution must be expelled before administration. Figure 14D-9, *A*, illustrates the Carpuject syringe; Figure 14D-9, *B*, shows the Tubex syringe. Prefilled syringes are also used in place of prefilled cartridges.

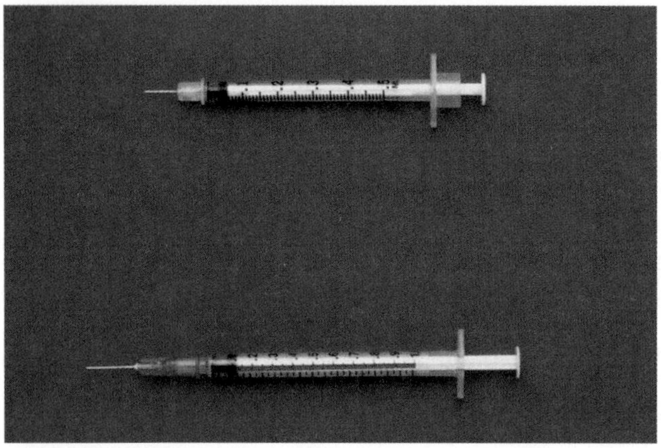

FIGURE 14D–6 Two types of tuberculin syringes. (Courtesy Becton-Dickinson Division, Franklin Lakes, New Jersey.)

Needles

Needle size has two components: **gauge** (diameter of the lumen) and length. The larger the gauge number, the smaller the diameter of the **lumen**, and the smaller the gauge, the larger the diameter of the lumen. The most common gauge numbers of needles range from 18 to 26. Needle length varies from $\frac{3}{8}$ inch to 2 inches. Table 14D-1 lists the needle gauges and lengths for use in subcutaneous and IM injections.

When choosing the needle length for an IM injection, the size of the patient and the amount of fatty tissue must be considered. A patient with minimal fatty (subQ) tissue may need a needle length of 1 inch. For a patient with more fatty tissue, the needle length for an IM injection would be $1\frac{1}{2}$ to 2 inches.

Many insulin syringes and prefilled cartridges have permanently attached needles. With other syringes, the needle can be changed to the desired needle size. Needle gauge and length are indicated on the syringe package or on the top cover of the syringe. It appears as gauge/length; for example, 20 g/$1\frac{1}{2}$.

Figure 14D-10 illustrates the parts of a needle.

Angles for Injections

For injections, the needle enters the skin at different angles. Intradermal injections are given at a 10- to 15-degree angle,

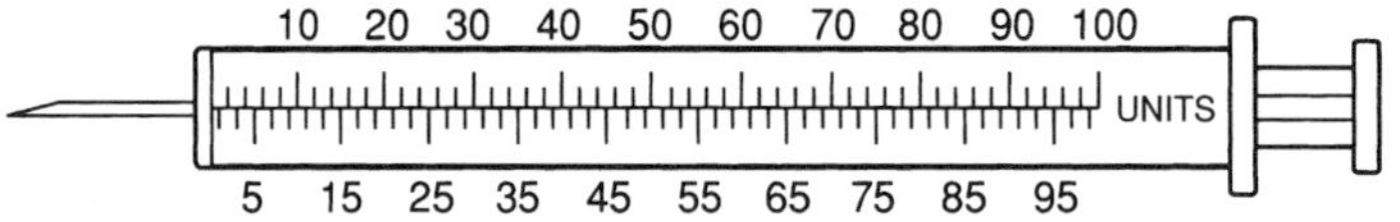

FIGURE 14D–7 Insulin syringe. (From Kee JL, Marshall SM: *Clinical calculations,* ed. 7, St. Louis, 2013, Elsevier.)

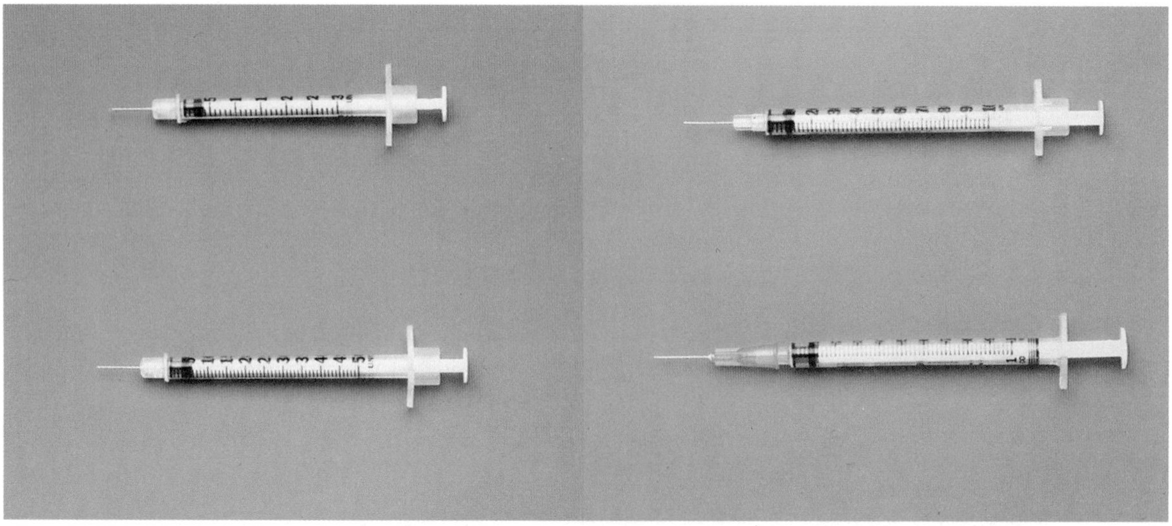

FIGURE 14D–8 Various types of insulin syringes. (Courtesy Becton-Dickinson Division, Franklin Lakes, New Jersey.)

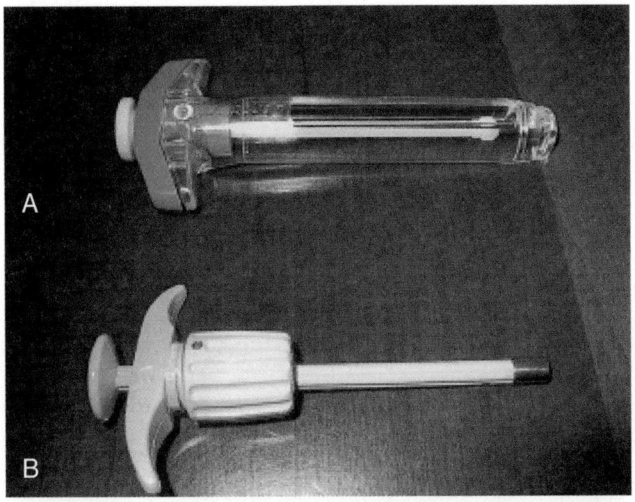

FIGURE 14D–9 **A,** Carpuject syringe. **B,** Tubex syringe.

TABLE 14D-1 NEEDLE SIZE AND LENGTH

TYPE OF INJECTION	NEEDLE GAUGE	NEEDLE LENGTHS (INCHES)
Intradermal	25, 26	3/8, 1/2, 5/8
Subcutaneous	23, 25, 26	3/8, 1/2, 5/8
Intramuscular	19, 20, 21, 22	1, 1 1/2, 2

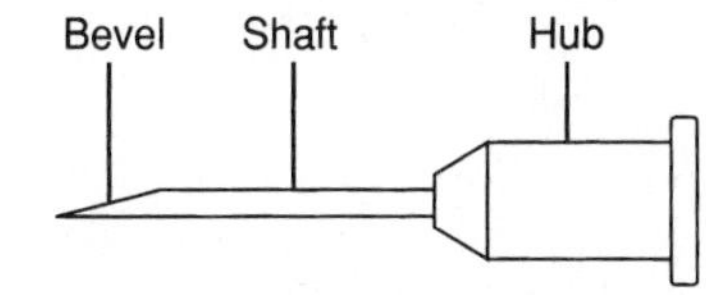

FIGURE 14D–10 Parts of a needle.

subQ injections at a 45- to 90-degree angle, and IM injections at a 90-degree angle. In Chapter 13, the angles for intradermal, subQ, and IM injections are illustrated.

PRACTICE PROBLEM 1

Syringes and Needles

Think through and answer each question. Correct answers are given at the end of the section.

1. To mix 4 mL of bacteriostatic water in a vial with a powdered drug, which size syringe should be used?
2. To give 0.4 mL of drug solution subQ, what type of syringe should be used?
3. Meperidine (Demerol) is available in a prefilled cartridge. Half of the drug solution is used. Should the remaining solution in the cartridge be saved for future use?
4. Which has a larger needle lumen, a 21-gauge needle or a 26-gauge needle?
5. Which needle has a length of 5/8 inch, a 21-gauge needle or a 25-gauge needle?
6. Which needle is used for an IM injection, a 20-gauge needle with a 1 1/2-inch length or a 25-gauge needle with a 5/8-inch length?

INTERPRETING INJECTABLE DRUG LABELS

Drugs for injections are stored in liquid and powder form in vials and ampules. If the drug is in liquid form, the drug dose with its equivalent in milliliters is printed on the drug label. However, drugs in powder form must be reconstituted (i.e., changed to liquid form before use). Usually the instructions for reconstitution are given on the drug label and drug instructions. If this is not the case, consult a pharmacist or the drug circular.

EXAMPLE

Nafcillin sodium is the generic name; there is no brand (trade) name. The drug is for IM or IV administration. Instructions on the drug label read: "When reconstituted with 6.6 mL of diluent, each vial contains 8 mL of solution."

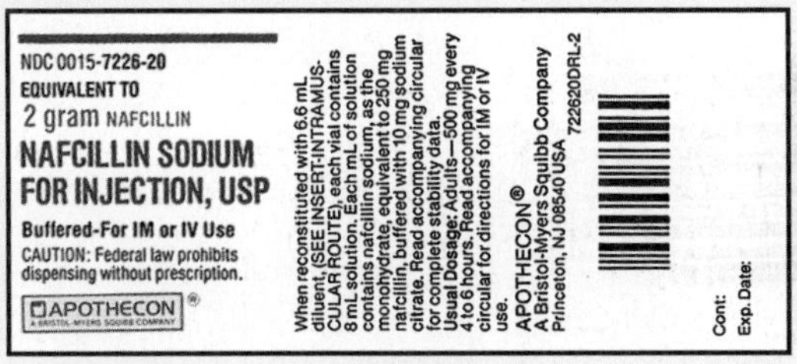

INTRADERMAL INJECTIONS

An **intradermal** injection is usually used for skin testing to diagnose the cause of an allergy or to determine the presence of a microorganism. The choice of syringe for intradermal testing is the tuberculin syringe with a 25-gauge needle.

The inner portion of the forearm is frequently used for diagnostic testing because there is less hair in the area and the test results are more visible. The upper back may also be used as a testing site. The needle is inserted with the **bevel** pointing upward at a 10- to 15-degree angle. Do *not* aspirate. Test results are read 48 to 72 hours after the intradermal injection. A reddened or raised area is a positive reaction.

SUBCUTANEOUS INJECTIONS

Drugs injected into the **subcutaneous (subQ)** or fatty tissue are absorbed slowly because there are fewer blood vessels in fatty tissue. The amount of drug solution administered subQ is generally 0.5 to 1 mL at a 45-, 60-, or 90-degree angle. Drug solutions that irritate fatty tissues are given IM because they can cause sloughing of the subQ tissue.

The two types of syringes used for subQ injections are the tuberculin syringe (1 mL), calibrated in 0.1 mL and 0.01 mL, and the 3-mL syringe, calibrated in 0.1 mL. The needle gauge commonly used is 25 or 26, and the length is 3/8 to 5/8 inch. Insulin is also administered subQ and is discussed later in this section.

Calculations: Subcutaneous Injections

To calculate dosages for subQ injections, use the basic formula of *D/H* × *V*, the ratio-and-proportion method, fractional equation, or dimensional analysis (see Section 14B). Heparin is a drug frequently administered subQ. It can be given at a 60- to 90-degree angle, depending on the amount of fatty tissue. The skin is lifted, and the heparin solution is injected into the subQ tissue. Do not aspirate or massage the injected site, because massage could cause small-vessel damage and bleeding.

Units should be written out as a word and not abbreviated as "U" only. When U is written, it may appear as O, and thus the patient could receive a higher dose of the drug.

EXAMPLE

Order: heparin 2500 units subQ
Available: heparin 10,000 units/mL in multiple-dose vial (10 mL)
Basic Formula:

$$\frac{D}{H} \times V = \frac{25\cancel{00}\text{ units}}{10{,}0\cancel{00}\text{ units}} \times 1\text{ mL} = \frac{25}{100} = 0.25\text{ mL}$$

Ratio-and-Proportion Method:

$$\begin{array}{ccccccc} H & : & V & :: & D & : & x \\ 10{,}000\text{ units} & : & 1\text{ mL} & :: & 2500\text{ units} & : & x\text{ mL} \end{array}$$

$$10{,}000\,x = 2500$$

$$x = \frac{25}{100} = 0.25\text{ mL}$$

Fractional Equation:

$$\frac{H}{V} = \frac{D}{x} = \frac{10{,}000\text{ units}}{1\text{ mL}} = \frac{2500\text{ units}}{x\text{ mL}}$$

$$10{,}000x = 2500$$

$$\text{(cross-multiply)} \qquad x = 0.25\text{ mL}$$

Answer: heparin 2500 units = 0.25 mL

Dimensional Analysis:

$$\text{mL} = \frac{1\text{ ml} \times \overset{1}{\cancel{2500}}\ \cancel{\text{units}}}{\underset{4}{\cancel{10{,}000}}\ \cancel{\text{units}} \times 1} = \frac{1}{4}\text{ or }0.25\text{ mL}$$

PRACTICE PROBLEM 2

Subcutaneous Injections

> Use the formula chosen for the calculation of drug dosages from Section 14B. The same formula should be used when calculating oral, subQ, IM, insulin, and IV dosages.

EXAMPLE

1. Order: heparin 7500 units subQ
   Available:

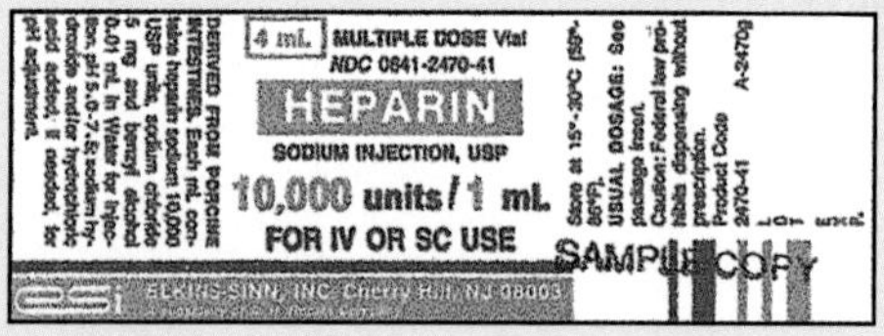

   How many milliliters should the patient receive?
2. Order: Lovenox (enoxaparin) 20 mg, subQ, q12h. Lovenox is a low–molecular weight heparin (LMWH).
   Available:

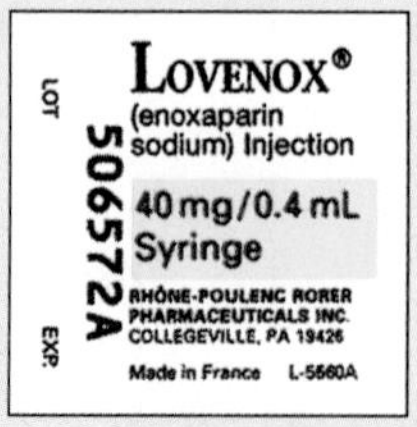

   How many milliliters would you give per dose?

3. Order: atropine sulfate 0.5 mg subQ
   Available:

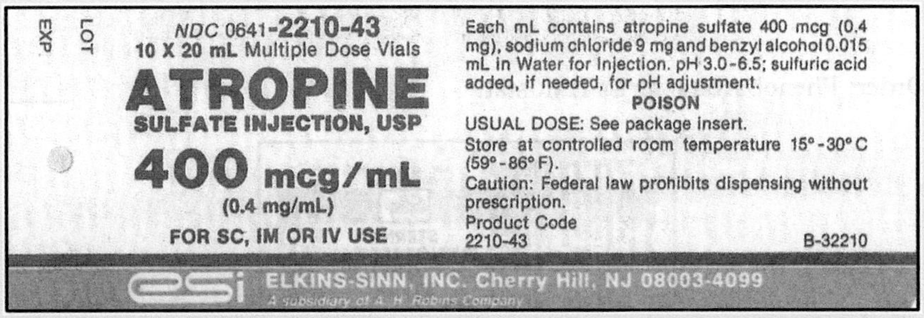

   How many milliliters should the patient receive?
4. Order: epinephrine (Adrenalin) 0.2 mg subQ, STAT
   Available: epinephrine (Adrenalin) 1 mg/mL (1 : 1000) in ampule
   What type of syringe should be used? ______
   How many milliliters should the patient receive? ______

INSULIN INJECTIONS

Insulin has been available since 1925, when it was extracted from beef and pork pancreases. In the 1980s, human insulin was synthetically produced and began replacing beef and pork insulin in the United States. Some individuals are allergic to beef insulin, so it has not been available since 1998. Pork insulin was more frequently prescribed because it has biologic properties similar to those of human insulin. Since December 2005, pork insulin has not been available in the United States. Some patients may be importing it. Now, insulin analogs have been developed and are currently in use.

Insulin is prescribed and measured in United States Pharmacopeia (USP) units. Most insulins are produced in concentrations of 100 units/mL. Insulin should be administered with an insulin syringe, which is calibrated to correspond with the 100 units of insulin. Insulin bottles and syringes are color-coded to avoid error. The 100 units/mL (or U-100) insulin bottle and the 100 units/mL syringe are coded orange. Administering insulin with a tuberculin syringe *should be avoided.*

Administration of medication requires attention to detail, and insulin is no exception. Insulin is ordered in units. For example, if the prescribed insulin dosage is 30 units, withdraw 30 units from a bottle of 100 units of insulin using a 100-unit calibrated insulin syringe (Figure 14D-11).

Insulin is administered subQ at a 45-, 60-, or 90-degree angle into the subQ tissue. The subQ absorption rate of insulin is slower because there are fewer blood vessels in the fatty tissue than in muscular tissue. The angle for administering insulin depends on the amount of fatty tissue. For an obese person, the angle may be 90 degrees; for a very thin person, the angle may be 45 to 60 degrees.

Types of Insulins

Insulins are clear (regular or crystalline insulin) and cloudy (NPH) because of the substance protamine, which is used to prolong the action of insulin in the body. Only clear (regular) insulin can be given IV as well as subQ. The source of insulin is human (Humulin).

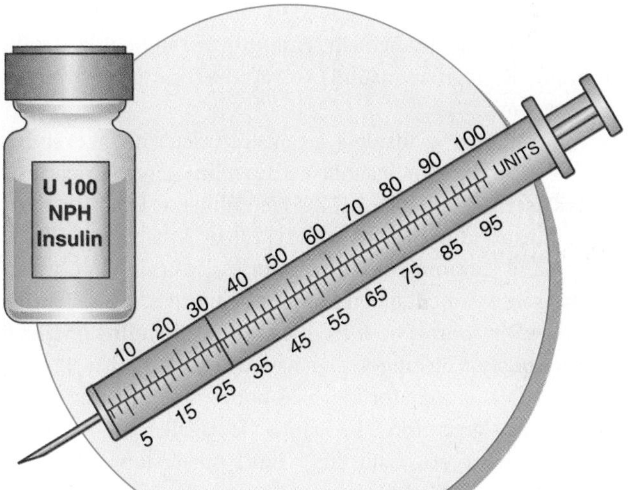

FIGURE 14D–11 Bottle of U 100 insulin and a U 100 calibrated insulin syringe. (From Kee JL, Marshall SM: *Clinical calculations,* ed. 7, St. Louis, 2013, Elsevier.)

Insulin is categorized as rapid-acting, fast-acting, intermediate- acting, long-acting, and commercial premixed insulin (see Figure 14D-12). The first rapid-acting insulin, Humalog (lispro insulin), was approved for use in 1996. Lispro and the new rapid-acting insulins, Aspart and Apidra, act faster than regular insulin and thus can be administered 5 to 15 minutes before mealtime, whereas regular insulin is given 30 minutes before meals. Rapid-acting insulins can become effective within 5 to 15 minutes of injection and last 3 to 5 hours. Lispro insulin (Humalog) is formed by reversing two amino acids in human regular insulin (Humulin R). Aspart insulin (NovoLog) is an analog of human insulin with a rapid onset. It is structured identically to human insulin except for one amino acid. Apidra (glulisine insulin), like Aspart insulin, is a synthetic analog of natural human insulin. **Rapid-acting (Humalog, Aspart, Apidra) and fast-acting (Humulin R) regular insulin can be given both intravenously and subcutaneously. Intermediate-acting and long-acting insulins can *only* be administered subcutaneously.**

Fast-acting insulin (regular or Humulin R insulin) is also clear but takes longer to start working compared with rapid-acting insulins. It is administered 15 to 30 minutes before meals and is effective for 6 to 8 hours. It is usually given before the meal, but it is sometimes given during or after the meal. Humulin R and Novolin R are brand names for fast-acting human insulin.

Intermediate-acting insulin (NPH, Humulin N, Novolin N) is administered 30 minutes before the meal (breakfast) and becomes effective in 1 to 2 hours. Its duration of action in the body is 12 to 18 hours. This type of insulin contains protamine, which prolongs the action in the body. It is cloudy because of the protamine added to the regular insulin. It can *only* be given subcutaneously. Humulin N can be mixed with Humulin R (regular insulin) or rapid-acting insulin in the same syringe.

The long-acting insulins are insulin determir (Levemir), an analog of human insulin, and insulin glargine (Lantus). Lantus is the first long-acting recombinant DNA (rDNA) human insulin for patients with type 1 or 2 diabetes mellitus. Lantus and Levemir are clear, colorless insulins that are to be given *only* subcutaneously and *not* intravenously. **Lantus and Levemir *cannot* be mixed with other insulins or given intravenously.** The long-acting insulin acts within 1 to 2 hours and lasts in the body for 18 to 24 hours. The Levemir vial is tall and has a green top. The Lantus vial is taller and narrower than the other types of insulin. It has a purple top and purple print on the label. Levemir is usually administered in the evening or at bedtime; however, it can be administered once or twice a day subcutaneously. Lantus is usually administered at bedtime, and the incidence of nocturnal hypoglycemia is not common. Some patients report more pain at the injection site with long-acting insulins than with Humulin N or NPH insulin.

The use of commercially premixed combination insulins has become popular for patients with diabetes who mix fast-acting and intermediate-acting insulins. Examples are two groups: the rapid-acting and intermediate-acting insulins are Novolog mix 70/30 and Humalog mix 75/25. The fast-acting and intermediate-acting insulins are Humulin 70/30, Novolin 70/30, and Humulin 50/50 (see Figure 14D-12). They are available in vials or pens that resemble a fountain pen (Figures 14D-12 and 14D-13). Some patients need less than 30 units of Humulin R and more Humulin N, so these combinations of insulins cannot be used. They must mix their insulins according to the prescribed units of insulin.

Mixing Insulins

Regular insulin is frequently mixed with insulin containing protamine (NPH, Humulin N). The following is an example of a method for mixing insulin. Remember that Lantus and Levemir insulins cannot be mixed with regular insulin.

EXAMPLE

Order: regular insulin 10 units and Humulin N insulin 35 units subQ every day at 7:00 AM

Available: regular insulin 100 units/mL and Humulin N insulin 100 units/mL. Insulin syringe: 100 units/mL

METHOD

1. Clean the rubber tops of the insulin bottles.
2. Draw up 35 units of air, and inject into the Humulin N insulin bottle. Avoid letting the needle contact the Humulin N insulin solution. Withdraw the needle.
3. Draw up 10 units of air, and inject into the regular insulin bottle.
4. First, withdraw 10 units of regular insulin. Regular insulin is always drawn up first.
5. Insert needle into Humulin N bottle, and withdraw 35 units of Humulin N insulin. The total is 45 units.
6. Administer the two insulins immediately after mixing. Do *not* allow the insulin mixture to stand, because unpredicted physical changes may occur.

Insulin pumps are discussed in Chapter 52.

INTRAMUSCULAR INJECTIONS

Muscle has more blood vessels than fatty tissue, so medications given by **intramuscular (IM)** injection are absorbed more rapidly than those given by subQ injection. The volume of solution for an IM injection is 0.5 to 3 mL, with the average being 1 to 2 mL. A volume of drug solution greater than 3 mL causes increased muscle tissue displacement and possible tissue damage. Occasionally 5 mL of selected drugs, such as magnesium sulfate, may be injected into a large muscle, such as the dorsogluteal. A dose greater than 3 mL is usually divided and given at two different sites.

The needle gauges for IM injections are 19 and 20 for thick solutions and 20 and 21 for thin solutions. IM injections are administered at a 90-degree angle. The needle length depends on the amount of adipose (fat) and muscle tissue; the average needle length is 1½ inches.

The discussion on IM injections is divided into three subsections: (1) drug solutions for injection, (2) powdered drug

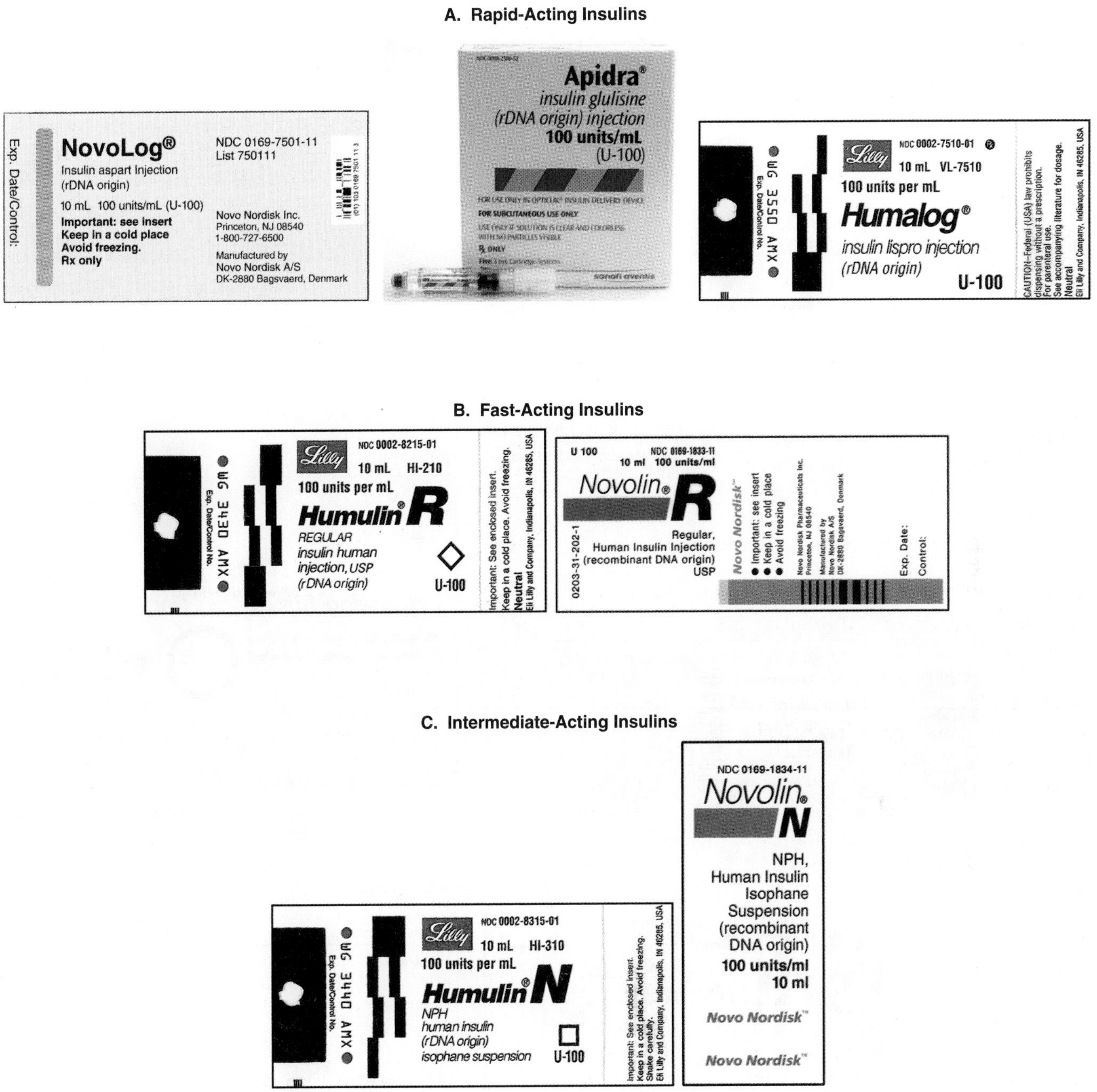

FIGURE 14D–12 Types of Insulin. **A,** Rapid-acting insulins. **B,** Fast-acting insulins. **C,** Intermediate-acting insulins.

Continued

reconstitution, and (3) mixing injectable drugs. An example is given for each subsection, and practice problems follow.

Sites of IM injections are shown in Chapter 13.

Drug Solutions for Injection

Commercially premixed drug solutions are stored in vials and ampules for ready use. The drug label on the container gives the drug dose by weight and its equivalent in milliliters.

Powdered Drug Reconstitution

Certain drugs lose their potency in liquid form; therefore manufacturers package these drugs in powdered form. They are reconstituted using a **diluent** (bacteriostatic water or saline) before administration. The drug label or the instructional insert (accompanying pamphlet) frequently gives the type and amount of diluent to use. If the type and amount

D. Long-Acting Insulin

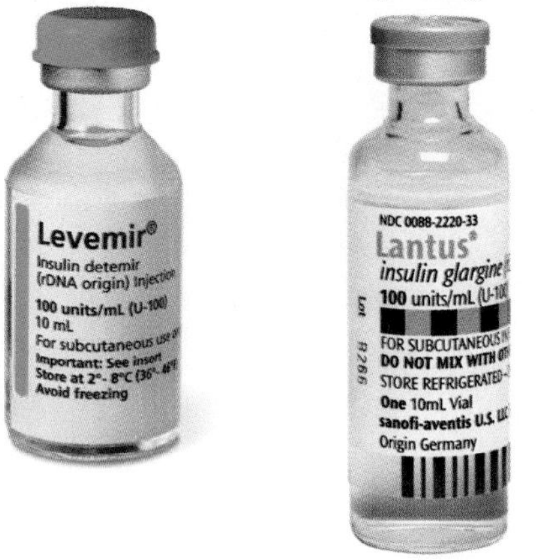

E. Combinations

E1. Rapid- and Intermediate-Acting Insulins

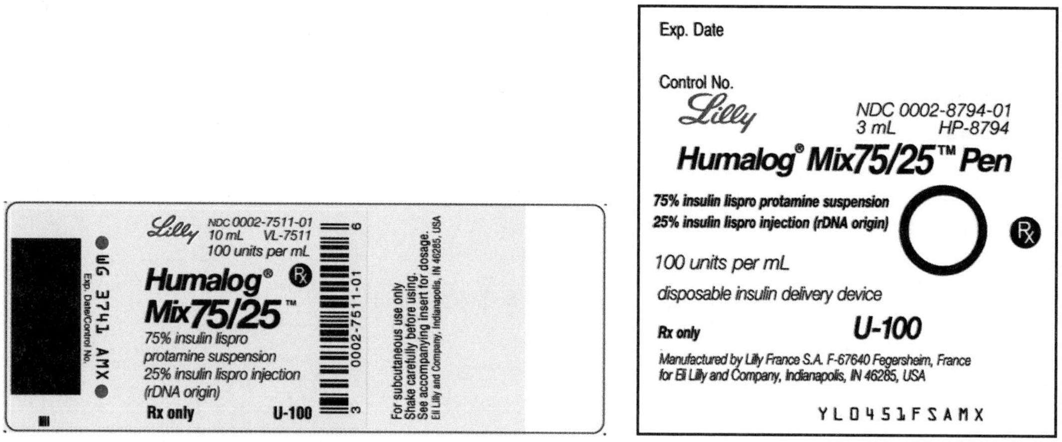

E2. Fast- and Intermediate-Acting Insulins

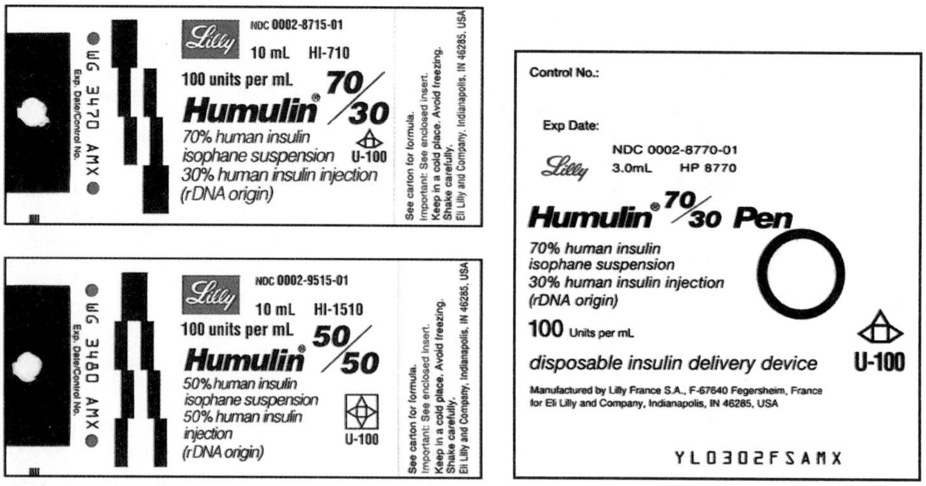

FIGURE 14D–12, cont'd **D,** Long-acting insulin. **E,** Combinations. *E-1,* Rapid and intermediate-acting insulins. *E-2,* Fast- and intermediate-acting insulins. (From Kee JL, Marshall SM: *Clinical calculations,* ed. 7, St. Louis, 2013, Elsevier.)

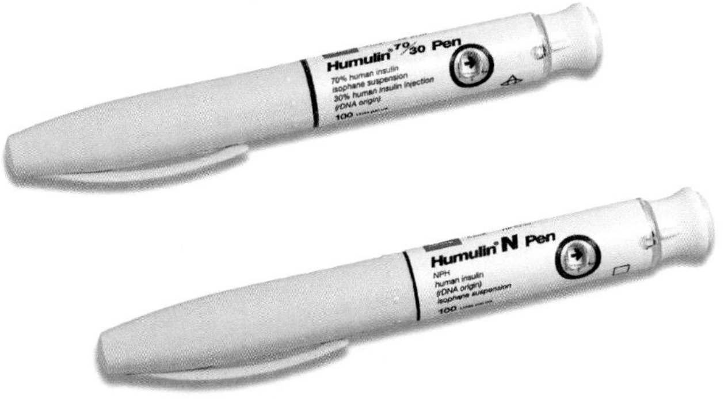

FIGURE 14D–13 Insulin pens. (From Eli Lilly and Company, Indianapolis, Indiana.)

PRACTICE PROBLEM 3

Insulins

Indicate on the insulin syringe the amount of insulin that should be withdrawn for each type of insulin.

1. Order: NPH insulin 45 units subQ

   Available: NPH insulin 100 units/mL and insulin syringe 100 units/mL

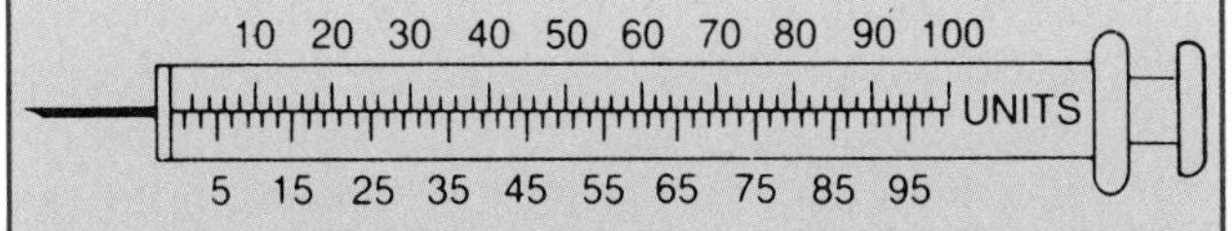

2. Order: regular insulin 15 units and Humulin N insulin 25 units subQ

   Available: regular insulin 100 units/mL and Humulin N insulin 100 units/mL, and insulin syringe 100 units/mL

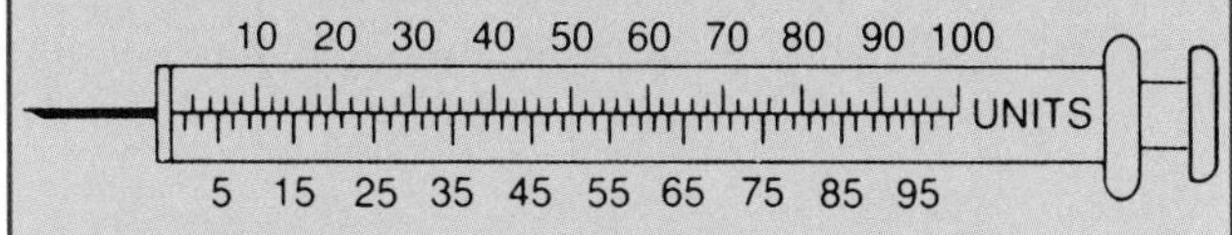

3. Order: regular insulin 6 units and Humulin N insulin 40 units

   Available: regular insulin 100 units/mL and Humlin N insulin 100 units/mL, and insulin syringe 100 units/mL

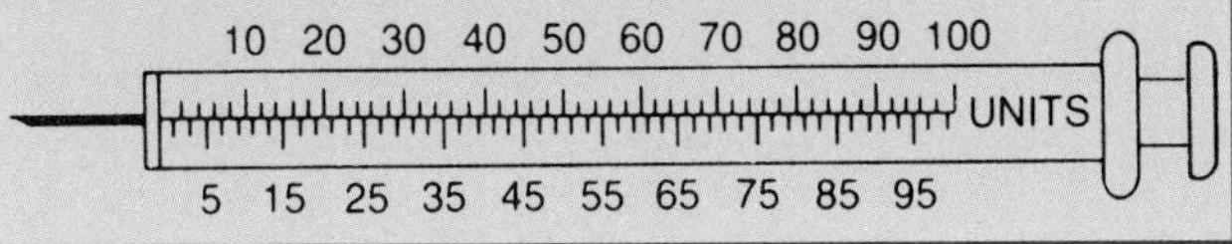

of diluent are not on the drug label or in the instructional insert, contact the pharmacist.

EXAMPLE

Order: gentamicin (Garamycin) 50 mg IM

Available: gentamicin 80 mg/2 mL in a vial

a. BF: $\frac{D}{H} \times V = \frac{50}{80} \times 2 = \frac{100}{80} = 1.25 \text{ mL}$

b. RP: $H : V :: D : x$

$$80 \text{ mg} : 2 \text{ mL} :: 50 \text{ mg} : x \text{ mL}$$

$$80x = 100$$

$$x = \frac{100}{80} = 1.25 \text{ mL}$$

c. FE: $\frac{H}{V} = \frac{D}{x}$ $\frac{80 \text{ mg}}{2 \text{ mL}} = \frac{50 \text{ mg}}{x}$

$$80x = 100$$

$$(\text{cross-multiply})\ x = 1.25 \text{ mL}$$

d. DA: $\text{mL} = \frac{2 \text{ mL} \times 50 \not{\text{mg}}}{80 \not{\text{mg}} \times 1} = \frac{100}{80} = 1.25 \text{ mL}$

Usually manufacturers determine the amount of diluent to mix with the drug powder to yield 1 to 2 mL/dose. The powdered drug occupies space; therefore the volume of the drug solution is increased. Once the powdered drug has been reconstituted, the unused drug solution should be dated and initialed on the drug label. Unused drug solutions in vials are refrigerated and may be used for 48 hours to 1 week according to the manufacturer's recommendation. Unused drug solutions in ampules are discarded.

Mixing Injectable Drugs

Drugs mixed together in the same syringe must be compatible to prevent precipitation. To determine drug compatibility, check drug reference texts or with a pharmacist. When in doubt about compatibility, do *not* mix drugs.

The three methods used for mixing drugs are (1) mixing two drugs in the same syringe from two vials, (2) mixing two drugs in the same syringe from one vial and one ampule, and (3) mixing two drugs in a prefilled cartridge from a vial.

Method 1: Mixing Two Drugs in the Same Syringe from Two Vials

1. Draw air into the syringe to equal the amount of solution to be withdrawn from the first vial, and inject the air into the first vial. Do not allow the needle to come into contact with the solution. Remove the needle.

EXAMPLE

Order: cefotetan disodium (Cefotan) 0.5 g IM, q12h

Available (NOTE: Circular states to add 2.6 mL of diluent to yield 3 mL of drug.):

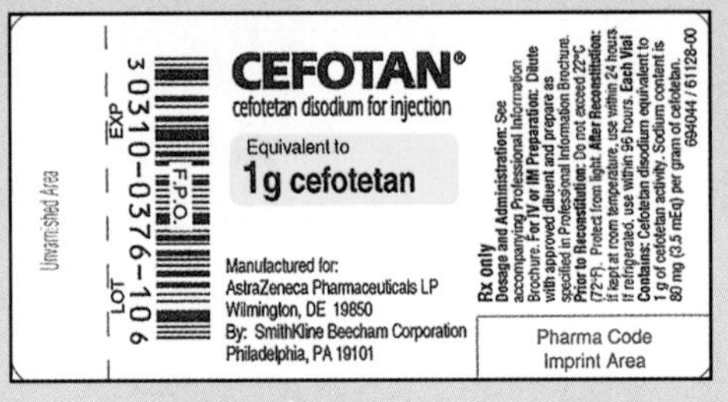

Add 2.6 mL of diluent; 1 g of cefotetan disodium = 3 mL

BF: $\frac{D}{H} \times V = \frac{0.5}{1} \times 3 \text{ mL} = 1.5 \text{ mL}$

$= 0.5$ g of cefotetan disodium

DA: $\text{mL} = \frac{3 \text{ mL} \times 0.5 \not{g}}{1 \not{g} \times 1} = 1.5 \text{ mL}$

No conversion is needed.

SECTION 14D

2. Draw air into the syringe to equal the amount of solution to be withdrawn from the second vial. Invert the second vial, and inject the air. Withdraw the desired amount of solution from the second vial.
3. Change the needle, unless the entire volume in the first vial will be used.
4. Invert the first vial, and withdraw the desired amount of solution.

Method 2: Mixing Two Drugs in the Same Syringe from One Vial and One Ampule

1. Inject air into the vial.
2. Remove the desired amount of solution from the vial.
3. Withdraw the desired amount of solution from the ampule.

Method 3: Mixing Two Drugs in a Prefilled Cartridge from a Vial

1. Check the drug dose and the amount of solution in the prefilled cartridge. If a smaller dose is needed, or if a prefilled drug syringe is used, expel the excess solution.
2. Draw air into the cartridge to equal the amount of solution to be withdrawn from the vial. Invert the vial, and inject the air.
3. Withdraw the desired amount of solution from the vial. Be sure that the needle remains in the fluid, and do not take more solution than needed.

Mixing Drugs in the Same Syringe

Order: meperidine (Demerol) 25 mg and atropine sulfate 0.4 mg IM

Available: meperidine in a Tubex cartridge labeled 50 mg/mL

Atropine sulfate in a multidose vial labeled 0.4 mg/mL

How many milliliters of each drug should be given, and how are they mixed? _____

1. Meperidine dose

a. $\frac{D}{H} \times V = \frac{25}{50} \times 1 = \frac{25}{50} = 0.5 \text{ mL}$

b. $H : V :: D : x$

$50 \text{ mg} : 1 \text{ mL} :: 25 \text{ mg} : x \text{ mL}$

$$50x = 25$$

$$x = \frac{1}{2} = 0.5 \text{ mL}$$

2. Atropine dose:

The label indicates 0.4 mg = 1 mL.

Answer: Give meperidine 0.5 mL and atropine 1 mL.

Procedure

Mix two drugs in the cartridge, with one drug from a vial and the other drug in the prefilled cartridge.

1. Check the drug dose and volume on the prefilled cartridge.
2. Expel 0.5 mL and any excess drug solution (meperidine) from the cartridge (0.5 mL remains in the cartridge). Have another nurse witness the waste of a narcotic.
3. Draw 1 mL of air into the cartridge, and inject the air into the vial that contains the atropine.
4. Withdraw 1 mL of atropine from the vial into the meperidine solution in the cartridge.

PRACTICE PROBLEM 4

Intramuscular Injections

1. Order: cefazolin (Ancef) 500 mg IM, q6h

Available:

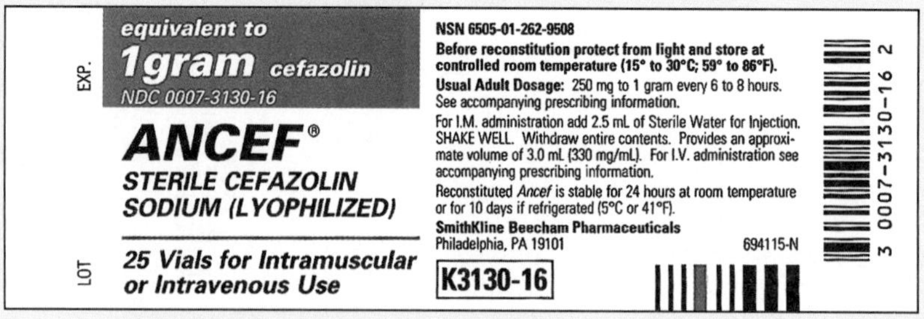

How many milliliters should be given? _____

SECTION 14D

2. Order: atropine sulfate 0.3 mg IM, STAT

   Available: atropine sulfate

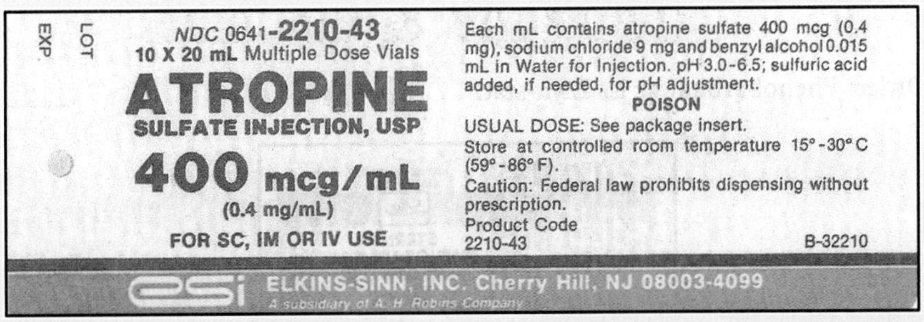

   How may milliliters of atropine should be given? ______

3. Order: oxacillin 250 mg IM q6h

   Available: (Drug label states to add 2.7 mL of diluent = 3 mL of drug solution)

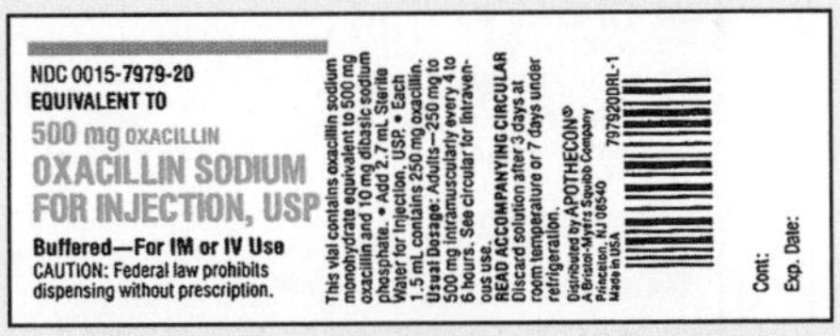

   How many milliliters should be given? ______ After the drug is reconstituted, how long can it be refrigerated? ______

4. Order: digoxin 0.25 mg IM daily

   Available: digoxin 0.5 mg/2 mL

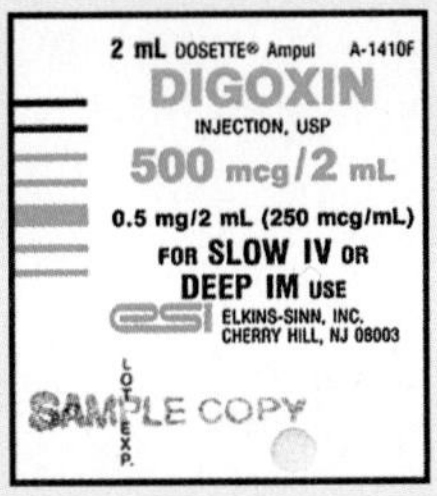

   How many milliliters should be given? ______ What should be done with the excess digoxin solution? ______ (Usually parenteral digoxin is administered IV.)

5. Order: chlorpromazine (Thorazine) 50 mg IM, STAT

   Available:

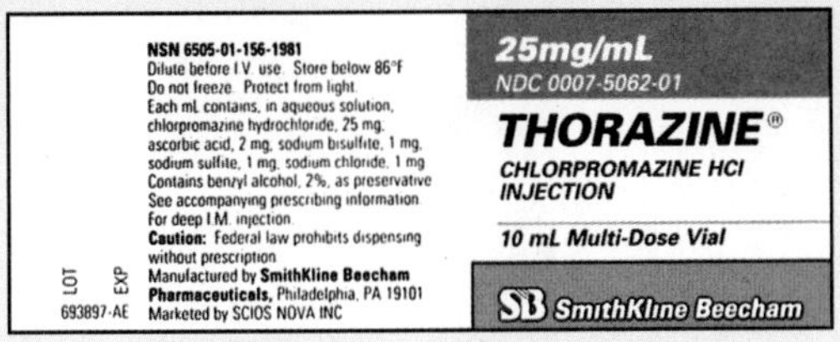

   How many milliliters should be given? ______ Can the vial be used again? ______

6. Order: meperidine 60 mg and hydroxyzine (Vistaril) 25 mg, IM. These two drugs are compatible.

   Available: Hydroxyzine 100 mg/2 mL in vial

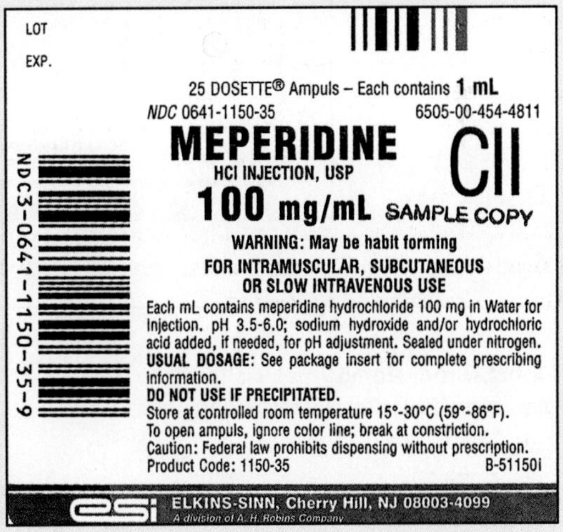

   How many milliliters of meperidine and how many milliliters of hydroxyzine should be given? ______

   Explain how the two drugs would be mixed.

7. Order: morphine SO_4 6 mg IM q4h, PRN

   Available:

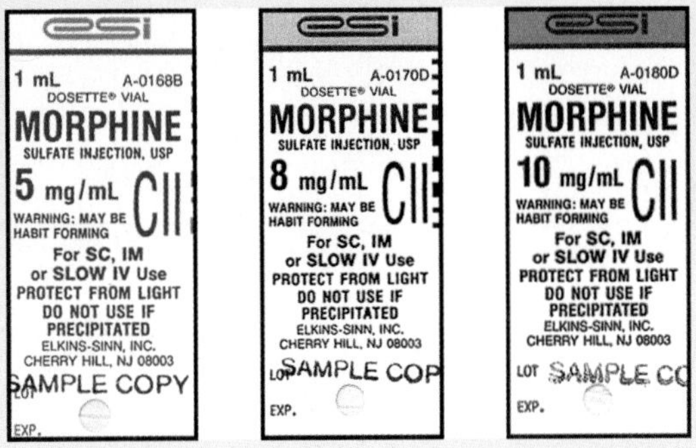

   a. Which morphine vial should be selected? ______ Explain your answer. ______

   b. How many milliliters of morphine should be administered per dose? ______ Explain your answer. ______

Continued

8. Order: cefotaxime NA (Claforan) 750 mg IM, b.i.d.

   Available:

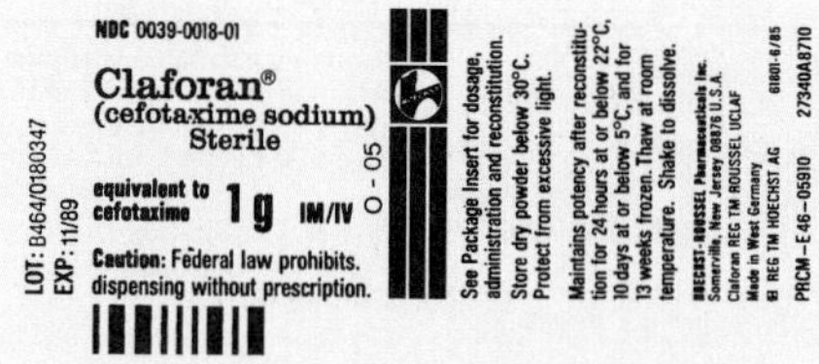

   Drug label: Pamphlet states to add 3 mL of diluent equal 3.4 mL

   a. 1 g = ______ mg

   b. How many milligrams (mg) should the patient receive per day? ______

   c. How many milliliters (mL) would you give per dose? ______

9. Order: diazepam (Valium) 6 mg IM, STAT, and repeat in 4 hours if necessary

   Available:

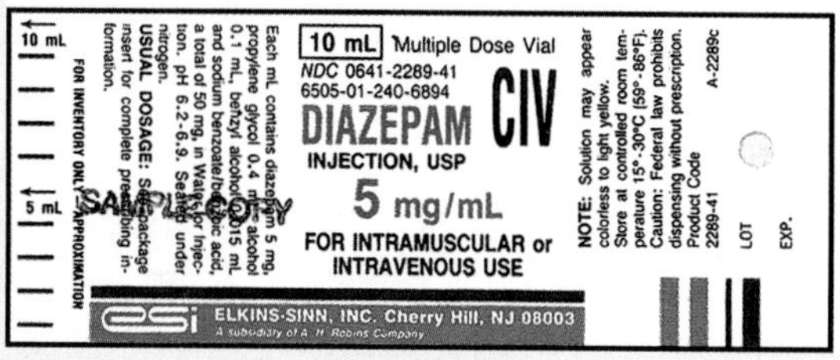

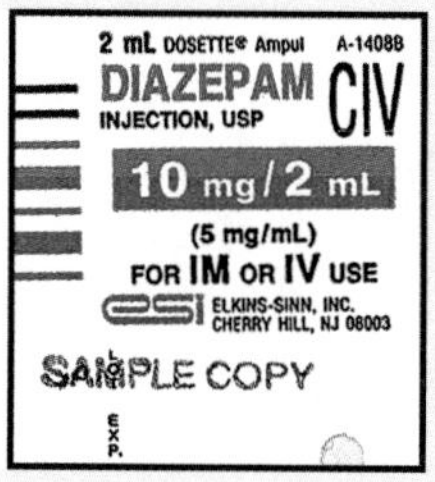

   a. Which ampule or vial of diazepam would you select? ______

   b. How many milliliters of diazepam should the patient receive? ______

Additional Dimensional Analysis (refer to Section 14B as needed)

10. Order: vitamin B_{12} (cyanocobalamin) 60 mcg IM, daily

    Available:

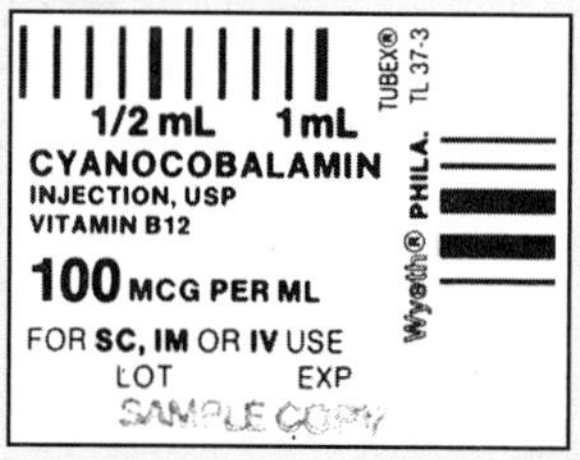

    Conversion factor: None (both are in micrograms).

    a. How many milliliters (mL) should the patient receive per day? ______

11. Order: Cefobid 500 mg IM, q12h

    Available (NOTE: Instructions state to add 1.6 mL of diluent to the vial; drug liquids in 1 g = 2 mL):

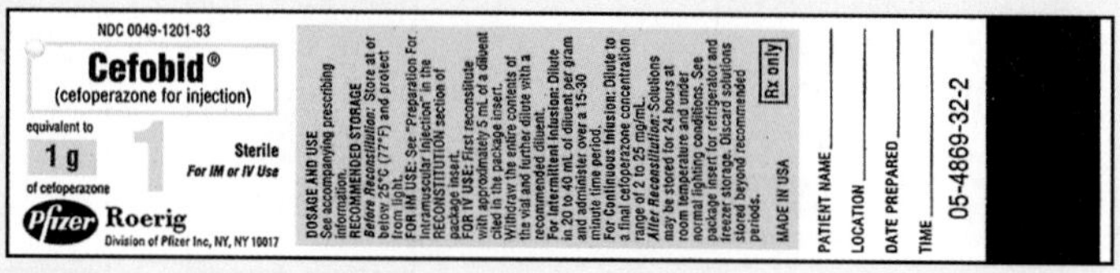

    Factors: 1 g = 2 mL (drug label and after reconstitution)

    Conversion factor: 1000 mg = 1 g

    How many milliliters should the patient receive per dose? ______

SECTION 14D

12. Order: meperidine (Demerol) 35 mg and promethazine (Phenergan) 10 mg, IM

Drugs available: meperidine 50 mg/mL in an ampule; promethazine 25 mg/mL in an ampule

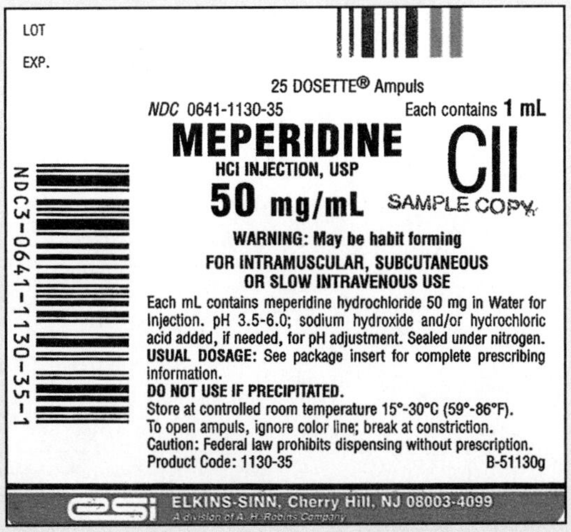

a. How many milliliters of meperidine would you give? ______

b. How many milliliters of promethazine would you give? ______

c. Explain how the two drugs would be mixed.

ANSWERS TO PRACTICE PROBLEMS

1 SYRINGES AND NEEDLES

1. 5-mL syringe
2. Tuberculin syringe (1 mL)
3. No, it should be discarded in the sink or toilet and witnessed by another RN or LPN, according to agency policy.
4. 21-gauge needle
5. 25-gauge needle
6. 20-gauge needle 1.5 ($1\frac{1}{2}$) inches in length

2 SUBCUTANEOUS INJECTIONS

1. 0.75 mL
2. Lovenox 0.2 mL for 20 mg
3. The drug label reads: 1.25 mL = 0.5 mg of atropine. Also, under the word "atropine," it reads 0.4 mg/mL

a. BF: $\frac{D}{H} \times V = \frac{0.5}{0.4} \times 1 = 1.25\,\text{mL}$

b. RP: H : V :: D : x

$$0.4\,\text{mg} : 1\,\text{mL} :: 0.5\,\text{mg} : x\,\text{mL}$$

$$0.4x = 0.5$$

$$x = \frac{0.5}{0.4} = 1.25\,\text{mL}$$

c. DA: $\text{mL} = \frac{1\,\text{mL} \times 0.5\,\cancel{\text{mg}}}{0.4\,\cancel{\text{mg}} \times 1} = 1.25\,\text{mL}$

4. A tuberculin syringe should be used.

a. BF: $\frac{D}{H} \times V = \frac{0.2}{1.0} \times 1 = 1.0\overline{)0.20}^{\,2.0} = 0.2\,\text{mL}$

b. RP: H : V :: D : x

$$1\,\text{mg} : 1\,\text{mL} :: 0.2\,\text{mg} : x\,\text{mL}$$

$$1.0x = 0.2$$

$$x = \frac{0.2}{1.0} = 0.2\,\text{mL}$$

Answer: epinepherine 0.2 mg = 0.2 mL

3 INSULINS

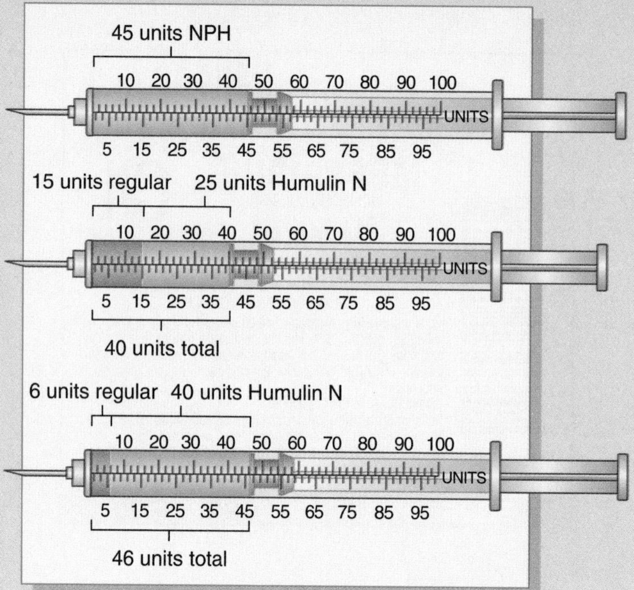

4 INTRAMUSCULAR INJECTIONS USING BASIC FORMULA, RATIO AND PROPORTION, FRACTIONAL EQUATION, OR DIMENSIONAL ANALYSIS

1. Instructions on the drug label read: Add 2.5 mL of sterile water. The drug solution equals 3.0 mL (drug powder is equal to 0.5 mL).

   Change 1 g to mg; 1 g = 1000 mg

   or Change 500 mg to g; 500 mg = 0.500 g (0.5 g)

   a. BF: $\frac{D}{H} \times V = \frac{0.5}{1\,g} \times 3\,mL = 1.5\,mL$

   b. RP: H : V :: D : x

   $1000\,mg : 3\,mL :: 500\,mg : x\,mL$

   $1000x = 1500$

   $x = 1.5\,mL$

   c. DA: $mL = \frac{3\,mL \times 1\,g \times \overset{1}{500\,mg}}{1\,g \times \underset{2}{1000\,mg} \times 1} = \frac{3}{2}$

   $= 1.5\,mL$

   Answer: cefazolin 500 mg = 1.5 mL

2. The atropine drug label is marked as 0.4 mg/mL. The approximate equivalent of 0.3 mg is 0.8 mL. If the 0.3 mg = 0.8 mL is unknown, the problem may be calculated using 0.4 mg = 1 mL

   BF: $\frac{D}{H} \times V = \frac{0.3}{0.4} \times 1 = \frac{0.3}{0.4} = 0.75$, or $0.8\,mL$

3. For oxacillin sodium, the drug label indicates that 2.7 mL of sterile water should be added to the vial containing 500 mg of drug. The total volume would be 3 mL.

   a. BF: $\frac{D}{H} \times V = \frac{250}{500} \times 3.0 = \frac{750}{500} = 1.5\,mL$

   b. FE: $\frac{H}{V} = \frac{D}{x}\ \frac{500\,mg}{3\,mL} = \frac{250\,mg}{x\,mL}$

   (cross-multiply) $500x = 750$

   $x = 1.5\,mL$

   c. DA: $mL = \frac{3\,mL \times \overset{1}{250\,mg}}{\underset{2}{500\,mg} \times 1} = 1.5\,mL$

4. BF: $\frac{D}{H} \times V = \frac{0.25}{0.50} \times 2 \times \frac{0.50}{0.50} = 1\,mL$

   Withdraw 1 mL from the ampule. Discard the remaining 1 mL of digoxin solution.

5. Thorazine 50 mg = 2 mL. Yes, the vial can be used for multiple doses.

6. Meperidine 60 mg = 0.6 mL; hydroxyzine 25 mg = 0.5 mL

   Meperidine

   BF: $\frac{D}{H} \times V = \frac{60}{100} \times 1 \times \frac{60}{100} = 0.6\,mL$

Hydroxyzine

$$\text{BF: } \frac{D}{H} \times V = \frac{25}{100} \times 2 \times \frac{50}{100} = 0.5\text{ mL}$$

Procedure

a. Withdraw 0.5 mL of hydroxyzine from the vial.

b. Meperidine is in a dosette ampule. Withdraw 0.6 mL of meperidine solution into the syringe containing hydroxyzine. Discard the balance of the solution in the ampule.

c. Total amount of the two drug solutions is 1.1 mL. Administer IM.

7. a. Morphine vials 8 mg/mL and 10 mg/mL. Morphine 5 mg/mL vial could not be used because it is a single-vial dose.

b. Morphine 8 mg/mL vial

$$\text{BF: } \frac{D}{H} \times V = \frac{6\,\cancel{mg}}{8\,\cancel{mg}} \times 1\text{ mL} = \frac{6}{8} = 0.75\text{ mL}$$

Morphine 10 mg/mL vial

$$\text{BF: } \frac{D}{H} \times V = \frac{6\,\cancel{mg}}{10\,\cancel{mg}} \times 1\text{ mL} = \frac{6}{10} = 0.6\text{ mL}$$

8. a. 1 g = 1000 mg

b. 750 mg × 2 (b.i.d.) = 1500 mg/day or 1.5 g/day

c. $$\frac{D}{H} \times V = \frac{\overset{3}{\cancel{750}}}{\underset{4}{\cancel{1000}}} \times 3.4\text{ mL} = \frac{3 \times 3.4}{4} = \frac{10.2}{4} = 2.55 \text{ or } 2.6\text{ mL of Claforan}$$

9. a. Either the ampule or the vial could be used. The diazepam 5 mg/mL is a multiple-dose vial that contains 10 mL of drug solution. The 10 mg/2 mL ampule is to be used one time; if not entirely used, it must be discarded.

$$\text{Vial: BF: } \frac{D}{H} \times V = \frac{6\,\cancel{mg}}{5\,\cancel{mg}} \times 1\text{ mL} = 1.2\text{ mL}$$

b. ***or***

Ampule: RP: H : V :: D : x

10 mg : 2 mL :: 6 mg : x mL

$10x = 12$

$x = 1.2$ mL

$$\text{Vial: DA: mL} = \frac{1\text{ mL} \times 6\,\cancel{mg}}{5\,\cancel{mg} \times 1} = \frac{6}{5} = 1.2\text{ mL}$$

$$\text{Ampule: FE: } \frac{H}{V} = \frac{D}{x} = \frac{10\text{ mg}}{2\text{ mL}} = \frac{6\text{ mg}}{x}$$

(cross-multiply) $10x = 12$

$x = 1.2$ mL

10. a. RP: H : V :: D : X

$100\text{ mcg} : 1\text{ mL} :: \overset{3}{\cancel{60}}\text{ mcg} : X$

$\underset{5}{\cancel{100}}\,X = 60$

X = 0.6 mL of cyanocobalamin

$$\text{DA: mL} = \frac{1 \times 60\text{ mcg}}{100\text{ mcg} \times 1} = \frac{3}{5} = 0.6\text{ mL of cyanocobalamin}$$

11. 1 mL per dose

$$\text{DA: mL} = \frac{2\text{ mL} \times 1\,\cancel{g} \times \overset{1}{\cancel{500}}\,\cancel{mg}}{1\,\cancel{g} \times \underset{2}{\cancel{1000}}\,\cancel{mg} \times 1} = \frac{2}{2} = 1\text{ mL}$$

12. a. meperidine:

$$\text{DA: mL} = \frac{1\text{ mL} \times \overset{7}{\cancel{35}}\,\cancel{mg}}{\underset{10}{\cancel{50}}\,\cancel{mg} \times 1} = \frac{7}{10} = 0.7\text{ mL}$$

b. promethazine

$$\text{DA: mL} = \frac{1\text{ mL} \times \overset{2}{\cancel{10}}\,\cancel{mg}}{\underset{5}{\cancel{25}}\,\cancel{mg} \times 1} = \frac{2}{5} = 0.4\text{ mL}$$

c. Procedure:

1. Obtain 0.7 mL of meperidine from the ampule and 0.4 mL of promethazine from the ampule.
2. Discard the remaining solutions within the ampules.

Section 14E: Calculations of Intravenous Fluids

OBJECTIVES

- Describe the differences between continuous intravenous infusion and intermittent intravenous infusion.
- Define macrodrip and microdrip sets, keep vein open (KVO), and to keep open (TKO).
- Calculate intravenous flow rate using one of the given formulas.
- Explain how intravenous drug solutions administered by secondary set are calculated.
- Differentiate between volumetric and nonvolumetric intravenous regulators and pump electronic regulators.

OUTLINE

KEY TERMS

Intravenous (IV) fluid therapy is used to administer fluids that contain water, dextrose, vitamins, electrolytes, and drugs. Today an increasing number of drugs are administered by the IV route for direct absorption and fast action. Some drugs are given by IV push (**bolus**). Many drugs administered IV irritate the veins, so these drugs are diluted in 50 to 100 mL of fluid. Other drugs are delivered in a large volume of fluid over a specific period, such as 4 to 8 hours.

Two methods are used to administer IV fluids and drugs: continuous IV infusion and intermittent IV infusion. Continuous IV infusion replaces fluid loss, maintains fluid balance, and serves as a vehicle for drug administration. Intermittent IV infusion is used primarily to give IV drugs.

Nurses have an important role in the preparation and administration of IV solutions and IV drugs. The nursing functions and responsibilities during drug preparation include the following:

- Knowing IV sets and their drop factors
- Calculating IV flow rates
- Mixing and diluting drugs in IV fluids
- Gathering equipment
- Knowing the drugs and the expected and untoward reactions

Nursing responsibilities continue with assessment of the patient for effectiveness and untoward effects of the therapy and assessment of the IV site.

CONTINUOUS INTRAVENOUS ADMINISTRATION

When IV solutions are required, the health care provider orders the type and amount of IV solution in liters over a 24-hour period or in milliliters per hour. The nurse calculates the IV flow rate according to the drop factor, the amount of fluids to be administered, and the time period.

Intravenous Sets

Various IV infusion sets are marketed by Abbott, Cutter, McGaw, and Travenol. The **drop factor**, the number of drops per milliliter, is normally printed on the packaging cover of the IV set. A set that delivers large drops per milliliter (10 to 20 gtt/mL) is called a **macrodrip set,** and one that delivers small drops per milliliter (60 gtt/mL) is called a **microdrip (minidrip) set.** Examples of drop factors, macrodrip sets, and microdrip sets are listed in Table 14E-1.

TABLE 14E-1 INTRAVENOUS SETS

MANUFACTURER	DROPS (gtt/mL)
Macrodrip Sets	
Abbott	15
Cutter	20
McGaw	15
Travenol	10
Microdrip Sets	
Travenol	60
Minidrip sets	60

In most instances, the nurse has the choice of using either the macrodrip or microdrip set. If the IV rate is to infuse at 100 mL/h or more, the macrodrip set is usually used. If the infusion rate is less than (<) 100 mL/h or the patient is a child, the microdrip set is preferred. Slow drip rates of <100 mL/h make macrodrip adjustment difficult.

At times, IV fluids are given at a slow rate to **keep vein open (KVO),** also called **to keep open (TKO)**. The reasons for ordering KVO include a suspected or potential emergency situation for rapid administration of fluids and drugs, and the need for an open line to give IV drugs at specified hours. For KVO, a microdrip set (60 gtt/mL) and a 250-mL IV bag may be used. KVO is usually regulated to deliver 10 mL/h.

Calculating Intravenous Flow Rate

Three different methods may be used to calculate IV flow rate (drops per minute, gtt/min). The nurse should select one method, memorize it, and consistently use it to calculate IV flow rate. Method II is usually the preferred method.

Method I: Three-Step

1. $\dfrac{\text{Amount of solution}}{\text{Hours to administer}} = \text{milliliters per hour (mL/h)}$
2. Milliliters per hour = milliliters per minute (mL/min)
3. Milliliters per minute × drops per milliliter of IV set = drops/minute (gtt/min)

Method II: Two-Step

1. $\dfrac{\text{Amount of fluid}}{\text{Hours to administer}} = \text{milliliters per hour (mL/h)}$
2. $\dfrac{\text{Milliliters per hour} \times \text{Drops per milliliter (IV set)}}{60 \text{ minutes}}$
   $= \text{drops/minute (gtt/min)}$

Method III: One-Step

1. $\dfrac{\text{Amount of fluid} \times \text{Drops per milliliter (IV set)}}{\text{Hours to administer} \times \text{Minutes per hours (60)}}$
   $= \text{drops/minute (gtt/min)}$

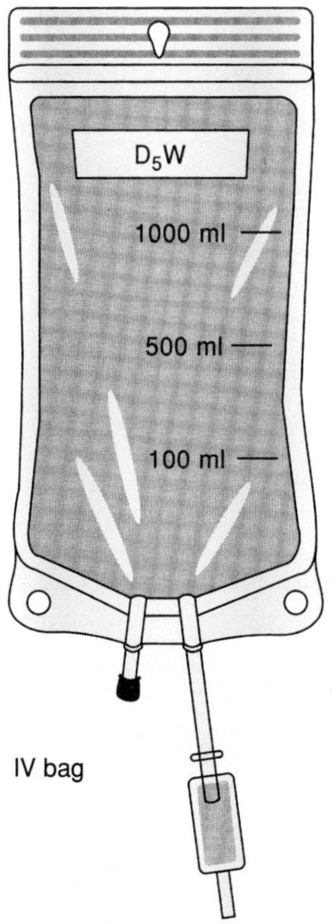

FIGURE 14E–1 Intravenous bag. (From Kee JL, Marshall SM: *Clinical calculations,* ed. 7, St. Louis, 2013, Elsevier.)

Mixing Drugs for Continuous Intravenous Administration

Drugs such as potassium chloride and vitamins are frequently added to the IV solution bag for continuous IV infusion. Drugs should be added to the bag or bottle immediately before administering the IV fluid. Inject the drug into the rubber stopper on the IV bag or bottle, and rotate the bag several times to ensure that the drug is dispersed throughout the solution (Figure 14E-1). *Do not add the drug while the infusion is running unless the bag is rotated.* A drug solution injected into an upright infusing IV solution concentrates the drug into the lower portion of the IV bag, preventing it from dispersing evenly. The patient receives a concentrated drug solution, which may be harmful, for example, if the drug is potassium chloride. If drugs are injected into the IV bag before use, the bag should be refrigerated to maintain drug potency.

Commercially prepared IV solutions contain various nutrients (e.g., dextrose) and electrolytes. The commonly used solutions are 5% dextrose in water (D_5W), normal saline (NSS), one-half normal saline (½ NSS), and lactated Ringer's (LR). Abbreviations for these types of solutions are listed in Table 14E-2.

INTERMITTENT INTRAVENOUS ADMINISTRATION

Some IV drugs are prescribed to be administered three to six times a day in a small volume of IV fluid (50 to 100 mL of

TABLE 14E-2 ABBREVIATIONS OF SOLUTIONS

INTRAVENOUS SOLUTIONS	ABBREVIATIONS
5% Dextrose in water	D_5W, 5% D/W
10% Dextrose in water	$D_{10}W$, 10% D/W
0.9% Sodium chloride, normal saline solution	0.9% NaCl, NSS
0.45% Sodium chloride, ½ normal saline solution	0.45% NaCl, ½ NSS
5% Dextrose in 0.9% sodium chloride	D_5NSS, 5% D/NSS, 5% D/0.9% NaCl
5% Dextrose in 0.45% sodium chloride or 5% Dextrose in ½ normal saline solution	D_5/½ NSS, 5% D/½ NSS
Lactated Ringer's solution	LR

D_5W or NSS 0.9% sodium chloride). The drug solution is usually infused over a period of 15 minutes to 1 hour. Separate tubing for IV drugs, the **secondary IV line set,** is inserted into a port (rubber stopper) of the IV connector on the continuous, or **primary IV line set.** This type of IV administration is called *intermittent IV therapy.*

EXAMPLE

Order: 1000 mL of 5% dextrose in water (D_5W) with potassium chloride (KCl) 20 mEq in 8 h

Available: 1000 mL of 5% dextrose in water. Potassium chloride 40 mEq/20 mL ampule. IV set labeled 10 gtt/mL

Drug calculation: Use the basic formula, the ratio-and-proportion method, fractional equation, or dimensional analysis (refer to Section 14B if needed).

a. BF: $\frac{D}{H} \times V = \frac{20}{40} \times 20 = \frac{400}{40} = 10 \text{ mL of KCl}$

b. RP: H : V :: D : x

40 mEq : 20 mL :: 20 mEq : x mL

$$40x = 400$$

$$x = 10 \text{ mL of KCl}$$

c. DA: $\text{mL} = \frac{20 \text{ mL} \times \overset{1}{\cancel{20}} \text{ mEq}}{\underset{2}{\cancel{40}} \text{ mEq} \times 1} = 10 \text{ mL of KCl}$

The calculation of IV flow rate is described using the three methods outlined previously. However, it is strongly recommended that only one method be selected to determine IV flow rate.

Method I

1. $\frac{1000 \text{ mL}}{8 \text{ h}} = 125 \text{ mL/h}$
2. $\frac{125 \text{ mL}}{60 \text{ min}} = 2.0 - 2.1 \text{ mL/h}$
3. $2.1 \times 10 = 21$ gtt/min

Method II

1. $1000 \div 8 = 125$ mL/h
2. $\frac{125 \text{ mL/h} \times \overset{1}{\cancel{10}} \text{ gtt/mL}}{\underset{6}{\cancel{60}} \text{ min}} = \frac{125}{6} = 20 - 21 \text{ gtt/min}$

Method III

1. $\frac{1000 \text{ mL} \times \overset{1}{\cancel{10}} \text{ gtt/mL}}{8 \text{ h} \times \underset{6}{\cancel{60}} \text{ min}} = \frac{1000}{48} = 20 \text{ or } 21 \text{ gtt/min}$

PRACTICE PROBLEM 1

Continuous Intravenous Flow Rates

Select one of the three methods to calculate IV flow rate.

1. Order: 1000 mL of D_5/½ NSS to infuse over 12 h

   Available: macrodrip set with 10 gtt/mL and a microdrip set with 60 gtt/mL
   a. Should a macrodrip or microdrip IV set be used? ______
   b. Calculate the IV flow rate in drops per minute according to the IV set that was selected. ______
2. Order: 3 L of IV solutions to infuse over 24 h

   1 liter of D_5W and 2 liters of D_5/½ NSS
   a. One liter is equal to how many milliliters? ______
   b. Each liter should infuse for how many hours? ______
   c. The institution uses a set with a drop factor of 15 gtt/mL. How many drops per minute should the patient receive? ______
3. Order: 250 mL of D_5W to KVO
   a. What type of IV set should be used? ______
   b. Determine how many drops per minute the patient should receive. ______
4. Order: 1000 mL of D_5/½ NSS, 1 vial of multiple vitamin (MVI), and 10 mEq of KCl (potassium chloride) in 10 h

   Available: 1000 mL of D_5/½ NSS; MVI: 1 vial; KCl 20 mEq/20-mL vial. Macrodrip set: 15 gtt/mL; microdrip set 60 gtt/mL
   a. How many milliliters of KCl should be injected into the IV bag? ______
   b. How many drops per minute should the patient receive using the macrodrip set and the microdrip set?

Secondary Intravenous Sets without IV Pumps

Two IV sets available to administer IV drugs are (1) the calibrated cylinder (chamber) with tubing, such as the Buretrol, Volutrol, and Soluset; and (2) the secondary IV set, which is similar to a regular IV set except the tubing is shorter (Figure 14E-2). The secondary IV line set is used mostly to infuse small volumes—50, 100, 250 mL and for children's IV solution. The chamber of the Buretrol, Volutrol, and Soluset holds 150 mL of solution. Medication is injected into the chamber and then diluted with solution. These methods of administering IV drugs are referred to as **IV piggyback (IVPB).**

Drugs for IV infusion are diluted before infusion. Clinical agencies frequently have their own protocols for dilutions; the

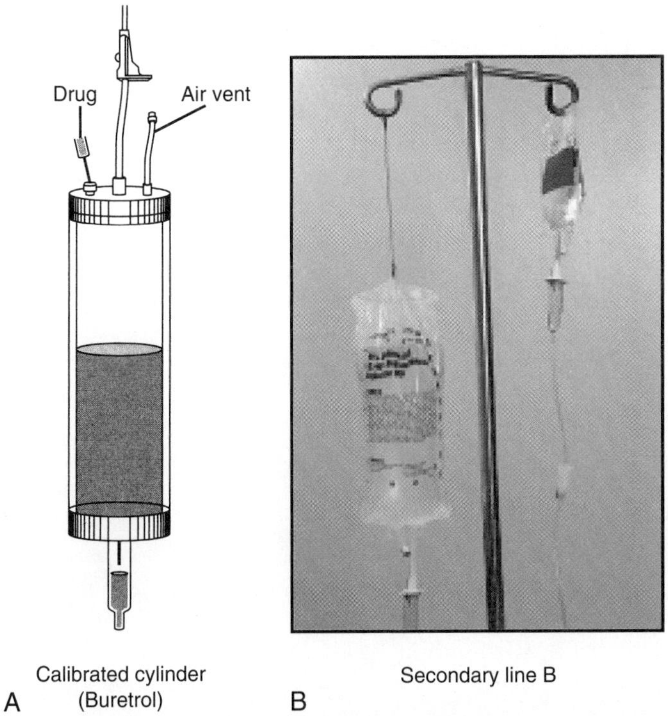

FIGURE 14E–2 **A,** The calibrated cylinder (Buretrol) is an example of a secondary intravenous (IV) device. **B,** An example of a secondary line containing medication. The primary IV bag is 6 inches below the secondary IV bag. (**A,** From Kee JL, Marshall SM: *Clinical calculations,* ed. 7, St. Louis, 2013, Elsevier. **B,** From Leahy JM, Kizilay PE: *Foundations of nursing practice: a nursing process approach,* Philadelphia, 1998, Saunders.)

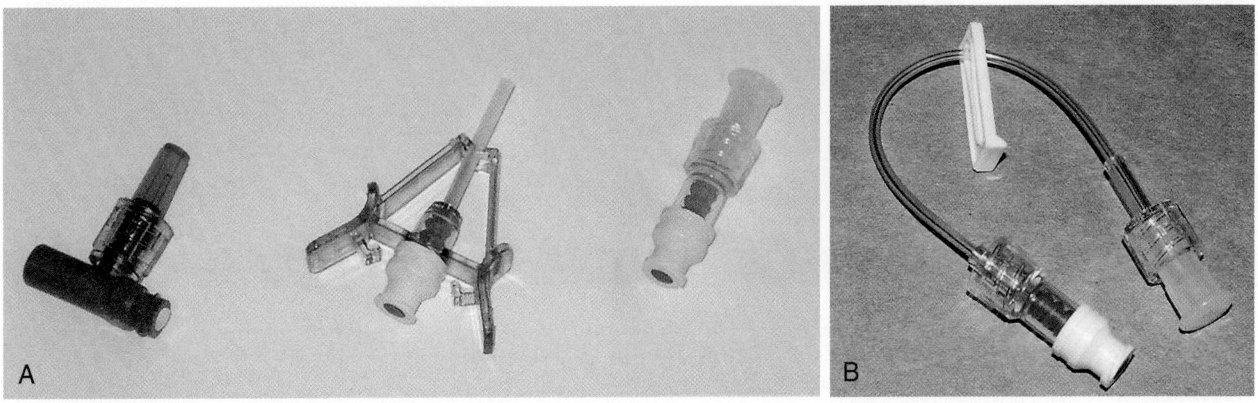

FIGURE 14E–3 Needleless infusion devices. Medication in a needleless syringe can be inserted into a needleless infusion device. (From Kee JL, Marshall SM: *Clinical calculations,* ed. 7, St. Louis, 2013, Elsevier.)

pharmacist and the drug circular are also resources for infusion guidelines. Guidelines and protocols help to prevent drug and fluid incompatibility.

The current trend to IV medication administration is the use of premixed IV drugs in 50- to 500-mL bags. These premixed IV medications are prepared by the manufacturer or by the hospital pharmacy. The problems of contamination and drug errors are decreased with the use of premixed IV medications. Each IV drug bag has separate tubing to prevent admixture. The cost is higher, but the risk is lower with the use of premixed IV drug bags. Because not all medication can be premixed in the solution, nurses will continue to prepare some drugs for IV administration.

Note: When using a calibrated cylinder such as the Buretrol, add 15 mL of IV solution to flush the drug out of the IV line after the drug infusion is completed. The flush volume is added to the patient's intake. Check hospital policy.

INTERMITTENT INFUSION ADAPTERS/DEVICES

When continuous IV fluid infusion is to be discontinued and intermittent drug therapy is to begin, an adapter is attached to the IV catheter or needle where the IV tubing was disconnected. Adapters have ports (stoppers) where needles, needleless, or IV tubing can be inserted as needed to continue drug therapy. The use of adapters increases the patient's mobility by not having an IV line "tagging along" and is cost-effective because less IV tubing, solution, and equipment are needed. Figure 14E-3 shows examples of needleless infusion devices.

DIRECT INTRAVENOUS INJECTIONS

Medications that are given by the IV injection route are calculated in the same manner as medications for intramuscular

(IM) injection. This route is often referred to as **IV push.** Clinically, it is the preferred route for patients with poor muscle mass or decreased circulation or for a drug that is poorly absorbed from the tissues. Medications administered by this route have a rapid onset of action, and calculation errors can have serious, even fatal, consequences. The nurse must read drug information inserts carefully and must give attention to the amount of drug that can be given per minute. If the drug is pushed into the bloodstream at a faster rate than specified in the drug literature, adverse reactions to the medication are likely to occur.

ELECTRONIC INTRAVENOUS REGULATORS

Pumps are **electronic intravenous (IV) regulators** used in hospitals and some community settings. The electronic IV regulators are set to deliver a prescribed rate of IV solution. If the flow rate is obstructed, an alarm sounds.

IV pumps deliver IV solution against resistance. The flow rate is set in milliliters per hour. Pumps do not recognize infiltration. The alarm does not sound until the pump has exerted its maximum pressure to overcome resistance.

EXAMPLE

Order: Lasix 80 mg, IV, STAT

Available: Lasix 10 mg/mL. IV infusion not to exceed 40 mg/min

a. RP: $H : V :: D : x$

$$10\text{ mg} : 1\text{ mL} :: 80\text{ mg} : x$$
$$10x = 80$$
$$x = 8\text{ mL of Lasix}$$

or

$$\text{DA: mL} = \frac{1\text{ mL} \times \overset{8}{\cancel{80}}\ \cancel{\text{mg}}}{\underset{1}{\cancel{10}}\ \cancel{\text{mg}} \times 1} = 8\text{ mL of Lasix}$$

b. known drug minutes : known minutes :: desired drug : desired minutes

$$40\text{ mg} : 1\text{ min} :: 80\text{ mg} : x$$
$$40x = 80$$
$$x = 2\text{ min}$$

PRACTICE PROBLEM 2

Direct IV Injection

1. Order: protamine sulfate 40 mg IV, STAT

   Available:

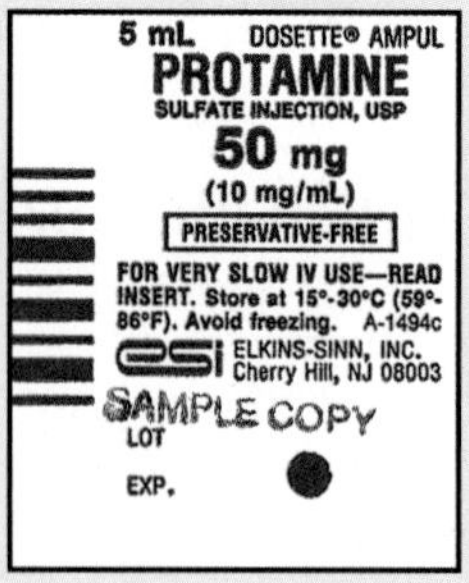

   IV infusion not to exceed 5 mg/min

   a. How many milliliters should the patient receive? ______

   b. For how many minutes should protamine be administered? ______

2. Order: morphine sulfate 5 mg IV, q3h, PRN

   Available:

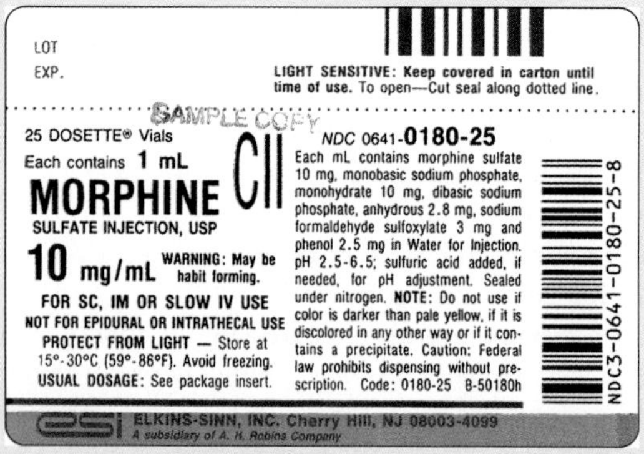

   IV infusion not to exceed 10 mg/4 min

   a. How many milliliters should the patient receive? ______

   b. For how many minutes should morphine be administered? ______

   Note: When giving drugs by direct IV infusion, always verify the compatibility of the IV solution and the drug, or precipitation can result. Incompatibility can be avoided if the IV tubing is flushed with compatible solution of either normal saline or sterile water before and after administration.

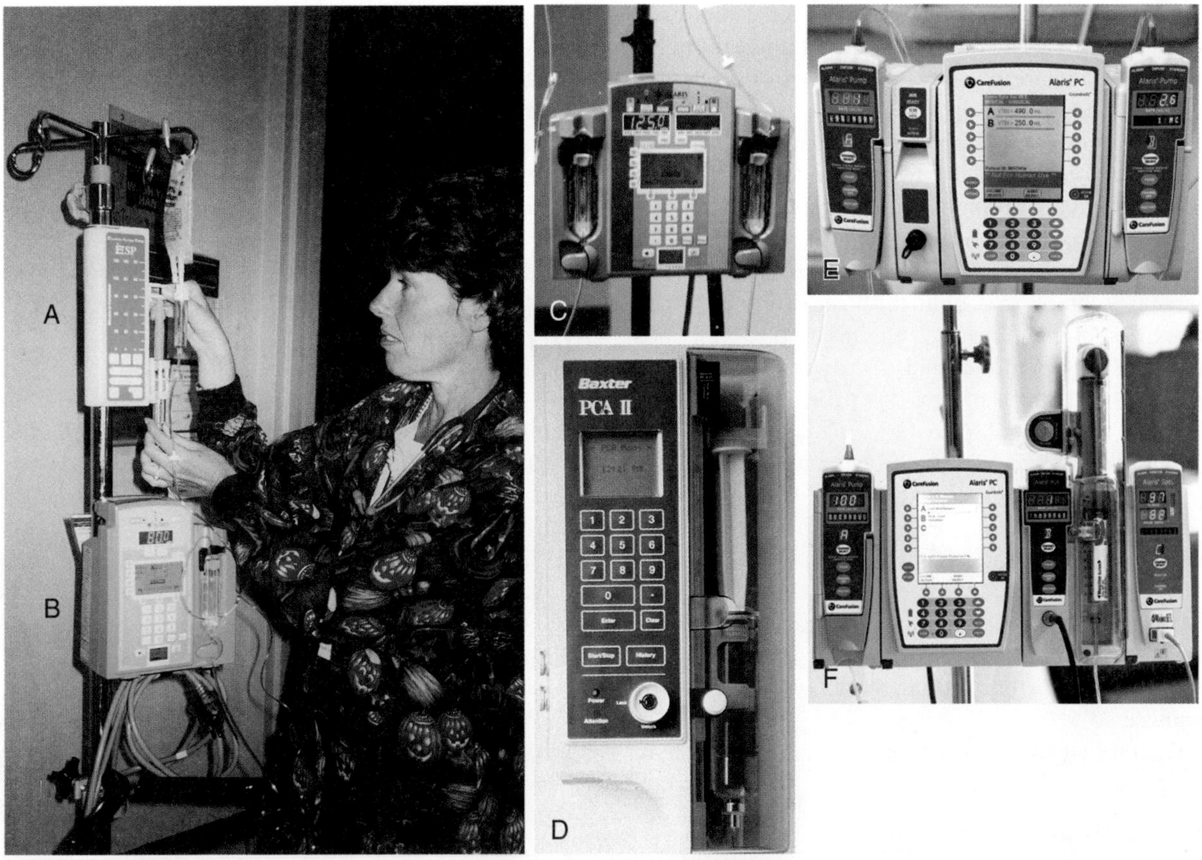

FIGURE 14E–4 Multichannel infusion pump. **A,** Syringe pump. **B,** Single-infusion pump. **C,** Dual-channel infusion pump. **D,** Patient-controlled analgesia (PCA) pump. **E,** Alaris System Large Volume Pump with PCA. **F,** Medley pump module attached to Medley programming module. (From Kee JL, Marshall SM: *Clinical calculations,* ed. 7, St. Louis, 2013, Elsevier.)

IV pumps are recommended for use with all central lines, such as femoral and subclavian sites, and peripheral lines. Ongoing nursing assessment is essential when using electronic IV regulators.

There are two types of flow control for electronic IV regulators: volumetric and nonvolumetric regulators. A **volumetric regulator** delivers a specific volume of fluid at a specific rate, in milliliters per hour. A **nonvolumetric regulator** is designed to infuse at a drop rate in drops per minute. To determine whether the machine is volumetric or nonvolumetric, check to see whether the panel display is calibrated for mL/h or gtt/min. Figure 14E-4 shows a variety of electronic IV regulators for the administration of IV fluids and drugs.

Safety Considerations for IV Use

All IV infusions should be checked every half-hour or hour, according to the policy of the institution. Common problems associated with IV infusions are kinked tubing, infiltration, and "free flow" IV rates. If IV tubing kinks, the flow is interrupted and the prescribed amount of fluid will not be given. The access site can clot. When infiltration occurs, IV fluid extravasates into the tissues and not into the vascular space. Trauma occurs to the tissues at the IV site. "Free flow" IV rate refers to a rapid infusion of IV fluids, thus faster than prescribed, causing fluid overload. Because of the possibility of free flow IV rate, electronic infusion pumps are commonly used today.

Electronic and volumetric infusion pumps are not without flaws. Mechanical problems can occur. Also, incorrectly programming an infusion pump can result in an incorrect infusion rate. Frequent monitoring of IV infusions can prevent complications of IV therapy such as fluid overload, thrombus formation, and infiltration.

Infusion Pumps

Various types of infusion pumps are shown in Figure 14E-4. Part A shows a syringe pump, Part B shows a single-infusion pump, and Part C shows a dual-channel infusion pump. Part D shows a patient-controlled analgesia (PCA) pump, Part E shows the Alaris System Large-Volume pump with PCA, and Part F shows the Medley pump module attached to the Medley programming module.

PATIENT-CONTROLLED ANALGESIA

Patient-controlled analgesia (PCA) is another method used to administer drugs IV. The objective of PCA is to provide a uniform serum concentration of drug(s), thus avoiding drug peaks and valleys. This method is designed to meet the needs of patients who require at least 24 to 48 hours of regular IM narcotic injections.

Several reasons for the use of PCA include (1) effective pain control without the patient feeling oversedated, (2) considerable reduction in the amount of narcotic used (approximately one half that of IM delivery), and (3) patients' feelings of having greater control over their pain.

There are choices available in the delivery of PCA. The pump is programmed to administer the prescribed medication (1) at patient demand, (2) continuously, and (3) continuously and supplemented by patient demand (see Chapter 13).

The health care provider's order must include the following:

- Drug ordered
- Loading dose: administered by the health care provider to obtain baseline serum concentration of analgesic
- PCA dose: amount to be administered each time patient activates the button
- Lockout interval: time during which PCA cannot be administered
- Dose limit: the maximum amount the patient can receive during a specified time

Patient Teaching

- Inform the patient that the pain should be tolerable, not necessarily absent.
- Advise the patient of the pump's safety features, including the alarms.
- Instruct the patient in the use of the control button (medication administered when button is *released*).
- Instruct the patient to report any side effects or adverse reactions to the medication.
- Have naloxone (Narcan) easily accessible.

CALCULATING FLOW RATES FOR INTRAVENOUS DRUGS

IV drug infusion rates depend on the drug dosing instructions, which indicate the amount of solution for dilution, and the length of infusion time. The nurse must first calculate the drug dose from the health care provider's order, and then calculate the flow rate.

1. *Secondary Sets:* To find drops per minute for IV drugs, use calibrated cylinders (Buretrol, Volutrol), 50- to 250-mL bag (Add-A-Line), or any other nonvolumetric regulator.
2. *Volumetric Regulators:* To find milliliters per hour (Infusion rate)

Problems for calculating IV drug dosage and IV flow rate in drops per minute and in milliliters per hour are given below.

EXAMPLE

Order: ceftazidime (Fortaz) 1.5 g IV q6h

Available:

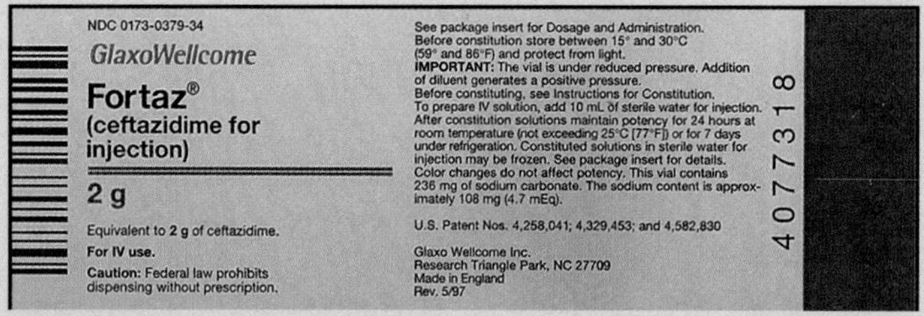

Set and solution: Cylinder set with drop factor of 60 gtt/mL; 500 mL of D_5W.

Instruction: Dilute ceftazidime 1.5 g in 100 mL of D_5W and infuse over 30 minutes.

1. Calculate drug dosage according to drug label.
2. Calculate drops per minute for drug solution.
3. Calculate milliliters per hour using volumetric infusion pump rate (mL/h).

Answer

1. Drug Calculation

Drug label states to add 10 mL of sterile water (2g = 10 mL)

$$\text{BF: } \frac{D}{H} \times V = \frac{1.5\,\text{g}}{2\,\text{g}} \times 10\,\text{mL} = \frac{15}{2} = 7.5\,\text{mL of ceftazidime}$$

$$\text{DA: mL} = \frac{10\,\text{mL} \times 1.5\,\cancel{\text{g}}}{2\,\cancel{\text{g}} \times 1} = \frac{15}{2} = 7.5\,\text{mL}$$

2. Secondary Set

$$\frac{\text{Amount of solution} \times \text{Drops per milliliter (set)}}{\text{Minutes to administer}} = \frac{100\text{ mL} \times \overset{2}{\cancel{60}}\text{ gtt}}{\underset{1}{\cancel{30}}\text{ min}} = 200\text{ gtt/min}$$

Inject 7.5 mL of ceftazidime in 100 mL of D_5W in the cylinder chamber.

Regulate IV flow rate to 200 gtt/min. It may be impossible to count 200 gtt/min. Instead of using the cylinder chamber, the nurse may use a secondary set that has a larger drop factor or a regulator. If the cylinder set is the only available secondary IV set, then the 200 gtt/min may be approximated.

3. Volumetric Infusion Pump Rate

$$\text{Amount of solution} \div \frac{\text{Minutes to administer}}{\text{60 minutes per hour}} = 100\text{ mL} + 7.5\text{ mL (drug)} \div \frac{30\text{ min}}{60\text{ min}} =$$

$$\text{(invert divisor and multiply) } 107.5\text{ mL} \times \frac{\overset{2}{\cancel{60}}}{\underset{1}{\cancel{30}}} = 215\text{ mL/h}$$

Set volumetric infusion rate at 215 mL/h to deliver drug in 30 min.

PRACTICE PROBLEM 3

Intermittent Intravenous Set

Solve the IV drug problems by (1) calculating the drug dosage according to the drug label or information given and (2) calculating drops per minute for the drug solution.

1. Order: kanamycin (Kantrex) 15 mg/kg/day in three divided doses (q8h) IV
   Patient weighs 50 kg.

   Available:

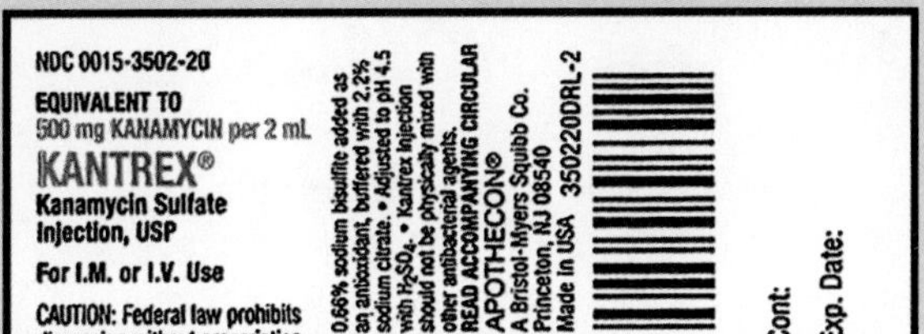

   Set and solution: Cylinder set with a drop factor of 60 gtt/mL; 500 mL D_5W

   Instruction: Dilute the drug in 75 mL of D_5W and infuse over 30 min.

   a. Drug dosage per day should be ______.
   b. Drug dosage per 8 hours ______; mL per dose ______.
   c. How many drops per minute should the patient receive? ______

2. Order: tobramycin (Nebcin) 50 mg IV q8h

   Drug parameters: 3 mg/kg/day in three divided doses. Patient weighs 65 kg.

   Available:

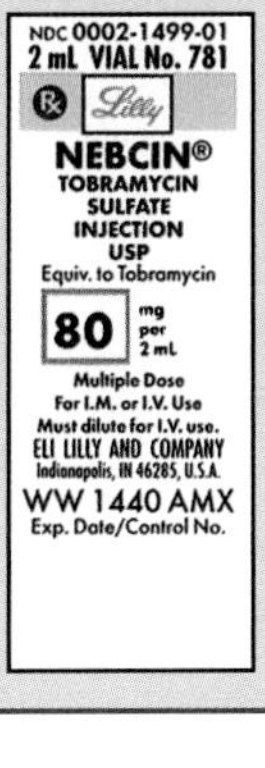

   Set and solution: Cylinder set with a drop factor of 60 gtt/mL; 500 mL D_5W

   Instruction: Dilute tobramycin in 100 mL of D_5W and infuse over 40 min.

   a. How many milliliters should the patient receive per dose? ______
   b. How may gtt/min? ______.
   c. Is the prescribed dose within safe drug parameters? ______ Explain your answer.

3. Order: ampicillin 500 mg IV q6h

   Available: Add 4.5 mL of diluent = 5 mL (2 g = 5 mL)

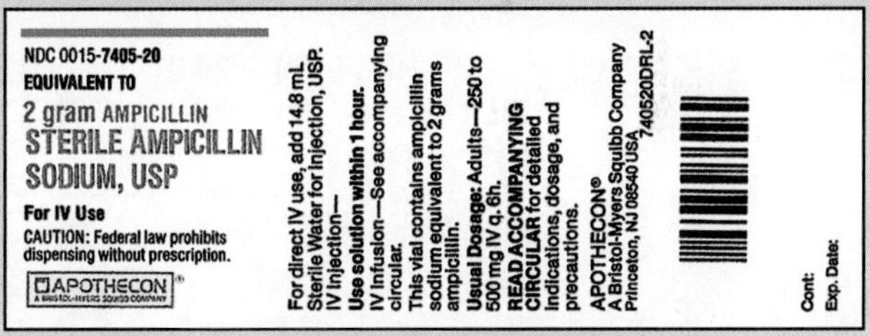

   Convert grams to milligrams.

   Set and solution: Cylinder set with a drop factor of 60 gtt/mL; 5 mL of D_5W.

   Instruction: Dilute ampicillin in 50 mL of D_5W and infuse over 15 min.

   a. How many mL should the patient receive per dose? ______
   b. How many gtt/min using the cylinder set? ______
   c. Determine the volumetric infusion rate. ______

4. Order: ticarcillin (Ticar) 750 mg IV q6h

   Available:

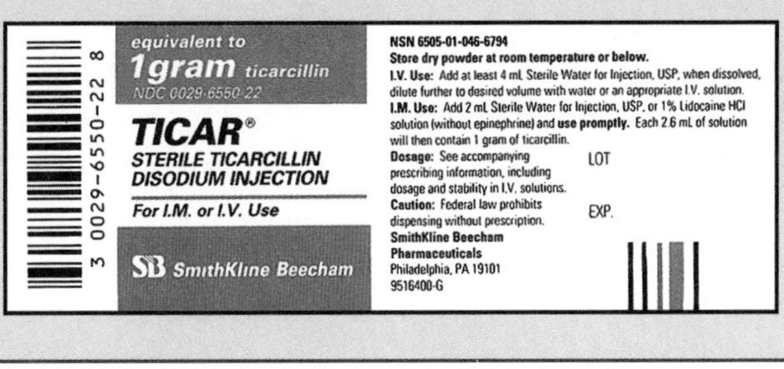

Continued

Set and solution: Cylinder IV set with drop factor of 60 gtt/mL; 500 mL D_5W

Instruction: Dilute ticarcillin in 20 mL of D_5W and infuse over 30 min.

a. How many mL should the patient receive per dose? ______

b. How many gtt/min should the patient receive? ______

c. Determine the volumetric infusion rate. ______

5. Order: ciprofloxacin (Cipro) 0.1 g IV q12h

Available:

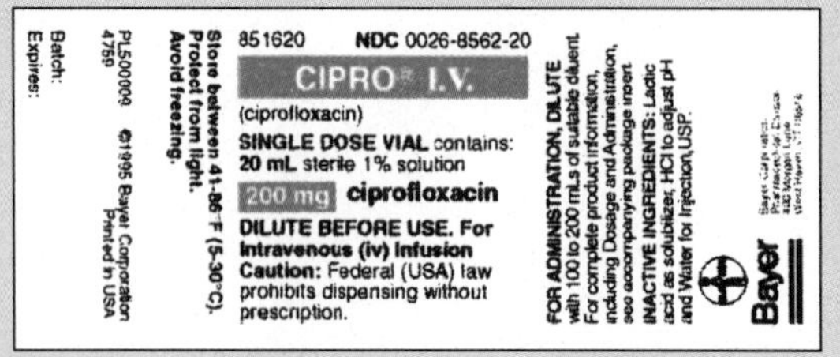

Set and solution: Secondary IV set with drop factor of 15 gtt/mL; 100 mL D_5W

Instruction: Dilute ciprofloxacin in 100 mL of D_5W and infuse over 60 min.

a. Change grams to milligrams. ______

b. How many milliliters (mL) of Cipro should be given per dose? ______

c. What is the IV flow rate in drops per minute? ______

d. Determine the volumetric infusion rate. ______

6. Order: Nitropress 40 mg in 250 mL of D_5W for 90 minutes

Drug parameter or range: 0.3 to 8 mcg/kg/min

Patient weighs: 75 kg

Available:

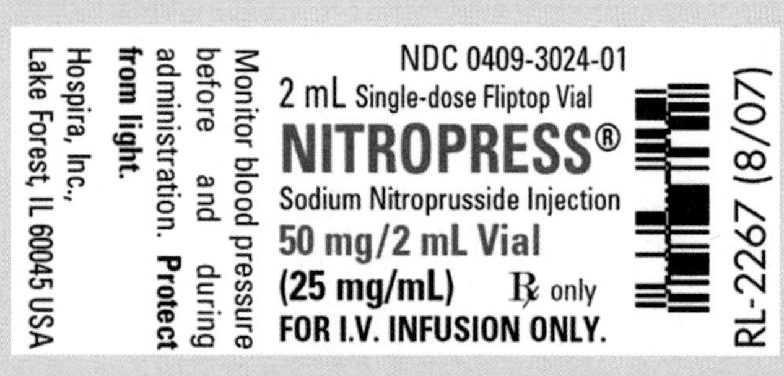

a. 1 mg = ______ mcg

b. What is the drug parameter/range? ______

b. Is the Nitropress dose within normal range? ______

c. Drug calculation ______

d. Determine the volumetric infusion rate. ______

7. Order: gentamicin 100 mg IV q8h

Patient weighs 165 pounds

Drug parameters: 3 to 5 mg/kg/day in 3 divided doses

Available: gentamicin 80 mg/2 mL vial

Set and Solution: Cylinder IV set with drop factor 60 gtt/mL; 250 mL of D_5W

Instruction: Dilute gentamicin in 75 mL of D_5W and infuse over 40 minutes.

a. How many kg does the patient weigh? ______

b. Is the prescribed dose within safe drug parameters? ______

c. How many milliliters (mL) of gentamicin should the patient receive per dose? ______

d. What is the IV flow rate? ______

e. Determine the volumetric infusion rate. ______

8. Order: etoposide (VePesid) 75 mg/m^2/day for 5 consecutive days q3-4wk. Patient's weight is 134 lb and height is 66 inches.

Use the nomogram to determine body surface areas (BSA, m^2) (Figure 14E-5)

Available:

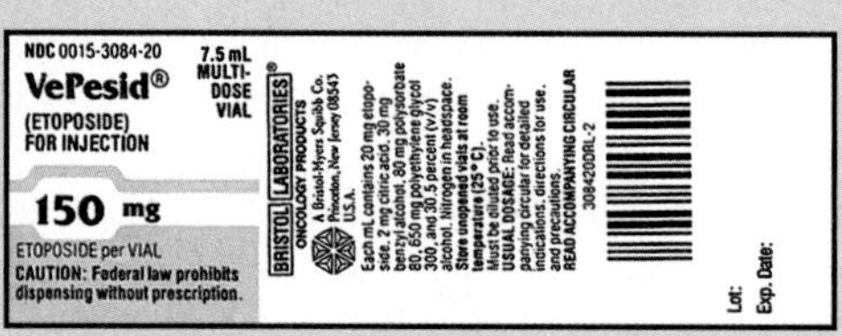

a. What is the patient's BSA? ______

b. How many milligrams should the patient receive? ______

c. How many milliliters of drug solution should the patient receive?

Set and Solution: Secondary set with 250 mL of D_5W to run for 60 min. Drop factor is 15 gtt/mL.

Determine the volumetric pump for this problem in addition to the drug and IV flow calculations.

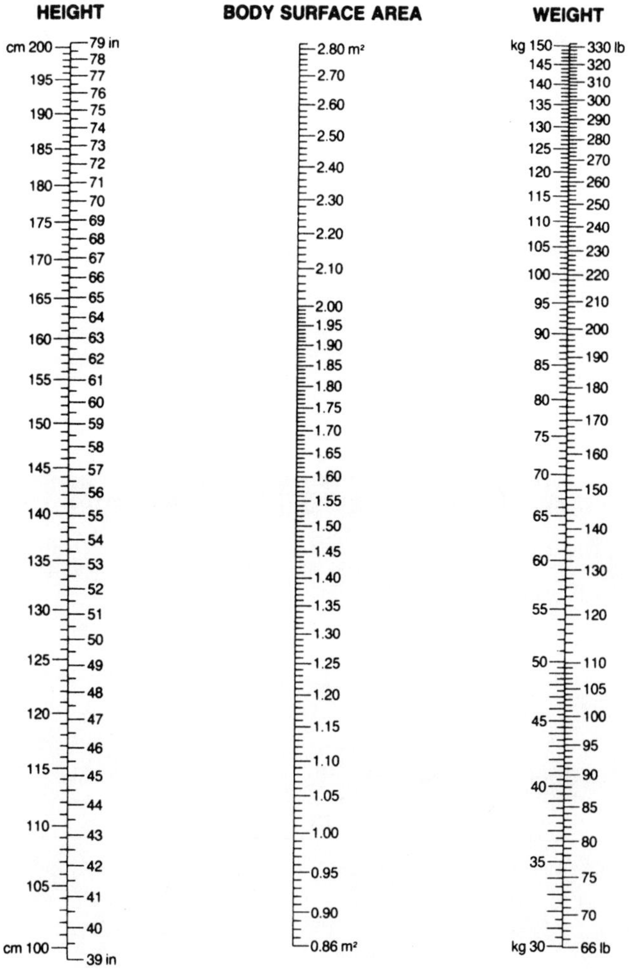

FIGURE 14E–5 Nomogram of body surface area for adults. Directions: (1) Find height. (2) Find weight. (3) Draw a straight line that connects the height and weight. (4) Where the line intersects on the body surface area column is the body surface area (m^2). (Sources: Deglin J, Vallerand A, Russin A: *Davis's drug guide for nurses,* ed. 2, Philadelphia, 1991, FA Davis; Lentner C (ed): *Geigy scientific tables,* ed. 8, vol. 1, Basle, Switzerland, 1981, Ciba-Geigy, pp. 226-227. In RE Behrman, RM Kliegman, HB Jensen: *Nelson textbook of pediatrics,* ed. 18, Philadelphia, 2007, Saunders.)

ANSWERS TO PRACTICE PROBLEMS

1 CONTINUOUS INTRAVENOUS FLOW RATES

1. a. Microdrip set because the patient is to receive 83 mL/h
   b. Two-step method: for continuous IV flow rate

   Step 1. $\frac{1000}{12} = 83 \text{ mL/h}$

   Step 2. $\frac{83 \text{ mL/h} \times \overset{1}{\cancel{60}} \text{ drobs}}{\underset{1}{\cancel{60}} \text{ min}} = 83 \text{ gtt/min}$

2. a. 1000 mL
   b. 8 h
   c. Step 1. $\frac{1000}{8} = 125 \text{ mL/h}$

   Step 2. $\frac{125 \text{ mL/h} \times \overset{1}{\cancel{15}} \text{ gtt}}{\underset{4}{\cancel{60}} \text{ min}} = \frac{125}{4} = 31 \text{ gtt/min}$

3. a. Microdrip set
   b. Step 1. $\frac{250}{44} = 10 \text{ mL/h}$

   Step 2. $\frac{10 \text{ mL/h} \times \overset{1}{\cancel{60}} \text{ gtt}}{\underset{1}{\cancel{60}} \text{ min}} = 10 \text{ gtt/min}$

4. a. KCl: BF: $\frac{D}{H} \times V = \frac{10}{20} \times 20 = \frac{200}{20} = 10 \text{ mL KCl}$
   b. $\frac{1000}{10} = 100 \text{ mL/h}$

   Macrodrip set $\frac{100 \times \overset{1}{\cancel{15}}}{\underset{4}{\cancel{60}} \text{ min}} = 25 \text{ gtt/min}$

   Microdrip set $\frac{100 \times \overset{1}{\cancel{60}}}{\underset{1}{\cancel{60}} \text{ min}} = 100 \text{ gtt/min}$

2 DIRECT IV INJECTION

1. a. BF: $\frac{D}{H} \times V = \frac{40\,\cancel{mg}}{10\,\cancel{mg}} \times 1\,mL = 4\,mL$

   DA: $mL = \frac{1\,mL \times 40\,\cancel{mg}}{10\,\cancel{mg} \times 1} = \frac{40}{10} = 4\,mL$

   b. known drug : known min :: desired drug : desired min

   $5\,mg : 1\,min :: 40\,mg : x$

   $5x = 40$

   $x = 8\,min$

2. a. RP: $H : V :: D : x$

   $10\,mg : 1\,mL :: 5\,mg : x$

   $10x = 5$

   $x = \frac{5}{10} = \frac{1}{2}$ or 0.5 mL drug

   b. known drug : known min :: desired drug : desired min

   $10\,mg : 4\,min :: 5\,mg : x$

   $10x = 20$

   $x = 2\,min$

3 INTERMITTENT INTRAVENOUS SET

1. a. 750 mg per day

   b. Drug calculation for q8h; 250 mg per dose.

   BF: $\frac{D}{H} \times V = \frac{250\,\cancel{mg}}{500\,\cancel{mg}} \times 2 = \frac{500}{500} = 1\,mL$ of kanamycin

   or

   RP: $H : V :: D : x$

   $500\,mg : 2\,mL :: 250\,mg : x\,mL$

   $500x = 500$

   $x = 1\,mL$ of kanamycin

   c. IV flow calculation: $\frac{75\,mL \times 60\,(set)}{30\,min} = \frac{4500}{30}$

   $= 150\,gtt/min$

2. a. Drag calculation: BF: $\frac{D}{H} \times V = \frac{50}{80} \times 2 = \frac{100}{80}$

   $= 1.25\,mL$ of tobramycin

   b. IV flow calculation: $\frac{100\,mL \times \cancel{60}^{3}\,gtt\,(set)}{\cancel{40}_{2}\,min}$

   $= \frac{300}{2} = 150\,gtt/min$

   c. Drug parameter: It is within safe parameters ($3\,kg \times 65 = 195$ mg/day)

   Patient is receiving $50\,mg \times 3 = 150$ mg/day (less than drug parameter)

3. a. Drug calculation: Convert to milligrams.

   $2\,g = 2{,}000\,mg$

   BF: $\frac{D}{H} \times V = \frac{500}{2000} \times 5 = \frac{5}{4} = 1.25\,mL$ of ampicillin

   or

   RP: $H : V :: D : x$

   $2000\,mg : 5\,mL :: 500\,mg : x\,mL$

   $2000x = 2500$

   $x = 1.25\,mL$ of ampicillin

   b. IV flow calculation:

   $\frac{50\,mL \times \cancel{60}^{4}\,gtt\,(set)}{\cancel{15}_{1}\,min} = \frac{200}{1} = 200\,gtt/min$

   c. Volumetric infusion pump rate:

   $50\,mL + 1.25\,mL \div \frac{15}{60} = 51.25\,mL \times \frac{\cancel{60}^{4}}{\cancel{15}_{1}} = 205\,mL/hr$

4. Drug label = Add 4 mL of sterile water.

   a. BF: $\frac{D}{H} \times V = \frac{750\,\cancel{mg}}{1000\,\cancel{mg}} \times 4\,mL = \frac{3000}{1000}$

   $= 3\,mL$ of Ticar

   or

   DA: $mL = \frac{4\,mL \times 1\,\cancel{g} \times \cancel{750}^{3}\,\cancel{mg}}{1\,\cancel{g} \times \cancel{1000}_{4}\,\cancel{mg} \times 1} = \frac{12}{4}$

   $= 3\,mL$ of Ticar

   b. IV flow calculation: $\frac{20\,mL \times \cancel{60}^{2}\,gtt\,(set)}{\cancel{30}_{1}\,min} = \frac{40}{1}$

   $= 40\,gtt/min$

c. Volumetric infusion pump rate:

$$20\text{ mL} + 3\text{ mL} + \frac{30}{60} = 23\text{ mL} \times \frac{\overset{2}{\cancel{60}}}{\underset{1}{\cancel{30}}} = 46\text{ mL/h}$$

(Increase in D_5W solution may be desired)

5. a. 0.1 g = 0.100 mg = 100 mg

b. $\text{BF: } \frac{D}{H} \times V = \frac{\overset{1}{\cancel{100}}\text{ mg}}{\underset{2}{\cancel{200}}\text{ mg}} \times 20\text{ mL} = \frac{20}{2} = 10\text{ mL}$

$$\text{DA: mL} = \frac{20\text{ mL} \times \overset{1}{\cancel{100}}\text{ mg}}{\underset{2}{\cancel{200}}\text{ mg} \times 1} = \frac{20}{2} = 10\text{ mL}$$

c. $\frac{10\text{ mL} + 100\text{ mL} \times 15\text{ gtt/mL (set)}}{60\text{ min to admin}} = \frac{100 \times \overset{1}{\cancel{15}}}{\underset{4}{\cancel{60}}} =$

27.5, or 28 gtt/min

d. $10\text{ mL} + 100\text{ mL} \div \frac{\overset{1}{\cancel{60}}\text{ min to admin}}{\underset{1}{\cancel{60}}\text{ min/h}} = 110\text{ mL/h}$

6. a. 1 mg = 1000 mcg

b. Drug parameters: 0.3 mcg × 75 kg = 22.5 mcg
OR 0.0225 or 0.023 mg/minutes
8 mcg × 75 kg = 600 mcg OR 0.600 mg/minutes
0.023 mg × 90 min = 2.07 mg per 90 minutes
0.600 mg × 90 min = 54 mg per 90 minutes

c. Yes. Range: 2.07 to 54 mg per 90 minutes is within range of 40 mg to administer.

d. Drug calculation:

$$\text{BF: } \frac{D}{H} \times V = \frac{40\text{ mg}}{50\text{ mg}} \times 2\text{ mL} = \frac{80}{50} = 1.6\text{ mL of Nitropress}$$

$$\text{FE: } \frac{H}{V} = \frac{D}{x} = \frac{50\text{ mg}}{2\text{ mL}} = \frac{40\text{ mg}}{x}$$

(cross-multiply) $50x = 80$
$x = 1.6$ mL of Nitropress to add to IV fluid

e. Infusion Pump Rate:

$$\text{Amount of solution} \div \frac{\text{minutes to administer}}{60\text{ minutes (hr)}} = \text{mL/hr}$$

$$250 \div \frac{90\text{ minutes}}{60\text{ minutes}} = \text{Invert divisor and multiple}$$

$$250 \times \frac{\overset{2}{\cancel{60}}}{\underset{3}{\cancel{90}}} = \frac{500}{3} = 166.66 \text{ or } 167\text{ mL/hr (round off to whole numbers)}$$

7. a. 165 pounds ÷ 2.2 = 75 kg

b. Yes, dose is within safe drug parameters.
3 mg × 75 kg = 225 mg divided by 3 doses = 75 mg
5 mg × 75 kg = 375 mg divided by 3 doses = 125 mg

c. $\text{BF: } \frac{D}{H} \times V = \frac{100\text{ mg}}{80\text{ mg}} \times 2\text{ mL} = \frac{200}{80} = 2.5\text{ mL}$

$$\text{DA: mL} = \frac{2\text{ mL} \times \overset{5}{\cancel{100}}\text{ mg}}{\underset{4}{\cancel{80}}\text{ mg} \times 1} = \frac{10}{4} = 2.5\text{ mL}$$

d. $\frac{75\text{ mL} \times \overset{3}{\cancel{60}}\text{ gtt/ mL (set)}}{\underset{2}{\cancel{40}}\text{ min to admin}} = \frac{225}{2} = 112.5\text{ gtt/min}$

e. $75\text{ mL} \div \frac{40\text{ min to admin}}{60\text{ min/h}} =$

(invert divisor and multiply) $75 \times \frac{\overset{3}{\cancel{60}}}{\underset{2}{\cancel{40}}} = \frac{225}{2}$

112.5, or 113 mL/h

8. a. Patient's BSA is 1.75.

b. 75 mg × 1.75 (BSA) = 131.25 or 131 mg

c. $\frac{D}{H} \times V = \frac{131}{150} \times 7.5\text{ mL} = \frac{982.5}{150} = 6.55\text{, or } 6.6\text{ mL}$

IV flow calculation with secondary set:

$$\frac{250\text{ mL} \times 15\text{ gtt (set)}}{60\text{ min}} = \frac{3750}{60} = 62.5\text{ gtt/nun}$$

Volumetric pump rate: 250 mL + 6.6 mL

$$(256.6 \text{ or } 257\text{ mL}) \div \frac{60}{60} = 257\text{ mL} \times \frac{\overset{1}{\cancel{60}}}{\underset{1}{\cancel{60}}}$$

= 257 mL/h

Section 14F: Pediatric Drug Calculations

OBJECTIVES

- Use one of the two primary methods to determine pediatric drug dosage.
- Describe the dosage inaccuracies that may occur with pediatric drug formulas.
- Identify the steps used to determine body surface area from a pediatric nomogram.
- Calculate the drug dosages correctly in the practice problems.

OUTLINE

KEY TERMS

body surface area (BSA) or m^2, p. 202
body weight (BW), p. 202

Pediatric drug dosages differ greatly from those for adults because of the physiologic differences between the two. Neonates and infants have immature kidney and liver function, which delays metabolism and elimination of many drugs. In neonates, drug absorption is different as a result of slow gastric emptying time. Decreased gastric acid secretion in children younger than 3 years of age contributes to altered drug absorption. Neonates and infants have a lower concentration of plasma proteins, which can cause toxicity with drugs that are highly bound to proteins. Young children have less total body fat and more body water; therefore lipid-soluble drugs require smaller doses when less-than-normal fat is present. Water-soluble drugs can require large doses because of a greater percentage of body water. It is the nurse's responsibility to ensure that a safe drug dosage is given and to closely monitor signs and symptoms of side effects and adverse drug reactions.

The purpose of learning how to calculate pediatric drug dosages is to ensure that children receive the correct dose within the approved therapeutic range. The two methods that are considered safe in the administration of drugs to children are the **body weight (BW)** (kg) and **body surface area (BSA)** or m^2 methods. Many manufacturers supply information in their literature concerning drug doses for children according to BW. Also, manufacturers frequently give drug parameters for safe dose ranges. It is the nurse's responsibility to check the dose ranges given by the pharmaceutic manufacturers to be certain that the prescribed dose is within the parameters.

ORAL

Oral pediatric drug delivery usually requires the use of a calibrated measuring device because most drugs for small children are in liquid form. The measuring device can be a small plastic cup, an oral dropper, a measuring spoon, or an oral syringe (Figure 14F-1). Some liquid medications come with their own calibrated droppers. The type of measuring device chosen depends on the age or the developmental level of the child. For infants and toddlers, the oral syringe and dropper can provide better drug delivery than a small cup. A young child who is cooperative is able to use a small cup or measuring spoon. The cup or spoon may be rinsed with water or juice to ensure that the child has received all of the drug. Avoid giving oral medications to a crying child or infant because the drug could be easily aspirated or the child could "spit out" the drug. For the older child, some drugs are available in chewable form. Children should be told not to chew drugs that are enteric-coated or in time-release form.

INTRAMUSCULAR

Intramuscular (IM) sites for drug administration are chosen on the basis of the age and muscle development of the child (Table 14F-1). All injections should be given in a manner that minimizes physical and psychosocial trauma. Explanations of injection administration should be given to children who can comprehend. With the very young child, distraction or brief restraint may be necessary. Comfort measures should immediately follow the injection.

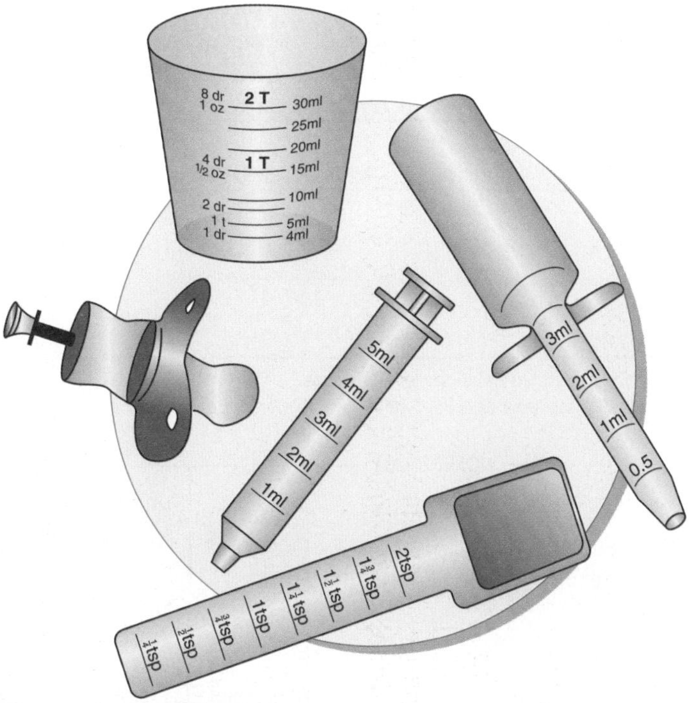

FIGURE 14F–1 Calibrated measuring devices. (From Kee JL, Marshall SM: *Clinical calculations,* ed. 7, St. Louis, 2013, Elsevier.)

PEDIATRIC DOSAGE PER BODY WEIGHT

EXAMPLE

Order: cefaclor (Ceclor) 50 mg q.i.d. Child weighs 15 lb or 6.8 kg (15 ÷ 2.2 = 6.8).

Child's drug dosage: 20 to 40 mg/kg/day in 3 divided doses

Available:

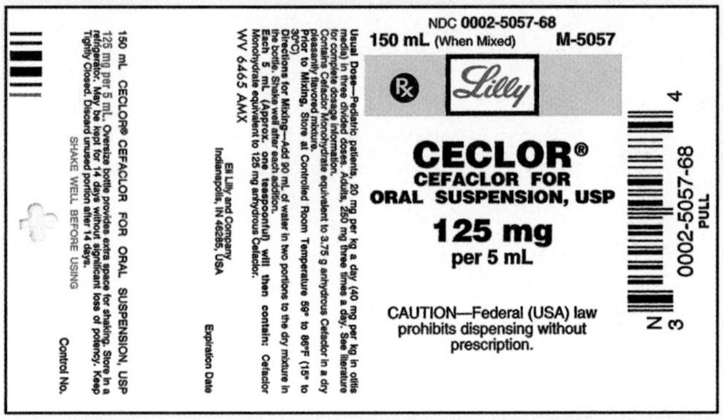

Is the prescribed dose safe? _____

Answer:

Drug parameters: 20 mg × 6.8 kg = 136 mg/day

40 mg × 6.8 kg = 272 mg/day

Dosage order: 50 mg × 4 = 200 mg/day

Dosage is within safe drug parameters.

a. BF: $\frac{D}{H} \times V = \frac{50}{125} \times 5 = \frac{250}{125} = 2\text{ mL}$

b. RP: H : V :: D : x

$125\text{ mg} : 5\text{ mL} :: 50\text{ mg} : x\text{ mL}$

$125x = 250$

$x = 2\text{ mL (cc)}$

c. FE: $\frac{H}{V} = \frac{D}{x} \quad \frac{125\text{ mg}}{5\text{ mL}} = \frac{50\text{ mL}}{x\text{ mL}}$

(cross-multiply) $125x = 250$

$x = 2\text{ mL}$

d. DA: $\text{mL} = \frac{5\text{ mL} \times \overset{2}{\cancel{50}}\,\cancel{\text{mg}}}{\underset{5}{\cancel{125}}\,\cancel{\text{mg}} \times 1} = \frac{10}{5} = 2\text{ mL}$

Cefaclor 50 mg = 2 mL. Give 2 mL 4 times a day.

PEDIATRIC DOSAGE PER BODY SURFACE AREA

To calculate pediatric dose by BSA, the child's height and weight are needed. Figure 14F-2 is the nomogram used to determine the BSA for infants and children. The square root formula may be used for BSA.

$$\text{BSA} = \frac{\sqrt{\text{height (in)} \times \text{weight (lb)}}}{3131\text{ (constant)}}$$

TABLE 14F-1 PEDIATRIC GUIDELINES FOR INTRAMUSCULAR INJECTIONS ACCORDING TO MUSCLE GROUP*

	AMOUNT BY MUSCLE GROUP (mL)					
	VASTUS LATERALIS	**RECTUS FEMORIS**	**VENTROGLUTEAL**	**DORSAL GLUTEAL**	**GLUTEUS MAXIMUS**	**DELTOID**
Neonates	0.5 mL	Not safe	Not safe	Not safe	Not safe	Not safe
Infants 1-12 months	0.5-1 mL	Not safe	Not safe	Not safe	Not safe	Not safe
Toddlers 1-2 years	0.5-2 mL	0.5-1 mL	Not safe	Not safe	Not safe	0.5-1 mL
Preschool to child 3-12 years	2 mL	2 mL	0.5-3 mL	0.5-2 mL	0.5-2 mL	0.5-1 mL
Adolescent 12-18 years	2 mL	2 mL	2-3 mL	2-3 mL	2 mL	1-1.5 mL

*The safe use of all sites is based on normal muscle development and size of the child. Follow institutional policies and procedures. In some institutions, the dorsal gluteal site is prohibited. (From Kee JL, Marshall SM: *Clinical calculations*, ed. 7, St. Louis, 2013, Elsevier.)

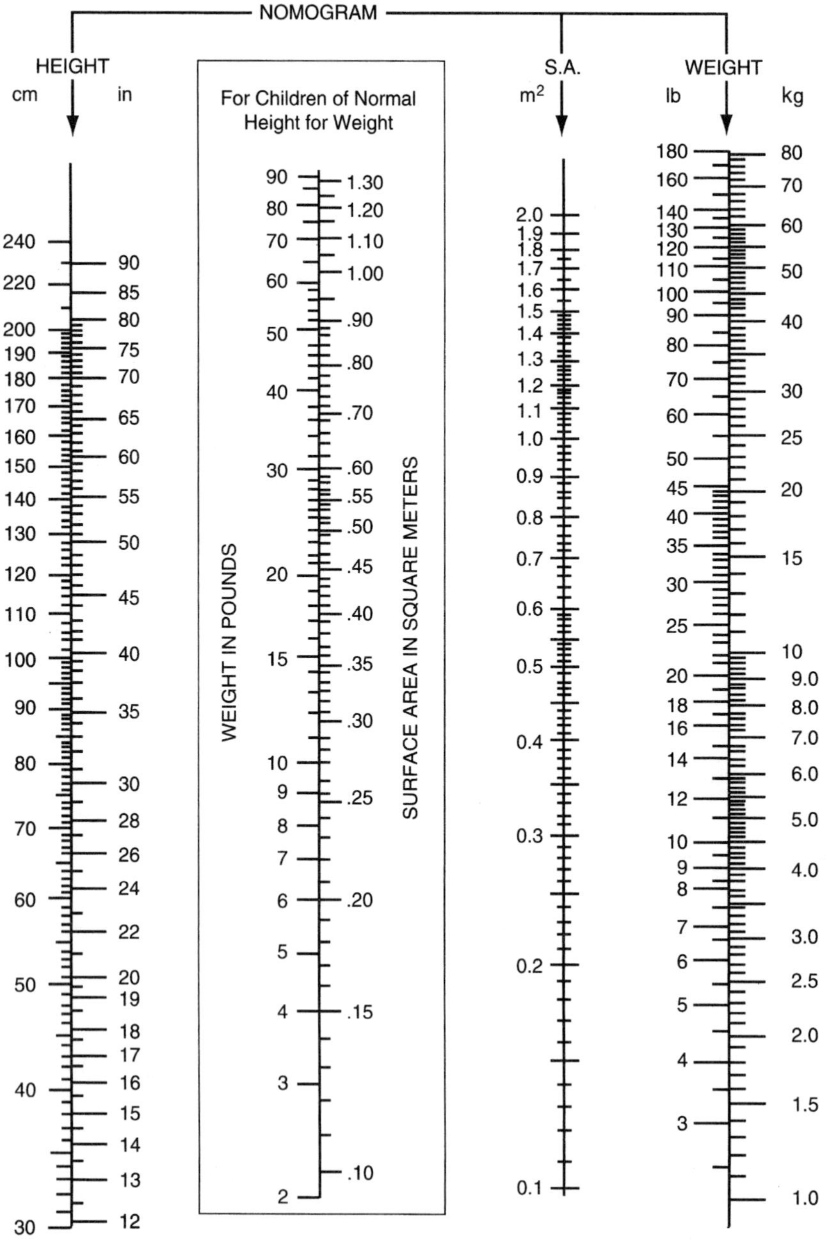

FIGURE 14F–2 Nomogram of body surface area for infants and children. Directions: (1) Find height. (2) Find weight. (3) Draw a straight line that connects the height and weight. (4) Where the line intersects on the body surface area column is the body surface area (m^2). (Sources: Deglin J, Vallerand A, Russin A: *Davis's drug guide for nurses,* ed. 2, Philadelphia, 1991, FA Davis; Lentner C (ed): *Geigy scientific tables,* ed. 8, vol. 1, Basle, Switzerland, 1981, Ciba-Geigy, pp. 226-227. In RE Behrman, RM Kliegman, HB Jensen: *Nelson textbook of pediatrics,* ed. 18, Philadelphia, 2007, Saunders.)

EXAMPLE

Order: methotrexate (Mexate) 50 mg weekly. Child's height is 54 inches and weight is 90 lb (41 kg).
Child's drug dosage: 25 to 75 mg/m²/week
Child's height and weight intersect at 1.3 m² (BSA).
Is the prescribed dose safe? _____

Answer:

Multiply the BSA, 1.3 m², by the minimum and maximum doses.

$$25\ \text{mg} \times 1.3\ \text{m}^2 = 32.5\ \text{mg}$$
$$75\ \text{mg} \times 1.3\ \text{m}^2 = 97.5\ \text{mg}$$

$$\text{BSA by square root: } \frac{\sqrt{54\ \text{in} \times 90\ \text{lb}}}{3131} = \text{m}^2 = 1.55$$
$$25\ \text{mg} \times 1.55\ \text{m}^2 = 38.5\ \text{mg}$$
$$75\ \text{mg} \times 1.55\ \text{m}^2 = 116.3\ \text{mg}$$

Dosage is considered safe within the parameters according to the child's BSA.

PRACTICE PROBLEM 1

Pediatric Dosing (Oral)

Solve the following problems using the BW or BSA method. The safe dosage is given in drug reference books.

1. Order: dicloxacillin sodium 100 mg q6h. Child weighs 55 lb (25 kg).
   Child's drug dosage range: Less than 40 kg, 12.5 to 25 mg/kg/day
   Available: dicloxacillin 62.5 mg per 5 mL
   a. Is the prescribed dose safe?______
   b. How many milliliters should be given for each dose? ______
2. Order: digoxin (Lanoxin) 35 mcg/kg/loading dose, PO
   Child weighs 10 kg
   Available: Lanoxin 50 mcg/mL (0.05 mg/mL)
   a. How many micrograms or milligrams should the child receive?______
   b. How many milliliters should be given for the loading dose?
3. Order: amoxicillin (Amoxil) 200 mg PO q8h. Child weighs 26 lb (12 kg).
   Child's drug dosage: 20 to 40 mg/kg/day in 3 divided doses
   Available:

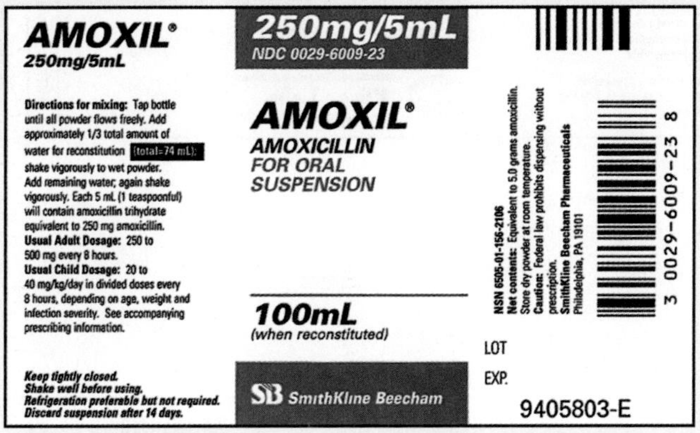

   a. Is the prescribed dose safe?______
   b. How many milliliters should be given every 8 hours? ______
4. Order: azithromycin (Zithromax), PO. First day: 10 mg/kg/day; next 4 days: 5 mg/kg/day.
   Child weighs 44 lb.
   Available:

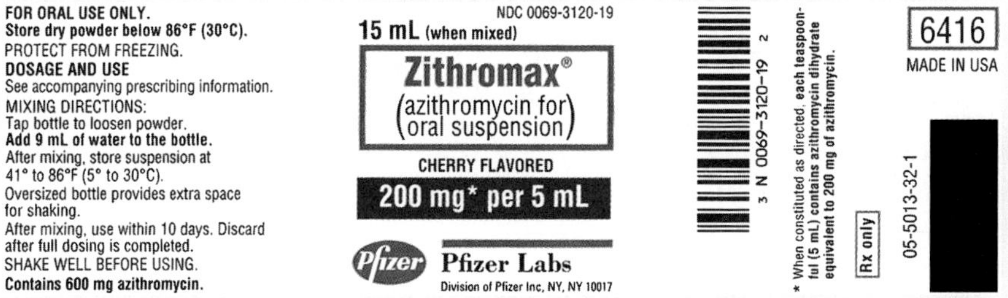

   a. How much does the child weigh in kilograms? ______
   b. How many milliliters should the child receive for the first day? ______
   c. How many milliliters should the child receive each day for the next 4 days (second to fifth days)? ______

Continued

SECTION 14F

5. Order: amoxicillin and clavulanate potassium (Augmentin) 100 mg PO q8h
   Child weighs 28 lb.
   Child's drug dosage: 20 to 40 mg/kg/day
   Available:

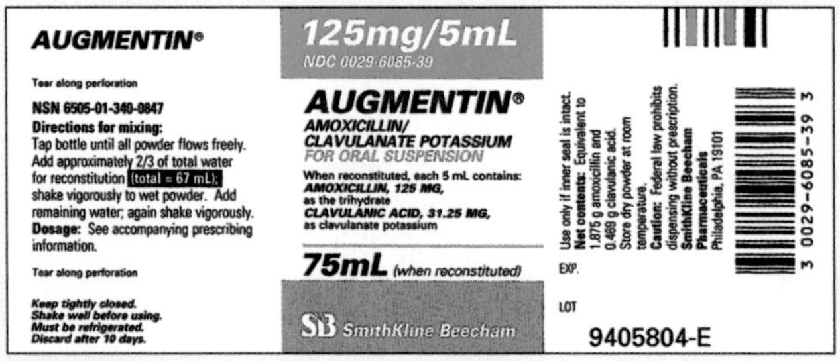

a. Is the prescribed dose within safe drug parameters? ______
b. How many milliliters should the child receive per dose? ______

6. Order: doxycycline (Vibramycin) 50 mg PO q12h
   Child is 10 years old and weighs 88 lb.
   Child's drug dosage: 2.2 to 4.4 mg/kg/day in 1-2 doses
   Available:

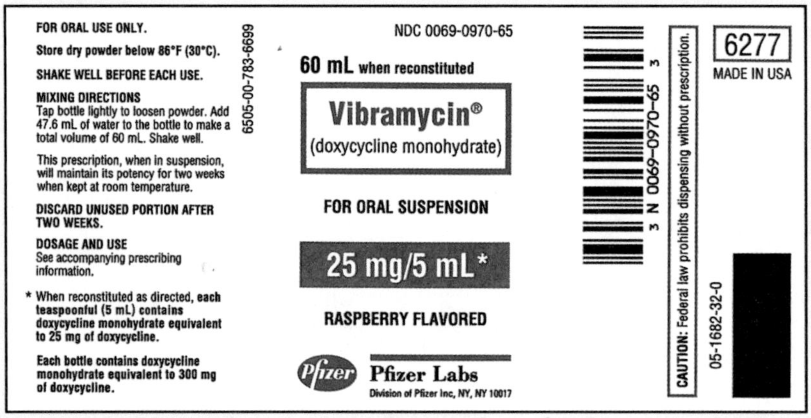

a. What would be the dosage parameter range for this child? ______
b. Is the prescribed dose within safe drug parameters? ______
c. How many milliliters should the child receive per dose? ______

7. Order: penicillin V potassium (Veetids) 400,000 units, PO, q6h
   Child's weight: 55 pounds
   Child's drug dosage: 25,000-90,000 units/kg/day in 3-6 divided doses
   Available:

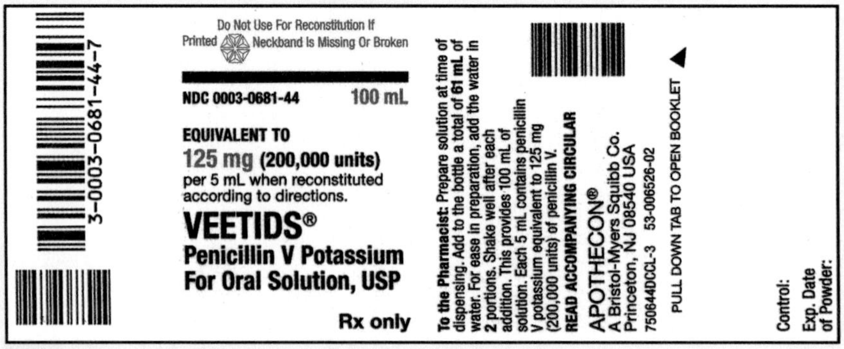

a. How many kilograms (kg) does the child weigh? ______
b. Is the prescribed dose within safe drug parameters? ______
c. How many milliliters (mL) of penicillin V should you give per dose? ______

8. Order: vinblastine (Velsar)
   Child's BSA is 1.2 m^2.
   Child's drug dosage: 2.5 mg/m^2
   How many milligrams should the child receive? ______

PEDIATRIC CALCULATIONS FOR INJECTABLES

The same methods used to calculate oral dosages for children are used to calculate injectable dosages. They are calculated from (1) BW (kg) and (2) BSA (m^2). Use the nomogram for BSA.

PRACTICE PROBLEM 2

Pediatric Injectables

Solve the following drug problems, and indicate whether the drug dose is within the safe drug parameters.

1. Order: tobramycin (Nebcin) 10 mg IM q8h
   Child weighs 10 kg.
   Child's drug dosage: 3 mg/kg/day in 3 divided doses
   Available:

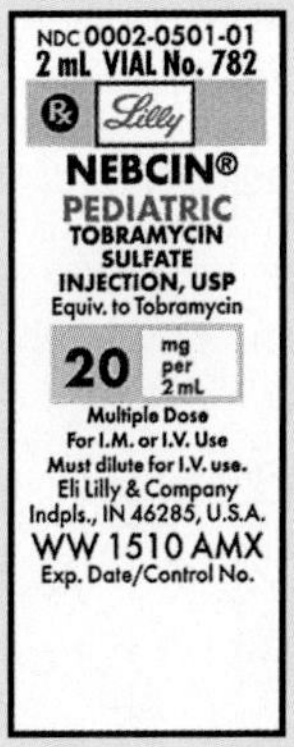

   b. Is the prescribed dose within safe drug parameters? ______
   c. How many milliliters should the child receive per dose? ______

2. Order: promethazine (Phenergan) 20 mg IM q6h
   Child weighs 45 kg.
   Child's drug dosage: 0.25 to 0.5 mg/kg/dose; repeat every 4-6 hours
   Available: Phenergan 25 mg/mL
   a. Is the prescribed dose within safe drug parameters? ______
   b. How many milliliters should the child receive per dose? ______

3. Order: naloxone 0.2 mg IM, STAT
   Child weighs: 44 pounds.
   Child's drug dosage: 0.01 mg/kg
   Available:

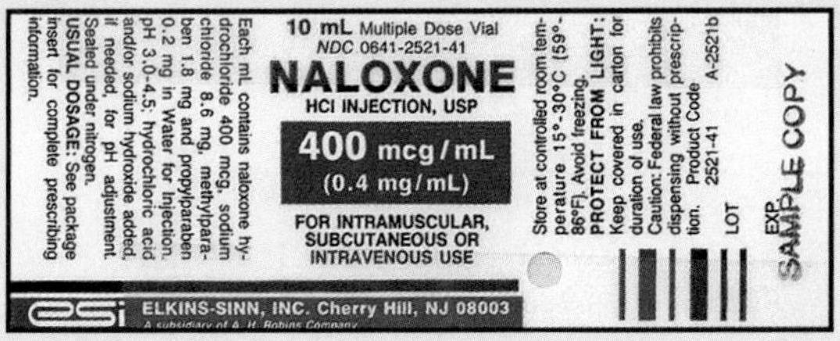

   a. How many kilograms (kg) does the child weigh? ______
   b. Is the prescribed dose within safe drug parameters? ______
   c. How many milliliters should the child receive? ______

4. Order: nafcillin sodium 200 mg IM q6h
   Child weighs 10 kg.
   Child's drug dosage: 100 to 300 mg/kg/day in divided doses
   Available: 1.8 mL of diluent = 2 mL

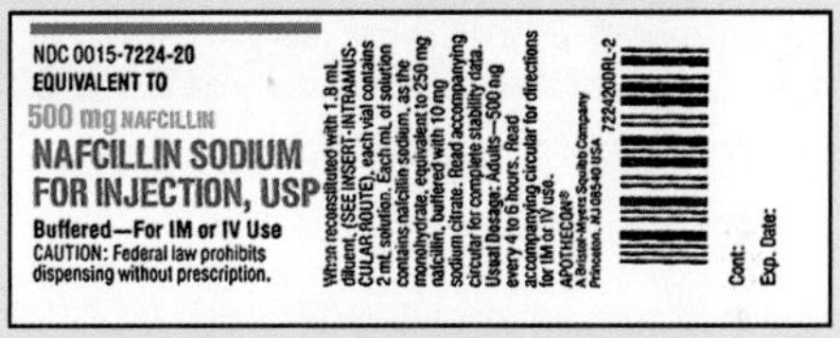

   a. How many milligrams will the child receive per day? ______
   b. Is the prescribed dose within safe drug parameters? ______
   c. How many milliliters should the child receive per dose? ______

5. Order: The newborn is to receive AquaMEPHYTON (vitamin K) 0.5 mg immediately after delivery.
   Available:

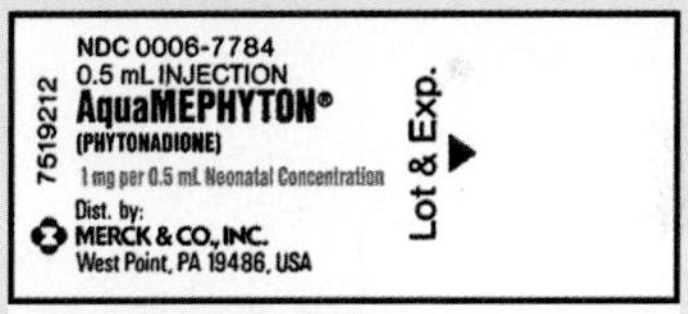

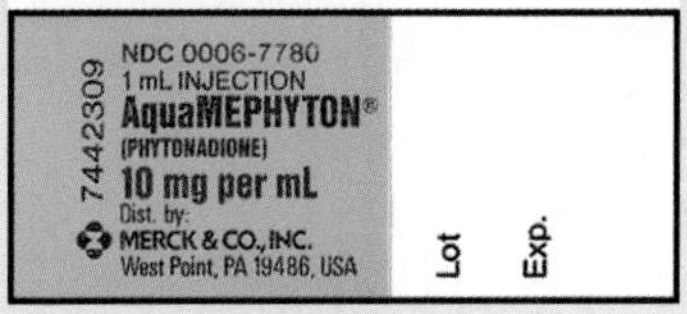

   a. Which AquaMEPHYTON container should be selected? ______
   b. How many milliliters should the newborn receive? ______

6. Order: cefazolin (Ancef) 125 mg IM q6h
   Child weighs 22 kg.
   Child's drug dosage: 25 to 50 mg/kg/day in 3-4 divided doses (up to 100 mg/kg/day)
   Available:

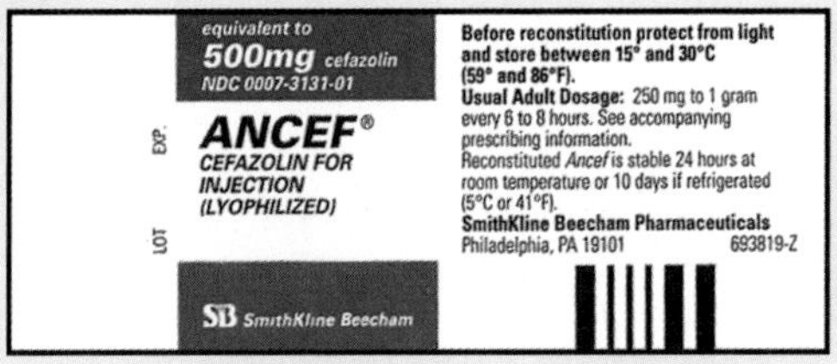

   a. How many milligrams should the child receive per day? ______
   b. Is the prescribed dose within safe drug parameters? ______

Continued

SECTION 14F

c. The drug label does not give the amount of diluent to add to the Ancef powder. Check the pamphlet insert. With 3.4 mL of diluent added, it is equivalent to 4 mL of drug solution.
d. How many milliliters of cefazolin should the child receive per dose? ______

7. Order: hydroxyzine (Vistaril) 50 mg IM
Child's height is 47 inches and weight is 45 lb.
Child's drug dosage: 30 mg/m^2
Available: Vistaril 25 mg/mL
a. Is the prescribed dose within safe drug parameters? _____

8. Order: methotrexate (Mexate) 50 mg IM weekly
Child's height is 56 inches and weight is 100 lb.
Child's drug dosage: 25 to 75 mg/m^2/wk
Available: methotrexate 2.5 mg/mL; 25 mg/mL; 100 mg/mL
a. Is the prescribed dose within safe drug parameters? ______
b. Which methotrexate should be selected? ______

ANSWERS TO PRACTICE PROBLEMS

1 PEDIATRIC DOSING (ORAL) USING BASIC FORMULA, RATIO AND PROPORTION, OR DIMENSIONAL ANALYSIS

1. a. Child weighs 25 kg (55 lb ÷ 2.2 = 25 kg)
Drug parameters:
12.5 mg × 25 kg = 312.5 mg/day
25 mg × 25 kg = 625 mg/day
Dosage order: 100 mg × 4 times a day (q6h) = 400 mg/day
Dosage is within safe drug parameters.

b. BF: $\frac{D}{H} \times V = \frac{100}{62.5} \times 5\,\text{mL} = \frac{500}{62.5} = 8\,\text{mL}$

RP: H : V :: D : x

$62.5\,\text{mg} : 5\,\text{mL} :: 100\,\text{mg} : x\,\text{mL}$

$62.5x = 500$

$x = 8\,\text{mL}$ of dicloxacillin

2. Child's drug dosage:
a. 35 mcg × 10 kg = 350 mcg, or 0.35 mg
350 mcg = 0.350 mg

b. BF: $\frac{D}{H} \times V = \frac{350\,\text{mcg}}{50\,\text{mcg}} \times 1\,\text{mL} = 7\,\text{mL}$ loading dose

or

BF: $\frac{0.35\,\text{mg}}{0.05\,\text{mg}} \times 1\,\text{mL} = 7\,\text{mL}$ loading dose

3. Drug parameters:
20 mg × 12 kg = 240 mg/day
40 mg × 12 kg = 480 mg/day
Dosage order: 200 mg x 3 (q8h) = 600 mg/day
Dosage is not within safe drug parameters. Dose exceeds the drug parameters. Do *not* give the medication. Notify the health care provider.

4. a. 20 kg
b. First day: 10 mg × 20 kg = 200 mg

BF: $\frac{D}{H} \times V = \frac{\overset{1}{\cancel{200}\,\cancel{\text{mg}}}}{\underset{1}{\cancel{200}\,\cancel{\text{mg}}}} \times 5\,\text{mL} = 5\,\text{mL}$

or

RP: H : V :: D : x

$200\,\text{mg} : 5\,\text{mL} :: 200\,\text{mg} : x$

$200x = 1000$

$x = 5\,\text{mL}$

or

$\text{DA: mL} = \frac{5\,\text{mL} \times \overset{1}{\cancel{200}\,\cancel{\text{mg}}}}{\underset{1}{\cancel{200}\,\cancel{\text{mg}}} \times 1} = 5\,\text{mL}$

First day give 5 mL.
c. Second to fifth days (next 4 days):
5 mg × 20 kg = 100 mg
Give 2.5 mL/day. Same answer worked out by BF, RP, and DA.

5. a. Drug parameters: (28 lb ÷ 2.2 = 12.7 kg)
20 mg × 12.7 kg = 254 mg/day
40 mg × 12.7 kg = 508 mg/day
Dosage order: 100 mg × 3 (q8h) = 300 mg/day
Dosage is within safe drug parameters.
b. 4 mL of Augmentin

6. a. Drug parameters: 88 mg to 176 mg/day
b. Dose is within safe drug parameters.
c. FE: $\frac{H}{V} = \frac{D}{x} \quad \frac{25\,\text{mg}}{5\,\text{mL}} = \frac{50\,\text{mL}}{x} = 10\,\text{mL}$ per dose of Vibramycin

(cross-multiply) $25x = 250$

$x = 10\,\text{mL}$

7. a. Child's weight 55 lbs ÷ 2.2 = 25 kg
b. 25,000 units × 25 = 625,000 units
90,000 units × 25 = 2,250,000 units
Child to receive 400,000 units × 4 (q6h) = 1,600,000 units per day
Yes, dose is within safe drug parameters
c. BF: $\frac{D}{H} \times V = \frac{40}{20} \times 5 = \frac{200}{20} = 10\,\text{mL}$ of Veetids per dose

8. Drug dosage: 2.5 mg × 1.2 m^2 = 3 mg
Administer 3 mg vinblastine.

2 PEDIATRIC INJECTABLES

1. a. Tobramycin parameter: 3 mg/kg/day ×10 kg = 30 mg/day in three divided doses
   Drug order: 10 mg × 3 (q8h) = 30 mg/day
   Dosage is within safe drug parameters.
   b. 10 mg = 1 mL/dose
   Child should receive 1 mL per dose.
2. a. Phenergan parameters:
   0.25 mg/kg/dose × 45 kg = 11.25 mg/dose
   0.50 mg/kg/dose × 45 kg = 22.5 mg/dose
   Drug order: Phenergan 20 mg IM per dose
   Dosage is within safe drug parameters.
   b. Phenergan 20 mg = 0.8 mL
3. a. Child weighs 44 lbs ÷ 2.2 = 20 kg
   b. 0.01 mg × 20 kg = 0.2 mg
   Yes, dosage is within safe drug parameters.
   c. RP: H : V :: D : x
   $$0.4\,\text{mg} : 1\,\text{mL} :: 0.2\,\text{mg} : x$$
   $$0.4x = 0.2$$
   $$x = \tfrac{1}{2} \text{ or } 0.5\,\text{mL of naloxone}$$
4. a. 200 mg × 4 (q6h) = 800 mg/day
   b. Dose per day is safe but not in therapeutic range. Notify health care provider.
   100 mg × 10 kg = 1000 mg
   300 mg × 10 kg = 3000 mg
   c. Add 1.8 mL diluent = 2 mL (500 g = 2 mL)
   RP: H : V :: D : x
   $$500 : 2 :: 200 : x$$
   $$500x = 400$$
   $$x = 0.8\,\text{mL}$$
   Nafcillin 200 mg = 0.8 mL per dose
5. a. Preferred selection is AquaMEPHYTON 1 mg = 0.5 mL.
   b. $$\frac{D}{H} \times V = \frac{0.5\,\cancel{mg}}{1.0\,\cancel{mg}} \times 0.5\,\text{mL} = \frac{0.25}{1.0} = 0.25\,\text{mL}$$
   AquaMEPHYTON 1 mg = 0.5 mL
   $$\frac{D}{H} \times V = \frac{0.5\,\cancel{mg}}{10\,\cancel{mg}} \times 1\,\text{mL} = \frac{0.5}{10} = 0.05\,\text{mL}$$
   For AquaMEPHYTON 1 mg = 0.5 mL. Give 0.25 mL. (Use a tuberculin syringe.)
   For AquaMEPHYTON 10 mg = 1 mL. Give 0.05 mL. (Use a tuberculin syringe; however, it would be difficult to give this small amount.)
6. a. 125 mg × 4 (q6h) = 500 mg
   b. Drug parameters: 22 kg. 25 mg/kg/day = 550 mg
   22 kg × 50 mg/kg/day = 1100 mg
   22 kg × 100 mg/kg/day = 2200 mg maximum (range: 550 to 2200 mg)
   Drug dose per day is below the suggested child's drug dose range. The nurse should contact the health care provider. The daily drug dose may need to be increased.
   c. Add 3.4 mL of diluent yielding 4 mL of drug solution.
   d. $$\text{DA: mL} = \frac{4\,\text{mL} \times \overset{1}{\cancel{125}}\,\cancel{mg}}{\underset{4}{\cancel{500}}\,\cancel{mg} \times 1} = 1\,\text{mL}$$
   Give 1 mL of cefazolin (Ancef) per dose.
7. Height and weight intersect at 0.82 m^2.
   Hydroxyzine parameter: 30 mg/m^2 × 0.82 m^2 = 24.6 mg, or 25 mg
   Drug order: hydroxyzine 50 mg IM
   Dosage is *not* within safe drug parameters. Dosage exceeds the drug parameters. Do not give the medication. Notify the health care provider.
8. Height and weight intersect at 1.38 m^2.
   Methotrexate parameters:
   25 mg/m^2/wk × 1.38 m^2 = 34.5 mg/wk
   75 mg/m^2/wk × 1.38 m^2 = 103.5 mg/wk
   Drug order: methotrexate 50 mg/wk IM
   Dosage is within safe drug parameters.
   (1) If methotrexate 25 mg/mL is used, give 2 mL (50 mg) **or** (2) If methotrexate 100 mg/mL is used, give 0.5 mL. Because of the amount of solution, it may be more desirable to give 0.5 mL of the 100 mg/mL solution.

UNIT IV

Nutrition and Electrolytes

Vitamins, minerals, and electrolytes are essential for cellular function. If significant lack of or imbalance of these chemical components occurs, replacement drug therapy is necessary, as is identifying and addressing any underlying causes for the lack or imbalance.

Both fat-soluble vitamins (vitamins A, D, E, and K) and water-soluble vitamins (vitamin B complex and C) are discussed in Chapter 15, Vitamin and Mineral Replacement. Iron is the primary mineral described in this chapter; other minerals discussed are copper, zinc, chromium, and selenium.

Body electrolytes are plentiful in extracellular and intracellular fluids and in the gastrointestinal mucosa. Potassium, sodium, calcium, and magnesium promote transmission and conduction of nerve impulses and contractility of muscles. Inadequate dietary intake and many disorders contribute to electrolyte imbalances. Chapter 16, Fluid and Electrolyte Replacement, discusses electrolyte replacement, and Chapter 17, Nutritional Support, discusses enteral and parenteral nutrition therapy.

CHAPTER

15

Vitamin and Mineral Replacement

evolve WEBSITE

http://evolve.elsevier.com/KeeHayes/pharmacology/

- Animations
- Content Updates
- Key Points
- Review Questions for the NCLEX® Examination
- References from the Textbook
- Unfolding Case Studies

OBJECTIVES

- Discuss the four justifications for the use of vitamin supplements.
- Differentiate between water-soluble and fat-soluble vitamins.
- Relate food sources and deficiency conditions associated with each vitamin.
- Explain the need for iron and foods that are high in iron content.
- Explain the uses for iron, copper, zinc, chromium, and selenium.
- Describe the nursing interventions, including patient teaching, related to vitamin and mineral uses.

OUTLINE

KEY TERMS

adequate intake, p. 212
estimated average requirement, p. 212
fat-soluble vitamins, p. 212
free radicals, p. 215
iron, p. 218
megavitamin therapy, p. 216
minerals, p. 218
recommended dietary allowance, p. 212
tolerable upper intake level, p. 212
water-soluble vitamins, p. 215

Vitamins and minerals are needed in correct portions for normal body function. Overuse of vitamins and minerals, particularly fat-soluble vitamins and iron, may lead to vitamin or iron toxicity.

VITAMINS

Vitamins are organic chemicals that are necessary for normal metabolic functions and for tissue growth and healing. The body needs only a small amount of vitamins daily, which can be obtained through one's diet. A well-balanced diet has all of the vitamins and minerals needed for body functioning. The intake of vitamins should be increased by those experiencing periods of rapid body growth, those who are pregnant or breastfeeding, those with a debilitating illness, those with malabsorptive issues (e.g., Crohn's disease), and those with inadequate diets (e.g., alcoholics, some geriatric patients). Children who have poor nutrient intake or are malnourished may need vitamin replacement. People on "fad" or restrictive diets may have vitamin deficiencies, as may those who are unable to afford or do not select a wide variety of foods.

The sale of vitamins in the United States is a multibillion-dollar business. Numerous vitamins and herbal medications are available for specialized needs such as cholesterol, memory, menopause, and prostate. Before purchasing these agents, the patient should discuss with the health care provider the health value and use of multiple vitamins and herbal medications. People may take vitamins to relieve tiredness or to improve general overall health; these are inappropriate indications for vitamin therapy. Vitamin supplements are not necessary if the individual is healthy and consumes a well-balanced daily diet on a regular basis; however, patients may take vitamins as a sort of "insurance" to be sure they are getting what they need.

The Food and Nutrition Board of the National Academy of Sciences has established the Dietary Reference Intakes (DRI).

The DRI nutrient recommendations include the following:

1. **Adequate intake (AI)** is the amount determined to be sufficient in the absence of scientific information. The AI is based on data about the levels of vitamin intake that seem to maintain a healthy status.
2. **Estimated average requirement (EAR)** is the amount thought to provide a sufficient intake in one half of healthy persons in a defined group.
3. **Recommended dietary allowance (RDA)** is the amount thought to provide the needs of 98% of well children and adults of specific age group and gender. RDAs were developed to prevent deficiencies and may not be reflective of all groups, such as older adults.
4. **Tolerable upper intake level (UL)** is the maximum amount considered not likely to be a risk for healthy persons in a specified group. This is not a recommended level to take.

Vitamin deficiencies can cause cellular and organ dysfunction that may result in slow recovery from illness. Vitamin supplements are necessary for the vitamin deficiencies described in Table 15-1, but vitamins are frequently taken prophylactically rather than therapeutically.

With the goal of facilitating better nutrition, the United States Department of Agriculture (USDA) has developed Choose My Plate, part of a communications initiative based on their *2010 Dietary Guidelines for Americans.* Available at www.ChooseMyPlate.gov, MyPlate is an interactive tool that helps Americans to eat more healthfully (Figure 15-1), and the SuperTracker assists in the planning, analyzing, and tracking of nutrition and physical activity. This website offers a variety of features, including both consumer and professional information.

The National Academy of Sciences Food and Nutrition Board publishes the U.S. RDA for daily dose requirements of each vitamin. The U.S Food and Drug Administration (FDA) requires that all vitamin products be labeled according to the amount of vitamin content and the proportion of the RDA provided by the vitamin product. Individuals should be encouraged to check the RDA listed on a vitamin container to determine whether the product provides the RDA dose requirements. The RDA may need to be modified for patients who are ill.

Megadoses of vitamins are available, advertised for specific health conditions; these high doses can be toxic. Patients should be advised to contact their health care provider before taking these products. Megadoses of fat-soluble vitamins (A, D, E, and K) may cause toxic effects. Megadoses of water-soluble vitamins are eliminated via the urine and thus are generally not toxic. Adverse reactions (kidney stones and nerve damage, respectively) have been reported from Vitamin C and Vitamin B_6. However, it is also claimed that B vitamins may positively influence metabolism in older adults.

Table 15-2 lists fat-soluble and water-soluble vitamins, their functions, suggested food sources, and selected deficiency conditions.

Fat-Soluble Vitamins

Vitamins fall into two general categories: fat-soluble and water-soluble. The **fat-soluble vitamins** are A, D, E, and K.

TABLE 15-1 JUSTIFICATION FOR VITAMIN SUPPLEMENTS

CATEGORIES	DEFICIENCIES
Malabsorption, diarrhea, infectious and inflammatory diseases (e.g., Crohn's disease, celiac disease)	
Inability to use vitamins	Liver disease (cirrhosis, hepatitis), renal disease, certain hereditary deficiencies
Increased vitamin losses	Fever from infectious process, hyperthyroidism, hemodialysis, cancer, starvation, crash diets
Increased vitamin requirements	Early childhood, pregnancy, debilitating disease (cancer, alcoholism), gastrointestinal surgery, special diets

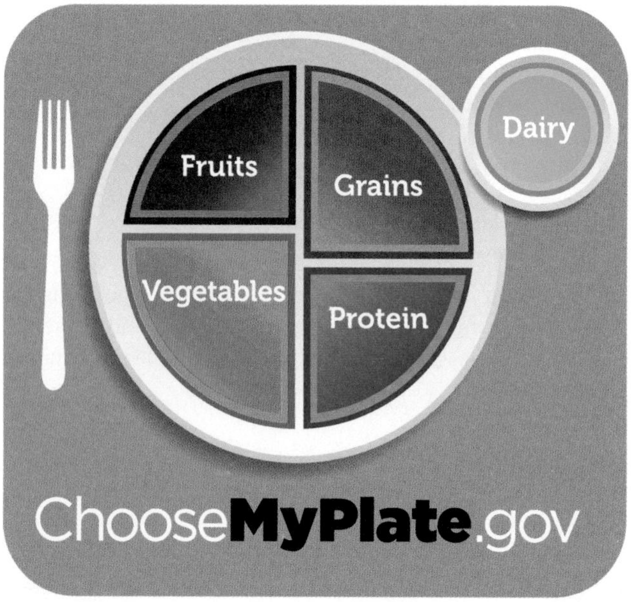

FIGURE 15–1 The U.S. Department of Agriculture's ChooseMyPlate.

TABLE 15-2 VITAMINS: FUNCTIONS, SUGGESTED FOOD SOURCES, AND SELECTED DEFICIENCY CONDITIONS

VITAMIN	FUNCTION	FOOD SOURCES	DEFICIENCY CONDITIONS
A (retinol)	Required for development and maintenance of healthy eyes, gums, teeth, skin, hair, and selected glands. Needed for fat metabolism.	Fortified milk, butter, eggs, leafy green and yellow vegetables and fruits. *Natural vitamin A, found only in animal sources: cod, halibut, shark, tuna	Dry skin, poor tooth development, night blindness
B_1 (thiamine)	Promotes use of sugars (energy). Required for good function of nervous system and heart.	Enriched breads and cereals, yeast, liver, pork, fish, milk, lentils, blackstrap molasses	Sensory disturbances, retarded growth, fatigue, anorexia
B_2 (riboflavin)	Promotes body's use of carbohydrates, proteins, and fats by releasing energy to cells. Required for tissue integrity.	Milk, enriched breads and cereals, liver, lean meat, eggs, almonds, wheat germ, soy, leafy green vegetables†	Visual defects such as blurred vision and photophobia; cheilosis; rash on nose; numbness of extremities
B_6 (pyridoxine)	Important in metabolism, protein synthesis, and formation of red blood cells.	Lean meat, leafy green vegetables, whole-grain cereals, yeast, bananas, salmon, soybeans, seeds, nuts, avocados, bananas, carrots	Neuritis, convulsions, dermatitis, anemia, lymphopenia
B_{12} (cobalamin)	Functions as a building block of nucleic acids and to form red blood cells. Facilitates functioning of nervous system.	Liver, kidney, fish, milk, eggs, chicken, turkey	Gastrointestinal disorders, poor growth, anemias
folic acid (folvite)	Helps in formation of genetic materials and proteins for the cell nucleus. Assists with intestinal functioning. Prevents selected anemias.	Leafy green vegetables, yellow fruits and vegetables, yeast, organ meats, black-eyed peas, lentils	Decreased white blood cell count and clotting factors, anemias, intestinal disturbances, depression
Pantothenic acid	Promotes body's use of carbohydrates, fats, and proteins. Essential for formation of specific hormones and nerve-regulating substances.	Eggs, leafy green vegetables, nuts, liver, kidney, skim milk, seeds, nuts, wheat germ, salmon	Natural deficiency unknown in humans
Niacin	In all body tissues. Necessary for energy-producing reactions. Assists nervous system.	Eggs, meat, liver, beans, peas, enriched bread and cereals	Retarded growth, pellagra, headache, memory loss, anorexia, insomnia
Biotin	Synthesis of fatty acids and energy production from glucose. Required by body chemical systems.	Eggs, milk, leafy green vegetables, liver, kidney	Natural deficiency unknown in humans
C (ascorbic acid)	Helps tissue repair and growth. Required in formation of collagen.	Citrus fruits, cantaloupe, tomatoes, leafy green vegetables, sweet red peppers, potatoes, strawberries, kiwi	Poor wound healing, bleeding gums, scurvy, predisposition to infection
D (calciferol)	Promotes use of phosphorus and calcium. Important for strong teeth and bones.	Vitamin D–fortified milk, egg yolk, tuna, salmon, liver	Rickets in children; osteomalacia in adults
E (alpha-tocopherol)	Protects fatty acids and promotes formation and functioning of red blood cells, muscle, and other tissues.	Whole-grain cereals, wheat germ, vegetable oils, lettuce, sunflower seeds, milk, eggs, meat, avocados, asparagus	Breakdown of red blood cells
K	Essential for blood clotting.	Leafy green vegetables, liver, cheese, egg yolk, vegetable oil, tomatoes	Increased clotting time, leading to increased bleeding and hemorrhage

*Yellow fruits and vegetables include apricots, cantaloupe, carrots, rutabaga, pumpkin, squash, and sweet potatoes.
†Leafy green vegetables include brussels sprouts, chard, broccoli, kale, spinach, and turnip and mustard greens.

They are metabolized slowly; can be stored in fatty tissue, liver, and muscle in significant amounts; and are excreted in the urine at a slow rate. Vitamins A and D are toxic if taken in excessive amounts over time. Current research shows that vitamin D toxicity is quite rare, and its symptoms are fairly nonspecific. Given that many people are found to be vitamin D deficient, it is not uncommon to see high-dose vitamin D therapy (e.g., 50,000 units/week). Historically, vitamins E and K were thought to be less toxic than vitamins A and D. Vitamin E was once considered a "wonder" drug, supposedly beneficial for the heart and brain, but it was later determined that vitamin E was an independent risk factor for the development of heart failure.

Foods rich in vitamin A, vitamin D, vitamin E, or vitamin K are shown in Table 15-2.

Vitamin A

Vitamin A is essential for bone growth and the maintenance of epithelial tissues, skin, eyes, and hair. It has been used for the treatment of skin disorders such as acne; however, excess doses can be toxic. During pregnancy, excessive amounts of vitamin A (>6000 international units) might have a teratogenic effect (birth defects) on the fetus. Prototype Drug Chart 15-1 describes the pharmacologic data on vitamin A. IM administration is used only in acutely ill patients or patients refractory to the oral route, such as those with gastrointestinal (GI) malabsorption syndrome.

Pharmacokinetics When a person is deficient in vitamin A, the vitamin is absorbed faster than when there is no deficiency or intestinal obstruction. A portion of vitamin A is stored in the liver, and this function can be inhibited with liver disease. Massive doses of vitamin A may cause hypervitaminosis A, symptoms of which are hair loss, peeling skin, anorexia, abdominal pain, lethargy, nausea, and vomiting.

The UL for vitamin A is 3000 mcg daily (3000 mcg daily = 10,000 international units). Excess use of vitamin A should be avoided unless warranted because this vitamin is stored in the liver, kidneys, and fat, and it is slowly excreted from the body. Excess vitamin A is stored in the liver for up to 2 years. Vitamin A toxicity affects multiple organs, especially the liver. To prevent the occurrence of vitamin A toxicity, the dose for healthy patients should not be greater than 7500 international units.

Mineral oil, cholestyramine, alcohol, and antilipemic drugs decrease the absorption of vitamin A. Vitamin A is excreted through the kidneys and feces.

Pharmacodynamics Vitamin A is necessary for many biochemical processes. It aids in the formation of the visual pigment needed for night vision. This vitamin is needed in bone growth and development, and it promotes the integrity of the mucosal and epithelial tissues. An early sign of vitamin A deficiency (hypovitaminosis A) is night blindness. This may progress to dryness and ulceration of the cornea and to blindness.

Vitamin A taken orally begins to take effect in 1 to 2 hours and peaks in 4 to 5 hours. Its duration of action is unknown. Because vitamin A is stored in the liver, the vitamin may be available to the body for days, weeks, or months.

Vitamin D

Vitamin D has a major role in regulating calcium and phosphorus metabolism and is needed for calcium absorption

PROTOTYPE DRUG CHART 15-1

Vitamin A

Drug Class Fat-soluble vitamin Trade Names: Acon, Aquasol A, Del-VI-A Pregnancy Category: A (X if doses are above RDA)	**Dosage** Severe deficiency: A and C >8 y: PO: 100,000-500,000 international units/d × 3 d; then 50,000 international units/d × 14 d (based on severity) C: Infant to 8 y: IM: 5000-15,000 international units/d × 10 d Maintenance: C: 4-8 y: IM: 5000-15,000 international units/d × 2 mo C: <4 y 10,000 international units/d × 2 mo
Contraindications Hypervitaminosis A, pregnancy (massive doses)	**Drug-Lab-Food Interactions** Drug: Mineral oil may decrease absorption of vitamin A, cholestyramine Lab: May increase BUN, calcium, cholesterol, triglycerides; may lower erythrocyte, leukocyte counts Food: None known
Pharmacokinetics Absorption: PO: 1 h Distribution: PB: UK Metabolism: t½: weeks-months Excretion: Urine	**Pharmacodynamics** PO: Onset: 1-2 h Peak: 4-5 h Duration: UK
Therapeutic Effects/Uses To treat vitamin A deficiency (biliary tract or pancreatic disease, colitis, cirrhosis, celiac disease, sprue), prevent night blindness, treat skin disorders, promote bone development Mode of Action: Essential for growth, bone and teeth development, vision, integrity of skin and mucous membranes, and reproduction	
Side Effects Headache, fatigue, drowsiness, irritability, anorexia, vomiting, diarrhea, dry skin, visual changes	**Adverse Reactions** Evident only with toxicity: leukopenia, aplastic anemia, papilledema, increased intracranial pressure, hypervitaminosis A, bulging fontanelles in infants, jaundice

A, Adult; *C,* child; *d,* day; *h,* hour; *IM,* intramuscular; *PB,* protein binding; *PO,* by mouth; *RDA,* recommended daily allowance; *t½,* half life; *UK,* unknown; *y,* year; <, less than; >, greater than.

from the intestines. Dietary vitamin D is absorbed in the small intestine and requires bile salts for absorption. There are two compounds of vitamin D: vitamin D_2, ergocalciferol (a synthetic fortified vitamin D), and vitamin D_3, cholecalciferol (a natural form of vitamin D influenced by ultraviolet sunlight through the skin). Over-the-counter vitamin D supplements usually contain vitamin D_3. Once absorbed, vitamin D is converted to calcifediol (also known as *25-hydroxycholecalciferol*) in the liver. Calcifediol is then converted to an active form, calcitriol, in the kidneys. Studies have suggested that vitamin D, taken with calcium, can reduce the incidence of fractures.

Calcitriol, the active form of vitamin D, functions as a hormone and, with parathyroid hormone (PTH) and calcitonin, regulates calcium and phosphorus metabolism. Calcitriol and PTH stimulate bone reabsorption of calcium and phosphorus. Excretion of vitamin D is primarily in bile; only a small amount is excreted in the urine. If serum calcium levels are low, more vitamin D is activated; when serum calcium levels are normal, activation of vitamin D is decreased.

Excess vitamin D ingestion (>40,000 international units) results in hypervitaminosis D and may cause hypercalcemia (an elevated serum calcium level). Anorexia, nausea, and vomiting are early symptoms of vitamin D toxicity.

Vitamin E

Vitamin E has antioxidant properties that protect cellular components from being oxidized and red blood cells from hemolysis. Vitamin E depends on bile salts, pancreatic secretion, and fat for its absorption. Vitamin E is stored in all tissues, especially the liver, muscle, and fatty tissue. About 75% of vitamin E is excreted in bile.

It has been reported that taking 400 to 800 international units of vitamin E per day reduces the number of nonfatal myocardial infarctions (MIs). Also, it has been stated that taking 200 international units per day for several years can reduce the risk of coronary artery disease (CAD), but the use of vitamin E for CAD is being questioned. However, many still state that this vitamin protects the heart and arteries and aids in the prevention of macular degeneration because of its antioxidant effects (i.e., it inhibits the oxidation of other compounds by blocking a group of harmful chemicals called **free radicals**). Many patients with Alzheimer's or Parkinson's disease take supplemental vitamin E for its antioxidant effects.

> **SAFETY: Preventing Medication Errors**
>
> **Do not confuse...**
>
> - **Aquasol A** or **Aquasol E** with **Anusol,** an antiinflammatory generally used to treat hemorrhoids

Side effects of large doses of vitamin E may include fatigue, weakness, nausea, GI upset, headache, and breast tenderness. Vitamin E may prolong the prothrombin time (PT). Patients taking warfarin should have their PT monitored closely. Iron and vitamin E should not be taken together because iron can interfere with the body's absorption and use of vitamin E.

Vitamin K

Vitamin K occurs in four forms. Vitamin K_1 (phytonadione) is the most active form; vitamin K_2 (menaquinone) is synthesized by intestinal flora; and vitamin K_3 (menadione) and vitamin K_4 (menadiol) have been produced synthetically. Vitamin K_2 is not commercially available. Vitamins K_1 and K_2 are absorbed in the presence of bile salts. Vitamins K_3 and K_4 do not need bile salts for absorption. After vitamin K is absorbed, it is stored primarily in the liver and in other tissues. Half of vitamin K comes from the intestinal flora, and the remaining portion comes from one's diet.

Vitamin K is needed for synthesis of prothrombin and the clotting factors VII, IX, and X. For oral anticoagulant overdose, vitamin K_1 (phytonadione) is the only vitamin K form available for therapeutic use and is most effective in preventing hemorrhage. The commercial drugs available for vitamin K_1 are called Mephyton and AquaMEPHYTON. Vitamin K is used for two reasons: (1) as an antidote for oral anticoagulant overdose and (2) to prevent and treat the hypoprothrombinemia of vitamin K deficiency. Spontaneous hemorrhage may occur with vitamin K deficiency due to lack of bile salts and malabsorption syndromes that interfere with vitamin K uptake (e.g., celiac disease). Newborns are vitamin K deficient; thus, a single dose of phytonadione is recommended immediately after delivery. This practice is common in the United States but controversial in other countries. This can elevate the bilirubin level and cause hyperbilirubinemia with a risk of kernicterus. There are oral and parenteral forms of phytonadione; IV administration is dangerous and may cause death.

Water-Soluble Vitamins

Water-soluble vitamins are the B-complex vitamins and vitamin C. This group of vitamins is not usually toxic unless taken in extremely excessive amounts. Water-soluble vitamins are not stored by the body, so consistent, steady supplementation is required. Water-soluble vitamins are readily excreted in the urine. Protein binding of water-soluble vitamins is minimal. Foods that are high in vitamin B are grains, cereal, bread, and meats. There are reports that B vitamins may promote a sense of well-being and increased energy as well as decreased anger, tension, and irritability. Citrus fruits and green vegetables are high in vitamin C. If the fruits and vegetables are cut or cooked, a large amount of vitamin C is lost.

Vitamin B Complex

Vitamin B_1 (thiamine), vitamin B_2 (riboflavin), vitamin B_3 (nicotinic acid, or niacin), and vitamin B_6 (pyridoxine) are four of the vitamin B-complex members. This B-complex group is water-soluble. It is a common group of vitamins administered in the clinical setting, especially to patients with alcoholism.

Thiamine deficiency can lead to the polyneuritis and cardiac pathology seen in beriberi or to Wernicke's encephalopathy that progresses to Korsakoff's syndrome, conditions most commonly associated with alcohol abuse. Wernicke-Korsakoff syndrome is a significant central nervous system disorder characterized by confusion, nystagmus, diplopia, ataxia, and loss of recent memory. If not treated, it may cause irreversible brain damage. IV administration of thiamine is recommended for treatment of Wernicke-Korsakoff syndrome. Thiamine must be given before giving any glucose to avoid aggravation of symptoms.

Riboflavin may be given to manage dermatologic problems such as scaly dermatitis, cracked corners of the mouth, and inflammation of the skin and tongue. To treat migraine headache, riboflavin is given in larger doses than for dermatologic concerns.

Niacin is given to alleviate pellagra and hyperlipidemia, for which large doses are required. Chapter 46 offers a discussion of niacin use to reduce cholesterol levels. However, large doses may cause GI irritation and vasodilation, resulting in a flushing sensation.

Pyridoxine is administered to correct vitamin B_6 deficiency. It may also help alleviate the symptoms of neuritis caused by isoniazid (INH) therapy for tuberculosis. Vitamin B_6 is an essential building block of nucleic acids, red blood cell formation, and synthesis of hemoglobin. Pyridoxine is used to treat vitamin B_6 deficiency caused by lack of adequate diet, inborn errors of metabolism, or drug-induced deficiencies secondary to INH, penicillamine, or cyclosporine (or hydralazine) therapy. It is also used to treat neonates with seizures refractive to traditional therapy. Vitamin B_6 deficiencies may occur in alcoholics along with deficiencies of other B-complex vitamins. Patients with diabetes or alcoholism may benefit from daily supplementation. Pyridoxine is readily absorbed in the jejunum and stored in the liver, muscle, and brain. It is metabolized in the liver and excreted in the urine.

SAFETY: Preventing Medication Errors

Do not confuse...
pyridoxine (vitamin B_6) with
- **paroxetine** (Paxil), an antidepressant
- **pralidoxime**, an antidote used to treat poisoning with organophosphate pesticides and chemicals that have anticholinesterase activity
- **phenazopyridine** (Pyridium), a urinary analgesic

Vitamin C

Vitamin C (ascorbic acid) is absorbed from the small intestine. Vitamin C aids in the absorption of iron and in the conversion of folic acid. Vitamin C is not stored in the body and is excreted readily in the urine. A high serum vitamin C level that results from excessive dosing of vitamin C is excreted by the kidneys unchanged.

The recommended daily dose of vitamin C for an adult is 50 to 100 mg/day. Some individuals take greater amounts to treat upper respiratory infections, cancer, or hypercholesterolemia. Massive doses of vitamin C can cause diarrhea and GI upset. Prototype Drug Chart 15-2 details pharmacologic data on vitamin C.

Pharmacokinetics Vitamin C is absorbed readily through the GI tract and is distributed throughout the body fluids. The kidneys completely excrete vitamin C, mostly unchanged.

Pharmacodynamics Vitamin C is needed for carbohydrate metabolism and protein and lipid synthesis. Collagen synthesis also requires vitamin C for capillary endothelium, connective tissue and tissue repair, and osteoid tissue of the bone. Large doses of vitamin C (>5 to 10 g) may decrease the effect of oral anticoagulants. Smoking decreases serum vitamin C levels. Vitamin C (in doses >500 mg) aids iron absorption.

The use of **megavitamin therapy,** massive doses of vitamins, is questionable at best. Megadoses of vitamins can cause toxicity and might result in minimal desired effect. Most authorities believe that vitamin C does not cure or prevent the common cold; rather, they believe that vitamin C has a placebo effect. Moreover, megadoses of vitamin C taken with aspirin or sulfonamides may cause crystal formation in the urine (crystalluria). Excessive doses of vitamin C can cause a false-negative occult (blood) stool result and false-positive sugar result in the urine when tested by the Clinitest method. If large doses of megavitamins are to be discontinued, a gradual reduction of dosage is necessary to avoid vitamin deficiency. Note: There is danger of children overdosing on adult or children's multivitamins containing iron.

Folic Acid (Folate)

Folic acid is absorbed from the small intestine, and the active form of folic acid (folate) is circulated to all tissues. One third of folate is stored in the liver, and the rest is stored in tissues. Eighty percent of folate is excreted in bile and 20% in urine.

Folic acid is essential for body growth. It is needed for deoxyribonucleic acid (DNA) synthesis, and without folic acid there is a disruption in cellular division. Chronic alcoholism, poor nutritional intake, malabsorption syndromes, pregnancy, and drugs that cause inadequate absorption (phenytoin, barbiturates) or folic acid antagonists (methotrexate, triamterene, trimethoprim) are causes of folic acid deficiencies. Symptoms of folic acid deficiencies include anorexia, nausea, stomatitis, diarrhea, fatigue, alopecia, and blood dyscrasias (megaloblastic anemia, leukopenia, thrombocytopenia). These symptoms are usually not noted until 2 to 4 months after folic acid storage is depleted.

Folic acid deficiency during the first trimester of pregnancy can affect the development of the central nervous system (CNS) of the fetus. This may cause neural tube defects (NTDs) such as spina bifida (defective closure of the bony structure of the spinal cord) or anencephaly (lack of brain mass formation). The U.S. Public Health Services recommends that all women who may become pregnant consume 400 mcg of supplemental folic acid each day—in addition to the folate they get with food. Synthetic folate is more stable than food; bioavailability is >85% and <59%, respectively. There is some evidence that 400 to 800 mcg (0.4 to 0.8 mg) of folic acid per day can decrease the incidence of coronary artery disease (CAD). It is thought that folic acid decreases the amino acid homocysteine in the blood, which may contribute to heart disease. Folic acid may also offer some protection from colorectal cancer.

PROTOTYPE DRUG CHART 15-2

Vitamin C

Drug Class Water-soluble vitamin Trade Names: Ascorbicap, Cecon, Cevalin, Solucap C, ♣ Apo-C, Ce-Vi-Sol, Redoxon Pregnancy Category: A (C if used in doses above RDA)	**Dosage** Prophylactic: A: PO: 45-60 mg/d C: PO: 20-50 mg/d Severe deficit: Scurvy A: PO: IM: IV: 150-250 mg/twice daily (larger doses have shown no additional benefit. C: PO: IM: IV: 100-300 mg/d × 2 wk; then 35 mg or more daily Chronic disease/fracture/wound healing: A: IM/IV/PO: 200-500 mg/d for 1-2 months C: IM/IV/PO: 100-200 mg/d for 1-2 months Pregnancy and lactation: A: PO: 160-80 mg/d
Contraindications Caution: Renal calculi, gout, anemia: sickle cell, sideroblastic, thalassemia	**Drug-Lab-Food Interactions** Decrease ascorbic acid uptake taken with salicylates; may decrease effect of oral anticoagulants; may decrease elimination of aspirins Lab: May decrease bilirubin, urinary pH; may increase uric acid, uric oxalate Food: None known
Pharmacokinetics Absorption: PO: quickly Distribution: PB: 25% Metabolism: t½: UK Excretion: In the urine; unchanged with high doses	**Pharmacodynamics** PO: Onset: >2 d Peak: UK Duration: UK
Therapeutic Effects/Uses To prevent and treat vitamin C deficiency (scurvy); to increase wound healing; for burns. Preserves integrity of blood vessels. Mode of Action: A water-soluble vitamin, essential for collagen formation and tissue repair (bones, skin, blood vessels); synthesis of lipids, protein, carnithine	
Side Effects Oral: Nausea, vomiting, diarrhea; heartburn; headache Parenteral: Flushing, headache, dizziness, soreness at injection site	**Adverse Reactions** Kidney stones, crystalluria, hyperuricemia. Hemolytic anemia with patients with G6PD deficiency. Life-threatening: Sickle cell crisis, deep vein thrombosis

A, Adult; *C*, child; *d*, day; *IM*, intramuscular; *IV*, intravenous; *PB*, protein binding; *PO*, by mouth; *t½*, half-life; *UK*, unknown; >, greater than; ♣, Canadian drug name.

SAFETY: Preventing Medication Errors

Do not confuse...

- **Folvite** with **Florvite,** a fluoride supplement added to the water supply.

Excessive doses of folic acid may mask signs of vitamin B_{12} deficiency, which is a risk in older adults. Patients taking phenytoin (Dilantin) to control seizures should be cautious about taking folic acid. This vitamin can lower the serum phenytoin level, which could increase the risk of seizures. The phenytoin dose would need to be adjusted in such patients. This is a complex interaction that is not fully understood, but it is thought that 1 mg or less per day of folic acid is safe in patients with controlled epilepsy.

Vitamin B_{12}

Vitamin B_{12}, like folic acid, is essential for DNA synthesis. Vitamin B_{12} aids in the conversion of folic acid to its active form. With active folic acid, vitamin B_{12} promotes cellular division. It is also needed for normal hematopoiesis (development of red blood cells in bone marrow) and to maintain nervous system integrity, especially the myelin.

The gastric parietal cells produce an intrinsic factor that is necessary for the absorption of vitamin B_{12} through the intestinal wall. Without the intrinsic factor, little or no vitamin B_{12} is absorbed. After absorption, vitamin B_{12} binds to the protein transcobalamin II and is transferred to the tissues. Most vitamin B_{12} is stored in the liver. Vitamin B_{12} is slowly excreted, and it can take 2 to 3 years for stored vitamin B_{12} to be depleted and a deficit noticed.

Vitamin B_{12} deficiency is uncommon unless there is a disturbance of the intrinsic factor and intestinal absorption. Pernicious anemia (lack of the intrinsic factor) is the major cause of vitamin B_{12} deficiency. Vitamin B_{12} deficiency can also develop in strict vegetarians who do not consume meat, fish, or dairy products. Other possible causes of vitamin B_{12}

deficiency include malabsorption syndromes (cancer, celiac disease, certain drugs), gastrectomy, Crohn's disease, and liver and kidney diseases. B_{12} deficiency is commonly seen with metformin and proton pump inhibitors (e.g., omeprazole). Symptoms may include numbness and tingling in the lower extremities, weakness, fatigue, anorexia, loss of taste, diarrhea, memory loss, mood changes, dementia, psychosis, megaloblastic anemia with macrocytes (overenlarged erythrocytes [red blood cells]) in the blood, and megaloblasts (overenlarged erythroblasts) in the bone marrow.

To correct vitamin B_{12} deficiency, cyanocobalamin in crystalline form can be given intramuscularly for severe deficits. It cannot be given intravenously because of possible hypersensitive reactions. Cyanocobalamin can be given orally and is commonly found in multivitamin preparations. It can also be given as a subcutaneous injection.

MINERALS

Various **minerals**, such as iron, copper, zinc, chromium, and selenium, are needed for body function.

Iron

Iron (ferrous sulfate, gluconate, or fumarate) is vital for hemoglobin regeneration. Sixty percent of the iron in the body is found in hemoglobin. One of the causes of anemia is iron deficiency. A normal diet contains 5 to 20 mg of iron per day. Foods rich in iron include liver, lean meats, egg yolks, dried beans, green vegetables (e.g., spinach), and fruit. Food and antacids slow the absorption of iron, and vitamin C increases iron absorption.

During pregnancy, an increased amount of iron is needed, but during the first trimester of pregnancy megadoses of iron are contraindicated because of its possible teratogenic effect on the fetus. Larger doses of iron are required during the second and third trimesters of pregnancy.

The dose of iron for infants and children 6 months to 2 years of age is 1.5 mg/kg of body weight. For the adult, 50 mg/day is needed for hemoglobin regeneration. The ferrous sulfate tablet is 325 mg, of which 65 mg is elemental iron. Therefore one tablet of ferrous sulfate is sufficient as a daily iron dose when indicated. Prototype Drug Chart 15-3 describes the pharmacologic data on iron.

Pharmacokinetics Iron is absorbed by the intestines and enters the plasma as heme, or it may be stored as ferritin. Although food decreases absorption by 25% to 50%, it may be necessary to take iron preparations with food to avoid GI discomfort. Vitamin C at doses > 500 mg may slightly increase iron absorption, whereas tetracycline, quinolone antibiotics (ciprofloxacin, levoflaxicin, etc.), and antacids can decrease absorption (Herbal Alert 15-1).

HERBAL ALERT 15-1

Iron

Chamomile, feverfew, peppermint, and St. John's wort interfere with the absorption of iron and other minerals.

Nursing Process

Patient-Centered Collaborative Care

Vitamins

Assessment

- Check patient for vitamin deficiency before start of therapy and regularly thereafter. Explore such areas as inadequate nutrient intake, debilitating disease, and GI disorders.
- Obtain 24- and 48-hour diet history analysis.

Nursing Diagnoses

- Imbalanced nutrition related to inadequate intake of food sources of vitamins
- Deficient knowledge related to food sources of vitamins
- Readiness for enhanced decision making related to food choices and vitamin supplementation

Planning

- Patient will eat a well-balanced diet.
- Patient with vitamin deficiency will take vitamin supplements as prescribed.
- Patient will demonstrate knowledge of food sources of vitamins.

Nursing Interventions

- Administer vitamins with food to promote absorption.
- Store drug in light-resistant container.
- Use the supplied calibrated dropper for accurate dosing when administering vitamins in drop form. Solution may be administered mixed with food or dropped into the mouth.
- Administer IM primarily for patients unable to take by PO route (e.g., GI malabsorption syndrome).
- Recognize need for vitamin E supplements for infants receiving vitamin A to avoid risk of hemolytic anemia.
- Monitor for vitamin A therapeutic serum levels (80 to 300 international units/mL).

Patient Teaching

General

- Advise patient to take prescribed amount of drug.
- Counsel patients to read vitamin labels to determine which vitamin is most appropriate for them.
- Advise patient to consult with health care provider/pharmacist regarding interactions with prescription and OTC medications.
- Discourage patient from taking megavitamins over a long period unless these are prescribed for a specific purpose by health care provider. To discontinue long-term megavitamin therapy, a gradual decrease in vitamin intake is advised to avoid vitamin deficiency.
- Inform patient that missing vitamins for 1 or 2 days is not a cause for concern, because deficiencies do not occur for some time.

PROTOTYPE DRUG CHART 15-3

Iron

Drug Class	Dosage
Mineral for antianemia Trade Names: ferrous sulfate (Feosol, Fer-Iron), ferrous gluconate (Fergon, Fertinic), ferrous fumarate (Feostat, Fumerin) Pregnancy Category: A	Sulfate: A: PO: 250-325 mg t.i.d. C: 6-12 y: PO 3/kg elemental iron per day in 1-2 divided doses Pregnancy: PO: 300-600 mg/d Gluconate: A: PO: 320-640 mg t.i.d./q.i.d. C: 6-12 y: PO: 3 mg/kg elemental iron per day C: < 6 y: PO: 100-300 mg/d
Contraindications	**Drug-Lab-Food Interactions**
Hemolytic anemia, hemosiderosis, peptic ulcer, ulcerative colitis Caution: Bronchial asthma, iron hypersensitivity	Increased effect of iron with vitamin C; decreased effect of tetracycline, antacids, penicillamine Lab: May increase bilirubin; may decrease calcium Food: None known
Pharmacokinetics	**Pharmacodynamics**
Absorption: PO: 10%-30% intestines Distribution: PB: UK Metabolism: t½: 6 h Excretion: Urine, feces, sweat	PO: Onset: 4 d Peak: 7-14 d Duration: 3-4 months
Therapeutic Effects/Uses	
To prevent and treat iron-deficiency anemia Mode of Action: Enables RBC development and oxygen transport via hemoglobin	
Side Effects	**Adverse Reactions**
Nausea, vomiting, diarrhea, constipation, epigastric pain; elixir may stain teeth	May aggravate existing GI conditions Pallor, drowsiness Life-threatening: Iron poisoning (mostly in children) and may result in cardiovascular collapse, metabolic acidosis Toxicity: Nausea, vomiting, diarrhea, (green then tarry stools), hematemesis, pallor, cyanosis, shock, coma

A, Adult; *C*, child; *d*, day; *GI*, gastrointestinal; *h*, hour; *PB*, protein binding; *PO*, by mouth; *t.i.d.*, three times a day; *q.i.d.*, four times a day; *RBC*, red blood cell; *t½*, half-life; *UK*, unknown; *y*, year; ≥, greater than or equal to.

- Advise patient to check expiration dates on vitamin containers before purchasing them. Potency of the vitamin is reduced after the expiration date.
- Counsel patient to avoid taking mineral oil with vitamin A on a regular basis, because it interferes with absorption of the vitamin; mineral oil also interferes with vitamin K absorption. If needed, take mineral oil at bedtime.
- Explain to patient that there is no scientific evidence that megadoses of vitamin C will cure a cold.
- Alert patient not to take megadoses of vitamin C with aspirin or sulfonamides because crystals may form in the kidneys and urine.
- Alert patient to avoid excessive intake of alcoholic beverages. Alcohol can cause vitamin B-complex deficiencies.

Diet

- Advise patient to eat a well-balanced diet. Vitamin supplements are not necessary if the person is healthy and receives proper nutrition on a regular basis.
- Educate patient about foods rich in vitamin A, including milk, butter, eggs, and leafy green and yellow vegetables. Foods rich in other vitamins are listed in Table 15-2.

Side Effects

- Advise patient that nausea, vomiting, headache, loss of hair, and cracked lips (symptoms of hypervitaminosis A) should be reported to the health care provider. Early symptoms of hypervitaminosis D are anorexia, nausea, and vomiting.

Cultural Considerations

- Food and food choices have strong cultural roots. Determine the patient's preferred and culturally meaningful foods, and incorporate them into food and supplement plan.
- Use interpreters as appropriate.
- G-6-PD deficiency is common among people of Arab or Chinese heritage.

Evaluation

- Evaluate patient's understanding of the purpose of vitamins and their correct use.
- Evaluate effectiveness of patient's diet for the inclusion of appropriate amounts and types of food. Have patient periodically keep a diet chart for a complete week to determine typical nutrition.
- Determine whether patient with malnutrition is receiving appropriate vitamin therapy.

Pharmacodynamics Iron replacement is given primarily to correct or control iron-deficiency anemia, which is diagnosed by a laboratory blood smear. Positive findings for this anemia are microcytic (small), hypochromic (pale) erythrocytes (red blood cells [RBCs]). Clinical signs and symptoms include fatigue, weakness, shortness of breath, pallor, and, in cases of severe anemia, increased GI bleeding. The dosage of ferrous sulfate for prophylactic use is 300 to 325 mg/day; for therapeutic use, the dosage is 600 to 1200 mg/day in divided doses.

The onset of action for iron therapy takes days, and its peak action does not occur for days or weeks; therefore the patient's symptoms are slow to improve. Increased hemoglobin and hematocrit levels occur within 3 to 7 days.

Iron toxicity is a serious cause of poisoning in children. As few as 10 tablets of ferrous sulfate (3 g) taken at one time can be fatal within 12 to 48 hours. Hemorrhage due to the ulcerogenic effects of unbound iron leads to shock. Parents should be cautioned against leaving iron tablets that look like candy (e.g., M&Ms) within a child's reach. Most iron products are distributed in bubble packs. There is also danger of children overdosing on adult or children's multivitamins containing iron.

Copper

Copper is needed for the formation of RBCs and connective tissues. Copper is a cofactor of many enzymes, and its function is in the production of the neurotransmitters norepinephrine and dopamine. Excess serum copper levels may be associated with Wilson's disease, which is an inborn error of metabolism that allows for large amounts of copper to accumulate in the liver, brain, cornea (brown or green Kayser-Fleischer rings), or kidneys.

A prolonged copper deficiency may result in anemia, which is not corrected by taking iron supplements. Abnormal blood and skin changes caused by a copper deficiency include a decrease in white blood cell count, glucose intolerance, and a decrease in skin and hair pigmentation. Mental retardation may also occur in the young.

The RDA for copper is 1.5 to 3 mg/day. Most adults consume about 1 mg/day. Foods rich in copper are shellfish (crab, oysters), liver, nuts, seeds (sunflower, sesame), legumes, and cocoa.

Zinc

Zinc is important to many enzymatic reactions and is essential for normal growth and tissue repair, wound healing, and taste and smell. The use of zinc has greatly increased in the past few years; some believe zinc can alleviate symptoms of the common cold and shorten its duration. Individuals may take as much as 200 mg/day. The adult RDA is 12 to 19 mg/day. Foods rich in zinc include beef, lamb, eggs, and leafy and root vegetables.

Large doses, more than 150 mg, may cause a copper deficiency, a decrease in high-density lipoprotein (HDL) cholesterol ("good" cholesterol), and a weakened immune response. Zinc can inhibit tetracycline absorption. Patients taking zinc and an antibiotic should not take them together; zinc should be taken at least 2 hours after taking an antibiotic. Patients on long-term parenteral nutrition are at risk for zinc deficiency. Serum zinc levels may not correlate with degree of deficiency.

Chromium

Chromium is said to be helpful in the control of type 2 diabetes (non–insulin-dependent diabetes). It is thought that this mineral helps to normalize blood glucose by increasing the effects of insulin on the cells. If a patient is taking large doses of chromium and an oral hypoglycemic agent or insulin, the glucose level should be monitored closely for a hypoglycemic reaction. The dose of an oral hypoglycemic drug or insulin may need to be decreased. Some patients with an impaired glucose tolerance or patients who do not have diabetes may benefit by taking chromium. In addition, chromium claims to promote weight loss and muscle building. Multivitamin and mineral preparations contain chloride salt of chromium.

There is no RDA for chromium; however, 50 to 200 mcg/day is considered within the normal range for adults and children older than 6 years of age. Foods rich in chromium include meats, whole-grain cereals, and brewer's yeast.

Selenium

Selenium acts as a cofactor for an antioxidant enzyme that protects protein and nucleic acids from oxidative damage. Selenium works with vitamin E. It is thought that selenium has an anticarcinogenic effect, and doses lower than 200 mcg may reduce the risk of lung, prostate, and colorectal cancer. Excess doses of more than 200 mcg might cause weakness, hair loss, dermatitis, nausea, diarrhea, and abdominal pain. Also, there may be a garlic-like odor from the skin and breath.

The RDA for selenium is 40 to 75 mcg (lower dose for women, higher dose for men). Foods rich in selenium include meats (especially liver), seafood, eggs, and dairy products.

Nursing Process
Patient-Centered Collaborative Care

Antianemia, Mineral: Iron

Assessment

- Obtain a drug history of current drugs and herbs patient is taking.
- Obtain a history of anemia or health problems that may lead to anemia.
- Assess patient for signs and symptoms of iron-deficiency anemia, such as fatigue, malaise, pallor, shortness of breath, tachycardia, and cardiac dysrhythmia.
- Assess the patient's RBC count, hemoglobin, hematocrit, iron level, and reticulocyte count before the start of and throughout therapy.

Nursing Diagnoses

- Imbalanced nutrition related to inadequate intake of food sources of iron
- Deficient knowledge of food sources of iron
- Readiness for enhanced decision making related to food choices and vitamin/mineral supplementation

Planning

- Patient will name at least six foods high in iron content.
- Patient will consume foods rich in iron.
- Patient with iron-deficiency anemia or with low hemoglobin will take iron replacement as recommended by health care provider, resulting in laboratory results within the desired range.

Nursing Interventions

- Encourage patient to eat a nutritious diet to obtain sufficient iron. Iron supplements are not needed unless the person is malnourished or pregnant or has abnormal menses.
- Store drug in light-resistant container.
- Administer IM injection of iron by the Z-track method to avoid leakage of iron into the subcutaneous tissue and skin, resulting in irritation and stains to the skin.

Patient Teaching

General

- Advise patient to take the tablet or capsule between meals with at least 8 ounces of juice or water to promote absorption. If gastric irritation occurs, instruct the patient to take with food.
- Advise patient to swallow the tablet or capsule whole.
- Encourage patient to maintain upright position for 30 minutes after taking oral iron preparation to prevent esophageal corrosion from reflux.
- Do not administer the iron tablet within 1 hour of ingesting antacid, milk, ice cream, or other milk products.
- Counsel patient that certain herbal drugs can decrease absorption of iron and other minerals (see Herbal Alert 15-1).
- Advise patient to increase fluids, activity, and dietary bulk to avoid or relieve constipation. Slow-release iron capsules decrease constipation and gastric irritation.
- Instruct adults not to leave iron tablets within reach of children. If a child swallows many tablets, induce vomiting and immediately call the local poison control center; the telephone number is in the front of most telephone books (include this number on emergency reference list).
- Encourage patient to take only the prescribed amount of drug to avoid iron poisoning. Be alert to iron in many multivitamin preparations.
- Be alert that iron content varies among iron salts; therefore do not substitute one for another.
- Advise patient that drug treatment for anemia is generally less than 6 months.

Diet

- Counsel patient to include iron-rich foods in diet, such as lean meats, egg yolk, dried beans, green vegetables, and fruit.

Side Effects

- Advise patient taking the liquid iron preparation to use a straw to prevent discoloration of tooth enamel.
- Alert patient that the drug turns stools a harmless black or dark green.
- Instruct patient about signs and symptoms of toxicity, including nausea, vomiting, diarrhea, pallor, hematemesis, shock, and coma, and report occurrence to health care provider.

Cultural Considerations

- Ask about cultural practices and incorporate them as appropriate.
- Use interpreter as needed.

Evaluation

- Evaluate the effectiveness of iron therapy by determining that patient is not fatigued or short of breath and that hemoglobin level is within desired range.

KEY WEBSITES

Center for Food Safety and Applied Nutrition: *www.cfsan.fda.gov*

Choose My Plate: *www.choosemyplate.gov/*

National Library of Medicine: *www.nlm.nih.gov*

CRITICAL THINKING CASE STUDY

AP is pregnant and is taking two 325-mg tablets of ferrous sulfate. She has a 2-year-old daughter.

1. What precautions should AP take in regard to the container of ferrous sulfate? Explain your answer.
2. If AP asks whether she should take more than two tablets of iron per day, how should the nurse respond?
3. AP states that she is constipated and wonders whether iron is the cause. How can this problem be alleviated? What would be an appropriate response?
4. Develop a safety plan with AP related to medication safety in the home with children.

NCLEX STUDY QUESTIONS

1. The nurse is reviewing a patient's laboratory test results and current medications and notes that the patient's prothrombin time is prolonged. The nurse checks the patient's medication list. What vitamin or mineral might be contributing to this?
   a. Vitamin A
   b. Selenium
   c. Vitamin D
   d. Vitamin E
2. A patient comes to the office with a chief complaint of hair loss and peeling skin. The nurse notes that many vitamins and minerals are on the list of medications that the patient reports using to treat liver disease. The patient's complaint may be caused by excess of what vitamin or mineral?
   a. Vitamin A
   b. Zinc
   c. Vitamin C
   d. Vitamin D
3. The nurse routinely includes health teaching about vitamins to patients. Vitamin D has a major role in which process?
   a. Ensuring night and color vision
   b. Regulating calcium and phosphorous metabolism
   c. Body growth
   d. DNA and prothrombin synthesis
4. The nurse is doing preconception counseling with a patient. Folic acid is included in the health teaching plan because it is known to prevent CNS anomalies and may offer protection from which disorder?
   a. Colorectal cancer
   b. Diabetes mellitus
   c. Celiac disease
   d. Migraine headaches
5. A prenatal patient tells the nurse that she is not taking vitamins because she heard that vitamins may cause damage to the fetus if she becomes pregnant. What is the nurse's best response?
   a. "Vitamins can only help you and your baby."
   b. "Take extra vitamins now to make up for missed doses."
   c. "Megadoses of vitamins can be harmful in the first trimester."
   d. "Taking above the RDA of any vitamin is not recommended."
6. A patient asks the nurse for information about fat-soluble vitamins. What is the nurse's best response?
   a. "Fat-soluble vitamins are metabolized rapidly."
   b. "Fat-soluble vitamins cannot be stored in the liver."
   c. "Fat-soluble vitamins are excreted slowly in urine."
   d. "Fat-soluble vitamins can never be toxic."
7. A patient complains of night blindness. The nurse correctly recommends which foods?
   a. Skim milk and peas
   b. Fortified milk and eggs
   c. Nuts and yeast
   d. Enriched bread and cereal
8. A patient diagnosed with alcoholism has questions about his medications. The nurse correctly explains that alcoholism can be associated with deficiency of which vitamin?
   a. A
   b. B_{12}
   c. D
   d. K
9. A patient complains of anorexia, nausea, and vomiting. The patient's list of medications includes multiple large doses of vitamins. The nurse notes that the patient's complaints may be related to early signs of toxicity of which vitamin?
   a. A
   b. B
   c. C
   d. D
10. A patient takes iron on a daily basis. Which comment from the patient suggests the need for health teaching related to iron?
    a. "I will swallow the tablet whole."
    b. "I take the tablet immediately before I go to bed."
    c. "I know that multivitamins might include iron."
    d. "I keep the tablets out of my children's reach."
11. A patient asks the nurse, "What does copper do for me? I think it must be bad for me." What is the nurse's best response?
    a. "Copper is needed for red blood cell formation."
    b. "Be sure to include nuts and seeds in your diet."
    c. "Why do you think copper is bad for you?"
    d. "Are you taking 5 mg of copper a day?"

Answers: 1, d; 2, a; 3, b; 4, a; 5, c; 6, c; 7, b; 8, b; 9, d; 10, b; 11, c.

CHAPTER

16

Fluid and Electrolyte Replacement

evolve WEBSITE

http://evolve.elsevier.com/KeeHayes/pharmacology/

- Animations
- Content Updates
- Key Points
- Review Questions for the NCLEX® Examination
- References from the Textbook
- Unfolding Case Studies

OBJECTIVES

- Describe osmolality and tonicity.
- Discuss normal range for serum osmolality and tonicity of intravenous solutions.
- Describe the classifications of intravenous fluids.
- Discuss the functions of major electrolytes.
- Differentiate between major intracellular and extracellular electrolytes.
- Explain the difference between cations and anions.
- Describe major signs and symptoms of deficiency and excess of potassium, sodium, calcium, magnesium, chloride, and phosphorus.
- Explain the methods used to correct potassium, calcium, and magnesium excess.
- Apply the nursing process to the care of the patient experiencing fluid, potassium, sodium, calcium, and magnesium imbalances.

OUTLINE

KEY TERMS

The authors gratefully acknowledge the work of Jane F. Marek, who updated this chapter for the eighth edition.

TABLE 16-1 ADULT BODY FLUID VOLUME

FLUID COMPARTMENT	PERCENTAGE
Intracellular fluid	40%
Extracellular fluid	20%
Interstitial fluid	15%
Intravascular fluid	5%
Transcellular fluid	Approximately 1-2 L total, but generally not included in calculations
Total body fluid	60%

TABLE 16-2 CATIONS AND ANIONS

CATIONS	ANIONS
Potassium (K^+)	Chloride (Cl^-)
Sodium (Na^+)	Bicarbonate (HCO_3^-)
Calcium (Ca^{2+})	Phosphate (PO_4^-)
Magnesium (Mg^{2+})	Sulfate (SO_4^-)

TABLE 16-3 ELECTROLYTE CONCENTRATION IN BODY FLUIDS

INTRACELLULAR FLUID	EXTRACELLULAR FLUID
Major Cations	**Major Cations**
Potassium	Sodium
Magnesium	Potassium
Sodium	Calcium
	Magnesium
Major Anions	**Major Anions**
Phosphorus	Chloride
	Phosphorus

Fluid and electrolyte balance is necessary to maintain homeostasis. Intake must equal output to maintain fluid balance, and the body constantly strives for equilibrium. The kidneys, with the respiratory, endocrine, gastrointestinal (GI), and integumentary systems, regulate fluid and electrolyte balance.

The total body water of a 70-kg man is approximately 60% (40 L). This percentage varies with age, gender, and percentage of body fat. Neonates have 70% to 80% water, whereas older adults have 45% to 55% water. Women tend to have less body water than men due to effects of hormones and to higher amount of adipose tissue, which contains very little water. Total body water is contained in two major compartments: the intracellular fluid (ICF) compartment and the extracellular fluid (ECF) compartment. The ECF compartment is composed of plasma (intravascular), intrastitial fluid (surrounding cells), and transcellular fluid, also known as the third-space (mucus and GI, cerebrospinal, pericardial, synovial, and ocular fluids). Table 16-1 shows the fluid compartments and percentage of total body water. Fluids move freely between the intracellular and extracellular compartments to maintain balance and homeostasis.

Electrolytes are substances that separate or dissociate into ions (charged particles) in solution; they are abundant in both ICF and ECF. Ions carry either a positive charge **(cation)** or a negative charge **(anion).** Major cations and anions are listed in Table 16-2. Electrolyte balance is essential for normal physiologic functioning and is closely linked with fluid balance. In addition, most electrolytes interact with hydrogen ions to maintain acid-base balance. Electrolyte balance must be kept within a narrow range to maintain homeostasis. Many illnesses and body system alterations cause electrolyte imbalances, which must be corrected quickly before serious sequelae ensue.

The major electrolytes in body fluids are sodium, potassium, calcium, magnesium, chloride, phosphorus, sulfate, hydrogen and bicarbonate ions, and many proteins. Electrolyte concentration differs in ICF and ECF. Table 16-3 lists the major cations and anions found in body fluid.

Administering intravenous (IV) fluids and electrolyte replacements may be thought of as "routine" nursing care but requires as much diligence and critical thinking as administration of any medication. This chapter describes fluid replacement strategies, pharmacologic management of specific electrolyte imbalances, and nursing care of patients with fluid and electrolyte imbalances.

HOMEOSTASIS

Two principles stand out when considering homeostasis and fluid and electrolyte balance. The first principle is that anions and cations must be balanced within each compartment and remain electrically neutral. The amount of fluid within each compartment remains constant. Compartments work continuously to maintain fluid balance and replace and exchange ions to maintain neutrality. The second principle is that the fluid compartments remain in osmotic equilibrium (except for transient changes).

Movement of fluid and particles between and within compartments is controlled by a number of processes, including osmosis, diffusion, membrane transport, hydrostatic pressure, membrane permeability, colloidal osmotic pressure (plasma proteins), and size of the particle (ion). The number of solutes in a solution is expressed as a unit of measurement called the **osmole,** which is particularly useful when referencing osmotic solutions.

Osmolality and osmolarity are two different terms of measurement used to describe the number of osmoles or solutes in a solution. In clinical practice, the difference between the absolute values of these two measurements is negligible. Hence, these terms are often used interchangeably. However, they are two separate measurements. **Osmolality** refers to the number of osmoles per kilogram of water and is expressed as mmol/kg (SI units) or mOsm/kg (conventional units). Osmolality is the concentration of fluid that affects the movement of water between compartments by osmosis. **Osmolarity** is the number of osmoles in 1 L of solution and is expressed as mmol/L (SI units) or mOsm/L (conventional units).

Osmolality

Osmolality refers to the number of particles dissolved in the serum, primarily sodium, urea (blood urea nitrogen [BUN]), and glucose. It also is a measure of the concentration of solutes per kilogram in urine. Normal serum osmolality ranges from 280 to 300 mOsm/kg. As the number of particles increases, the concentration of the solution also increases. The change in the concentration of particles will affect chemical behavior and movement of water. Sodium is the primary electrolyte in the ECF and keeps water in this compartment.

The following three types of fluid concentration are based on the osmolality of body fluids:

1. **Iso-osmolar** fluid has the same proportion of weight of particles (e.g., sodium, glucose) and water.
2. **Hypo-osmolar** fluid contains fewer particles than water.
3. **Hyperosmolar** fluid contains more particles than water. The plasma/serum osmolality (concentration of circulating body fluids) can be calculated if the serum sodium level is known or the sodium, glucose, and BUN levels are known.

Hypo-osmolality of body fluid may be the result of excess water intake or fluid overload (edema) caused by an inability to excrete excess water. Hyperosmolality of body fluid could be caused by severe diarrhea, increased salt and solutes (protein) intake, inadequate water intake, diabetes, ketoacidosis, or sweating.

Osmolality and Tonicity

The terms *osmolality* and *tonicity* have been used interchangeably; they are similar but not identical. Osmolality refers to the concentration of particles in a solution and is used in reference to body fluids. **Tonicity** is used primarily as a measurement of the concentration of IV solutions compared with the osmolality of body fluids.

FLUID REPLACEMENT

General Considerations

All routes of fluid intake and loss must be considered when assessing fluid balance. General guidelines can be used as the basis for establishing fluid needs. The recommended water intake for a healthy adult is 3.7 L for a man and 2.7 L for a woman, or approximately 30 to 40 mL/kg/d. Patients lose water daily through various routes: about 350 mL through respiration; 450 mL through skin in perspiration and evaporation; 1400 mL in urine; and 200 mL in feces. Insensible losses (water lost via the lungs, skin, and feces) are not measurable. The minimum urinary output for an adult is 0.5 to 1 mL/kg/h or 35 to 70 mL/h for the 70-kg patient.

Daily water requirements differ according to the patient's age and medical problems. Fluid maintenance needs for the NPO (nothing by mouth) patient can be calculated as follows: 4 mL/kg/h for first 10 kg of weight; 2 mL/kg/h for second 10 kg of weight; 1 mL/kg/h for every kg of weight thereafter. Using this formula, a 70-kg patient would require 110 mL/h of IV fluid (IVF), or 2640 mL/d.

IVFs are ordered based on an evaluation of the patient's fluid and electrolyte balance, fluid requirements, and fluid needs. Several questions must be addressed. Is the purpose of IV therapy replacement or maintenance? What are the patient's water, electrolyte, and protein requirements? The patient's weight, caloric needs, and body surface area are other important considerations. Illness and surgery increase the amount of fluids lost and affect fluid and electrolyte needs. Ongoing assessment and monitoring the patient's responses to fluid and electrolyte therapy is vital for patients with fluid and electrolyte imbalances.

Intravenous Solutions

With fluid volume deficit (FVD) from the extracellular body compartment, fluid is lost from the interstitial and vascular spaces. Different types and concentrations of IVFs are available to replace body fluid losses.

Types of Intravenous Solutions

The three general classifications of IV solutions used for fluid replacement are crystalloids (with and without added electrolytes), colloids, and blood and blood products.

Crystalloids

Crystalloid solutions contain fluids and electrolytes and are able to freely cross capillary walls. They do not contain any proteins, which are necessary to maintain the colloidal oncotic pressure that prevents water from leaving the intravascular space. Crystalloids are used to treat dehydration and electrolyte imbalances and as short-term maintenance fluids. Crystalloids cause early plasma expansion but have a shorter duration of action than colloid solutions.

Crystalloid IVFs are classified by their total osmolality when compared with the osmolality of serum. The three major classifications of crystalloid IVF are isotonic, hypotonic, and hypertonic (Table 16-4):

- **Isotonic** solutions have the same approximate osmolality as ECF or plasma. Because of the osmotic equilibrium, water does not enter or leave the cell; therefore, there is no effect on red blood cells (RBCs). Isotonic solutions are primarily used for hydration and to expand ECF volume, because the fluid remains in the intravascular space.
- **Hypotonic** solutions exert less osmotic pressure than ECF, which allows water to move into the cell. IV infusions of hypotonic solutions result in an increased solute concentration in the intravascular space, causing fluid to move into the intracellular and interstitial spaces. Excessive infusion of hypotonic solutions may cause hemolysis, decreased blood pressure, and decreased IVF volume.
- **Hypertonic** solutions exert greater osmotic pressure than ECF, resulting in a higher solute concentration than the serum. When administered, hypertonic IVF fluids pull water from the interstitial space to the ECF via osmosis and cause cell shrinkage. Patients receiving hypertonic solutions must be monitored carefully for signs of circulatory overload (because of the increase in ECF volume).

TABLE 16-4 TONICITY OF INTRAVENOUS SOLUTIONS

TONICITY OF SOLUTION AND OSMOLALITY (mOsm/kg)	EXAMPLES OF IVF AND APPROXIMATE* OSMOLARITY (mOsm/L)	GENERAL INDICATIONS AND CAUTIONS FOR USE
Isotonic (280-300)	Lactated Ringer's solution (275) Ringer's solution (275) Normal saline (308) 5% Dextrose and water (250) (may be classified as hypotonic and isotonic; initially isotonic, then metabolized to hypotonic) Plasma-Lyte (294)	Lactated Ringer's solution provides electrolytes (balanced electrolyte solution). Cautious use in patients with renal failure (contains K^+) and in patients with alkalosis; liver converts Lactated Ringer's solution to bicarbonate **Hydration** Corrects dehydration and sodium depletion Replaces gastrointestinal losses Dextrose provides some calories Caution with use in patients with cardiac or renal disease; risk for fluid volume overload Do not administer isotonic solutions to patients with known or suspected increased intracranial pressure (ICP)
Hypotonic (<280)	0.45% Normal saline (154) 0.33% NaCl (103) 2.5% Dextrose and water (126)	Replaces cellular fluid; treats intracellular dehydration (diabetic ketoacidosis, hyperosmolar hyperglycemic state) Provides free water to allow excretion of body wastes Dextrose provides some calories Do not administer hypotonic solutions to patients with known or suspected ICP or patients with liver disease, shock, trauma, or burns (risk of depleting intravascular volume) Monitor for signs of FVD; monitor for worsening hypovolemia due to decrease in vascular volume
Hypertonic >300	3% Sodium chloride (513) 5% Dextrose and 0.45% normal saline (408) 5% Dextrose and normal saline (560) 5% Dextrose in Lactated Ringer's (525) 10% Dextrose and water (505) 50% Dextrose and water (2526)	Increases serum osmolality Corrects severe hyponatremia; decreases ICP in patients with cerebral edema Dextrose provides some calories Cautious use, may cause intravascular volume overload and pulmonary edema; administer slowly and carefully with infusion control device; for use only in critical care areas and constant monitoring; monitor electrolytes and for signs of FVE Avoid prolonged use Contraindicated for patients with cardiac or renal disease and those with dehydration or diabetic ketoacidosis Higher concentrations of dextrose (>10%) must be given through a central venous access device; may be added to amino acid solutions as total parenteral nutrition

*Refer to manufacturer's label on individual bags of IVF for exact osmolarity.

Parenteral solutions containing dextrose are available in different concentrations and in combination with other solutions, such as normal saline and lactated Ringer's solution. Dextrose solutions provide hydration and some calories and increase glucose levels in the blood. Dextrose solutions are also used to dilute IV medications for administration after compatibility between IVF and the medication has been verified. Dextrose may also affect the stability of some medications; a pharmacist should be consulted if there are questions regarding admixtures. The addition of dextrose to an IV solution affects the tonicity of the solution after it is infused. Five-percent dextrose solutions are hypertonic when added to normal saline or lactated Ringer's solution, but the remaining solution is isotonic because the dextrose is quickly metabolized to carbon dioxide and water.

The Infusion Nursing Society's Practice Guidelines recommend that dextrose solutions higher than 10% should be given via a central vein. An exception is 50% dextrose, which may be given in small amounts via a peripheral vein to correct hypoglycemia. Dextrose can be irritating to veins due to the pH of the solution (3.4 to 4). If hypertonic solutions are not diluted and given peripherally, there is a risk of vein irritation, damage, and thrombosis. Long-term use of hypertonic solutions may result in electrolyte depletion, increased intravascular volume, fluid overload, water intoxication, and pulmonary edema. Rapid infusions of dextrose solutions may cause hyperglycemia, which can lead to osmotic diuresis and fluid and electrolyte imbalance. Hypertonic IV solutions should be administered in a critical care unit, where the staffing ratio allows continuous monitoring for complications. To decrease medication errors with hypertonic solutions, hospitals may limit access of these solutions and dispense them only directly from the pharmacy.

Sodium solutions are available in various concentrations and tonicities. Isotonic solutions are primarily used for hydration to expand the ECF and during blood product transfusions. Rapid infusion of isotonic saline solutions may lead to hypernatremia, fluid volume excess (FVE), and electrolyte depletion. Long-term use should also be avoided, as normal saline provides no calories. Hypotonic solutions are also used for hydration and to treat hyperosmolar diabetes. Hypertonic saline solutions are used to treat severe hyponatremia or hypochloremia; careful monitoring of electrolyte levels is important to avoid excess replacement.

Balanced electrolyte solutions, such as lactated Ringer's solution and Ringer's solution, contain electrolytes (no magnesium) and minimal calories with the addition of dextrose. Their primary use is hydration and electrolyte replacement. However, they do not provide adequate electrolytes for maintenance therapy for patients with limited or no oral intake. Lactated Ringer's solution is similar in electrolyte content to plasma. Lactate is added as a buffering agent and is metabolized to bicarbonate. Complications of infusions of Ringer's and lactated Ringer's include fluid overload, excess electrolytes, and metabolic acidosis with long-term therapy. Because lactate is metabolized in the liver, lactated Ringer's is contraindicated for patients with liver disease.

Colloids

Colloid solutions contain protein or other large molecular substances that increase osmolarity without dissolving in the solution. Because of their size, the particles are unable to pass through the semipermeable membranes of the capillary walls and stay within the intravascular compartment; thus, colloids are also known as plasma expanders. They act by increasing the colloidal oncotic pressure and pulling fluids from the interstitial space into the plasma, increasing blood volume. The composition of colloid solutions includes proteins, carbohydrates, and lipids. Colloids typically have small and large particles, except albumin, whose particles are all one size. Commonly used colloids are shown in Table 16-5.

Blood and Blood Products

Blood and blood products include whole blood and the components that can be processed through centrifugation methods. Blood products include packed RBCs (PRBCs), plasma, platelets, and cryoprecipitate. Plasma can be further processed into volume expanders, coagulation factor concentrates, and immune globins. A unit of PRBCs contains concentrated RBCs with most of the plasma and platelets removed; approximate volume is 350 mL/unit. The approximate volume of a unit of whole blood is 500 mL/unit. Advantages of infusing PRBCs over whole blood are that infusing packed cells allows an increase in oxygen-carrying capacity with a smaller volume, and other portions of the blood can be processed for other therapies. One unit of whole blood elevates the hemoglobin by approximately 0.5 to 1 g/dL, and one unit of packed RBCs elevates the hematocrit by three points.

It is critical for nurses to understand the specific blood component to be infused *before* beginning the infusion. Reducing errors and increasing patient safety during blood and blood product transfusions is a focus of the Joint Commission on Accreditation of Health Care Organizations and is one of the 2013 National Patient Safety Goals. The National Healthcare Safety Network's Hemovigilance Module was developed to increase patient safety and decrease costs associated with transfusion-related adverse events.

The maximum rate of infusion is 4 hours per unit, beginning with removal of the unit from the refrigerator. Loop diuretics are often prescribed to patients receiving whole blood or PRBCs to prevent circulatory overload, particularly in patients who are at risk for developing pulmonary edema and FVE. For patients receiving multiple blood transfusions, the serum ionized calcium level should be monitored. Both PRBCs and whole blood are processed using sodium citrate and citric acid for anticoagulation; multiple blood transfusions can result in a decrease in the plasma ionized (free) calcium levels. Practice guidelines are available from the American Red Cross (see Key Websites).

IV lipid emulsions are indicated for patients who are unable to tolerate oral or enteral feedings for 7 days or more. Lipids can supply up to 30% of the patient's caloric intake. Parenteral nutrition provides essential nutrients intravenously, including proteins, carbohydrates, electrolytes, trace minerals, and vitamins. Lipids are often added to parenteral nutrition formulas; these formulas are referred to as total nutrient admixture. The patient must have a centrally or peripherally inserted vascular access device to receive parenteral nutrition formulas (see Chapter 17).

Nursing Process
Patient-Centered Collaborative Care

Fluid Imbalance

Assessment

- Identify patient at risk for FVD and FVE. Contributing factors for FVD include prolonged inadequate intake, lack of access or inability to obtain fluids, excessive losses due to bleeding or trauma, and GI losses. Contributing factors for FVE include heart failure, liver disease, kidney failure, excessive sodium intake, and excessive or too rapid infusion of IVF.
- Assess patient's history to identify factors that may contribute to FVD and FVE.
- Differentiate between causes of deficient fluid volume, including hypovolemia and dehydration.
- Assess vital signs and patient's usual baseline values. Report abnormal findings.

TABLE 16-5 COMMON COLLOID SOLUTIONS

COMMON SOLUTIONS	INDICATIONS	NURSING IMPLICATIONS	ADVERSE EFFECTS AND CONTRAINDICATIONS
High–molecular-weight dextran (6% dextran 70 and 75) (synthetic colloids)	Treatment of shock caused by hemorrhage, burns, or trauma Maximum volume-expansion effect 1 hour after administration With normal renal functioning, increased volume is excreted within 24 hours	Administer colloid solutions with an 18-g or larger needle Dextran solutions are not a substitute for blood products and have no oxygen-carrying capacity Can be used emergently if cross-matching or blood products are unavailable May interfere with laboratory testing for typing and cross-matching; draw necessary blood samples before administration Increased volume may cause dilutional hemoglobin and hematocrit Assess fluid volume status, may cause circulatory overload Monitor for signs and symptoms of FVE	Wheezing, urticaria, chest tightness, nausea, and vomiting Anaphylactoid reactions are rare, but potentially fatal Contraindicated for patients with renal disease, heart failure, and bleeding disorders
Low–molecular-weight dextran 40 (6%) (synthetic colloids)	Intraoperative prophylaxis of venous and pulmonary embolism Early fluid replacement and treatment of hypovolemic shock	Same as for high–molecular-weight dextran	Same as for high–molecular-weight dextran
Hydroxyethyl starch (Hetastarch) 6% (synthetic polymer closely related to human albumin)	Early fluid replacement and treatment of hypovolemic shock, burns Maximum volume expansion shortly after infusion completed; duration of action 24-36 hours	Hetastarch 6% with 0.9% NaCl is isotonic (310 mOsm/L) Hetastarch 6% with 7.2% NaCl is hypertonic Does not interfere with blood typing and cross-matching Assess fluid volume status, may cause circulatory overload	Severe anaphylactic reaction Interferes with platelet function, increases bleeding time Contraindicated for patients with bleeding disorders and renal, cardiac, and liver disease
Albumin (5% and 25%) Prepared from human blood and blood products; considered a blood product	Regulates plasma volume and tissue fluid balance 5% solution is isotonic; used to treat hypovolemia 25% solution is hypertonic; generally used for patients with fluid and sodium restrictions	Assess fluid volume status, may cause circulatory overload	Contraindicated in patients with heart failure or severe anemia Hold ACEI at least 24 hours before administering albumin due to the risk of adverse reactions including hypotension and flushing

- Assess patient's laboratory values. Plasma or serum osmolality is the primary indicator of patient's hydration status
- Determine adequate urine output for patient based on weight and renal function.
- Obtain urine specific gravity (SG). Normal range is 1.005 to 1.030.
- Check types of IVF ordered per day, including amount to be infused, hourly rate, and solution for tonicity and electrolyte content. Consider if fluid ordered is appropriate for patient's history and clinical condition; collaborate with licensed provider to determine appropriate fluid replacement for patient. Excessive administration of IVF containing sodium to patients with altered regulatory mechanisms may precipitate FVE.
- Assess patient's usual weight.

Nursing Diagnoses

- Deficient fluid volume related to fluid loss and/or inadequate fluid intake, failure of regulatory mechanisms
- FVE related to altered regulatory mechanisms and excess fluid or sodium intake

Planning

- Patient will exhibit balanced fluid volume.
- Patient will have balanced intake and output over 24-hour period.
- Patient will be hydrated as evidenced by moist mucous membranes, elastic skin turgor, vital signs; adequate urine output; urine SG between 1.005 and 1.010; stable weight; and no changes in mental status.
- Patient will not exhibit signs of circulatory overload.
- Patient and family will verbalize understanding of teaching and factors related to FVD and FVE.

Nursing Interventions

General

- Monitor and record vital signs; assess trends and deviation from patient's baseline. Report significant changes to health care provider.
- Measure and record intake and output every 1 to 4 hours, including all forms of output. Measure urine SG.
- Monitor types of fluids patient is receiving. Report if only one type of IVF is prescribed daily. This can cause fluid imbalance.
- Use strict aseptic technique when inserting IV access devices. Check IV site for patency and signs of complications such as phlebitis and infiltration. Adhere to agency policy regarding site rotation and dressing and tubing changes. Avoid contamination when administering IV medications. Follow evidence-based practice guidelines, and implement interventions to decrease central line–associated infections.
- Monitor IV infusion at least hourly; ensure that prescribed amount infuses hourly. Set IV pump correctly, and validate correct drip rate.
- Measure patient's weight daily at the same time, using the same scale, with the same amount of clothing. A gain of 1 kg (2.2 to 2.5 lb) is equivalent to 1 L of fluid.

FVD

- Administer isotonic IVF as ordered.
- Monitor strict intake and output hourly. Encourage frequent oral intake if patient is able. Provide oral care if patient is unable to perform independently. Moisturize skin to prevent dryness; reposition patient every 2 hours, padding bony prominences; and monitor frequently for skin breakdown and pressure.
- Monitor for signs and symptoms of FVD as a result of dehydration, including excess thirst (mild dehydration). Marked thirst, dry mucous membranes, poor skin turgor, decreased urine output, tachycardia, changes in mental status, and slightly decreased systolic blood pressure are indicators of marked dehydration. Dehydration can also result from third-spacing of fluid; although the central volume is low, the patient may exhibit weight gain and generalized edema, atypical of the usual presentation of FVD.
- Monitor vital signs for indications of FVD including increased temperature, weak pulse, tachycardia, hypotension, and tachypnea. Assess for orthostatic hypotension, which can occur with hypovolemia. Use safety precautions when transferring the patient from bed to chair, avoiding abrupt changes in position. Other signs and symptoms of FVD include flattened neck veins; weight loss; decreased skin turgor; dry mucous membranes; oliguria; concentrated urine; decreased capillary refill; pale, cool, clammy skin; and muscle weakness.
- Monitor laboratory values associated with FVD daily, including increased hemoglobin and hematocrit; urine SG >1.030; and increased sodium, BUN, and serum osmolality. When evaluating increased BUN, it is important to review serum creatinine results. Elevated BUN can indicate dehydration, but BUN may also be elevated for other reasons, including excessive protein breakdown. Assessing serum creatinine will determine degree of renal impairment. Evaluate electrolyte levels for imbalances.

FVE

- Monitor and record vital signs indicating FVE, including tachycardia, bounding pulse, tachypnea, increased blood pressure, and increased pulse pressure. Other signs and symptoms of FVE include altered mental status; generalized edema; anasarca; constant, irritated cough; dyspnea; orthopnea; crackles; pulmonary congestion; muffled heart sounds; fatigue; weight gain; increased central venous pressure; jugular vein distention; and increased urine output.
- Monitor laboratory results associated with FVE daily, including elevated BUN, hemoglobin and hematocrit, sodium, serum osmolality, and urine SG <1.010. Monitor electrolytes for imbalances, and creatinine and albumin levels. Chest x-ray may reveal pulmonary congestion.
- Administer diuretics as ordered; implement fluid and sodium restrictions. Recommend a nutritionist consult if warranted. Position patient with head of bed elevated to facilitate ease of respiration, and provide additional pillows if necessary. Monitor edematous areas for signs of pressure and altered skin integrity. Provide meticulous skin care, and reposition patient at least every 2 hours.

Patient Teaching

- Instruct patient that thirst means a mild ECF deficit. Oral fluid intake is the best means of fluid replacement. Increasing fluid intake is important; older patients' thirst mechanisms are frequently decreased. The nurse should offer fluids frequently on a scheduled basis to older adults.
- Advise patient to report frequent vomiting or diarrhea. When vomiting and diarrhea occur constantly or over several days, severe fluid volume and electrolyte imbalance can result.
- Assist patient to plan a typical 24-hour intake based on individual fluid needs. Encourage patient to monitor fluid intake and output. Advise patient to report to the health care provider any abnormal findings, such as changes in urination patterns, fatigue, shortness of breath, weight gain (>2 lb/d or >5 lb/wk) or loss, peripheral edema, or tight shoes and rings. Encourage patient to drink adequate fluids daily, and involve family for support.

Cultural Considerations

- Use an interpreter as appropriate.
- Involve the extended family in health teaching and support.
- Incorporate food choices that are culturally acceptable.

Evaluation

- Patient's vital signs remain within normal limits.
- Fluid intake is balanced with output. Urine output is adequate for age, weight, and history.
- Patient and family understand treatment plan and expected outcomes.
- IVFs are administered as ordered without complications or harm to patient.

ELECTROLYTES

Potassium

Potassium (K^+) is the major intracellular cation; 98% of the body's potassium is found within the cells, and 2% is found in the ECF. Potassium is essential for neuromuscular activity and cellular metabolism. Potassium levels affect cardiac and skeletal muscle activity.

Potassium moves in and out of the cells under the influence of the potassium-sodium pump. Acid-base balance also influences potassium levels. Acidotic conditions tend to pull potassium out of cells; alkalotic conditions tend to put potassium back into cells. Normal renal functioning is needed to maintain potassium balance; the majority is excreted via the kidneys, although the kidneys do not regulate excretion of potassium as well as they conserve sodium. Aldosterone also plays a role in the excretion of potassium.

Daily dietary intake is necessary because potassium is poorly stored in the body. Recommended potassium intake is about 40 to 60 mEq daily, either in potassium-rich foods or as potassium supplements. Foods rich in potassium include tuna fish and fruits and vegetables such as mangoes, avocados, tomatoes, cucumbers, spinach, and bananas.

Functions

Potassium is necessary for transmission and conduction of nerve impulses and for contraction of skeletal, cardiac, and smooth muscles. It is also necessary for normal kidney function and for the enzyme action used to change carbohydrates to energy (glycolysis) and amino acids to protein. Potassium promotes glycogen storage in hepatic cells, regulates the osmolality of cellular fluids, and plays a role in acid-base balance.

Hypokalemia

Hypokalemia, or potassium deficit, occurs with serum levels <3.5 mEq/L. Most cases of hypokalemia are caused by excessive loss rather than deficient intake. Whenever cells are damaged from trauma, injury, surgery, or shock, potassium leaks from the cells into the intravascular fluid and is excreted by the kidneys. With cellular loss of potassium, potassium shifts from the blood plasma into the cell to restore the cellular potassium balance; hypokalemia usually results. GI sources of potassium loss include vomiting, diarrhea, suctioning, recent ileostomy formation, and draining fistulae. Between 80% and 90% of potassium in the body is excreted in the urine; 8% is excreted in the feces. Major causes of potassium loss are vomiting, diarrhea, or as a result of diuretic therapy. Other causes include burns, total parenteral nutrition therapy, alkalosis, prolonged laxative use, excessive licorice consumption, corticosteroid use, increased aldosterone levels, and decreased magnesium levels.

Hypokalemia may not be symptomatic until potassium levels are <3.0 mEq/L. It is important to recognize early signs and symptoms to prevent severe hypokalemia, which can result in cardiac arrest and death. Early clinical manifestations include fatigue, muscle weakness, anorexia, nausea, and vomiting. Muscle weakness does not usually occur until potassium levels are <2.5 mEq/L. Weakness usually begins in the lower extremities, progresses cephalad to the trunk, and may result in paralysis; respiratory muscle involvement may result in respiratory arrest. Quadricep weakness may be one of the earliest signs. Severe signs and symptoms include paresthesias, leg cramps, decreased bowel motility and paralytic ileus, confusion, rhabdomyolysis and myoglobinuria, atrial and ventricular dysrhythmias, and cardiac arrest. Electrocardiogram (ECG) changes include flattened or inverted T waves and depressed ST segments. Patients at risk for hypokalemia-induced dysrhythmias include older adults, those with heart disease or co-existing hypomagnesemia, and those on digoxin or other antiarrhythmics. Certain drugs, such as potassium-wasting diuretics and cortisone preparations, promote potassium loss. Patients receiving these drugs should increase their potassium intake by consuming foods rich in potassium or taking potassium supplements as prescribed by their health care provider. Serum potassium levels should be monitored periodically for abnormalities.

Treatment for hypokalemia due to excessive potassium loss depends on the severity of the deficit. Patients with low-normal serum potassium levels may be advised to consume additional foods high in potassium. Usual dietary potassium intake for adults is 50 to 100 mEq daily; typically, a loss of 200 mEq or more is sufficient to cause hypokalemia. Management goals for patients with hypokalemia include preventing and treating life-threatening complications, replacing potassium and returning levels to normal, and diagnosing and correcting the cause of the deficiency.

Potassium replacements can be given orally or intravenously (Box 16-1). Table 16-6 lists the potassium preparations used to treat hypokalemia, and Prototype Drug Chart 16-1 compares the pharmacokinetics and pharmacodynamics of oral and IV potassium preparations.

Pharmacodynamics Potassium maintains neuromuscular activity. Onset of action of oral potassium may be within 30 minutes; for IV potassium, it is immediate. Duration of action of potassium is not known; however, it may vary according to the dose taken. ECG and serum potassium levels should be closely monitored when large doses are administered.

BOX 16-1 ORAL AND IV POTASSIUM PREPARATIONS

Oral Potassium Preparations

- Potassium bicarbonate: Indicated for use in patients with hypokalemia and metabolic acidosis. (Potassium acetate available for IV administration.)
- Potassium phosphate: Found primarily in food. Indicated for patients with hypokalemia and hypophosphatemia.
- Potassium gluconate: available as elixir or tablet
- Potassium chloride: All other indications, including hypokalemic alkalosis. Raises serum K^+ level faster than potassium bicarbonate. Available as liquid, powder, tablet, capsule, crystalline (salt substitute), controlled-release microencapsulated tablets, wax-matrix–extended-release tablets, enteric-coated tablets, and effervescent tablets for solution.

Nursing Implications for Oral Preparations

- Liquid forms are inexpensive but not palatable. Must be diluted in water or juice; follow manufacturer's instructions (minimum amount for dilution 90 mL). Follow with a large glass of water to enhance esophageal peristalsis. Dilute liquid forms before administering via enteral feeding tube.
- Administer medication with food and while patient is sitting up to prevent esophagitis. Instruct patient to remain upright at least 30 minutes after administration. Any form may cause nausea and vomiting. Large tablets may be difficult to swallow.
- Advise patient not to suck on tablets to avoid oral ulceration. Extended-release forms may not be crushed or chewed.
- Enteric-coated tablets are associated with small bowel ulceration; wax-matrix tablets may cause small bowel ulceration, stricture, and perforation. Advise patient that wax-matrix casing may be visible in stool. Risk of gastrointestinal side effects lowest with microencapsulated preparations.
- Assess potassium levels after 60 mEq of K^+; if immediate-acting form is given, draw K^+ level after 60 minutes; for sustained-release forms, draw K^+ level after 3 hours. Patients on maintenance doses should have periodic levels drawn by the primary care provider.

Nursing Implications for Intravenous Potassium Administration

- IV therapy is indicated for patients unable to tolerate oral therapy or in addition to oral therapy for patients with severe hypokalemia.
- Only *diluted* potassium chloride may be administered IV; concentrated KCl is *never* administered IV; KCl is *never* given by direct injection into the vein.*
- Monitor IV site and infusion carefully, avoid extravasation and infiltration.
- Too rapid infusion may cause fatal hyperkalemia.
- Administer via peripheral or central vein. *Must be administered with a calibrated infusion device. Refer to individual institution's policy for administration.* Pain is associated with peripheral infusion; administer via central vein whenever possible. Recommended maximum concentration for peripheral administration is 10 mEq/100 mL or 40 mEq/1000 mL; maximum infusion rate for adults with serum K^+ >2.5 mEq/L is 10 mEq/h or 200 mEq/24 h. Rates higher than 10 mEq/h require continuous ECG monitoring and serum K^+ level determination. For urgent use or if serum K^+ is <2 mEq/L, infusion rates up to 40/mEq/h or 400 mEq/d are admissible with continuous ECG monitoring and frequent serum K^+ level measurements.
- Administration via central venous access device: Preferred route for patients with severe hypokalemia. Recommended infusion rate is 10 to 20 mEq/h, except for emergencies and patients with severe hypokalemia.
- Potassium chloride should be diluted in saline solution, not dextrose, for administration. Dextrose solutions stimulate insulin release, which will cause extracellular K^+ to shift into cells, reducing already low K^+ levels.

*Potassium chloride concentrate for injection is an ISMP High-Alert medication. Potassium chloride injection has been removed from general floor stock on noncritical care units in most U.S. hospitals as a result of recommendations from the ISMP and Institute for Healthcare Improvement. Despite the limited access, errors involving administration of IV KCl still occur. To reduce errors, the following precautions should be followed: KCl vials should not be stocked on nursing units. The pharmacy should prepare admixtures prior to dispensing to patient-care units or dispense only premixed solutions to reduce the risk of patients receiving undiluted potassium. Never add KCl to an existing IV infusion.

TABLE 16-6 POTASSIUM SUPPLEMENTS

PREPARATION	DRUG
Oral liquid	Potassium chloride: 10% = 20 mEq/15 mL, 20% = 40 mEq/15 mL (Kay Ciel, Kaochlor 10%, Kaon-Cl 20%)
Oral tablet or capsule	Potassium chloride: enteric-coated tablet (Kaon, Kaon-Cl, Slow-K, 8 mEq Kaochlor, K-Lyte, effervescent tablet K-Lyte/Cl, K-Dur, Micro-K, Ten-K, K-Tab)
Intravenous potassium	Potassium chloride in clear liquid in multidose vial or ampule (2 mEq/mL)

Hyperkalemia

Hyperkalemia is defined as a serum potassium level >5.3 mEq/L; causes include excessive intake, decreased excretion, or shift from intracellular to extracellular space. The most common causes are renal failure and medications that interfere with potassium excretion. Renal disease or kidney failure results in potassium accumulating in the intravascular fluid and hyperkalemia. Persons at risk for developing hyperkalemia include premature infants, older adults, and those with a history of genitourinary disease, adrenal insufficiency, cancer, poorly controlled diabetes, or polypharmacy. Hyperkalemia manifests primarily as cardiac and neuromuscular symptoms. Signs and symptoms include cardiac dysrhythmias, including characteristic ECG changes—early tachycardia followed by bradycardia; paresthesias of face, tongue, hands, and feet; and GI hyperactivity, including nausea, diarrhea, and abdominal cramping. Metabolic acidosis may also be present.

Management goals are to eliminate the cause of the excess, shift potassium back into the cells, increase potassium excretion, decrease potassium intake, and prevent further episodes of hyperkalemia. For mild hyperkalemia, foods rich in potassium are usually restricted. Treatment strategies for hyperkalemia are outlined in Box 16-2.

PROTOTYPE DRUG CHART 16-1

Potassium

Drug Class	Dosage
Electrolyte Trade Names: Kaochlor, Kaon Cl, Kay Ciel, Micro K, K Dur Pregnancy Category: A	A: Prevention of hypokalemia: 20 mEq daily in 1-2 divided doses. A: Replacement: 40 to 100 mEq daily in divided doses A: IV: 10-60 mEq/100 mL of solution; *max:* 200-400 mEq/d; doses >10 mEq/h require continuous ECG monitoring
Contraindications	**Drug-Lab-Food Interactions**
Renal insufficiency or failure, Addison's disease, hyperkalemia, severe dehydration, acidosis, potassium-sparing diuretics	Drug: Increases serum potassium levels: ACE inhibitors, potassium-sparing diuretics, NSAIDs, beta-adrenergic blockers, heparin, salt substitutes. Decreases serum potassium levels: thiazide and loop diuretics, amphotericin B, antacids, insulin, fluconazole, theophylline, and laxatives Caution: Cardiac and renal disease, burns Food: Excessive intake of licorice may cause hypokalemia and sodium retention; salt substitutes contain potassium
Pharmacokinetics	**Pharmacodynamics**
Absorption: PO: rapidly absorbed, 95% in body fluids Distribution: PB: UK Metabolism: t½: UK Excretion: 80%-90% in urine; 10% in feces	PO: Onset: 30 min Peak: 1-2 h Duration: UK IV: Onset: Rapid Peak: 1-1.5 h Duration: UK
Therapeutic Effects/Uses	
To correct potassium deficit; strengthen cardiac and muscular activities; prevent hypokalemia in at-risk patients; treat hypokalemic alkalosis. Mode of Action: Transmits and conducts nerve impulses; contracts skeletal, smooth, and cardiac muscles.	
Side Effects	**Adverse Reactions**
Nausea, vomiting, diarrhea, abdominal cramps, irritability, rash (rare); phlebitis with IV administration	Hyperkalemia (older adults with renal impairment); oliguria, ECG changes (peaked T waves, widened QRS complex, prolonged PR interval), GI ulceration Life-threatening: Cardiac dysrhythmias, respiratory distress, ventricular fibrillation, cardiac arrest

A, Adult; *ACE,* angiotensin-converting enzyme; *ECG,* electrocardiogram; *GI,* gastrointestinal; *h,* hour; *IV,* intravenous; *PB,* protein-binding; *PO,* by mouth; *t ½,* half-life; *UK,* unknown; >, greater than.

BOX 16-2 HYPERKALEMIA: TREATMENTS AND RATIONALES

Potassium Restriction

- Restriction of potassium intake will slowly lower serum level.
- For mild hyperkalemia (slightly elevated K^+ levels) (5.4 to 5.6 mEq/L, potassium restriction is normally effective).

Intravenous Sodium Bicarbonate

- By elevating pH level, potassium moves back into cells and lowers serum level.
- Temporary treatment

10% Calcium Gluconate

- Decreases irritability of myocardium resulting from hyperkalemia.
- Temporary treatment; does not promote K^+ loss.
- Caution: Administering to patient on digitalis can cause digitalis toxicity.

Insulin and Glucose (10%-50%)

- Moves potassium back into cells.
- Temporary treatment; effective for approximately 6 hours and not always as effective when repeated.

Kayexalate (Sodium Polystyrene) and Sorbitol 70%

- Kayexalate is used as a cation exchange for severe hyperkalemia; may cause hypocalcemia and hypomagnesemia and sodium retention.
- Can be administered orally or rectally.
- Approximate dosages:

Oral Administration

- Kayexalate: 10-20 g, 3-4 times daily
- Sorbitol 70%: 20 mL with each dose

Rectal Administration

- Kayexalate: 30-50 g as warm emulsion, enema given high into sigmoid colon
- Sorbitol 70%: 50 mL; mix with 100-150 mL of water

Constipation is a common adverse effect; assess bowel function daily; monitor for fecal impaction. A mild laxative may be prescribed.

Effect of Drugs on Potassium Balance

Potassium-wasting diuretics are a major cause of hypokalemia. Diuretics are divided into two categories: potassium-wasting (kaliuretic) and potassium-sparing (antikaliuretic) drugs. Potassium-wasting diuretics excrete potassium and other electrolytes such as sodium and chloride in the urine. Potassium-sparing diuretics retain potassium but excrete sodium and chloride in the urine.

Laxatives, corticosteroids, antibiotics, and potassium-wasting diuretics are the major drug classifications that can cause hypokalemia. Other drug classifications that may cause hyperkalemia include oral and IV potassium salts, central nervous system (CNS) agents, and potassium-sparing diuretics. Tables 16-7 and 16-8 list drugs that affect potassium balance.

Nursing Process
Patient-Centered Collaborative Care

Potassium

Assessment

- Assess for signs and symptoms of potassium imbalance. Symptoms of hypokalemia include nausea, vomiting, polyuria, cardiac dysrhythmias, abdominal distention, and soft, flabby muscles. Symptoms of hyperkalemia include oliguria, nausea, abdominal cramps, tachycardia and later bradycardia, weakness, and numbness or tingling in the extremities.
- Assess serum potassium level; normal level is 3.5 to 5.3 mEq/L. Report serum potassium deficit or excess to the health care provider.
- Obtain baseline vital signs and ECG readings. Report abnormal findings. Vital signs and ECG results can be compared with future readings.
- Check patient for signs and symptoms of digitalis toxicity when receiving a digitalis preparation and a potassium-wasting diuretic or a cortisone preparation. Decreased serum potassium level enhances the action

TABLE 16-7 DRUGS CAUSING HYPOKALEMIA

SUBSTANCES	RATIONALE
Laxatives Enemas (hyperosmolar)	Abuse can cause potassium depletion.
Corticosteroids	
Cortisone	Ion-exchange agent
Prednisone	Steroids promote potassium loss and sodium retention.
Kayexalate	Exchanges potassium ion for a sodium ion.
Levodopa/L-dopalithium	Increase potassium loss via urine.
Antibiotic I: amphotericin B, polymyxin B, gentamicin, neomycin, amikacin, tobramycin, cisplatin	Have a toxic effect on renal tubules and thus decrease potassium reabsorption.
Antibiotic II: penicillin, ampicillin, carbenicillin, ticarcillin, nafcillin, piperacillin, azlocillin	Enhance potassium excretion by the presence of nonabsorbable anions.
Alpha-adrenergic blockers Insulin and glucose	Promote movement of potassium into cells, thus lowering the serum potassium level.
Beta$_2$-agonists: terbutaline, albuterol Estrogen	Promote potassium loss.

TABLE 16-8 DRUGS CAUSING HYPERKALEMIA

SUBSTANCES	RATIONALE
potassium chloride (oral or IV) potassium salt substitutes potassium penicillin (pen-vee K) KPO_4 enema	Excess ingestion or infusion can cause potassium excess.
Angiotensin-converting enzyme inhibitors: captopril (Capoten), quinapril HCl (Accupril), ramipril (Altace)	Increase the state of hypoaldosteronism (decrease sodium and increase potassium) and impair renal potassium excretion.
Angiotensin II receptor antagonists Losartan potassium (Cozaar)	Decrease adrenal synthesis of aldosterone; potassium is retained and sodium is excreted.
Beta-adrenergic blockers: propranolol (Inderal), nadolol (Corgard)	Decrease cellular uptake of potassium, and decrease Na-K-ATPase function.
Digoxin	Therapeutic dose is not affected; however, with overdose, potassium excess may occur.
Heparin	Inhibits adrenal aldosterone production.
Low–molecular-weight heparin	Suppresses aldosterone
	Decreases potassium homeostasis; renal excretion of potassium is reduced.
Immunosuppressive drugs: cyclosporine, tacrolimus, cyclophosphamide	Reduce potassium excretion by induction of hypoaldosteronism; loss of potassium from cells.
Nonsteroidal antiinflammatory drugs: ibuprofen, indomethacin	Impair potassium homeostasis and block cellular potassium uptake.
Succinylcholine	Allows for leakage of potassium out of cells.
CNS agents: barbiturates, sedatives, opioids, heroin, amphetamines	Usually characterized by muscle necrosis and cellular shift of potassium from cells to serum.

of digitalis, increasing the likelihood of digitalis toxicity. Signs and symptoms of digitalis toxicity are nausea, vomiting, anorexia, bradycardia (pulse rate <60 or markedly decreased), cardiac dysrhythmias, and visual disturbances.

Nursing Diagnoses

- Deficient knowledge related to inadequate knowledge of medications and foods affecting potassium levels
- Risk for decreased cardiac output related to excess serum potassium
- Activity intolerance related to muscle weakness

Planning

- Patient's serum potassium level will be within normal range.
- Patient will verbalize understanding of the potassium imbalance and state methods to decrease recurrence. Patient with hypokalemia will eat potassium-rich foods. Patient with hyperkalemia will avoid potassium-rich foods.

Nursing Interventions

- Give oral potassium with sufficient amount of water or juice (at least 3 to 8 oz) and with meals. Potassium is extremely irritating to the gastric mucosa.
- Hang IV solutions containing potassium to be infused only with an infusion-control device; monitor infusion at least hourly.
- Potassium cannot be given intramuscularly. Potassium should never be given as an IV bolus or push. Giving IV potassium directly into the vein causes cardiac dysrhythmias and cardiac arrest.
- Check amount of urine output. Potassium accumulation occurs if patient is receiving potassium and urine output is <25 mL/h or <600 mL/d. Remember: 80% to 90% of potassium is excreted in the urine. Report results to the health care provider.
- Monitor serial potassium levels frequently as well as serum creatinine, BUN, glucose, electrolytes, and arterial blood gases. Report abnormal results to health care provider.
- Monitor ECG. With hypokalemia, there is a flat or inverted T wave, a depressed ST segment, and a prolonged QT interval. With hyperkalemia, there is a narrow and peaked T wave, widened QRS complex, prolonged PR interval, flattened or absent T waves, and depressed ST segment.
- Monitor patient's response to activity, and plan frequent rest periods due to muscle weakness associated with potassium imbalances.
- Check IV site for infiltration if patient is receiving IV potassium. Potassium can cause extravasation and tissue necrosis if it infiltrates into subcutaneous tissue. Discontinue IV immediately if infiltration occurs.
- Monitor patients receiving medications for hyperkalemia for signs and symptoms of continuing hyperkalemia or iatrogenic hypokalemia.

Patient Teaching

General

- Advise patient to have serum potassium level checked at regular intervals as prescribed by primary health care provider when taking medications that affect potassium levels.
- Instruct patient to drink a full glass of water or juice when taking oral potassium supplements. Potassium preparations can be taken during or after a meal. Explain to patient that potassium is very irritating to the stomach.
- Encourage patient to comply with prescribed potassium dose, regular laboratory tests, and medical follow-up related to the health problem and drug regimen.
- Instruct patient to report signs and symptoms of hypokalemia and hyperkalemia.

Diet

- Instruct patients who are taking medications promoting potassium loss to eat potassium-rich foods.
- Instruct patients at risk for potassium imbalances regarding dietary sources of potassium and potassium content of foods.

Cultural Considerations

- Use an interpreter as appropriate.
- Involve the extended family in health teaching and support.
- Incorporate food choices that are culturally acceptable.

Evaluation

- Evaluate patient's serum potassium level and ECG. Cardiac rhythm should return to patient's normal baseline without dysrhythmias. Serum potassium level remains within normal range. Report to the health care provider if the level remains abnormal. Potassium replacements and diet may need modification.

Sodium

Sodium is the major cation in the ECF. The normal serum or plasma sodium level is 135 to 145 mEq/L. A serum sodium level <135 mEq/L is called **hyponatremia,** and a serum sodium level >145 mEq/L is called **hypernatremia.** Sodium and chloride imbalances typically occur together. The most serious problems associated with serum sodium deficit or excess are cerebral dehydration, seizures, and coma.

The dietary requirement for sodium is 2 to 4 g/d. Sodium-rich foods include bacon, luncheon meats, corned beef, decaffeinated coffee, ham, tomato juice, pickles, and soda crackers.

Functions

Sodium is found in most body fluids, plays a major role in fluid volume balance, and is the primary determinant of plasma osmolality. Sodium combines readily with chloride (Cl^-) or bicarbonate (HCO_3^-) to promote acid-base balance. Sodium promotes the transmission and conduction of nerve impulses and is part of the sodium/potassium pump. There is rapid sodium influx into cells during depolarization as potassium shifts out of cells to maintain water balance and neuromuscular activity. When sodium shifts into the cell, depolarization occurs. Repolarization of the cell occurs when the cell membrane is primarily permeable to potassium with the shift of potassium out of the cell due to the diffusion gradient. Sodium imbalance is usually accompanied by water imbalance due to its effects on fluid volume balance.

Hyponatremia

Hyponatremia is caused by sodium loss, deficient intake, or water gain. Sodium loss can result from vomiting, diarrhea, nasogastric suctioning, burns, wound drainage, trauma, renal failure, heart failure, third-spacing, syndrome of inappropriate antidiuretic hormone secretion, excessive hypertonic or sodium-free IVF, surgery, and thiazide diuretics. Hyponatremia may occur with hypovolemia and hypervolemia. Presenting symptoms depend on the onset and degree of deficit. Signs and symptoms of hyponatremia due to water shifting into cells are primarily neuromuscular and GI and include muscle weakness; decreased deep tendon reflexes; headaches; lethargy; confusion; seizures; coma; abdominal cramps; nausea and vomiting; tachycardia and hypotension; pale skin; and dry mucous membranes. Signs of hyponatremia associated with decreased ECF (hypovolemia) include tachycardia; weak, thready pulse; and decreased blood pressure progressing to orthostatic hypotension. If hyponatremia is caused by increased ECF (hypervolemia), signs and symptoms include jugular vein distention, weight gain, edema, and increased blood pressure.

Oral sodium replacement is the preferred treatment if the patient is able or if the deficit is mild. Sodium may also be replaced via enteral feeding tubes. For a serum sodium level between 125 and 135 mEq/L, IV normal saline (0.9% sodium chloride) may increase sodium content in vascular fluid. For a serum sodium level <120 mEq/L, a hypertonic 3% or 5% saline solution may be necessary.

Hypernatremia

Hypernatremia can be caused by sodium gain, sodium retention, or water loss. Causes include excessive oral sodium intake, deficient water intake, hypertonic tube feedings, hypertonic IVF, hyperaldosteronism, Cushing's syndrome, corticosteroid use, and acute kidney failure. Other causes include vomiting, diarrhea, burns, diabetes insipidus, and mineralocorticoid excess.

Signs of fluid imbalance depend on the cause; water loss presents with symptoms of FVD, while sodium gain presents with symptoms of FVE. Signs and symptoms of hypernatremia are dry, sticky mucous membranes; flushed, dry skin; agitation; elevated body temperature; rough, edematous, dry tongue; nausea and vomiting; anorexia; tachycardia; hypertension; muscle twitching; hyperreflexia; seizures; and coma. Thirst is usually the first symptom of sodium deficit.

Management of hypernatremia depends on the cause and severity of the deficit. Frequent monitoring of sodium levels is necessary while the underlying cause is being treated. When the serum sodium level is elevated >145 mEq/L, sodium restriction is indicated. Treatments include administration of IVF and diuretics.

Nursing Process
Patient-Centered Collaborative Care

Sodium

Assessment

- Assess patient for signs and symptoms of sodium imbalance. Symptoms of hyponatremia are muscle weakness, headaches, lethargy, confusion, seizures, abdominal cramps, nausea and vomiting, tachycardia and hypotension, pale skin, and dry mucous membranes. Symptoms of hypernatremia are flushed, dry skin; agitation; elevated body temperature; rough, dry tongue; nausea and vomiting; anorexia; tachycardia; hypertension; muscle twitching; and hyperreflexia.
- Check serum sodium level. Report abnormally low sodium levels (<125 mEq/L), because prompt medical care is required.
- Obtain history of health problems that may lead to sodium loss or excess.

Nursing Diagnoses

- Risk for imbalanced (excess) fluid volume related to water retention
- Readiness to learn about sodium-rich foods

Planning

- Patient's serum sodium level will be within normal range in 3 to 5 days.
- Edema will be decreased in patient with sodium retention.

Nursing Interventions

- Monitor prescribed medical regimen for correction of hyponatremia—for example, water restriction, IV normal saline (0.9% sodium chloride), or 3% saline solution to correct serum sodium levels <115 mEq/L.
- Monitor serum sodium levels. Report abnormal levels.

Patient Teaching

- Instruct patient with hypernatremia to avoid foods high in sodium. Instruct patient to avoid using salt when cooking and adding salt to food at the table.

- Emphasize importance of reading labels on food products.

Cultural Considerations
- Use interpreter as appropriate.
- Involve extended family in health teaching and support.
- Incorporate food choices that are culturally acceptable.

Evaluation
- Evaluate patient's serum sodium level. Report if sodium imbalance continues.
- Assess patient's fluid volume balance. Monitor intake and output carefully; monitor daily weights.
- Assess patient for signs of circulatory overload and deficit.

Calcium

Calcium is found in approximately equal proportions in ICF and ECF. The serum calcium range is 4.5 to 5.5 mEq/L, or 8.5 to 10.5 mg/dL. A calcium deficit (<4.5 mEq/L) is called **hypocalcemia,** and a calcium excess (>5.5 mEq/L) is called **hypercalcemia.** Over 90% of the body's calcium is found in bones and teeth. Of the remaining calcium found in the blood, about 50% is bound to protein, primarily albumin. The remaining 50% is free, ionized calcium (iCa) and can leave the vascular space and be active in cellular functions. Serum levels are measures of both ionized and protein-bound calcium.

The normal serum iCa range is 2.2 to 2.5 mEq/L, or 4.25 to 5.25 mg/dL. Calcium levels are affected by acid-base balance and plasma albumin levels. When an individual is acidotic, calcium is released from serum protein, which increases serum iCa level. During alkalosis, calcium is bound to protein, and there is less iCa. If serum albumin levels are decreased, there is more free circulating calcium, even when the serum calcium level is decreased. There are formulas to correct the serum calcium levels in patients with hypoalbuminemia.

Functions

Calcium promotes normal nerve and muscle contraction and plays a role in cardiac excitability. This cation also maintains normal cellular permeability and promotes blood clotting by converting prothrombin into thrombin. Calcium is also needed for formation of bone and teeth. Calcium levels are regulated by parathyroid hormone and calcitonin. Calcium functions are closely related to magnesium and phosphorus. Calcium and phosphorus have an inverse relationship; that is, increased calcium levels result in decreased phosphorus levels.

Vitamin D is needed for calcium absorption from the GI tract. Aspirin and anticonvulsants can alter vitamin D, affecting calcium absorption. Loop or high-ceiling diuretics (see Chapter 43), steroids (cortisone), magnesium preparations, and phosphate preparations promote calcium loss. Conversely, thiazide diuretics increase serum calcium levels.

Hypocalcemia

Inadequate calcium intake causes calcium to leave bone to maintain a normal serum calcium level. Because of calcium loss from bones (bone demineralization), pathological fractures may occur if calcium deficit persists. Hyperphosphatemia, acute pancreatitis, widespread bony metastases, hypoparathyroidism, alkalosis, diarrhea, alcoholism, malnutrition, use of loop diuretics, vitamin D deficiency, and multiple blood transfusions are common causes of hypocalcemia.

Signs and symptoms of hypocalcemia reflect calcium's role in nerve transmission and heart and muscle function. Neurologic and neuromuscular symptoms include anxiety, irritability, and tetany; twitching; hyperactive deep tendon reflexes; carpopedal spasm; spasmodic contractions; laryngeal spasm; and seizures. Positive Chvostek's and Trousseau's signs are classic signs of hypocalcemia associated with tetany. Cardiovascular manifestations include decreased cardiac output; dysrhythmias; and ECG changes including prolonged QT interval, elongated ST segment, and ventricular tachycardia (torsades de pointes). Hypocalcemia also causes a diminished response to digitalis; other signs are dry, brittle nails and dry hair and skin.

If metabolic acidosis is present with hypocalcemia, tetany symptoms are absent because calcium leaves protein sites during an acidotic state; thus, more iCa is available. During an alkalotic state, more calcium binds with protein. There is less iCa, and tetany symptoms usually result.

Many calcium preparations can be administered orally or IV. The treatment depends on the cause, degree of deficit, and clinical condition of the patient. IV calcium replacement should be administered only to acutely symptomatic patients. Oral calcium preparations are available in tablets, capsules, and powders. Calcium preparations are combined with various salts such as chloride, carbonate, gluconate, gluceptate, and lactate. IV calcium is available as calcium chloride (CaCl) (10%) and calcium gluconate (10%); both can be used for acute hypocalcemia and during cardiac resuscitation. Calcium gluconate may be given subcutaneously or intramuscularly. Both preparations deliver 20 mg of elemental calcium per mEq. Calcium gluconate has the same action on the heart as digitalis: it increases the force of systolic contractions. Prototype Drug Chart 16-2 describes the pharmacokinetics and pharmacodynamics of calcium preparations.

The patient's renal functioning should be assessed before administering IV CaCl; this solution contains aluminum, which can be toxic if renal insufficiency exists. IV calcium should be administered cautiously in patients who take digitalis because an increase in serum calcium increases the risk of digitalis toxicity. Concentrated calcium solutions (10% CaCl) require a central line for administration. The solution should be administered slowly via an infusion-control device,

PROTOTYPE DRUG CHART 16-2

Calcium

Drug Class Electrolyte Pregnancy Category: C Drug Forms: Tablet, capsule, liquid, injection	**Dosage** Tetany: A: IV: 4-16 mEq C: IV: 0.5-0.7 mEq/kg t.i.d., q.i.d. Hypocalcemia: A: PO: 500 mg/d in divided doses
Contraindications Hypercalcemia, renal calculi, digitalis toxicity, ventricular fibrillation Caution: Renal insufficiency, renal stones, dehydration, diarrhea, respiratory acidosis, or respiratory failure	**Drug-Lab-Food Interactions** Drug: Increase digitalis toxicity: digoxin; decrease calcium channel blockers, verapamil; decrease absorption of tetracycline; increase serum calcium level: thiazide diuretics Lab: May increase gastrin, pH; may decrease phosphate, potassium
Pharmacokinetics Absorption: PO: 35% absorbed, requires vitamin D Distribution: PB: UK Metabolism: t½: UK Excretion: 20% in urine, 70% in feces, some in saliva	**Pharmacodynamics** PO: Onset: UK Peak: UK Duration: 2-4 h IV: Onset: Rapid Peak: UK Duration: 2-3 h
Therapeutic Effects/Uses To correct calcium deficit or tetany symptoms, prevent osteoporosis Mode of Action: Transmits nerve impulses, contracts skeletal and cardiac muscles, maintains cellular permeability; promotes strong bone and teeth growth	
Side Effects PO: Nausea, vomiting, constipation, pain, drowsiness, headache, muscle weakness	**Adverse Reactions** Hypercalcemia, ECG changes (shortened QT interval), metabolic alkalosis, heart block, rebound hyperacidity Life-threatening: Renal failure, cardiac dysrhythmias, cardiac arrest

A, Adult; *C,* child; *d,* day; *ECG,* electrocardiogram; *GI,* gastrointestinal; *h,* hour; *IV,* intravenous; *PB,* protein binding; *PO,* by mouth; *q.i.d.,* four times a day; *t ½,* half-life; *t.i.d.,* three times a day; *UK,* unknown.

and the patient should be monitored frequently. Too rapid an infusion may cause cardiac syncope and decreased blood pressure from peripheral vasodilation. Use of a small-bore needle in a large vein minimizes venous irritation. The patient may report a burning sensation with higher infusion rates. It is essential to ascertain that the IV is in the vein and not infiltrated. Local extravasation may cause tissue necrosis and sloughing. Refer to agency policy if infiltration occurs.

Patients with hypocalcemia should be assessed for hypomagnesemia, hypokalemia, and acid-base imbalances, and any abnormalities should be corrected. Hypomagnesemia should be corrected first; low magnesium levels may render the patient refractory to treatment for hypocalcemia.

Pharmacokinetics Vitamin D promotes calcium absorption from the GI tract; phosphorus inhibits calcium absorption. The pH affects the amount of free iCa. When pH is decreased (acidic), there is more free iCa, because it has been released from protein-binding sites. With an increased pH (alkalosis), more calcium is bound to protein.

Hypercalcemia

Elevated serum calcium may be a result of hyperparathyroidism, malignancy, hypophosphatemia, excessive calcium intake, prolonged immobilization, multiple fractures, and drugs such as thiazide diuretics and steroids. Signs and symptoms of hypercalcemia are fatigue, muscle weakness, depressed deep tendon reflexes, confusion, impaired memory, anorexia, nausea, vomiting, constipation, and kidney stones of calcium composition. ECG changes include shortened QT interval and ST segment; the patient may exhibit decreased heart rate and dysrhythmias.

Effect of Drugs on Calcium Balance

Phosphate preparations, corticosteroids, loop diuretics, aspirin, anticonvulsants, magnesium sulfate, and mithramycin are some of the drug groups that can lower serum calcium levels. Excess calcium salt ingestion or infusion and thiazide and chlorthalidone diuretics can all contribute to an increased serum calcium level. Table 16-9 lists drugs that affect calcium balance.

Clinical Management of Calcium Imbalance

Clinical management of hypocalcemia consists of oral supplements and IV calcium. Table 16-10 lists oral and IV preparations of calcium salts, their dosages, and drug forms. Calcium carbonate can cause GI upset because it produces carbon dioxide. For better calcium absorption, calcium supplements should contain vitamin D, and oral calcium should be taken 30 minutes before meals.

TABLE 16-9 DRUGS AFFECTING CALCIUM BALANCE

SUBSTANCES	RATIONALE
Drugs Causing Hypocalcemia	
Magnesium sulfate Propylthiouracil (Propacil) Colchicine Plicamycin (Mithracin) Neomycin Excessive sodium citrate	Inhibit parathyroid hormone/PTH secretion and decrease serum calcium level.
Acetazolamide Aspirin Anticonvulsants Glutethimide (doriden) Estrogens Aminoglycosides: gentamicin, amikacin, tobramycin	Can alter vitamin D metabolism needed for calcium absorption.
Phosphate preparations: oral, enema, intravenous; sodium phosphate; potassium phosphate	Can increase serum phosphorus level and decrease serum calcium level.
Corticosteroids: cortisone, prednisone	Decrease calcium mobilization and inhibit calcium absorption.
Loop diuretics: furosemide (Lasix)	Reduce calcium absorption from renal tubules.
Drugs Causing Hypercalcemia	
Calcium salts Vitamin D	Excess ingestion of calcium and vitamin D and infusion of calcium can increase serum calcium level.
IV lipids	Can increase serum calcium level.
Androgens	Can induce hypercalcemia.
Diuretics: thiazides, chlorthalidone (Hygroton)	
Lithium	Increases parathyroid hormone/PTH secretion.

TABLE 16-10 CALCIUM PREPARATIONS

CALCIUM NAME	DRUG FORM	DRUG DOSE
Orals		
calcium carbonate	650- to 1500-mg tablets	400 mg/g*
calcium citrate	950-mg tablet	211 mg/g*
calcium gluconate	500- to 1000-mg tablets	90 mg/g*
Intravenous		
calcium chloride	10 mL	272 mg/g*; 13.5 mEq
calcium gluconate	10 mL	90 mg/g*; 4.5 mEq

*Elemental calcium is 1 g.

The goal for managing hypercalcemia is to correct the underlying cause of serum calcium excess. Drugs such as calcitonin or IV saline solution administered rapidly and followed by a loop diuretic can be used to promote rapid urinary excretion of calcium.

Nursing Process
Patient-Centered Collaborative Care

Calcium

Assessment

- Assess patient for signs and symptoms of calcium imbalance. Signs and symptoms of hypocalcemia are tetany, muscle cramps, bleeding tendencies, and weak cardiac contractions. Signs and symptoms of hypercalcemia are flabby muscles, pain over bony areas, and kidney stones of calcium composition.
- Assess for Trousseau's sign (muscular spasm of hand and wrist when pressure applied to vessels and nerves of upper arm) and Chvostek's sign (spasm of facial muscles resulting from tap on facial nerve).
- Check serum calcium levels. Report abnormal test results. Serum iCa (normal: 2.2 to 2.5 mEq/L or 4.25 to 5.25 mg/dL) indicates free, circulating calcium and is more accurate for determining calcium imbalance.
- Assess for albumin levels, and correct for serum calcium level.
- Obtain vital signs and ECG readings. Report abnormal findings. Vital signs and ECG results can be compared with future readings.
- Gather current drug history for patient. Calcium enhances the effect of digoxin. Elevated serum calcium level can cause digitalis toxicity. Signs and symptoms of digitalis toxicity include nausea, vomiting, anorexia, bradycardia (pulse rate <60 or markedly decreased), cardiac dysrhythmias, and visual disturbances. Thiazide diuretics can increase the serum calcium level. Drugs that decrease the effect of calcium are calcium channel blockers, tetracycline, and sodium chloride.

Nursing Diagnoses

- Imbalanced nutrition less than body requirements related to GI discomfort
- Impaired tissue integrity related to numbness and tingling of hands
- Readiness to learn about calcium-rich foods

Planning

- Patient's serum calcium level will be within normal range.
- Tetany symptoms will cease. Patient will eat calcium-rich foods or take calcium supplements as ordered.
- Patient with hypercalcemia will avoid calcium-rich foods.

Nursing Interventions

- Monitor vital signs. Report abnormal findings. Compare with baseline vital signs. Monitor pulse rate if patient is taking digoxin. Bradycardia is a sign of digitalis toxicity.

- Administer IVFs slowly with 10% calcium gluconate or chloride. Calcium should not be added to solutions containing bicarbonate, because rapid precipitation occurs.
- Check IV site for infiltration if patient is receiving calcium in IVFs. Calcium can cause tissue necrosis and sloughing if it infiltrates into subcutaneous tissue. CaCl preparations should be administered through a central line only. Calcium gluceptate is the only calcium preparation that can be given IM.
- Monitor serum calcium and iCa levels.
- Monitor ECGs. With hypocalcemia, ST segment is lengthened and QT interval is prolonged. With hypercalcemia, ST segment is decreased and QT interval is shortened.

Patient Teaching

General

- Instruct patient to avoid overuse of antacids and chronic use of laxatives. Overuse of certain antacids may cause alkalosis, decreasing calcium ionization. Chronic use of laxatives decreases calcium absorption from the GI tract. Suggest high-fiber foods for improving bowel elimination.
- Encourage patient taking calcium supplements to check that the calcium tablet is absorbable. To do this, put one tablet into 1 oz of white vinegar. Stir every 3 minutes. The tablet should break up or dissolve within 30 minutes.
- Advise patient to take oral calcium supplements with meals or after meals to increase absorption.

Diet

- Suggest that patient consume high-calcium foods such as milk and dairy products. Protein and vitamin D are needed to enhance calcium absorption.
- Side Effects
- Instruct patient to report symptoms related to calcium excess or hypercalcemia, including muscle weakness, pain over bony areas, ECG changes, and renal (calcium composition) stones.

Cultural Considerations

- Use an interpreter as appropriate.
- Involve extended family in health teaching and support.
- Incorporate food choices that are culturally acceptable.

Evaluation

- Evaluate patient's serum calcium and electrolyte levels. Report if calcium imbalance continues.
- Monitor patient for neuromuscular and cardiac manifestations of calcium imbalance.

Magnesium

Magnesium is most plentiful in the ICF. Magnesium deficit often occurs with hypokalemia and hypocalcemia. Normal serum magnesium level is 1.5 to 2.5 mEq/L or 1.8 to 3 mg/dL. Magnesium deficit is called **hypomagnesemia,** and magnesium excess is called **hypermagnesemia.** Daily magnesium requirement is 8 to 20 mEq.

Functions

Magnesium promotes transmission of neuromuscular activity; it is an important mediator of neural transmission in the CNS. Like potassium, it promotes contraction of the myocardium. Magnesium activates many enzymes for metabolism of carbohydrates and protein and is responsible for transportation of sodium and potassium across cell membranes.

Serum magnesium deficit increases the release of acetylcholine from the presynaptic membrane of the nerve fiber, which increases neuromuscular excitability. Serum magnesium excess has a sedative effect on the neuromuscular system, which can result in loss of deep tendon reflexes. Cardiac (ventricular) dysrhythmias, hypotension, and heart block can occur as a result of hypomagnesemia.

Hypomagnesemia is probably the most undiagnosed electrolyte deficiency. This is most likely because hypomagnesemia is asymptomatic until the serum magnesium level approaches 1 mEq/L. Total serum magnesium concentration is not representative of the cellular magnesium levels.

To correct severe hypomagnesemia, IV magnesium sulfate is usually given. For hypermagnesemia, calcium gluconate may be given to decrease the serum magnesium level.

Effect of Drugs on Magnesium Balance

Sodium inhibits tubular absorption of magnesium and calcium. Long-term administration of saline infusions may result in losses of magnesium and calcium. Diuretics, certain antibiotics, laxatives, and steroids are drug groups that promote magnesium loss. Hypomagnesemia, like hypokalemia, enhances the action of digitalis and causes digitalis toxicity.

Magnesium sulfate corrects hypomagnesemia and symptoms of digitalis toxicity. It is common practice after bypass surgery or myocardial infarction for patients to be given magnesium sulfate orally, even when blood levels are normal, to prevent ventricular arrhythmias in the perioperative period.

Excess intake of magnesium salts is the major cause of serum magnesium excess. Commonly used medications that may cause hypermagnesemia include laxatives and antacids. Patient teaching regarding prolonged or frequent use of laxatives, particularly in older adults, is an important intervention in preventing electrolyte imbalance. Table 16-11 lists drugs that affect magnesium balance.

TABLE 16-11 DRUGS AFFECTING MAGNESIUM BALANCE

DRUGS	RATIONALE
Drugs Causing Hypomagnesemia	
Diuretics: furosemide (Lasix), ethacrynic acid (Edecrin), mannitol	Promote urinary loss of magnesium.
Antibiotics: gentamicin, tobramycin, carbenicillin, capreomycin, neomycin, polymyxin B, amphotericin B, digitalis, calcium gluconate, insulin	Can cause magnesium loss via kidney.
Laxatives: cisplatin	Abuse can cause magnesium loss via gastrointestinal tract.
Corticosteroids: cortisone, prednisone	Can decrease serum magnesium level.
Drugs Causing Hypermagnesemia	
Magnesium salts (Oral and enema: magnesium hydroxide [milk of magnesia]), magnesium sulfate (Epsom) salt, magnesium citrate, magnesium sulfate (maternity)	Excessive use can increase serum magnesium level. Use of excessive magnesium sulfate in treatment of toxemia can cause hypermagnesemia.
Lithium	Associated with hypermagnesemia.

Nursing Process
Patient-Centered Collaborative Care

Magnesium

Assessment

- Assess patient for signs and symptoms of magnesium imbalance. Signs and symptoms of hypomagnesemia are tetany-like symptoms caused by hyperexcitability (tremors, twitching of the face) and ventricular tachycardia that leads to ventricular fibrillation and hypertension. Signs and symptoms of hypermagnesemia are lethargy, drowsiness, weakness, paralysis, loss of deep tendon reflexes, hypotension, and heart block.
- Check serum magnesium levels for magnesium imbalance. Symptoms of magnesium deficit may not be seen until serum level is <1 mEq/L.
- Observe patients receiving digitalis preparations for digitalis toxicity. Magnesium deficit, like potassium deficit, enhances the action of digitalis, causing digitalis toxicity.

Nursing Diagnoses

- Imbalanced nutrition less than body requirements related to insufficient intake of magnesium-rich foods
- Decreased cardiac output related to hypomagnesemia or hypermagnesemia
- Readiness to learn about signs and symptoms of magnesium imbalance

Planning

- Patient's serum magnesium level will be within normal range.
- Patient will not experience life-threatening symptoms of magnesium imbalance.
- Patient will have normal serum electrolyte levels.

Nursing Interventions

- Report to health care provider if patient is NPO and receiving IVFs without magnesium salts for a prolonged period. Slowly administer IV magnesium sulfate in solution to prevent hot or flushed feeling. Monitor vital signs.
- Monitor urinary output. Most of the body's magnesium is excreted by the kidneys. Report if urine output is <600 mL/d.
- Monitor for digitalis toxicity (e.g., nausea, vomiting, bradycardia) in patients who have hypomagnesemia and are taking digoxin. Magnesium deficit enhances the action of digitalis preparations.
- Monitor vital signs. Report abnormal findings to health care provider.
- Monitor serum electrolyte results. Report low serum potassium or serum calcium levels. Low serum magnesium levels may be attributed to hypokalemia or hypocalcemia. When correcting a potassium deficit, potassium is not replaced in cells until magnesium is replaced. Serum magnesium level of 1 mEq/L or less can cause cardiac arrest.
- Check for Trousseau's and Chvostek's signs of severe hypomagnesemia. Tetany symptoms occur in both magnesium and calcium deficits.
- Have IV calcium gluconate available for emergency reversal of hypermagnesemia from overcorrection of a magnesium deficit.

Patient Teaching

- Advise patient with hypomagnesemia to eat foods rich in magnesium (green vegetables, fruits, fish, grains, nuts).
- Instruct patient with hypermagnesemia to avoid routine use of laxatives and antacids that contain magnesium. Suggest that patient check drug labels.

Cultural Considerations

- Use an interpreter as appropriate.
- Involve extended family in health teaching and support.
- Incorporate food choices that are culturally acceptable.

Evaluation

- Evaluate patient's serum magnesium level. Report if magnesium imbalance continues.
- Determine whether signs and symptoms caused by prior magnesium imbalance are absent.

Chloride

Chloride is the principal anion of ECF. The chloride ion is a major contributor to acid-base balance, gastric juice acidity, and the osmolality of ECF. Normal serum chloride level is 95 to 108 mEq/L. **Hypochloremia** is a decreased serum chloride level, and **hyperchloremia** is an elevated level. With increased serum osmolality (>300 mOsm/kg), there are more sodium and chloride ions proportional to the water. Sodium and chloride frequently work in combination. For example, during sodium retention, chloride is also frequently retained, resulting in increased water retention. Clinical manifestations of hypochloremia include tremors, twitching, and slow, shallow breathing. With severe chloride loss, decreased blood pressure is seen. Clinical manifestations of hyperchloremia include weakness; lethargy; deep, rapid breathing; and eventual unconsciousness.

Phosphorus

Phosphorus is found in both ICF and ECF but is the primary anion in ICF. Similar to calcium and magnesium, serum phosphorus levels are not reflective of the true concentration of the body's phosphorus. The majority of the body's phosphorus is found as phosphate; these two terms are used interchangeably.

Both phosphorus and calcium levels are regulated by parathyroid hormone (PTH) and need vitamin D for absorption from the GI tract. Serum phosphorus levels are decreased by PTH stimulation of the renal tubules to excrete phosphorus (and concomitantly increase serum calcium levels by causing calcium to leave bone). Normal serum phosphorus level is 1.7 to 2.6 mEq/L. Fifty-five percent is ionized (free), and 45% is protein bound.

Phosphorus is essential in bone and teeth formation and for neuromuscular activity. Phosphorus is an important component of nucleic acids (DNA and RNA) and assists in energy transfer in cells, helps maintain cellular osmotic pressure, and supports the acid-base balance of body fluids. Clinical manifestations of **hypophosphatemia** include muscle weakness, tremors, paresthesia, bone pain, hyporeflexia, seizures, hyperventilation, anorexia, and dysphagia. Symptoms of **hyperphosphatemia** are similar to those of hypocalcemia, including hyperreflexia, tetany, positive Chvostek's and Trousseau's signs, flaccid paralysis, muscular weakness, tachycardia, nausea, diarrhea, and abdominal cramps. Phosphorus-rich foods include whole-grain cereals, nuts, milk, and meat. Phosphorus deficiency can result from decreased intestinal absorption, malnutrition, alcoholism, vomiting, diarrhea, use of concentrated glucose solutions, respiratory alkalosis, glycosuria, hypokalemia, hypomagnesemia, or use of thiazide diuretics. Hypophosphatemia may lead to hemolytic anemia, platelet dysfunction, and reduced oxygen transport. Hyperphosphatemia is most often related to chronic kidney disease. Increased intake in the form of laxatives may also increase serum levels.

Treatment of phosphorus imbalance is aimed at eliminating or reducing the cause. Monitoring phosphorus, calcium, and magnesium levels and assessing the patient for signs of electrolyte and acid-base balance are important nursing interventions. Phosphorus replacement is guided by degree of deficit, onset, and patient presentation. Oral intake is the preferred route of replacement. IV phosphorus is available for treatment of patients who are unable to tolerate oral replacements or patients with severe deficits. Potassium phosphate is an Institute for Safe Medication Practices (ISMP) high-alert medication used for IV phosphorus replacement. Potassium phosphate must be diluted before use and infused slowly using an infusion-control device. Too-rapid infusion may cause potassium toxicity in patients with severe renal or adrenal insufficiency. The IV insertion site must be monitored for infiltration; potassium phosphate may cause tissue necrosis and sloughing if infiltration occurs. Phosphorus, potassium, and calcium levels and renal function should be monitored during and after infusion. Use of potassium phosphate is contraindicated in patients with hyperkalemia or hypocalcemia.

Hyperphosphatemia in patients with chronic kidney disease is treated with restriction of dietary phosphorus, phosphorus-binding medications such as calcium acetate (Phoslo), or dialysis. Hyperphosphatemia can lead to secondary hyperparathyroidism and osteodystrophy.

KEY WEBSITES

American Red Cross Practice Guidelines: *arcblood.redcross.org/new_site/pdfs/Practice_Guidelines_for_Blood_Transfusion.pdf*

National Healthcare Safety Network's Hemovigilance Module: *www.cdc.gov/nhsn/bio.html*

CRITICAL THINKING CASE STUDY

JS, 72 years of age, has had vomiting and diarrhea for 2 days. JS takes digoxin, 0.25 mg/d, and hydrochlorothiazide, 50 mg/d. His serum potassium level is 3.2 mEq/L. He complains of being dizzy. His blood pressure is slightly lower than usual. The nurse assesses his physiologic status and notes that his muscles are weak and flabby, his abdomen is distended, and peristalsis is diminished.

1. What signs and symptoms indicate that JS is in potassium imbalance?
2. What contributing factors caused JS's potassium imbalance?

3. What interventions should be performed for alleviating this potassium imbalance?
4. How much potassium chloride would be needed to elevate JS's serum potassium by 1 mEq?

JS is ordered IV infusions of 1 L of 5% dextrose in water with 30 mEq of potassium chloride (KCl) and 1 L of 5% dextrose in 0.45% NaCl (½ normal saline). He is also prescribed oral KCl 15 mEq, three times per day for 2 days. Oral KCl is available in 15 mEq/10 mL.

5. Explain the method for diluting KCl in IVFs. Can KCl be given intramuscularly, subcutaneously, or as an IV bolus (push)? Explain your answer.
6. What instructions should the nurse give JS for taking oral potassium supplements?
7. What happens if JS's urine output decreases while he is receiving IV and oral potassium? What would be the nurse's responsibility?
8. Because JS is taking a diuretic and digoxin, what should the nurse include with client teaching? Give examples.

NCLEX STUDY QUESTIONS

1. A patient is postoperative day 3 after a total colectomy and ileostomy. He has a nasogastric tube to continuous suction and a Foley catheter to continuous drainage. The night nurse reports a high output from the ileostomy. The patient's pulse is irregular, and he reports leg weakness. Based on this situation, the nurse would correctly suspect what type of imbalance?
   a. Hypokalemia
   b. Hyperkalemia
   c. Hyponatremia
   d. Hypercalcemia
2. A patient is receiving IV potassium supplements. What is the most important nursing implication when administering this drug?
   a. IV potassium supplements may only be administered via a central vascular access device.
   b. IV potassium must be diluted before administration.
   c. IV potassium must be chilled before administration.
   d. IV potassium preparations do not contain preservatives.
3. A patient is receiving 10 mEq of KCl in 100 mL of NS to infuse over 1 hour IVPB. The patient has a #22-gauge peripheral IV in his right forearm. The patient reports pain at the insertion site; the nurse notes that the site is reddened, warm, and tender to the touch. Which action would the nurse take?
   a. Aspirate and check for blood return, and then slow the IV rate.
   b. Discontinue the IV, and then have a central line inserted to administer the potassium.
   c. Stop the infusion, and discontinue the IV immediately.
   d. Apply warm compresses to the IV site.
4. The health care provider orders a hypertonic crystalloid IV solution for a 70-year-old patient with cerebral edema. Which assessment should the nurse report immediately to the provider?
   a. Improved blood pressure, increased urinary output, and stable vital signs
   b. Hyperglycemia, decreased urinary output, and increased level of consciousness
   c. Thirst, dry mouth, cool extremities, and decreased urinary output
   d. Headache, irritability, confusion, widening pulse pressure, and decreased level of consciousness
5. A patient is receiving fluid replacement. The nurse's health teaching with this patient includes which suggestions? (Select all that apply.)
   a. Measure weight daily.
   b. Know that thirst means a mild fluid deficit.
   c. Monitor fluid intake.
   d. Avoid the use of calcium supplements.
   e. Monitor output.
6. A patient gained 10 lb in 2 days. It is determined that the weight gain is caused by fluid retention. The nurse correctly estimates that the weight gain may be equivalent to approximately how much fluid?
   a. 2 L
   b. 4 L
   c. 10 L
   d. 11 L
7. A patient has hypernatremia. Which components are appropriate to include in the nursing care plan? (Select all that apply.)
   a. Seizure precautions
   b. Need to keep appointments for laboratory tests and with health care provider
   c. Signs and symptoms of hypernatremia (muscle cramps, weakness, fatigue)
   d. Need for fluid restrictions
   e. Need to read food labels
8. The nurse is reviewing the medication list of a patient with hypokalemia. Which products may be contributing to the cause of this imbalance? (Select all that apply.)
   a. Cortisone
   b. Licorice
   c. Azithromycin
   d. Estrogen
   e. Digoxin

Answers: 1, a; 2, b; 3, c; 4, d; 5, a, b, c, e; 6, b; 7, a, b, d, e; 8, a, b, e.

CHAPTER

17

Nutritional Support

evolve WEBSITE

http://evolve.elsevier.com/KeeHayes/pharmacology/

- Animations
- Content Updates
- Key Points
- Review Questions for the NCLEX® Examination
- References from the Textbook
- Unfolding Case Studies

OBJECTIVES

- Explain the differences between enteral nutrition and parenteral nutrition.
- Describe the routes for enteral feedings.
- Discuss examples of enteral solutions, and explain the differences.
- Explain the advantages and differences of the methods used to deliver enteral nutrition.
- Describe the complications that may occur with use of enteral nutrition and parenteral nutrition.
- Discuss the nursing interventions for patients receiving enteral nutrition and parenteral nutrition.

OUTLINE

KEY TERMS

bolus, p. 245
continuous feedings, p. 246
cyclic method, p. 246
enteral nutrition, p. 244
gastrostomy tube, p. 244
hyperalimentation, p. 244
intermittent enteral feedings, p. 245
intermittent infusion, p. 246
jejunostomy tube, p. 244
nasogastric tube, p. 244
nutritional support, p. 244
parenteral nutrition, p. 244
total parenteral nutrition, p. 244
Valsalva maneuver, p. 249

Nutrients are needed for cell growth, cellular function, enzyme activity, carbohydrate-fat-protein synthesis, muscular contraction, wound healing, immune competence, and gastrointestinal (GI) integrity. Inadequate nutrient intake can result from surgery, trauma, malignancy, and other catabolic illnesses. Without adequate nutritional support, protein catabolism (breakdown), malnutrition, and diminished organ functioning will affect the GI, hepatic, renal, cardiac, and respiratory systems. The functioning of the immune system also is decreased.

Patients who are well nourished can usually tolerate a lack of nutrients for 14 days without major health problems. However, patients who are critically ill may only tolerate a lack of nutrient support for a short period (a few days to a week) before signs of impaired organ function, infection, or morbidity result. If nutritional support is started within hours of an injury, as in the cases of severe trauma or burns, recovery is more rapid. When injury is a result of minor surgery, no severe bodily harm results from lack of nutritional support for days. For both the critically ill and for patients with major injuries, early nutritional support improves intestinal and hepatic blood flow and function, enhances wound healing, decreases the occurrence of infection, and improves the general outcome of the health situation. "Early fed" injured patients have a positive nitrogen balance and less chance for bacterial infections; thus, they also have a decrease in institutional length of stay.

Dextrose 5% in water (D_5W), normal saline, and lactated Ringer's solution are not forms of nutritional support (supporting healthy tissue growth and wellness), although these solutions do provide fluids and some electrolytes. A patient requires 2000 calories per day; critically ill patients may require 3000 to 5000 calories per day. For individuals with extensive burns, the caloric need could be even greater. Patients who receive nothing by mouth (NPO) for an extended period become malnourished. Delayed nutritional support by as little as 5 days for a patient experiencing trauma or neurologic damage (e.g., cervical fracture) could hamper wound healing and increase the risk for developing an infection.

There are two routes for administering **nutritional support**: enteral and parenteral. **Enteral nutrition,** which involves the GI tract, can be given orally or by feeding tubes (tube feeding). If the patient can swallow, nutrient preparations can be taken by mouth; if the patient is unable to swallow, a tube is inserted into the stomach or small intestine. **Parenteral nutrition** involves administering high-caloric nutrients through large veins, for example, the subclavian vein. This method is called **total parenteral nutrition (TPN), hyperalimentation (HA), or** *intravenous hyperalimentation* (IVH). Parenteral nutrition is more costly (approximately three times more expensive) than enteral nutrition, and the benefits are not significant. In fact with TPN there is a higher infection rate than with enteral nutrition. The use of TPN does not promote effective GI integrity, hepatic function, or body weight gain, as enteral nutrition does. Enteral feedings require a functioning GI tract. TPN becomes necessary when the GI tract is incapacitated due to uncontrolled vomiting, malabsorption, or intestinal obstruction. TPN may also be necessary in patients with a high risk for aspiration or to supplement inadequate oral intake. TPN is also used for GI rest from exacerbations of Crohn's disease and ulcerative colitis; elemental nutrition absorbed by the duodenum and jejunum may be used for exacerbation of Crohn's disease involving the terminal ilium or ascending colon. TPN is also needed in conjunction with enteral feedings for patients with multiple trauma, including burn patients, when metabolic demand exceeds the number of calories that can be delivered by the GI system.

Solutions for enteral nutrition and parenteral nutrition include amino acids, carbohydrates, electrolytes, fats, trace elements, and vitamins.

ENTERAL NUTRITION

Enteral nutrition requires adequate small bowel function with digestion, absorption, and GI motility. To determine whether there is a lack of GI motility, the nurse assesses for abdominal distention and a decrease or absence of bowel sounds and notes if the patient has a bowel movement.

In critically ill patients, frequently there is a decrease or absence in gastric emptying time; then TPN may be necessary. The preferred method for nutritional support is enteral feedings for patients with intact gastric emptying and with a decreased risk of aspiration.

Routes for Enteral Feedings

The routes for enteral feedings include: oral, gastric by **nasogastric tube** or **gastrostomy tube,** and small intestinal by nasoduodenal/nasojejunal or **jejunostomy tube**. Use of a nasogastric tube through oral (mouth) or nasal cavities is the most common route for short-term enteral feedings. The gastrostomy, nasoduodenal/nasojejunal, and jejunostomy tubes are used for long-term enteral feedings. Figure 17-1 displays the four types of GI tubes used for enteral feedings. If aspiration is a concern, the small intestinal route is suggested.

Enteral Solutions

Several types of liquid formulas are available for enteral feedings. These solutions differ according to their various nutrients, caloric values, and osmolality. The three groups of solutions for enteral nutrition are blenderized; polymeric (milk-based and lactose-free); and elemental or monomeric. Examples of commercial preparations are listed according to their groups in Table 17-1. Components of the enteral solutions include (1) carbohydrates in the form of dextrose, sucrose, lactose, starch, or dextrin (the first three are simple sugars that can be absorbed quickly); (2) protein in the form of intact proteins, hydrolyzed proteins, or free amino acids; and (3) fat in the form of corn oil, soybean oil, or safflower oil (some have a higher oil content than others). With all enteral nutrition, sufficient water to maintain hydration is essential.

Blended formulas for enteral solutions are liquid in consistency, so they are able to pass through the tube. These are individually prepared based on the patient's nutritional need. Frequently, baby food is used with liquid added. If food particles are too large, the tube can become clogged.

The two groups of polymeric solutions are milk based and lactose free. Most milk-based polymeric preparations come in powdered form to be mixed with milk or water. Many of these solutions do not provide complete nutritional requirements unless given in large amounts. Frequently they are used as a supplement to meet nutritional needs. Lactose-free polymeric solutions are commercially prepared in liquid form for replacement feedings. Many of these solutions are isotonic (300 to 340 mOsm/kg water), and the breakdown of nutrients includes 50% carbohydrates, 15% protein, 15% fat, and 20% other nutrients. Examples of polymeric solutions include

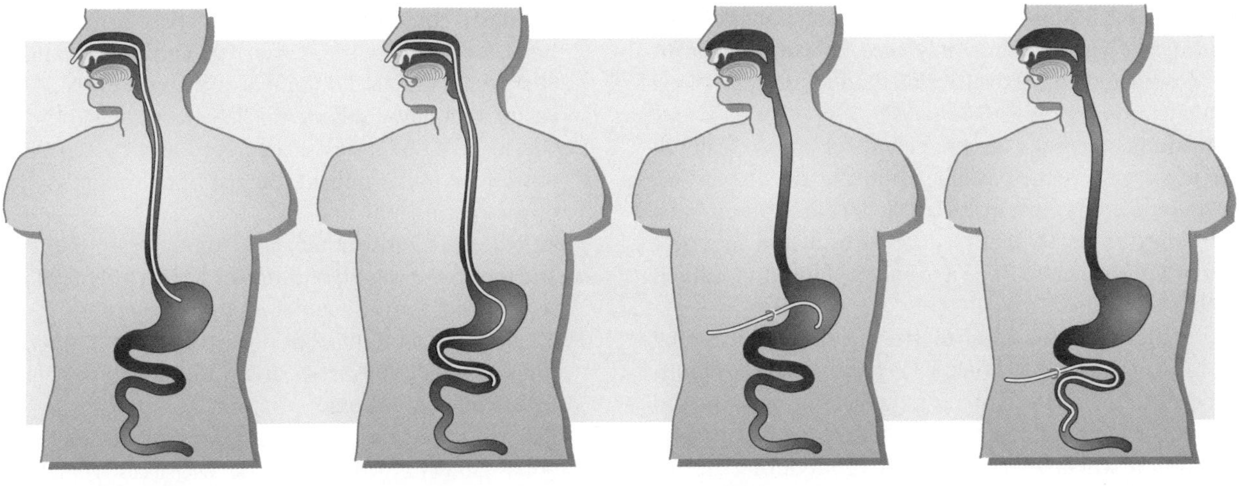

FIGURE 17–1 Types of gastrointestinal tubes used for enteral feedings. A nasogastric tube is passed from the nose into the stomach. A weighted nasoduodenal/nasojejunal tube is passed through the nose into the duodenum/jejunum. A gastrostomy tube is introduced through a temporary or permanent opening on the abdominal wall (stoma) into the stomach. A jejunostomy tube is passed through a stoma directly into the jejunum.

TABLE 17-1 COMMERCIAL PREPARATIONS FOR ENTERAL FEEDING

TYPE OF FORMULA	COMMERCIAL PREPARATION	DESCRIPTION
Blenderized	Compleat	Blended natural foods Formulas come ready to use
Polymeric Milk-based Lactose-free	Meritene Sustacal Boost Ensure Entrition Fibersource Isocal Osmolite Resource Ultracal	Supplements prescribed for patients who have normal or near-normal gastrointestinal function Usually taste good Most commonly prescribed formula May be used as tube feeding, meal replacement, or oral supplement Contains protein, carbohydrates, and fat Adequate quantities meet reference daily intakes for vitamins and minerals
Elemental (monomeric)	Criticare HN Peptamen Liquid Vital HN Vivonex TEN	Partially digested nutrients for feeding Contains nitrogen (free amino acids), carbohydrates (glucose polymers), and minimal fat (long-chain triglycerides) Used for various gastrointestinal diseases

Ensure, Isocal, and Osmolite. These solutions provide 1 calorie per milliliter of feeding.

Characteristics of the formula may be targeted to treat a specific group of disorders. For those with diabetes mellitus, Glucerna and Diabetic Resource (low-carbohydrate, high-fat, lactose-free products) are most helpful. NutriHep (low-fat, lactose-free product) is recommended to treat hepatic disorders. For individuals with pulmonary disorders, Pulmocare or Respalor (low-carbohydrate, high-fat products) are commonly prescribed. Nepro and Novasource Renal (low-fat amino acids, water-soluble vitamins) are used to treat those with renal disorders.

For partial GI tract dysfunction, the elemental or monomeric solutions are useful (e.g., Peptinex DT). They are available in powdered and liquid forms. The nutrients from these solutions are rapidly absorbed in the small intestine. They are more expensive than the other enteral solutions.

Methods for Delivery

Enteral feedings may be given by **bolus,** intermittent drip or infusion, continuous drip, or cyclic infusion. The bolus method was the first method used to deliver enteral feedings. With the bolus method, 250 to 400 mL of solution is rapidly administered through a syringe or funnel into the tube four to six times a day. This method takes about 10 minutes each feeding, and may not be tolerated well by the patient because a massive volume of solution is given in a short period. This method can cause nausea, vomiting, aspiration, abdominal cramping, and diarrhea, but a healthy patient can normally tolerate the rapidly infused solution. This method is usually reserved for ambulatory patients.

Intermittent enteral feedings are administered every 3 to 6 hours over 30 to 60 minutes by gravity drip or pump infusion. At each feeding, 300 to 400 mL of solution is usually given. A feeding bag is commonly used. **Intermittent infusion** is considered an inexpensive method for administering enteral nutrition.

Continuous feedings are prescribed for the critically ill or for those who receive feedings into the small intestine. The enteral feedings are given by an infusion pump such as the Kangaroo set to control the flow at a slow rate over 24 hours. Approximately 50 to 125 mL of solution is infused per hour.

The **cyclic method** is another type of continuous feeding that is infused over 8 to 16 hours daily (day or night). Administration during daytime hours is suggested for patients who are restless or for those who have a greater risk for aspiration. The nighttime schedule allows more freedom during the day for patients who are ambulatory.

Complications

Dehydration can occur if an insufficient amount of water is given with or between feedings. Some enteral solutions are hyperosmolar and can draw water out of the cells to maintain serum iso-osmolality.

Aspiration pneumonitis is the major complication of enteral nutrition and may occur if the patient is fed while lying down or is unconscious. The head of the bed should be elevated at least 30 to 45 degrees. The nurse should check for gastric residual by gently aspirating the stomach contents before administering the next enteral feeding and every 4 hours minimum between feedings.

One of the major problems of enteral feeding is diarrhea. This could be caused by rapid administration of feeding, high caloric solutions, malnutrition, GI bacteria *(Clostridium difficile)*, and drugs. Antibacterials and drugs that contain magnesium (e.g., antacids [Maalox], sorbitol [used as filler for certain drugs]) are associated with the occurrence of diarrhea. Many oral liquid drugs are hyperosmolar and tend to pull water into the GI tract and cause diarrhea.

Diarrhea can usually be managed or corrected by decreasing the rate of infusion of the enteral solution, diluting the solution, changing the solution, discontinuing the drug, increasing the patient's daily water intake, or administering enteral solution containing fiber.

Monitoring is essential when the patient is receiving enteral nutrition. Recommended parameters to monitor include: blood chemistry; BUN, creatinine, and electrolytes; glucose; triglycerides; serum proteins; I&O; and weight. Frequency of monitoring is patient dependent and more frequent at initiation of enteral nutrition.

Enteral Safety

The American Society for Parenteral and Enteral Nutrition (ASPEN) initiated the Be A.L.E.R.T. campaign to promote safe tube feeding:

Aseptic technique: For preparation and delivery of enteral formula, practice good hand-washing technique, wear gloves when handling feeding tube, and avoid touching can tops, container openings, spike, and spike port.

Label enteral equipment: Label with patient name (and location), formula name and rate, date and time of initiation, and nurse's initials. Equipment is changed every 24 hours; ensure that new equipment is labeled.

Elevate head of bed at least 30 degrees: Elevate when clinically possible, as it may mitigate the risk of reflux and aspiration of gastric content.

Right patient, right formula, right tube: Match the formula and rate to the patient's feeding order; verify enteral tubing set; connect formula container to feeding tube.

Trace all lines and tubing back to patient: avoid misconnections; trace all lines from origin to patient; only enteral-to-enteral connections.

Refer to the Agency for Healthcare Research and Quality National Guideline Clearinghouse website at *guideline.gov/content.aspx* for practice recommendations on initiation and advancement of enteral feedings; enteral feeding pumps; patient positioning; flushes; enteral misconnections; and special considerations for preterm infants.

Enteral Medications

Pancreatic enzymes such as pancreatin (Creon) and pancrelipase (Viokase) are products used by individuals with pancreatic enzyme deficiency resulting from conditions such as pancreatectomy, pancreatic obstruction, and cystic fibrosis. Both these preparations promote digestion and absorption of foods normally accomplished by natural amylase, lipase, and protease. Best given before meals, these artificial enzymes promote digestion and absorption of food.

Most drugs that can be administered orally can also be given via enteral tube. The drug must be in liquid form or dissolved into a liquid. Drugs that cannot be dissolved are time-release forms, enteric-coated forms, sublingual forms, and bulk-forming laxatives.

Liquid medication must be properly diluted when administered through the feeding tube. The drug dose is usually given as a bolus and then followed with water. Most liquid medications are hyperosmolar (>1000 mOsm/kg water) compared with the osmolality of the secretions of the GI tract (130 to 350 mOsm/kg water). Although the hyperosmolality of liquid medication was once thought to be well tolerated by the GI tract, abdominal distention and cramping, vomiting, and diarrhea can result from the administration of undiluted hyperosmolar liquid medications and electrolyte solutions. Liquid medication should be diluted with water to reduce the osmolality to 500 mOsm/kg H_2O (mildly hypertonic) and thus decrease GI intolerance. Table 17-2 lists the osmolalities of various commercial drug suspensions and solutions.

It is essential to know the importance of temporarily stopping the infusion when certain types of medications are administered. Some medications require that the feeding be stopped for as long as 30 minutes to allow for adequate absorption. For example, absorption of phenytoin suspension (Dilantin) is significantly reduced in the presence of protein, so it is important to stop the feeding for 1 hour before and after administering this drug. The phenytoin order may be changed to an injectable form to avoid the tube

TABLE 17-2 OSMOLALITY OF SELECTED DRUG SUSPENSIONS AND SOLUTIONS

DRUG	AVERAGE mOsm/kg
acetaminophen elixir, 65 mg/mL	5400
amoxicillin suspension, 50 mg/mL	2250
cephalexin (Keflex) suspension, 50 mg/mL	1950
cimetidine (Tagamet) solution, 60 mg/mL	5500
digoxin elixir, 50 mcg/mL	1350
docusate sodium (Colace) syrup, 3.3 mg/mL	3900
furosemide (Lasix) solution, 10 mg/mL	2050
lithium citrate syrup, 1.6 mEq/mL	6850
milk of magnesia suspension	1250
potassium chloride liquid, 10%	3550
prochlorperazine syrup, 1 mg/mL	3250
theophylline solution, 5.33 mg/mL	800

feeding being off for 2 hours at a time, especially if the patient is diabetic and requires insulin while on enteral feeding. The therapeutic effect of a drug may be affected as well. Sucralfate (Carafate), a treatment for gastric ulcers, may lose its effectiveness if the feeding is not held for 30 minutes after administering the medication.

Nursing Process
Patient-Centered Collaborative Care

Enteral Nutrition

Assessment
- Confirm that the feeding tube is securely in place.
- Assess patient's tolerance to enteral feeding, including possible GI disturbance (nausea, cramping, diarrhea).
- Determine urine output, and record for future comparison.
- Obtain patient's weight to be used for future comparisons.
- Listen for bowel sounds. Report diminished or absent bowel sounds immediately to health care provider. Also palpate abdomen for distention and percuss.
- Assess baseline laboratory values. Compare with future laboratory results.

Nursing Diagnoses
- Deficient fluid volume related to inadequate fluid intake or excess fluid loss
- Diarrhea related to ingredients in enteral feedings
- Risk for aspiration related to enteral feedings via nasogastric tube
- Imbalanced nutrition, less than body requirements, related to inability to absorb nutrients or tolerate oral intake

Planning
- Patient will not aspirate during enteral feedings (especially with nasogastric tube route).
- Patient will receive adequate nutritional support through enteral feedings.
- Complication of diarrhea related to enteral feedings will be managed.

Nursing Interventions
- Check tube placement by aspirating gastric secretion or injecting air into tube to listen by stethoscope for air movement in the stomach. (However, injecting air to check for placement may be misleading, because the tube may be in the base of the lung and air flow there produces similar sounds as when the tube is placed in the stomach.) For placement of the tube for small intestine route, confirmation by x-ray may be needed.
- Determine gastric residual before enteral feeding. A residual of more than 50% of previous feeding indicates delayed gastric emptying. Notify health care provider. Usual residual is 0 to 100 mL.
- Check continuous route for gastric residual every 2 to 4 hours. If residual is more than 50 mL, stop infusion for 30 minutes to 1 hour and then recheck.
- Raise head of bed to a 30- to 45-degree angle at all times during infusion of tube feedings. If elevating head of bed is contraindicated, then position patient on right side.
- Deliver enteral feeding according to method ordered: bolus, gastric, or small intestine.
- Flush feeding tube accordingly: intermittent feeding, 30 mL before and after; continuous feeding, every 4 hours; medications, 30 mL before and after. If tube obstruction occurs, flush with warm water or cola.
- Monitor adverse effects of enteral feedings such as diarrhea. To manage or correct diarrhea, decrease enteral feeding flow rate, and as diarrhea lessens gradually increase feeding rate. Enteral solution may be diluted and then gradually increased to full strength. However, diluted solution can decrease nutrient intake. Determine whether drugs could be causing diarrhea.
- Dilute drug solution's osmolality to 500 mOsm when giving liquid medication through the tube. Consult with health care provider.
- Monitor vital signs. Report abnormal findings.
- Give additional water during the day to prevent dehydration. Consult with health care provider.
- Weigh patient to determine weight gain or loss. Compare with baseline weight. Patient should be weighed at the same time each day with same scale and same amount of clothing.
- Change feeding bag daily. Do not add new solution to old solution in feeding bag. Nutritional solution should be room temperature.

Patient Teaching

- Instruct patient to report any problems related to enteral feedings such as diarrhea, sore throat, and abdominal cramping.

Cultural Considerations

- Respect cultural beliefs concerning refusal to receive enteral nutrition or TPN. Explain the need for adequate nutrition, and find ways that nutritional needs can be met.
- Communicate, verbally or in writing, how enteral nutrition is used by various cultural groups such as those in developing countries.
- Use an interpreter as appropriate.

Evaluation

- Determine that patient is receiving prescribed nutrients daily and is free of complications associated with enteral feedings.

PARENTERAL NUTRITION

Total Parenteral Nutrition

TPN is the primary method for providing complete nutrients by the parenteral or IV route. TPN is an infusion of hyperosmolar glucose, amino acids, vitamins, electrolytes, minerals, and trace elements; it can meet a patient's total nutritional needs. TPN is indicated for patients with severe burns who are in negative nitrogen balance; patients with GI disorders whose GI tract needs a complete rest; patients with absorption problems such as pancreatitis, Crohn's disease, and ulcerative colitis; and patients with debilitating diseases such as metastatic cancer or acquired immunodeficiency syndrome (AIDS).

The nutritional content of TPN generally includes water 30 to 40 mL/kg/d; energy 30 to 60 kcal/kg/d; amino acids 1 to 2 g/kg/d; essential fatty acids; vitamins; and minerals. Solutions differ for pediatric patients, who have varied fluid needs and require more energy and amino acids per kg/d.

The average percentage of dextrose in TPN is 25%. This high glucose concentration is mixed with commercially prepared protein and lipid sources. Fat emulsion supplement therapy provides an increased number of calories and is a carrier of fat-soluble vitamins. Vitamins and electrolytes are added before administration. Electrolytes are frequently added immediately before the infusion based on assessments of the patient's serum electrolyte levels. High glucose concentrations are irritating to peripheral veins, so TPN is administered through central venous lines, such as the subclavian or internal jugular, or through PICC lines.

Enteral feedings should be considered before TPN. Enteral feeding poses less risk of sepsis, maintains GI integrity, and is less costly. When enteral nutrition cannot be used because of severe GI disorders, TPN should be prescribed. TPN enhances wound healing and provides the necessary nutrients to prevent cellular catabolism.

The nurse must be familiar with the specific equipment used in caring for the patient on TPN. A variety of "setups" are available for administration. Some tubings have antireflux valves, and others have clamps. Each has implications for the administration of medications. Parenteral preparations must be administered by infusion pump to ensure accurate flow rate.

Management of patients requiring parenteral and enteral nutrition is best accomplished by an interdisciplinary team approach, including a nurse, physician, dietician, and pharmacist. Policies and procedures for TPN therapy may vary by region and institution and must be researched and followed accordingly.

Complications

Complications associated with TPN can result from catheter insertion and TPN infusion. Table 17-3 lists the complications associated with TPN.

To prevent air embolism, all central lines should have slide clamps on them to be closed completely when the solution bag and tubing are changed. Strict asepsis is necessary when changing IV tubing and dressings at the insertion site. Gloves, masks, and antibacterial ointment are usually necessary. TPN solution is an excellent medium for organism growth. Hypertonic dextrose in a protein hydrolysate solution promotes yeast and bacterial growth. It has been reported that these organisms do not grow as rapidly in the preferred crystalline amino acid solution as they do in a protein hydrolysate solution. Refrigerate prepared solutions, and administer within 24 hours. Most TPN solutions are prepared by the pharmacist with the use of a laminar airflow hood.

Hyperglycemia occurs primarily as a result of the hypertonic dextrose solution of 20% or greater when TPN is initiated. This may be transient until the pancreas adjusts to the hyperglycemic load. Hyperglycemia also occurs when the infusion rate for TPN is too rapid. In some cases, insulin is added to the TPN solution, which tends to be more effective than administering the insulin subcutaneously. Usually 1 L of solution is ordered for the first 24 hours when initiating TPN therapy. This allows the pancreas to accommodate to the increased glucose concentration of the solution. Additional daily increases of 500 to 1000 mL are ordered until the desired daily volume of 2.5 to 3 L is reached.

Sudden interruption of TPN therapy can cause hypoglycemia. After the glucose level is decreased, the insulin level remains, causing a hypoglycemic state. It is suggested that an isotonic dextrose solution be administered for 12 to 24 hours after TPN therapy is discontinued. A gradual decrease in the hourly infusion rate of TPN may also be used to discontinue TPN therapy. This process decreases the possibility of a hypoglycemic reaction.

TPN solutions and tubing should be changed every 24 hours. Dressing changes are required every 48 to 72 hours, varying by agency policy. In some institutions, the dressing is changed every 24 hours for the first 7 to 10 days.

TABLE 17-3 COMPLICATIONS OF TOTAL PARENTERAL NUTRITION

COMPLICATION	CAUSES	SYMPTOMS
Catheter Insertion		
Pneumothorax	Accidental puncture of the pleural cavity	Sharp chest pain, decreased breath sounds
Hemothorax	Catheter damages the large vein	Same as pneumothorax
Hydrothorax	Catheter perforates the vein, releasing solution into the chest	Same as pneumothorax
Total Parenteral Nutrition Infusion		
Air embolism	Intravenous (IV) tubing disconnected. Catheter not clamped. Injection port fell off. Improper changing of IV tubing (no **Valsalva maneuver**).	Coughing, shortness of breath, chest pain, cyanosis
Infection	Poor aseptic technique when catheter inserted. Contamination when changing tubing, mixing solution, or changing dressing.	Temperature >100° F (37.7° C). Tachycardia; chills; sweating; redness; swelling; drainage at insertion site; neck, arm, or shoulder pain; lethargy
Hyperglycemia	Fluid infused too rapidly. Insufficient insulin coverage. Infection.	Nausea, headache, weakness, thirst, elevated blood glucose
Hypoglycemia	Fluids stopped abruptly. Too much insulin infused.	Pallor; cold, clammy skin; increased pulse rate; "shaky feeling"; headache; blurred vision
Fluid overload hypervolemia	Increased IV rate. Fluids shift from cellular to vascular spaces because of hypertonic solutions.	Cough, dyspnea, neck vein engorgement, chest rales, metabolic complications

Nursing Process
Patient-Centered Collaborative Care

Total Parenteral Nutrition

Assessment
- Obtain baseline vital signs for future comparison.
- Confirm baseline weight.
- Determine laboratory results (electrolytes, glucose, protein [pre-albumin], and white blood cell levels frequently change during TPN therapy). Early laboratory results are useful for future comparison.
- Check urine output. Report abnormal findings.
- Read the label on TPN solution. Compare solution with order.
- Assess TPN insertion site for erythema, leaking, and edema.

Nursing Diagnoses
- Risk for imbalanced fluid volume related to excess fluid infusion or renal dysfunction or osmotic diuresis resulting from hyperosmolar TPN solution
- Risk for imbalanced nutrition related to altered type of nutritional support
- Risk for infection related to TPN solution that has a high glucose concentration
- Ineffective breathing pattern related to complication from insertion of subclavian line
- Deficient knowledge related to TPN therapy

Planning
- Patient's nutrient needs will be met via TPN.
- Infection will be avoided.

Nursing Interventions
- Check vital signs, and report changes.
- Determine body weight, and compare with baseline weight.
- Monitor laboratory results and report abnormal findings, especially electrolytes, protein, and glucose. Compare laboratory changes with baseline findings.
- Measure intake and output. Fluid volume deficit or excess could occur. Because the TPN solution is hyperosmolar, fluid shift occurs, which can cause osmotic diuresis.
- Monitor temperature changes for possible infection or febrile state. Use aseptic technique when changing dressings and solution bottles or bags.
- Check blood glucose level periodically. When TPN therapy is started, there may be a transient elevated glucose level until pancreatic beta cells adjust to secretion of insulin. If this occurs, the flow rate for TPN should be started slowly and gradually increased as blood glucose level decreases. Regular insulin may be added to TPN fluids to correct elevated glucose levels.
- Refrigerate TPN solution that is not in use. High glucose concentration is an excellent medium for bacterial growth.

- Monitor flow rate of TPN. Start with 60 to 80 mL/h, and increase slowly to the ordered level to avoid hyperglycemia.
- Hang dextrose 10% if TPN finishes before the next time it is to be administered.
- Have patient perform Valsalva maneuver (taking deep breath, holding it, and bearing down) in the absence of clamp to close tubing completely during solution bag/tubing change to prevent air embolus. Valsalva maneuver may cause dysrhythmias, so monitor cardiac status.
- Check for signs and symptoms of overhydration: coughing, dyspnea, neck vein engorgement, or chest rales. Report findings.
- Follow the agency policy for changing dressing and tubing. Usually tubing is changed daily, and dressing is changed every 24 hours for first 10 days and every 48 hours thereafter.
- Do not draw blood, give medications, or check central venous pressure via TPN line. Results could be invalid.

Patient Teaching

- Provide emotional support to patient and family before and during TPN therapy.
- Be available to discuss patient concerns, or refer patient to appropriate health care provider.
- Instruct patient to notify health care provider immediately if experiencing discomfort or reactions.
- Keep patient informed of progress and effectiveness of TPN.

Cultural Considerations

- Respect patient's cultural beliefs about refusing TPN.
- Explain reasons for adequate nutrition, and find ways to meet nutritional needs.
- Use an interpreter as appropriate.

Evaluation

- Evaluate patient's positive and negative response to TPN therapy.
- Determine periodically whether patient's serum electrolytes, protein, and glucose levels are within desired ranges.
- Evaluate nutritional status by weight changes, energy level, feeling of well-being, symptom control, or healing.
- Evaluate patient and family's understanding of purpose and possible complications of TPN therapy.

TRANSITIONAL FEEDING: PARENTERAL TO ENTERAL

The first stage of transitioning from parenteral to enteral feeding is determining a patient's GI tolerance, accomplished by giving a small amount of enteral feeding at a slow rate of about 25 to 40 mL/h. As the enteral rate is increased every 8 to 24 hours by increments of 25 to 40 mL, the parenteral preparation is reduced by the appropriate amount. Parenteral nutrition is typically discontinued when about 75% to 80% of a patient's nutritional needs are being met through enteral feeding.

KEY WEBSITES

American Society for Parenteral and Enteral Nutrition: *www.nutritioncare.org*

Infusion Nurses Society: *www.ins1.org*

CRITICAL THINKING CASE STUDY

MM had abdominal surgery and received D_5W and D_5 0.45% NaCl for 4 days. A nasogastric tube was inserted for enteral nutrition. It was determined that the function of MM's GI tract was intact.

1. Why would MM receive enteral nutrition? Is enteral nutrition needed for short-term or long-term therapy?
2. Differentiate between Ensure solution and other forms of enteral solutions.
3. MM is at risk for complications related to enteral nutrition. Discuss potential complications, and give specific nursing interventions for each.
4. Differentiate methods of delivery of enteral nutrition. Describe nursing interventions related to each method.
5. Give the rationale for changing MM's enteral nutrition from bolus method to intermittent method.

NCLEX STUDY QUESTIONS

1. The nurse is determining a patient's gastric residual before administering an enteral feeding; the last feeding was 240 mL. The patient will be discharged on enteral feedings. It is important to include in the health teaching plan that a residual of more than which amount would indicate delayed gastric emptying (based on last feeding)?
   a. 100 mL
   b. 125 mL
   c. 150 mL
   d. 175 mL
2. The nurse is assisting a patient with self-administration of an enteral feeding. It is important to include in the health teaching plan that the feeding should be administered at which temperature?
   a. Slightly warmed
   b. Chilled
   c. Ice cold
   d. Room temperature
3. The nurse is reviewing the plan of care for a patient receiving enteral therapy. What is the most common complication of enteral therapy?
   a. Aspiration
   b. Constipation
   c. Diarrhea
   d. Muscle weakness
4. Which is appropriate nursing care for a patient receiving total parenteral nutrition (TPN) in an acute care setting? (Select all that apply.)
   a. Monitor blood glucose levels periodically.
   b. Measure intake and output each shift.
   c. Administer blood products through the TPN line.
   d. Monitor TPN insertion site for erythema, leaking, or edema.
   d. Monitor the patient's weight monthly for significant changes.
5. A patient has been on TPN for 1 month, and there is an order to discontinue TPN tomorrow. The nurse contacts the health care provider because sudden interruption of TPN therapy may cause which condition?
   a. Dehydration
   b. Tremors
   c. Urinary retention
   d. Hypoglycemia
6. A patient is receiving TPN at home. The visiting nurse assists the family with the care plan, which includes changing the TPN solution and tubing. What is the recommended initial frequency for changing the tubing?
   a. Every 24 hours
   b. Every 36 hours
   c. Every 48 hours
   d. Every 72 hours
7. The visiting nurse has a caseload of adult and pediatric patients receiving TPN at home and is checking all orders for TPN solutions. Which order (all have appropriate amounts of essential fatty acids, vitamins, and minerals) requires the nurse to contact the health care provider?
   a. Adults: water 32 mL/kg/d; energy 32 kcal/kg/d; amino acids 1.2 g/kg/d
   b. Adults: energy 34 kcal/kg/d; amino acids 2 g/kg/d
   c. Children: water 32 mL/kg/d; energy 120 kcal/kg/d; amino acids 2.5 g/kg/d
   d. Children: water 38 mL/kg/d; energy 58 kcal/kg/d; amino acids 2 g/kg/d
8. The nurse is reviewing the care plan with a patient using enteral nutrition. Which interventions by the nurse are appropriate for this strategy? (Select all that apply.)
   a. Check continuous route for gastric residual every 2-4 hours.
   b. Raise head of bed to a 30- to 45-degree angle before administering.
   c. Change the feeding bag every 3 days.
   d. Report diminished or absent bowel sounds to health care provider.
   e. Explain that any diarrhea the patient experiences is related to the nutrition.
9. The nurse is to administer enteral medications to a patient who cannot swallow and is receiving continuous enteral feedings. Which is correct concerning administration of the enteral medications?
   a. Ordered medications are added to the enteral feeding solution.
   b. Liquid medications are diluted, given as a bolus, and followed with water.
   c. Extra amounts of water are used to dissolve time-release medications.
   d. Undiluted hyperosmolar medications may be given to a patient on a fluid restriction.

Answers: 1, b; 2, d; 3, c; 4, a, b, d; 5, d; 6, a; 7, b; 8, a, b, d; 9, b.

UNIT V

Autonomic Nervous System Agents

The central nervous system (CNS) is the body's primary nervous system, consisting of the brain and spinal cord. The peripheral nervous system (PNS), located outside the brain and spinal cord, is made up of two divisions: the autonomic and the somatic. After interpretation by the CNS, the PNS receives stimuli and initiates responses to these stimuli.

The autonomic nervous system (ANS), also called the visceral system, acts on smooth muscles and glands. Its functions include control and regulation of the heart, respiratory system, gastrointestinal tract, bladder, eyes, and glands. The ANS is an involuntary nervous system over which we have little or no control. We breathe, our hearts beat, and peristalsis continues without our realizing it. However, unlike the ANS, the somatic nervous system is a voluntary system that innervates skeletal muscles over which there is control.

The two sets of neurons in the autonomic component of the PNS are the (1) afferent (sensory) neurons and the (2) efferent (motor) neurons. The afferent neurons send impulses to the CNS, where they are interpreted. The efferent neurons receive the impulses (information) from the brain and transmit these impulses through the spinal cord to the effector organ cells. The efferent pathways in the ANS are divided into two branches: the sympathetic and the parasympathetic nerves. Collectively, these two branches are called the sympathetic nervous system and the parasympathetic nervous system (Figure V-1).

The sympathetic and parasympathetic nervous systems act on the same organs but produce opposite responses to provide homeostasis (balance) (Figure V-2). Drugs act on the sympathetic and parasympathetic nervous systems by either stimulating or depressing responses.

SYMPATHETIC NERVOUS SYSTEM

The sympathetic nervous system is also called the adrenergic system because at one time it was believed that *adrenaline* was the neurotransmitter that innervated smooth muscle. The neurotransmitter, however, is norepinephrine.

The adrenergic receptor organ cells are of four types: $alpha_1$, $alpha_2$, $beta_1$, and $beta_2$ (Figure V-3). Norepinephrine is released from the terminal nerve ending and stimulates the cell receptors to produce a response.

PARASYMPATHETIC NERVOUS SYSTEM

The parasympathetic nervous system is called the cholinergic system because the neurotransmitter at the end of the neuron that innervates the muscle is acetylcholine.

The cholinergic receptors at organ cells are either nicotinic or muscarinic, meaning that they are stimulated by the alkaloids nicotine and muscarine, respectively (see Figure V-3). Acetylcholine stimulates the receptor cells to produce a response, but the enzyme acetylcholinesterase may inactivate acetylcholine before it reaches the receptor cell.

Drugs that mimic the neurotransmitters norepinephrine and acetylcholine produce responses opposite to each other in the same organ. (Table V-1 lists the organ responses from drugs that act on these systems.) For example, an adrenergic drug (sympathomimetic) increases the heart rate, whereas a cholinergic drug (parasympathomimetic) decreases the heart rate (see Figure V-2). However, a drug that mimics the sympathetic nervous system and a drug that blocks the parasympathetic nervous system can cause similar responses in the organ. For instance, the sympathomimetic and the parasympatholytic (block impulses from PNS) drugs both increase heart rate; the adrenergic blockers and the cholinergic drugs both decrease heart rate.

Many name classifications are given to drugs that mimic or block both the sympathetic nervous system and the parasympathetic nervous system (Table V-2). The nurse must become familiar with these names. Drug names and specific actions are discussed in Chapter 18, Adrenergic Agonists and Adrenergic Blockers, and Chapter 19, Cholinergic Agonists and Anticholinergics.

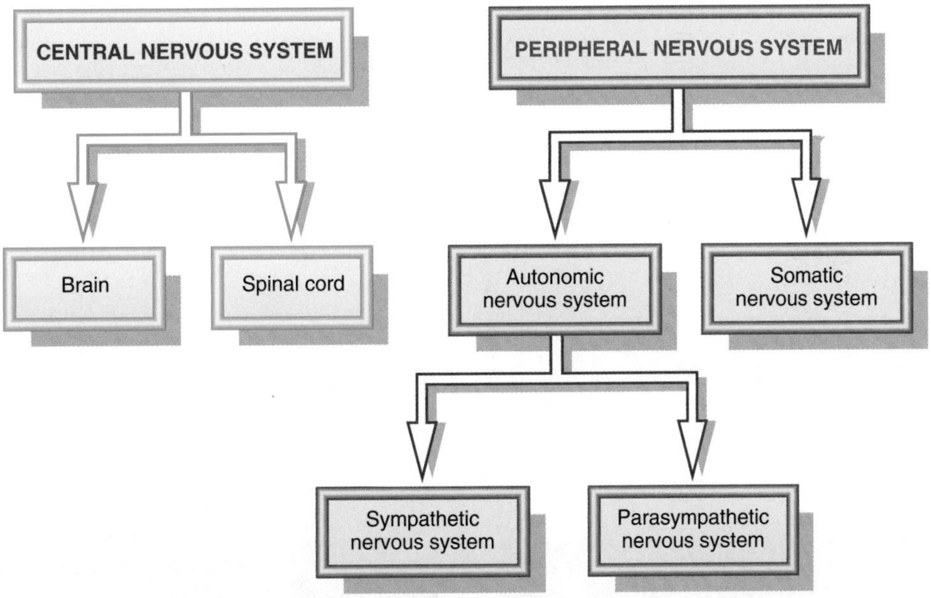

FIGURE V–1 Subdivisions of the peripheral nervous system.

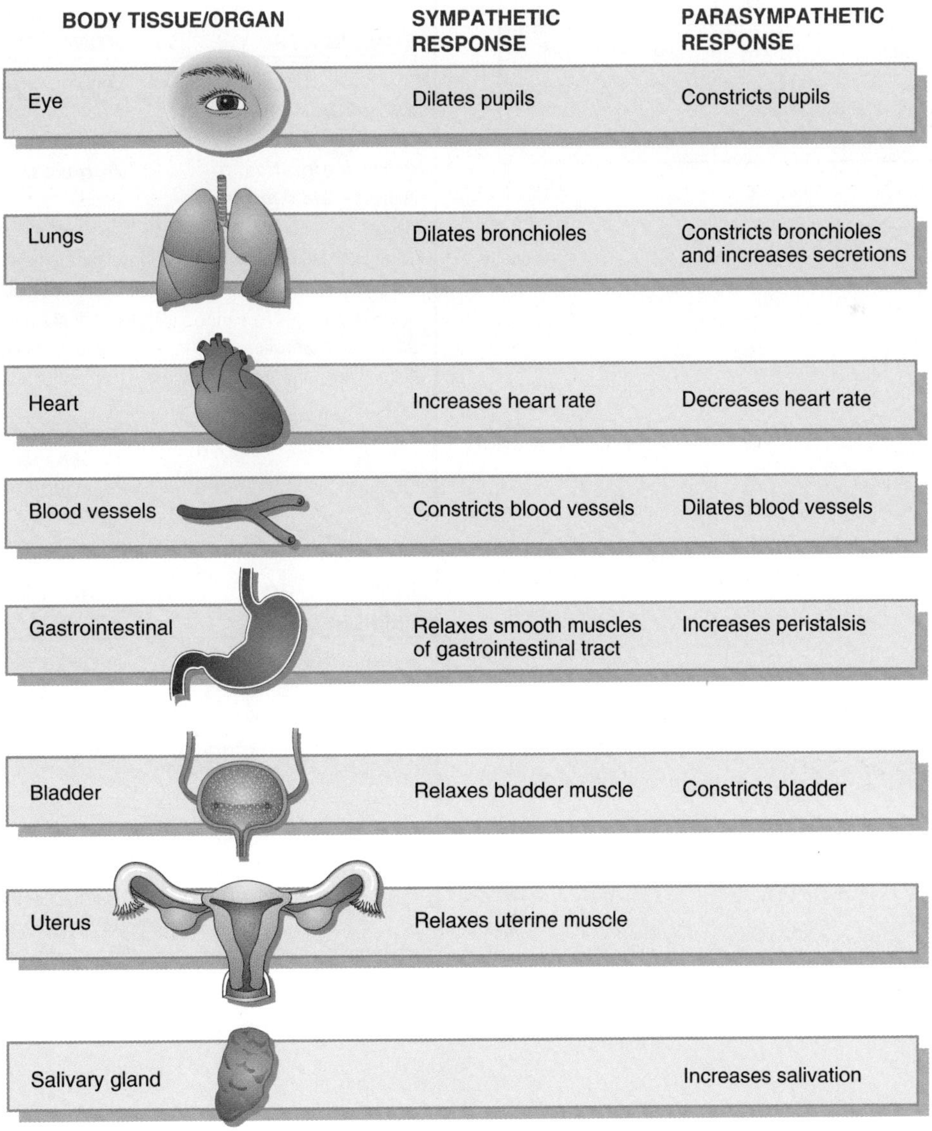

FIGURE V–2 Sympathetic and parasympathetic effects on body tissues. The sympathetic and parasympathetic nervous systems have opposite responses on body tissues and organs.

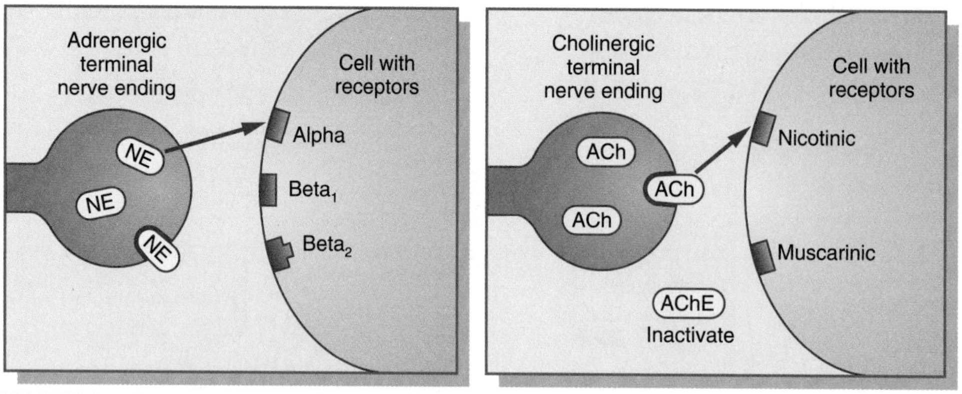

FIGURE V–3 Sympathetic and parasympathetic transmitters and receptors. *ACh,* Acetylcholine; *AChE,* acetylcholinesterase; *NE,* norepinephrine.

TABLE V-1 SYMPATHETIC AND PARASYMPATHETIC RESPONSES TO DRUGS

SYMPATHETIC	PARASYMPATHETIC	RESPONSE
Sympathomimetic	Parasympathomimetic	Opposite response
Sympatholytic	Parasympatholytic	Opposite response
Sympathomimetic	Parasympatholytic	Similar response
Sympatholytic	Parasympathomimetic	Similar response

TABLE V-2 AUTONOMIC NERVOUS SYSTEMS: SYMPATHETIC AND PARASYMPATHETIC

SYMPATHETIC STIMULANTS	PARASYMPATHETIC STIMULANTS
Sympathomimetics (Adrenergics, Adrenomimetics, or Adrenergic Agonists) *Action:* Increase blood pressure Increase pulse rate Relax bronchioles Dilate pupils of eyes Relax uterine muscles Increase blood sugar	**Direct-Acting** ***Parasympathomimetics (Cholinergics or Cholinergic Agonists)*** *Action:* Decrease blood pressure Decrease pulse rate Constrict bronchioles Constrict pupils of eyes Increase urinary contraction Increase peristalsis **Indirect-Acting** ***Cholinesterase Inhibitors (Anticholinesterase)*** *Action:* Increase muscle tone
SYMPATHETIC DEPRESSANTS	**PARASYMPATHETIC DEPRESSANTS**
Sympatholytics (Adrenergic Blockers, Adrenolytics, or Adrenergic Antagonists) *Action:* Decrease pulse rate Decrease blood pressure Constrict bronchioles	***Parasympatholytics (Anticholinergics, Cholinergic Antagonists, or Antispasmodics)*** *Action:* Increase pulse rate Decrease mucous secretions Decrease gastrointestinal motility Increase urinary retention Dilate pupils of eyes

CHAPTER

18

Adrenergic Agonists and Adrenergic Blockers

evolve WEBSITE

http://evolve.elsevier.com/KeeHayes/pharmacology/

- Animations
- Content Updates
- Key Points
- Review Questions for the NCLEX® Examination
- References from the Textbook
- Unfolding Case Studies

OBJECTIVES

- Explain major responses to stimulation of adrenergic receptors.
- Differentiate between selective and nonselective adrenergic agonists.
- Contrast the uses of alpha blockers and beta blockers.
- Compare general side effects of adrenergic agonists and adrenergic blockers.
- Describe nursing interventions, including patient teaching, associated with adrenergic agonists and adrenergic blockers.
- Apply the nursing process for the patient taking beta-adrenergic blockers.
- Compare the indications of adrenergic agonists and adrenergic blockers.

OUTLINE

KEY TERMS

adrenergic blockers, p. 262
adrenergic neuron blockers, p. 263
adrenergic receptor, p. 255
alpha blockers, p. 262
beta blockers, p. 263
catecholamines, p. 258
nonselective, p. 258
selective, p. 258
sympatholytics, p. 255
sympathomimetics, p. 255

This chapter discusses two groups of drugs that affect the sympathetic nervous system: adrenergic agonists (**sympathomimetics**) and adrenergic blockers (**sympatholytics**), along with their dosages and uses.

ADRENERGIC AGONISTS

Drugs that stimulate the sympathetic nervous system are called *adrenergics, adrenergic agonists,* or *sympathomimetics,* because they mimic the sympathetic neurotransmitters norepinephrine and epinephrine. They act on one or more **adrenergic receptor** sites located in the effector cells of muscles, such as the heart, bronchiole walls, gastrointestinal (GI) tract, urinary bladder, and ciliary muscle of the eye. There are many adrenergic receptors. The four main receptors are $alpha_1$, $alpha_2$, $beta_1$, and $beta_2$, which mediate the major responses described in Table 18-1 and illustrated in Figure 18-1.

TABLE 18-1 EFFECTS OF ADRENERGIC AGONISTS AT RECEPTORS

RECEPTOR	PHYSIOLOGIC RESPONSES
$Alpha_1$	Increases force of heart contraction; vasoconstriction increases blood pressure; mydriasis (dilation of pupils) occurs; decreases secretion in salivary glands; increases urinary bladder relaxation and urinary sphincter contraction
$Alpha_2$	Inhibits release of norepinephrine; dilates blood vessels; produces hypotension; decreases gastrointestinal motility and tone
$Beta_1$	Increases heart rate and force of contraction; increases renin secretion, which increases blood pressure
$Beta_2$	Dilates bronchioles; promotes gastrointestinal and uterine relaxation; promotes increase in blood sugar through glycogenolysis in liver; increases blood flow in skeletal muscles

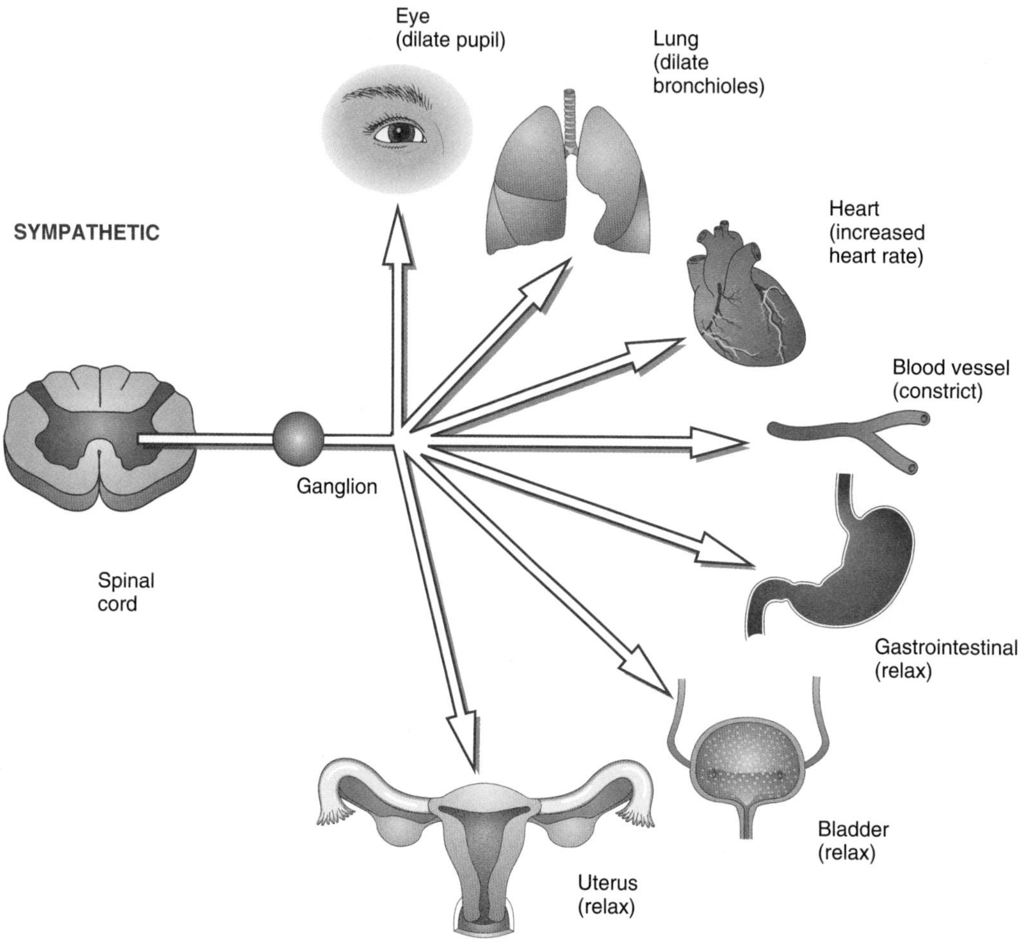

FIGURE 18–1 Sympathetic responses. Stimulation of the sympathetic nervous system or use of sympathomimetic (adrenergic agonist) drugs can cause the pupils and bronchioles to dilate; heart rate to increase; blood vessels to constrict; and muscles of the gastrointestinal tract, bladder, and uterus to relax, thereby decreasing contractions.

The alpha-adrenergic receptors are located in blood vessels, eye, bladder, and prostate. When the $alpha_1$ receptors in vascular tissues (vessels) of muscles are stimulated, the arterioles and venules constrict, increasing peripheral resistance and blood return to the heart. Circulation is improved, and blood pressure is increased. When there is too much stimulation, blood flow is decreased to the vital organs.

The $alpha_2$ receptors are located in the postganglionic sympathetic nerve endings. When stimulated, they inhibit the release of norepinephrine, leading to a decrease in vasoconstriction. This results in vasodilation and a decrease in blood pressure.

The $beta_1$ receptors are located in the kidney but primarily in the heart. Stimulation of the $beta_1$ receptor increases myocardial contractility and heart rate.

The $beta_2$ receptors are found mostly in the smooth muscles of the lung and gastrointestinal tract, the liver, and the uterine muscle. Stimulation of the $beta_2$ receptor causes (1) relaxation of the smooth muscles of the lungs, resulting in bronchodilation; (2) a decrease in gastrointestinal tone and motility; (3) activation of glycogenolysis in the liver and increased blood glucose; and (4) relaxation of the uterine muscle, resulting in a decrease in uterine contraction (Figure 18-2; see also Table 18-1).

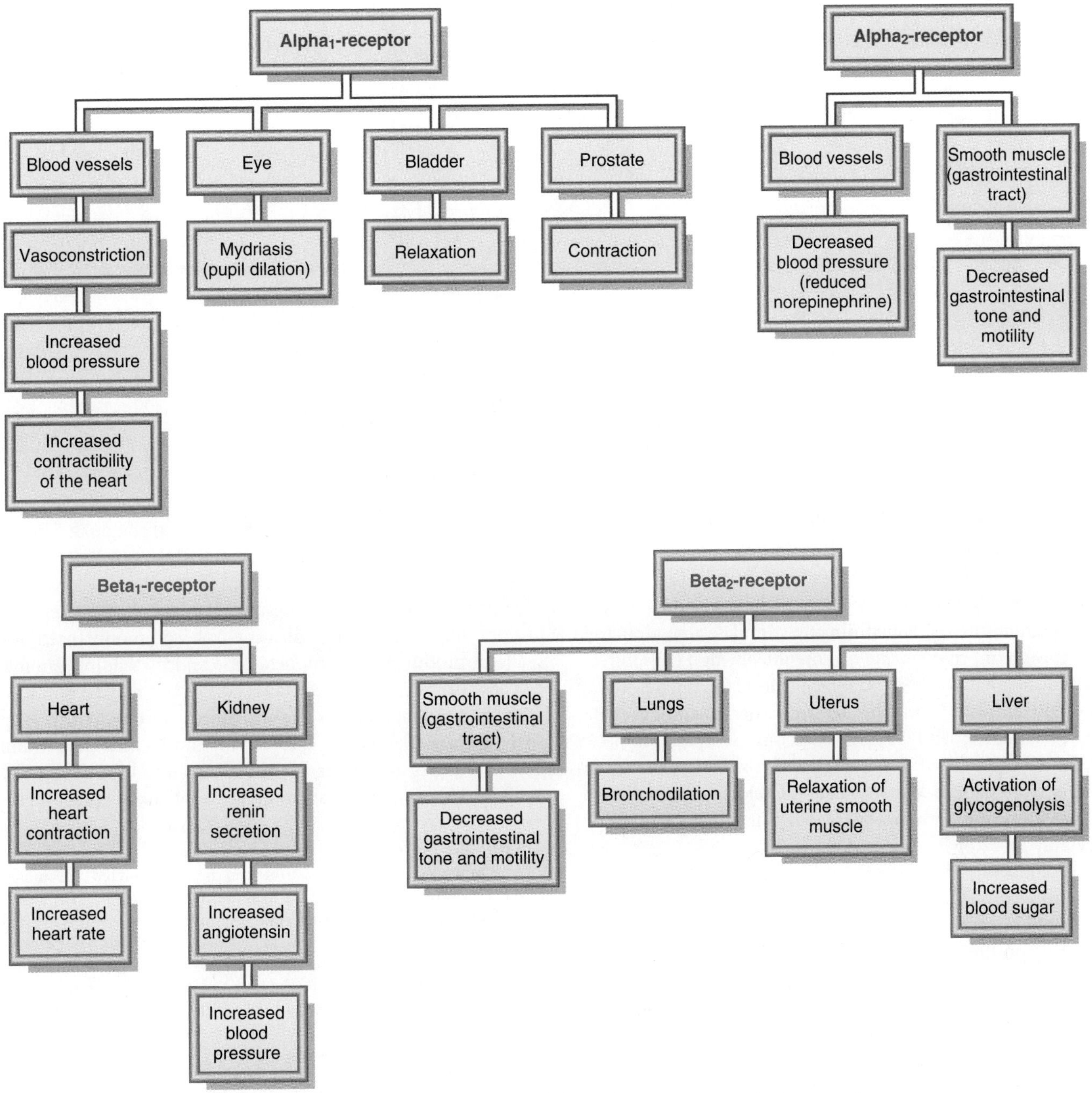

FIGURE 18–2 Effects of activation of alpha$_1$, alpha$_2$, beta$_1$, and beta$_2$ receptors.

Another adrenergic receptor is dopaminergic and is located in the renal, mesenteric, coronary, and cerebral arteries. When this receptor is stimulated, the vessels dilate and blood flow increases. Only dopamine can activate this receptor.

Inactivation of Neurotransmitters

After the neurotransmitter (e.g., norepinephrine) has performed its function, the action must be stopped to prevent prolonging the effect. Transmitters are inactivated by (1) reuptake of the transmitter back into the neuron (nerve cell terminal), (2) enzymatic transformation or degradation, and (3) diffusion away from the receptor. The mechanism of norepinephrine reuptake plays a more important role in inactivation than the enzymatic action. Following the reuptake of the transmitter in the neuron, the transmitter may be degraded or reused. The two enzymes that inactivate norepinephrine are (1) monoamine oxidase (MAO), which is inside the neuron; and (2) catechol-O-methyltransferase (COMT), which is outside of the neuron.

Drugs can prolong the action of the neurotransmitter (e.g., norepinephrine) by either (1) inhibiting the norepinephrine reuptake, which prolongs the action of the transmitter or (2) inhibiting the degradation of norepinephrine by enzyme action.

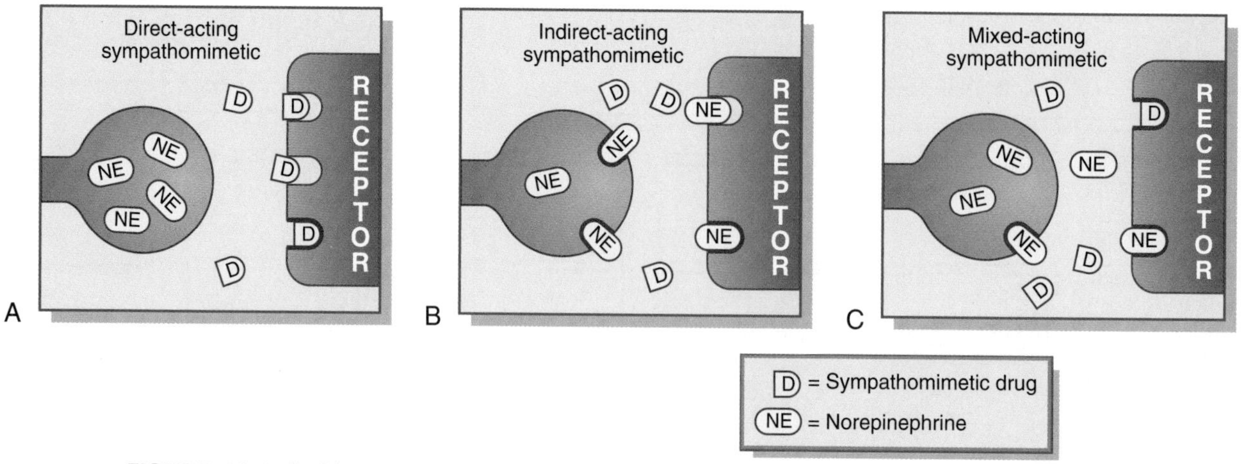

FIGURE 18–3 **A,** Direct-acting sympathomimetics; **B,** indirect-acting sympathomimetics; and **C,** mixed-acting sympathomimetics.

Classification of Sympathomimetics

The sympathomimetic drugs that stimulate adrenergic receptors are classified into three categories according to their effects on organ cells. Categories include (1) direct-acting sympathomimetics, which directly stimulate the adrenergic receptor (e.g., epinephrine or norepinephrine); (2) indirect-acting sympathomimetics, which stimulate the release of norepinephrine from the terminal nerve endings (e.g., amphetamine); and (3) mixed-acting sympathomimetics (both direct and indirect acting), which stimulate the adrenergic receptor sites and stimulate the release of norepinephrine from the terminal nerve endings (e.g., ephedrine) (Figure 18-3).

Pseudoephedrine is an example of a mixed-acting sympathomimetic. This drug acts indirectly by stimulating the release of norepinephrine from the nerve terminals and acts directly on the $alpha_1$ and $beta_1$ receptors. Pseudoephedrine, like epinephrine, increases heart rate. It is not as potent a vasoconstrictor as epinephrine, and there is less risk of hemorrhagic stroke and hypertensive crisis. Pseudoephedrine is helpful to relieve nasal and sinus congestion without rebound congestion.

Catecholamines are the chemical structures of a substance (either endogenous or synthetic) that can produce a sympathomimetic response. Examples of endogenous catecholamines are epinephrine, norepinephrine, and dopamine. The synthetic catecholamines are isoproterenol and dobutamine. Noncatecholamines (e.g., phenylephrine, metaproterenol, albuterol) stimulate the adrenergic receptors. Most noncatecholamines have a longer duration of action than the endogenous or synthetic catecholamines.

Many of the adrenergic agonists stimulate more than one of the adrenergic receptor sites. An example is epinephrine (Adrenalin), which acts on $alpha_1$-, alpha $_2$-, $beta_1$-, and $beta_2$-adrenergic receptor sites. The responses from these receptor sites include increase in blood pressure, pupil dilation, increase in heart rate (tachycardia), and bronchodilation. In anaphylactic shock, epinephrine is useful because it increases blood pressure, heart rate, and airflow through the lungs. Because epinephrine affects different adrenergic receptors, it is **nonselective.** Additional side effects result when more responses occur than are desired. Pseudoephedrine, ephedrine, and phenylpropanolamine are commonly used for illegal production of amphetamine and methamphetamine. These drugs are considered OTC drugs but may be obtained in limited amounts per month. Stores are required to keep these drugs behind the counter or in a locked cabinet and keep a log of purchases for at least 2 years. Prototype Drug Chart 18-1 lists the pharmacologic behavior of epinephrine.

Epinephrine

Pharmacokinetics Epinephrine can be administered subcutaneously, intravenously, topically, or by inhalation, intracardiac, and instillation methods. It is not given orally, because it is rapidly metabolized in the GI tract and liver resulting in unstable serum levels. The percentage by which the drug is protein-bound and its half-life are unknown. Epinephrine is metabolized by the liver and excreted in the urine.

Pharmacodynamics Epinephrine is frequently used in emergencies to treat anaphylaxis, which is a life-threatening allergic response. Epinephrine is a potent inotropic (strengthens myocardial contraction) drug that increases cardiac output, promotes vasoconstriction and systolic blood pressure elevation, increases heart rate, and produces bronchodilation. High doses can result in cardiac dysrhythmias necessitating electrocardiogram (ECG) monitoring. Epinephrine can also cause renal vasoconstriction, thereby decreasing renal perfusion and urinary output.

The onset of action and peak concentration times are rapid. The use of decongestants with epinephrine has an additive effect. When epinephrine is administered with digoxin, cardiac dysrhythmias may occur. Beta blockers can antagonize the action of epinephrine. Tricyclic antidepressants and monoamine oxidase inhibitors (MAOIs) allow epinephrine's effects to be intensified and prolonged. Epinephrine is also discussed in Chapter 59 as one of the drugs used during emergencies.

Albuterol

Albuterol sulfate (Proventil), a $beta_2$-adrenergic agonist, is **selective** for $beta_2$-adrenergic receptors, so the response is relaxation of bronchial smooth muscle and bronchodilation. A patient with asthma may tolerate albuterol better than isoproterenol (which activates $beta_1$ and $beta_2$ receptors) because

PROTOTYPE DRUG CHART 18-1

Epinephrine

Drug Class	Dosage
Sympathomimetic: adrenergic agonist Trade Name: Adrenalin Pregnancy Category: C	Anaphylaxis: A: subQ: 0.3-0.5 mL of 1:1000 PRN IV: 0.1-0.25 mg of 1:10,000 infused slowly over 5-10 min A: subQ/IM: 0.3 mg EpiPen autoinjector
Contraindications	**Drug-Lab-Food Interactions**
Cardiac tachydysrhythmias, cerebral arteriosclerosis, pregnancy, narrow-angle glaucoma, cardiogenic shock Caution: Hypertension, prostatic hypertrophy, hyperthyroidism, pregnancy, diabetes mellitus (hyperglycemia could result)	Drug: Increased effects with tricyclic antidepressants and MAOIs. Methyldopa and beta blockers antagonize epinephrine effects. Digoxin may cause dysrhythmias with epinephrine. Lab: Increase blood glucose, serum lactic acid
Pharmacokinetics	**Pharmacodynamics**
Absorption: subQ/IM/IV: Rapidly; inactivated in GI tract Distribution: PB: UK Metabolism: t½: UK Excretion: In urine and breast milk	subQ: Onset: 5-15 min Peak: 20 min Duration: 1-4 hours IV: Onset: Immediate Peak: 2-5 min Duration: 5-10 min Inhal: Onset: 1-5 min Peak: 3-5 min Duration: 1-3 hours
Therapeutic Effects/Uses	
To treat allergic reaction, anaphylaxis, asthma, bronchospasm, severe hypotension, cardiac arrest Mode of Action: Acts on alpha and beta receptors; promotion of CNS and cardiac stimulation and bronchodilation; strengthens cardiac contraction, increases cardiac rate and cardiac output; reduces mucosal congestion by inhibiting histamine release; reverses anaphylactic reactions	
Side Effects	**Adverse Reactions**
Anorexia, nausea, vomiting, nervousness, tremors, agitation, sweating, headache, pallor, insomnia, weakness, dizziness	Palpitations, tachycardia, hypertension, dyspnea. Necrosis and gangrene of IV site upon infiltration Life-threatening: Ventricular fibrillation, pulmonary edema

A, Adult; *CNS,* central nervous system; *IM,* intramuscular; *Inhal,* inhalation; *IV,* intravenous; *min,* minute; *PB,* protein-binding; *PRN,* as needed; *subQ,* subcutaneous; *t½,* half-life; *UK,* unknown.

albuterol's action is more selective (activates only the $beta_2$ receptors). By using selective sympathomimetics, fewer undesired adverse effects will occur. However, high dosages of albuterol may affect $beta_1$ receptors, causing an increase in heart rate. Prototype Drug Chart 18-2 lists the drug data related to albuterol.

Pharmacokinetics Albuterol sulfate (Proventil, Ventolin) is well absorbed from the GI tract and is extensively metabolized by the liver. The half-life of the drug differs slightly according to the route of administration (oral route is 2.7 to 6 hours; inhalation route is 3.5 hours).

Pharmacodynamics The primary use of albuterol is to prevent and treat bronchospasm. With inhalation, the onset of action of albuterol is faster than with oral administration, though the duration of action is the same for both oral and inhalation preparations.

Tremors, restlessness, and nervousness may occur when albuterol is taken. Tremors and nervousness are the most common side effects of oral or inhalation albuterol. If albuterol is taken with an MAOI, hypertensive crisis can result. Beta blockers may inhibit the action of albuterol. Albuterol and the $beta_2$ drugs are also discussed in Chapter 41 and 44, respectively.

CENTRAL-ACTING ALPHA AGONISTS

Clonidine and Methyldopa

Clonidine (Catapres) is a selective $alpha_2$-adrenergic agonist (sympathomimetic) used primarily to treat hypertension. $Alpha_2$ drugs act by decreasing the release of norepinephrine from sympathetic nerves and decreasing peripheral adrenergic receptor activation. $Alpha_2$ drugs also produce vasodilation by stimulating $alpha_2$ receptors in the central nervous system (CNS), leading to a decrease in blood pressure (see Chapter 44).

Methyldopa (Aldomet) is an alpha-adrenergic agonist (sympathomimetic) that acts within the CNS. This drug is taken up into the brainstem neurons and converted to methylnorepinephrine, which is an $alpha_2$-adrenergic agonist that leads to $alpha_2$ activation. The decrease of sympathetic outflow from the CNS causes vasodilation and a reduction in blood pressure (see Chapter 44).

PROTOTYPE DRUG CHART 18-2

Albuterol

Drug Class $Beta_2$-adrenergic agonist Trade Names: Proventil, Ventolin Pregnancy Category: C	**Dosage** A: PO: 2-4 mg, t.i.d./q.i.d.; *max:* 32 mg/d in 4 divided doses SR: 4-8 mg, q12h Inhal: 1-2 puffs q4-6h PRN Nebulizer: 0.5 mL of 0.5% sol in 3 mL of 0.9% NaCl in 5-15 min 2 to 6 y: PO: 0.1-0.2 mg/kg/t.i.d.; *max:* 4 mg/dose 6 to 12 y: PO: 2 mg, t.i.d./q.i.d. 6 to 12 y: Inhal: 1-2 puffs q4-6h PRN
Contraindications Cardiac dysrhythmias, coronary artery disease Caution: Severe cardiac disease, hypertension, hyperthyroidism, diabetes mellitus, renal dysfunction, older adults, pregnancy	**Drug-Lab-Food Interactions** Drug: Increase effect with other sympathomimetics; may increase effect with MAOIs and tricyclic antidepressants Antagonize effect with beta-adrenergic blockers (beta blockers) Lab: May increase glucose level slightly; may decrease serum potassium level
Pharmacokinetics Absorption: Well absorbed from the GI tract after oral administration; well absorbed from respiratory tract after inhalation Distribution: PB: UK Metabolism: $t\frac{1}{2}$: PO: 2.7-6 h; Inhal: 3.5 h Excretion: 75% excreted in the urine	**Pharmacodynamics** PO: Onset: 30 min Peak: 2-3 h Duration: 4-6 h Inhal: Onset: 5-15 min Peak: 0.5-2 h Duration: 2-6 h
Therapeutic Effects/Uses To treat bronchospasm, asthma, bronchitis, and other COPD Mode of Action: Stimulates $beta_2$-adrenergic receptors in the lungs, which relaxes the bronchial smooth muscle, thus causing bronchodilation	
Side Effects Tremor, dizziness, nervousness, restlessness, sweating, blurred vision, flushing, headache, hoarseness, pharyngitis, nasal congestion, insomnia, weakness, nausea, diarrhea	**Adverse Reactions** Palpitations, tachycardia, hypertension, hallucinations, seizures, hyperglycemia Life-threatening: Cardiac dysrhythmias, Stevens-Johnson syndrome

A, Adult; *C,* child; *COPD,* chronic obstructive pulmonary disease; *d,* day; *GI,* gastrointestinal; *h,* hour; *Inhal,* inhalation; *MAOI,* monoamine oxidase inhibitor; *min,* minute; *PB,* protein-binding; *PO,* by mouth; *PRN,* as needed; *q.i.d.,* four times a day; *SR,* sustained release; *sol,* solution; *t½,* half-life; *t.i.d.,* three times a day; *UK,* unknown; *y,* year.

Side Effects and Adverse Reactions

Additional undesired side effects frequently result when the drug dosage is increased or the drug is nonselective. Side effects commonly associated with adrenergic agonists include hypertension, tachycardia, palpitations, restlessness, tremors, dysrhythmias, dizziness, urinary retention, nausea, vomiting, dyspnea, and pulmonary edema.

Names of adrenergic drugs, the receptors they activate, dosage information, and common uses are listed in Table 18-2.

Nursing Process

Patient-Centered Collaborative Care

Adrenergic Agonist

Assessment

- Record baseline vital signs for future comparison.
- Assess the patient's drug history.
- Determine patient's health history. Most adrenergic agonists are contraindicated if the patient has cardiac dysrhythmias, narrow-angle glaucoma, or cardiogenic shock.
- Determine baseline glucose level.

Nursing Diagnoses

- Disturbed sleep pattern related to adverse drug effect of insomnia
- Deficient knowledge related to drug administration

Planning

- Patient's vital signs will be within acceptable ranges.
- Patient will experience therapeutic effects by improved blood pressure, breathing pattern, and cardiac output.

Nursing Interventions

- Administer epinephrine 1 mg (10 mL of a 1:10,000 concentration per AHA guidelines) IV for cardiac

TABLE 18-2 ADRENERGIC AGONISTS (ALPHA$_1$, BETA$_1$, AND BETA$_2$)

GENERIC (BRAND)	ROUTE AND DOSAGE	USES AND CONSIDERATIONS
epinephrine (Adrenalin Chloride) Alpha$_1$, beta$_1$, and beta$_2$	See Prototype Drug Chart 18-1.	
ephedrine HCl, ephedrine sulfate (Pretz-D) I Alpha$_1$, beta$_1$, and beta$_2$	A: PO: 25-50 mg t.i.d./q.i.d. subQ/IM/IV: 12.5-50 mg; *max:* 150 mg/24 h C: >2 y: PO: 2-3 mg/kg/d in 4-6 divided doses; *max:* 3 mg/kg/24 h	To treat hypotensive states, bronchospasm, nasal congestion. Also may be used to treat mild cases of asthma. Drug resistance may occur with prolonged use of ephedrine. If this occurs, stop drug for 3-5 d, and then resume. Pregnancy category: C; PB: UK; $t_{1/2}$: 3-6 h
norepinephrine bitartrate (Levophed) Alpha$_1$ and beta$_1$	A: IV: 4 mg in 500-1000 mL of D$_5$W or D$_5$NS infused initially 8-12 mcg/min, then titrated to maintain blood pressure; monitor blood pressure	To treat shock by potent vasoconstriction. Increases blood pressure and cardiac output. Monitor blood pressure and rhythm every 2-5 min during infusion. Pregnancy category: C; PB: UK; $t_{1/2}$: UK
dopamine HCl (Intropin) Alpha$_1$ and beta$_1$	A: IV/INF: 2-5 mcg/kg/min initially; gradually increase 5-10 mcg/kg/min; *max:* 50 mcg/kg/min C: IV: 1-5 mcg/kg/min; increase 2.5-5 mcg/kg/min; *max:* 20 mcg/kg/min	To correct hypotension. Does not decrease renal function in doses <5 mcg/kg/min. Pregnancy category: C; PB: UK; $t_{1/2}$: 2 min
midodrine (ProAmatine) Alpha$_1$	A: PO: 10 mg t.i.d.; *max:* 30 mg/d	To treat symptomatic orthostatic hypotension. Blood pressure may increase by 15-30 mm Hg in 1 h with 1 10-mg dose. Pregnancy category: C; PB: UK; $t_{1/2}$: 3-4 h
phenylephrine HCl (12-hour spray, Afrin 4 hrNeo-Synephrine) Alpha	Nasal decongestant: A: 2-3 sprays q4h PRN Hypotension: A: IM/subQ: 1-5 mg initially, then 1-10 mg q10-15min PRN	To treat nasal congestion; acts as a decongestant. Used for patients with common cold, sinusitis, allergic rhinitis. Have patient blow nose before drug is administered. Nasal decongestant therapy should not exceed 3 days. Pregnancy category: C; PB: UK; $t_{1/2}$: 2.5 h
pseudoephedrine HCl (Sudafed) Alpha and beta$_1$	Nasal decongestant: A: PO: 60 mg q4-6h; PO/SR: 120 mg q12h; *max:* 240 mg/d C: >2 y: PO: 15 mg q4-6h; *max:* 60 mg/d C: 6-12 y: PO: 30 mg q4-6h; *max:* 120 mg/d	To treat nasal congestion. OTC drug but controlled by placement behind counter or locked up. Check label for contraindications. Avoid taking with a history of hypertension, cardiac disease, or diabetes mellitus. Pregnancy category: C; PB: UK; $t_{1/2}$: 9-16 h
albuterol (Proventil, Ventolin) Beta$_2$	See Prototype Drug Chart 18-2.	
metaproterenol sulfate (Alupent) Beta$_2$	A and C: >9 y: PO: 20 mg q6-8h Older adults: 10 mg initially; may increase to 20 mg q6-8h C: 6 to 9 y: PO: 10 mg t.i.d./q.i.d. A and C: >12 y: Inhal: 2-3 puffs q3-4h; *max:* 12 puffs/d	To treat bronchospasm by bronchodilation. Pregnancy category: C; PB: UK; $t_{1/2}$: UK
dobutamine HCl (Dobutrex) Beta$_1$	A and C: IV: 0.5-1 mcg/kg/min initially; increase dose gradually; *max:* 40 mcg/kg/min	To treat cardiac decompensation (which may result from cardiogenic shock or cardiac surgery) by enhancing myocardial contractility, stroke volume, and cardiac output. Pregnancy category: C; PB: UK; $t_{1/2}$: 2 min
terbutaline sulfate Beta$_2$	Bronchodilator: A: PO: 2.5-5 mg t.i.d.; SC: 0.25 mg initially; no more than 0.5 mg in 4 h	Used primarily to correct bronchospasm. Pregnancy category: C; PB: 25%; $t_{1/2}$: 3-4 h

A, Adult; *C*, child; *d*, day; *FDA*, U.S Food and Drug Administration; *gtt*, drops; *h*, hour; *IM*, intramuscular; *inf*, infusion; *inhal*, inhalation; *IPPB*, intermittent positive pressure breathing; *IV*, intravenous; *min*, minute; *NSS*, normal saline solution; *OTC*, over-the-counter; *PB*, protein-binding; *PO*, by mouth; *PRN*, as needed; *q.i.d.*, four times a day; *SL*, sublingual; *sol*, solution; *SR*, sustained release; *subQ*, subcutaneous; $t_{1/2}$, half-life; *t.i.d.*, three times a day; *UK*, unknown; *y*, year; >, greater than; <, less than.

resuscitation; may repeat q3-5 min. Follow each dose with 20-mL saline flush to ensure proper delivery. Normally, epinephrine is administered 1 mg IV over 1 minute or more; however, in cardiac arrest, it may be given more rapidly.

- Monitor IV site frequently when administering norepinephrine bitartrate (Levarterenol) or dopamine (Intropin) because extravasation of these drugs causes tissue necrosis. These drugs should be diluted sufficiently in IV fluids.

- Administer antidote, phentolamine mesylate (Regitine) 5 to 10 mg, diluted in 10 to 15 mL of saline infiltrated into the area for IV extravasation of norepinephrine (Levophed) and dopamine.
- Record patient's vital signs. Report signs of increasing blood pressure and increasing heart rate. If patient receives an alpha-adrenergic agonist intravenously for shock, check the blood pressure q3-5min or as indicated to avoid severe hypertension.
- Monitor ECG for dysrhythmias when given IV.
- Report side effects of adrenergic drugs: tachycardia, palpitations, tremors, dizziness, and increased blood pressure.
- Check patient's urinary output, and assess for bladder distention. Urinary retention can result from high drug dose or continuous use of adrenergic agonists.
- Offer food to patient when giving adrenergic agonists to avoid nausea and vomiting.
- Evaluate blood glucose levels in patients with diabetes mellitus because they may be increased.

Patient Teaching

General

- Advise patient to read labels on all over-the-counter (OTC) drugs for cold symptoms and diet pills. Many of these have properties of sympathetic (adrenergic agonists, sympathomimetics) drugs and should not be taken if patient is hypertensive or has diabetes mellitus, cardiac dysrhythmias, or coronary artery disease.
- Explain to patient that continuous use of nasal sprays or drops that contain adrenergic agonists may result in rebound (inflamed and congested tissue) nasal congestion.

Self-Administration

- Encourage patient to take medication as prescribed.
- Advise patient and family on proper administration of drug and allow return demonstration. Cold medications by spray or drops in the nostrils should be used with the head in an upright position. Use of nasal spray while lying down can cause systemic absorption. Coloration of nasal spray or drops might indicate deterioration.
- Notify health care provider if EpiPen is needed more than twice a week.
- Encourage patient to have EpiPen readily available at all times and to store additional medication in a cool, dark place (refrigeration is not recommended).
- Teach patient and family that EpiPen must be taken immediately upon the initial occurrence of difficulty breathing, wheezing, hoarseness, hives, itching, or swelling of lips and tongue.
- Teach patient to administer EpiPen properly. Inspect solution for particles or discoloration prior to administration. Do not use if particles are pink to brown in color. Take care to inject subcutaneously and not intradermally, and to apply sufficient pressure to activate EpiPen while holding device in place for 5 to 10 seconds. The EpiPen should be inserted into outer thigh. After administration, massage injection site for 10 seconds to promote absorption and reduce vasoconstriction and tissue irritation.

Side Effects

- Encourage patient to report side effects (e.g., rapid heart rate, palpitations, rash, itching, flushing, chest pain, irregular heartbeat, vomiting, numbness of fingers and toes) to a health care provider as dose may require adjustment.

Cultural Considerations

- Decrease language barriers for patients with language difficulties and for those who do not work in the health care field by decoding the jargon of the health care environment.

Evaluation

- Evaluate patient's response to the adrenergic agonist.
- Evaluate patient's vital signs, and report abnormal findings. Epinephrine stimulates $alpha_1$ (increases blood pressure), $beta_1$ (increases heart rate), and $beta_2$ (dilates bronchial tubes) receptors. Albuterol (Proventil) stimulates $beta_2$ receptors.
- Report possible drug-drug interactions. Beta blockers decrease the effect of epinephrine and albuterol. Over-the-counter cold and allergy drugs, caffeine, alcohol, herbs, and dietary supplements may lead to interactions.

ADRENERGIC BLOCKERS (ANTAGONISTS)

Drugs that block the effects of adrenergic neurotransmitters are called **adrenergic blockers,** adrenergic antagonists, or sympatholytics. They act as antagonists to adrenergic agonists by blocking the alpha and beta receptor sites. Most adrenergic blockers block either the alpha receptor or the beta receptor. They block the effects of the neurotransmitter either directly by occupying the receptors or indirectly by inhibiting the release of the neurotransmitters norepinephrine and epinephrine. Table 18-3 lists the effects of alpha blockers and beta blockers at receptors.

Alpha-Adrenergic Blockers

Drugs that block or inhibit a response at the alpha-adrenergic receptor site are called alpha-adrenergic blockers or **alpha blockers.** Alpha-blocking agents are divided into two groups: selective alpha blockers that block $alpha_1$, and nonselective alpha blockers that block $alpha_1$ and $alpha_2$. Because alpha-adrenergic blockers can cause orthostatic hypotension and reflex tachycardia, many of these drugs are not as frequently prescribed as beta blockers.

TABLE 18-3 EFFECTS OF ADRENERGIC BLOCKERS AT RECEPTORS

RECEPTOR	RESPONSES
$Alpha_1$	Vasodilation: decreases blood pressure; reflex tachycardia might result; miosis (constriction of pupil) occurs; suppresses ejaculation; reduces contraction of smooth muscle in bladder neck and prostate gland
$Beta_1$	Decreases heart rate; reduces force of contractions
$Beta_2$	Constricts bronchioles; contracts uterus; inhibits glycogenolysis, which can decrease blood sugar

Alpha blockers promote vasodilation, causing a decrease in blood pressure. If vasodilation is long-standing, orthostatic hypotension can result. Dizziness may also be a symptom of a drop in blood pressure. As blood pressure decreases, pulse rate usually increases to compensate for the low blood pressure and inadequate blood flow. Alpha blockers can be used to treat peripheral vascular disease (e.g., Raynaud's disease). Vasodilation occurs, permitting more blood flow to the extremities. These drugs are also helpful in decreasing symptoms of benign prostatic hypertrophy. Alpha blockers are also discussed in Chapter 44.

Beta-Adrenergic Blockers

Beta-adrenergic blockers, commonly called **beta blockers,** decrease heart rate, and a decrease in blood pressure usually follows. Some beta blockers are nonselective, blocking both $beta_1$ and $beta_2$ receptors. Not only does the heart rate decrease because of $beta_1$ blocking, but bronchoconstriction also occurs. Nonselective beta blockers (block both $beta_1$ and $beta_2$) should be used with extreme caution in any patient who has chronic obstructive pulmonary disease (COPD) or asthma.

Propranolol hydrochloride (Inderal) was the first beta blocker prescribed to treat angina, cardiac dysrhythmias, hypertension, and heart failure. This medication is given for migraine prophylaxis. Although it is still prescribed today, propranolol has many side effects, partly because of its nonselective response in blocking both $beta_1$ and $beta_2$ receptors.

A selective adrenergic blocker has a greater affinity for certain receptors. If the desired effect is to decrease pulse rate and blood pressure, then a selective $beta_1$ blocker such as atenolol (Tenormin) or metoprolol tartrate (Lopressor) may be ordered.

Intrinsic sympathomimetic activity (ISA) is the ability of certain beta blockers to bind with a beta receptor to prevent strong agonists from binding to that receptor producing complete activation. Nonselective beta blockers (block both $beta_1$ and $beta_2$) that have ISA include carteolol, carvedilol, penbutolol, and pindolol. The selective blocker (blocks $beta_1$ only) that has ISA is acebutolol. These agents may be recommended for patients experiencing bradycardia.

Atenolol (Tenormin), a selective $beta_1$ blocker, is one of the most frequently prescribed drugs in the United States. Atenolol decreases sympathetic outflow to the periphery and suppresses the renin-angiotensin-aldosterone system response, It is contraindicated in bradycardia, heart block, cardiogenic shock, pulmonary edema, acute bronchospasm, and pregnancy. Prototype Drug Chart 18-3 describes the pharmacologic behavior of atenolol.

Beta blockers are useful in treating mild to moderate hypertension, angina pectoris, and myocardial infarction. The use of beta blockers as antihypertensives, antidysrhythmics, and drugs for angina is discussed in Chapters 42 and 44. Table 18-4 lists the alpha and beta blockers and their dosages, uses, and considerations.

Pharmacokinetics Atenolol is 50% absorbed from the GI tract. It does not readily cross the blood-brain barrier. It has a half-life of 3 to 6 hours and is eliminated in urine and feces.

Pharmacodynamics By blocking $beta_1$ receptors, atenolol decreases the heart rate, peripheral vascular resistance, force of cardiac contractions, cardiac output, as well as systolic and diastolic blood pressure. It is available in tablets and for intravenous administration. The onset of action of the oral preparation is 1 hour; peak time is 2 to 4 hours, and duration of action is 24 hours. This drug is effective for dosing once a day, especially for patients who do not adhere to schedules with drug doses of several times a day.

Drug Interactions

Many drugs interact with atenolol. Nonsteroidal antiinflammatory drugs (NSAIDs) decrease the hypotensive effect of atenolol. Hypotension can be potentiated if atenolol is taken with another antihypertensive, though this may be the desired result. When atenolol is given concurrently with atropine and other anticholinergics, absorption is increased. The risk of hypoglycemia is increased when the patient is taking insulin and sulfonylureas.

Side Effects and Adverse Reactions

The side effects commonly associated with beta blockers are bradycardia, hypotension, headache, dizziness, cold extremities, hypoglycemia, and bronchospasm. General side effects of beta-adrenergic blockers include cardiac dysrhythmias, flushing, hypotension, weakness, impotence or decreased libido, depression, and pulmonary edema. Usually the side effects are dose related.

Adrenergic Neuron Blockers

Drugs that block the release of norepinephrine from the sympathetic terminal neurons are called **adrenergic neuron blockers,** which are classified as a subdivision of the adrenergic blockers. The clinical use of neuron blockers is to decrease blood pressure. (Herbal Alert 18-1) Reserpine, an example of an adrenergic neuron blocker, is an

HERBAL ALERT 18-1

Reserpine

St. John's wort may antagonize the hypotensive effects of reserpine.

PROTOTYPE DRUG CHART 18-3

Atenolol

Drug Class $Beta_1$-adrenergic blocker Trade Name: Tenormin Pregnancy Category: D	**Dosage** Hypertension, angina: A: PO: Initially 25-50 mg/d; may increase to 100 mg/d Older adults: PO: 25-50 mg/d Myocardial infarction: A: PO: Initially 50 mg/d
Contraindications Sinus bradycardia, heart block >first-degree, cardiogenic shock, pulmonary edema, acute bronchospasm, uncompensated cardiac failure, pregnancy, lactation Caution: Renal dysfunction, diabetes mellitus	**Drug-Lab-Food Interactions** Drug: *Increased* absorption with atropine and other anticholinergics, *decreased* effects with NSAIDs, *increased* risk of hypoglycemia with insulin and sulfonylureas, *increased* hypotension with prazosin and terazosin, *increased* lidocaine and verapamil levels with toxicity
Pharmacokinetics Absorption: 50% absorbed in GI tract Distribution: PB: 6%-16% Metabolism: $t\frac{1}{2}$: 6-7 h Excretion: Urine and feces	**Pharmacodynamics** PO: Onset: 1 h Peak: 2-4 h Duration: 24 h
Therapeutic Effects/Uses To treat hypertension, angina pectoris, myocardial infarction, and heart failure Mode of Action: Selectively blocks $beta_1$-adrenergic receptor sites, decreases sympathetic outflow to the periphery, suppresses renin-angiotensin-aldosterone system	
Side Effects Drowsiness, dizziness, fainting, depression, alopecia, weakness, nausea, vomiting, diarrhea, cool extremities, impotence, decreased libido	**Adverse Reactions** Bradycardia, hypotension, heart failure, masking of hypoglycemia Life-threatening: Bronchospasm, pulmonary edema, dysrhythmias, thrombocytopenia

A, Adult; *COPD,* chronic obstructive pulmonary disease; *GI,* gastrointestinal; *h,* hour; *IV,* intravenously; *min,* minute; *NSAID,* nonsteroidal antiinflammatory drug; *PB,* protein-binding; *PO,* by mouth; $t\frac{1}{2}$, half-life; *UK,* unknown.

TABLE 18-4 ADRENERGIC BLOCKERS

GENERIC (BRAND)	ROUTE AND DOSAGE	USES AND CONSIDERATIONS
phentolamine mesylate (Regitine) $Alpha_1$	Treat catecholamine extravasation: A: Intradermal: 5-10 mg in 10 mL NS infiltrated into affected area within 12 h of extravasation	Antidote for dopamine, dobutamine, phenylephrine, epinephrine, and norepinephrine infiltration to prevent dermal necrosis. Redness and tissue warmth are signs of effective treatment. Pregnancy category: C; PB: UK; $t\frac{1}{2}$: 20 min
doxazosin mesylate (Cardura) $Alpha_1$	A: PO: 1 mg/d initially *max:* 16 mg/d for hypertension; *max:* 8 mg/d for BPH	To treat mild to moderate hypertension and BPH. Check for orthostatic hypotension. Dizziness, headache, syncope may occur. Pregnancy category: C; PB: 98%; $t\frac{1}{2}$: 22 h
prazosin HCl (Minipress) $Alpha_1$	A: PO: 1 mg h.s. initially 2-3 times/d; *max:* 20 mg/d C: 5 mcg/kg q6h; *max:* 15 mg/d	To manage mild to moderate hypertension. May be used in combination with other antihypertensive drugs. Pregnancy category: C; PB: 97%; $t\frac{1}{2}$: 2-4 h
terazosin HCl (Hytrin) $Alpha_1$	A: PO: initially 1 mg h.s., maint: 1-5 mg/d in 2 divided doses; *max:* 20 mg/d	To treat hypertension. May be used in combination with a diuretic or with other antihypertensive drugs. Also used to treat BPH. May cause dizziness, headache, edema, orthostatic hypotension. Pregnancy category: C; PB: 90%-94%; $t\frac{1}{2}$: 12 h
carvedilol (Coreg) $Alpha_1$, $beta_1$, and $beta_2$	A: PO: 6.25 mg b.i.d.; *max:* 50 mg/d	To treat hypertension and heart failure. Can be used alone or with a thiazide diuretic. Pregnancy category: C; PB: 98%; $t\frac{1}{2}$: 7-10 h

TABLE 18-4 **ADRENERGIC BLOCKERS—cont'd**

GENERIC (BRAND)	ROUTE AND DOSAGE	USES AND CONSIDERATIONS
labetalol (Normodyne, Trandate) Alpha$_1$, beta$_1$, and beta$_2$	A: PO: 100 mg b.i.d.; dose may be increased q2-3d; *max:* 2400 mg/d; IV: 20 mg; repeat 20-80 mg at 10-min interval; *max:* 300 mg/d	To treat mild to severe hypertension. Pregnancy category: C; PB: 50%; t½: 2.5-8 h
penbutolol (Levatol) Beta$_1$ and beta$_2$	A: PO: 20 mg/d; *max:* 80 mg/d	To treat mild to moderate hypertension in patients with angina, prior MI, or heart failure. Patients with asthma should avoid taking the drug. Pregnancy category: C; PB: 80%-98%; t½: 5 h
propranolol HCl (Inderal) Beta$_1$ and beta$_2$	A: PO: Initially: 40 mg b.i.d.; increase q3-7d up to 160-480 mg/d in 2-3 divided doses; *max:* 640 mg/d	To manage hypertension, angina pectoris, and dysrhythmias. To prevent myocardial infarction and migraines. Pregnancy category: C; PB: 93%; t½: 2-6 h
nadolol (Corgard) Beta$_1$ and beta$_2$	A: PO: 40-80 mg/d; *max:* 320 mg/d for hypertension and 240 mg/d for angina	To manage hypertension and angina pectoris. Contraindicated in bronchial asthma and severe COPD because it blocks beta$_2$ receptors. Pregnancy category: C; PB: 30%; t½: 10-24 h
pindolol (Visken) Beta$_1$ and beta$_2$	A: PO: 5 mg b.i.d; maint: 10-30 mg in divided doses; *max:* 60 mg/d in divided doses	To manage hypertension. Contraindicated in asthma, COPD, and second- and third-degree heart block. Pregnancy category: B; PB: 40%; t½: 3-4 h
sotalol (Betapace) Beta$_1$ and beta$_2$	A: PO: 80 mg b.i.d.; may increase gradually. Average: 240-320 mg/d	To treat life-threatening ventricular arrhythmias. Correct hypokalemia and hypomagnesemia before initiating therapy. Pregnancy category: B; PB: 0%; t½: 12 h
timolol maleate (Blocadren) Beta$_1$ and beta$_2$	A: PO: Initially 10 mg b.i.d.; maint: 20-40 mg/d in 2 divided doses; *max:* 60 mg/d	To manage mild to moderate hypertension and dysrhythmias, and to prevent reinfarction after MI. For ophthalmic use to treat IOP. Unlabeled use: prophylaxis for migraine headache and stable angina. Use with caution in patients with asthma or COPD. Pregnancy category: C; PB: <10%; t½: 3-4 h
Selective Beta-Adrenergic Blockers		
metoprolol tartrate (Lopressor) Beta$_1$	Hypertension: A: PO: 50-100 mg/d in 1-2 divided doses; may increase weekly; *max:* 450 mg/d in divided doses Myocardial infarction: A: IV: 5 mg q2min in 3 doses, then PO 50-100 mg b.i.d.	To manage hypertension, angina pectoris, and postmyocardial infarction. Bradycardia, dizziness, and gastrointestinal distress may occur. Pregnancy category: C; PB: 12%; t½: 3-4 h
atenolol (Tenormin)Beta$_1$	See Prototype Drug Chart 18-3.	
acebutolol HCl (Sectral) Beta$_1$	A: PO: Initially: 200-400 mg/d; maint: 200-800 mg/d in 1 to 2 divided doses; *max:* 1200 mg/d Older adults: *max:* 800 mg/d	To treat mild to moderate hypertension, angina pectoris, and dysrhythmias. Check apical pulse; do not give if <60 beats/min. Pregnancy category: B; PB: 26%; t½: 3-4 h
betaxolol (Betoptic) Beta$_1$	Hypertension: A: PO: 5-10 mg/d; *max:* 20 mg/d	To treat hypertension and chronic open angle glaucoma. Ophthalmic preparation is used to decrease IOP. Pregnancy category: C; PB: 50%; t½: 15 h
bisoprolol fumarate (Zebeta) Beta$_1$	A: PO: Initially: 2.5-5 mg/d; *max:* 20 mg/d	To treat hypertension. Unlabeled use: angina pectoris. Long-acting beta blocker. May decrease heart rate and blood pressure. Pregnancy category: C; PB: 30%-36%; t½: 10-12 h
esmolol HCl (Brevibloc) Beta$_1$	A: IV: Loading dose: 500 mcg/kg/min for 1 min; then 50 mcg/kg/min for 4 min; *max:* 500 mcg/kg/min/loading dose; 200 mcg/kg/min for IV maintenance infusion	To treat supraventricular tachydysrhythmias. Unlabeled use: hypertension. Contraindications: heart block, bradycardia, cardiogenic shock, uncompensated heart failure. Pregnancy category: C; PB: 55%; t½: 9 min

A, Adult; *b.i.d.*, two times a day; *BPH*, benign prostatic hypertrophy; *C*, child; *COPD*, chronic obstructive pulmonary disease; *d*, day; *h*, hour; *IM*, intramuscular; *IOP*, intraocular pressure; *IV*, intravenous; *PB*, protein-binding; *PO*, by mouth; *PRN*, as necessary; *t½*, half-life; *UK*, unknown; >, greater than; <, less than.

antihypertensive agent. Effects of this drug closely resemble those of alpha- and beta-adrenergic blockers. Reserpine also reduces the serotonin and catecholamine transmitters. Depletion of these neurotransmitters may lead to severe mental depression. Reserpine is discussed in more detail in Chapter 44.

Nursing Process
Patient-Centered Collaborative Care

Adrenergic Neuron Blockers

Assessment
- Obtain baseline vital signs and electrocardiogram for future comparison. Bradycardia and decrease in blood pressure are common cardiac effects of adrenergic neuron blockers.
- Determine the drugs that the patient currently takes. Report if any are diuretics, NSAIDs, digoxin, MAOIs, or CNS depressants.
- Obtain patient's health history. Depression, peptic ulcer, and heart failure may result from taking an adrenergic neuron blocker, and these drugs could potentiate pre-existing conditions.

Nursing Diagnoses
- Decreased cardiac output related to hypotension and bradycardia
- Risk for falls related to dizziness
- Fatigue related to medication adverse effects
- Sexual dysfunction related to adverse effects of erectile and ejaculatory dysfunction
- Noncompliance related to undesired adverse effects of erectile dysfunction

Planning
- Patient will adhere to the drug regimen.
- Patient's vital signs will be within the desired range.

Nursing Interventions
- Monitor patient's vital signs. Report marked changes such as marked decrease in blood pressure and heart rate.
- Report any complaints of excessive dizziness, lightheadedness, early morning insomnia, mental depression, or chest pain.
- Assist patient with ambulation to avoid falls from orthostatic hypotension, which is more common with high doses.
- Note any complaint of stuffy nose, because vasodilation may result and nasal congestion can occur.

Patient Teaching
General
- Encourage patient to adhere to the drug regimen.
- Advise patient that therapeutic effects of reserpine may not occur for 2 to 3 weeks after initiation of therapy.

Self-Administration
- Teach patient and family how to take pulse and blood pressure.
- Encourage patient to take reserpine at the same time every day and not to discontinue without permission of health care provider.

Side Effects
- Encourage patient to avoid orthostatic (postural) hypotension by slowly rising from supine or sitting positions to standing.
- Inform patient and family of possible mood changes when taking reserpine due to catecholamine depletion. Mood changes can include depression, detachment, inability to concentrate, nightmares, and suicidal tendencies.
- Warn patient that reserpine may cause impotence or decreased libido, which is usually dose related.
- Advise patient not to drive or engage in operation of dangerous equipment until the drug response is known.

Cultural Considerations
- Obtain interpreter when necessary. Do not rely on family members, who may not fully disclose because of honor or shame.
- Discuss ethnicity of interpreter, as well as the language desired when translation is needed. Provide an interpreter with the same ethnic background and gender if possible, especially when sensitive topics are being addressed.

Evaluation
- Evaluate effectiveness of the adrenergic neuron blocker. Vital signs must be stable within the desired range.

KEY WEBSITES

Information on albuterol: *www.medicinenet.com/albuterol/article.htm*

Information on anaphylaxis: *www.drugs.com/mtm/epinephrine-injection.html*

CRITICAL THINKING CASE STUDY

An older adult patient has asthma. An adrenergic agonist is selected for treatment.

1. What are the drug advantages and disadvantages associated with the use of an adrenergic agonist, such as ephedrine, metaproterenol, or albuterol, for this patient? Explain your answer.
2. Is age a factor in drug selection? Explain your answer.

An older adult patient has hypertension and asthma. An adrenergic blocker is selected for treatment.

1. What are the drug advantages and disadvantages associated with the use of doxazosin, prazosin, propranolol, metoprolol, and atenolol for this patient? Explain your answer.
2. What needs to be included when teaching this patient about the use of an adrenergic blocker?

NCLEX STUDY QUESTIONS

1. The nurse will monitor the patient taking albuterol (Proventil) for which conditions? (Select all that apply.)
   a. Palpitations
   b. Hypertension
   c. Hypoglycemia
   d. Bronchospasm
   e. Uterine contractions
2. Nadolol (Corgard) is prescribed for a patient. The nurse realizes that this drug is a beta-adrenergic blocker and that this drug classification is contraindicated for patients with which condition?
   a. Hypothyroidism
   b. Angina pectoris
   c. Bronchial asthma
   d. Liver dysfunction
3. The nurse realizes that $beta_1$ receptor stimulation is differentiated from $beta_2$ stimulation in that stimulation of $beta_1$ receptors leads to which condition?
   a. Increased bronchodilation
   b. Decreased uterine contractility
   c. Increased myocardial contractility
   d. Decreased blood flow to skeletal muscles
4. A patient is given epinephrine (Adrenalin), an adrenergic agonist (sympathomimetic). The nurse should monitor the patient for which condition?
   a. Decreased pulse
   b. Pupil constriction
   c. Bronchial constriction
   d. Increased blood pressure
5. A patient who is taking epinephrine is also taking several other medications. The nurse should realize that there is a possible drug interaction with which drugs? (Select all that apply.)
   a. albuterol (Proventil)
   b. metoprolol (Lopressor)
   c. propranolol (Inderal)
   d. digoxin (Lanoxin)
   e. methyldopa (Aldomet)
6. A patient is prescribed metoprolol (Lopressor) to treat hypertension. It is important for the nurse to monitor the patient for which condition? (Select all that apply.)
   a. Bradycardia
   b. Hypotension
   c. Ankle edema
   d. Decreased respirations
   e. Increased respirations
7. The nurse is administering atenolol (Tenormin) to a patient. Which concurrent drugs does the nurse expect to most likely cause an interaction? (Select all that apply.)
   a. ginseng supplement
   b. An NSAID, such as aspirin
   c. atropine, an anticholinergic
   d. haloperidol (Haldol)
   e. methyldopa (Aldomet)

Answers: 1, a, b; 2, c; 3, c; 4, d; 5, b, c, d; 6, a, b; 7, b, c.

CHAPTER

19

Cholinergic Agonists and Anticholinergics

evolve WEBSITE

http://evolve.elsevier.com/KeeHayes/pharmacology/

- Animations
- Content Updates
- Key Points
- Review Questions for the NCLEX® Examination
- References from the Textbook
- Unfolding Case Studies

OBJECTIVES

- Compare the responses of cholinergic agonists and anticholinergic drugs.
- Differentiate between direct-acting and indirect-acting cholinergic agonists.
- Contrast the major side effects of cholinergic agonists and anticholinergics.
- Differentiate the uses of cholinergic agonists and anticholinergics.
- Apply the nursing process, including patient teaching associated with cholinergic agonists and anticholinergics.
- Apply the nursing process for the patient taking neostigmine, a reversible cholinesterase inhibitor.

OUTLINE

KEY TERMS

The two groups of drugs that affect the parasympathetic nervous system are the (1) cholinergic agonists (parasympathomimetics) and the (2) *anticholinergics* (parasympatholytics). The Unit V opener offers a discussion and comparison of the parasympathetic nervous system (parasympathomimetics and parasympatholytics) and the sympathetic nervous system.

CHOLINERGIC AGONISTS

Drugs that stimulate the parasympathetic nervous system are called **cholinergic agonists,** or **parasympathomimetics,** because they mimic the parasympathetic neurotransmitter acetylcholine. Cholinergic agonists are also called *cholinomimetics or cholinergic stimulants.* **Acetylcholine (ACh)** is the

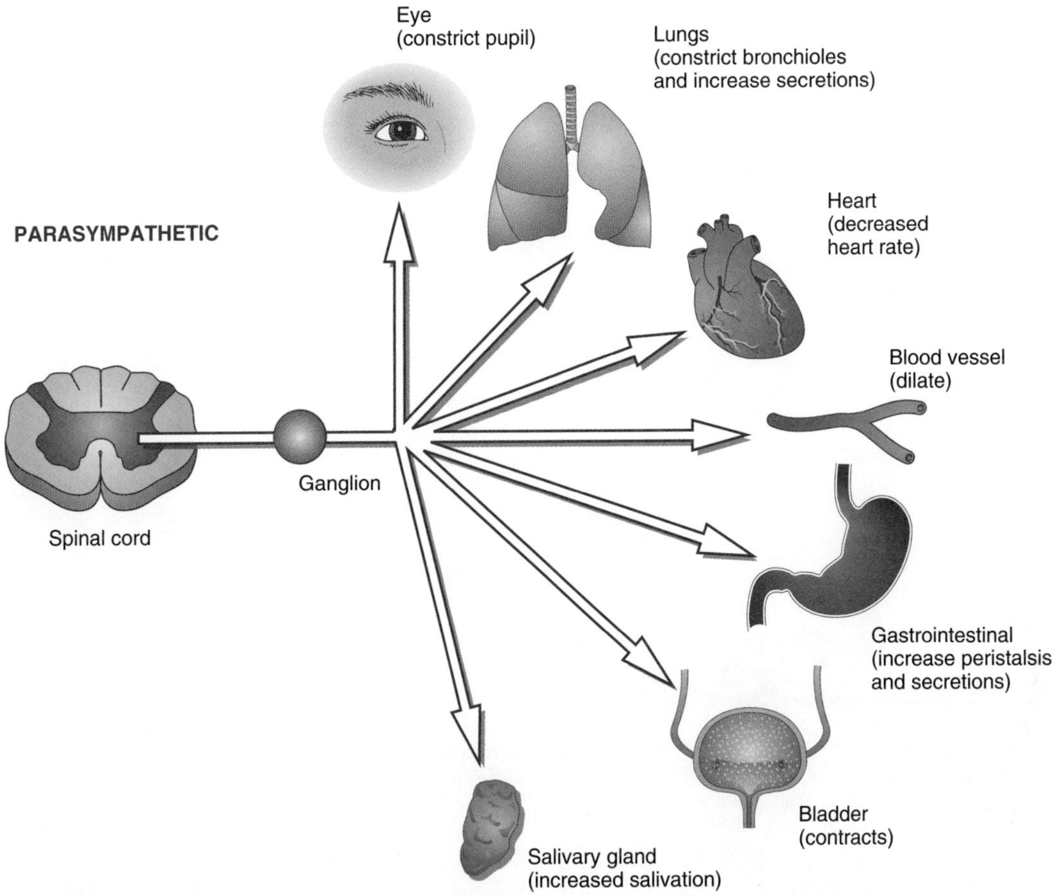

FIGURE 19–1 Parasympathetic responses. Stimulation of the parasympathetic nervous system or use of parasympathomimetic drugs will cause the pupils to constrict, bronchioles to constrict and bronchial secretions to increase, heart rate to decrease, blood vessels to dilate, peristalsis and gastric secretions to increase, the bladder muscle to contract, and salivary glands to increase salivation.

neurotransmitter located at the ganglions and the parasympathetic terminal nerve endings. It innervates cholinergic receptors in organs, tissues, and glands. The two types of cholinergic receptors are (1) **muscarinic receptors,** which stimulate smooth muscle and slow the heart rate; and (2) **nicotinic receptors** (neuromuscular), which affect the skeletal muscles. Many cholinergic agonists are nonselective because they can affect both the muscarinic and nicotinic receptors. However, there are selective cholinergic agonists for the muscarinic receptors that do *not* affect the nicotinic receptors. Figure 19-1 illustrates the effects of parasympathetic or cholinergic stimulation.

There are **direct-acting cholinergic agonists** and indirect-acting cholinergic agonists. *Direct-acting cholinergic agonists* act on receptors to activate a tissue response (Figure 19-2, *A*). *Indirect-acting cholinergic agonists* inhibit the action of the enzyme **cholinesterase (ChE)** (acetylcholinesterase) by forming a chemical complex, thus permitting acetylcholine to persist and attach to the receptor (Figure 19-2, *B*). Drugs that inhibit cholinesterase are called *cholinesterase inhibitors, acetylcholinesterase (AChE) inhibitors,* or **anticholinesterases.** Cholinesterase may destroy acetylcholine before it reaches the receptor or after it has attached to the site. By inhibiting or destroying the enzyme cholinesterase, more acetylcholine is available to stimulate the receptor and remain in contact with it longer.

Cholinesterase inhibitors (anticholinesterases) can be separated into reversible inhibitors and irreversible inhibitors. The reversible inhibitors bind the enzyme cholinesterase for several minutes to hours, and the irreversible inhibitors bind the enzyme permanently. The resulting effects vary with how long the cholinesterase is bound.

The major responses of cholinergic agonists are to stimulate bladder and gastrointestinal (GI) tone, constrict the pupils of the eyes **(miosis),** and increase neuromuscular transmission. Other effects of cholinergic agonists include decreased heart rate and blood pressure and increased salivary, GI, and bronchial glandular secretions. Table 19-1 lists the functions of direct- and indirect-acting cholinergic agonists.

Direct-Acting Cholinergic Agonists

Many drugs classified as **direct-acting cholinergic agonists** are primarily selective to the muscarinic receptors but are

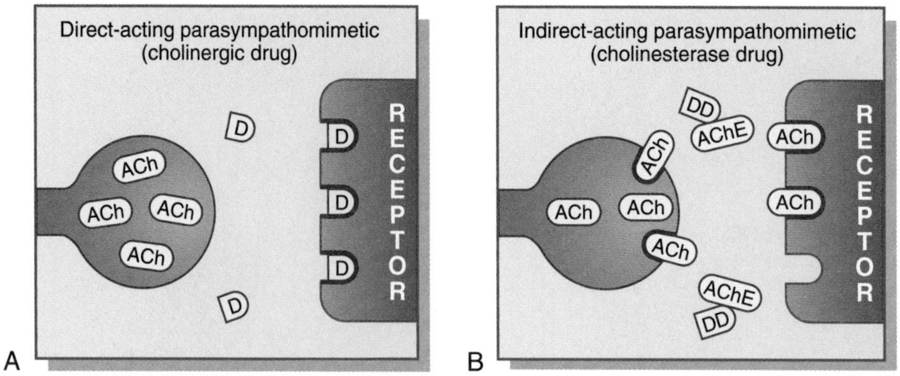

FIGURE 19–2 *A,* Direct-acting parasympathomimetic (cholinergic agonist). Cholinergic agonists resemble acetylcholine and act directly on the receptor. *B,* Indirect-acting parasympathomimetic (cholinesterase inhibitor). Cholinesterase inhibitors inactivate the enzyme acetylcholinesterase (cholinesterase), thus permitting acetylcholine to react to the receptor. *ACh,* Acetylcholine; *AChE,* acetylcholinesterase or cholinesterase; *D,* cholinergic agonist; *DD,* cholinesterase inhibitor (anticholinesterase).

TABLE 19-1 EFFECTS OF CHOLINERGIC AGONISTS

BODY TISSUE	RESPONSE
Cardiovascular*	Decreases heart rate, lowers blood pressure because of vasodilation, and slows conduction of atrioventricular node.
Gastrointestinal†	Increases tone and motility of smooth muscle of stomach and intestine. Increases peristalsis and relaxes sphincter muscles.
Genitourinary	Contracts muscles of the urinary bladder, increases tone of ureters, and relaxes bladder's sphincter muscles. Stimulates urination.
Ocular†	Increases pupillary constriction, or miosis (pupil becomes smaller) and increases accommodation (flattening or thickening of eye lens for distant or near vision).
Glandular*	Increases salivation, perspiration, and tears.
Bronchial (lung)*	Stimulates bronchial smooth muscle contraction and increases bronchial secretions.
Striated muscle†	Increases neuromuscular transmission and maintains muscle strength and tone.

*Tissue responses to large doses of cholinergic agonists.
†Major tissue responses to normal doses of cholinergic agonists.

nonspecific because the muscarinic receptors are located in the smooth muscle of the GI and genitourinary tracts, glands, and heart. Bethanechol chloride (Urecholine), a direct-acting cholinergic agonist, acts on the muscarinic (cholinergic) receptor and is used primarily to increase micturition (urination) in the treatment of urinary retention and neurogenic bladder. Metoclopramide HCl (Reglan) is a direct-acting cholinergic agonist that is usually prescribed to treat gastroesophageal reflux disease (GERD). Metoclopramide accelerates gastric emptying time. Prototype Drug Chart 19-1 details the pharmacologic behavior of bethanechol, which is a classic cholinergic agonist.

Pharmacokinetics Bethanechol chloride (Urecholine) is poorly absorbed from the GI tract. The percentage of protein-binding and the half-life are unknown. The drug is most likely excreted in the urine.

Pharmacodynamics The principal use of bethanechol is to promote micturition by stimulating the muscarinic cholinergic receptors in the detrusor muscle to contract the bladder and produce urine output. The patient voids approximately 30 minutes to 1.5 hours after taking an oral dose of bethanechol because of the increased tone of the detrusor muscle. Bethanechol also increases peristalsis in the GI tract. The drug should be taken on an empty stomach. It should not be administered by injection.

Side Effects and Adverse Reactions

Mild to severe side effects of most muscarinic agonists such as bethanechol include hypotension, bradycardia, blurred vision, excessive salivation, increased gastric acid secretion, abdominal cramps, diarrhea, bronchoconstriction, and, in some cases, cardiac dysrhythmias. This group of agents should be prescribed cautiously for patients with low blood pressure and heart rates. Muscarinic agonists are contraindicated for patients with intestinal or urinary tract obstruction, severe bradycardia, and for those with active asthma.

Direct-Acting Cholinergics: Eye

Pilocarpine is a direct-acting cholinergic agonist that constricts the pupils of the eyes, thus opening the canal of Schlemm to promote drainage of aqueous humor (fluid). This drug is used to treat glaucoma by relieving fluid (intraocular) pressure in the eye and to promote miosis in eye surgery and examinations. An oral form of pilocarpine is used to relieve xerostomia (dry mouth). Pilocarpine also acts on the nicotinic receptor, as does carbachol. Both agents are discussed in more detail in Chapter 49.

Indirect-Acting Cholinergic Agonists

The **indirect-acting cholinergic agonists** do not act on receptors; instead they inhibit or inactivate the enzyme cholinesterase, permitting acetylcholine to accumulate at the receptor sites (see Figure 19-2, *B*). This action gives them

PROTOTYPE DRUG CHART 19-1

Bethanechol Chloride

Drug Class Cholinergic: parasympathomimetic Trade Names: Urecholine Pregnancy Category: C	**Dosage** A: PO: 10-50 mg t.i.d./q.i.d.; *max:* 200 mg/d
Contraindications Contraindicated: Intestinal or urinary tract obstruction, severe bradycardia, hypotension, COPD, asthma, peptic ulcer, parkinsonism.	**Drug-Lab-Food Interactions** Drug: Decreases bethanechol effect with antidysrhythmics (e.g., procainamide); ganglionic blocking agents (e.g., mecamylamine) cause significant hypotension and false test results (amylase, lipase); atropine counteracts bethanechol action Lab: Increases AST, bilirubin, amylase, lipase
Pharmacokinetics Absorption: PO: Poorly absorbed Distribution: PB: UK Metabolism: t½: UK Excretion: In urine	**Pharmacodynamics** PO: Onset: 0.5-1.5 h Peak: 1-2 h Duration: 4-6 h
Therapeutic Effects/Uses To treat urinary retention Mode of Action: Stimulates the cholinergic (muscarinic) receptors; promotes contraction of the bladder; increases GI secretions and peristalsis, pupillary constriction, and bronchoconstriction	
Side Effects Nausea, vomiting, diarrhea, abdominal cramps, salivation, sweating, flushing, frequent urination, blurred vision, miosis	**Adverse Reactions** Orthostatic hypotension, bradycardia, muscle weakness Life-threatening: Acute asthma attack, heart block, circulatory collapse, cardiac arrest

A, Adult; *AST,* aspartate aminotransferase; *b.i.d.,* two times a day; *COPD,* chronic obstructive pulmonary disease; *d,* day; *GI,* gastrointestinal; *h,* hour; *IM,* intramuscular; *IV,* intravenous; *min,* minute; *PB,* protein-binding; *PO,* by mouth; *PRN,* as needed; *q.i.d.,* four times a day; *subQ,* subcutaneous; *t½,* half-life; *t.i.d.,* three times a day; *UK,* unknown.

the name *cholinesterase (ChE) inhibitors, acetylcholinesterase (AChE) inhibitors,* or *anticholinesterases,* of which there are two types: reversible and irreversible.

Nursing Process
Patient-Centered Collaborative Care

Cholinergic Agonist, Direct Acting: Bethanechol (Urecholine)

Assessment
- Assess baseline vital signs for future comparison.
- Assess urine output (should be >1500 mL/d).
- Obtain patient history of health problems such as peptic ulcer, urinary obstruction, or asthma. Cholinergic agonists can aggravate symptoms of these conditions.

Nursing Diagnoses
- Impaired urinary elimination related to urinary retention
- Anxiety related to wheezing
- Risk for impaired skin integrity related to rash
- Ineffective breathing pattern related to excess mucous secretions in lungs

Planning
- Patient will have increased bladder tone after taking cholinergic agonists.

Nursing Interventions
- Monitor patient's vital signs. Heart rate and blood pressure decrease when large doses of cholinergics are taken. Orthostatic hypotension is a side effect of a cholinergic agonist such as bethanechol.
- Record fluid intake and output. Decreased urinary output should be reported because it may be related to urinary obstruction.
- Give cholinergic agonists 1 hour before or 2 hours after meals. If patient complains of gastric pain, the drug may be given with meals.
- Check serum amylase, lipase, aspartate aminotransferase, and bilirubin levels. These laboratory values may increase slightly when taking cholinergic agonists.
- Observe patient for side effects such as gastric pain or cramping, diarrhea, increased salivary or bronchial secretions, bradycardia, and orthostatic hypotension.

- Auscultate breath sounds for rales (cracking sounds from fluid congestion in lungs) or rhonchi (rough sounds resulting from mucous secretions in lungs). Cholinergic agonists can increase bronchial secretions.
- Have IV atropine sulfate (0.6 mg to 1.2 mg) available as an antidote for cholinergic overdose. Early signs of overdosing include flushing, salivation, sweating, nausea, and abdominal cramps.
- Increase bathing frequency and linen change when needed. Diaphoresis (excessive perspiration) may occur.
- Monitor for possible cholinergic crisis (overdose) including symptoms of muscular weakness and increased salivation.

Patient Teaching

- Teach patient to take the cholinergic agonist as prescribed. Compliance with the drug regimen is essential.
- Direct patient to report severe side effects, such as profound dizziness or a decrease in heart rate below 60 beats/min.
- Teach patient to arise from a lying position slowly to avoid dizziness. This is most likely a result of orthostatic hypotension.
- Encourage patient to maintain effective oral hygiene if excess salivation occurs.
- Advise patient to report any difficulty in breathing as a result of respiratory distress.

Cultural Considerations

- Use both hands to show respect when offering a prescription, instructions, or pamphlets to Asians and Pacific Islanders.
- Recognize the importance of including women in decision making and disseminating health information. The extended family structure is important for teaching health strategies and providing support.

Evaluation

- Determine the effectiveness of the cholinergic agonist or anticholinesterase drug.
- Evaluate the stability of patient's vital signs, and note the presence of side effects or adverse reactions.

The function of the enzyme cholinesterase is to break down into choline and acetic acid. A small amount of cholinesterase can break down a large amount of acetylcholine in a short period. A cholinesterase inhibitor drug binds with cholinesterase, allowing acetylcholine to activate the muscarinic and nicotinic cholinergic receptors. This action permits skeletal muscle stimulation, which increases the force of muscular contraction. Because of this action, cholinesterase inhibitors are useful to increase muscle tone for patients with myasthenia gravis (a neuromuscular disorder). By increasing acetylcholine, additional effects occur, such as increase in GI motility, bradycardia, miosis, bronchial constriction, and increased micturition.

The primary use of reversible cholinesterase inhibitors is to treat myasthenia gravis; another use is to treat Alzheimer's disease. The primary clinical indication for irreversible cholinesterase inhibitors is glaucoma.

Reversible Cholinesterase Inhibitors

Reversible cholinesterase inhibitors are used (1) to produce pupillary constriction in the treatment of glaucoma and (2) to increase muscle strength in patients with myasthenia gravis. Drug effects persist for several hours. Drugs used to increase muscular strength in myasthenia gravis include neostigmine (Prostigmin [short-acting]), pyridostigmine bromide (Mestinon [moderate-acting]), ambenonium chloride (Mytelase [long-acting]), and edrophonium chloride (Tensilon [short-acting for diagnostic purposes]). These drugs are discussed in more detail in Chapter 24. A reversible anticholinesterase drug is physostigmine (Antilirium) or ophthalmic form (Isopto Eserine). Physostigmine is used as an antidote for atropine to reverse anticholinergic toxicity. Ophthalmic agents are further discussed in Chapter 49.

Side Effects

Caution for reversible cholinesterase inhibitors is required for patients who have bradycardia, asthma, peptic ulcers, or hyperthyroidism. Cholinesterase inhibitors are contraindicated for patients with intestinal or urinary obstruction.

Irreversible Cholinesterase Inhibitors

Irreversible cholinesterase inhibitors are potent agents because of their long-lasting effect. The enzyme cholinesterase must be regenerated before the drug effect diminishes—a process that may take days or weeks. These drugs are used to produce pupillary constriction.

Table 19-2 lists examples of cholinergic drugs and their standard dosages and common uses.

ANTICHOLINERGICS

Drugs that inhibit the actions of acetylcholine by occupying the acetylcholine receptors are called **anticholinergics** or **parasympatholytics.** Other names used for anticholinergics are **cholinergic blocking agents,** *cholinergic or muscarinic antagonists, antiparasympathetic agents, antimuscarinic agents,* and *antispasmodics.* The major body tissues and organs affected by the anticholinergic group of drugs are the heart, respiratory tract, GI tract, urinary bladder, eyes, and exocrine glands. By blocking the parasympathetic nerves, the sympathetic (adrenergic) nervous system dominates. Anticholinergics and adrenergic agonists produce many of the same responses.

Anticholinergic and cholinergic agonists have opposite effects. The major responses to anticholinergics are a decrease in GI motility, a decrease in salivation, dilation of pupils **(mydriasis),** and an increase in pulse rate. Other effects of

TABLE 19-2 CHOLINERGIC AGONISTS

GENERIC (BRAND)	ROUTE AND DOSAGE	USES AND CONSIDERATIONS
Direct-Acting Cholinergic Agonists		
bethanechol Cl (Urecholine)	See Prototype Drug Chart 19-1.	
metoclopramide HCl (Reglan)	A: PO: 5-10 mg q8h PRN	For GERD, gastroparesis, and nausea. Central dopamine receptor antagonist. Increases gastric emptying time. Pregnancy category: B; PB: 30%; $t_{1/2}$: 2.5-6 h
carbachol (Miostat)	Ophthalmic: 0.75%-3%, 1-2 gtt, 3 daily	To reduce IOP, miosis. See Chapter 49.
pilocarpine HCl (Pilocar)	Ophthalmic: 0.5%-4%, 1 gt	To reduce IOP, miosis. See Chapter 49.
Cholinesterase Inhibitor		
donepezil HCl (Aricept); rivastigmine (Exelon)	See Chapter 23, Table 23-6.	
Indirect-Acting Cholinergics or Cholinesterase Inhibitors for the Eye		
demecarium bromide (Humorsol)	0.125%-0.25%, 1 gt q12-48h	To reduce IOP in glaucoma; long-acting miotic. See Chapter 49.
echothiophate iodide (Phospholine Iodide)	0.03%-0.25%, 1 gt daily or b.i.d.	To reduce IOP; long-acting miotic. See Chapter 49.
isoflurophate (Floropryl)	0.25%, ointment q8-72h	To treat glaucoma. Apply to the conjunctival sac. See Chapter 49.
Reversible Cholinesterase Inhibitors: Myasthenia Gravis		
ambenonium Cl (Mytelase)	A: PO: 2.5-5 mg t.i.d./q.i.d.; dose may be increased; maint: 50-75 mg t.i.d./q.i.d.	To increase muscle strength in myasthenia gravis; long-acting. May be used with glucocorticoids. Pregnancy category: C; PB: UK; $t_{1/2}$: UK
edrophonium Cl (Tensilon)	A: IV: 2 mg; then 8 mg if no response IM: 10 mg; may repeat with 2 mg in 30 min C: <34 kg: IV: 1 mg; repeat in 30-45 sec if no response; *max:* 5 mg C: >34 kg: IV: 2 mg; repeat with 1 mg if no response; *max:* 10 mg	To diagnose myasthenia gravis; very short-acting. Pregnancy category: C; PB: UK; $t_{1/2}$: 1.2-2 h
neostigmine methylsulfate (Prostigmin)	A: 15 mg t.i.d.; gradually increase to maintenance dose of 150 mg; *max:* 375 mg/d A: IM/IV: 0.5-2.5 mg q1-3h; *max:* 10 mg/d C: IM/IV: 0.01-0.04 mg/kg q2-4h	To increase muscle strength in myasthenia gravis; short-acting. Used also to prevent or treat postoperative urinary retention. Pregnancy category: C; PB: 15%-25%; $t_{1/2}$: 1-1.5 h
physostigmine salicylate (Antilirium); (Isopto Eserine Salicylate-ophthalmic form)	A: IV/IM: 0.5-2 mg/dose, repeat q10-30min PRN; C: IV: 0.02 mg/kg/dose, repeat q5-10 min PRN; *max:* 2 mg total A: 0.25% to 0.5%, 1-2 gtt daily or q.i.d.; max: 8 gtt/d	To reverse anticholinergic toxicity and to reduce IOP, miosis; short-acting. Pregnancy category: C; PB: UK; $t_{1/2}$: 15-40 min
pyridostigmine bromide (Mestinon)	A: PO: 60-120 mg t.i.d./q.i.d.; maint: 600 mg/d in 3-4 divided doses; SR: 180-540 mg daily or b.i.d. IM/IV: 2 mg q2-3h C: PO: 7 mg/kg/d in 5-6 divided doses	To increase muscle strength in myasthenia gravis. Prevents destruction of the neurotransmitter acetylcholine. Pregnancy category: C; PB: 10%; $t_{1/2}$: 3-4 h
Antidote for Irreversible and Reversible Cholinesterase Inhibitors		
pralidoxime Cl (Protopam)	A: IV: 1-2 g in 100 mL of saline solution infused over 15-30 min; follow with 250 mg q5min PRN	To treat overdose of a cholinesterase inhibitor for myasthenia gravis and to treat overdose of organophosphate pesticides that cause muscle paralysis. Pregnancy category: C; PB: UK; $t_{1/2}$: 1-2.7 h

A, Adult; *a.c.,* before meals; *b.i.d.,* two times a day; *C,* child; *d,* day; *GERD,* gastroesophageal reflux disease; *GI,* gastrointestinal; *gt,* drop; *gtt,* drops; *h,* hour; *IM,* intramuscular; *IOP,* intraocular pressure; *IV,* intravenous; *maint,* maintenance; *PB,* protein-binding; *p.c.,* after meals; *PO,* by mouth; *PRN,* as needed; *q.i.d.,* four times a day; *sec,* second; *SR,* sustained-release; $t_{1/2}$, half-life; *t.i.d.,* three times a day; *UK,* unknown; >, greater than; <, less than.

anticholinergics include decreased bladder contraction, which can result in urinary retention, and decreased rigidity and tremors related to neuromuscular excitement. An anticholinergic can act as an antidote to the toxicity caused by cholinesterase inhibitors and organophosphate ingestion. The various effects of anticholinergics are described in Table 19-3.

Muscarinic receptors are a type of *cholinergic receptor* involved in tissue and organ responses to anticholinergics, because anticholinergics inhibit the actions of acetylcholine by occupying these receptor sites. Figure 19-3 illustrates this action of anticholinergic drugs. Anticholinergic drugs may also block the effect of direct-acting parasympathomimetics such as bethanechol and pilocarpine and of indirect-acting parasympathomimetics such as physostigmine and neostigmine.

TABLE 19-3 EFFECTS OF ANTICHOLINERGIC DRUGS

BODY TISSUES	RESPONSES
Cardiovascular	Increases heart rate with large doses. Small doses can decrease heart rate.
Gastrointestinal (GI)	Relaxes smooth muscle tone of GI tract, decreasing GI motility and peristalsis. Decreases gastric and intestinal secretions.
Urinary tract	Relaxes bladder detrusor muscle and increases constriction of internal sphincter. Urinary retention can result.
Ocular	Dilates pupils (mydriasis) and paralyzes ciliary muscle (cycloplegia), causing a decrease in accommodation.
Glandular	Decreases salivation, perspiration, and bronchial secretions.
Bronchial	Dilates the bronchi, and decreases bronchial secretions.
Central nervous system	Decreases tremors and rigidity of muscles. Drowsiness, disorientation, and hallucinations can result from large doses.

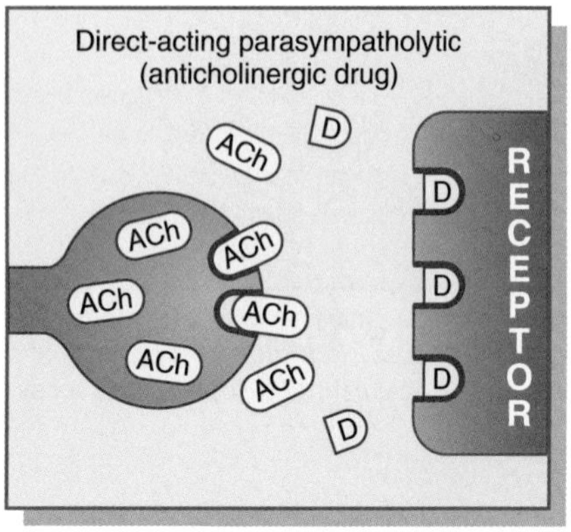

FIGURE 19–3 Anticholinergic response. The anticholinergic drug occupies the receptor sites, blocking acetylcholine. *ACh,* Acetylcholine; *D,* anticholinergic drug.

Atropine

Atropine sulfate, first derived from the belladonna plant *(Atropa belladonna)* and purified in 1831, is a classic anticholinergic, or muscarinic antagonist drug. Scopolamine was the second belladonna alkaloid produced. Atropine and scopolamine act on muscarinic receptors, but they have little effect on nicotinic receptors. Atropine is useful primarily (1) as a preoperative medication to decrease salivary secretions and (2) as an agent to increase heart rate when bradycardia is present. Atropine or auto-injector (Atropen) can also be used as an antidote for muscarinic agonist poisoning caused by an overdose of a cholinesterase inhibitor or a muscarinic drug such as bethanechol. However, if a patient takes atropine or an atropine-like drug (e.g., antihistamine), side effects can occur. Prototype Drug Chart 19-2 details the pharmacologic behavior of atropine.

Synthetic anticholinergic drugs are also used as antispasmodics to treat peptic ulcers and intestinal spasticity. One example is propantheline bromide (Pro-Banthine), which has been available for several decades. It decreases gastric secretions and GI spasms. Since the introduction of the histamine (H_2) blockers, anticholinergic agents such as propantheline are rarely used to decrease gastric secretions.

Pharmacokinetics Atropine sulfate is well absorbed orally and parenterally. It crosses the blood-brain barrier and exerts its effect on the central nervous system (CNS). The protein binding is unknown. It crosses the placenta. Atropine has a short half-life, so there is little cumulative effect. Most of the absorbed atropine is excreted in the urine (75% to 95%).

Pharmacodynamics Atropine sulfate blocks acetylcholine by occupying the muscarinic receptor. It increases the heart rate by blocking vagus stimulation and promotes dilation of the pupils by paralyzing the iris sphincter. The two most frequent uses of atropine are to decrease salivation and respiratory secretions preoperatively and to treat sinus bradycardia by increasing the heart rate. Atropine also is used ophthalmically for mydriasis and cycloplegia before eye exams and to treat inflammation of the iris (iritis) and uveal tract.

Its onset of action orally is between 0.5 to 1 hour and peaks at 1 hour. For the IM route, the onset of action is 10 to 30 minutes and peaks at 30 minutes. The duration for oral and IM routes is 4 hours; via the IV route, the onset of action is immediate and peak action is at 2 to 4 minutes.

Side Effects and Adverse Reactions

The common side effects of atropine and atropine-like drugs include dry mouth, decreased perspiration, blurred vision, tachycardia, constipation, and urinary retention. Other side effects and adverse reactions are nausea, headache, dry skin, abdominal distention, hypotension or hypertension, impotence, photophobia (intolerance of bright light), and coma.

Antiparkinson-Anticholinergic Drugs

At one time atropine was given to patients with Parkinson's disease to decrease salivation and drooling. It was also found to have some effect on the motor manifestation of this disease by decreasing tremors and rigidity. Additional studies indicate that anticholinergic (antimuscarinic) agents affect the CNS as well as the parasympathetic nervous system. These anticholinergic drugs affect the CNS by suppressing the

PROTOTYPE DRUG CHART 19-2

Atropine

Drug Class Anticholinergic: parasympatholytic Trade Name: Atropine Pregnancy Category: C	**Dosage** To treat bradycardia: A: IV: 0.5-1 mg, repeat q5min PRN up to 2 mg C: IV: 0.01-0.03 mg/kg/dose; *max:* 0.4 mg/dose Preoperatively: A: PO: 2 mg 30-60 min before anesthesia C >20 kg: IV/IM: 0.2-1 mg before anesthesia
Contraindications Narrow-angle glaucoma, obstructive GI disorders, paralytic ileus, ulcerative colitis, tachycardia, benign prostatic hypertrophy, myasthenia gravis, myocardial ischemia, hypersensitivity Caution: Renal or hepatic disorders, COPD, heart failure	**Drug-Lab-Food Interactions** Drug: Increases anticholinergic effect with phenothiazines, antihistamines, tricyclic antidepressants, amantadine, quinidine; high-dose anticholinergics may decrease effects of carbidopa/levodopa by delaying GI absorption; anticholinergics may enhance therapeutic effects at therapeutic doses.
Pharmacokinetics Absorption: PO/IM: Well absorbed Distribution: PB: UK; crosses the placenta Metabolism: $t\frac{1}{2}$: 2-3 h Excretion: 75% excreted in urine	**Pharmacodynamics** PO: Onset: 0.5-1 h Peak: 1 h Duration: 4 h IM: Onset: 10-30 min Peak: 0.5 h Duration: 4 h IV: Onset: Immediate Peak: 5 min Duration: UK Instill: Onset: 20-30 min Peak: 30-40 min Duration: days
Therapeutic Effects/Uses Preoperative medication to reduce salivation, to increase heart rate for bradycardia, and to dilate pupils for ocular diagnostic exams Mode of Action: Inhibits acetylcholine by occupying the receptors; increases heart rate by blocking vagus stimulation; promotes pupil dilation by blocking iris sphincter muscle	
Side Effects Dry mouth, nausea, headache, constipation, dry skin, flushing, mydriasis, blurred vision, anxiety, photophobia, palpitations, urinary retention	**Adverse Reactions** Tachycardia, hypotension Life-threatening: Ventricular fibrillation, Stevens-Johnson syndrome, coma

A, Adult; *C,* child; *COPD,* chronic obstructive pulmonary disease; *GI,* gastrointestinal; *h,* hour; *IM,* intramuscular; *instill,* instillation; *IV,* intravenous; *MAOI,* monoamine oxidase inhibitor; *min,* minute; *PB,* protein-binding; *PO,* by mouth; *PRN,* as needed; $t\frac{1}{2}$, half-life; *UK,* unknown; >, greater than.

tremors and muscular rigidity of parkinsonism, but they have little effect on mobility and muscle weakness. As a result of these findings, several anticholinergic drugs were developed for the treatment of Parkinson's disease (e.g., trihexyphenidyl hydrochloride [Artane], biperiden [Akineton], and benztropine [Cogentin]). These drugs can be used alone in early stages of parkinsonism. They may be used in combination with levodopa/carbidopa to control parkinsonism or used alone to treat pseudoparkinsonism, which results from the side effects of the phenothiazines in antipsychotic drugs. Drugs used to treat parkinsonism are described in more detail in Chapter 23. Prototype Drug Chart 19-3 lists the drug data related to benztropine (Cogentin), which is used for parkinsonism.

Pharmacokinetics Benztropine is well absorbed from the GI tract. Its protein-binding percentage and half-life are unknown. It is excreted in the urine.

Pharmacodynamics Benztropine decreases involuntary movement and diminishes the signs and symptoms of tremors and muscle rigidity that occur with Parkinson's disease and pseudoparkinsonism. It is available as an oral tablet and as parenteral intramuscular and intravenous injections. Alcohol and other CNS depressants potentiate sedation. Anticholinergics, phenothiazines, and tricyclic antidepressants may increase the anticholinergic effects of benztropine. The side effects are similar to other anticholinergic drugs.

Nursing Process
Patient-Centered Collaborative Care

Anticholinergic Drugs: Atropine

Assessment

- Obtain baseline vital signs for future comparison. Tachycardia is a side effect that occurs with large doses of anticholinergics such as atropine sulfate.

PROTOTYPE DRUG CHART 19-3

Benztropine

Drug Class	Dosage
Antiparkinson: anticholinergic agent Trade Names: Cogentin Pregnancy Category: C	Parkinsonism: A: PO: 0.5-6 mg/d h.s.; *max:* 8 mg/d Extrapyramidal symptoms except tardive dyskinesia (drug induced) A: PO: 1-4 mg q.d./b.i.d.
Contraindications	**Drug-Lab-Food Interactions**
Closed-angle glaucoma, tardive dyskinesia, psychosis, dementia, myasthenia gravis Caution: Tachycardia, cardiac disease, autonomic neuropathy, benign prostatic hypertrophy, children younger than 3 years of age	Drug: Increases anticholinergic effect with phenothiazines, tricyclic antidepressants, and other anticholinergics
Pharmacokinetics	**Pharmacodynamics**
Absorption: PO: Well absorbed Distribution: PB: UK Metabolism: $t\frac{1}{2}$: UK Excretion: In urine	PO: Onset: 1 h Peak: 2-3 h Duration: 6-10 h
Therapeutic Effects/Uses	
To decrease involuntary symptoms of parkinsonism or drug-induced parkinsonism Mode of Action: Blocks cholinergic (muscarinic) receptors, thus decreasing acetylcholine to reduce excess cholinergic activity (involuntary movements). Also, blocks dopamine reuptake to prolong dopamine effects and decrease involuntary movement.	
Side Effects	**Adverse Reactions**
Nausea, vomiting, dry mouth, constipation, restlessness, flushing, dizziness, blurred vision, photophobia, pupil dilation, amnesia, confusion, depression, hallucinations, anhidrosis (decreased sweating), weakness, hyperthermia, paresthesia	Tachycardia, palpitations, urinary retention Life-threatening: Paralytic ileus

A, Adult; *b.i.d.*, two times a day; *d*, day; *GI*, gastrointestinal; *h*, hour; *IM*, intramuscular; *IV*, intravenous; *min*, minute; *PB*, protein-binding; *PO*, by mouth; *q.d.*, once daily; $t\frac{1}{2}$, half-life; *UK*, unknown.

- Assess urine output. Urinary retention may occur.
- Check patient's medical history. Atropine and atropine-like drugs are contraindicated if patient has narrow-angle glaucoma, obstructive GI disorder, paralytic ileus, ulcerative colitis, benign prostatic hypertrophy, or myasthenia gravis.
- Obtain patient's drug history. Phenothiazines and antidepressants increase the effect of anticholinergics.

Nursing Diagnoses

- Impaired urinary elimination related to urinary retention
- Impaired oral mucous membranes related to decreased oral secretions
- Risk for injury related to acute confusion
- Risk for constipation related to decreased peristalsis secondary to atropine side effects.

Planning

- Patient's secretions will be decreased before surgery.
- Patient will not have side effects that may become a health problem.

Nursing Interventions

- Monitor patient's vital signs. Report if tachycardia occurs.
- Determine fluid intake and output. Encourage patient to void before taking the medication. Report decreased urine output. Anticholinergics can cause urinary retention. Maintain adequate fluid intake.
- Assess bowel sounds. Absence of bowel sounds may indicate paralytic ileus resulting from a decrease in GI motility (peristalsis).
- Examine for constipation caused by decrease in GI motility. Encourage patient to ingest foods that are high in fiber, to drink adequate amounts of fluids, and to exercise if able.
- Use bed alarms for patients who are confused and debilitated. Atropine could cause central nervous system stimulation (excitement, confusion) or drowsiness.
- Provide mouth care. Atropine decreases oral secretions and can cause dryness.
- Administer IV atropine undiluted or prefer diluted in 10 mL of sterile water. Rate of administration is 1 mg or fraction thereof/min.

Patient Teaching

General

- Direct patient to avoid hot environments and excess physical exertion. Elevations in body temperature can result from diminished sweat gland activity.
- Teach patient with narrow-angle glaucoma to avoid atropine-like drugs. Anticholinergics cause mydriasis and increase intraocular pressure. Instruct patient to check labels on over-the-counter (OTC) drugs to determine whether they are contraindicated for glaucoma.
- Instruct patient not to drive a motor vehicle or participate in activities that require alertness. Drowsiness is common.
- Tell patient with mydriasis following an eye examination to use sunglasses in bright light because of photophobia.

Side Effects

- Advise patient of common side effects such as dry mouth, decrease in urination, and constipation that occur as a result of anticholinergic use.
- Direct patient to increase fluid intake and consumption of high-fiber foods to prevent constipation when taking anticholinergics for a prolonged period.
- Instruct patient to urinate before taking the anticholinergic. Urinary retention can be a problem.
- Advise patient to report a marked decrease in urine output.
- Suggest that patient use hard candy, ice chips, or chewing gum. Maintain effective oral hygiene if patient's mouth is dry. Anticholinergics decrease salivation.
- Encourage patient to use eye drops to moisten dry eyes that result from decreased lacrimation (tearing).

Cultural Considerations

- Obtain an interpreter when necessary. Do not rely on family members, who may not fully disclose because of honor, guilt, or lack of understanding of medical terminology.
- Ask open-ended questions, and have patients demonstrate rather than verbalize their understanding of treatments. Because politeness may prevail, do not assume that a positive response means a definite yes.

Evaluation

- Evaluate patient's response to the anticholinergic.
- Determine whether constipation, urinary retention, or increased pulse rate is or remains a problem.

PROTOTYPE DRUG CHART 19-4

Tolterodine Tartrate

Drug Class Antimuscarinic agent: anticholinergic Trade Names: Detrol, Detrol LA Pregnancy Category: C	**Dosage** A: PO: 2 mg b.i.d. or 4 mg/day SR
Contraindications Hypersensitivity, urinary retention, gastric retention, uncontrolled narrow-angle glaucoma, lactation Caution: Controlled narrow-angle glaucoma, cardiovascular disease, urinary bladder outflow obstruction, pyloric stenosis or other GI obstructive disorders, paralytic ileus, ulcerative colitis, renal or hepatic dysfunction	**Drug-Lab-Food Interactions** Drug: Increased effects with amantadine, amoxapine, bupropion, clozapine, cyclobenzaprine, disopyramide, maprotiline, olanzapine, orphenadrine, H_1 blockers, phenothiazines, and tricyclic antidepressants; decreased effects with azole antifungals (e.g., ketoconazole) or macrolide antibiotics (e.g., erythromycin), cyclosporine, and fluoxetine Food: Grapefruit juice may increase drug levels
Pharmacokinetics Absorption: GI absorption decreased with food Distribution: PB: 96% Metabolism: $t\frac{1}{2}$: 2-4 h Excretion: Urine and feces	**Pharmacodynamics** PO: Onset: UK Peak: 1-2 h Duration: UK
Therapeutic Effects/Uses To decrease urinary frequency, urgency, and incontinence Mode of Action: Blocks cholinergic (muscarinic) receptors selectively in urinary bladder	
Side Effects Dry mouth, eyes, and skin; headache, dizziness, vertigo, nervousness, nausea, vomiting, diarrhea, abdominal pain, constipation, dyspepsia, flatulence, dysuria, weight gain, arthralgia, urinary retention	**Adverse Reactions** Bronchitis, visual abnormalities, chest pain, hypertension

A, Adult; *b.i.d.,* two times a day; *GI,* gastrointestinal; *H1,* histamine 1; *h,* hour; *PB,* protein binding; *PO,* by mouth; *SR,* sustained-release; $t\frac{1}{2}$, half-life; *UK,* unknown; *URI,* upper respiratory tract infection; *UTI,* urinary tract infection.

TABLE 19-4 ANTICHOLINERGICS

GENERIC (BRAND)	ROUTE AND DOSAGE	USES AND CONSIDERATIONS
Anticholinergics: Gastrointestinal or Cholinergic Blockers		
atropine sulfate	See Prototype Drug Chart 19-2.	
dicyclomine HCl (Bentyl)	A: PO: 20-40 mg q.i.d.; *max:* 160 mg/d IM: 10-20 mg q6h; *max:* 80 mg/d C >2 y: PO: 10 mg t.i.d./q.i.d.; *max:* 40 mg/d	Treatment of IBS. Avoid use in patients with narrow-angle glaucoma, severe ulcerative colitis, and paralytic ileus. Pregnancy category: B; PB: UK; t½: 9-10 h
glycopyrrolate (Robinul)	GI disorders: A: PO: 1-2 mg b.i.d./t.i.d.; *max:* 6 mg/d IM/IV: 0.1-0.2 mg t.i.d./q.i.d. Preoperative: A: IM: 4 mcg/kg 30 min-1 h before surgery	Presurgery to reduce secretions and for peptic ulcer. Contraindicated in patients with narrow-angle glaucoma, obstructive GI tract, and ulcerative colitis. Pregnancy category: B; PB: UK; t½: 0.5-2 h
hyoscyamine SO_4 (Cystospaz, Anaspaz)	A: PO/SL: 0.125-0.25 mg q4h PRN SR: 0.375-0.75 mg/q12h subQ/IM/IV: 5 mcg/kg 30-60 min preop C: 2-10 y: 0.0625-0.125 mg q4h PRN	Treatment of peptic ulcer and IBS. Controls gastric secretion and spastic bladder. Contraindicated in patients with narrow-angle glaucoma and severe ulcerative colitis. Pregnancy category: C; PB: 50%-60%; t½: 3.5 h
methscopolamine bromide (Pamine)	A: PO: 2.5-5 mg a.c. and h.s.; *max:* 12.5 mg/d	Has been used in treatment of peptic ulcer, IBS. Now used to relieve allergic rhinitis, sinusitis, and common cold. Avoid use in patients with prostatic hypertrophy and ileus. Pregnancy category: C; PB: UK; t½: UK
propantheline bromide (Pro-Banthine)	A: PO: 15 mg a.c. t.i.d.; 30 mg h.s. Older adults: 7.5 mg a.c. t.i.d.	Antispasmodic for peptic ulcer. Contraindicated in glaucoma, myasthenia gravis, and prostatic hypertrophy. Pregnancy category: C; PB: UK; t½: 9 h
scopolamine (Transderm Scōp)	Preoperative: subQ/IM/IV: 0.3-0.6 mg C: subQ: 0.1-0.3 mg; Motion sickness: A: PO: 250-800 mcg 1 h before needed; transdermal patch: 1.5 mg patch behind ear q72h	For preanesthetic drug, IBS, motion sickness, and delirium. Contraindicated in patients with narrow-angle glaucoma, obstructive GI disease, severe ulcerative colitis, and paralytic ileus. Pregnancy category: C; PB: 30%; t½: 8 h
Cholinergic Antagonists: Eye		
cyclopentolate HCl (Cyclogyl)	0.5%-2% sol, 1-2 gtt	For mydriasis and cycloplegia for eye examination. See Chapter 49.
homatropine (Isopto Homatropine)	2%-5% sol, 1-2 gtt	For mydriasis and cycloplegia (paralysis of ciliary muscle resulting in loss of accommodation) for eye examination. See Chapter 49.
tropicamide (Mydriacyl Ophthalmic)	0.5%-1% sol, 1-2 gtt	For mydriasis and cycloplegia for eye examination. See Chapter 49.
Anticholinergic-Antiparkinson Drugs		
benztropine mesylate (Cogentin)	See Prototype Drug Chart 19-3.	
biperiden lactate (Akineton)	Parkinsonism: A: PO: 2 mg t.i.d./q.i.d.; *max:* 16 mg/d	Treatment of parkinsonism and drug-induced extrapyramidal syndrome. Pregnancy category: C; PB: UK; t½: 6-10 h; See Chapter 23.
trihexyphenidyl HCl (Artane)	Parkinsonism: A: PO: 1 mg initially, increase to 6-10 mg/d, usually t.i.d with meals and h.s. A: PO: Extended-release: 5-10 mg after breakfast Drug-induced extrapyramidal syndrome: A: PO: 1 mg/d, increase to 5-15 mg/d in divided doses	Treatment of parkinsonism and drug-induced extrapyramidal syndrome. Pregnancy category: C; PB: UK; t½: UK; see Chapter 23.
Anticholinergic–Antimuscarinic Drugs		
tolterodine tartrate (Detrol, Detrol LA)	See Prototype Drug Chart 19-4.	
Others		
ipratropium bromide (Atrovent)	A: Inhal: 2 inhal q.i.d.; *max:* 12 inhal/d	Anticholinergic bronchodilator to treat chronic obstructive pulmonary disease by blocking action of acetylcholine at bronchial smooth muscle sites, promoting bronchodilation. Pregnancy category: B; PB: UK; t½: 2 h. See Chapter 41.

A, Adult; *a.c.,* before meals; *b.i.d.,* two times a day; *C,* child; *d,* day; *EPR,* extrapyramidal reaction; *GI,* gastrointestinal; *gtt,* drops; *h,* hour; *h.s. at bedtime, IBS,* irritable bowel syndrome; *IM,* intramuscular; *inhal,* inhalation; *IV,* intravenous; *maint,* maintenance; *min,* minute; *PB,* protein-binding; *p.c.,* after meals; *PO,* by mouth; *PRN,* as needed; *q.d.,* once daily; *q.i.d.,* four times a day; *subQ,* subcutaneous; *SL,* sublingual; *sol,* solution; *SR,* sustained-release; *t½,* half life; *t.i.d.,* three times a day; *UK,* unknown; >, greater than; <, less than.

Anticholinergics for Treating Motion Sickness

The effects of anticholinergics on the CNS benefit patients who are prone to motion sickness. An example of such an anticholinergic, classified as an antihistamine for motion sickness, is scopolamine. It is available topically as a skin patch (Transderm Scōp) that is placed behind the ear. Prevention of motion sickness is also provided via wrist bands and ginger, including ginger gum or candy. Transdermal scopolamine is delivered over 3 days and is frequently prescribed for activities such as flying, cruising on the water, and bus or automobile trips. Other drugs classified as antihistamines for motion sickness are dimenhydrinate (Dramamine), cyclizine (Marzine), and meclizine hydrochloride (Antivert). Most of these drugs can be purchased OTC, with the exception of Transderm Scōp.

Examples of anticholinergic drugs and their dosages and common uses are found in Table 19-4. Dosages may vary according to age, sex, and weight. Because anticholinergic drugs can increase intraocular pressure, they should not be administered to patients diagnosed with glaucoma (Prototype Drug Chart 19-4).

Side Effects and Adverse Reactions

Side effects of antihistamines used as anticholinergics include dry mouth, visual disturbances (especially blurred vision resulting from pupillary dilation), constipation secondary to decreased GI peristalsis, urinary retention related to decreased bladder tone, tachycardia (when taken in large doses), hypotension, skin rash, muscle weakness, and flushing.

KEY WEBSITES

Anticholinergics: *www.cnsonline.org/www/archive/ms/ms-6c.html*

Beers Criteria Guidelines: *www.americangeriatrics.org/health_care_professionals/clinical_practice/clinical_guidelines_recommendations/2012*

Cholinergics: *www.cnsonline.org/www/archive/ms/ms-6a.html*

CRITICAL THINKING CASE STUDY

JS, a 56-year-old man, is scheduled for surgery to remove gallstones. He has been in good health, and his only other clinical problem is glaucoma. Preoperative medications, meperidine 75 mg and atropine sulfate 0.4 mg, were given intramuscularly 1 hour before surgery.

1. What are the advantages of giving atropine sulfate before surgery?
2. What are some contraindications of atropine sulfate?
3. If this patient received an atropine-like drug for several months, what assessments should be made related to its effects?
4. How does atropine sulfate differ from bethanechol chloride?

   This patient receives ophthalmic pilocarpine drops to control glaucoma.
5. How does pilocarpine differ from physostigmine? Explain your answer.
6. What patient teaching should the nurse include related to the use of pilocarpine?

NCLEX STUDY QUESTIONS

1. A patient is receiving bethanechol (Urecholine). The nurse realizes that the action of this drug is to treat which condition?
   a. Glaucoma
   b. Urinary retention
   c. Delayed gastric emptying
   d. Gastroesophageal reflux disease
2. The nurse teaches the patient receiving atropine (Atreza) to expect which side effect?
   a. Diarrhea
   b. Bradycardia
   c. Blurred vision
   d. Frequent urination
3. When benztropine (Cogentin) is ordered for a patient, the nurse acknowledges that this drug is an effective treatment for which condition?
   a. Parkinsonism
   b. Paralytic ileus
   c. Motion sickness
   d. Urinary retention
4. Dicyclomine (Bentyl) is an anticholinergic, which the nurse realizes is given to treat which condition?
   a. Mydriasis
   b. Constipation
   c. Urinary retention
   d. Irritable bowel syndrome

5. The nurse realizes that cholinergic agonists mimic which parasympathetic neurotransmitter?
   a. dopamine
   b. acetylcholine
   c. cholinesterase
   d. monoamine oxidase
6. The nurse is administering bethanechol (Urecholine), a cholinergic agonist, and should know that the expected cholinergic effects include which of the following?
   a. Increased heart rate
   b. Decreased peristalsis
   c. Decreased salivation
   d. Increased pupil constriction
7. When a patient has a cholinergic overdose from excessive dosing of bethanechol (Urecholine), the nurse anticipates administration of which drug as the antidote?
   a. atropine
   b. tolterodine
   c. benztropine
   d. metoclopramide

Answers: 1, b; 2, c; 3, a; 4, d; 5, b; 6, d; 7, a.

UNIT VI

Neurologic and Neuromuscular Agents

The nervous system is composed of all nerve tissues: brain, spinal cord, nerves, and ganglia. The purpose of the nervous system is to receive stimuli and transmit information to nerve centers for an appropriate response. There are two types of nervous system: the central nervous system and the peripheral nervous system.

The central nervous system (CNS), composed of the brain and spinal cord, regulates body functions (Figure VI-1). The CNS interprets information sent by impulses from the peripheral nervous system (PNS) and returns the instruction through the PNS for appropriate cellular actions. Stimulation of the CNS may either increase nerve cell (neuron) activity or block nerve cell activity.

The PNS consists of two divisions: the somatic nervous system (SNS) and the autonomic nervous system (ANS). The SNS is voluntary and acts on skeletal muscles to produce locomotion and respiration. The ANS, also called the visceral system, is involuntary and controls and regulates the functioning of the heart, respiratory system, gastrointestinal system, and glands. The ANS, a large nervous system that functions without our conscious control, has two subdivisions: the sympathetic and the parasympathetic nervous systems.

The sympathetic nervous system of the ANS is called the adrenergic system because its neurotransmitter is norepinephrine. The parasympathetic nervous system is called the cholinergic system because its neurotransmitter is acetylcholine. Because organs are innervated by both the sympathetic and the parasympathetic systems, they can produce opposite responses. The sympathetic response is excitability, and the parasympathetic response is inhibition.

The sympathetic and the parasympathetic nerve pathways originate from different locations in the spinal cord. These nervous systems send information by two types of nerve fibers, the preganglionic and the postganglionic, and by the ganglion between these fibers (Figure VI-2). The preganglionic nerve fiber carries messages from the CNS to the ganglion, and the postganglionic fiber transmits impulses from the ganglion to body tissues and organs.

The sympathetic nervous system is also called the thoracolumbar division of the ANS, because the preganglionic fibers originate from the thoracic (T1 to T12) and the upper lumbar (L1 and L2) segments of the spinal cord. The sympathetic preganglionic fibers are short from the spinal cord to the ganglion, and the sympathetic postganglionic fibers are long from the ganglion to the body cells. Figure VI-3 illustrates the sympathetic preganglionic fibers from the spinal cord.

The parasympathetic nervous system is called the craniosacral division of the ANS, because the preganglionic fibers

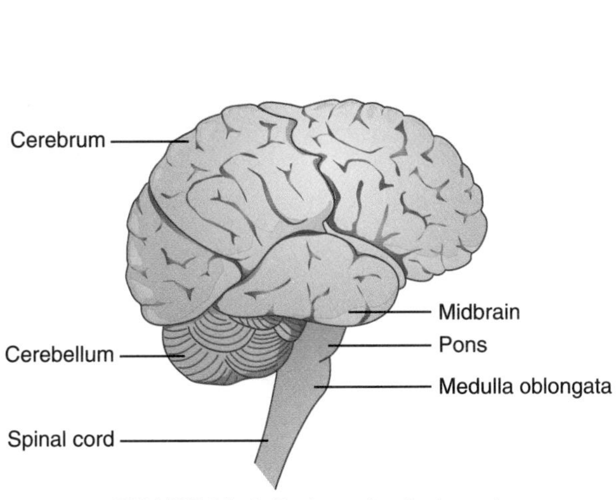

FIGURE VI–1 Brain and spinal cord.

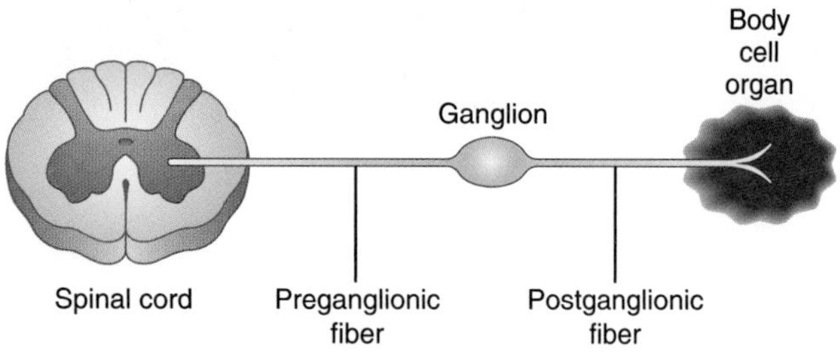

FIGURE VI–2 Preganglionic and postganglionic nerve fibers.

originate with cranial nerves III, VII, IX, and X from the brainstem and sacral segments S2, S3, and S4 of the spinal cord. The parasympathetic preganglionic fibers are long from the spinal cord to the ganglion, and the parasympathetic postganglionic fibers are short from the ganglion to the body cells. Figure VI-4 illustrates the parasympathetic preganglionic fibers from the spinal cord.

Drugs that stimulate and depress the CNS are discussed in Chapter 20, Central Nervous System Stimulants, and Chapter 21, Central Nervous System Depressants. Drugs used to control convulsions (Chapter 22, Anticonvulsants) are considered CNS depressants. Drugs used to treat neuromuscular disorders, such as parkinsonism, myasthenia gravis, multiple sclerosis, and Alzheimer's disease, have varying effects on the nervous system and muscles (Chapter 23, Drugs for Neurologic Disorders: Parkinsonism and Alzheimer's Disease; and Chapter 24, Drugs for Neuromuscular Disorders: Myasthenia Gravis, Multiple Sclerosis, and Muscle Spasms).

Figure VI-5 shows a schematic breakdown of the nervous systems in the body.

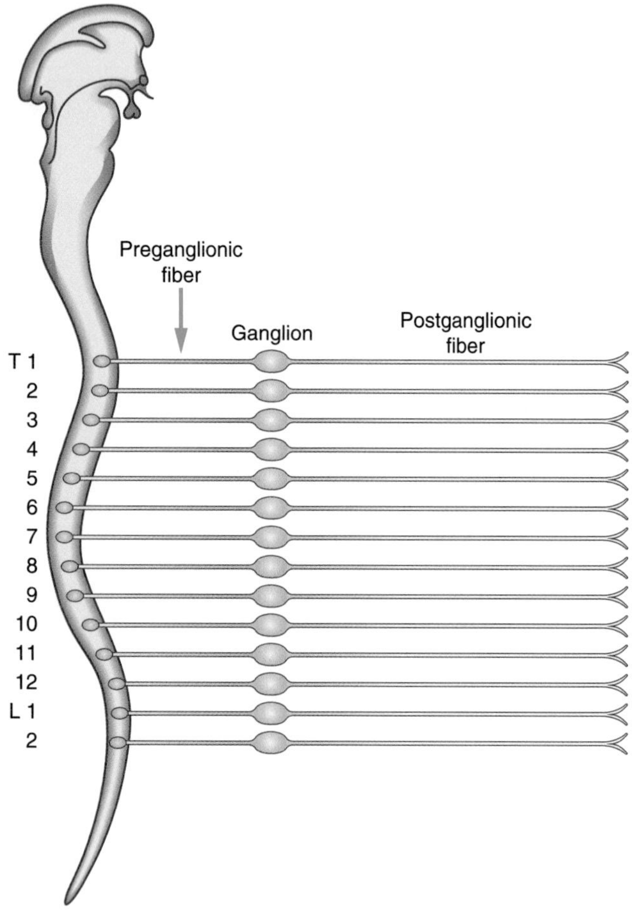

FIGURE VI–3 Sympathetic nerve fibers.

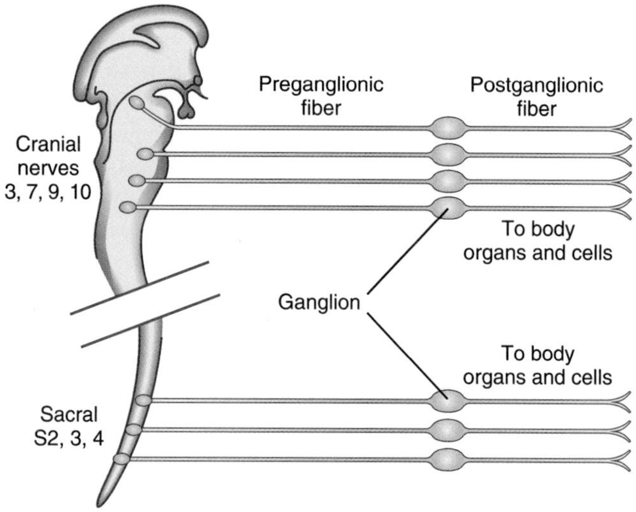

FIGURE VI–4 Parasympathetic nerve fibers.

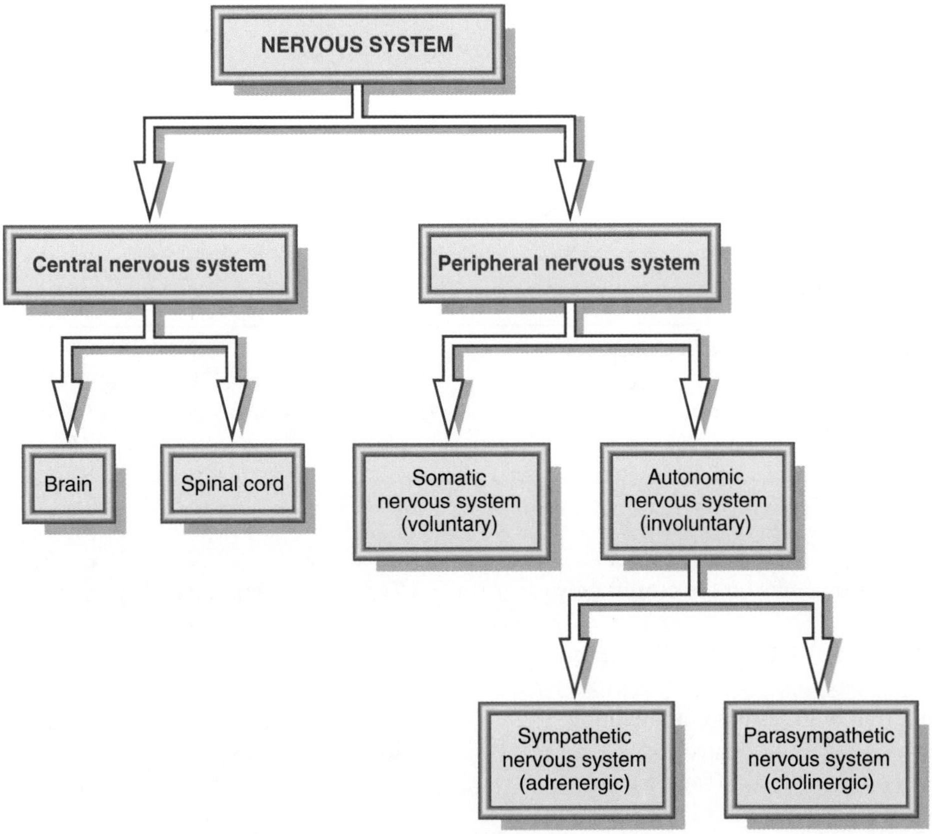

FIGURE VI–5 The body's nervous system.

CHAPTER

20

Central Nervous System Stimulants

evolve WEBSITE

http://evolve.elsevier.com/KeeHayes/pharmacology/

- Animations
- Content Updates
- Key Points
- Review Questions for the NCLEX® Examination
- References from the Textbook
- Unfolding Case Studies

OBJECTIVES

- Explain the effects of stimulants on the central nervous system (CNS).
- Compare attention deficit/hyperactivity disorder and narcolepsy.
- Differentiate the action of drugs used for attention deficit/hyperactivity disorder and narcolepsy.
- Contrast the common side effects of amphetamines, anorexiants, analeptics, doxapram, and caffeine.
- Compare the pharmacology of drugs used in the treatment of migraine headaches.
- Apply the nursing process for the patient taking CNS stimulants.
- Apply the nursing process for the patient taking doxapram (Dopram).

OUTLINE

KEY TERMS

Numerous drugs can stimulate the **central nervous system (CNS),** which involves the brain and spinal cord that regulates body functions. Medically approved use of CNS stimulants is limited to the treatment of attention deficit/hyperactivity disorder (ADHD) in children, narcolepsy, and the reversal of respiratory distress. The major group of CNS stimulants includes amphetamines and caffeine, which stimulate the cerebral cortex of the brain; analeptics and caffeine, which act on the brainstem and medulla to stimulate respiration; and anorexiants such as diethylpropion, which are thought to suppress appetite by stimulating the satiety center in the hypothalamic and limbic areas of the brain. Amphetamines and related anorexiants are greatly abused. Long-term use of amphetamines can produce psychological **dependence** or **tolerance**, a condition in which larger and larger doses of a drug are needed to reproduce the initial response. These medications are recommended for short-term use only (up to 12 weeks). Gradually increasing a drug dose and then abruptly stopping the drug may result in depression and withdrawal symptoms.

Drugs used to treat migraine and cluster headaches include analgesics, ergot alkaloids, and selective serotonin$_1$ receptor agonists (triptans). **Migraine headaches** generally cause severe throbbing pain. They are often preceded by an aura (visual, smells, tingling, vertigo warning). The cause is not definitive but is thought to be due to changes in the brainstem, which activates the trigeminal nerve. Low serotonin levels may also be involved by triggering the trigeminal system to release neuropeptides, which cause pain. Triggering factors for migraines include certain foods (beer, red wine, aged cheese, chocolate, caffeine, monosodium glutamate), skipping meals, intense physical exertion, female hormonal changes, bright lights, stress, weather changes, and certain medications (oral contraceptives, vasodilators). The cause of **cluster headaches** is unknown, but they are generally considered to be caused by the hypothalamus activating the trigeminal nerve. These headaches recur 1 to 3 times per day in a period lasting from approximately 2 weeks to 3 months. Cluster headaches do not typically have triggers, but once a cluster headache begins, alcohol, nicotine, and nitroglycerin immediately lead to a severe headache.

PATHOPHYSIOLOGY

Attention deficit/hyperactivity disorder (ADHD) might be caused by a dysregulation of the transmitters serotonin, norepinephrine, and dopamine. ADHD occurs primarily in children, usually before the age of 7 years, and may continue through the teenage years. In some cases, it may not be identified until early adulthood. The incidence of ADHD is three to seven times more common in boys than in girls. Characteristic behaviors of the various types of ADHD include inattentiveness, inability to concentrate, restlessness (fidgety), hyperactivity (excessive and purposeless activity), inability to complete tasks, and impulsivity.

The child with ADHD may display poor coordination, and there may be abnormal electroencephalographic (EEG) findings. Intelligence is usually not affected, but learning disabilities are often present. This disorder has also been called *minimal brain dysfunction, hyperactivity in children, hyperkinesis,* and *hyperkinetic syndrome with learning disorder.* Some professionals state that ADHD is often incorrectly diagnosed, resulting in many children receiving unnecessary treatment for months or years.

Narcolepsy is characterized by falling asleep during normal waking activities such as driving a car or talking with someone. Sleep paralysis, the condition of muscle paralysis that is normal during sleep, usually accompanies narcolepsy and affects the voluntary muscles. The narcoleptic is unable to move and may collapse.

AMPHETAMINES

Amphetamines stimulate the release of **neurotransmitters**—norepinephrine and dopamine—from the brain and sympathetic nervous system (peripheral nerve terminals). Amphetamines ordinarily cause euphoria and alertness, but they can also cause sleeplessness, restlessness, tremors, and irritability. Cardiovascular problems such as increased heart rate, palpitations, cardiac dysrhythmias, and increased blood pressure can result from continuous use of amphetamines.

The half-life of amphetamines varies from 4 to 30 hours. Amphetamines are prescribed for narcolepsy and in some cases for ADHD, when amphetamine-like drugs are ineffective. Amphetamine (Adderall) has been effective for controlling ADHD. Dextroamphetamine (Dexedrine) and methamphetamine (Desoxyn) may also be prescribed for some ADHD patients.

Side Effects and Adverse Reactions

Amphetamines can cause adverse effects in the central nervous system and the cardiovascular, gastrointestinal (GI), and endocrine systems. Side effects and adverse reactions include restlessness, insomnia, tachycardia, hypertension, heart palpitations, dry mouth, anorexia, weight loss, diarrhea, constipation, and impotence.

Amphetamine-Like Drugs for ADHD and Narcolepsy

Methylphenidate (Ritalin) and dexmethylphenidate (Focalin), classed as amphetamine-like drugs, are given to increase a child's attention span and cognitive performance (e.g., memory, reading) and to decrease impulsiveness, hyperactivity, and restlessness. Methylphenidate is also used to treat narcolepsy. There may be potential abuse of methylphenidate; thus it is classified as a controlled-substance schedule (CSS) II drug. Prototype Drug Chart 20-1 illustrates the pharmacokinetics, pharmacodynamics, and therapeutic effects of methylphenidate in the treatment of ADHD and narcolepsy. Amphetamine and amphetamine-like drugs should not be taken in the evening or before bedtime, because insomnia may result.

Modafinil (Provigil) is another drug prescribed for narcolepsy. It increases the amount of time patients with narcolepsy feel awake. Its mechanism of action is not fully known.

Methylphenidate is the most frequently prescribed drug used to treat ADHD. Table 20-1 lists the amphetamines and amphetamine-like drugs and their dosages, uses, and considerations.

Pharmacokinetics Methylphenidate is well absorbed from the GI mucosa. Methylphenidate is usually administered to children twice a day before breakfast and lunch. Because food affects its absorption rate, this drug should be given 30 to 45 minutes before meals. Methylphenidate should be given 6 hours or more before sleep, because it may cause insomnia. Transdermal patches may be worn for 9 hours. This drug is excreted in the urine; 40% of methylphenidate is excreted unchanged.

Pharmacodynamics Methylphenidate helps to correct ADHD by decreasing hyperactivity and improving attention span. This drug may also be prescribed for treating narcolepsy. Amphetamine-like drugs are considered more effective in treating ADHD than amphetamines, except for Adderall. Amphetamines are generally avoided because they have a higher potential for abuse, habituation, and tolerance. Sympathomimetics (e.g., pseudoephedrine) and psychostimulants (e.g., caffeine) taken concurrently with methylphenidate increase stimulatory effects of irritability, nervousness, tremors, and insomnia. Concurrent MAO inhibitors may cause hypertensive crisis. Methylphenidate potentiates the action of CNS stimulants, such as caffeine, and inhibits the metabolism

PROTOTYPE DRUG CHART 20-1

Methylphenidate

Drug Class	Dosage
Amphetamine-like drug: CNS stimulant Trade Names: Ritalin, Ritalin SR, Concerta, Daytrana transdermal patch, Quillivant XR CSS II Pregnancy Category: C	Attention deficit/hyperactivity disorder (ADHD): C >6 y: PO: 5-10 mg before breakfast and lunch; if necessary, increase dosage weekly by 5-10 mg; *max:* 60 mg/d A: PO: 20-30 mg/d in divided doses before breakfast and lunch; *max:* 60 mg/d A: PO: Sustained-release: 18-36 mg once daily; *max:* 72 mg/d C: PO: Sustained-release: 18 mg/d; *max:* 2 mg/kg/d Narcolepsy: A: PO: 10-60 mg/d, in 2-3 divided doses 30 min before meals
Contraindications	**Drug-Lab-Food Interactions**
Hyperthyroidism, anxiety, history of seizures, coronary artery disease, hypertension, Tourette's syndrome, glaucoma, psychosis, mental depression Caution: Not to be used in children <6 y, depression, substance abuse, pregnancy	Drug: May increase stimulatory effects of sympathomimetics and psychostimulants; may reduce effect of antihypertensives Increases effects of oral anticoagulants, barbiturates, anticonvulsants, tricyclic antidepressants; increases hypertensive crisis with MAOIs Food: Caffeine may increase effects
Pharmacokinetics	**Pharmacodynamics**
Absorption: Well absorbed from GI tract Distribution: PB: 10%-33% Metabolism: t½: 1.3-7.7 h Excretion: 40% excreted unchanged in urine	PO: Onset: 0.5-1 h Peak: 2 h Sustained-release: 5 h; transdermal: 8 h Duration: 3-6 h; Sustained-release: 8 h Sustained-release: 4-8 h
Therapeutic Effects/Uses	
To correct hyperactivity caused by ADHD, increase attention span, and control narcolepsy Mode of Action: Research suggests modulation of serotonergic pathways by affecting changes in dopamine transport	
Side Effects	**Adverse Reactions**
Anorexia, vomiting, diarrhea, insomnia, dizziness, nervousness, restlessness, irritability, tremors, euphoria, blurred vision, headache, increased hyperactivity, abdominal pain, anemia, upper respiratory infection	Tachycardia, hypertension, growth suppression, palpitations, seizures, transient weight loss in children; life-threatening: Exfoliative dermatitis, stroke, thrombocytopenia, hepatotoxicity

A, Adult; *ADHD,* attention deficit/hyperactivity disorder; *C,* child; *CD,* controlled dose; *CNS,* central nervous system; *CSS,* Controlled Substances Schedule; *d,* day; *GI,* gastrointestinal; *h,* hour; *MAOI,* monoamine oxidase inhibitor; *min,* minute; *PB,* protein-binding; *PO,* by mouth; *t½,* half life; *UK,* unknown; *y,* year.

of some barbiturates, such as phenobarbital, leading to increased blood levels and potential toxicity.

Nursing Process
Patient-Centered Collaborative Care

Central Nervous System Stimulant: Methylphenidate HCl (Ritalin)

Assessment

- Determine whether patient has a history of heart disease, hypertension, hyperthyroidism, parkinsonism, or glaucoma; in such cases, the drug is usually contraindicated.
- Assess vital signs to be used for future comparisons. Closely monitor patients with cardiac disease, because the drug may reverse effects of antihypertensives.
- Assess patient's mental status (e.g., mood, affect, aggressiveness).
- Evaluate height, weight, and growth of children.
- Assess complete blood count (CBC), differential white blood cells (WBCs), and platelets before and during therapy.

Nursing Diagnoses

- Risk-prone health behavior (e.g., impulsiveness, short attention span, distractibility) that interferes with peer relationships, learning, and discipline related to hyperactivity adverse effect
- Interrupted family processes related to dysfunctional behavior
- Risk for delayed development related to treatment regimen
- Deficient knowledge related to inexperience with Ritalin drug regimen

TABLE 20-1 AMPHETAMINES AND AMPHETAMINE-LIKE DRUGS

GENERIC (BRAND NAME)	ROUTE AND DOSAGE	USES AND CONSIDERATIONS
Amphetamines		
amphetamine sulfate (Adderall, Adderall XR) CSS II	Narcolepsy: A: PO: 5-60 mg/d in divided doses; *max:* 60 mg/d C: 6-12 y: PO: 5 mg q.d. or b.i.d., increase 5 mg/d weekly until desired response ADHD: C: >12 y: 5 mg b.i.d., increase 10 mg/d weekly until desired response C: 6-12 y: PO: 2.5 mg/d, increase 5 mg/d weekly until desired response; *max:* 40 mg/d	For narcolepsy, ADHD. Dosage should be minimal to control symptoms in ADHD. CNS and cardiac toxicity may occur. Pregnancy category: C; PB: UK; $t_{1/2}$: 10 h
dextroamphetamine sulfate (Dexedrine) CSS II	ADHD: C: 3-5 y: PO: 2.5 mg/d or b.i.d. C: 6-12 y: PO: 5 mg/d or b.i.d., *max:* 40 mg/d	Uses similar to amphetamines. Has been used for weight loss and narcolepsy. May cause psychosis, aggression, and cardiac events. May cause sudden death in patients with structural cardiac abnormalities. Pregnancy category: C; PB: UK; $t_{1/2}$: 10-12 h
lisdexamfetamine dimesylate (Vyvanse) CSS II	ADHD: A/C: >12 y: PO: 30 mg/d in morning, may increase 10-20 mg/d weekly, *max:* 70 mg/d	For ADHD. May cause anorexia, insomnia, headache, and irritability. May cause psychosis, aggression, and cardiac events. May cause sudden death in patients with structural cardiac abnormalities. Pregnancy category: C; PB: UK; $t_{1/2}$: 10-12 h
Amphetamine-Like Drugs		
methylphenidate HCl (Ritalin) CSS II	See Prototype Drug Chart 20-1.	
modafinil (Provigil) CSS IV	A: PO: 200 mg/d in the morning Older adults: PO: 100 mg/d in the morning	For narcolepsy. Does not disrupt nighttime sleep. Common side effects include headache, nausea, diarrhea, and nervousness. Pregnancy category: C; PB: 60%; $t_{1/2}$: 15 h
dexmethylphenidate (Focalin)	Immediate-release A and C: >6 y: PO: 2.5 mg b.i.d.; increase 2.5-5 mg/d at weekly intervals; *max:* 20 mg/d Extended-release: A: PO: 10 mg/d, may increase 10 mg/wk; *max:* 40 mg/d C: >6: PO: 5 mg/d, may increase 5 mg/wk; *max:* 30 mg/d	For ADHD. May cause psychosis, aggression, and cardiac events. May cause sudden death in patients with structural cardiac abnormalities. Pregnancy category: C; PB: UK; $t_{1/2}$: 2.2 h
armodafinil (Nuvigil)	A and C: >16 y: PO: 150-250 mg q.d. in morning	For narcolepsy. Pregnancy category: C; PB: 60%; $t_{1/2}$: 15 h

A, Adult; *ADHD,* attention deficit/hyperactivity disorder; *C,* child; *CNS,* central nervous system; *CSS,* Controlled Substances Schedule; *d,* day; *h,* hour; *PB,* protein binding; *PO,* by mouth; $t_{1/2}$, half life; *UK,* unknown; *y,* year; >, greater than.

Planning

- Patient's hyperactivity will be decreased.
- Patient will increase attention span.
- Patient's blood pressure and heart rate will be within normal limits.
- Patient will behave in a calm manner.

Nursing Interventions

- Monitor vital signs. Report irregularities.
- Evaluate height, weight, and growth of children.
- Observe patient for withdrawal symptoms (e.g., nausea, vomiting, weakness, headache).
- Monitor patient for side effects (e.g., insomnia, restlessness, nervousness, tremors, irritability, tachycardia, elevated blood pressure). Report findings.

Patient Teaching

General

- Teach patient to take drug before meals.
- Advise patient to avoid alcohol consumption.
- Encourage use of sugarless gum to relieve dry mouth.
- Teach patient to monitor weight twice a week and report weight loss.
- Advise patient to avoid driving and using hazardous equipment when experiencing tremors, nervousness, or increased heart rate.
- Teach patient not to abruptly discontinue the drug; dose must be tapered off to avoid withdrawal symptoms. Consult health care provider before modifying dose.
- Encourage patient to read labels on over-the-counter (OTC) products, because many contain caffeine. A high plasma caffeine level could be fatal.

- Teach nursing mothers to avoid taking all CNS stimulants (e.g., caffeine). These drugs are excreted in breast milk and can cause hyperactivity or restlessness in infants.
- Direct family to seek counseling for children with attention deficit/hyperactivity disorder. Drug therapy alone is not an appropriate therapy program. Notify school nurse of drug therapy regimen.
- Explain to patient and family that long-term use may lead to drug abuse.

Diet
- Advise patient to avoid foods that contain caffeine.
- Encourage parents to provide children with a nutritious breakfast because the drug may have anorexic effects.

Side Effects
- Teach patient about drug side effects and the need to report tachycardia and palpitations. Monitor children for onset of Tourette's syndrome.

Cultural Considerations
- Decrease language barriers by decoding the jargon of the health care environment for those who have language difficulties or are not in the health care field.

Evaluation
- Evaluate effectiveness of drug therapy, level of hyperactivity, and presence of adverse effects.
- Monitor weight, sleep patterns, and mental status.
- Evaluate patient's knowledge of Ritalin therapy.

ANOREXIANTS, LIPASE INHIBITORS, ANALEPTICS, AND RESPIRATORY STIMULANTS

Anorexiants

Amphetamines were once freely prescribed as **anorexiants** (appetite suppressants) for short-term use (4 to 12 weeks), but because of tolerance, psychological dependence, and abuse, they are no longer recommended for use as appetite suppressants. The U.S. Food and Drug Administration (FDA) has ordered the removal of phenylpropanolamine from OTC weight-loss drugs and cold remedies. There is increased risk of hemorrhagic stroke in young women who take drugs containing phenylpropanolamine and a 16-times greater risk in women who take the drugs as appetite suppressants. (This drug has not been associated with an increased risk of stroke in men.) It has been suggested that phenylpropanolamine might also cause renal failure, psychosis, hypertension, and cardiac dysrhythmias. Topical use of the drug has not been associated with systemic effects. Most of the anorexiants used to suppress appetite (Table 20-2) do not have the serious side effects associated with amphetamines. For weight-loss attempts, emphasis should be placed on nutritious diet, exercise, and behavior modification. Reliance on appetite suppressants should be discouraged. Individuals who take anorexiants should be under the care of a health care provider.

Side Effects and Adverse Reactions

Children younger than 12 years should not be given anorexiants, and self-medication with anorexiants should be discouraged. Long-term use of these drugs frequently results in such severe side effects as nervousness, restlessness, irritability, insomnia, heart palpitations, and hypertension.

Lipase Inhibitors

Lipase inhibitors have replaced anorexiants as the drug of choice for weight loss. They decrease GI absorption of dietary fats. The fats are excreted in feces, leading to weight loss. Side effects from lipase inhibitors include oily spotting, fecal urgency and incontinence, steatorrhea, flatus with discharge, headache, nausea, vomiting, and abdominal cramping. Hypoglycemia may occur in diabetic patients.

Analeptics

Analeptics, which are CNS stimulants, mostly affect the brainstem and spinal cord but also affect the cerebral cortex. The primary use of an analeptic is to stimulate respiration. One subgroup of analeptics is the xanthines (methylxanthines), of which caffeine and theophylline are the main drugs. Depending on the dose, caffeine stimulates the CNS, and large doses stimulate respiration. Newborns with respiratory distress might be given caffeine to increase respiration. Theophylline is used mostly to relax the bronchioles; however, it has also been used to increase respiration in newborns. Refer to Chapter 41 for further discussion of theophylline. Table 20-2 lists the analeptics and their dosages, uses, and considerations.

Side Effects and Adverse Reactions

Side effects from caffeine are similar to those from anorexiants: nervousness, restlessness, tremors, twitching, palpitations, and insomnia. Other side effects include diuresis (increased urination), GI irritation (e.g., nausea, diarrhea), and, rarely, tinnitus (ringing in the ear). More than 300 mg of caffeine affects the CNS and heart (i.e., dysrhythmias, convulsions). High doses of caffeine in coffee, chocolate, and cold-relief medications can cause psychological dependence. The half-life of caffeine is approximately 5 hours; however, the half-life is prolonged in patients with liver disease and in patients who are taking oral contraceptives or are pregnant. Caffeine is contraindicated during pregnancy, because its effect on the fetus is unknown.

TABLE 20-2 ANOREXIANTS AND ANALEPTICS

DRUG	ROUTE AND DOSAGE	USES AND CONSIDERATIONS
Anorexiants		
benzphetamine HCl (Didrex) CSS III	A: PO: 25-50 mg daily to t.i.d; *max:* 150 mg/d	Short-term (8-12 wk) treatment for weight loss. Similar to amphetamines. Potential for abuse. Avoid during pregnancy. Pregnancy category: X; PB: UK, $t\frac{1}{2}$: 6-10 h
diethylpropion HCl (Tenuate) CSS IV	A: PO: 25 mg t.i.d. 30-60 min a.c. Sustained-release: 75 mg/d; *max:* 75 mg/d	For appetite suppression by stimulating the appetite control center in the hypothalamus. For short-term use. Pregnancy category: B; PB: UK; $t\frac{1}{2}$: 4-8 h
phentermine HCl (Suprenza) CSS IV	A/Adol: >16 y: PO: 15-37.5 mg/d in the morning	For short-term appetite suppression. Pregnancy category: X; PB: UK; $t\frac{1}{2}$: 19-24 h
phentermine-topiramate (Qsymia)	Extended-release: A: PO: 3.75/23 mg phentermine-topiramate q.d. for 14 d in the morning, then 7.5/46 mg/d; *max:* 15/92 mg	For short-term weight management when patient has at least one comorbid condition (hypertension, dyslipidemia, type 2 diabetes). May increase suicidal risk. Evaluate weight loss in 12 weeks. Pregnancy category: X; PB: 15%-41%; $t\frac{1}{2}$: 20-65 h
phendimetrazine (Bontril)	A: PO: 17.5-35 mg b.i.d. or t.i.d. 1 h a.c. Extended-release: A: PO: 105 mg/d 30-60 min a.c.	For short-term appetite suppression. Pregnancy category: X; PB: UK; $t\frac{1}{2}$: 2-10 h
Serotonin 2C Receptor Agonist		
lorcaserin (Belviq)	A: PO: 10 mg q12h	For short-term weight management when patient has at least one comorbid condition (hypertension, dyslipidemia, type 2 diabetes). May increase suicidal risk. Discontinue if 5% weight loss not achieved in 12 weeks. Pregnancy category: X; PB: 70%; $t\frac{1}{2}$: 11 h
Analeptics		
Methylxanthines		
caffeine citrate (Cafcit, NoDoz)	Neonatal apnea: Infant: PO/IV: 20-25 mg/kg loading dose, then after 24 hr, 5-10 mg/kg/d	Used as a CNS and respiratory stimulant. Used for newborns with apnea to stimulate respiration; increases heart rate and blood pressure. Given by NGT or IV. Pregnancy category: C; PB: 36%; $t\frac{1}{2}$: A: 3-7 h
OTC drugs: caffeine (NoDoz, Vivarin), coffee	A: 100-200 mg q3-4h PRN	Restores mental alertness. Brewed coffee contains 60-250 mg caffeine per cup. Black tea brewed 4 min has 40-100 mg caffeine.
theophylline	Infants: PO/IV: 0.5 mg/kg	Used for newborns with apnea to stimulate respiration. Given by NGT or PO. Pregnancy category: C; PB: 40%; $t\frac{1}{2}$: A: 6.5-10.5 h, neonate: 6.5-10.5 h
Respiratory Stimulants		
doxapram HCl (Dopram)	A: IV: 0.5-1 mg/kg, may repeat to total of 2 mg/kg; infusion: 5 mg/min, then reduce to 1-3 mg/min; *max:* 4 mg/kg	Used for respiratory depression. Can increase blood pressure. Pregnancy category: B; PB: UK; $t\frac{1}{2}$: A: 2.5-4 h, neonate: 7-10 h

Adol, Adolescent; *A,* adult; *a.c.,* before meals; *C,* child; *CSS,* Controlled Substances Schedule; *d,* day; *FDA,* U.S. Food and Drug Administration; *h,* hour; *IM,* intramuscular; *IV,* intravenous; *MAOI,* monoamine oxidase inhibitor; *max,* maximum; *min,* minute; *NGT,* nasogastric tube; *OTC,* over the counter; *PB,* protein binding; *PO,* by mouth; *subQ,* subcutaneous; $t\frac{1}{2}$, half-life; *t.i.d.,* three times a day; *UK,* unknown.

Respiratory Stimulants

Doxapram (Dopram), a CNS and respiratory stimulant, is used to treat respiratory depression caused by drug overdose, preanesthetic and postanesthetic respiratory depression, and chronic obstructive pulmonary disease (COPD). It should be used with caution for the treatment of neonatal apnea. It is administered intravenously, and its onset of action is within 20 to 40 seconds with a peak action within 2 minutes. Side effects are infrequent; however, with an overdose, hypertension, tachycardia, tremors, spasticity, and hyperactive reflexes may occur. Mechanical ventilation is more effective than doxapram for treating patients who experience respiratory depression as a result of using certain drugs.

KEY WEBSITES

Methylphenidate drug information: *www.drugs.com/methylphenidate.html*

NIDA InfoFacts: Methylphenidate (Ritalin): *www.nida.nih.gov/Infofacts/Ritalin.html*

CRITICAL THINKING CASE STUDY

MP, a 67-year-old man, wants to lose 30 pounds. He wants to take an OTC diet pill but does not want to be on a calorie-restricted diet.

1. Would you recommend a diet pill? Why or why not?
2. What do you need to assess concerning this patient's physical status before suggesting a diet pill or an exercise program?
3. What behavior modifications might you suggest related to attempted weight loss?
4. In what ways could diet modification and exercise help this patient? Explain your answer.
5. Would you suggest a commercial weight-loss program? Why or why not?

NCLEX STUDY QUESTIONS

1. When a 12-year-old child is prescribed methylphenidate, which is most important for the nurse to monitor?
   a. Temperature
   b. Respirations
   c. Intake and output
   d. Height and weight
2. Several children are admitted for diagnosis with possible attention deficit/hyperactivity disorder. Which is most important for the nurse to observe?
   a. A girl who is lethargic
   b. A girl who lacks impulsivity
   c. A boy with smooth coordination
   d. A boy with an inability to complete tasks
3. The nurse monitoring a patient for methylphenidate withdrawal should observe the patient for which condition?
   a. Tremors
   b. Insomnia
   c. Weakness
   d. Tachycardia
4. The nurse is teaching a patient to self-administer medications. The nurse knows that which drug is used to treat narcolepsy?
   a. modafinil
   b. atomoxetine
   c. lisdexamfetamine
   d. methylphenidate
5. A newborn patient is in respiratory distress. The nurse anticipates preparation for which medication to be given?
   a. modafinil
   b. armodafinil
   c. theophylline
   d. amphetamine

Answers: 1, d; 2, d; 3, c; 4, a; 5, c.

CHAPTER 21

Central Nervous System Depressants

evolve WEBSITE

http://evolve.elsevier.com/KeeHayes/pharmacology/

- Animations
- Content Updates
- Key Points
- Review Questions for the NCLEX® Examination
- References from the Textbook
- Unfolding Case Studies

OBJECTIVES

- Differentiate the types and stages of sleep.
- Explain several nonpharmacologic ways to induce sleep.
- Differentiate among these adverse effects: hangover, dependence, tolerance, withdrawal symptoms, and rapid eye movement (REM) rebound.
- Discuss the uses of benzodiazepines.
- Apply the nursing process for the patient taking benzodiazepines for hypnotic use.
- Differentiate nursing interventions related to barbiturates, benzodiazepines, nonbenzodiazepines, and melatonin agonist hypnotics.
- Compare the stages of anesthesia.
- Explain the uses for topical anesthetics.
- Differentiate general and local anesthetics and their major side effects.

OUTLINE

KEY TERMS

anesthetics, p. 299
balanced anesthesia, p. 299
caudal block, p. 301
dependence, p. 293
epidural block, p. 301
hangover, p. 293
hypnotic effect, p. 292
insomnia, p. 292
nerve block, p. 301
nonrapid eye movement (NREM) sleep, p. 292
rapid eye movement (REM) sleep, p. 292
saddle block, p. 302
sedation, p. 292
spinal anesthesia, p. 301
spinal block, p. 301
tolerance, p. 293
withdrawal symptoms, p. 293

Drugs that are central nervous system (CNS) depressants cause varying degrees of depression (reduction in functional activity) within the CNS. The degree of depression depends primarily on the drug and the amount of drug taken. The broad classification of CNS depressants includes sedative-hypnotics, general anesthetics, analgesics, opioid and nonopioid analgesics, anticonvulsants, antipsychotics, and antidepressants. The last five groups of depressant drugs are presented in separate chapters. Sedative-hypnotics and general anesthetics are discussed in this chapter.

TYPES AND STAGES OF SLEEP

Sleep disorders such as **insomnia** (inability to fall or remain asleep) occur in 10% to 30% of Americans. Insomnia occurs more frequently in women and increases with age.

People spend approximately one third of their lives, or as much as 25 years, sleeping. Normal sleep is composed of two definite phases: **rapid eye movement (REM) sleep** and **nonrapid eye movement (NREM) sleep.** Both REM and NREM occur cyclically during sleep at about 90- minute intervals (Figure 21-1). The four succeedingly deeper stages of NREM sleep end with an episode of REM sleep, and the cycle begins again. If sleep is interrupted, the cycle begins again with stage 1 of NREM sleep. Individuals perform better during their waking hours if they experience all types and stages of sleep.

It is during the REM sleep phase that individuals experience most of their recallable dreams. Children have few REM sleep periods and have longer periods of stage 3 and 4 NREM sleep. Older adults experience a decrease in stages 3 and 4 NREM sleep and have frequent waking periods.

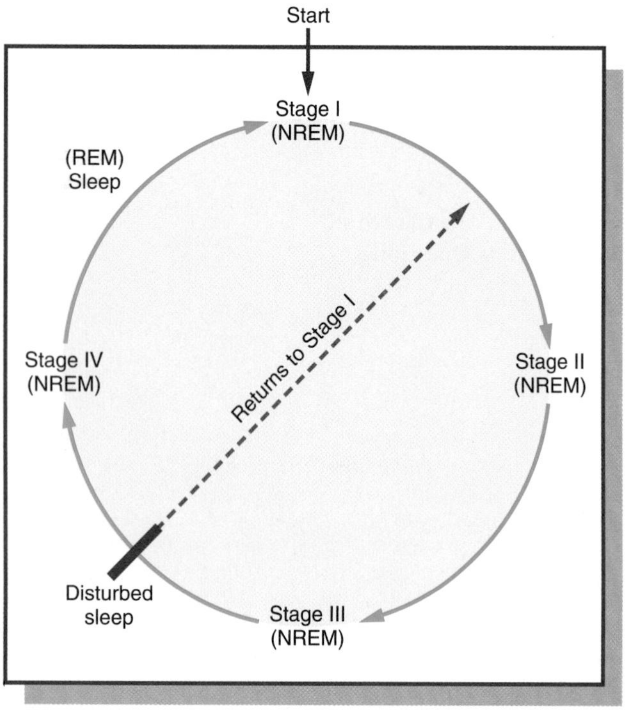

FIGURE 21–1 Types and stages of sleep. *NREM,* Nonrapid eye movement (four stages); *REM,* rapid eye movement (dreaming).

It is difficult to rouse a person during REM sleep. The period of REM sleep episodes becomes longer during the sleep process. Frequently if a person is roused from REM sleep, a vivid, bizarre dream may be recalled. If these dreams are unpleasant, they may be called *nightmares.* Sleep-walking or nightmares that occur in children take place during NREM sleep.

NONPHARMACOLOGIC METHODS

Before using sedative-hypnotics or over-the-counter (OTC) sleep aids, various nonpharmacologic methods should be used to promote sleep. Once the nurse discovers why the patient cannot sleep, the following ways to promote sleep may be suggested:

1. Arise at a specific hour in the morning.
2. Take few or no daytime naps.
3. Avoid drinks that contain caffeine and alcohol 6 hours before bedtime. Also avoid smoking nicotine 6 hours before bedtime.
4. Avoid heavy meals or strenuous exercise before bedtime.
5. Take a warm bath, listen to quiet music, or perform other soothing activities before bed.
6. Decrease exposure to loud noises.
7. Avoid drinking copious amounts of fluids before sleep.
8. Drink warm milk before bedtime.

SEDATIVE-HYPNOTICS

Sedative-hypnotics are commonly ordered for treatment of sleep disorders. The mildest form of CNS depression is **sedation,** which diminishes physical and mental responses at lower dosages of certain CNS depressants but does not affect consciousness. Sedatives are used mostly during the daytime. Increasing the drug dose can produce a **hypnotic effect**—not hypnosis but a form of "natural" sleep. Sedative-hypnotic drugs are sometimes the same drug; however, certain drugs are used more often for their hypnotic effect. With very high doses of sedative-hypnotic drugs, anesthesia may be achieved. An example of an ultrashort-acting barbiturate used to produce anesthesia is thiopental sodium (Pentothal).

Sedatives were first prescribed to reduce tension and anxiety. Barbiturates were initially used for their antianxiety effect until the early 1960s, when benzodiazepines were introduced. Because of the many side effects of barbiturates and their potential for physical and mental dependency, they are now less frequently prescribed.

More than $35 million is spent each year on OTC sleep aids such as Nytol, Sominex, Sleep-Eze, and Tylenol PM. The primary ingredient in OTC sleep aids is an antihistamine such as diphenhydramine (not barbiturates or benzodiazepines).

There are short-acting hypnotics and intermediate-acting hypnotics. Short-acting hypnotics are useful in achieving sleep, because they allow the patient to awaken early in the

TABLE 21-1 COMMON SIDE EFFECTS AND ADVERSE REACTIONS OF SEDATIVE-HYPNOTICS

SIDE EFFECTS AND ADVERSE REACTIONS	EXPLANATION OF THE EFFECTS
Hangover	A hangover is residual drowsiness resulting in impaired reaction time. The intermediate- and long-acting hypnotics are frequently the cause of drug hangover. The liver biotransforms these drugs into active metabolites that persist in the body, causing drowsiness.
REM rebound	REM rebound, which results in vivid dreams and nightmares, frequently occurs after taking a hypnotic for a prolonged period then abruptly stopping. However, it may occur after taking only one hypnotic dose.
Dependence	Dependence is the result of chronic hypnotic use. Physical and psychological dependence can result. Physical dependence results in the appearance of specific withdrawal symptoms when a drug is discontinued after prolonged use. The severity of withdrawal symptoms depends on the drug and dosage. Symptoms may include muscular twitching and tremors, dizziness, orthostatic hypotension, delusions, hallucinations, delirium, and seizures. Withdrawal symptoms start within 24 hours and can last for several days.
Tolerance	Tolerance results when there is a need to increase the dosage over time to obtain the desired effect. It is mostly caused by an increase in drug metabolism by liver enzymes. The barbiturate drug category can cause tolerance after prolonged use. Tolerance is reversible when the drug is discontinued.
Excessive depression	Long-term use of a hypnotic may result in CNS depression, which is characterized by lethargy, sleepiness, lack of concentration, confusion, and psychological depression.
Respiratory depression	High doses of sedative-hypnotics can suppress the respiratory center in the medulla.
Hypersensitivity	Skin rashes and urticaria can result when taking barbiturates. Such reactions are rare.

REM, Rapid eye movement.

morning without experiencing lingering side effects. Intermediate-acting hypnotics are useful for sustaining sleep; however, after using one the patient may experience residual drowsiness, or **hangover**, in the morning. This may be undesirable if the patient is active and requires mental alertness. The ideal hypnotic promotes natural sleep without disrupting normal patterns of sleep and produces no hangover or undesirable effect. Table 21-1 lists the common side effects and adverse reactions associated with sedative-hypnotic use and abuse.

Hypnotic drug therapy should usually be short-term to prevent drug **dependence** and drug **tolerance.** Interrupting hypnotic therapy can decrease drug tolerance, but abruptly discontinuing a high dose of hypnotic taken over a long period can cause **withdrawal symptoms.** In such cases, the dose should be tapered to avoid withdrawal symptoms. As a general rule, the lowest dose should be taken to obtain sleep. Patients with severe respiratory disorders should avoid hypnotics, which could cause an increase in respiratory depression. Usually hypnotics are contraindicated during pregnancy. Ramelteon (Rozerem) is the only major sedative-hypnotic approved for long-term use. This drug may be used for treating chronic insomnia.

The category of sedative-hypnotics includes barbiturates, benzodiazepines, and nonbenzodiazepines, among others. Each category is discussed separately. Prototype drug charts are included for benzodiazepines and nonbenzodiazepines.

Barbiturates

Barbiturates were introduced as a sedative in the early 1900s. They are classified as long-acting, intermediate-acting, short-acting, and ultrashort-acting.

- The *long-acting* group includes phenobarbital and mephobarbital and is used to control seizures in epilepsy.
- The *intermediate-acting* barbiturates, such as butabarbital (Butisol), are useful as sleep sustainers for maintaining long periods of sleep. Because these drugs take approximately 1 hour for the onset of sleep, they are not prescribed for those who have trouble getting to sleep. Vital signs should be closely monitored in persons who take intermediate-acting barbiturates.
- The *short-acting* barbiturates secobarbital (Seconal) and pentobarbital (Nembutal) are used primarily for sedation preoperatively. Vital signs should be closely monitored in persons who take short-acting barbiturates.
- The *ultrashort-acting* barbiturate, thiopental sodium (Pentothal), is used as a general anesthetic.

Barbiturates should be restricted to short-term use (2 weeks or less) because of their numerous side effects, including tolerance to the drug. In the United States, barbiturates are classified in the schedule of the Controlled Substances Act as class II for short-acting, class III for intermediate-acting, and class IV for long-acting. In Canada, barbiturates are classified as schedule G. Barbiturates are listed in Table 21-2.

Pharmacokinetics Pentobarbital (Nembutal) has been available for nearly half a century and was the hypnotic of choice until the introduction of benzodiazepines in the 1960s. It has a slow absorption rate and is moderately protein-bound. The long half-life is mainly because of the formation of active metabolites resulting from liver metabolism.

Pharmacodynamics Pentobarbital and secobarbital are used primarily for short-term treatment of insomnia. Other uses include control of seizures, preoperative anxiety, and sedation induction. They have a rapid onset with a short duration of action and are considered short-acting barbiturates. The onset of action of pentobarbital is slower when administered intramuscularly (IM) than when administered orally (PO).

TABLE 21-2 SEDATIVE-HYPNOTICS: BARBITURATES AND OTHERS

GENERIC (BRAND)	ROUTE AND DOSAGE	USES AND CONSIDERATIONS
Barbiturates: Short-Acting		
pentobarbital sodium (Nembutal Sodium) CSS II	Insomnia: A: PO: 100-200 mg h.s.; IM: 150-200 mg C: PO/IM: 2-6 mg/kg h.s.; *max:* 100 mg/d Preoperative: A: PO/IM: 100-200 mg in 2 divided doses Older adults: PO/IM: 100 mg in 2 divided doses C: PO/IM: 2-6 mg/kg	For sedation, sleep, or preanesthesia. May cause sleep-related behaviors and suicidal ideation. Pregnancy category: D; PB: 35%-45%; t½: 4-50 h
secobarbital sodium (Seconal Sodium) CSS II	Preoperative sedation: A: PO: 100-300 mg 1-2 h before surgery C: PO: 2-6 mg/kg 1-2 h before surgery	For preoperative sedation; may lead to sleep-related behaviors and suicidal ideation. Pregnancy category: D; PB: UK; t½: 15-40 h
Barbiturates: Intermediate-Acting		
butabarbital sodium (Butisol Sodium) CSS III	Sedative: A: PO: 15-30 mg t.i.d./q.i.d. C: PO: 2 mg/kg/dose t.i.d. Hypnotic: A: PO: 50-100 mg h.s. Preoperative sedative: A: PO: 50-100 mg, 1-1.5 h before surgery C: 2-6 mg/kg; *max:* 100 mg/d	To relieve anxiety and as short-term (less than 14 days) hypnotic for insomnia. Avoid alcohol with all barbiturates. May cause sleep-related behaviors. May cause abnormal thinking and angioedema. No longer accepted for use in older adults or debilitated adult patients for insomnia. Pregnancy category: D; PB: 50%; t½: 100 h
Barbiturates: Long-Acting		
mephobarbital (Mebaral) CSS IV	Sedative: A: PO: 32-100 mg t.i.d./q.i.d. C: PO: <5 y: 16-32 mg t.i.d./q.i.d. C: PO: >5 y: 32-64 mg t.i.d./q.i.d.	To control convulsive episodes, agitation, anxiety, suicidal ideation, and delirium tremens. Pregnancy category: D; PB: UK; t½: 11-67 h
phenobarbital (Luminal) CSS IV	A: PO: 30-200 mg/d for less than 14 days	Used more for seizure control, preoperative sedation, and anxiety. Need to monitor for respiratory depression. Pregnancy category: D; PB: 20%-45%; t½: 50-140 h

A, Adult; *b.i.d.*, two times a day; *C*, child; *CSS*, Controlled Substances Schedule; *d*, day; *h*, hour; *h.s.*, at bedtime; *IM*, intramuscular; *IV*, intravenous; *max*, maximum; *PB*, protein-binding; *p.c.*, after meals; *PO*, by mouth; *PR*, rectally; *PRN*, as needed; *q.i.d.*, four times a day; *t½*, half-life; *t.i.d.*, three times a day; *UK*, unknown; *wk*, week; <, less than; >, greater than.

SAFETY: Preventing Medication Errors

Do not confuse ...

- **phenobarbital** (a long-acting barbiturate used to control seizures) with **pentobarbital** (an ultrashort-acting barbiturate used as a general anesthetic).

Many drug interactions are associated with barbiturates. Alcohol, narcotics, and other sedative-hypnotics used in combination with barbiturates may further depress the CNS. Pentobarbital increases hepatic enzyme action, causing an increased metabolism and decreased effect of drugs such as oral anticoagulants, glucocorticoids, tricyclic antidepressants, and quinidine. Pentobarbital may cause hepatotoxicity if taken with large doses of acetaminophen.

Benzodiazepines

Selected benzodiazepines (minor tranquilizer or anxiolytic) were introduced with chlordiazepoxide (Librium) in the 1960s as antianxiety agents. This drug group is ordered as sedative-hypnotics for inducing sleep. Several benzodiazepines marketed as hypnotics include flurazepam (Dalmane), alprazolam (Xanax) (Prototype Drug Chart 21-1), temazepam (Restoril), triazolam (Halcion), estazolam (ProSom), and quazepam (Doral) (Table 21-3). Increased anxiety might be the cause of insomnia for some patients, so lorazepam (Ativan) and diazepam (Valium) can be used to alleviate the anxiety. These drugs are classified as schedule IV according to the Controlled Substances Act. The benzodiazepines increase the action of the inhibitory neurotransmitter gamma-aminobutyric acid (GABA) to the GABA receptors. Neuron excitability is reduced.

Nursing Process

Patient-Centered Collaborative Care

Sedative-Hypnotic: Benzodiazepines

Assessment

- Obtain drug history of current drugs and herbs patient is taking, especially CNS depressants, which would

PROTOTYPE DRUG CHART 21-1

Alprazolam

Drug Class	Dosage
Sedative-hypnotic: benzodiazepine Trade name: Xanax CSS: IV Pregnancy Category: D	A: PO: Initially 0.25-0.5 mg h.s.; *max:* 10 mg/d
Contraindications	**Drug-Lab-Food Interactions**
Respiratory depression, acute alcohol intoxication, psychotic reactions, recent respiratory depressants, hypersensitivity Caution: Older adults, sleep apnea, renal or liver dysfunction, depression, suicidal ideation, drug abuse	Drug: Decreases respiration with alcohol, CNS depressants; azole antifungals (ketoconazole), antibiotics (erythromycin), aprepitant, cimetidine, diltiazem, verapamil increase blood levels of alprazolam; rifabutin, rifampin, cortisone, phenytoin decrease blood levels; alprazolam increases digoxin and lithium levels Food: Grapefruit increases alprazolam levels; green tea decreases alprazolam effects
Pharmacokinetics	**Pharmacodynamics**
Absorption: PO: 90% absorbed from GI tract Distribution: PB: 80%-90% Metabolism: $t\frac{1}{2}$: 11-16 h Excretion: In urine as metabolites	PO: Onset: UK Peak: 1-2 h (immediate-release); 9 h (extended-release); 1.5-2 h (disintegrating tablet) Duration: UK
To Treat Anxiety and Panic Disorders	
Mode of Action: CNS depression, binds receptors in limbic system and reticular formation, increases GABA to GABA receptors, shift of chloride ions leads to less excitability and stabilizes neuronal membranes	
Side Effects	**Adverse Reactions**
Lethargy, drowsiness, dizziness, headache, constipation, memory impairment, increased appetite, blurred vision, decreased libido, paradoxical reactions	Depression, impaired coordination

A, Adult; *C,* child; *CNS,* central nervous system; *CSS,* Controlled Substances Schedule; *d,* day; *GI,* gastrointestinal; *h,* hour; *h.s.,* at bedtime; *MAOIs,* monoamine oxidase inhibitors; *min,* minute; *PB,* protein binding; *PO,* by mouth; $t\frac{1}{2}$, half-life; *UK,* unknown.

potentiate respiratory depression and hypotensive effects.

- Assess baseline vital signs for future comparison.
- Determine if there is a history of insomnia or anxiety disorders.
- Assess renal function. Urine output should be 1500 mL/day. Renal impairment could prolong drug action by increasing half-life of the drug.

Nursing Diagnoses

- Sleep deprivation related to adverse effect of insomnia
- Risk for injury related to dizziness and hypotension
- Ineffective breathing pattern related to CNS depression
- Ineffective sexuality pattern related to adverse effect of erectile dysfunction

Planning

- Patient will receive adequate sleep when taking benzodiazepine.

Nursing Interventions

- Monitor vital signs, especially respirations and blood pressure.
- Use bed alarm for older adults and patients receiving a hypnotic for the first time. Confusion may occur, and injury may result.
- Observe patient for adverse reactions, especially an older adult or a debilitated patient.
- Examine patient's skin for rashes. Skin eruptions may occur in patients taking benzodiazepines.

Patient Teaching

General

- Teach patient to use nonpharmacologic ways to induce sleep (taking a warm bath, listening to quiet music, drinking warm fluids, avoiding drinks with caffeine for 6 hours before bedtime).
- Encourage patient to avoid alcohol and antidepressant, antipsychotic, and opioid drugs while taking benzodiazepines. Respiratory depression may occur when these drugs are combined.
- Warn patient that certain herbs (Herbal Alert 21-1) may interact with benzodiazepines. Herbal supplement may need to be discontinued or prescription drug dose may need to be modified.

TABLE 21-3 SEDATIVE-HYPNOTICS: BENZODIAZEPINES AND NONBENZODIAZEPINES

GENERIC (BRAND)	ROUTE AND DOSAGE	USES AND CONSIDERATIONS
Benzodiazepines		
alprazolam (Xanax) CSS IV	See Prototype Drug Chart 21-1.	
estazolam (ProSom) CSS IV	A: PO: 1-2 mg h.s. Older adults: PO: 0.5-1 mg h.s.	For treatment of insomnia. Should not be used longer than 6 wk. Decreases frequency of nocturnal awakening. May cause sleep-driving behaviors. Pregnancy category: X; PB: 93%; $t\frac{1}{2}$: 10-24 h
lorazepam (Ativan) CSS IV	Insomnia: A: PO: 2-4 mg h.s. Older adults: PO: 1-2 mg h.s.	Used as a preoperative sedative and to reduce anxiety. Pregnancy category: D; PB: 91%; $t\frac{1}{2}$: 12-14 h
temazepam (Restoril) CSS IV	Hypnotic: A: PO: 15-30 mg h.s. Older adults: PO: 7.5 mg h.s.	To treat insomnia. Also has sedative effects. May cause sleep-related behavior. Pregnancy category: X; PB: 98%; $t\frac{1}{2}$: 8-15 h
triazolam (Halcion) CSS IV	Hypnotic: A: PO: 0.125-0.25 mg h.s. (*max:* 0.5 mg/d) Older adults: PO: 0.0625-0.125 mg h.s.	For management of insomnia. Should not be used longer than 7-10 d at a time to avoid tolerance. Avoid alcohol and smoking when taking triazolam. May cause sleep-related behavior. Pregnancy Category: X; PB: 90%; $t\frac{1}{2}$: 1.5-5.5 h
Benzodiazepine Antagonists		
flumazenil (Romazicon)	A: IV: 0.2 mg over 30 sec; may repeat with 0.3 mg in 30 sec; *max:* 3 mg total dose	Management of benzodiazepine overdose or reversal of sedative effects of benzodiazepine with general anesthesia. Pregnancy category: C; PB: 50%; $t\frac{1}{2}$: 54 min
Nonbenzodiazepines		
zolpidem tartrate (Ambien) CSS IV	See Prototype Drug Chart 21-2.	
eszopiclone (Lunesta) CSS IV	Insomnia: A: PO: 2-3 mg h.s. Older adults: PO: 1-2 mg h.s.	To treat insomnia. May cause sleep-related behavior, worsening of preexisting depression, and suicidal ideation. Pregnancy category: C; PB: 52%-59%; $t\frac{1}{2}$: 6 h
zaleplon (Sonata) CSS IV	Insomnia: A: PO: 10 mg h.s.; *max:* 20 mg h.s. Older adults: PO: 5 mg h.s.; *max:* 10 mg h.s.	For ultrashort-term treatment of insomnia. May cause sleep-related behavior. Pregnancy category: C; PB: 60%; $t\frac{1}{2}$: 1 h
Melatonin Agonist		
ramelteon (Rozerem)	A: PO: 8 mg with 30 minutes of bedtime	For treatment of insomnia by regulating circadian rhythm. May be used long-term for chronic insomnia. Pregnancy category: C; PB: 82%; $t\frac{1}{2}$: 1-2.5 h

A, Adult; *CSS,* Controlled Substances Schedule; *d,* day; *h,* hour; *h.s.,* at bedtime; *IV,* intravenous; *max,* maximum; *PB,* protein binding; *PO,* by mouth; *sec,* second; $t\frac{1}{2}$, half-life; *UK,* unknown; *wk,* week.

- Advise patient not to drive a motor vehicle or operate machinery. Caution is always encouraged.
- Encourage patient to check with health care provider about OTC sleeping aids. Drowsiness may result from taking these drugs; therefore, caution while driving is advised.

Side Effects

- Advise patient to report adverse reactions such as cognitive changes and paradoxical reactions to health care provider. Drug selection or dosage might need to be changed.
- Teach patient that benzodiazepines should be gradually withdrawn, especially if it has been taken for several weeks. Abrupt cessation may result in withdrawal symptoms (e.g., tremors, muscle twitching).

Cultural Considerations

- Use an interpreter as needed, and involve extended family in health teaching and support.
- Provide written instruction (or videos) in patient's preferred language.

Evaluation

- Assess the effectiveness of benzodiazepines.
- Evaluate respiratory status to ensure that respiratory depression has not occurred.

SAFETY: Preventing Medication Errors

Do not confuse ...

- **Lorazepam** (a benzodiazepine used to reduce anxiety) with **alprazolam** (a benzodiazepine used to treat anxiety and insomnia).

Benzodiazepines (except for temazepam) can suppress stage 4 of NREM sleep, which may result in vivid dreams or nightmares and can delay REM sleep. Benzodiazepines are effective for sleep disorders for several weeks longer than

HERBAL ALERT 21-1

Sedatives

- Kava kava should not be taken in combination with CNS depressants such as barbiturates and opioids. This herb may increase the sedative effect.
- Valerian, when taken with alcohol and other CNS depressants such as barbiturates, may increase the sedative effects of the prescribed drug.

other sedative-hypnotics; to prevent *REM rebound,* however, they should not be used for longer than 3 to 4 weeks.

Triazolam (Halcion) is a short-acting hypnotic with a half-life of 2 to 5 hours. It does not produce any active metabolites. Complaints of adverse reactions to prolonged use of triazolam (e.g., loss of memory) led to its removal from the market in Great Britain, but a British advisory group is recommending that the legislative body reinstate triazolam. Its use is under review by the U.S. Food and Drug Administration (FDA). Currently, it is seldom prescribed.

Small doses of benzodiazepines are recommended for patients with renal or hepatic dysfunction. For benzodiazepine overdose, the benzodiazepine antagonist flumazenil (Romazicon) may be prescribed. Benzodiazepines prescribed as antianxiety drugs are discussed in Chapter 27.

Pharmacokinetics Benzodiazepines are well absorbed through the gastrointestinal (GI) mucosa. They are rapidly metabolized in the liver to active metabolites. Alprazolam has an intermediate half-life of 11 to 16 hours. Benzodiazepines are highly protein bound, and more free drug is available when taken with other highly protein-bound drugs, which increases the risk for adverse effects.

Pharmacodynamics Benzodiazepines are used to treat insomnia by inducing and sustaining sleep. They have a rapid onset of action and intermediate- to long-acting effects. The normal recommended dose of a benzodiazepine may be too much for the older adult, so half the dose is recommended initially to prevent overdosing.

Alcohol or opioids taken with a benzodiazepine may cause an additive depressive CNS response. Most benzodiazepines may have an adverse effect of sleep-related behaviors (eating, driving, or telephoning during sleep).

Nonbenzodiazepines

Zolpidem (Ambien) is a nonbenzodiazepine that differs in chemical structure from benzodiazepines. It is used for short-term treatment (less than 10 days) of insomnia. Its duration of action is 6 to 8 hours with a short half-life of 2 to 4.5 hours. Zolpidem is metabolized in the liver to three inactive metabolites and is excreted in bile, urine, and feces. When zolpidem is prescribed for older adults, the dose should be decreased. Table 21-3 lists the benzodiazepines and nonbenzodiazepines used as sedative-hypnotics and their dosages, uses, and considerations. Zolpidem is described in Prototype Drug Chart 21-2.

Melatonin Agonists

Ramelteon (Rozerem) is in the newest category of sedative/hypnotics, called melatonin agonists. Ramelteon is the first FDA-approved hypnotic that is not classified as a controlled substance. This drug acts by selectively targeting melatonin receptors to regulate circadian rhythm in the treatment of insomnia. Ramelteon has not been shown to decrease REM sleep. This new drug has a half life of 1 to 3 hours. Adverse effects of ramelteon include drowsiness, dizziness, fatigue, headache, nausea, and suicidal ideation. Ramelteon is also used as an antianxiety drug.

Sedatives and Hypnotics for Older Adults

Identifying the cause of insomnia in an older adult should be the first diagnostic consideration, and nonpharmacologic methods should be used before sleep medications are prescribed. Because of physiologic changes in older adults, the use of hypnotics can cause a variety of side effects.

Barbiturates increase CNS depression and confusion in older adults and should not be taken for sleep. The short- to intermediate-acting benzodiazepines such as estazolam (ProSom), temazepam (Restoril), and triazolam (Halcion) are considered safer than barbiturates. Long-acting hypnotic benzodiazepines such as flurazepam, quazepam (Doral), and diazepam (Valium) should be avoided. In many cases, older adults should be instructed to take the prescribed benzodiazepine no more than four times a week to avoid side effects and drug dependency. They can choose selected nights to take the hypnotic.

The main sleep problem experienced by older adults is frequent nighttime awakening. Reports have shown that older women experience more troublesome sleep patterns than men. Sleep disturbance may be caused by discomfort or pain. Occasionally a nonsteroidal antiinflammatory drug (NSAID) such as ibuprofen may alleviate the discomfort that prevents sleep.

Nursing Process
Patient-Centered Collaborative Care

Sedative-Hypnotic: Nonbenzodiazepines

Assessment
- Assess baseline vital signs and laboratory tests (e.g., AST, ALT, bilirubin) for future comparisons.
- Obtain drug history. Taking CNS depressants with nonbenzodiazepine hypnotics can depress respirations.
- Ascertain patient's problem with sleep disturbance.

Nursing Diagnoses
- Sleep deprivation related to anxiety
- Fatigue related to insomnia
- Risk for injury related to adverse effect sleep-related behaviors

Planning
- Patient will remain asleep for 6 to 8 hours.

PROTOTYPE DRUG CHART 21-2

Zolpidem Tartrate

Drug Class	Dosage
Sedative-hypnotic: nonbenzodiazepine Trade names: Ambien, Ambien CR (extended release), Edluar (sublingual), Intermezzo (sublingual) CSS: IV Pregnancy Category: C	A: PO: 5-10 mg h.s.; *max:* 10 mg/d Older adults: PO: 5 mg h.s.; *max:* 5-10 mg/d
Contraindications	**Drug-Lab-Food Interactions**
Hypersensitivity to benzodiazepine, respiratory depression, lactation Caution: Renal or liver dysfunction; mental depression, suicidal ideation; pregnancy; children, older adults, and debilitated individuals	Drug: Decreases CNS function with alcohol, CNS depressants, anticonvulsants, and phenothiazines; increased levels with azole antifungals; decreased levels with rifampin Food: Decreases absorption
Pharmacokinetics	**Pharmacodynamics**
Absorption: PO: well absorbed Distribution: PB: 92% Metabolism: t½: 2-4.5 h Excretion: In bile, urine, and feces	PO: Onset: 7-27 min Peak: 0.5-2.3 h Duration: 6-8 h
Therapeutic Effects/Uses	
To treat insomnia Mode of Action: CNS depression, neurotransmitter inhibition	
Side Effects	**Adverse Reactions**
Drowsiness, lethargy, headache, hot flashes, hangover (residual sedation), irritability, dizziness, ataxia, visual disturbances, anxiety, mental depression, nausea and vomiting, erectile dysfunction	Tolerance, psychological or physical dependence; sleep-related behaviors, hypotension, angioedema, dysrhythmias, suicidal ideation

A, Adult; *CNS,* central nervous system; *CSS,* Controlled Substances Schedule; *d,* day; *h,* hour; *h.s.,* at bedtime; *min,* minute; *PB,* protein-binding; *PO,* by mouth; *t½,* half-life.

Nursing Interventions

- Monitor vital signs. Check for signs of respiratory depression (slow, irregular breathing patterns).
- Use bed alarm for older adults or patients receiving nonbenzodiazepines for the first time. Confusion may occur, and injury may result.
- Observe patient for side effects of nonbenzodiazepines (e.g., hangover [residual sedation], lightheadedness, dizziness, confusion).

Patient Teaching

General

- Teach patient to use nonpharmacologic ways to induce sleep (taking a warm bath, listening to music, drinking warm fluids such as milk, avoiding drinks with caffeine after dinner).
- Encourage patient to avoid alcohol, antidepressant, antipsychotic, and narcotic drugs while taking nonbenzodiazepines. Severe respiratory depression may occur when these drugs are combined.
- Advise patient to take nonbenzodiazepine before bedtime. Alprazolam takes effect within 15 to 30 minutes.
- Suggest that patient urinate before taking nonbenzodiazepine to prevent sleep disruption.
- Encourage patient to check with health care provider about OTC sleeping aids.
- Drowsiness may result from taking these drugs, so caution while driving is advised.

Side Effects

- Advise patient to report adverse reactions such as hangover to health care provider. Drug selection or dosage may need to be changed if hangover occurs.

Cultural Considerations

- Ask patient about methods family members have used to promote sleep.
- Suggest nonpharmacologic alternatives that may be effective in inducing sleep.

Evaluation

- Evaluate effectiveness of sedative-hypnotic in promoting sleep.
- Determine whether side effects such as hangover occur after several days of taking sedative-hypnotic. Another hypnotic may be prescribed if side effects persist.

ANESTHETICS

Anesthetics are classified as *general* and *local*. General anesthetics depress the CNS, alleviate pain, and cause a loss of consciousness. The first anesthetic, nitrous oxide ("laughing gas"), was used for surgery in the early 1800s. It is still an effective anesthetic and is frequently used in dental procedures and surgery.

Pathophysiology

Several theories exist regarding how inhalation anesthetics cause CNS depression and a loss of consciousness. The differing theories suggest the following about inhalation anesthetics:

1. The lipid structure of cell membranes is altered, resulting in impaired physiologic functions.
2. The inhibitory neurotransmitter gamma-aminobutyric acid (GABA) is activated to the GABA receptor that pushes chloride ions into the neurons. This greatly decreases the fire action potentials of the neurons.
3. The ascending reticular activating system is altered, and the neurons cease to transmit information (stimuli) to the brain.

Balanced Anesthesia

Balanced anesthesia is a combination of drugs that are frequently used in general anesthesia. Balanced anesthesia may include the following:

1. A hypnotic given the night before
2. Premedication with an opioid analgesic or benzodiazepine (e.g., midazolam [Versed]) plus an anticholinergic (e.g., atropine) given about 1 hour before surgery to decrease secretions
3. A short-acting barbiturate such as thiopental sodium (Pentothal)
4. An inhaled gas—often a combination of nitrous oxide and oxygen
5. A muscle relaxant given as needed

Balanced anesthesia minimizes cardiovascular problems, decreases the amount of general anesthetic needed, reduces possible postanesthesia nausea and vomiting, minimizes the disturbance of organ function, and decreases pain. Because the patient does not receive large doses of general anesthetics, fewer adverse reactions occur. Recovery is enhanced by allowing quicker mobility.

Stages of General Anesthesia

General anesthesia proceeds through four stages (Table 21-4). The surgical procedure is usually performed during the third stage. If an anesthetic agent is given immediately before inhalation anesthesia, the third stage can occur without the early stages of anesthesia being observed. However, if the drug is given slowly, all stages of anesthesia are usually observed.

TABLE 21-4 STAGES OF ANESTHESIA

STAGE	NAME	DESCRIPTION
1	Analgesia	Begins with consciousness and ends with loss of consciousness. Speech is difficult; sensations of smell and pain are lost. Dreams and auditory and visual hallucinations may occur. This stage may be called the *induction stage*.
2	Excitement or delirium	Produces a loss of consciousness caused by depression of the cerebral cortex. Confusion, excitement, or delirium occur. Short induction time.
3	Surgical	Surgical procedure is performed during this stage. There are four phases. The surgery is usually performed in phase 2 and upper phase 3. As anesthesia deepens, respirations become more shallow and respiratory rate is increased.
4	Medullary paralysis	Toxic stage of anesthesia. Respirations are lost, and circulatory collapse occurs. Ventilatory assistance is necessary.

Assessment before Surgery

The patient's response to anesthesia may differ according to variables related to the health status of the individual. These variables include age (young and older adult), a current health disorder (e.g., renal, liver), pregnancy, history of heavy smoking, and frequent use of alcohol and drugs. These problems must be identified *before* surgery because the type and amount of anesthetic required might need adjustment.

Inhalation Anesthetics

During the third stage of anesthesia, inhalation anesthetics (i.e., gas or volatile liquids administered as gas) are used to deliver general anesthesia. Certain gases, notably nitrous oxide, are absorbed quickly, have a rapid action, and are eliminated rapidly. Cyclopropane was a popular inhalation anesthetic from 1930 to 1960, but because of its highly flammable state as ether, it is no longer used. In the late 1950s, halothane (Fluothane) was introduced as a nonflammable alternative. Other inhalation drugs used as anesthetics include methoxyflurane, enflurane (Ethrane), isoflurane (Forane), desflurane (Suprane), and sevoflurane (Ultane).

Inhalation anesthetics typically provide smooth induction. Upon discontinuing administration of halothane, isoflurane, and enflurane, recovery of consciousness usually occurs in approximately 1 hour. Recovery from desflurane and sevoflurane is within minutes. Inhalation anesthetics are usually combined with a barbiturate (e.g., thiopental), a strong analgesic (e.g., morphine), and a muscle relaxant (e.g., pancuronium) for surgical procedures.

Adverse effects from inhalation anesthetics include respiratory depression, hypotension, dysrhythmias, and hepatic dysfunction. In patients at risk, these drugs may trigger malignant hyperthermia. The newer drugs primarily cause less nausea and vomiting than the older anesthetics.

Intravenous Anesthetics

IV anesthetics may be used for general anesthesia or for the induction stage of anesthesia. For outpatient surgery of short duration, an intravenous anesthetic might be the preferred form of anesthesia. Previously thiopental sodium (Pentothal), an ultrashort-acting barbiturate, was the general anesthetic used for short-term surgery. It is still used for the rapid induction stage of anesthesia and in dental procedures. Presently droperidol (Innovar), etomidate (Amidate), and ketamine hydrochloride (Ketalar) are also used intravenously as general anesthetics. IV anesthetics have rapid onsets and short durations of action. Table 21-5 describes the inhalation and intravenous anesthetics used for general anesthesia.

Midazolam (Versed) and propofol (Diprivan) are commonly administered for the induction and maintenance of anesthesia or conscious sedation for minor surgery or procedures like mechanical ventilation or intubation. Patients are sedated and relaxed but responsive to commands.

Adverse effects from IV anesthetics include respiratory and cardiovascular depression. Propofol supports microbial

TABLE 21-5 INHALATION AND INTRAVENOUS ANESTHETICS

DRUG	INDUCTION TIME	CONSIDERATIONS
Inhalation: Volatile Liquids		
halothane (Fluothane)	Rapid	Highly potent anesthetic. Rapid recovery. Could decrease blood pressure. Has a bronchodilator effect. Contraindicated in obstetrics.
methoxyflurane (Penthrane)	Slow	Used during labor. Drug dose is usually less than other anesthetics and does not suppress uterine contraction. Could cause hypotension. Contraindicated in renal disorders.
enflurane (Ethrane)	Rapid	Can depress respiratory function; ventilatory support may be necessary. Not to be used during labor because it could suppress uterine contractions. Avoid in patients with seizure disorders.
isoflurane (Forane)	Rapid	Frequently used in inhalation therapy. Has a smooth and rapid induction of anesthesia and rapid recovery. Could cause hypotension and respiratory depression. Not to be used during labor because it suppresses uterine contractions. Has minimal cardiovascular effect.
desflurane (Suprane)	Rapid	Volatile liquid anesthetic. Rapid recovery after anesthetic administration has ceased. Could cause hypotension and respiratory depression.
sevoflurane (Ultane)	Rapid	For induction and maintenance during surgery. May be given alone or combined with nitrous oxide.
Inhalation: Gas		
nitrous oxide (laughing gas)	Very rapid	Rapid recovery. Has minimal cardiovascular effect. Should be given with oxygen. Low potency.
Intravenous (Ultrashort-Acting Barbiturates)		
thiopental sodium (Pentothal)	Rapid	Has short duration of action. Used for rapid induction of general surgery. Keep patient warm; shivering and tremors may occur. Can depress respiratory center; ventilatory assistance might be necessary.
methohexital sodium (Brevital sodium)	Rapid	Has short duration. Frequently used for induction and with other drugs as part of balanced anesthesia. An inhalation anesthesia usually follows.
thiamylal sodium (Surital)	Rapid	Used for induction of anesthesia and as anesthesia for electroshock therapy.
Benzodiazepines		
diazepam (Valium)	Moderate to rapid	For induction of anesthesia. No analgesic effect.
midazolam (Versed)	Rapid	For induction of anesthesia and for endoscopic procedures. IV drug can cause conscious sedation. Avoid if cardiopulmonary disorder is present.
Others		
droperidol and fentanyl (Innovar)	Moderate to rapid	A neuroleptic analgesic when combined with fentanyl (potent opiate narcotic). Frequently used with a general anesthetic. Can also be used as a preanesthetic drug. Also used for diagnostic procedures. May cause hypotension and respiratory depression.
etomidate (Amidate)	Rapid	Used for short-term surgery, for induction of anesthesia, or with a general anesthetic to maintain the anesthetic state.
ketamine hydrochloride (Ketalar)	Rapid	Used for short-term surgery or induction of anesthesia. Increases salivation, blood pressure, and heart rate. May be used for diagnostic procedures. Avoid with history of psychiatric disorders.
propofol (Diprivan)	Rapid	For induction of anesthesia; may be used with general anesthesia. Short duration of action. May cause hypotension and respiratory depression. Pain can occur at injection site, so may be mixed with a local anesthetic (lidocaine) to decrease pain.
fospropofol (Lusedra)	Rapid	For induction and maintenance of anesthesia. May cause hypotension and respiratory depression.

growth and may increase the risk for bacterial infection. Discarding opened vials within 6 hours is a necessary precaution in the prevention of sepsis.

Topical Anesthetics

Use of topical anesthetic agents is limited to mucous membranes, broken or unbroken skin surfaces, and burns. Topical anesthetics come in different forms: solution, liquid spray, ointment, cream, gel, and powder. Topical anesthetics decrease the sensitivity of nerve endings in the affected area.

Local Anesthetics

Local anesthetics block pain at the site where the drug is administered, allowing consciousness to be maintained. Local anesthetics are useful in dental procedures, suturing skin lacerations, short-term (minor) surgery at a localized area, blocking nerve impulses (nerve block) below the insertion of a spinal anesthetic, and diagnostic procedures such as lumbar puncture and thoracentesis.

Most local anesthetics are divided into two groups, the esters and the amides, according to their basic structures. The amides have a very low incidence of allergic reaction.

The first local anesthetic used was cocaine hydrochloride in the late 1800s. Procaine hydrochloride (Novocain), a synthetic of cocaine, was discovered in the early 1900s. Lidocaine hydrochloride (Xylocaine) was developed in the mid-1950s to replace procaine, except in dental procedures. Lidocaine has a rapid onset and a long duration of action, is more stable in solution, and causes fewer hypersensitivity reactions than procaine. Since the introduction of lidocaine, many local anesthetics have been marketed. Table 21-6 describes the various types of local anesthetics according to short-, moderate-, and long-acting effects.

Orthopedic joint surgeries, mastectomy, cesarean section, hysterectomy, hernia repair, and cholecystectomy frequently use the postoperative pain control provided by an anesthetic pump. For example, the patient who has a bilateral hernia repair has a catheter inserted into deep fascia of the lower abdominal area. A continuous flow of bupivacaine (Marcaine), a local anesthetic, is delivered via a Y-connector to both sides at a flow rate of approximately 2 mL/h. By controlling pain with this delivery method, the patient is allowed increased mobility, reduced opioid use (which reduces associated drowsiness and nausea), and reduced hospital stay.

Spinal Anesthesia

Spinal anesthesia requires that a local anesthetic be injected in the subarachnoid space at the third or fourth lumbar space. If the local anesthetic is given too high in the spinal column, the respiratory muscles could be affected, and respiratory distress or failure could result. Headaches might result following spinal anesthesia (a "spinal"), possibly because of a decrease in cerebrospinal fluid pressure caused by a leak of fluid at the needle insertion point. Encouraging the patient to remain flat following surgery with spinal anesthesia and to take increased fluids usually decreases the likelihood of leaking spinal fluid. Hypotension also can result following spinal anesthesia due to predisposing factors including sensory block location, history of hypertension, and chronic alcohol intake.

Various sites of the spinal column can be used for a **nerve block** with a local anesthetic (Figure 21-2). A **spinal block** is the penetration of the anesthetic into the subarachnoid membrane, the second layer of the spinal cord. An **epidural block** is the placement of the local anesthetic in the outer covering of the spinal cord, or the dura mater. A **caudal block**

TABLE 21-6 LOCAL ANESTHETICS

ANESTHETICS	TYPE	USES AND CONSIDERATIONS
Short-Acting (½ to 1 Hour)		
chloroprocaine (Nesacaine)	Ester	For infiltration, caudal, and epidural anesthesia. Onset of action is 6 to 12 minutes.
procaine HCl (Novocain)	Ester	For nerve block, infiltration, epidural, and spinal anesthesia. Useful in dentistry. Caution in use for patients allergic to ester-type anesthetics
Moderate-Acting (1 to 3 Hours)		
lidocaine (Xylocaine)	Amide	For nerve block, infiltration, epidural, and spinal anesthesia. Allergic reaction is rare. Used to treat cardiac dysrhythmias (see Chapter 42).
mepivacaine HCl (Carbocaine HCl, Isocaine, Polocaine)	Amide	For nerve block, infiltration, caudal, and epidural anesthesia. May be used in dentistry.
prilocaine HCl (Citanest)	Amide	For peripheral nerve block, infiltration, caudal, and epidural anesthesia. May be used in dentistry.
Long-Acting (3 to 10 Hours)		
bupivacaine (Marcaine, Sensorcaine)	Amide	For peripheral nerve block, infiltration, caudal, and epidural anesthesia.
dibucaine HCl (Nupercainal)	Amide	For topical use (creams and ointment) to affected areas.
etidocaine (Duranest)	Amide	For peripheral nerve block, infiltration, caudal, and epidural anesthesia.
tetracaine HCl (Pontocaine)	Ester	For spinal anesthesia (high and low saddle block). Also for topical use to affected areas such as the eye to anesthetize the cornea, the nose and throat for bronchoscopy, and the skin for relief of pain and pruritus (itching).

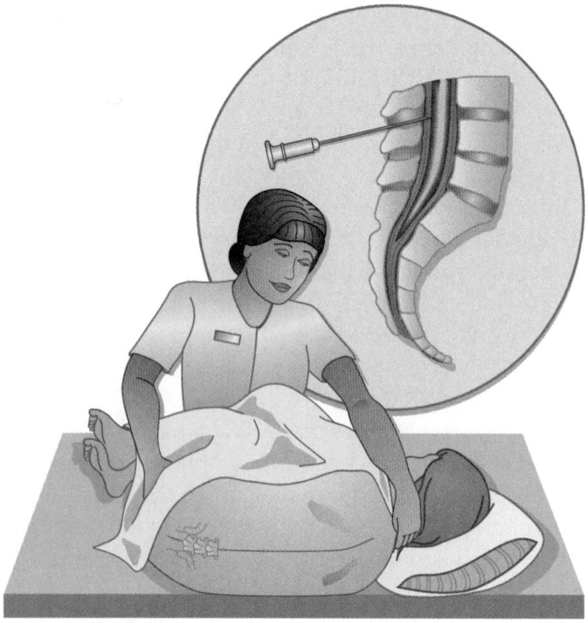

FIGURE 21–2 Positioning a patient for a spinal anesthetic.

is placed near the sacrum. A **saddle block** is given at the lower end of the spinal column to block the perineal area. Blood pressure should be monitored during administration of these types of anesthesia, because a decrease in blood pressure resulting from the drug and procedure might occur. A saddle block is frequently used for women in labor during childbirth. Further discussion of labor and delivery drugs may be found in Chapter 54.

Nursing Process
Patient-Centered Collaborative Care

Anesthetics

Assessment
- Assess baseline vital signs.
- Obtain a drug and health history, noting drugs that affect the cardiopulmonary systems.

Nursing Diagnoses
- Acute pain related to injury
- Ineffective breathing pattern related to central nervous system depression

Planning
- Patient will participate in preoperative preparation and understand postoperative care.
- Patient's vital signs will remain stable following surgery.

Nursing Interventions
- Monitor patient's postoperative state of sensorium. Report if patient remains excessively nonresponsive or confused.
- Observe preoperative and postoperative urine output. Report deficit of hourly or 8-hour urine output.
- Monitor vital signs following general and local anesthesia; hypotension and respiratory depression may result.
- Administer an analgesic or a narcotic-analgesic with caution until patient fully recovers from anesthetic. To prevent adverse reactions, dosage might need to be adjusted if patient is under the influence of anesthetic.

Patient Teaching
- Explain to patient the preoperative preparation and postoperative nursing assessment and interventions.

Cultural Considerations
- Allow adequate time for information processing for the patient whose first language is not English to avoid an inaccurate response or no response. Allow time for patients and their families to respond to questions, especially when there is a language barrier.
- Speak clearly and slowly, giving time for translation. Obtain an interpreter if necessary.

Evaluation
- Evaluate patient's response to the anesthetics. Continue to monitor patient for adverse reactions.

Nurses play an important role in patient assessment before and after general and local anesthesia is administered. Preparing the patient for surgery by explaining the preparations and completing the preoperative orders, including premedications, is necessary to enhance the safety and effectiveness of anesthesia and surgery.

KEY WEBSITES

Information on lorazepam: *www.drugs.com/lorazepam.html*

Information of eszopiclone: *www.Lunesta.com*

CRITICAL THINKING CASE STUDY

JZ, a 72-year-old woman, has difficulty staying asleep. She asks the nurse whether she should take Nytol or Sominex before bedtime.

1. Before JZ takes any sleep aid or hypnotic, what nursing assessments should be made?
2. Describe a nursing plan that may help alleviate JZ's sleep disturbance.
3. Would JZ be a candidate for taking a benzodiazepine? Explain your answer.
4. What follow-up plan should the nurse have related to JZ's sleep problem?

NCLEX STUDY QUESTIONS

1. It is important for the nurse teaching the patient regarding secobarbital (Seconal) to include which information about the drug?
   a. It is a short-acting drug that may cause one to awaken early in the morning.
   b. It is an intermediate-acting drug that frequently causes REM rebound.
   c. It is an intermediate-acting drug that frequently causes a hangover effect.
   d. It is a long-acting drug that is frequently associated with dependence.
2. A patient taking lorazepam (Ativan) asks the nurse how this drug works. The nurse should respond by stating that it is a benzodiazepine that acts by which mechanism?
   a. Depressing the central nervous system (CNS), leading to a loss of consciousness
   b. Depressing the CNS, including the motor and sensory activities
   c. Increasing the action of the inhibitory neurotransmitter gamma-aminobutyric acid (GABA) to GABA receptors
   d. Creating an epidural block by placement of the local anesthetic in the outer covering of the spinal cord
3. A patient is taking zolpidem (Ambien) for insomnia. The nurse prepares a care plan that includes monitoring of the patient for side effects/adverse reactions of this drug. Which is a side effect of zolpidem?
   a. Insomnia
   b. Headache
   c. Laryngospasm
   d. Blood dyscrasias
4. A patient received spinal anesthesia. Which is most important for the nurse to monitor?
   a. Loss of consciousness
   b. Hangover effects and dependence
   c. Hypotension and headaches
   d. Excitement or delirium
5. A nurse is teaching a patient about zolpidem. Which is important for the nurse to include in the teaching of this drug?
   a. The maximum dose is 20 mg/d.
   b. It may lead to psychological dependence.
   c. For older adults, the dose is 15 mg at bedtime.
   d. The drug should only be used for 21 days or less.
6. A patient is taking triazolam (Halcion). Which instructions about this drug are important for the nurse to include?
   a. It may be used as a barbiturate for only 4 weeks.
   b. Use as a nonbenzodiazepine to reduce anxiety.
   c. This drug does not lead to vivid dreams or nightmares.
   d. Avoid alcohol and smoking while taking this drug.
7. A patient is to receive conscious sedation for a minor surgical procedure. Which drug administration should the nurse expect? (Select all that apply.)
   a. Propofol (Diprivan) to sustain natural sleep
   b. Lidocaine (Xylocaine) to provide local anesthesia
   c. Midazolam (Versed) to promote sedation and following of commands
   d. Ketamine (Ketalar) for rapid induction and prolonged duration of action
   e. Phenobarbital (Luminal) for short-acting duration of sleep

Answers: 1, a; 2, c; 3, b; 4, c; 5, b; 6, d; 7, a, c.

CHAPTER

22

Anticonvulsants

evolve WEBSITE

http://evolve.elsevier.com/KeeHayes/pharmacology/

- Animations
- Content Updates
- Key Points
- Review Questions for the NCLEX® Examination
- References from the Textbook
- Unfolding Case Studies

OBJECTIVES

- Contrast the two international classifications of seizures with characteristics of each type.
- Differentiate between the types of seizures.
- Summarize the pharmacokinetics, side effects and adverse reactions, therapeutic plasma phenytoin level, contraindications for use, and drug interactions of phenytoin (Dilantin).
- Compare the actions of hydantoins, long-acting barbiturates, succinimides, oxazolidones, benzodiazepines, iminostilbenes, and valproate.
- Apply the nursing process to anticonvulsants including patient teaching.

OUTLINE

KEY TERMS

anoxia, p. 304
anticonvulsants, p. 305
atonic seizure, p. 305
clonic seizure, p. 305
convulsion, p. 304
electroencephalogram, p. 304
gingival hyperplasia, p. 306
grand mal, p. 305
hydantoins, p. 306
idiopathic, p. 304
nystagmus, p. 306
petit mal, p. 305
psychomotor, p. 305
seizure, p. 304
seizure threshold, p. 306
sloughing, p. 306
status epilepticus, p. 306
teratogenic, p. 306
tonic seizure, p. 305

Millions of people in the United States have active epilepsy, a seizure disorder. The **seizure** associated with epilepsy results from abnormal electric discharges from the cerebral neurons and is characterized by a loss or disturbance of consciousness and usually by a **convulsion** (involuntary paroxysmal muscular contractions). The **electroencephalogram (EEG)**, computed tomography (CT), and magnetic resonance imaging (MRI) are useful in diagnosing epilepsy. The EEG records abnormal electric discharges of the cerebral cortex. Of all seizure cases, 75% are considered to be primary, or **idiopathic** (of unknown cause), and the remaining are secondary to brain trauma, brain **anoxia** (absence of oxygen), infection, or cerebrovascular disorders (e.g., cerebrovascular accident, stroke). Epilepsy is a chronic, usually lifelong, disorder. The majority of persons with seizures had their first seizure before 20 years of age.

Seizures that are not associated with epilepsy could result from fever, hypoglycemic reaction, electrolyte imbalance (hyponatremia), metabolic imbalance (acidosis or alkalosis), and alcohol or drug use. When these conditions are corrected, the seizures cease. Recurrent seizures may result from birth and perinatal injuries, head trauma, congenital malformations, neoplasms (tumors), and idiopathic or unknown causes.

INTERNATIONAL CLASSIFICATION OF SEIZURES

There are various types of seizures, such as **grand mal** (tonic-clonic), **petit mal** (absence), and **psychomotor**. The international classification of seizures (Table 22-1) describes two categories of seizure: generalized and partial. A person may also have mixed (more than one type) seizures.

ANTICONVULSANTS

Drugs used for epileptic seizures are called **anticonvulsants** or antiepileptic drugs (AEDs). Anticonvulsant drugs stabilize nerve cell membranes and suppress the abnormal electric impulses in the cerebral cortex. These drugs prevent seizures but do not eliminate the cause or provide a cure. Anticonvulsants are classified as central nervous system (CNS) depressants.

With the use of anticonvulsants, seizures are controlled in approximately 70% of patients. Anticonvulsants are usually taken throughout the person's lifetime. In some cases, the health care provider might discontinue the anticonvulsant if no seizures have occurred in the past 3 to 5 years.

There are many types of anticonvulsants used to treat seizures, including the hydantoins (phenytoin), long-acting barbiturates (phenobarbital, mephobarbital, primidone), succinimides (ethosuximide), benzodiazepines (diazepam, clonazepam), carbamazepine, and valproate (valproic acid). Anticonvulsants are not indicated for all types of seizures. For example, phenytoin is effective in treating grand mal (tonic-clonic) seizures and psychomotor seizures but is not effective in treating petit mal (absence) seizures.

Pharmacophysiology: Action of Anticonvulsants

The anticonvulsant drugs work in one of three ways: (1) by suppressing sodium influx through the drug binding to the sodium channel when it is inactivated, prolonging the channel inactivation and thereby preventing neuron firing; (2) by suppressing the calcium influx, preventing the electric current generated by the calcium ions to the T-type calcium channel; or (3) by increasing the action of gamma-aminobutyric acid (GABA), which inhibits neurotransmitter throughout the brain. The drugs that suppress sodium influx are phenytoin,

TABLE 22-1 INTERNATIONAL CLASSIFICATION OF SEIZURES

CATEGORY	CHARACTERISTICS
Generalized Seizures	Convulsive and nonconvulsive; involve both cerebral hemispheres of the brain
Tonic-clonic seizure	Also called *grand mal seizure;* most common form of seizure. In the tonic phase, skeletal muscles contract or tighten in a spasm lasting 3 to 5 seconds. In the clonic phase, there is a dysrhythmic muscular contraction, or jerkiness, of legs and arms lasting 2 to 4 minutes
Tonic seizure	Sustained muscle contraction
Clonic seizure	Dysrhythmic muscle contraction
Absence seizure	Also called *petit mal seizure;* brief loss of consciousness lasting less than 10 seconds; fewer than three spike waves on the electroencephalogram (EEG) printout; usually occurs in children
Myoclonic seizure	Isolated clonic contraction or jerks lasting 3 to 10 seconds; may be limited to one limb (focal myoclonic) or involve the entire body (massive myoclonic); may be secondary to a neurologic disorder such as encephalitis or Tay-Sachs disease
Atonic seizure	Head drop; loss of posture; sudden loss of muscle tone. If lower limbs are involved, patient could collapse
Infantile spasms	Muscle spasm
Partial Seizures	Involve one hemisphere of the brain. No loss of consciousness in simple partial seizures, but there is a loss of consciousness in complex partial seizures
Simple seizure	Occurs in motor, sensory, autonomic, and psychic forms; no loss of consciousness
Motor	Formerly called the *Jacksonian seizure;* involves spontaneous movement that spreads; can develop into a generalized seizure
Sensory	Visual, auditory, or taste hallucinations
Autonomic response	Paleness, flushing, sweating, or vomiting
Psychological	Personality changes
Complex seizure	Loss of consciousness. Patient does not recall behavior immediately before, during, and immediately after seizure
Psychomotor	Complex symptoms: automatisms (repetitive behavior such as chewing or swallowing motions), behavioral changes, and motor seizures
Cognitive	Confusion or memory impairment
Affective	Bizarre behavior
Compound	May lead to generalized seizures such as tonic-clonic, tonic

fosphenytoin, carbamazepine, oxcarbazepine, valproic acid, topiramate, zonisamide, and lamotrigine. Valproic acid and ethosuximide are examples of drugs that suppress calcium influx. Examples of drug groups that enhance the action of GABA are barbiturates, benzodiazepines, and tiagabine. Gabapentin promotes GABA release.

Hydantoins

The first anticonvulsant used to treat seizures was phenytoin, a hydantoin discovered in 1938 that is still the most commonly used drug for controlling seizures. **Hydantoins** act by inhibiting sodium influx, stabilizing cell membranes, reducing repetitive neuronal firing, and limiting seizures. By increasing the electrical stimulation threshold in cardiac tissue, it also acts as an antidysrhythmic. It has a small effect on general sedation, and it is nonaddicting. However, this drug should not be used during pregnancy because it can have a **teratogenic** effect on the fetus.

> **SAFETY: Preventing Medication Errors**
>
> **Do not confuse...**
> **Cerebyx** (hydantoin anticonvulsant) with **Celebrex** (nonsteroidal antiinflammatory drug). The names of these drugs look and sound alike but are different in their pharmacology.

Drug dosage for phenytoin and other anticonvulsants is age related. Newborns, persons with liver disease, and older adults require a lower dosage because of a decrease in metabolism resulting in more available drug. Conversely, individuals with an increased metabolic rate, such as children, may require an increased dosage. The drug dosage is adjusted according to the therapeutic plasma or serum level. Phenytoin has a narrow therapeutic range of 10 to 20 mcg/mL. The benefits of an anticonvulsant become apparent when the serum drug level is within the therapeutic range. Typically, if the drug level is below the desired range, the patient is not receiving the required drug dosage to control seizure activity. If the drug level is above the desired range, drug toxicity may result. Monitoring the therapeutic serum drug range is of utmost importance to ensure drug effectiveness. Prototype Drug Chart 22-1 lists the pharmacologic data associated with phenytoin.

Pharmacokinetics Phenytoin is slowly absorbed from the small intestine. It is a highly protein-bound (90% to 95%) drug; a decrease in serum protein or albumin can increase the free phenytoin serum level. With a small to average drug dose, the half-life of phenytoin is approximately 24 hours, but the range can be from 7 to 42 hours. Phenytoin is metabolized to inactive metabolites, and this portion is excreted in the urine.

Pharmacodynamics The pharmacodynamics of orally administered phenytoin include onset of action within 30 minutes to 2 hours, peak serum concentration in 1.5 to 6 hours, steady state of serum concentration in 7 to 10 days, and a duration of action dependent on the half-life of up to 45 hours. Oral phenytoin is most commonly ordered as a sustained-release (SR) capsule. The peak SR concentration time is 4 to 12 hours.

Intravenous (IV) infusion of phenytoin should be administered by direct injection into a large vein via a central line or peripherally inserted central catheter. The drug may be diluted in saline solution; however, dextrose solution should be avoided because of drug precipitation. The manufacturer recommends administration of phenytoin via Y-tube or three-way stopcock rather than continuous IV infusion to avoid precipitation. IV phenytoin 50 mg, or a fraction thereof, should be administered over 1 minute for adults and at a rate of 25 mg/min when the patient is older. Infusion rates of more than 50 mg/min may cause hypotension or cardiac dysrhythmias, especially with older and debilitated patients. Local irritation at the injection site may be noted, and **sloughing** (formation of dead tissue that separates from living tissue) may occur. The IV line should always be flushed with saline before and after each dose to reduce venous irritation. Intramuscular (IM) injection of phenytoin irritates tissues and may cause damage. For this reason and because of its erratic absorption rate, phenytoin is not given by the IM route.

Side Effects and Adverse Reactions

The severe side effects of hydantoins include neurologic and psychiatric effects (i.e., slurred speech, confusion, depression), thrombocytopenia (low platelet count), leukopenia (low white blood cell count), and **gingival hyperplasia** (overgrowth of the gum tissues or reddened gums that bleed easily). Patients on hydantoins for long periods might have an elevated blood sugar (hyperglycemia) that results from the drug inhibiting the release of insulin. Less severe side effects include nausea, vomiting, constipation, drowsiness, headaches, alopecia, hirsutism, and **nystagmus** (constant, involuntary, cyclical movement of the eyeball).

Drug-Drug Interactions

Drug interaction is common with hydantoins, because they are highly protein-bound. Hydantoins compete with other drugs (e.g., anticoagulants, aspirin) for plasma protein-binding sites. The hydantoins displace anticoagulants and aspirin, causing more free-drug availability and increasing their activity. Barbiturates, rifampin, and a chronic ingestion of ethanol increase hydantoin metabolism. Drugs like sulfonamides and cimetidine (Tagamet) can increase the action of hydantoins by inhibiting liver metabolism, which is necessary for drug excretion. Antacids, calcium preparations, sucralfate (Carafate), and antineoplastic drugs also decrease the absorption of hydantoins. Antipsychotics and certain herbs can lower the **seizure threshold** (level at which seizure may be induced) and increase seizure activity (Herbal Alert 22-1). The patient should be closely monitored for seizure occurrence.

Barbiturates

Phenobarbital, a long-acting barbiturate, is still prescribed to treat partial seizures, grand mal seizures, and acute episodes of **status epilepticus** seizures (rapid succession of epileptic

> **HERBAL ALERT 22-1**
>
> ***Anticonvulsants***
>
> - Evening primrose and borage may lower seizure threshold when these herbs are taken with anticonvulsants. The anticonvulsant dose may need modification.
> - Ginkgo may decrease phenytoin effectiveness.

PROTOTYPE DRUG CHART 22-1

Phenytoin

Drug Class Anticonvulsant: hydantoin Trade Name: Dilantin Pregnancy Category: D	**Dosage** A: PO: 4-7 mg/kg/d IV: LD: 15-20 mg/kg/d; *max:* 30 mg/kg C: 5 mg/kg/d in 2-3 divided doses; Therapeutic serum range: 10-20 mcg/mL Toxic level: 30-50 mcg/mL
Contraindications Hypersensitivity, heart block, bradycardia, psychiatric disorders, pregnancy Caution: Hyponatremia, hypotension, hypoglycemia, suicidal ideation, myasthenia gravis, systemic lupus erythematosus	**Drug-Lab-Food Interactions** Drug: Increase effects with cimetidine, isoniazid, chloramphenicol; decrease effects with folic acid, calcium, antacids, sucralfate, vinblastine, cisplatin Decrease effects of anticoagulants, oral contraceptives, antihistamines, corticosteroids, theophylline, cyclosporin, quinidine, dopamine, rifampin Food: Decreased effects of folic acid, calcium, and vitamin D as absorption is decreased by phenytoin
Pharmacokinetics Absorption: PO: Slowly absorbed; IM: Erratic rate of absorption Distribution: PB: 90-95% Metabolism: t½: 7-42 h; average: 24 h Excretion: In urine, small amount; in bile and feces, moderate amounts	**Pharmacodynamics** PO: Onset: 0.5-2 h Peak: 1.5-6 h Duration: 6-12 h IV: Onset: Within minutes to 1 h Peak: 2 h moderate amount Duration: >12 h
Therapeutic Effects/Uses To prevent tonic-clonic (grand mal) and complex partial seizures Mode of Action: Reduces motor cortex activity by altering ion transport	
Side Effects Headache, diplopia, confusion, dizziness, sluggish, decreased coordination, ataxia, slurred speech, rash, anorexia, nausea, vomiting, hypotension (after IV administration), pink-red/brown discoloration of urine	**Adverse Reactions** Leukopenia, hepatitis, depression, gingival hyperplasia, nystagmus, hirsutism, osteoporosis Life-threatening: Aplastic anemia, thrombocytopenia, agranulocytosis, Stevens-Johnson syndrome, hypotension, ventricular fibrillation, encephalopathy, suicidal ideation

A, Adult; *C,* child; *d,* day; *h,* hour; *IM,* intramuscular; *IV,* intravenous; *LD,* loading dose; *max,* maximum; *min,* minute; *PB,* protein-binding; *PO,* by mouth; *q.i.d.,* four times a day; *t ½,* half-life; *t.i.d.,* three times a day; >, greater than; <, less than.

seizures); meningitis; toxic reactions; and eclampsia. Barbiturates reduce seizures by enhancing the activity of GABA, which is an inhibitory neurotransmitter. Possible teratogenic effects and other side effects related to phenytoin are less pronounced with phenobarbital. The therapeutic serum range of phenobarbital is 20 to 40 mcg/mL. Risks associated with the use of phenobarbital include sedation and patient tolerance to the drug. Discontinuance of phenobarbital should be gradual to avoid recurrence of seizures.

Succinimides

The succinimide drug group is used to treat absence or petit mal seizures, and it may be used in combination with other anticonvulsants to treat such seizures. Ethosuximide (Zarontin) is the succinimide of choice. Succinimides act by decreasing calcium influx through the T-type calcium channels. The therapeutic serum range of ethosuximide is 40 to 100 mcg/mL. Adverse affects include blood dyscrasias, renal and liver impairment, and systemic lupus erythematosus.

Benzodiazepines

The three benzodiazepines that have anticonvulsant effects are clonazepam, clorazepate dipotassium, and diazepam. Clonazepam is effective in controlling petit mal (absence) seizures, but tolerance may occur 6 months after drug therapy starts, and consequently clonazepam dosage must be adjusted. Clorazepate dipotassium is frequently administered in adjunctive therapy for treating partial seizures.

Diazepam is primarily prescribed for treating acute status epilepticus and must be administered IV to achieve the desired response. The drug has a short-term effect; thus other anticonvulsants such as phenytoin or phenobarbital need to be given during or immediately after administration of diazepam.

Iminostilbenes

Carbamazepine, an iminostilbene, is effective in treating refractory seizure disorders that have not responded to other anticonvulsant therapies. It is used to control grand mal and partial seizures and a combination of these seizures.

Carbamazepine is also used for psychiatric disorders (e.g., bipolar disease), trigeminal neuralgia (as an analgesic), and alcohol withdrawal. The therapeutic serum range of carbamazepine is 5 to 12 mcg/mL.

An interaction may occur when grapefruit juice is taken with carbamazepine (Tegretol), causing possible toxicity. Therefore drug concentrations must be monitored carefully.

Valproate

Valproic acid has been prescribed for petit mal, grand mal, and mixed types of seizures. The safety and efficacy of this drug has not been established for children younger than 2 years of age. Care should be taken when giving this drug to very young children and to patients with liver disorders, because hepatotoxicity is one of the possible adverse reactions. Liver enzymes should be monitored. The therapeutic serum range for a patient with seizures is 50 to 100 mcg/mL. The FDA has approved divalproex sodium (Depakote) for treatment of manic episodes associated with bipolar disorder.

Table 22-2 lists the various anticonvulsants and their dosages, uses, and considerations. Table 22-3 lists selected anticonvulsants that are frequently prescribed to treat seizure disorders.

Anticonvulsant dosages usually start low and gradually increase over a period of weeks until the serum drug level is within therapeutic range or the seizures cease. Serum anticonvulsant drug levels should be closely monitored to prevent toxicity.

Anticonvulsants and Pregnancy

During pregnancy, seizure episodes increase 25% in women with epilepsy. Hypoxia that may occur during seizures places both the pregnant woman and her fetus at risk.

Many anticonvulsant drugs have teratogenic properties that increase the risk for fetal malformations. Phenytoin and carbamazepine have been linked to fetal anomalies such as cardiac defects and cleft lip and palate. It has been reported that valproic acid is known to cause major congenital malformation in infants in 4% to 8% of pregnant women who take the drug. As expected, the highest incidence of birth defects occurs when the woman takes combinations of anticonvulsant drugs.

Anticonvulsant drugs tend to act as inhibitors of vitamin K, contributing to hemorrhage in infants shortly after birth. Frequently, pregnant women taking anticonvulsants are given an oral vitamin K supplement during the last week or 10 days of the pregnancy, or vitamin K is administered to the infant soon after birth.

Anticonvulsants also increase the loss of folate (folic acid) in pregnant women. Thus, pregnant individuals should take daily folate supplements.

Anticonvulsants and Febrile Seizures

Seizures associated with fever usually occur in children between 3 months and 5 years of age. Epilepsy develops in approximately 2.5% of children who have had one or more febrile seizures. Prophylactic anticonvulsant treatment such as phenobarbital or diazepam may be indicated for high-risk patients. Valproic acid should not be given to children younger than 2 years of age because of its possible hepatotoxic effect.

Nursing Process
Patient-Centered Collaborative Care

Anticonvulsants: Phenytoin

Assessment

- Obtain a health history including current drugs and herbs patient uses. Report and document any probable drug-drug or herb-drug interactions.
- Assess patient's knowledge regarding medication regimen.
- Check urinary output to determine whether adequate (>1500 mL/d).
- Determine laboratory values related to renal and liver function. If both BUN and creatinine levels are elevated, a renal disorder should be suspected. Elevated serum liver enzymes (alkaline phosphatase, alanine aminotransferase, gamma-glutamyl transferase, 59-nucleotidase) indicate a hepatic disorder.

Nursing Diagnoses

- Risk for injury related to decreased coordination
- Impaired oral mucous membranes related to blood dyscrasias
- Imbalanced nutrition: less than body requirements related to anorexia
- Risk for falls related to dizziness secondary to phenytoin side effect

Planning

- Patient will be free of seizures.
- Patient will adhere to anticonvulsant therapy.
- Patient's side effects from phenytoin will be minimal.

Nursing Interventions

- Monitor serum drug levels of anticonvulsant to determine therapeutic range (10 to 20 mcg/mL).
- Encourage patient's compliance to medication regimen.
- Monitor patient's CBC levels for early detection of blood dyscrasias.
- Use seizure precautions (environmental protection from sharp objects, such as table corners) for patients at risk for seizures.
- Determine whether patient is receiving adequate nutrients; phenytoin may cause anorexia, nausea, and vomiting.

TABLE 22-2 ANTICONVULSANTS

GENERIC (BRAND)	ROUTE AND DOSAGE	USES AND CONSIDERATIONS
Barbiturates		
mephobarbital (Mebaral) CSS IV	A: PO: 200-600 mg/d in 2-4 divided doses; *max:* 600 mg/d for seizures C: 6-12 mg/kg/d in 2-4 divided doses	For grand mal and petit mal (absence) seizures. May be used in combination with other anticonvulsants. Also used to manage delirium tremens. May cause drowsiness, dizziness, suicidal ideation. Pregnancy category: D; PB: UK; $t\frac{1}{2}$: 11-67 h
phenobarbital (generic) CSS IV	Status epilepticus: A/C: IV: 15-18 mg/kg; *max:* 30 mg/kg Maintenance: A/C: PO: 1-3 mg/kg/d in 2 divided doses; Therapeutic serum range: 20-40 mcg/mL	Long-acting barbiturate. Used for grand mal (tonic-clonic) seizures, partial seizures, and to control status epilepticus. May be used in combination with phenytoin. High doses for adults may lead to coma and respiratory depression. High doses for older adults or children may cause confusion, depression, irritability. Adverse effects include suicidal ideation. Long-term use with high doses could cause physical dependence. Pregnancy category: D; PB: 20%-45%; $t\frac{1}{2}$: A: 50-120 h; C: 35-75 h
primidone (Mysoline)	A: PO: 125-250 mg/d; *max:* 2 g/d C: <8 y: PO: 50-125 mg/d; *max:* 25 mg/kg/d Therapeutic serum range: 5-12 mcg/mL	Barbiturate-like drug. Used to manage grand mal and psychomotor seizures. Take with food if drug causes GI distress. Pregnancy category: D; PB: 20%-45%; $t\frac{1}{2}$: 10-12 h
Benzodiazepines (Anxiolytics)		
clonazepam (Klonopin) CSS IV	A: PO: 1.5 mg/d; gradually increase dose q3d until seizures controlled; *max:* 20 mg/d C: PO: 0.01-0.03 mg/kg/d; *max:* 0.05 mg/kg/d	For petit mal (absence), myoclonus, and status epilepticus. May be used when petit mal seizures are refractory to succinimides or valproic acid. Pregnancy category: D; PB: 85%; $t\frac{1}{2}$: 25-40 h
clorazepate (Tranxene) CSS IV	A: PO: 7.5 mg t.i.d.; *max:* 90 mg/d C: >9 y: PO: 3.75-7.5 mg b.i.d.; *max:* 60 mg/d	May be used for partial seizures and as adjunctive therapy for seizures. Also treats anxiety and acute alcohol withdrawal. Pregnancy category: D; PB: 97%; $t\frac{1}{2}$: 48 h
diazepam (Valium) CSS IV	Status epilepticus: A: IV: 5-10 mg; repeat if needed at 10- to 15-min intervals; *max:* 30 mg C: <5 y: IV: 0.2-0.5 mg over 2-5 min; *max:* 5 mg C: >5 y: IV 1 mg/kg q2-5 min slowly; repeat if needed: *max:* 10 mg	For status epilepticus (drug of choice). Administer IV slowly to avoid respiratory depression and hypotension, and repeat q10-15min up to 30 mg PRN; then q2-4h PRN. Also treats anxiety and substance abuse withdrawal. Pregnancy category: D; PB: 98%; $t\frac{1}{2}$: 30-60 h
lorazepam (Ativan) CSS IV	Status epilepticus: A: IV: 4 mg over 2-5 min; *max:* 10 mg/d; may repeat in 10-15 min Anxiety: A: PO: 2-3 mg/d in 2-3 divided doses Older adult: PO: 1-2 mg/d in 2-3 divided doses; *max:* 2 mg/d for skilled nursing facility residents	To control status epilepticus. Infusion rate should not exceed 2 mg/min. Also treats anxiety and substance abuse withdrawal. Pregnancy category: D; PB: 91%; $t\frac{1}{2}$: 12-14 h
Hydantoins		
fosphenytoin (Cerebyx)	A: IV: LD: 10-20 mg PE/kg Maintenance: 4-6 mg PE/kg/d Status epilepticus: IV: LD: 15-20 mg PE/kg infused at 100-150 mg PE/min	For grand mal seizures, complex partial seizures, and status epilepticus. Decreases sodium and calcium ion influx in the neurons. Converts to phenytoin. Dilute in D_5W or 0.9% NaCl. Pregnancy category: D; PB: 95%-99%; $t\frac{1}{2}$: 8-15 min
phenytoin (Dilantin)	See Prototype Drug Chart 22-1.	
Iminostilbene		
carbamazepine (Tegretol)	A: PO: 200 mg b.i.d.; increasing doses as needed C: >6 y: PO: 10 mg/kg/d in divided doses; *max:* 35 mg/kg/d C: 6-12 y: 100 mg b.i.d.; *max:* 1g/d Therapeutic serum range: 5-12 mcg/mL	For tonic-clonic, partial, simple, and complex seizures. Used in treating seizures unresponsive to other anticonvulsants. Now approved to treat bipolar disorder. Pregnancy category: D; PB: 76%; $t\frac{1}{2}$: 12-17 h after repeated dosing
oxcarbazepine (Trileptal, Oxtellar XR)	A: PO: 300 mg b.i.d.; increase to 2400 mg/d C: 4-16 y: PO: 8-10 mg/kg Extended release: A: PO: Initially 600 mg qd; may increase 600 mg/d to target range of 1200-2400 mg qd	To control refractory partial seizures as monotherapy. Can be used for generalized tonic-clonic seizures and as adjunctive therapy for partial seizures. Blocks the sodium channel. Less adverse effects than carbamazepine; drug-level monitoring is usually not necessary. Pregnancy category: C; PB: 40%; $t\frac{1}{2}$: 2 h
Succinimides		
ethosuximide (Zarontin)	A: PO: 250 mg b.i.d.; increase dose gradually *max:* 1.5 g/d C: 3-6 y: PO: Initially 15 mg/kg/d; may increase to 40 mg/kg/d Therapeutic serum range: 40-100 mcg/mL	For petit mal (absence) and myoclonic seizures. Gastric irritation is common; may take with food. Pregnancy category: C; PB: UK; $t\frac{1}{2}$: A: 50-60 h, C: 25-30 h

Continued

TABLE 22-2 ANTICONVULSANTS—cont'd

GENERIC (BRAND)	ROUTE AND DOSAGE	USES AND CONSIDERATIONS
Valproate		
valproate, valproic acid, divalproex Na (Depakote)	A/C: PO: 10-15 mg/kg/d in divided doses; Increase 5-10 mg/kg/d weekly until seizures controlled; *max:* 60 mg/kg/d Therapeutic serum range: 50-100 mcg/mL	For psychomotor, myoclonic, absence, and tonic-clonic seizures. Also approved for bipolar disorder and migraine prophylaxis. Avoid during pregnancy. Pregnancy category: D; PB: 90%; t½: 6-16 h
Miscellaneous		
acetazolamide (Diamox)	Commonly used with other anticonvulsants: A: PO: 8-30 mg/kg/d in divided doses; *max:* 1 g/d	For grand mal, petit mal (absence), and focal seizures. Maintain adequate fluid intake to prevent renal impairment. Pregnancy category: C; PB: 90%; t½: 10-15 h
gabapentin (Neurontin)	Adjunctive therapy for partial seizures: A: PO: 300-1200 mg/d in 3 divided doses; max time between doses: 12 h; *max:* 3600 mg/d C: 3-12 y: 10-15 mg/kg/d; *max:* 50 mg/kg/d	Used as adjunctive therapy for partial seizures. Promotes GABA release. To avoid GI upset, give drug with food. High doses are limited to short-term. If drug is discontinued, gradually reduce dose to avoid occurrence of seizures. Pregnancy category: C; PB: 3%; t½: 5-7 h
lamotrigine (Lamictal)	A: PO: Initially: 50 mg/d for 2 wk; then 50 mg b.i.d. for 2 wk; increase by 100 mg/d q1-2wk up to recommended maintenance dose of 250 mg b.i.d.	For partial and tonic-clonic seizures. Also used for treatment of Lennox-Gastaut syndrome in adults and children. Blocks sodium influx. May be given with other anticonvulsants. Discontinue if rash appears as may develop life-threatening Stevens-Johnson syndrome. Pregnancy category: C; PB: 55%; t½: 25-30 h
levetiracetam (Keppra)	A: PO: 500 mg b.i.d.; may increase dose q2wk by 1000 mg/d; *max:* 3000 mg/d in divided doses	For complex partial seizures. For adjunctive and monotherapy. Unlikely to cause drug interactions. Pregnancy category: C; PB: <10%; t½: 6-8 h
tiagabine (Gabitril)	A: PO: 4 mg/d; may increase by 4-8 mg/d; *max:* 56 mg/d C: 12-18 y: PO: 4 mg/d; may increase by 4-8 mg; *max:* 32 mg/d	For partial seizures as adjunctive therapy. Increases GABA levels. Pregnancy category: C; PB: 96%; t½: 7-9 h
topiramate (Topamax)	A: PO: 50 mg/d in 2 divided doses; may increase 50 mg/d by weekly increment; *max:* 1600 mg/d C: 2-16 y: PO: Initially 25 mg/d h.s.; may increase 25 mg/d by weekly increment; *max:* 9 mg/kg/d	For partial seizures and generalized tonic-clonic seizures. Inhibits calcium channels and increases action of GABA. Older adults can take adult dose. Pregnancy category: D; PB: 15%-41%; t½: 21 h
zonisamide (Zonegran)	A/C: >16 y: PO: 100 mg/d for 2 wk; may increase 100 mg/d at 2 wk intervals; *max:* 400 mg/d	For adjunctive treatment of partial seizures. Blocks sodium and calcium channels. Does not affect serum levels of phenytoin or valproic acid. Contraindicated if sensitive to sulfonamides. Pregnancy category: C; PB: 40%; t½: 60 h
magnesium sulfate	Preeclampsia or eclampsia: A: IV: Initially 4 g over 3-4 min, follow with 1-3 g/h via infusion pump; *max:* 40 g/d Hypomagnesemic seizures: A: IV/IM: 1 to 2 g q6h for 4 doses based on blood levels, then 60 mg/kg/d	To control seizures in toxemia of pregnancy caused by eclampsia or preeclampsia. Pregnancy category: A; PB: UK; t½: UK
pregabalin (Lyrica)	Adjunctive therapy for partial seizures: A: PO: Initially 150 mg/d in 2-3 divided doses; *max:* 600 mg/d Fibromyalgia: A: PO: Initially 75 mg b.i.d.; may increase to 150 mg b.i.d. within 1 week; *max:* 450 mg/d	For partial seizures and neuralgia. Binds $alpha_2$-delta receptor sites affecting calcium channels in CNS tissues. Pregnancy category: C; PB: 0%; t½: 6 h
lacosamide (Vimpat)	A: PO: 50 mg b.i.d.; maintenance: 200-400 mg/d	For partial seizures. Side effects include blurred vision, dizziness, fatigue, suicidal ideation. Pregnancy category: C; PB: 15%; t½: 13 h
ezogabine (Potiga)	A: PO: Initially 100 mg t.i.d.; increase up to 200-400 mg t.i.d.; *max:* 1200 mg t.i.d. Older adult: PO: Initially 50 mg t.i.d.; increase up to 250 mg t.i.d.; *max:* 750 mg t.i.d.	For partial seizures. Side effects include blurred vision, nystagmus, dizziness, appetite stimulation, leukopenia, neutropenia, suicidal ideation. Pregnancy category: C; PB: 80%; t½: 7-11 h
perampanel (Fycompa)	A/C: >12 y: PO: Initially 2 mg at bedtime; increase by 2 mg/d on weekly basis to 4-8 mg qHS; *max:* 12 mg/d	For partial seizures. Common side effects include dizziness, drowsiness, headache, fatigue, and irritability. Has black box warning of life-threatening psychiatric and behavioral reactions, such as aggression, hostility, anger, and homicidal ideation. Notify health care provider if any changes in mood, behavior, or personality occur. Pregnancy category: C; PB: 95%-96%; t½: 105 h

A, Adult; *b.i.d.,* twice a day; *C,* child; *CNS,* central nervous system; *CSS,* Controlled Substances Schedule; *GABA,* gamma aminobutyric acid; *GI,* gastrointestinal; *d,* day; *h,* hour; *IM,* intramuscular; *IV,* intravenous; *LD,* loading dose; *max,* maximum; *min,* minute; *PB,* protein-binding; *PE,* phenytoin equivalents; *PO,* by mouth; *PRN,* as needed; *q.i.d.,* four times a day; *sol,* solution; *SR,* sustained-release; *t½,* half-life; *UK,* unknown; *y,* year; *>,* greater than; *<,* less than.

TABLE 22-3 SELECTED ANTICONVULSANTS FOR SEIZURE DISORDERS

SEIZURE DISORDER	DRUG THERAPY
Tonic-clonic (grand mal)	phenytoin carbamazepine fosphenytoin valproic acid lamotrigine primidone phenobarbital
Partial (complex-secondarily generalized)	phenytoin carbamazepine oxcarbazepine levetiracetam primidone phenobarbital tiagabine topiramate zonisamide
Absence (petit mal)	ethosuximide valproic acid lamotrigine clonazepam
Myoclonic, atonic, atypical absence	valproic acid lamotrigine clonazepam
Status epilepticus	diazepam fosphenytoin lorazepam phenytoin

- Advise female patients who are taking oral contraceptives and anticonvulsants to use an additional contraceptive method.

Patient Teaching

General

- Teach patient to shake suspension form thoroughly before use to adequately mix medication and assure accurate dosage.
- Advise patient not to drive or perform other hazardous activities when initiating anticonvulsant therapy as drowsiness may occur.
- Counsel female patients contemplating pregnancy to consult with health care provider, because phenytoin and valproic acid may have a teratogenic effect.
- Monitor serum phenytoin levels closely during pregnancy, because seizures tend to become more frequent due to increased metabolic rates.
- Warn patient to avoid alcohol and other CNS depressants, because they can cause an added depressive effect on the body.
- Explain to patient that certain herbs can interact with an anticonvulsant drug (see Herbal Alert 22-1) and dose adjustment may be required.
- Encourage patient to obtain medical alert identification card, medical alert bracelet, or tag that indicates health diagnosis and drug regimen.
- Teach patient not to abruptly stop drug therapy, but rather to withdraw the prescribed drug gradually under medical supervision to prevent seizure rebound (recurrence of seizures) and status epilepticus (continuous seizure state).

TABLE 22-4 SELECTED ANTICONVULSANTS: PHARMACOKINETICS, PHARMACODYNAMICS, AND THERAPEUTIC RANGES

	PHARMACOKINETICS			PHARMACODYNAMICS			
DRUG	PROTEIN-BINDING (%)	t½	EXCRETION	PO ONSET	PEAK TIME (h)	DURATION OF ACTION (h)	THERAPEUTIC SERUM RANGE
phenytoin (Dilantin)	95	6-45 h (average 22 h)	Kidneys, bile, and GI	30 min to 2 h	1.5-3	6-12	10-20 mcg/mL
phenobarbital	20-45	2-6 d	50%-75% in urine	30-60 min	8-12	6-24	20-40 mcg/mL
ethosuximide (Zarontin)	UK	A: 50-60 h C: 25-30 h	25% in urine unchanged	UK	>4	12-60	50-150 mcg/mL
clonazepam (Klonopin)	85	25-40 h	Kidneys and feces	20-60 min	1-2	6-12	20-80 ng/mL
carbamazepine (Tegretol)	75-90	15-30 h	75% in urine, 25% in feces	Varies	4-7	6-12	5-12 mcg/mL
valproic acid (Depakene)	90	6-16 h	Kidneys	20-30 min	1-4	24	40-100 mcg/mL

A, Adult; *C*, child; *d*, day; *GI*, gastrointestinal; *h*, hour; *min*, minute; *PO*, by mouth; *t½*, half-life; *UK*, unknown; >, greater than.

- Counsel patient about the need for preventive dental checkups.
- Warn patient to take prescribed anticonvulsant, get laboratory tests as ordered, and keep follow-up visits with health care provider.
- Teach patient not to self-medicate with over-the-counter (OTC) drugs without first consulting health care provider.
- Advise patient with diabetes to monitor serum glucose levels more closely than usual because phenytoin may inhibit insulin release, causing an increase in glucose level.
- Inform patient of the existence of national, state, and local associations that provide resources, current information, and support for persons with epilepsy.

Diet
- Coach patient to take anticonvulsant at the same time every day with food or milk.

Side Effects
- Tell patient that urine may be a harmless pinkish red or reddish brown.
- Advise patient to maintain good oral hygiene and to use a soft toothbrush to prevent gum irritation and bleeding.
- Teach patient to report symptoms of sore throat, bruising, and nosebleeds, which may indicate a blood dyscrasia.
- Encourage patient to inform health care provider of adverse reactions such as gingivitis, nystagmus, slurred speech, rash, and dizziness. Stevens-Johnson syndrome begins with a rash.

Cultural Considerations
- Communicate respect for cultural beliefs concerning refusal or reluctance to take anticonvulsant medications daily for life; use an interpreter and the extended family as needed to help patient understand importance of keeping to a prescribed drug regimen.
- Use a written drug schedule in patient's preferred language to support adherence to prescribed drug regimen.
- Encourage patient's compliance with follow-up by a community nurse.
- When language barriers exist, videos and pictures showing patient's own cultural group may help strengthen compliance with health interventions.

Evaluation
- Evaluate effectiveness of drug in controlling seizures.
- Continue to monitor serum phenytoin levels to determine whether they are within desired range. High serum levels of phenytoin are frequently indicators of phenytoin toxicity.
- Monitor patient for hydantoin overdose. Initial symptoms are nystagmus and ataxia (impaired coordination). Later symptoms are hypotension, unresponsive pupils, and coma. Respiratory and circulatory support, as well as hemodialysis, are usually used in the treatment of phenytoin overdose.

Anticonvulsants and Status Epilepticus

Status epilepticus, a continuous seizure state, is considered a medical emergency. If treatment is not begun immediately, death could result. The choices of pharmacologic agents are diazepam (Valium) administered IV or lorazepam (Ativan) followed by IV administration of phenytoin (Dilantin). For continued seizures, midazolam (Versed) or propofol (Diprivan) and then high-dose barbiturates are used. These drugs should be administered slowly to avoid respiratory depression.

The pharmacologic behavior of specific anticonvulsants is summarized in Table 22-4.

KEY WEBSITES

Management of status epilepticus: *www.emedicine.medscape.com/article/1164462-overview*

Phenytoin: *www.drugs.com/phenytoin.html/*

Seizure disorders in the older adult: *www.epilepsyfoundation.org/livingwithepilepsy/seniors/*

CRITICAL THINKING CASE STUDY

SS, a 26-year-old woman, takes phenytoin 100 mg t.i.d. to control grand mal seizures. SS and her husband are contemplating starting a family.

1. What action should the nurse take in regard to patient family planning?
   SS complains of frequent "upset stomach" and "bleeding gums" when brushing her teeth.
2. To decrease GI distress, what can be suggested?
3. To alleviate bleeding gums, what patient teaching for SS may be included?
4. The nurse checks SS's serum phenytoin level. What are the indications of an abnormal serum level? What appropriate actions should be taken?

NCLEX STUDY QUESTIONS

1. The nurse witnesses a patient's seizure involving generalized contraction of the body followed by jerkiness of the arms and legs. The nurse reports that this is which type of seizure?
   a. Myoclonic
   b. Petit mal
   c. Tonic clonic
   d. Psychomotor
2. Phenytoin has been prescribed for a patient with seizures. The nurse should include which appropriate nursing intervention in the plan of care?
   a. Report an abnormal phenytoin level of 18 mcg/mL.
   b. Monitor CBC levels for early detection of blood dyscrasias.
   c. Encourage the patient to brush teeth vigorously to prevent plaque buildup.
   d. Teach the patient to stop the drug immediately when passing pinkish-red or reddish-brown urine.
3. When administering phenytoin, the nurse realizes more teaching is needed if the patient makes which statement?
   a. "I must shake the oral suspension very well before pouring it in the dose cup."
   b. "I cannot drink alcoholic beverages when taking phenytoin."
   c. "I should take phenytoin 1 hour before meals."
   d. "I will need to get periodic dental checkups."
4. A patient is having absence (petit mal) seizures. Which of the following does the nurse expect to be prescribed for this type of seizures? (Select all that apply.)
   a. phenytoin (Dilantin)
   b. phenobarbital (Luminal)
   c. valproic acid (Depakote)
   d. clonazepam (Klonopin)
   e. ethosuximide (Zarontin)
5. A patient is admitted to the emergency department with status epilepticus. Which drug should the nurse most likely prepare to administer to this patient? (Select all that apply.)
   a. diazepam (Valium)
   b. midazolam (Versed)
   c. gabapentin (Neurontin)
   d. levetiracetam (Keppra)
   e. topiramate (Topamax)
6. The nurse should monitor the patient receiving phenytoin for which adverse effect?
   a. Psychosis
   b. Nosebleeds
   c. Hypertension
   d. Gum erosion
7. The nurse is administering valproic acid (Depakote) to a patient. The nurse checks the laboratory values and finds a serum range for valproic acid of 200 mcg/ml. What should the nurse do?
   a. Increase the daily dose to get the patient's level to a therapeutic range.
   b. Hold the morning dose but give the other scheduled dosages for the day.
   c. Ask the patient if he is having any adverse effects from the medication.
   d. Hold the medication and notify the health care provider.

Answers: 1, c; 2, b; 3, c; 4, c, d, e; 5, a, b; 6, b; 7, d.

CHAPTER

23

Drugs for Neurologic Disorders: Parkinsonism and Alzheimer's Disease

evolve WEBSITE

http://evolve.elsevier.com/KeeHayes/pharmacology/

- Animations
- Content Updates
- Key Points
- Review Questions for the NCLEX® Examination
- References from the Textbook
- Unfolding Case Studies

OBJECTIVES

- Summarize the pathophysiology of parkinsonism and Alzheimer's disease.
- Contrast the actions of anticholinergics, dopaminergics, dopamine agonists, MAO-B inhibitors, and COMT inhibitors in the treatment of parkinsonism.
- Compare the side effects of various antiparkinsonism drugs.
- Apply the nursing process to anticholinergics, dopaminergics, and acetylcholinesterase inhibitors.
- Differentiate the phases of Alzheimer's disease with corresponding symptoms.
- Compare the side effects/adverse effects of acetylcholinesterase inhibitors that are used to treat Alzheimer's disease.

OUTLINE

KEY TERMS

acetylcholinesterase inhibitors, p. 322
Alzheimer's disease, p. 314
bradykinesia, p. 314
dopamine agonists, p. 315
dyskinesia, p. 321
dystonic movement, p. 317
parkinsonism, p. 314
pseudoparkinsonism, p. 315

Parkinsonism (Parkinson's disease) is a chronic neurologic disorder that affects the extrapyramidal motor tract (which controls posture, balance, and locomotion). It is considered a syndrome (combination of symptoms) because of its three major features: rigidity, **bradykinesia** (slow movement), and tremors. Rigidity (abnormally increased muscle tone) increases with movement. Postural changes caused by rigidity and bradykinesia include the chest and head thrust forward with the knees and hips flexed, a shuffling gait, and the absence of arm swing. Other characteristic symptoms are masked facies (no facial expression), involuntary tremors of the head and neck, and pill-rolling motions of the hands. The tremors may be more prevalent at rest.

Alzheimer's disease is a chronic, progressive, neurodegenerative condition with marked cognitive dysfunction. Various theories exist as to the cause of Alzheimer's disease: neuritic plaques, degeneration of the cholinergic neurons, and deficiency in acetylcholine.

PARKINSONISM

In 1817, Dr. James Parkinson described six patients as having "shaking palsy." Three symptoms were described by Parkinson: (1) involuntary tremors of the limbs, (2) rigidity of muscles, and (3) slowness of movement. In the United States, there are approximately one million persons with **parkinsonism,** and 50,000 new cases are diagnosed each year. Because parkinsonism generally affects patients 50 years of age and older, many consider the health problem to be part of the aging process caused by loss of neurons. The three cardinal symptoms are rigidity, tremors, and bradykinesia. Normally the symptoms have a gradual onset and are usually mild and unilateral in the beginning.

There are different types of parkinsonism. **Pseudoparkinsonism** frequently occurs as an adverse reaction to antipsychotic drugs, especially the phenothiazines. In addition, parkinsonism symptoms could result from poisons (e.g., carbon monoxide, manganese), arteriosclerosis, and Wilson's disease (hepatolenticular degeneration).

Nonpharmacologic Measures

Symptoms of parkinsonism can be lessened through the use of nonpharmacologic measures such as patient teaching, exercise, nutrition, and group support. Exercise can improve mobility and flexibility; the patient with parkinsonism should enroll in a therapeutic exercise program tailored to this disorder. A balanced diet with fiber and fluids helps prevent constipation and weight loss. Patients with parkinsonism and their family members should be encouraged to attend a support group to help cope with and understand this disorder.

Pathophysiology

Parkinsonism is caused by an imbalance of the neurotransmitters dopamine (DA) and acetylcholine (ACh). It is marked by degeneration of neurons of the extrapyramidal motor tract. The reason for the degeneration of neurons is unknown.

There are two neurotransmitters within neurons of the striatum of the brain: dopamine, an inhibitory neurotransmitter, and acetylcholine, an excitatory neurotransmitter. Dopamine is released from the dopaminergic neurons; acetylcholine is released from the cholinergic neurons. Dopamine normally maintains control of acetylcholine and inhibits its excitatory response. In parkinsonism, there is an unexplained degeneration of the dopaminergic neurons, and an imbalance between dopamine and acetylcholine occurs. With less dopamine production, the excitatory response of acetylcholine exceeds the inhibitory response of dopamine. An excessive amount of acetylcholine stimulates neurons that release GABA. With increased stimulation of GABA, the symptomatic movement disorders of parkinsonism occur.

By the time early symptoms of parkinsonism appear, 80% of the striatal dopamine has already been depleted. The remaining striatal neurons synthesize dopamine from levodopa and release dopamine as needed. Before the next dose of levodopa, symptoms (e.g., slow walking, loss of dexterity) return or worsen, but within 30 to 60 minutes of receiving a dose, the patient's functioning is much improved.

Drugs used to treat parkinsonism reduce the symptoms or replace the dopamine deficit. These drugs fall into five categories: (1) anticholinergics, which block cholinergic receptors; (2) dopamine replacements, which stimulate dopamine receptors; (3) **dopamine agonists,** which stimulate dopamine receptors; (4) MAO-B inhibitors, which inhibit the monoamine oxidase-B (MAO-B) enzyme that interferes with dopamine; and (5) COMT inhibitors, which inhibit the catechol *O*-methyltransferase enzyme that inactivates dopamine. Table 23-1 compares the various parkinsonism drugs.

Anticholinergics

Anticholinergic drugs reduce the rigidity and some of the tremors characteristic of parkinsonism but have minimal effect on bradykinesia. The anticholinergics are parasympatholytics that inhibit the release of acetylcholine. Anticholinergics are still used to treat drug-induced parkinsonism, or pseudoparkinsonism, a side effect of the antipsychotic drug group phenothiazines. Examples of anticholinergics used for parkinsonism include trihexyphenidyl (Artane), benztropine (Cogentin), and biperiden (Akineton).

SAFETY: Preventing Medication Errors

Do not confuse ...

- **Artane** with **Altace**

Diphenhydramine (Benadryl), an antihistamine, has similar anticholinergic properties. It is sometimes used to treat mild parkinsonism and for older adults who may not be able to tolerate the dopamine agonist group of drugs.

HERBAL ALERT 23-1

Orphenadrine Citrate

Valerian and kava kava potentiate sedation.

Nursing Process

Patient-Centered Collaborative Care

Antiparkinson: Anticholinergic Agent

Assessment

- Obtain patient's health history. Report if patient has a history of glaucoma, GI dysfunction, urinary retention, angina pectoris, or myasthenia gravis. All anticholinergics are contraindicated if patient has glaucoma.

TABLE 23-1 COMPARISON OF DRUGS USED TO TREAT PARKINSON'S DISEASE

DRUG	PURPOSE
Dopaminergics	
carbidopa-levodopa	Decreases symptoms of parkinsonism. Carbidopa, a decarboxylase inhibitor, permits more levodopa to reach the striatum nerve terminals (where levodopa is converted to dopamine). With the use of carbidopa, less levodopa is needed.
Dopamine Agonists	
amantadine	First used as an antiviral drug for influenza A. Decreases symptoms of parkinsonism. Can be used for early treatment of Parkinson's disease, which could delay the necessity of levodopa. Is effective in treating drug-induced parkinsonism, and has fewer side effects than anticholinergics.
bromocriptine	A D_2-dopamine receptor agonist. Can be used for early treatment of Parkinson's disease. With increasing motor symptoms, can be given with levodopa therapy.
pramipexole (Mirapex), ropinirole HCl (Requip)	D_2- and D_3-dopamine receptor agonists. Can be used in combination with levodopa. Fewer side effects than older dopamine agonists.
MAO-B Inhibitors	
selegiline HCl (Eldepryl)	Inhibits catabolic enzymes of dopamine. Extends action of dopamine. Can be used for early treatment of Parkinson's disease. If given with levodopa, dosage of levodopa is usually decreased.
rasagiline (Azilect)	Inhibits breakdown of dopamine at synapses in the brain. Allows neurons to reabsorb more dopamine for use later.
COMT Inhibitors	
entacapone (Comtan), tolcapone (Tasmar)	Inhibits COMT enzyme, increasing concentration of levodopa. Used in combination with levodopa-carbidopa (Sinemet). With COMT inhibitors, smaller dose of levodopa is needed.
Anticholinergics; Antiparkinson	
	First group of drugs used to treat Parkinson's disease before levodopa and dopamine agonists were introduced. Useful in decreasing tremors related to Parkinson's disease. The major use of these agents currently is to treat drug-induced parkinsonism. Treatment starts with low dosages, and then dose is gradually increased. Older adults are more susceptible to the many side effects of anticholinergics. Patients with memory loss or dementia should not be on anticholinergic therapy.

COMT, Catechol *O*-methyltransferase; *MAO-B,* monoamine oxidase-B.

- Obtain a drug history. Report any probable drug-drug interaction, such as phenothiazines, tricyclic antidepressants, and antihistamines, which increase the effect of trihexyphenidyl.
- Assess baseline vital signs for future comparison. Pulse rate may increase.
- Assess patient's knowledge regarding medication regimen.
- Determine usual urinary output as a baseline for comparison. Urinary retention may occur with continuous use of anticholinergics.

Nursing Diagnoses
- Impaired physical mobility related to muscle rigidity, tremors, and bradykinesia
- Impaired urinary elimination related to urinary retention
- Knowledge deficit related to unfamiliarity with drug regimen

Planning
- Patient will have decreased involuntary symptoms caused by parkinsonism or drug-induced parkinsonism.

Nursing Interventions
- Monitor vital signs, urine output, and bowel sounds. Increased pulse rate, urinary retention, and constipation are side effects of anticholinergics.
- Observe for involuntary movements.

Patient Teaching
General
- Advise patient to avoid alcohol, cigarettes, caffeine, and aspirin to decrease gastric acidity.

Side Effects
- Encourage patient to relieve dry mouth with hard candy, ice chips, or sugarless chewing gum. Anticholinergics decrease salivation.
- Suggest that patient use sunglasses in direct sunlight because of possible photophobia.
- Advise patient to void before taking the drug to minimize urinary retention.
- Counsel patient who takes an anticholinergic for control of symptoms of parkinsonism to have routine eye examinations because patients who have glaucoma should not take anticholinergics.

Diet

- Encourage patient to ingest foods high in fiber and increase fluid intake to prevent constipation.

Cultural Considerations

- Assess personal beliefs of patient or family, and modify communications to meet cultural needs; use an interpreter and community nurse follow-up as needed.

Evaluation

- Evaluate patient's response to trihexyphenidyl or benztropine mesylate to determine whether parkinsonism symptoms are controlled.

Table 23-2 lists the anticholinergics and their dosages, uses, and considerations. Anticholinergics used to treat parkinsonism are also discussed in Chapter 19.

Dopaminergics

Carbidopa and Levodopa

The first dopaminergic drug was levodopa (L-dopa), which was introduced in 1961 but is no longer available in the United States. When introduced, levodopa was effective in diminishing symptoms of Parkinson's disease and increasing mobility, because the blood-brain barrier admits levodopa but not dopamine. The enzyme dopa decarboxylase converts levodopa to dopamine in the brain, but this enzyme is also found in the peripheral nervous system and allows 99% of levodopa to be converted to dopamine *before* it reaches the brain. Therefore only about 1% of levodopa taken is available to be converted to dopamine once it reaches the brain, and large doses are needed to achieve a pharmacologic response. These high doses could cause many side effects, including nausea, vomiting, dyskinesia, orthostatic hypotension, cardiac dysrhythmias, and psychosis.

Because of the side effects of levodopa and the fact that so much levodopa is metabolized before reaching the brain, an alternative drug, carbidopa, was developed to inhibit the enzyme dopa decarboxylase. By inhibiting the enzyme in the peripheral nervous system, more levodopa reaches the brain. The carbidopa is combined with levodopa in a ratio of 1 part carbidopa to 10 parts levodopa. Figure 23-1 illustrates the comparative action of levodopa and carbidopa-levodopa.

The advantages of combining levodopa with carbidopa are as follows:

- More dopamine reaches the basal ganglia.
- Smaller doses of levodopa are required to achieve the desired effect.

The disadvantage of the carbidopa-levodopa combination is that with more available levodopa, more side effects may be noted. Side effects may include nausea, vomiting, **dystonic movement** (involuntary abnormal movement), and psychotic behavior. The peripheral side effects of levodopa are not as prevalent; however, cardiac dysrhythmia, palpitations, and orthostatic hypotension may occur. The carbidopa-levodopa combination is usually not used to treat drug-related pseudoparkinsonism. Prototype Drug Chart 23-1 lists the pharmacologic behavior of carbidopa-levodopa.

Dopamine Agonists

Other dopaminergics called **dopamine agonists** stimulate the dopamine receptors. For example, amantadine hydrochloride (Symmetrel) is an antiviral drug that acts on the dopamine receptors. It may be taken alone or in combination with carbidopa-levodopa or an anticholinergic drug. Initially, amantadine produces improvement in symptoms of

TABLE 23-2 ANTIPARKINSON DRUGS: ANTICHOLINERGICS

GENERIC (BRAND)	ROUTE AND DOSAGE	USES AND CONSIDERATIONS
benztropine mesylate (Cogentin)	Parkinsonism: A: PO/IM: Initially 0.5-1 mg/d h.s. *maint:* 6 mg/d in 2 divided doses; *max:* 8 mg/d Extrapyramidal syndrome: A: PO: 1-4 mg q.d./b.i.d.	For parkinsonism and drug-induced parkinsonism to reduce dystonia. May be taken with other antiparkinson drugs. Contraindicated in glaucoma, GI obstruction, severe ulcerative colitis, prostatic hypertrophy, myasthenia gravis. Pregnancy category: C; PB: UK; t½: UK
biperiden HCl (Akineton)	Parkinsonism: A: PO: 2 mg t.i.d./q.i.d.; *max:* 16 mg/d EPS: A: PO/IM: 2 mg q.d./b.i.d.; *max:* 8 mg/d C: IM: 40 mcg/kg, may repeat q30min; *max:* 4 mg/d	For parkinsonism and drug-induced parkinsonism (EPS). With prolonged use, drug tolerance may occur. Similar contraindications as benztropine. Avoid taking drug with alcohol or CNS depressants. Dry mouth, blurred vision, drowsiness, muscle weakness, and constipation may occur. Pregnancy category: C; PB: UK; t½: UK
trihexyphenidyl HCl (Artane)	Parkinsonism: A: PO: 1 mg initially, increase by 2 mg q3-5d up to 6-10 mg/d; *max:* 15 mg/d EPS: A: PO: 1 mg initially, increase to 5-15 mg/d in divided doses	For treating involuntary movement symptoms of parkinsonism and drug-induced pseudoparkinsonism. Does not treat drug-induced tardive dyskinesia. Pregnancy category: C; PB: UK; t½: 5-10 h

A, Adult; *b.i.d.*, two times a day; *C*, child; *CNS*, central nervous system; *d*, day; *EPS*, extrapyramidal symptoms; *GI*, gastrointestinal; *GU*, genitourinary; *h*, hour; *h.s.*, at bedtime; *IM*, intramuscular; *IV*, intravenous; *min*, minute; *PB*, protein-binding; *p.c.*, after meals; *PO*, by mouth; *PRN*, as needed; *q.i.d.*, four times a day; *t½*, half-life; *t.i.d.*, three times a day; *UK*, unknown.

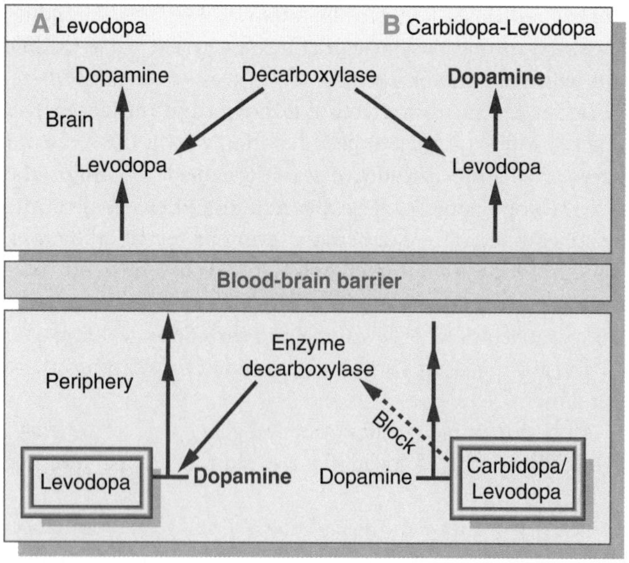

FIGURE 23–1 A, When levodopa is used alone, only 1% reaches the brain because 99% converts to dopamine while in the peripheral nervous system. **B**, By combining carbidopa with levodopa, carbidopa can inhibit the enzyme decarboxylase in the periphery, thereby allowing more levodopa to reach the brain.

parkinsonism in approximately two thirds of patients, but this improvement is usually not sustained, because drug tolerance develops. Amantadine can also be used to treat drug-induced parkinsonism.

Bromocriptine mesylate (Parlodel) acts directly on dopamine receptors in the central nervous system (CNS), cardiovascular system, and gastrointestinal (GI) tract. Bromocriptine is more effective than amantadine and the anticholinergics; however, it is not as effective as carbidopa-levodopa in alleviating parkinsonism symptoms. Patients who do not tolerate carbidopa-levodopa are frequently given bromocriptine.

SAFETY: Preventing Medication Errors

Do not confuse ...
- **Symmetrel** with **Synthroid**
- **Parlodel** with **pindolol**
- **Mirapex** with **MiraLax**

MAO-B Inhibitors

The enzyme monoamine oxidase-B (MAO-B) causes catabolism (breakdown) of dopamine. Selegiline inhibits MAO-B, thus prolonging the action of levodopa. It may be ordered for

PROTOTYPE DRUG CHART 23-1

Carbidopa-Levodopa

Drug Class Antiparkinson: dopamine replacement Trade Name: Sinemet Pregnancy Category: C	**Dosage** A: PO: Initially 1 tablet containing 10 or 25 carbidopa/100 levodopa t.i.d./q.i.d.; maint: 25/250 mg t.i.d./q.i.d.; *max:* 8 tablets/d Extended-release: 50 mg carbidopa/200 mg levodopa b.i.d.
Contraindications Narrow-angle glaucoma; severe cardiac, renal, hepatic disease; suspicious skin lesions (activates malignant melanoma) Caution: Peptic ulcer, psychiatric disorders, seizure disorder, suicidal ideation	**Drug-Lab-Food Interactions** Drug: Increase hypertensive crisis with MAOIs Decrease levodopa effect with anticholinergics, antipsychotics Lab: May increase BUN, AST, ALT, ALP, LDH
Pharmacokinetics Absorption: PO: Well absorbed Distribution: PB: Carbidopa: 36%; levodopa: UK Metabolism: t½: 1-2 h Excretion: In urine as metabolites	**Pharmacodynamics** PO: Onset: 15 min; ER: onset: 4-6 h Peak: 1-3 h Duration: 5-2 h
Therapeutic Effects/Uses To treat parkinsonism; to relieve tremors and rigidity Mode of Action: Transmission of levodopa to brain cells for conversion to dopamine; carbidopa blocks the conversion of levodopa to dopamine in the intestine and peripheral tissues	
Side Effects Anorexia, nausea, vomiting, dysphagia, fatigue, dizziness, headache, dry mouth, bitter taste, twitching, blurred vision, insomnia, dark urine	**Adverse Reactions** Involuntary movements, palpitations, orthostatic hypotension, urinary retention, priapism, psychosis, severe depression with suicidal ideation, hallucinations Life-threatening: Agranulocytosis, hemolytic anemia, thrombocytopenia, cardiac dysrhythmias, neuroleptic malignant syndrome

A, Adult; *ALP,* alkaline phosphatase; *ALT,* alanine aminotransferase; *AST,* aspartate aminotransferase; *b.i.d.,* two times a day; *BUN,* blood urea nitrogen; *h,* hour; *LDH,* lactic dehydrogenase; *maint,* maintenance; *MAOIs,* monoamine oxidase inhibitors; *min,* minute; *PB,* protein-binding; *PO,* by mouth; *q.i.d.,* four times a day; *t½,* half-life; *t.i.d.,* three times a day; *UK,* unknown.

newly diagnosed patients with parkinsonism. The use of selegiline could delay carbidopa-levodopa therapy by 1 year. It decreases "on-off" fluctuations. Rasagiline (Azilect) is an MAO-B inhibitor used for the treatment of parkinsonism.

Large doses of selegiline may inhibit MAO-A, an enzyme that promotes metabolism of tyramine in the GI tract. If they are not metabolized by MAO-A, ingestion of foods high in tyramine (aged cheese, red wine, and bananas) can cause a hypertensive crisis. Severe adverse drug interactions can occur between selegiline and various tricyclic antidepressants (TCA) or selective serotonin reuptake inhibitors (SSRIs).

COMT Inhibitors

The enzyme catechol *O*-methyltransferase (COMT) inactivates dopamine. When taken with a levodopa preparation, COMT inhibitors increase the amount of levodopa concentration in the brain. Tolcapone (Tasmar) was the first COMT inhibitor taken with levodopa for advanced parkinsonism. This drug can affect liver cell function; therefore serum liver enzymes should be closely monitored. Entacapone (Comtan) does not affect liver function. In 2003, the FDA approved a combination drug of dopaminergics (carbidopa and levodopa) and a COMT inhibitor (entacapone) called Stalevo. With various dosage strengths available, Stalevo provides greater dosing flexibility and individualization to the patient. This combination of three drugs lessens the "wearing off" effects of levodopa that are sometimes experienced prior to the next dose.

Table 23-3 lists dopaminergics, dopamine agonists, MAO-B inhibitors, and COMT inhibitors with their dosages, uses, and considerations.

TABLE 23-3 ANTIPARKINSON: DOPAMINERGICS

GENERIC (BRAND)	ROUTE AND DOSAGE	USES AND CONSIDERATIONS
Dopaminergics		
carbidopa-levodopa (Sinemet)	See Prototype Drug Chart 23-1.	
Dopamine Agonists		
amantadine HCl (Symmetrel)	Parkinsonism: A: PO: 100 mg b.i.d.; may increase dose; *max:* 400 mg/d	For early-onset parkinsonism, drug-induced parkinsonism, and influenza A respiratory virus. Effective for rigidity and bradykinesia; less effective for decreasing tremors. May be used alone or in combination. Has fewer side effects than anticholinergic drugs. Pregnancy category: C; PB: 60%-70%; $t\frac{1}{2}$: 11-15 h
bromocriptine mesylate (Parlodel)	A: PO: Initially 1.25-2.5 mg/d; may gradually increase dose; maint: 30-60 mg/d in 3 divided doses; *max:* 100 mg/d	To treat parkinsonism. Response is better than with amantadine. Can be taken in adjunct with levodopa or carbidopa-levodopa. Hypotension, lightheadedness, and syncope are major side effects. Initially, small doses are given and then gradually increased over several weeks. Pregnancy category: B; PB: 90%-96%; $t\frac{1}{2}$: 6-8 h; terminal phase: 50 h
pramipexole dihydrochloride (Mirapex)	A: PO: Initially: 0.125 mg t.i.d.; maint: 1.5 mg t.i.d.; *max:* 4.5 mg/d	To treat parkinsonism. Stimulates dopamine receptors in striatum. May cause dizziness, postural hypotension, hallucinations. Pregnancy category: C; PB: 15%; $t\frac{1}{2}$: 8-12 h
ropinirole HCl (Requip)	A: PO: Initially: 0.25 mg t.i.d.; *max:* 24 mg/d	To treat parkinsonism. Stimulates dopamine receptors in striatum. May cause nausea, fatigue, somnolence. Pregnancy category: C; PB: 40%; $t\frac{1}{2}$: 6 h
MAO-B Inhibitors		
selegiline HCl (Eldepryl)	A: PO: 5 mg b.i.d.; *max:* 10 mg/d	For early-onset parkinsonism. May delay use of levodopa therapy by 1 y. Can be given with levodopa preparations; dose of levodopa would need to be decreased. May cause suicidal ideation. Pregnancy category: C; PB: 85%; $t\frac{1}{2}$: 2-20 h
rasagiline (Azilect)	A: PO: 0.5-1 mg/d	For treatment of Parkinsonism. Pregnancy category: C; PB: 88%-94%; $t\frac{1}{2}$: 3 h
COMT Inhibitors		
tolcapone (Tasmar)	A: PO: 100 mg t.i.d.; *max:* 600 mg/d	For treatment of parkinsonism. Potentiates dopamine activity by inhibiting COMT. Used in conjunction with levodopa-carbidopa (Sinemet); prolongs action of levodopa. Monitor liver enzymes frequently as may cause fatal hepatotoxicity. Pregnancy category: C; PB: 99%; $t\frac{1}{2}$: 2-3 h
entacapone (Comtan)	A: PO: 200 mg with each dose of levodopa-carbidopa; *max:* 1600 mg/d	Used in combination with levodopa-carbidopa. Prevents peripheral COMT; thus more levodopa reaches the brain. Prolongs half-life of levodopa and decreases "on-off" fluctuations. Levodopa dose should be decreased when taken with a COMT inhibitor. Pregnancy category: C; PB: 98%; $t\frac{1}{2}$: 1-2 h

A, Adult; *COMT*, catechol *O*-methyltransferase; *d*, day; *GI*, gastrointestinal; *h*, hour; *max*, maximum; *PB*, protein-binding; *PO*, by mouth; *t½*, half-life; *t.i.d.*, three times a day; *UK*, unknown; >, greater than.

Nursing Process
Patient-Centered Collaborative Care

Antiparkinson: Dopaminergic Agent: Carbidopa-Levodopa

Assessment
- Obtain patient's vital signs to use for future comparison.
- Assess patient for signs and symptoms of parkinsonism, including stooped forward posture, shuffling gait, masked facies, and resting tremors.
- Obtain a history from patient of glaucoma, heart disease, peptic ulcers, kidney or liver disease, and psychosis.
- Obtain a drug history. Report if drug-drug interaction is probable. Drugs that should be avoided or closely monitored are levodopa, bromocriptine, and anticholinergics.

Nursing Diagnoses
- Impaired physical mobility related to dizziness
- Risk for activity intolerance related to fatigue
- Risk for falls related to shuffling gait
- Knowledge deficit related to unfamiliar medications

Planning
- Patient's symptoms of parkinsonism will be decreased or absent after 1 to 4 weeks of drug therapy.

Nursing Interventions
- Monitor patient's vital signs and electrocardiogram. Orthostatic hypotension may occur during early use of levodopa and bromocriptine. Instruct patient to rise slowly to avoid faintness.
- Observe for weakness, dizziness, or syncope, which are symptoms of orthostatic hypotension.
- Administer carbidopa-levodopa (Sinemet) with low-protein foods. High-protein diets interfere with drug transport to the CNS.
- Observe for symptoms of parkinsonism.

Patient Teaching
General
- Urge patient not to abruptly discontinue the medication. Rebound parkinsonism (increased symptoms of parkinsonism) can occur.
- Inform patient that urine may be discolored and will darken with exposure to air. Perspiration also may be dark. Explain that both are harmless but clothes may be stained.
- Advise patient to avoid chewing or crushing extended-release tablets.

Side Effects
- Encourage patient to report side effects and symptoms of dyskinesia. Explain to patient that it may take weeks or months before symptoms are controlled.

Diet
- Suggest to patient that taking levodopa with food may decrease GI upset, but food will slow the drug absorption rate.
- Urge patient who takes high doses of selegiline to avoid foods high in tyramine (e.g., aged cheese, red wine, cream, yogurt, chocolate, bananas, raisins) to prevent hypertensive crisis.

Amantadine and Bromocriptine
- Urge patient taking amantadine to report any signs of skin lesions, seizures, or depression. A history of these health problems should have been previously reported to health care provider.
- Advise patient taking bromocriptine to report symptoms of lightheadedness when changing positions (a symptom of orthostatic hypotension).
- Warn patient to avoid alcohol when taking bromocriptine.
- Teach patient to check heart rate and report changes in rate or irregularity.
- Counsel patient not to abruptly stop the drug without first notifying health care provider.

Cultural Considerations
- Recognize that various cultural groups will need guidance in understanding the disease process of parkinsonism. Support patient and family member who may be dismayed about the symptoms of parkinsonism and lack knowledge of the disease process.
- Secure an interpreter for patient who speaks little or no English to support understanding of drug doses and schedules and recognition of severe side effects that need to be reported to health care provider.

Evaluation
- Evaluate effectiveness of drug therapy in controlling symptoms of parkinsonism.
- Determine if there is an absence of side effects.

Determine if patient and family has increased knowledge of drug regimen.

Precautions for Drugs Used to Treat Parkinsonism
Side Effects and Adverse Reactions
The common side effects of anticholinergics include dry mouth and dry secretions, urinary retention, constipation, blurred vision, and an increase in heart rate. Mental effects

such as restlessness and confusion may occur in the older adult.

The side effects of carbidopa-levodopa are numerous. GI disturbances are common because dopamine stimulates the chemoreceptor trigger zone (CTZ) in the medulla, which stimulates the vomiting center. Taking the drug with food can decrease nausea and vomiting, but food slows the absorption rate. **Dyskinesia** (impaired voluntary movement) may occur with high levodopa dosages. Cardiovascular side effects include orthostatic hypotension and increased heart rate during early use of levodopa. Cardiac dysrhythmias may occur as carbidopa-levodopa dosages are increased. Nightmares, mental disturbances, and suicidal tendencies may occur.

Amantadine has few side effects, but they can intensify when the drug is combined with other antiparkinson drugs. Orthostatic hypotension, confusion, urinary retention, and constipation are common side effects of amantadine.

Side effects from bromocriptine are more common than from amantadine. These include GI disturbances (nausea), orthostatic hypotension, palpitations, chest pain, lower extremity edema, nightmares, delusions, and confusion. If bromocriptine is taken with carbidopa-levodopa, usually the drug dosages are reduced and side effects and drug intolerance decrease.

Pramipexole (Mirapex) and ropinirole (Requip) can cause nausea, dizziness, somnolence, weakness, and constipation. These drugs intensify the dyskinesia and hallucinations caused by levodopa. In 2006, pramipexole was FDA approved for treatment of restless legs syndrome.

Large doses of selegiline (Eldepryl) may inhibit MAO-A. Hypertensive crisis might occur if foods high in tyramine such as aged cheese, red wine, and bananas are ingested concurrently.

Tolcapone (Tasmar) may cause severe liver damage. Patients with liver dysfunction should not take this drug. Entacapone (Comtan) is not known to affect liver function. With entacapone, the urine can be dark yellow to orange; with tolcapone, the urine can be bright yellow. Both tolcapone and entacapone can intensify the adverse reactions of levodopa (e.g., hallucinations, orthostatic hypotension, constipation, dizziness) because these drugs prolong the effect of levodopa.

Contraindications

Anticholinergics or any drugs that have anticholinergic effects are contraindicated for persons with glaucoma. Persons with severe cardiac, renal, or psychiatric health problems should avoid levodopa drugs because of adverse reactions. Patients with chronic obstructive lung diseases such as emphysema can have dry, thick mucous secretions caused by large doses of anticholinergic drugs.

Drug-Drug Interactions

Antipsychotic drugs block the receptors for dopamine. Carbidopa-levodopa taken with a monoamine oxidase inhibitor (MAOI) antidepressant can cause a hypertensive crisis.

ALZHEIMER'S DISEASE

Alzheimer's disease is an incurable dementia illness characterized by chronic, progressive neurodegenerative conditions with marked cognitive dysfunction. Onset usually occurs between 45 and 65 years of age.

Pathophysiology

Many physiologic changes contribute to Alzheimer's disease. Currently, theories related to the changes that cause Alzheimer's disease include the following:

- Degeneration of the cholinergic neuron and deficiency in acetylcholine
- Neuritic plaques that form mainly outside of the neurons and in the cerebral cortex
- Apolipoprotein E_4 (apo E_4) that promotes formation of neuritic plaques, which binds beta-amyloid in the plaques
- Beta-amyloid protein accumulation in high levels that may contribute to neuronal injury
- Presence of neurofibrillary tangles with twists inside the neurons

Figure 23-2 illustrates the normal neuron and the neuron affected by Alzheimer's disease. The etiology of Alzheimer's disease is unknown. Factors thought to influence the occurrence of Alzheimer's disease are genetic predisposition, virus, infection, or inflammation that attacks brain cells, as well as nutritional, environmental, and immunologic.

Symptoms of Alzheimer's disease include memory loss, confusion, inability to communicate, aggressive behavior, depression, and psychoses (Table 23-4). With memory loss,

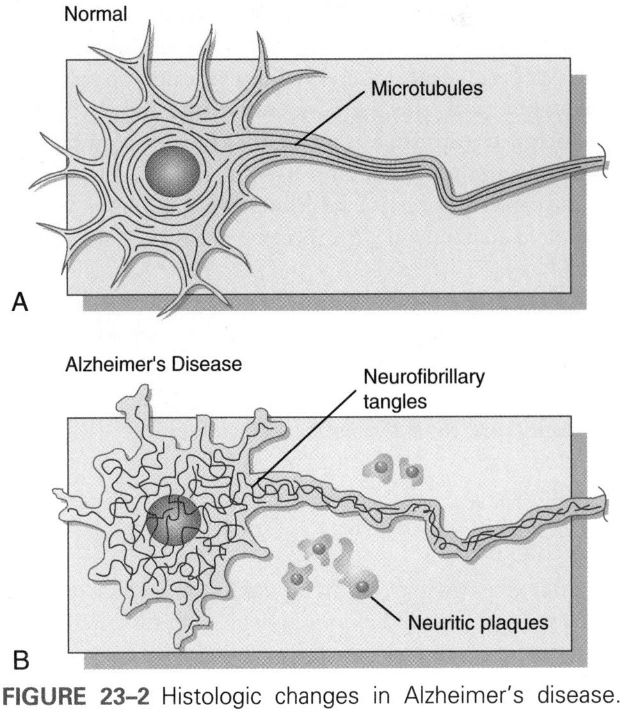

FIGURE 23–2 Histologic changes in Alzheimer's disease. **A**, Healthy neuron. **B**, Neuron affected by Alzheimer's disease showing characteristic neuritic plaques and cellular neurofibrillary tangles.

TABLE 23-4 STAGES OF COGNITIVE DECLINE DUE TO ALZHEIMER'S DISEASE

STAGE	CLINICAL PHASE	SYMPTOMS
1	Normal	No change in cognition
2	Very mild	Forgets object location; some deficit in word-finding
3	Mild (early confusion)	Early cognitive decline in one or more areas, memory loss, decreased ability to function in work situation, name-finding deficit, some decrease in social functioning, recall difficulties, anxiety
4	Moderate	Unable to perform complex tasks such as managing personal finances, planning a dinner party, concentrating, and knowing current events
5	Moderately severe (early dementia)	Usually needs assistance for survival, reminders to bathe, help in selecting clothes and other daily functions; may be disoriented as to time and recent events, although this can fluctuate; may become tearful
6	Severe (dementia)	Needs assistance with dressing, bathing, and toilet functions (e.g., flushing); may forget names of spouse, family, or caregivers and details of their personal lives; generally unaware of their surroundings; incontinence of urine and feces may occur; CNS disturbances such as agitation, delusions, paranoia, obsessive anxiety, and potential for violent behavior may increase
7	Very severe (late dementia)	Unable to speak (speech limited to five words or fewer); may scream or make other sounds; unable to ambulate, sit up, smile, or feed self; unable to hold head erect; ultimately slips into stupor or coma

logical thinking and judgment and time disorientation is also lost. As the disease progresses, memory loss becomes more severe; personality changes occur; and hyperactivity, hostility, paranoia, tendency to wander, and the inability to speak or express oneself result. Custodial care becomes necessary.

Acetylcholinesterase Inhibitors/Cholinesterase Inhibitors

There is no known cure for Alzheimer's disease. FDA-approved medications to treat Alzheimer's disease symptoms include **acetylcholinesterase (AChE) inhibitors.** (AChE is an enzyme responsible for breaking down ACh and is also known as *cholinesterase.*) The AChE inhibitors are tacrine (Cognex); donepezil (Aricept); and rivastigmine (Exelon), drug that permits more acetylcholine in the neuron receptors. Rivastigmine has effective penetration into the CNS; thus, cholinergic transmission is increased. These AChE inhibitors increase cognitive function for patients with mild to moderate Alzheimer's disease. A reversible AChE inhibitor used to treat mild to moderate Alzheimer's disease is galantamine (Razadyne).

Several drugs for treating Alzheimer's disease are under investigation. Some of these are certain nonsteroidal antiinflammatory drugs (piroxicam, indomethacin), calcium channel blockers, MAO-B inhibitors (selegiline), serotonin antagonists, CNS stimulants (methylphenidate [Ritalin]), angiotensin-converting enzyme (ACE) inhibitors, and Vitamin E.

Rivastigmine

Rivastigmine (Exelon), an AChE inhibitor, is prescribed to improve cognitive function for patients with mild to moderate Alzheimer's disease (Prototype Drug Chart 23-2). This drug increases the amount of ACh at the cholinergic synapses. Rivastigmine tends to slow the disease process. Rivastigmine has fewer drug interactions than donepezil. Table 23-5 lists the AChE inhibitors used to treat Alzheimer's disease.

Pharmacokinetics Rivastigmine is absorbed faster through the GI tract without food. It has a relatively short half-life and is given twice a day. The dose is gradually increased. The protein-binding power is average.

Pharmacodynamics Rivastigmine has been successful in improving memory in mild to moderate Alzheimer's disease. The onset of action is 0.5 to 1.0 hour for topical application; peak action is 8 to 16 hours. When given orally, the peak is 1 hour. This drug is contraindicated for patients with liver disease because hepatotoxicity may occur. Cumulative drug effect is likely to occur in older adults and in patients with liver and renal dysfunction.

Nursing Process
Patient-Centered Collaborative Care

Drug Treatment for Alzheimer's Disease: Rivastigmine

Assessment

- Assess patient's mental and physical abilities. Note limitation of cognitive function and self-care.
- Obtain a history of liver or renal disease or dysfunction.
- Assess for memory and judgment losses. Elicit from family members a history of behavioral changes (e.g., memory loss, declining interest in people or home, difficulty in following through with simple activities, and tendency to wander from home).
- Observe for signs of behavioral disturbances such as hyperactivity, hostility, and wandering.
- Examine patient for signs of aphasia or difficulty in speech.
- Note patient's motor function.
- Determine family members' ability to cope with patient's mental and physical changes.

PROTOTYPE DRUG CHART 23-2

Rivastigmine

Drug Class Acetylcholinesterase inhibitor Trade Name: Exelon Pregnancy Category: B	**Dosage** A: PO: Initially: 1.5 mg b.i.d.; increase gradually Maintenance: 3-6 mg b.i.d.; *max:* 12 mg/d
Contraindications Liver and renal diseases, urinary tract obstruction, orthostatic hypotension, bradycardia Caution: Asthma, COPD, seizures, peptic ulcer disease	**Drug-Lab-Food Interactions** Drug: Increase effect of theophylline, general anesthetics; TCAs decrease effect; increase effect with cimetidine; NSAIDs increase GI effects; tobacco increases clearance of rivastigmine Lab: Increase ALT, AST
Pharmacokinetics Absorption: PO: Food decreases absorption rate Distribution: PB: 40% Metabolism: t½: 1 h Excretion: In urine	**Pharmacodynamics** PO: Onset: UK Peak: 1 h Duration: UK
Therapeutic Effects/Uses Improves memory loss Mode of Action: Elevates acetylcholine concentration	
Side Effects Anorexia, nausea, vomiting, diarrhea, constipation, abdominal pain, gastrointestinal bleeding, dizziness, depression, peripheral edema, dry mouth, dehydration, restless legs syndrome, nystagmus	**Adverse Reactions** Seizures, bradycardia, orthostatic hypotension, cataracts, myocardial infarction, heart failure Life-threatening: Hepatotoxicity, suicidal ideation, Stevens-Johnson syndrome

A, Adult; *ALP,* alkaline phosphatase; *ALT,* alanine aminotransferase; *AST,* aspartate aminotransferase; *b.i.d.,* two times a day; *BUN,* blood urea nitrogen; *h,* hour; *LDH,* lactic dehydrogenase; *maint,* maintenance; *MAOIs,* monoamine oxidase inhibitors; *min,* minute; *PB,* protein-binding; *PO,* by mouth; *q.i.d.,* four times a day; *t½,* half-life; *t.i.d.,* three times a day; *UK,* unknown.

TABLE 23-5 ACETYLCHOLINESTERASE (ACHE) INHIBITORS FOR ALZHEIMER'S DISEASE

GENERIC (BRAND)	ROUTE AND DOSAGE	USES AND CONSIDERATIONS
donepezil (Aricept)	A: PO: 5-10 mg h.s.	Increases acetylcholine by inhibiting AChE to treat mild to moderate phase of Alzheimer's disease. Pregnancy category: C; PB: 96%; t½: 70 h
rivastigmine (Exelon)	See Prototype Drug Chart 23-2.	
tacrine HCl (Cognex)	A: PO: Initially 10 mg q.i.d.; after 4 wk, increase every other wk; *max:* 160 mg/d in 4 divided doses.	To treat mild to moderate Alzheimer's disease. AChE inhibitor. Has increased incidence of peripheral cholinergic side effects. Pregnancy category: C; PB: UK; t½: 1.5-4 h
memantine (Namenda)	A: PO: 5 mg/d, may increase dose in 5-mg increments every week to 10 mg/d; *max:* 20 mg/d	To treat mild to severe Alzheimer's disease. Neurotransmitter inhibitor. Pregnancy category: B; PB: 45%; t½: 60-80 h
galantamine (Razadyne)	A: PO: Initially 4 mg b.i.d., may increase 4 mg every 4 wk if well tolerated; maint: 12 mg b.i.d.; *max:* 24 mg/d	To treat mild to moderate Alzheimer's disease. Reversible AChE inhibitor. Pregnancy category: B; PB: 18%; t½: 7 h

A, Adult; *AChE,* acetylcholinesterase; *b.i.d.,* twice a day; *d,* day; *GI,* gastrointestinal; *h,* hour; *h.s.,* at bedtime; *max,* maximum; *PB,* protein-binding; *PO,* by mouth; *t½,* half-life; *UK,* unknown; *wk,* week.

Nursing Diagnoses

- Feeding self-care deficit related to memory loss
- Bathing self-care deficit related to memory loss
- Toileting self-care deficit related to memory loss
- Chronic confusion related to memory loss
- Interrupted family processes related to decreased cognition
- Compromised family coping related to overwhelming disruption of lifestyle
- Risk for injury related to hyperactivity and dizziness

- Imbalanced nutrition related to anorexia, nausea, and vomiting

Planning
- Patient's memory will be improved.
- Patient will maintain self-care of body functions with assistance.

Nursing Interventions
- Maintain consistency in care.
- Assist patient in ambulation and activity.
- Monitor for side effects related to continuous use of AChE inhibitors.
- Record vital signs periodically. Note signs of bradycardia and hypotension.
- Observe patient's behavioral changes, and record improvement or decline

Patient Teaching
General
- Explain to patient and family the purpose for prescribed drug therapy.
- Clarify time for drug dosing and schedule for increasing drug dosing to family member responsible for patient's medications.
- Teach family member about safety techniques (e.g., removing obstacles from patient's path so that patient can avoid injury when wandering).
- Inform family member of available support groups such as the Alzheimer's Disease and Related Disorders Association.

Side Effects
- Inform patient and family member that patient should rise slowly to avoid dizziness and loss of balance.
- Monitor routine liver function tests, as hepatotoxicity is an adverse effect.

Diet
- Inform family member about foods that may be prepared for patient's consumption and tolerance.

Cultural Considerations
- Recognize that various cultural groups may need guidance in understanding the disease process of Alzheimer's disease.
- Communicate respect for variant cultural beliefs and practices; help family members understand that their family member has a neurologic problem that may be part of the aging process. Explain how symptoms may become more progressive.

Evaluation
- Evaluate effectiveness of drug regimen by determining if patient's mental and physical status shows improvement from drug therapy

KEY WEBSITES

Information on tacrine: *www.nlm.nih.gov/medlineplus/druginfo/medmaster/a693039.html*

Information on Parkinson's disease: *www.nwpf.org/AboutParkinsons.aspx?gclid=CI25lpjLlpsCFYZM5Qod4l5jqA*

Information on Alzheimer's disease: *www.ninds.nih.gov/disorders/alzheimersdisease/alzheimersdisease.htm*

CRITICAL THINKING CASE STUDY

TR, a 79-year-old man, was diagnosed with Parkinson's disease 10 years ago. During his early treatment, he took selegiline. The drug dosage was increased to alleviate symptoms.

1. How does selegiline alleviate symptoms of parkinsonism?
2. What dietary changes should be made during the time TR takes selegiline?

Because TR developed numerous side effects and adverse reactions to selegiline, the health care provider changed the drug to carbidopa-levodopa (Sinemet). TR asks the nurse why the drug was changed.

3. What are the similarities and differences between selegiline and Sinemet?
4. What are the advantages of carbidopa-levodopa?

TR's family says they know a person with Parkinson's disease who takes the antiviral drug amantadine (Symmetrel). The family asks whether Symmetrel is the same as Sinemet and, if so, whether TR can take that drug instead of a drug containing carbidopa-levodopa.

5. What is the effect of amantadine on symptoms of parkinsonism?
6. What would be an appropriate response to the family's question concerning the use of Symmetrel for TR?
7. What are the uses for dopamine agonists and COMT inhibitors?
8. Certain anticholinergic drugs may be used to control parkinsonism symptoms. What is the action of these drugs, and what are their side effects? These anticholinergic drugs are usually prescribed for parkinsonism symptoms resulting from what?

NCLEX STUDY QUESTIONS

1. Which of the following assessment findings could the nurse see in a patient with parkinsonism? (Select all that apply.)
   a. An abrupt onset of symptoms
   b. Muscle rigidity
   c. Involuntary tremors
   d. Bradykinesia
   e. Bilateral muscle weakness
2. A patient is receiving carbidopa-levodopa for parkinsonism. What should the nurse know about this drug?
   a. Carbidopa-levodopa may lead to hypertension.
   b. Carbidopa-levodopa may lead to excessive salivation.
   c. Dopaminergic and anticholinergic therapy may lead to drowsiness and sedation.
   d. Dopaminergics and anticholinergics are contraindicated in patients with glaucoma.
3. The nurse has initiated teaching for a family member of a patient with Alzheimer's disease. The nurse realizes more teaching is needed if the family member makes which statement?
   a. As the disease gets worse, the memory loss will get worse.
   b. There are several theories about the cause of the disease.
   c. Personality changes and hostility may occur.
   d. It may take several medications to cure the disease.
4. A patient is taking rivastigmine (Exelon). The nurse should teach the patient and family which information about rivastigmine?
   a. That hepatotoxicity may occur
   b. That the initial dose is 6 mg t.i.d.
   c. That GI distress is a common side effect
   d. That weight gain may be a side effect
5. Which is a nursing intervention for a patient taking carbidopa-levodopa for parkinsonism?
   a. Encourage the patient to adhere to a high-protein diet.
   b. Inform the patient that perspiration may be dark and stain clothing.
   c. Advise the patient that glucose levels should be checked with urine testing.
   d. Warn the patient that it may take 4 to 5 days before symptoms are controlled.
6. What would the nurse teach a patient who is taking anticholinergic therapy for parkinsonism? (Select all that apply.)
   a. Avoid alcohol, cigarettes, and caffeine.
   b. Relieve dry mouth with hard candy or ice chips.
   c. Use sunglasses to reduce photophobia.
   d. Urinate 2 hours after taking the drug.
   e. Receive routine eye examinations.
7. A patient is taking rivastigmine (Exelon) to improve cognitive function. What should the nurse teach the patient/family member to do? (Select all that apply.)
   a. Rise slowly to avoid dizziness.
   b. Remove obstacles from pathways to avoid injury.
   c. Closely follow the drug dosing schedule.
   d. Have frequent checks for hypertension.
   e. Receive regular liver function tests.

Answers: 1, b, c, d; 2, d; 3, d; 4, c; 5, b; 6, a, b, c, e; 7, a, b, c.

CHAPTER

24

Drugs for Neuromuscular Disorders: Myasthenia Gravis, Multiple Sclerosis, and Muscle Spasms

evolve WEBSITE

http://evolve.elsevier.com/KeeHayes/pharmacology/

- Animations
- Content Updates
- Key Points
- Review Questions for the NCLEX® Examination
- References from the Textbook
- Unfolding Case Studies

OBJECTIVES

- Contrast the pathophysiology of myasthenia gravis and multiple sclerosis.
- Discuss the drug group used to treat myasthenia gravis.
- Compare the treatment strategies for the three phases of multiple sclerosis.
- Differentiate between the muscle relaxants used for spasticity and those used for muscle spasms.
- Apply the nursing process to drugs used to treat myasthenia gravis and muscle spasms.

OUTLINE

KEY TERMS

Myasthenia gravis (MG), a lack of nerve impulses and muscle responses at the myoneural (nerves in muscle endings) junction, causes fatigue and muscular weakness of the respiratory system, facial muscles, and extremities. Because of cranial nerve involvement, ptosis (drooping eyelid) and difficulty in chewing and swallowing occur. Respiratory arrest may result from respiratory muscle paralysis. The symptoms of MG are caused by autoimmune destruction of acetylcholine (ACh) receptor sites and a resultant decrease in neuromuscular transmission.

The neuromuscular disorder **multiple sclerosis** (MS) attacks the myelin sheath of nerve fibers, causing lesions known as *plaques.* While there are no definitive diagnostic tests, the sclerotic plaques are usually detected and measured by magnetic resonance imaging (MRI). Pharmacologic treatment is necessary to control the symptoms of this disorder.

Muscle spasms have various causes, including injury or motor neuron disorders that lead to conditions such as cerebral palsy, MS, spinal cord injuries (paraplegia [paralysis of

The authors gratefully acknowledge the work of Marilyn Herbert-Ashton, who updated this chapter for the eighth edition.

the legs]), cerebral vascular accident (stroke), or hemiplegia (paralysis of one side of the body). Spasticity of muscles can be reduced with the use of skeletal **muscle relaxants**.

MYASTHENIA GRAVIS

MG is a chronic autoimmune neuromuscular disease that affects approximately 14 in 100,000 persons. It can occur at any age; however, MG occurs more commonly in women younger than 30 years and in men older than 50 years. It is not a genetic disorder, but there can be a familial tendency.

Pathophysiology

MG results from a lack of ACh receptor sites. This autoimmune disorder involves an antibody response against an alpha subunit of the acetylcholine receptor (AChR) site at the neuromuscular junction. Antibodies attack AChR sites, obstructing the binding of ACh and eventually destroying receptor sites. When AChR sites are reduced, ACh molecules are prevented from binding to receptors and stimulating normal neuromuscular transmission. The result is ineffective muscle contraction and muscle weakness. About 90% of patients with MG have anti-acetylcholine antibodies that can be detected through serum testing.

The thymus gland is involved in systemic immunity that is active during infancy and early childhood, but the gland normally shrinks during adulthood. Approximately 60% of MG patients have thymic hyperplasia. It has been suggested in some cases that if the thymus gland is removed during the early onset of MG, clinical symptoms are greatly decreased. Thymectomy has been an option for patients younger than 50 years.

MG is characterized primarily by weakness and fatigue of the skeletal (voluntary) muscles. Other characteristics of MG include dysphagia (difficulty chewing and swallowing), dysarthria (slurred speech), and respiratory muscle weakness. Early symptoms of MG are ptosis (drooping eyelids) and diplopia (double vision).

The group of drugs used to control MG is the AChE inhibitors, also called *cholinesterase inhibitors* and *anticholinesterase;* they inhibit the action of the enzyme. As a result of this action, more acetylcholine is available to activate the cholinergic receptors and promote muscle contraction. The AChE inhibitors are classified as parasympathomimetics.

When muscular weakness of the patient with MG becomes generalized, **myasthenic crisis** may occur. This complication is a severe generalized muscle weakness and may involve the muscles of respiration, such as the diaphragm and intercostal muscles. Triggers of myasthenic crisis include inadequate dosing of AChE inhibitors, infection, emotional stress, menses, pregnancy, surgery, trauma, hypokalemia, temperature extremes, and alcohol intake. Myasthenic crisis can also occur three to four hours after taking certain medications (e.g., aminoglycoside and fluoroquinolone antibiotics, calcium channel blockers, phenytoin [Dilantin], and psychotropics). If muscle weakness remains untreated, death could result from paralysis of the respiratory muscles. Neostigmine (Prostigmin), a fast-acting AChE inhibitor, can relieve myasthenia crisis.

Overdosing with AChE inhibitors may cause another complication of MG called **cholinergic crisis,** which is an acute exacerbation of symptoms. A cholinergic crisis usually occurs within 30 to 60 minutes after taking anticholinergic medications. This complication is due to continuous depolarization of postsynaptic membranes that create neuromuscular blockade. The patient with cholinergic crisis often has severe muscle weakness that can lead to respiratory paralysis and arrest. Accompanying symptoms include **miosis** (abnormal pupil constriction), pallor, sweating, vertigo, excess salivation, nausea, vomiting, abdominal cramping, diarrhea, bradycardia, and **fasciculations** (involuntary muscle twitching).

Acetylcholinesterase Inhibitors/Cholinesterase Inhibitors

The first drug used to manage MG was neostigmine. It is a short-acting **acetylcholinesterase (AChE) inhibitor** with a half-life of 0.5 to 1 hour. The drug is given every 2 to 4 hours and must be given on time to prevent muscle weakness. The AChE inhibitor pyridostigmine bromide (Mestinon) has an intermediate action and is given every 3 to 6 hours. Ambenonium chloride (Mytelase) is a long-acting AChE inhibitor and is usually prescribed when the patient does not respond to neostigmine or pyridostigmine. Prototype Drug Chart 24-1 presents drug data related to pyridostigmine. Table 24-1 lists the AChE inhibitors. Cholinesterase inhibitors are discussed in Chapter 23.

Pharmacokinetics Pyridostigmine is poorly absorbed from the GI tract. Half of the sustained-release capsule is absorbed readily, but the balance is poorly absorbed. The duration of oral pyridostigmine is 3.5 to 4 hours; when given intravenously (IV), it is 2 hours. Because of its short half-life, pyridostigmine must be administered several times a day. The drug is metabolized by the liver and excreted in the urine.

Pharmacodynamics Pyridostigmine increases muscle strength of patients with muscular weakness resulting from MG. The onset of action of oral preparations is 0.5 to 1 hour. The duration of action is longer with the sustained-release drug capsule. One thirtieth of the oral dose of pyridostigmine can be administered IV. Overdosing of pyridostigmine can result in signs and symptoms of cholinergic crisis (i.e., extreme muscle weakness; increased salivation, tears, sweating; miosis); the antidote atropine sulfate should be available. This crisis requires emergency medical intervention because of respiratory muscle weakness.

Patients who do not respond to AChE inhibitors may require prednisone, plasma exchange, intravenous immune globulin (IVIG), or immunosuppressive drugs. Prednisone decreases MG symptoms and promotes remission, but long-term use can cause adverse dermatologic effects.

The immunosuppressive agent azathioprine (Imuran) can be used in conjunction with a lower dose of prednisone. With azathioprine, the white blood cell (WBC) count and liver enzymes should be closely monitored to avoid leukopenia and hepatotoxicity.

Overdosing and underdosing of AChE inhibitors have similar symptoms: muscle weakness, dyspnea (difficulty breathing), and dysphagia (difficulty swallowing). Additional symptoms that may be present with overdosing are increased salivation (drooling), bradycardia, abdominal cramping, and increased tearing and sweating. All doses of AChE inhibitors should be administered *on time,* because late administration of the drug could result in muscle weakness.

Underdosing can result in myasthenia crisis, and overdosing can result in cholinergic crisis. Edrophonium chloride (Tensilon) is an

PROTOTYPE DRUG CHART 24-1

Pyridostigmine

Drug Class	Dosage
Cholinesterase inhibitor Trade Name: Mestinon Pregnancy Category: C	A: PO: 60-120 mg in 5 to 6 doses per day; *max:* 600 mg/d in divided doses SR: 180-540 mg q.d./b.i.d., with at least 6 hours between doses; *max:* 1.5 g/d A: IM/IV: 2 mg q2-3h C: PO: 7 mg/kg/d in 5-6 divided doses C: IV/IM: 0.05-0.15 mg/kg; *max single dose:* 10 mg
Contraindications	**Drug-Lab-Food Interactions**
GI and GU mechanical obstruction, severe renal disease, ileus Caution: Asthma, hypotension, bradycardia, seizure disorder, peptic ulcer, cardiac dysrhythmias, renal dysfunction, hyperthyroidism, pregnancy, breastfeeding	Drug: Decrease pyridostigmine effect with atropine, corticosteroids, muscle relaxants, antidysrhythmics, aminoglycosides, anesthetics, magnesium, fluoroquinolones; increase toxicity with cholinesterase inhibitors, insecticides, atropine, tetracyclines, polymyxin B
Pharmacokinetics	**Pharmacodynamics**
Absorption: PO: Poorly absorbed; SR: 50% absorbed Distribution: PB: UK Metabolism: t½: PO: 3.5-4 h; IV: 2 h Excretion: In urine	PO: Onset: 30-45 min Peak: UK Duration: 3-6 h PO SR: Onset: 0.5-1 h Peak: UK Duration: 6-12 h IM: Onset: 15 min Peak: UK Duration: 2-4 h IV: Onset: 2-5 min Peak: UK Duration: 2-3 h
Therapeutic Effects/Uses	
To control and treat myasthenia gravis. Also used as a nondepolarizing muscle relaxant antagonist, and as an anti–nerve gas agent for U.S. military personnel for use in the immediate threat of the nerve gas Soman Mode of Action: Transmission of neuromuscular impulses by preventing destruction of acetylcholine	
Side Effects	**Adverse Reactions**
Nausea, vomiting, diarrhea, headache, blurred vision, dizziness, abdominal cramps, excess saliva and sweating, rash, miosis	Hypotension, bradycardia Life-threatening: Dyspnea, bronchospasm, cardiac dysrhythmias, seizures

A, Adult; *ALP,* alkaline phosphatase; *ALT,* alanine aminotransferase; *AST,* aspartate aminotransferase; *b.i.d.,* twice a day; *BUN,* blood urea nitrogen; *C,* child; *d,* day; *GI,* gastrointestinal; *GU,* genitourinary; *h,* hour; *IM,* intramuscular; *IV,* intravenous; *LDH,* lactic dehydrogenase; *MAOIs,* monoamine oxidase inhibitors; *max,* maximum; *min,* minute; *PB,* protein-binding; *PO,* by mouth; *q.d.,* every day; *q.i.d.,* four times a day; *SR,* sustained release; *t ½,* half-life; *t.i.d.,* three times a day; *UK,* unknown.

ultra–short-acting AChE inhibitor that may be used to distinguish between myasthenia crisis and cholinergic crisis. These two different crises have a similar major symptom: severe muscle weakness. After edrophonium is administered, if the symptoms are alleviated because of an increase in ACh, the cause is myasthenia crisis. However, if the muscle weakness becomes more severe, the cause is cholinergic crisis due to drug overdosing.

Edrophonium may also be used to diagnose MG. Its ultra-short duration of 5 to 20 minutes increases muscle strength immediately. If ptosis is immediately corrected after administration of this drug, the diagnosis is most likely MG.

Side Effects and Adverse Reactions

Side effects and adverse reactions of AChE inhibitors include GI disturbances (nausea, vomiting, diarrhea, abdominal cramps) and increased salivation and tearing. Other side effects include miosis (constricted pupil of the eye), blurred vision, bradycardia, and hypotension.

Nursing Process
Patient-Centered Collaborative Care

Drug Treatment for Myasthenia Gravis: Pyridostigmine (Mestinon)

Assessment

- Obtain a drug history of drugs patient currently takes. Report if a drug-drug interaction is likely. Patient should avoid atropine, atropine-like drugs, and muscle relaxants.
- Record baseline vital signs for future comparison.
- Assess patient for signs and symptoms of myasthenia crisis such as muscle weakness with difficulty breathing and swallowing.

TABLE 24-1 ACETYLCHOLINESTERASE (ACHE) INHIBITORS: MYASTHENIA GRAVIS

GENERIC (BRAND)	ROUTE AND DOSAGE	USES AND CONSIDERATIONS
Ambenonium (Mytelase)	A: PO: 2.5-5.0 mg t.i.d./q.i.d.; dose may be increased; *maint:* 15-100 mg/d	For myasthenia gravis. A long-acting AChE inhibitor. Six times more potent than neostigmine. Frequently used when patient cannot take neostigmine or pyridostigmine because of the bromide component. Can be taken in adjunct with glucocorticoid drug. Pregnancy category: C; PB: UK; t½: UK
Edrophonium (Tensilon)	A: IV 2 mg; then 8 mg if no response A: IM: 10 mg; if cholinergic reaction occurs, retest after 30 min with 2 mg to rule out false-negative. C <34 kg: IV: 1 mg, repeat in 45 sec if no response; *max:* 5 mg C >34 kg: IV: 2 mg, repeat with 1 mg if no response; *max:* 10 mg	For diagnosing myasthenia gravis. Ptosis should be absent in 1-5 min. Ultrashort-acting drug. Pregnancy category: C; PB: UK; t½: 1.2-2 h
neostigmine (Prostigmin)	A: PO: 15 mg t.i.d., may increase to 375 mg/d A: IV/IM/subQ: 0.5-2.5 mg q1-3h; *max:*10 mg/d C: PO: 0.033 mg/kg every 3-4 h C: IV/IM/subQ: 0.01-0.04 mg/kg every 2-4 h	For controlling myasthenia gravis. Must be given on time to prevent myasthenia crisis. Parenteral route is used if chewing, swallowing, and breathing are affected. Overdose can cause cholinergic reaction, nausea, abdominal cramps, excessive salivation, and sweating. Pregnancy category: C; PB: 15%-25%; t½: 42-60 min
pyridostigmine (Mestinon)	See Prototype Drug Chart 24-1.	

A, Adult; *C*, child; *d*, day; *h*, hour; *IM*, intramuscular; *IV*, intravenous; *PB*, protein-binding; *PO*, by mouth; *PRN*, as needed; *q.i.d.*, four times a day; *t½*, half-life; *t.i.d.*, three times a day; *UK*, unknown; <, less than; >, greater than.

Nursing Diagnoses
- Ineffective breathing pattern related to weak respiratory muscles
- Risk for activity intolerance related to fatigue
- Anxiety related to possible recurrence of myasthenia crisis and dyspnea
- Knowledge deficit related to unfamiliar medications

Planning
- Patient's symptoms of muscle weakness and difficulty breathing and swallowing caused by MG will be eliminated or reduced in 2 to 3 days.

Nursing Interventions
- Monitor effectiveness of drug therapy (acetylcholinesterase inhibitors). Muscle strength should be increased. Both depth and rate of respirations should be assessed and maintained within normal range.
- Administer pyridostigmine IV undiluted at rate of 0.5 mg/min. *Do not add the drug to IV fluids.*
- Observe patient for signs and symptoms of cholinergic crisis caused by overdosing (muscle weakness, increased salivation, sweating, tearing, miosis).
- Have readily available an antidote for cholinergic crisis (atropine sulfate).

Patient Teaching

General
- Teach patient to take drugs as prescribed to avoid recurrence of symptoms.
- Encourage patient to wear a medical identification bracelet or necklace that indicates health problem and drugs taken.

Side Effects
- Advise patient to report to health care provider recurrence of symptoms of MG. Drug therapy may need to be modified.

Diet
- Inform patient to take drug before meals for best drug absorption. If gastric irritation occurs, take drug with food.

Cultural Considerations
- Use simple and clear instructions. Involve family members in teaching about prescriptive therapies and disease process.
- Communicate respect for the patient's and family's culture and beliefs.
- Accommodate cultural values, and assess whether the patient and family are accustomed to not taking all of medication as ordered or using medicines prescribed for other people. Stress that medications need to be taken as prescribed; medications are ordered specifically for each ailment; unused drugs should be discarded; and use of medications by individuals other than the intended may have serious consequences.

Evaluation

- Evaluate effectiveness of the drug therapy to maintain muscle strength.
- Determine the absence of respiratory distress.
- Evaluate correct use of drug by patient.

MULTIPLE SCLEROSIS

MS is an autoimmune disorder that attacks the myelin sheath of nerve fibers in the brain and spinal cord, causing lesions that are called *plaques.* In the United States, MS affects approximately 300,000 persons (age 20 to 40 years), and most are Caucasian women. It is uncommon in African and Asian populations. Onset of MS is usually slow. It is a condition in which there are remissions and exacerbations of multiple symptoms (sensory and cerebellar), such as diplopia, weakness in the extremities, or spasticity. MS is difficult to diagnose because there is no specific diagnostic test, although the McDonald Criteria, revised in 2010, can be used to aid in the diagnosis. Laboratory tests that may suggest MS include elevated immunoglobulin G (IgG) in the cerebrospinal fluid, increased IgG/albumin ratio, and multiple lesions observable through MRI. Scheduling regular treatment protocols to avoid clinical MS attacks is not recommended, because of the side effects of the drugs (e.g., glucocorticoids) used.

There are treatment strategies for three types or phases of MS: the acute attack, remission-exacerbation, and chronic progressive MS. Table 24-2 describes these three phases. Goals for treatment strategies are to decrease the inflammatory process of nerve fibers and improve conduction of demyelinating axons.

SKELETAL MUSCLE RELAXANTS

Muscle relaxants relieve muscular spasms and pain associated with traumatic injuries and spasticity from chronic debilitating disorders (e.g., MS, stroke [cerebrovascular accident], cerebral palsy, head and spinal cord injuries). Spasticity results from increased muscle tone from hyperexcitable neurons caused by increased stimulation from the cerebral neurons or lack of inhibition in the spinal cord or at the skeletal muscles. The centrally acting muscle relaxants depress neuron activity in the spinal cord or brain or enhance neuronal inhibition on the skeletal muscles.

Centrally Acting Muscle Relaxants

The mechanism of action of centrally acting muscle relaxants is not fully known. Centrally acting muscle relaxants are used in cases of spasticity to suppress hyperactive reflex and for muscle spasms that do not respond to antiinflammatory agents, physical therapy, or other forms of therapy. The centrally acting muscle relaxants are described in Table 24-3. Prototype Drug Chart 24-2 gives the drug data for the centrally acting muscle relaxant cyclobenzaprine (Flexeril).

HERBAL ALERT 24-1

Diazepam

Kava kava and valerian may potentiate central nervous system depression.

TABLE 24-2 TREATMENT STRATEGIES FOR THE THREE PHASES OF MULTIPLE SCLEROSIS

PHASE	CHARACTERISTICS	TREATMENT STRATEGIES
Acute attack	Fatigue; motor weakness; optic neuritis	Glucocorticoids Corticotropin (Acthar Gel) 80-120 units IM qd for 2-3 weeks
Remission-exacerbation	Recurrence of clinical MS symptoms; spasticity	Biologic (immune) response modifiers (BRMs); see Chapter 39. Interferon-β (IFN-β) (Betaseron): 25 mcg (8 million international units) subQ every other day. Reduces spasticity and improves muscle movement. Also, interferon β-1a includes Rebif (given subQ in doses of 22 or 44 mcg 3 times per week) and Avonex (given IM in doses of 30 mcg every week), which are used in relapsing forms of MS. Glatiramer acetate (Copaxone) 20 mg subQ once daily; mitoxantrone (Novantrone), an antineoplastic, 12 mg/m^2 IV every 3 months with a lifetime cumulative dose of no more than 140 mg/m^2; and fingolimod (Gilenya), an S1P receptor modulator, 0.5 mg/d PO for adults Teriflunomide (Aubagio) given PO 7-14 mg/d Dimethyl fumarate (Tecfidera) given PO 120-240 mg b.i.d.
Chronic progressive	Progressive MS symptoms (using wheelchair)	Immunosuppressant cyclophosphamide (Cytoxan)

b.i.d., Twice a day; *d,* day; *IM,* intramuscular; *IV,* intravenous; *WBC,* white blood cell.

TABLE 24-3 MUSCLE RELAXANTS

GENERIC (BRAND)	ROUTE AND DOSAGE	USES AND CONSIDERATIONS
Anxiolytics		
diazepam (Valium) CSS IV	A: PO: 2 to 10 mg b.i.d./q.i.d. Older adults: PO: 2 to 2.5 mg qd/b.i.d. Infants >6 months: PO: 1 to 2.5 mg t.i.d./q.i.d. A/C >5 y: IM/IV: 5 to 10 mg q3-4h PRN C <5 y: IM/IV: 1 to 2 mg q3-4h PRN	Diazepam has many uses, one of which is to relieve muscle spasms associated with paraplegia and cerebral palsy. Contraindicated in narrow-angle glaucoma. Pregnancy category: D; PB: 98%; t½: 30 to 60 h
Muscle Relaxants		
Spasticity (Centrally Acting)		
baclofen (Lioresal)	A: PO: Initially 5 mg t.i.d.; increase gradually; *max:* 80 mg/d	For muscle spasms caused by MS and spinal cord injury. Overdose may cause CNS depression. Drowsiness, dizziness, nausea, and hypotension may occur. Pregnancy category: C; PB: 30%; t½: 2.5 to 4 h
tizanidine (Zanaflex)	A: PO: 8 mg q6-8h PRN; *max:* 12 mg single dose or 36 mg/d	To manage spasticity, especially for spinal cord injury and multiple sclerosis. Pregnancy category: C; PB: 30%; t½: 2.5 h
Spasticity (Direct Acting)		
dantrolene sodium (Dantrium)	A: PO: Initially 25 mg/d; increase gradually; *maint:* 100 mg b.i.d./q.i.d. C >5 y: PO: Initially 0.5 mg/kg/d; increase dose gradually by 0.5 mg/kg t.i.d./q.i.d.; *max:* 100 mg q.i.d	For chronic neurologic disorders causing spasms: spinal cord injuries, stroke, MS. Start with low doses and increase every 4 to 7 d. Avoid taking with alcohol or CNS depressants. Pregnancy category: C; PB: 95%; t½: 8 h
Centrally Acting Muscle Relaxants		
carisoprodol (Soma)	A: PO: 250-350 mg t.i.d/q.i.d.	For relaxation of skeletal muscles. Has CNS depressant effects. Avoid taking with alcohol or CNS depressants. Should only be used on short-term basis (2 to 3 weeks).Pregnancy category: C; PB: UK; t½: 2.4 h
chlorzoxazone (Parafon forte DSC)	A: PO: 250 to 500 mg t.i.d./q.i.d.; *max:* 3 g/d	For acute or severe muscle spasms. Not effective for cerebral palsy. Take with food to decrease GI upset. Pregnancy category: C; PB: UK; t½: 1 h
methocarbamol (Robaxin)	A: PO: Initially 1.5 g q.i.d.; *maint:* 4 to 4.5 g/d in 3 to 6 divided doses; *max:* 8 g/d A: IM/IV 1 g q8 h up to 3 consecutive days Not to exceed 3 mL/min IV or inject more than 5 mL IM into each gluteal muscle	For acute muscle spasms; drug used for treatment of tetanus. Has CNS depressant effects (sedation). Avoid taking with alcohol or CNS depressants. Urine may be green, brown, or black. Drowsiness that may occur usually decreases with continued drug use. Pregnancy category: C; PB: UK; t½: 1 to 2 h
metaxalone (Skelaxin)	A: PO: 800 mg t.i.d./q.i.d.; *max:* 3200 mg/d	For acute painful muscle spasticity Pregnancy category: UK; PB: UK; t½: 9 h
orphenadrine citrate (Norflex)	A: PO: 100 mg b.i.d.; *max:* 200 mg/d A: IM/IV: 60 mg q12h; *max:* 120 mg/d	For acute muscle spasm. Can be toxic with a mild overdose. Used in combination with aspirin and caffeine (Norgesic). Pregnancy category: C; PB: <20%; t½: 14 h
Depolarizing Muscle Relaxants (Adjunct to Anesthesia)		
succinylcholine (Anectine)	A/C: IM: 2.5 to 4 mg/kg; *max:* 150 mg; A: IV: 0.3 to 1.1 mg/kg	For surgical skeletal muscle relaxation. Also used in endoscopy and intubation. Pregnancy category: C; PB: UK; t½: UK
Nondepolarizing Muscle Relaxants (Adjunct to Anesthesia)		
pancuronium bromide (Pavulon)	A/C >1 month: IV: 0.04 to 0.1 mg/kg; then 0.01 mg/kg every 30 to 60 min PRN	Used in surgery for relaxation of skeletal muscle (e.g., abdominal wall). Considered to be five times as potent as tubocurarine chloride. Does not cause hypotension or bronchospasm. Pregnancy category: C; PB: 30% to 87%; t½: 2 h
vecuronium (Norcuron)	A/C >10 y: IV: 80 to 100 mcg/kg	For surgical skeletal muscle relaxation. Can be used for patients with asthma, renal disease, or limited cardiac reserve. Given after general anesthesia has been started. Pregnancy category: C; PB: 60% to90%; t½: 1 h

A, Adult; *b.i.d.*, twice a day; *C*, child; *CNS*, central nervous system; *CSS*, Controlled Substances Schedule; *d*, day; *GI*, gastrointestinal; *h*, hour; *IM*, intramuscular; *IV*, intravenous; *MS*, multiple sclerosis; *PB*, protein-binding; *PO*, by mouth; *PRN*, as needed; *q.i.d.*, four times a day; *t½*, half-life; *t.i.d.*, three times a day; *UK*, unknown; *y*, year; >, greater than; <, less than.

PROTOTYPE DRUG CHART 24-2

Cyclobenzaprine

Drug Class Centrally acting muscle relaxant Trade Name: Flexeril Pregnancy Category: B	**Dosage** A: P.O. 5-10 mg; *max:* 30 mg/d
Contraindications Acute myocardial infarction, AV blocks, bundle-branch block, cardiac arrhythmias, heart failure, hyperthyroidism, paralytic ileus, concurrent use of monoamine oxidase inhibitors or within 14 days after discontinuation. Caution: Seizure disorder, alcohol, CNS depressants, glaucoma, prostatic hypertrophy, urinary retention, hepatic dysfunction, breastfeeding	**Drug-Lab-Food Interactions** Drug: Increased CNS depression with alcohol, kava kava, valerian, barbiturates, tricyclic antidepressants, and other CNS depressants. Take with food or milk to decrease GI upset.
Pharmacokinetics Absorption: PO: Well absorbed Distribution: PB: 93% Metabolism: t½: 8-37 h Excretion: In urine	**Pharmacodynamics** PO: Onset: 1 h Peak: 3-8 h Duration: 12-24 h
Therapeutic Effects/Uses For short-term treatment of muscle spasms. Mode of Action: Relieves muscle spasms through a central action, possibly at the brain stem level.	
Side Effects Anticholinergic effects (blurred vision, constipation, dry mouth, tachycardia, urinary retention); drowsiness; dizziness; headache; fever; abdominal pain; vomiting; diarrhea; flatulence; erectile dysfunction	**Adverse Reactions** Allergic reactions, angioedema, myocardial infarction, seizures, ileus

A, Adult; *CNS,* central nervous system; *d,* day; *h,* hour; *max,* maximum; *PB,* protein-binding; *PO,* by mouth; *t½,* half-life; *UK,* unknown; >, greater than.

Spasticity

Skeletal muscle spasticity is muscular hyperactivity that causes contraction of the muscles, resulting in pain and limited mobility. Centrally acting muscle relaxants act on the spinal cord. Examples of centrally acting muscle relaxants used to treat spasticity are baclofen (Lioresal), dantroene (Dantrium), and tizanidine (Zanaflex). Diazepam (Valium), a benzodiazepine, has also been effective for treating spasticity.

SAFETY: Preventing Medication Errors

Do not confuse…

- **baclofen** (skeletal muscle relaxant) with **Bactroban** (topical antibacterial) or **Beclovent** (corticosteroid inhalant).

Muscle Spasms

Various centrally acting muscle relaxants are used for muscle spasm to decrease pain and increase range of motion. They have a sedative effect and should not be taken concurrently with CNS depressants such as barbiturates, narcotics, and alcohol. These agents, with the exception of cyclobenzaprine, can cause drug dependence. In addition, dizziness and drowsiness are common side effects. Examples of this group of centrally acting muscle relaxants are carisoprodol (Soma), chlorzoxazone (Parafon forte DSC), cyclobenzaprine (Flexeril), metaxalone (Skelaxin), methocarbamol (Robaxin), and orphenadrine citrate (Norflex).

Pharmacokinetics Cyclobenzaprine is well absorbed from the GI tract, and its half-life is moderate. The protein-binding percentage for cyclobenzaprine is 93%. Cyclobenzaprine is metabolized in the liver and excreted in urine.

Pharmacodynamics Cyclobenzaprine alleviates muscle spasm associated with acute painful musculoskeletal conditions. When cyclobenzaprine is taken with alcohol, kava kava, valerian, sedative-hypnotics, barbiturates, or tricyclic antidepressants (TCAs), increased central nervous system (CNS) depression occurs. The onset of action, peak concentration time, and duration of action for cyclobenzaprine is short.

Side Effects and Adverse Reactions

The side effects from centrally acting muscle relaxants include drowsiness, dizziness, lightheadedness, headaches, and occasional GI sensitivity (e.g., nausea, vomiting, abdominal distress). Cyclobenzaprine and orphenadrine have anticholinergic effects.

Nursing Process
Patient-Centered Collaborative Care

Muscle Relaxant: Cyclobenzaprine

Assessment

- Collect medical history. Cyclobenzaprine is contraindicated if patient has cardiovascular disorders,

hyperthyroidism, or hepatic impairment, or is taking concurrent MAOIs.
- Obtain baseline vital signs for future comparison.
- Secure patient's health history to identify the cause of muscle spasm and determine whether it is acute or chronic.
- Gather a drug history. Report if a drug-drug interaction is probable.
- Note if there is a history of narrow-angle glaucoma or MG. Cyclobenzaprine and orphenadrine are contraindicated with these health problems.

Nursing Diagnoses
- Impaired physical mobility related to dizziness and hyperactive reflexes
- Activity intolerance related to drowsiness and hyperactive reflexes

Planning
- Patient will be free of muscular pain within 1 week.

Nursing Interventions
- Monitor serum liver enzyme levels of patients taking dantrolene and carisoprodol. Report elevated levels of liver enzymes such as alkaline phosphatase (ALP), alanine aminotransferase (ALT), and gamma-glutamyl transferase (GGT).
- Record vital signs. Report abnormal results.
- Observe for CNS side effects (e.g., dizziness).

Patient Teaching

General
- Teach patient that the muscle relaxant should not be abruptly stopped. Drug should be tapered over 1 week to avoid rebound spasms.
- Advise patient not to drive or operate dangerous machinery when taking muscle relaxants. These drugs have a sedative effect and can cause drowsiness.
- Inform patient that most of the centrally acting muscle relaxants for acute spasms are usually taken for no longer than 3 weeks.
- Teach patient to avoid alcohol and CNS depressants. If muscle relaxants are taken with these drugs, CNS depression may be intensified.
- Advise patient that these drugs must be used cautiously for pregnant or nursing patients. Check with health care provider.

Side Effects
- Encourage patient to report side effects of the muscle relaxant: nausea, vomiting, dizziness, fainting, headache, and diplopia. Dizziness and fainting are most likely caused by orthostatic (postural) hypotension.

Diet
- Advise patient to take muscle relaxants with food to decrease gastrointestinal upset.

Cultural Considerations
- Use both hands to show respect when offering a prescription, instructions, or pamphlets to Asians and Pacific Islanders.
- Demonstrate respect by addressing patient formally until told otherwise, and do not ask private questions in public.

Evaluation
- Evaluate effectiveness of muscle relaxant to determine whether patient's muscular pain or spasms have decreased or disappeared.

KEY WEBSITES

McDonald Criteria: *www.va.gov/MS/articles/Diagnosing_MS_Using_the_McDonald_Criteria.asp*

Myasthenia Gravis Foundation of America: *www.myasthenia.org*

National Multiple Sclerosis Society: *www.nationalmssociety.org/index.aspx*

CRITICAL THINKING CASE STUDY

FR, a 29-year-old woman, was diagnosed with myasthenia gravis (MG) 2 years ago. She is receiving pyridostigmine (Mestinon) 120 mg t.i.d. Last evening, FR was involved in an automobile accident. She was taken to the emergency department unconscious and missed two evening doses of pyridostigmine.

1. How does pyridostigmine alleviate the symptoms of MG?
2. What are the potential side effects and adverse effects of pyridostigmine?
3. What problems are likely to develop following delayed pyridostigmine dosing?

FR is scheduled for surgery to repair a fractured right femur suffered in the accident. During surgery, FR develops bradycardia.

1. What medications may lead to drug interactions with pyridostigmine?
2. What problems may develop from pyridostigmine overdosing?
3. What are the similarities between myasthenia crisis and cholinergic crisis?

NCLEX STUDY QUESTIONS

1. When the nurse explains the pathophysiology of myasthenia gravis to a patient, which is the best explanation?
   a. Degeneration of cholinergic neurons and a deficit in acetylcholine lead to neuritic plaques and neurofibrillary tangles.
   b. Decreased amount of acetylcholine to cholinergic receptors produces weak muscles and reduced nerve impulses.
   c. Myelin sheaths of nerve fibers in brain and spinal cord develop lesions or plaques.
   d. Imbalance of dopamine and acetylcholine leads to degeneration of neurons in midbrain and extrapyramidal motor tracts.
2. The nurse is teaching a patient recently diagnosed with multiple sclerosis (MS) about the disease. Which statement is not correct concerning multiple sclerosis?
   a. The disease has periods of exacerbations and remissions.
   b. Goals of treatment are to decrease the inflammation in the nervous system.
   c. Patients with MS should avoid calcium channel blockers.
   d. A tapering course of glucocorticoids can be used to treat an acute attack.
3. A patient has spasticity following a spinal cord injury. The nurse anticipates that which drug will be prescribed to treat the patient's spasticity?
   a. tacrine (Cognex)
   b. ropinirole (Requip)
   c. cyclobenzaprine (Flexeril)
   d. pyridostigmine (Mestinon)
4. The nurse anticipates that the health care provider will prescribe which medication to treat a patient with multiple sclerosis in the chronic progressive phase?
   a. ambenonium (Mytelase)
   b. interferon β-1a (Avonex, Rebif)
   c. glatiramer acetate (Copaxone)
   d. cyclophosphamide (Cytoxan)
5. The nurse is providing medication instructions to a patient with acute muscle spasms who has been prescribed cyclobenzaprine (Flexeril). Which statement indicates to the nurse that the patient understands the instructions?
   a. "I plan to take this medication with a glass of milk."
   b. "Cyclobenzaprine should be taken once daily at bedtime."
   c. "I will only drink one glass of wine per day."
   d. "I will not be able to drink grapefruit juice while taking this drug."
6. Which instructions will the nurse include in the teaching plan for a patient who is taking pyridostigmine (Mestinon)? (Select all that apply.)
   a. Pyridostigmine bromide must be taken on time.
   b. Take two times per day.
   c. Underdosing can result in myasthenic crisis.
   d. Overdosing can result in cholinergic crisis.
   e. Report the adverse effect of tachycardia to the health care provider.
7. A patient is beginning to take cyclobenzaprine (Flexeril) for treatment of acute back spasms. Which interventions will the nurse include in the care of this patient? (Select all that apply.)
   a. Advise the patient to take this drug on an empty stomach.
   b. Inform the patient that muscular pain is usually relieved within 1 week.
   c. Tell the patient to report dizziness and double vision to the health care provider.
   d. Advise the patient to avoid alcohol.
   e. Taking narcotics at the same time can cause serious side effects.
8. The nurse is reviewing a patient's medication history for a patient who has just been prescribed cyclobenzaprine (Flexeril) for treatment of back spasms. The nurse plans to contact the health care provider if the patient is taking which medication?
   a. atorvastatin calcium (Lipitor)
   b. conjugated estrogen (Premarin)
   c. phenelzine (Nardil)
   d. penicillin G procaine (Crysticillin, Wycillin)
9. The nurse is caring for a patient who is diagnosed with myasthenia gravis. The patient is experiencing muscle weakness, dyspnea, bradycardia, and diaphoresis. The nurse anticipates that the health care provider will order which medication to distinguish between myasthenia crisis and cholinergic crisis?
   a. adrenocorticotropic hormone (ACTH) (H.P. Acthar)
   b. diazepam (Valium)
   c. edrophonium chloride (Tensilon)
   d. mitoxantrone (Novantrone)

Answers: 1, b; 2, a, d; 3, c; 4, d; 5, a; 6, a, c, d; 7, b, c, d, e; 8, c; 9, c.

Pain and Inflammation Management Agents

Inflammation is a reaction to tissue injury caused by the release of chemical mediators that trigger both a vascular response and the migration of fluid and cells (leukocytes, or white blood cells) to the injured site. The chemical mediators are (1) histamines, (2) kinins, and (3) prostaglandins. Histamine, the first mediator in the inflammatory process, causes dilation of the arterioles and increases capillary permeability, allowing fluid to leave the capillaries and flow into the injured area. Kinins, such as bradykinin, also increase capillary permeability and the sensation of pain. Prostaglandins are released, causing an increase in vasodilation, capillary permeability, pain, and fever. The antiinflammatory drugs, such as nonsteroidal antiinflammatory drugs (NSAIDs) and steroids (cortisone preparations), inhibit chemical mediators, thus decreasing the inflammatory process. Figure VII-1 illustrates the process of chemical mediators acting on injured tissues. The five responses to tissue injury are called the cardinal signs of inflammation: redness, swelling, pain, heat, and loss of function.

Inflammation may or may not be the result of an infection; only a small percentage of inflammations are caused by infections. Other causes of inflammation include trauma, surgical interventions, extreme heat or cold, and caustic chemical agents. Antiinflammatory drugs reduce fluid migration and pain, lessening loss of function and increasing the patient's mobility and comfort.

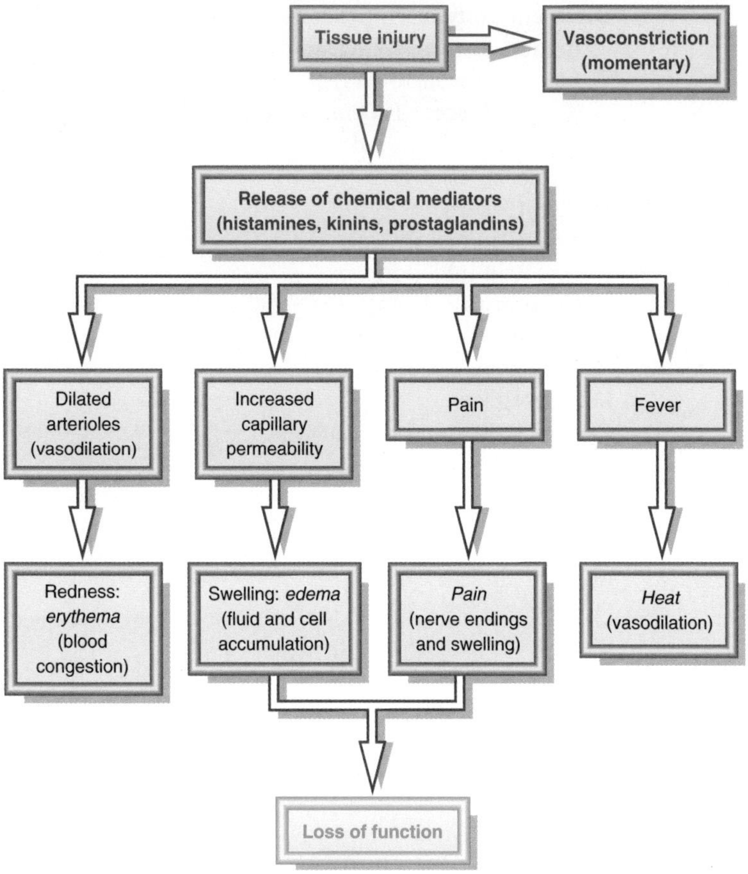

FIGURE VII–1 Chemical mediator response to tissue injury.

CHAPTER

25

Antiinflammatory Drugs

evolve WEBSITE

http://evolve.elsevier.com/KeeHayes/pharmacology/

- Animations
- Content Updates
- Key Points
- Review Questions for the NCLEX® Examination
- References from the Textbook
- Unfolding Case Studies

OBJECTIVES

- Explain the pathophysiologic basis of five cardinal signs of inflammation.
- Compare the action of various nonsteroidal antiinflammatory drugs (NSAIDs).
- Explain the use of disease-modifying antirheumatic drugs (DMARDs).
- Differentiate between the side effects and adverse reactions of NSAIDs and DMARDs.
- Correlate the nursing processes associated with NSAIDs and corticosteroids, including patient teaching.
- Apply the nursing process to the patient taking DMARDs.
- Compare the action of various antigout medications.

OUTLINE

Pathophysiology
Antiinflammatory Agents
Nonsteroidal Antiinflammatory Drugs
- Salicylates
- Nursing Process: Patient-Centered Collaborative Care: Salicylate: Aspirin
- *Para*-Chlorobenzoic Acid
- Phenylacetic Acid Derivatives
- Propionic Acid Derivatives
- Fenamates
- Oxicams
- Nursing Process: Patient-Centered Collaborative Care: Nonsteroidal Antiinflammatory Drug: Ibuprofen
- Selective COX-2 Inhibitors (Second-Generation NSAIDs)
- Use of NSAIDs in Older Adults

Corticosteroids
Disease-Modifying Antirheumatic Drugs
- Immunosuppressive Agents
- Immunomodulators
- Nursing Process: Patient-Centered Collaborative Care: Infliximab (Remicade)
- Antimalarials

Antigout Drugs
- Antiinflammatory Gout Drug: Colchicine
- Uric Acid Inhibitor
- Uricosurics
- Nursing Process: Patient-Centered Collaborative Care: Antigout: Allopurinol

Key Websites
Critical Thinking Case Study
NCLEX Study Questions

KEY TERMS

cyclooxygenase, p. 337
COX-2 inhibitors, p. 340
disease-modifying antirheumatic drugs, p. 345
gout, p. 348
immunomodulators, p. 345
immunosuppressives, p. 345
infection, p. 337
inflammation, p. 337
nonsteroidal antiinflammatory drugs, p. 337
prostaglandins, p. 337
uricosurics, p. 348

Inflammation is a response to tissue injury and infection. When the inflammatory process occurs, a vascular reaction takes place in which fluid, elements of blood, leukocytes (white blood cells [WBCs]), and chemical mediators accumulate at the injured tissue or infection site. The process of inflammation is a protective mechanism in which the body attempts to neutralize and destroy harmful agents at the site of injury and to establish conditions for tissue repair.

Although there is a relationship between inflammation and infection, these terms should *not* be used interchangeably. **Infection** is caused by microorganisms and results in inflammation, but *not* all inflammations are caused by infections.

PATHOPHYSIOLOGY

The five characteristics of inflammation, called *the cardinal signs of inflammation,* are redness, swelling (edema), heat, pain, and loss of function. Table 25-1 gives the description and explanation of the cardinal signs of inflammation. The two phases of inflammation are the *vascular phase,* which occurs 10 to 15 minutes after an injury, and the *delayed phase.* The vascular phase is associated with vasodilation and increased capillary permeability, during which blood substances and fluid leave the plasma and go to the injured site. The delayed phase occurs when leukocytes infiltrate the inflamed tissue.

Various chemical mediators are released during the inflammation process. Prostaglandins that have been isolated from the exudate at inflammatory sites are among them. **Prostaglandins** (chemical mediators) have many effects: vasodilation, relaxation of smooth muscle, increased capillary permeability, and sensitization of nerve cells to pain.

TABLE 25-1 CARDINAL SIGNS OF INFLAMMATION

SIGNS	DESCRIPTION AND EXPLANATION
Erythema (redness)	Redness occurs in the first phase of inflammation. Blood accumulates in the area of tissue injury because of the release of the body's chemical mediators (kinins, prostaglandins, and histamine). Histamine dilates the arterioles.
Edema (swelling)	Swelling is the second phase of inflammation. Plasma leaks into the interstitial tissue at the injury site. Kinins dilate the arterioles, increasing capillary permeability.
Heat	Heat at the inflammatory site can be caused by increased blood accumulation and may result from pyrogens (substances that produce fever) that interfere with the temperature-regulating center in the hypothalamus.
Pain	Pain is caused by tissue swelling and the release of chemical mediators.
Loss of function	Function is lost because of the accumulation of fluid at the tissue injury site and because of pain, which decreases mobility at the affected area.

Cyclooxygenase (COX) is the enzyme responsible for converting arachidonic acid into prostaglandins and their products. This synthesis of prostaglandins causes inflammation and pain at a tissue injury site. There are two enzyme forms of cyclooxygenase: COX-1 and COX-2. COX-1 protects the stomach lining and regulates blood platelets, and COX-2 triggers inflammation and pain.

ANTIINFLAMMATORY AGENTS

Drugs such as aspirin inhibit the biosynthesis of prostaglandin and are therefore called *prostaglandin inhibitors.* Because prostaglandin inhibitors affect the inflammatory process, they are more commonly called *antiinflammatory agents.*

Antiinflammatory agents also relieve pain (analgesic), reduce elevated body temperature (antipyretic), and inhibit platelet aggregation (anticoagulant). Aspirin is the oldest antiinflammatory drug, but it was first used for its analgesic and antipyretic properties. As a result of searching for a more effective drug with fewer side effects, many other antiinflammatory agents, or prostaglandin inhibitors, have been discovered. Although these drugs have potent antiinflammatory effects that mimic the effects of corticosteroids (cortisone), they are *not* chemically related to corticosteroids and therefore are called **nonsteroidal antiinflammatory drugs (NSAIDs).** Most NSAIDs are used to decrease inflammation and pain for patients who have some type of arthritic condition.

NONSTEROIDAL ANTIINFLAMMATORY DRUGS

NSAIDs are aspirin and aspirin-like drugs that inhibit the enzyme COX, which is needed for the biosynthesis of prostaglandins. Chapters 26 and 45 present expanded discussions of NSAIDs in their roles as analgesics and anticoagulants, respectively. These drugs may be called *prostaglandin inhibitors* with varying degrees of analgesic and antipyretic effects, but they are used primarily as antiinflammatory agents to relieve inflammation and pain. Their antipyretic effect is less than their antiinflammatory effect. With several exceptions, NSAID preparations are not suggested for use in alleviating mild headaches and mildly elevated temperature. Preferred drugs for headaches and fever are aspirin, acetaminophen, and ibuprofen (given to children and adults with high fever). NSAIDs are more appropriate for reducing swelling, pain, and stiffness in joints.

NSAIDs cost more than aspirin. Other than aspirin, the only NSAIDs that can be purchased over-the-counter (OTC) are ibuprofen (Motrin, Advil) and naproxen (Aleve). Ibuprofen is also available in generic form in 200-mg tablets or capsules. All other NSAIDs require a prescription. Examples of prescription products on the market that contain NSAID contents alone or in combination include Anaprox, Celebrex, Clinoril, Daypro, Equagesic, Naprosyn, Percodan, Relafen, Soma Compound, Talwin, and Toradol. If a patient can take aspirin for the inflammatory process without gastrointestinal (GI) upset, salicylate products are usually recommended.

There are seven groups of NSAIDs:

1. Salicylates
2. *Para*-chlorobenzoic acid derivatives, or indoles
3. Phenylacetic acids
4. Propionic acid derivatives
5. Fenamates
6. Oxicams
7. Selective COX-2 inhibitors

The first six NSAID groups on the list are known as *first-generation NSAIDs,* and the COX-2 inhibitors are called *second-generation NSAIDs.*

Table 25-2 provides dosage information and considerations for use for the most commonly used NSAIDs. The half-lives of NSAIDs differ greatly—some have a short half-life, and others have a moderate to long half-life with a general range of 8 to 24 hours. Aspirin should not be taken with an NSAID because of the side effects. In addition, combined therapy does not increase effectiveness.

Salicylates

Aspirin comes from the family of salicylates derived from salicylic acid. Aspirin is also called *acetylsalicylic acid (ASA)* after the acetyl group used in the composition of aspirin. The abbreviation frequently used for aspirin is ASA.

TABLE 25-2 ANTIINFLAMMATORY AGENTS: NONSTEROIDAL

GENERIC (BRAND)	ROUTE AND DOSAGE	USES AND CONSIDERATIONS
First-Generation NSAIDs		
Salicylates		
aspirin (ASA, Bayer, Ecotrin)	See Prototype Drug Chart 25-1.	
diflunisal (Dolobid)	A: PO: 250-500 mg b.i.d.; *max:* 1500 mg/d	Relief of mild to moderate pain; used to treat osteoarthritis and rheumatoid arthritis. Acts by inhibiting prostaglandin synthesis. Avoid if hypersensitive to aspirin. Do not use during third trimester of pregnancy. Pregnancy category: C; PB: 99%; t½: 8-12 h
Salicylate Derivatives		
olsalazine sodium (Dipentum)	A: PO: 500 mg q12h; may increase dose every 2-4 wk; *max:* 3 g/d in divided doses	For inflammatory bowel disease, especially ulcerative colitis. Excreted mainly in feces as 5-ASA. Pregnancy category: C; PB: 99%; t½: 5-10 h
sulfasalazine (Azulfidine)	A: PO: 0.5-1 g/d initially, then 2 g/d in divided doses; *max:* 3 g/d C >6 y: PO: 30-50 mg/kg/d in 4 divided doses; *max:* 2 g/d	For ulcerative colitis and rheumatoid arthritis. Avoid if allergic to sulfonamides or aspirin. Pregnancy category: B; PB: 99%; t½: 5-10 h
Para-Chlorobenzoic Acid (Indoles)		
indomethacin (Indocin)	A: PO: 75-150 mg/d in 3-4 divided doses with food for 7-14 d; *max:* 200 mg/d; SR: 75 mg daily/b.i.d.; *max:* 150 mg/d	For moderate to severe arthritic conditions. GI upset and ulceration are common. Take with food. Avoid if allergic to aspirin. Pregnancy category: C; PB: 99%; t½: 4.5 h
sulindac (Clinoril)	A: PO: 150-200 mg b.i.d.; *max:* 400 mg/d	For acute and chronic arthritis, bursitis, and tendinitis. Not as potent as indomethacin. Take with food. Pregnancy category: C; PB: 93%; t½: 7.8 h
tolmetin	A: PO: Initially: 400 mg t.i.d.; *maint:* 600-1800 mg/d in divided doses; *max:* 1.8 g/d C >2 y: PO: 20 mg/kg/d in divided doses; *max:* 30 mg/kg/d	For acute and chronic arthritis, including juvenile rheumatoid arthritis. Less potent than indomethacin; more effective than aspirin. Take with food. Pregnancy category: C (D, third trimester); PB: 90%-99%; t½: 1-2 h
Phenylacetic Acid		
diclofenac sodium (Voltaren XR)	A: PO: 25-50 mg t.i.d./q.i.d.; SR: 100 mg/d	For rheumatoid arthritis, osteoarthritis, and spondylitis. Also for acute gout, juvenile rheumatoid arthritis, bursitis, and tendinitis. Take with food to avoid GI upset. Pregnancy category: C (D, third trimester); PB: 90%-99%; t½: 2 h
etodolac (Lodine)	A: PO: 600-1000 mg/d in 2-4 divided doses PRN; *max:* 1200 mg/d	For acute pain, rheumatoid arthritis, and osteoarthritis. Take with food or antacid to avoid GI upset. Pregnancy category: C (D, third trimester); PR: 99%; t½: 6-7 h
ketorolac tromethamine (Toradol)	A: PO: 20 mg q6h PRN; *max:* 40 mg/d IM/IV: 30 mg q6h PRN; *max:* 120 mg/d Older adults: PO: 5-10 mg q6h PRN; *max:* 40 mg/d IM/IV: 15 mg q6h PRN; *max:* 60 mg/d	First injectable NSAID. For short-term pain management of 5 days or less. Also available for ophthalmic use to relieve itching caused by allergic conjunctivitis. Pregnancy category: C (D, third trimester); PB: 99%; t½: 4-6 h

TABLE 25-2 ANTIINFLAMMATORY AGENTS: NONSTEROIDAL—cont'd

GENERIC (BRAND)	ROUTE AND DOSAGE	USES AND CONSIDERATIONS
Propionic Acid		
fenoprofen calcium (Nalfon)	A: PO: 300-600 mg t.i.d./q.i.d.; *max:* 3200 mg/d	For mild to moderate pain. Also for arthritic conditions. Most effective after 2-3 wk of therapy. Take with food. Pregnancy category: C (D, third trimester); PB: 90%-99%; t½: 3 h
flurbiprofen sodium (Ansaid)	A: PO: 200-300 mg/d in 2-4 divided doses; *max:* 300 mg/d	For acute and chronic arthritis. Take with food. Pregnancy category: C (D, third trimester); PB: 99%; t½: 5 h
ibuprofen (Motrin, Advil)	See Prototype Drug Chart 25-2.	
ketoprofen (Nexcede)	Arthritis: A: PO: Initially 50 mg q.i.d. or 75 mg t.i.d.; *max:* 300 mg/d SR: A: PO: 200 mg q.d.; *max:* 200 mg/d SR: Older adult: PO: 100-150 mg/d; *max:* 200 mg/d Mild to moderate pain: A: PO: 12.5-50 mg q6-8h PRN; *max:* 300 mg/d	Relief of mild to moderate pain and acute and chronic arthritis. Take with food or 8 ounces of water to avoid GI upset. Pregnancy category: C (D, third trimester); PB: 99%; t½: 2-4 h
naproxen (Naprosyn, Aleve)	A: PO: 250-500 mg b.i.d.; *max:* 1500 mg/d C >2y: PO: 5-10 mg/kg q12h; *max:* 1000 mg/d	Relief of mild to moderate pain. Also for arthritic, gout, and bursitis conditions, and dysmenorrhea. OTC drug: Aleve. Take with food or with a full glass of water. Pregnancy category: C (D, third trimester); PB: 99%; t½: 12-17 h
oxaprozin (Daypro)	A: PO: 600-1200 mg/d; *max:* 1800 mg/d in divided doses	Treatment of acute and chronic arthritis. Take with food to avoid GI upset.. Pregnancy category: C (D, third trimester); PB: 99%; t½: 40 h
Anthranilic Acids (Fenamates)		
meclofenamate	A: PO: 200-400 mg/d in 3-4 divided doses; *max:* 400 mg/d	For acute and chronic arthritis. GI symptoms can be severe. Used when other NSAIDs are not effective. Take with food to avoid GI upset. Pregnancy category: C (D, at term); PB: 99%; t½: 2 h
mefenamic acid (Ponstel)	A: PO: Initially: 500 mg; then 250 mg q6h PRN; *max:* 1250 mg/d	For acute and chronic arthritis. Diarrhea is a common problem. Usually discontinued after 7 days. Pregnancy category: C (D, third trimester); PB: 90%; t½: 2 h
Oxicams		
piroxicam (Feldene)	A: PO: 10-20 mg q.d.; *max:* 20 mg/d	For arthritic conditions. Long half-life; effective at 2 weeks. GI upset may occur. Pregnancy category: C (D, third trimester); PB: 99%; t½: 50 h
meloxicam (Mobic)	A: PO: 7.5-15 mg/d; *max:* 15 mg/d	For osteoarthritis. Some COX-2 selectivity. Pregnancy category: C (first and second trimester), D (third trimester); PB: 99%; t½: 15-20 h
Naphthylalkanones		
nabumetone (Relafen)	A: PO: 500-1000 mg q.d./b.i.d.; *max:* 2000 mg/d	For chronic inflammation and pain, especially for arthritic conditions such as rheumatoid arthritis and osteoarthritis. Inhibits cyclooxygenase, particularly COX-2 more than COX-1; fewer GI problems. Pregnancy category: C (D, third trimester); PB: 99%; t½: 24 h
COX-2 Inhibitors (Second-Generation NSAIDs)		
celecoxib (Celebrex)	See Prototype Drug Chart 25-3.	

A, Adult; *b.i.d.,* twice a day; *C,* child; *d,* day; *GI,* gastrointestinal; *h,* hour; *IM,* intramuscular; *maint,* maintenance; *max,* maximum; *NSAID,* nonsteroidal antiinflammatory drug; *OTC,* over-the-counter; *PB,* protein-binding; *PO,* by mouth; *PRN,* as needed; *q.i.d.,* four times a day; *sol,* solution; *SR,* sustained-release; *t½,* half-life; *t.i.d.,* three times a day; *UK,* unknown; *wk,* week; *y,* year; >, greater than; <, less than.

Aspirin was developed in 1899 by Adolph Bayer, making it the oldest antiinflammatory agent. It was the most frequently used antiinflammatory agent before the introduction of ibuprofen. Aspirin is a prostaglandin inhibitor that decreases the inflammatory process. It is also considered an antiplatelet drug for patients with cardiac or cerebrovascular disorders; aspirin decreases platelet aggregation, and thus blood clotting is decreased. Because high doses of aspirin are usually needed to relieve inflammation, gastric distress is a common problem. In such cases, enteric-coated (EC) tablets

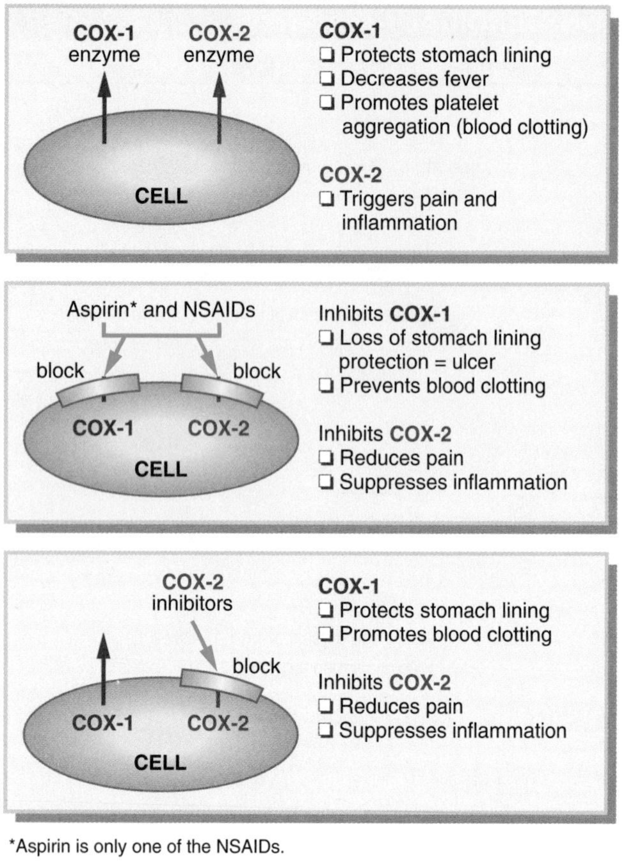

FIGURE 25–1 Uses of COX-1 and COX-2 inhibitors.

may be used. Aspirin should *not* be taken with other NSAIDs because it decreases the blood level and effectiveness of NSAIDs.

Aspirin and other NSAIDs relieve pain by inhibiting the enzyme COX, which is needed for the biosynthesis of prostaglandins. There are two enzyme forms of cyclooxygenase, symbolized as COX-1 and COX-2 (Figure 25-1). COX-1 protects the stomach lining and regulates blood platelets, promoting blood clotting. COX-2 triggers pain and inflammation at the injured site. Usually NSAIDs inhibit or block both COX-1 and COX-2. Inhibition of COX-1 produces the desirable effect of decreasing platelet aggregation, but the undesirable effect of decreasing protection to the stomach lining. Stomach bleeding and ulcers may occur with aspirin and NSAID agents. When COX-2 is inhibited, pain and fever are reduced and inflammation is suppressed, but COX-2 inhibitors do not cause gastric ulceration and have no effect on platelet function.

New NSAIDs, called **COX-2 inhibitors,** block only COX-2 and not COX-1. These drugs leave protection for the stomach lining intact (no gastric bleeding and ulcers), but still deliver relief for pain and inflammation.

A COX-2 inhibitor approved by the U.S. Food and Drug Administration (FDA) is celecoxib (Celebrex). Drugs similar to COX-2 inhibitors include meloxicam (Mobic) and nabumetone (Relafen), which allow some stomach protection. Patients at risk for stroke or heart attack who take aspirin to prevent blood clotting (decrease platelet aggregation) would not benefit from COX-2 inhibitors. If the COX-1 enzyme was not blocked, increased blood clotting would remain even though the stomach lining is protected.

Many researchers believe that COX-2 inhibitors may prevent some types of cancer (e.g., colon cancer). Fruits and vegetables block COX-2 enzyme naturally, protecting the colon from malignant growths.

Pharmacokinetics Aspirin is well absorbed from the GI tract (Prototype Drug Chart 25-1). It can cause GI upset, so it should be taken with water, milk, or food. The EC or buffered form can decrease gastric distress. EC tablets should not be crushed or broken.

Aspirin has a short half-life. It should not be taken during the last trimester of pregnancy, because it could cause premature closure of the ductus arteriosus in the fetus. Aspirin should not be taken by children with flu symptoms, because it may cause the potentially fatal Reye syndrome.

Pharmacodynamics Aspirin, like other NSAIDs, inhibits prostaglandin synthesis by inhibiting COX-1 and COX-2; thus it decreases inflammation and pain. The onset of action for aspirin is within 30 minutes. It peaks in 1 to 2 hours, and the duration of action is an average of 4 to 6 hours. The action for the rectal preparation of aspirin can be erratic because of blood supply and fecal material in the rectum; it may take a week or longer for a therapeutic antiinflammatory effect.

Hypersensitivity to Salicylate Products

Patients may be hypersensitive to aspirin. Tinnitus (ringing in the ears), vertigo (dizziness), and bronchospasm—especially in asthmatic patients—are symptoms of aspirin overdose or hypersensitivity to aspirin. Patients should not take diflunisal if they are hypersensitive to aspirin. Diflunisal is a derivative of salicylic acid, although it is not converted to salicylic acid in the body.

Salicylates are present in numerous foods (e.g., prunes, raisins, licorice) and in spices (e.g., curry powder, paprika).

Nursing Process
Patient-Centered Collaborative Care

Salicylate: Aspirin

Assessment

- Determine a medical history. Ask patient if there is any history of gastric upset, gastric bleeding, or liver disease. Aspirin can cause gastric irritation. It prolongs bleeding time by inhibiting platelet aggregation.
- Obtain a drug history. Report if a drug-drug interaction is probable.

Nursing Diagnoses

- Risk for injury related to vertigo
- Chronic pain related to tissue swelling of rheumatoid arthritis

Planning

- The patient's pain will be reduced within 12 to 24 hours.
- The patient's inflammation will be reduced within 1 week.

PROTOTYPE DRUG CHART 25-1

Aspirin

Drug Class	Dosage
Analgesic: antiinflammatory drug Trade Names: ASA, Bayer, Ecotrin, ♣ Astrin Pregnancy Category: D	Analgesic: A: PO: 325-650 mg q4h PRN; *max:* 4 g/d C: PO: 10-15 mg/kg in 4 to 6 divided doses; *max:* 4 g/d TIA and thromboembolic condition: A: PO: 81-325 mg/d Arthritis: A: PO: 3 g/d in divided doses TDM: 15-30 mg/dL; 150 to 300 mcg/mL
Contraindications	**Drug-Lab-Food Interactions**
Hypersensitivity to salicylates or NSAIDs, flu or virus symptoms in children, anticoagulant therapy, GI bleeding, bone marrow suppression, third trimester of pregnancy Caution: Renal or hepatic disorders gout, alcoholism Lab: Decrease cholesterol and potassium, T3, T4 levels; increase PT, bleeding time, uric acid	Drug: Increase risk of bleeding with anticoagulants and other NSAIDs; increase risk of hypoglycemia with oral hypoglycemic drugs; increase ulcerogenic effect with glucocorticoids
Pharmacokinetics	**Pharmacodynamics**
Absorption: PO: 80%-100% Distribution: PB: 80%-90%, crosses placenta Metabolism: t½: 2-3 h (low dose); 15-20 h (high dose) Excretion: 50% in urine	PO: Onset: 15-30 min Peak: 1-2 h Duration: 4-6 h PR: Onset: 1-2 h Peak: 3-5 h Duration: 4-7 h
Therapeutic Effects/Uses	
To reduce pain and inflammatory symptoms; to decrease body temperature; to inhibit platelet aggregation Mode of Action: Inhibition of prostaglandin synthesis, inhibition of hypothalamic heat-regulator center	
Side Effects	**Adverse Reactions**
Anorexia, nausea, vomiting, diarrhea, dizziness, confusion, hearing loss, heartburn, rash, abdominal pain, drowsiness	Tinnitus, urticaria, ulceration, GI bleeding Life-threatening: Agranulocytosis, hemolytic anemia, bronchospasm, anaphylaxis, thrombocytopenia, Reye's syndrome, hepatotoxicity, leukopenia

A, Adult; *ASA,* acetylsalicylic acid; *b.i.d.,* two times a day; *C,* child; *d,* day; *h,* hour; *max,* maximum; *min,* minute; *NSAIDs,* nonsteroidal antiinflammatory drugs; *PB,* protein binding; *PO,* by mouth; *PR,* per rectum; *PRN,* as necessary; *PT,* prothrombin time; *t ½,* half-life; *TDM,* therapeutic drug monitoring; *TIA,* transient ischemic attack; ♣, Canadian drug name.

Nursing Interventions

- Monitor serum salicylate (aspirin) level when patient takes high doses of aspirin for chronic conditions such as arthritis. Normal therapeutic range is 15 to 30 mg/dL. Mild toxicity occurs at serum level of >30 mg/dL, and severe toxicity occurs at >50 mg/dL.
- Observe patient for signs of bleeding such as dark (tarry) stools, bleeding gums, petechiae (round red spots), ecchymosis (excessive bruising), and purpura (large red spots) when patient takes high doses of aspirin.

Patient Teaching

General

- Advise patient not to take aspirin with alcohol or with drugs that are highly protein-bound, such as the anticoagulant warfarin (Coumadin). Aspirin displaces drugs like warfarin from the protein-binding site, causing increased anticoagulant levels.
- Suggest that patient inform the dentist before a dental visit if taking high doses of aspirin.
- Instruct patient to discontinue aspirin 3 to 7 days before surgery to reduce risk of bleeding (with the health care provider's approval).
- Keep aspirin bottle out of reach of children.
- Educate parent to call poison control center immediately if a child has taken a large or unknown amount of aspirin (or acetaminophen).
- Warn patient not to administer aspirin for virus or flu symptoms in children. Reye's syndrome (vomiting, lethargy, delirium, and coma) has been linked with aspirin and viral infections. Acetaminophen is usually prescribed for cold and flu symptoms.
- Inform patient that aspirin tablets can cause GI distress.

- Inform patient with dysmenorrhea to take acetaminophen instead of aspirin 2 days before and during the first 2 days of the menstrual period.

Side Effects

- Direct patient to report side effects such as drowsiness, tinnitus (ringing in the ears), headaches, flushing, dizziness, GI symptoms (bleeding, heartburn), visual changes, and seizures.

Diet

- Instruct patient to take aspirin (also ibuprofen) with food, at mealtime, or with plenty of fluids. EC aspirin helps prevent GI disturbance.

Cultural Considerations

- Do not misunderstand loud voice volume as necessarily reflecting anger or agitation; patients may be merely expressing their thoughts in a dynamic manner.

Evaluation

- Evaluate the effectiveness of aspirin in relieving pain. If pain persists, another analgesic such as ibuprofen may be prescribed.
- Determine whether patient has any side effects to aspirin.

Para-Chlorobenzoic Acid

One of the first NSAIDs introduced was indomethacin (Indocin), a *para*-chlorobenzoic acid. It is used for rheumatoid arthritis, gouty arthritis, and osteoarthritis and is a potent prostaglandin inhibitor. It is highly protein bound (90%) and displaces other protein-bound drugs, resulting in potential toxicity. It has a moderate half-life (4.5 hours). Indomethacin is very irritating to the stomach and should be taken with food.

Two other *para*-chlorobenzoic acid derivatives—sulindac (Clinoril) and tolmetin (Tolectin)—produce less severe adverse reactions than indomethacin. Tolmetin is not as highly protein-bound as indomethacin and sulindac, and it has a short half-life. This group of NSAIDs may cause sodium and water retention and increased blood pressure.

Phenylacetic Acid Derivatives

Diclofenac sodium (Voltaren-XR), a phenylacetic acid derivative, has a plasma half-life of 1.2 to 2 hours. Its analgesic and antiinflammatory effects are similar to those of aspirin, but it has minimal to no antipyretic effects. It is indicated for rheumatoid arthritis, osteoarthritis, and ankylosing spondylitis. Diclofenac is available in PO, extended-release, and topical 1% gel preparations. Adverse reactions are similar to those of other NSAIDs.

Ketorolac (Toradol), another phenylacetic acid derivative, is the first injectable NSAID. Like other NSAIDs, it inhibits prostaglandin synthesis, but it has greater analgesic properties than other antiinflammatory agents. Ketorolac is recommended for short-term management of pain. For postsurgical pain, it has shown analgesic efficacy equal or superior to that of opioid analgesics. It is administered intramuscularly in doses of 30 to 60 mg every 6 hours for adults. Ketorolac is also available in PO, IV, and intranasal preparations.

Propionic Acid Derivatives

The propionic acid group is a relatively new group of NSAIDs. These drugs are aspirin-like but have stronger effects and create less GI irritation. Drugs in this group are highly protein-bound, so drug interactions might occur, especially when given with another highly protein-bound drug. Propionic acid derivatives are better tolerated than other NSAIDs. Gastric upset occurs, but it is not as severe as with aspirin and indomethacin. Severe adverse reactions such as blood dyscrasias are not frequently seen. Ibuprofen (Motrin) is the most widely used propionic acid NSAID, and it may be purchased OTC in lower doses (200 mg). Prototype Drug Chart 25-2 details the pharmacologic behavior of ibuprofens. Six other propionic acid agents are fenoprofen calcium (Nalfon), naproxen (Naprosyn), ketoprofen (Orudis), flurbiprofen (Ansaid), and oxaprozin (Daypro).

Pharmacokinetics Ibuprofens are well absorbed from the GI tract. These drugs have a short half-life but are highly protein-bound. If ibuprofen is taken with another highly protein-bound drug, severe side effects may occur. The drug is metabolized in the liver to inactivate metabolites and is excreted as inactive metabolites in the urine.

Pharmacodynamics Ibuprofens inhibit prostaglandin synthesis and are therefore effective in alleviating inflammation and pain. They have a short onset of action, peak concentration time, and duration of action. It may take several days for the antiinflammatory effect to be evident.

There are many drug interactions associated with ibuprofen. It can increase the effects of warfarin (Coumadin), sulfonamides, many of the cephalosporins, and phenytoin. When taken with aspirin, its effect can be decreased. Hypoglycemia may result when ibuprofen is taken with insulin or an oral hypoglycemic drug. There is a high risk of toxicity when ibuprofen is taken concurrently with calcium channel blockers.

Fenamates

The fenamate group includes potent NSAIDs used for acute and chronic arthritic conditions. Like most NSAIDs, gastric irritation is a common side effect of fenamates, and patients with a history of peptic ulcer should avoid taking this group of drugs. Other side effects include edema, dizziness, tinnitus, and pruritus. Two fenamates are meclofenamate sodium monohydrate (Meclomen) and mefenamic acid (Ponstel).

Oxicams

Piroxicam (Feldene), an oxicam, is indicated for long-term arthritic conditions such as rheumatoid arthritis and osteoarthritis. It too can cause gastric problems such as ulceration and epigastric distress, but the incidence is lower than for some other NSAIDs. It is well tolerated, and its major advantage over other NSAIDs is its long half-life, which allows it to be taken only once daily.

Full clinical response to piroxicam may take 1 to 2 weeks. This drug is also highly protein-bound and may interact with

PROTOTYPE DRUG CHART 25-2

Ibuprofen

Drug Class Nonsteroidal antiinflammatory drug: propionic acid derivative Trade Names: Motrin, Advil Pregnancy Category: C (D, third trimester)	**Dosage** A: PO: 200-800 mg t.i.d./q.i.d.; *max:* 2400 mg/d
Contraindications Severe renal or hepatic disease, asthma, peptic ulcer, anticoagulant therapy Caution: Bleeding disorders, pregnancy, lactation, systemic lupus erythematosus	**Drug-Lab-Food Interactions** Drug: Increase bleeding time with oral anticoagulants; increase effects of phenytoin, sulfonamides, warfarin; decrease effect with aspirin; may increase severe side effects of lithium
Pharmacokinetics Absorption: PO: Well absorbed Distribution: PB: 90%-99% Metabolism: t½: 2-4 h Excretion: In urine, mostly as inactive metabolites; some in bile	**Pharmacodynamics** PO: Onset: 1 h Peak: 2-4 h Duration: 4-6 h
Therapeutic Effects/Uses To reduce inflammatory process; to relieve pain; antiinflammatory effect for arthritic conditions; to reduce fever Mode of Action: Inhibition of prostaglandin synthesis, thus relieving pain and inflammation	
Side Effects Anorexia, nausea, vomiting, diarrhea, edema, rash, purpura, tinnitus, fatigue, dizziness, lightheadedness, anxiety, confusion, fluid retention with edema	**Adverse Reactions** GI bleeding Life-threatening: Blood dyscrasias, cardiac dysrhythmias, nephrotoxicity, anaphylaxis

A, Adult; *C,* child; *d,* day; *GI,* gastrointestinal; *h,* hour; *max,* maximum; *PB,* protein-binding; *PO,* by mouth; *q.i.d.,* four times a day; *t ½,* half-life; *t.i.d.,* three times a day; *y,* year; <, less than; >, greater than.

another highly protein-bound drug if taken together. Piroxicam should not be taken with aspirin or other NSAIDs.

General Side Effects and Adverse Reactions for First-Generation NSAIDs

Most NSAIDs tend to have fewer side effects than aspirin when taken at antiinflammatory doses, but gastric irritation is still a common problem when NSAIDs are taken without food. In addition, sodium and water retention may occur. Alcoholic beverages consumed with NSAIDs may increase gastric irritation and should be avoided.

Nursing Process
Patient-Centered Collaborative Care

Nonsteroidal Antiinflammatory Drug: Ibuprofen

Assessment

- Check patient's history of allergy to NSAIDs such as ibuprofen. If an allergy is present, notify health care provider.
- Obtain a drug and herbal history, and report any possible drug-drug or herb-drug interactions. NSAIDs can increase the effects of phenytoin (Dilantin), sulfonamides, and warfarin. Most NSAIDs are highly protein-bound and can displace other highly protein-bound drugs like warfarin (Coumadin).
- Determine medical history. NSAIDs are contraindicated if patient has severe renal or liver disease, peptic ulcer, or bleeding disorder.
- Assess patient for GI upset and peripheral edema, which are common side effects of NSAIDs.

Nursing Diagnoses

- Risk for injury related to dizziness
- Risk for activity intolerance related to fatigue

Planning

- The patient's inflammatory process will subside in 1 to 3 weeks.

Nursing Interventions

- Observe patient for bleeding gums, petechiae, ecchymoses, or black (tarry) stools. Bleeding time can be prolonged when NSAIDs are taken, especially with a highly protein-bound drug such as warfarin (anticoagulant).
- Report if patient has GI discomfort. Administer NSAIDs at mealtime or with food to prevent GI upset.
- Monitor vital signs and check for peripheral edema, especially in the morning.

- Do not give directions such as "take one blue pill" at a specified time. Instead, provide name and dosage of medication.

Patient Teaching

General

- Inform patient not to take aspirin and acetaminophen with NSAIDs. Taking an NSAID with aspirin could cause GI upset and possible GI bleeding.
- Inform patient to avoid alcohol when taking NSAIDs. GI upset or gastric ulcer may result.
- Alert patient that many herbal products may interact with NSAIDs and could cause bleeding. Doses of NSAIDs and/or herbs may need to be modified to avoid possible bleeding occurrence (Herbal Alert 25-1).
- Direct patient to inform the dentist or surgeon before a procedure when taking ibuprofen or other NSAIDs for a continuous period.
- Warn female patients not to take NSAIDs 1 to 2 days before menstruation to avoid heavy menstrual flow. If discomfort occurs, acetaminophen is usually prescribed.
- Advise pregnant patients to avoid NSAIDs. Congenital abnormalities may occur when NSAIDS are taken during early pregnancy, and excess bleeding might occur during delivery.
- Inform patient that it may take several weeks to experience desired drug effect of some NSAIDs and disease-modifying antirheumatic drugs (DMARDs).

Side Effects

- Educate patient of the common side effects of NSAIDs. Nausea, vomiting, peripheral edema, GI upset, purpura or petechiae, or dizziness might occur. Report occurrences of side effects.

Diet

- Advise patient to take NSAIDs with meals or snacks to reduce GI upset.

Cultural Considerations

- Recognize that patients from various cultural backgrounds respond to pain and inflammation in various ways. In some cultures, the use of drugs to alleviate pain and inflammation is not acceptable. Herbal medicine and acupuncture may be used to alleviate pain.
- Be supportive of patient's methods for pain control. Explain the purpose of medications and their actions and side effects.

Evaluation

- Evaluate the effectiveness of the drug therapy, such as a decrease in pain and in swollen joints and an increase in mobility.

HERBAL ALERT 25-1

NSAIDs

Dong quai, feverfew, garlic, ginger, and ginkgo may cause bleeding when taken with nonsteroidal antiinflammatory drugs (NSAIDs).

Selective COX-2 Inhibitors (Second-Generation NSAIDs)

COX-2 inhibitors became available in the last several years to decrease inflammation and pain. Most NSAIDs are nonselective inhibitors that inhibit COX-1 and COX-2. By inhibiting COX-1, protection of the stomach lining is decreased and clotting time is also decreased, which may benefit the patient with cardiovascular or coronary artery disease (CAD). Selective COX-2 inhibitors are drugs of choice for patients with severe arthritic conditions who need high doses of an antiinflammatory drug, because large doses of NSAIDs may cause peptic ulcer and gastric bleeding.

Currently there is one drug, celecoxib (Celebrex), classified as a COX-2 inhibitor. Nabumetone (Relafen) is a similar drug that can be used; however it is not considered a "true" COX-2 inhibitor. Nabumetone inhibits COX-2 more than COX-1. Celecoxib is described in Prototype Drug Chart 25-3.

SAFETY: Preventing Medication Errors

Do not confuse...

- **Celebrex** (COX-2 inhibitor) with **Celexa** (selective serotonin reuptake inhibitor for depression) or **Cerebyx** (hydantoin anticonvulsant).

Use of NSAIDs in Older Adults

Older adults frequently use NSAIDs to treat pain associated with inflammation caused by osteoarthritis, rheumatoid arthritis, and neuromuscular-skeletal disorders. As older adults age, the number of drugs taken daily increases; therefore drug interactions are more common, especially when numerous drugs are taken with NSAIDs. With the use of NSAIDs, GI distress (including ulceration) is four times more common in older adults; hospitalization is often necessary.

The introduction of COX-2 inhibitors (second-generation NSAIDs) has decreased the incidence of GI problems associated with NSAID use; however, edema is likely to occur. Renal function should be evaluated, and older adults should increase their fluid intake for adequate hydration. To decrease possible complications, the NSAID dose should be lowered.

CORTICOSTEROIDS

Corticosteroids such as prednisone, prednisolone, and dexamethasone are frequently used as antiinflammatory agents. This group of drugs controls inflammation by suppressing or preventing many of the components of the inflammatory process at the injured site. Corticosteroids have been widely prescribed for arthritic conditions, and although they are not the drug of choice for arthritis because of their numerous side effects, they are frequently used to control arthritic flareups.

PROTOTYPE DRUG CHART 25-3

Celecoxib

Drug Class	Dosage
Nonsteroidal antiinflammatory: COX-2 inhibitor Trade Name: Celebrex Pregnancy Category: C (first and second trimester), D (third trimester)	Arthritis: A: PO: 100 mg b.i.d. or 200 mg daily Dysmenorrhea: A: PO: 400 mg first dose, follow with 200 mg same day if needed, and then 200 mg b.i.d. PRN
Contraindications	**Drug-Lab-Food Interactions**
Hypersensitivity, advanced renal disease, severe hepatic failure, anemia, concurrent use of diuretics and ACE inhibitors Caution: Renal or hepatic dysfunction, hypertension, fluid retention, heart failure, infection, history of GI bleeding or ulceration, concurrent anticoagulant therapy, steroids, or alcohol use	Drug: Decrease effect of ACE inhibitors, increased INR and GI bleeding with warfarin, may increase toxicity with lithium, fluconazole increases celecoxib levels.
Pharmacokinetics	**Pharmacodynamics**
Absorption: Well-absorbed in GI tract Distribution: PB: 97% Metabolism: t½: 11.2 h Excretion: Primarily in feces	PO: Onset: UK Peak: 3 h Duration: UK
Therapeutic Effects/Uses	
To treat osteoarthritis and rheumatoid arthritis, to relieve dysmenorrhea Mode of Action: Inhibits COX-2 (which normally promotes prostaglandin synthesis and inflammatory response) but does not inhibit COX-1	
Side Effects	**Adverse Reactions**
Headache, dizziness, sinusitis, nausea, flatulence, diarrhea, rash	Peripheral edema

A, Adult; *ACE,* angiotensin-converting enzyme; *b.i.d.,* twice a day; *COX,* cyclooxygenase; *GI,* gastrointestinal; *h,* hour; *INR,* international normalized ratio; *PB,* protein-binding; *PO,* by mouth; *PRN,* as needed; *t½,* half-life; *UK,* unknown.

The half-life of a corticosteroid is long (greater than 24 hours), and it is administered once a day in a large prescribed dose. When discontinuing steroid therapy, the dosage should be tapered over a period of 5 to 10 days. Steroids are discussed in more detail in Chapter 51.

DISEASE-MODIFYING ANTIRHEUMATIC DRUGS

When NSAIDs do not control immune-mediated arthritic disease sufficiently, other drugs, although more toxic, can be prescribed to alter the disease process. The **disease-modifying antirheumatic drugs (DMARDs)** include immunosuppressive agents, immunomodulators, and antimalarials. DMARDs help alleviate the symptoms of rheumatoid arthritis for the 2 million persons in the United States affected by the disorder. DMARDs are described in Table 25-3.

Immunosuppressive Agents

Immunosuppressives are used to treat refractory rheumatoid arthritis (arthritis that does not respond to antiinflammatory drugs). In low doses, selected immunosuppressive agents have been effective in the treatment of rheumatoid arthritis. Drugs such as azathioprine (Imuran), cyclophosphamide (Cytoxan), and methotrexate (Mexate), primarily used to suppress cancer growth and proliferation, might be used to suppress the inflammatory process of rheumatoid arthritis when other treatments fail. In one study of patients receiving cyclophosphamide, few new erosions of joint cartilage were present, suggesting that the disease process was not active.

Immunomodulators

Immunomodulators treat moderate to severe rheumatoid arthritis by disrupting the inflammatory process and delaying disease progression. Interleukin (IL-1) receptor antagonists and tumor necrosis factor (TNF) blockers are two groups of drugs classified as immunomodulators.

Anakinra (Kineret), an IL-1 receptor antagonist, blocks activity of IL-1 by inhibiting it from binding to interleukin receptors located in cartilage and bone. IL-1 is a proinflammatory cytokine that contributes to synovial inflammation and joint destruction. Anakinra is administered subcutaneously. The peak is 3 to 7 hours, and the half-life is 6 hours.

TNF blockers bind to TNF and block it from attaching to TNF receptors on synovial cell surfaces. By neutralizing TNF, a contributor to synovitis, inflammatory disease process is delayed. Etanercept (Enbrel) was the first TNF blocker developed and is administered subcutaneously. The peak half-life is 115 hours. Signs and symptoms of rheumatoid arthritis are suppressed rapidly with etanercept therapy but reappear if the drug is discontinued. Other TNF blockers include infliximab (Remicade), adalimumab (Humira), and leflunomide (Arava). Infliximab is administered intravenously (IV) over at least 2 hours, adalimumab is administered subcutaneously,

TABLE 25-3 ANTIINFLAMMATORY DRUGS: DMARDs

GENERIC (BRAND)	ROUTE AND DOSAGE	USES AND CONSIDERATIONS
golimumab (Simponi)	A: subQ: 50 mg every month	For treatment of rheumatoid arthritis. Adverse effects include blood dyscrasias. Pregnancy category: B; PB: UK; t½: 2 weeks
anakinra (Kineret)	A: subQ: 100 mg daily	For treatment of rheumatoid arthritis unresponsive to other DMARDs. Pregnancy category: B; PB: UK; t½: 4 to 6 h
etanercept (Enbrel)	A: subQ: 25 mg 2 times/wk or 50 mg/wk; *max:* 100 mg/wk C >4 y: subQ: 0.4 mg/kg 2 times/wk; *max:* 50 mg/wk	For treatment of rheumatoid arthritis unresponsive to other DMARDs. Pregnancy category: B; PB: UK; t½: 102 h
infliximab (Remicade)	See Prototype Drug Chart 25-4.	
rituximab (Rituxan)	A: IV: 1000 mg on day 1 and day 15 with methotrexate, then q16-24wks	For treatment of moderate to severe rheumatoid arthritis. Give methylpresnisolone 100 mg prior to each dose to decrease infusion reactions. Pregnancy category: C; PB: UK; t½: 60 to 174 h
adalimumab (Humira)	A: subQ: 40 mg every 2 wk	For treatment of rheumatoid arthritis unresponsive to other DMARDs. Pregnancy category: B; PB: UK; t½: 10 to 20 d
tocilizumab (Actemra)	A: IV: 4 mg/kg over 1 hour every 4 weeks; *max:* 800 mg/dose	For treatment of moderate to severe rheumatoid arthritis. Approved in 2010. Adverse effects include infection, GI perforation, hypertension. Pregnancy category: C; PB: UK; t½: 11 to 13 d
leflunomide (Arava)	A: PO: 100 mg/d for 3 d initially, then 20 mg/d	For treatment of rheumatoid arthritis unresponsive to other DMARDs. Pregnancy category: X; PB: 99%; t½: 19 d
abatacept (Orencia)	A: IV: 500 mg for <60 kg; 750 mg for 60 to 100 kg; 1 gram for >100 kg q2wk; initial dose followed by additional doses at 2- and 4-week intervals, then q4wk	For moderate to severe rheumatoid arthritis. Pregnancy category: C; PB: UK; t½: 13 d
tofacitinib (Xeljanz)	A: PO: 5 mg b.i.d.	For treatment of moderate to severe rheumatoid arthritis. Adverse effects include infection, headache, and hypertension. Pregnancy category: C; PB: 40%; t½: 3 h
tocilizumab (Actemra)	A: IV: 4 mg/kg q4wk initially; may increase to 8 mg/kg q4wk; *max:* 800 mg/dose q4wk	For treatment of moderate to severe rheumatoid arthritis unresponsive to other DMARDs. Adverse effects include gastritis, mouth ulcerations, upper abdominal pain, and hypertension. Pregnancy category: C; PB: UK; t½: up to 3 days

A, Adult; *C,* child; *d,* day; *DMARD,* disease-modifying antirheumatic drug;*GI,* gastrointestinal; *h,* hour; *IM,* intramuscular; *maint,* maintenance; *max,* maximum; *PB,* protein-binding; *PO,* by mouth; *PRN,* as needed; *t½,* half-life; *TD,* transdermal; *UK,* unknown; *wk,* week; *y,* year; >, greater than; <, less than.

and leflunomide is administered orally. Infliximab is described in Prototype Drug Chart 25-4.

Both IL-1 receptor antagonists and TNF blockers predispose the patient to severe infections; they are contraindicated in active infection and should be discontinued when an infection occurs. Immunomodulators are usually very expensive.

Nursing Process
Patient-Centered Collaborative Care

Infliximab (Remicade)

Assessment
- Determine a medical history. Ask patient if there is any history of seizures, diabetes mellitus, multiple sclerosis, or kidney or liver disease. Aspirin can cause gastric irritation. It prolongs bleeding time by inhibiting platelet aggregation.
- Obtain baseline renal and liver function tests.

Nursing Diagnoses
- Impaired physical mobility related to severe pain
- Chronic pain related to tissue swelling from rheumatoid arthritis

Planning
- The patient's pain will be reduced within 12 to 24 hours.
- The patient's inflammation will be reduced within 1 week.

Nursing Interventions
- Obtain negative tuberculosis skin test prior to initiating infliximab therapy.
- Monitor patient for signs and symptoms of infection. If a serious infection occurs while receiving infliximab therapy, antibiotic therapy should be initiated and infliximab discontinued.
- Monitor laboratory tests for blood dyscrasias (CBC), and renal and liver function (BUN, serum creatinine, ALP, AST, ALT).

PROTOTYPE DRUG CHART 25-4

Infliximab

Drug Class	Dosage
Immunomodulator: tumor necrosis factor blocker Trade Name: Remicade Pregnancy Category: B	Rheumatoid arthritis: A: IV: 3 mg/kg over 2 h; then 3 mg/kg on wk 2 and 6; and then q8wk Crohn's disease: A: IV: 5 mg/kg over 2 h initially and on wk 2 and 6, and then q8wk
Contraindications	**Drug-Lab-Food Interactions**
Hypersensitivity, heart failure Caution: Renal or hepatic dysfunction, bone marrow suppression, diabetes mellitus, immunosuppression, multiple sclerosis, seizures, older adults	Drug: May decrease effectiveness of vaccines; concurrent immunosuppressives may increase risk for infection or adverse effects
Pharmacokinetics	**Pharmacodynamics**
Absorption: UK Distribution: UK Metabolism: t½: 8-9.5 d Excretion: UK	IV: Onset: UK Peak: UK Duration: UK
Therapeutic Effects/Uses	
To treat moderate to severe rheumatoid arthritis and Crohn's disease Mode of Action: Binds to TNF and blocks it from attaching to TNF receptors on synovial cell surfaces. Reduces infiltration of inflammatory cells, and delays inflammatory process.	
Side Effects	**Adverse Reactions**
Headache, dizziness, coughing, fatigue, chills, hot flashes, anxiety, insomnia, depression, nausea, vomiting, diarrhea, constipation, flatulence, weight loss, rash, alopecia, dry skin, urinary frequency	Severe infections, chest pain, hypotension, hypertension, bradycardia, seizures, increased hepatic enzymes, neutropenia, pancytopenia, Stevens-Johnson syndrome

A, Adult; *d*, day; *IV*, intravenous; *t ½*, half-life; *UK*, unknown; *wk*, week.

- Flush IV tubing with normal saline before and after administration. Deliver IV medication through a 1.2 micron or less filter.
- Administer each dose over a minimum of 2 hours.
- Discontinue IV dose of infliximab if the patient develops acute infusion reaction (e.g., chest pain, fever, chills, dyspnea, pruritus, urticaria, hypotension or hypertension).
- Monitor patient up to 2 hours post-infusion for acute infusion reaction.

Patient Teaching

General

- Encourage patient to keep medical appointments and have regular scheduled laboratory tests for renal, liver, and complete blood count functions for early detection of blood dyscrasias and renal and liver damage.
- Advise patient to avoid live vaccine while taking infliximab.

Side Effects

- Teach patient to report dizziness, chills, depression, dyspnea, severe infections, seizures, fatigue, or rash immediately.
- Teach patient to report severe infections immediately.

Cultural Considerations

- Provide additional explanation as needed related to the disease process and the purpose of the drug and its side effects.
- Identify conflicts in values and beliefs.
- Suggest follow-up by a community health nurse to determine patient's compliance to the drug regimen and the effectiveness of the prescribed drug therapy.

Evaluation

- Evaluate patient's response to the DMARD. If pain persists, drug regimen may need modification.
- Determine the presence of adverse reactions. Drug therapy for pain may need to be changed.

Antimalarials

Antimalarial drugs may be used to treat rheumatoid arthritis when other methods of treatment fail. The mechanism of action of antimalarials in suppressing rheumatoid arthritis is unclear. The effect may take 4 to 12 weeks to become apparent, and antimalarials are usually used in combination with NSAIDs in patients whose arthritis is not under control.

ANTIGOUT DRUGS

Gout is an inflammatory condition that attacks joints, tendons, and other tissues. It may be called *gouty arthritis.* The most common site of acute gouty inflammation is at the joint of the big toe. Gout is characterized by a uric acid metabolism disorder and a defect in purine (products of certain proteins) metabolism, which results in an increase in urates (uric acid salts) and an accumulation of uric acid (hyperuricemia) or an ineffective clearance of uric acid by the kidneys. Uric acid solubility is poor in acid urine, and urate crystals may form, causing urate calculi. Gout may appear as bumps, or *tophi,* in the subcutaneous tissue of earlobes, elbows, hands, and the base of the large toe. In addition to tophi, the complications of untreated or prolonged periods of gout include gouty arthritis, urinary calculi, and gouty nephropathy.

Fluid intake should be increased while taking antigout drugs to promote uric acid excretion and prevent renal calculi. Foods high in purine (e.g., organ meats, sardines, salmon, gravy, herring, liver, meat soups) and alcohol (especially beer) should be avoided. Alcohol causes both an overproduction and underexcretion of uric acid. Acetaminophen should be taken for discomfort instead of aspirin (salicylic acid) to reduce acidity.

Antiinflammatory Gout Drug: Colchicine

The first drug used to treat gout was colchicine, introduced in 1936. This antiinflammatory gout drug inhibits the migration of leukocytes to the inflamed site. It is effective in alleviating acute symptoms of gout, but it is not effective in decreasing inflammation occurring in other inflammatory disorders. Colchicine does not inhibit uric acid synthesis and does not promote uric acid excretion. It should not be used if the patient has a severe renal, cardiac, or GI problem. Gastric irritation is a common problem, so colchicine should be taken with food. With high doses, nausea, vomiting, diarrhea, or abdominal pain occurs in approximately 75% of patients taking the drug.

Colchicine is well absorbed in the GI tract, and its peak concentration time is within 2 hours. Most of the drug is excreted in the feces, but 10% to 20% is excreted in the urine.

Uric Acid Inhibitor

Allopurinol (Zyloprim), first marketed in 1963, is not an antiinflammatory drug; instead, it inhibits the final steps of uric acid biosynthesis and therefore lowers serum uric acid levels, preventing the precipitation of an attack. This drug is frequently used as a prophylactic to prevent gout. It is a drug of choice for patients with chronic tophaceous gout. Allopurinol is also indicated for gout patients with renal impairment. It is useful for patients who have renal obstructions caused by uric acid stones and for patients with blood disorders such as leukemia and polycythemia vera. It is also given to patients who do not respond well to uricosuric drugs such as probenecid. Increased fluid intake is recommended to promote diuresis and alkalinization of the urine. Prototype Drug Chart 25-5 presents the pharmacologic behavior of allopurinol.

Pharmacokinetics Eighty percent of allopurinol is absorbed from the GI tract. Biosynthesis of uric acid occurs in the liver in pure form and active metabolites. The half-life of the drug itself is 2 to 3 hours and 20 to 24 hours for its active metabolites. The protein-binding percentage is unknown. Approximately 80% to 100% of allopurinol and its metabolites are excreted in urine.

Pharmacodynamics Allopurinol inhibits the production of uric acid by inhibiting the enzyme xanthine oxidase, which is needed in the synthesis of uric acid. Allopurinol also improves the solubility of uric acid. Its onset of action occurs within 30 to 60 minutes; its peak time averages 2 to 4 hours. Allopurinol has a long duration of action.

Alcohol, caffeine, and thiazide diuretics increase the uric acid level. Use of ampicillin or amoxicillin with allopurinol increases the risk of rash formation. Allopurinol can increase the effect of warfarin (Coumadin) and oral hypoglycemic drugs.

Uricosurics

Uricosurics increase the rate of uric acid excretion by inhibiting its reabsorption. These drugs are effective in alleviating chronic gout, but they should not be used during acute attacks. Probenecid (Benemid) is a uricosuric that has been available since 1945. It blocks the reabsorption of uric acid and promotes its excretion. Probenecid can be taken with colchicine. To begin initial therapy for relieving symptoms of gout and inhibiting uric acid reabsorption, small doses of colchicine should be given before adding probenecid. If gastric irritation occurs, probenecid should be taken with meals. It has an average half-life of 8 to 10 hours and is 85% to 95% protein-bound. Use caution when administering this drug with other highly protein-bound drugs.

Another uricosuric is sulfinpyrazone (Anturane). This drug is a metabolite of phenylbutazone and is more potent than probenecid. Sulfinpyrazone should be taken with meals or with antacids to prevent gastric irritation. Severe blood dyscrasias might occur, especially in patients with a history of blood dyscrasia. Table 25-4 gives dosages and considerations for the commonly used antigout drugs.

Side Effects and Adverse Reactions

Side effects may include flushed skin, sore gums, and headache. Kidney stones resulting from the uric acid could be prevented by increasing water intake and maintaining a urine pH above 6. Blood dyscrasias occur rarely. Aspirin use should be avoided, because it causes uric acid retention.

Nursing Process
Patient-Centered Collaborative Care

Antigout: Allopurinol

Assessment

- Obtain medical history from patient of any gastric, renal, cardiac, or liver disorders. Antigout drugs are excreted via kidneys, so sufficient renal function is needed. Drug dosage and drug selection might need to be changed.

PROTOTYPE DRUG CHART 25-5

Allopurinol

Drug Class Antigout: uric acid biosynthesis inhibitor Trade Names: Zyloprim, Aloprim, ♣ Apo-Allopurinol Pregnancy Category: C	**Dosage** A: PO: Initially: 100 mg/d, may increase; 200-300 mg/d (for mild gout); 400-600 mg/d (for severe gout); *max:* 800 mg/d C ≤10 y: PO: 10 mg/kg/d in 2-3 divided doses; *max:* 300 mg/dose
Contraindications Hypersensitivity, severe renal disease Caution: Hepatic disorder	**Drug-Lab-Food Interactions** Drug: Increase effect of warfarin, phenytoin, theophylline, anticancer drugs, ACE inhibitors; increase rash with ampicillin, amoxicillin; increase toxicity with thiazide diuretics; decrease allopurinol effect with antacids Lab: Increase AST, ALT, BUN
Pharmacokinetics Absorption: PO: 80% absorbed Distribution: PB: UK Metabolism: t½: 1-2 h Excretion: 80%-100% in urine	**Pharmacodynamics** PO: Onset: 0.5-1 h Peak: 2-4 h Duration: 18-30 h
Therapeutic Effects/Uses To treat gout and hyperuricemia; prevent urate calculi Mode of Action: Reduction of uric acid synthesis	
Side Effects Anorexia, nausea, vomiting, diarrhea, stomatitis, dizziness, headache, rash, pruritus, malaise, metallic taste, diaphoresis, edema, erectile dysfunction, peripheral neuropathy	**Adverse Reactions** Cataracts, retinopathy, bradycardia, depression Life-threatening: Bone marrow depression, aplastic anemia, thrombocytopenia, neutropenia, agranulocytosis, leukopenia

A, Adult; *ACE*, angiotensin-converting enzyme; *ALT*, alanine aminotransferase; *AST*, aspartate aminotransferase; *BUN*, blood urea nitrogen; *C*, child; *d*, day; *h*, hour; *max*, maximum; *PB*, protein-binding; *PO*, by mouth; *t½*, half-life; *UK*, unknown; *y*, year; ≤, less than or equal to; ♣, Canadian drug name.

TABLE 25-4 ANTIGOUT DRUGS

GENERIC (BRAND)	ROUTE AND DOSAGE	USES AND CONSIDERATIONS
Antiinflammatory Gout Drugs		
colchicine (Colcrys)	Acute gout attack: A: PO: Initially: 0.6-1.2 mg; 0.6 mg in 1 h; *max:* 2.4 mg/d Prophylaxis: A: PO: 0.6 mg q.d./b.i.d.; *max:* 1.2 mg/d	For acute gout and prophylaxis of recurrent gouty arthritis. Not for patients with renal or gastric disorders. Take with food. Pregnancy category: C; PB: 34%-44%; t½: 26.6-31.2 h
Uric Acid Biosynthesis Inhibitors		
allopurinol (Zyloprim)	See Prototype Drug Chart 25-5.	
febuxostat (Uloric)	A: PO: 40-80 mg/d; *max:* 120 mg/d	For hyperuricemia in gout. Blocks metabolism of xanthines to uric acid. Is more selective for xanthine oxidase than allopurinol. Side effects include GI distress and dysrhythmias. Pregnancy category: C; PB: 99.2%; t½: 5-8 h
Uricosurics		
probenecid	A: PO: First week: 250 mg b.i.d.; *maint:* 500 mg b.i.d.; *max:* 2 g/d C <50 kg: PO: 25-40 mg/kg/d in 4 divided doses	For hyperuricemia; promotes urinary excretion of uric acid. For gout and gouty arthritis. Alkaline urine helps prevent renal stones. Increase fluid intake. Pregnancy category: B; PB: 75%-95%; t½: 3-12 h
sulfinpyrazone (Anturane)	A: PO: Week 1: 100-200 mg b.i.d.; *maint:* 200-400 mg b.i.d.; may reduce to 200 mg/d; *max:* 800 mg/d	Management of hyperuricemia; decreases gouty attacks. May cause GI distress. Take with food. Pregnancy category: C; PB: 98%-99%; t½: 4 h

A, Adult; *b.i.d.*, twice a day; *C*, child; *d*, day; *GI*, gastrointestinal; *h*, hour; *IV*, intravenous; *maint*, maintenance; *max*, maximum; *min*, minute; *PB*, protein-binding; *PO*, by mouth; *PRN*, as needed; *t½*, half-life; <, less than.

- Obtain drug history. Report possible drug-drug interactions (see Prototype Drug Chart 25-2).
- Assess serum uric acid value for future comparison.
- Record urine output. Use initial urine output for future comparison.
- Check laboratory tests (e.g., blood urea nitrogen [BUN], serum creatinine, alkaline phosphatase [ALP], aspartate aminotransferase [AST], alanine aminotransferase [ALT], lactate dehydrogenase [LDH]), and compare with future laboratory test results.

Nursing Diagnoses

- Impaired tissue integrity related to inflammation of great toe
- Acute pain related to tissue swelling

Planning

- Patient's pain from gout will be absent or controlled without side effects.

Nursing Interventions

- Report GI symptoms, gastric pain, nausea, vomiting, or diarrhea when taking antigout drugs. Take these drugs with food to alleviate gastric distress.
- Record patient's urine output. Because the drugs and uric acid are excreted through the urine, kidney stones might occur, so both water intake and urine output should be increased.
- Monitor laboratory tests for renal and liver function (BUN, serum creatinine, ALP, AST, ALT).

Patient Teaching

General

- Encourage patient to keep medical appointments and have regular scheduled laboratory tests for renal, liver, and complete blood count functions. Some antigout drugs may cause blood dyscrasias; blood tests should be monitored.
- Instruct patient to increase fluid intake; it will increase drug and uric acid excretion.

Side Effects

- Inform patient to report to health care provider side effects of antigout drugs: anorexia, nausea, vomiting, diarrhea, stomatitis, dizziness, rash, pruritus, and metallic taste.
- Advise patient to have a yearly eye examination because visual changes can result from prolonged use of allopurinol.

Diet

- Warn patient to avoid alcohol and caffeine because they can increase uric acid levels.
- Suggest to patient not to take large doses of vitamin C while taking allopurinol; kidney stones may occur.
- Tell patient not to ingest foods high in purine content (e.g., organ meats, salmon, sardines, gravy, legumes). Purine foods increase uric acid levels.
- Direct patient to report any gastric distress. Encourage patient to take antigout drugs with food or at mealtime.

Cultural Considerations

- Provide additional explanation as needed related to the disease process and the purpose of the drug and its side effects.
- Identify conflicts in values and beliefs.
- Suggest follow-up by a community health nurse to determine patient's compliance to the drug regimen and the effectiveness of the prescribed drug therapy.

Evaluation

- Evaluate patient's response to the antigout drug. If pain persists, drug regimen may need modification.
- Determine the presence of adverse reactions. Drug therapy for gout pain may need to be changed.

KEY WEBSITES

Information on aspirin: *www.nlm.nih.gov/medlineplus/druginfo/medmaster/a682878.html*

Information on colchicine: *www.rxlist.com/cgi/generic2/colch.htm*

CRITICAL THINKING CASE STUDY

PQ, a 72-year-old woman, had taken 650 mg of aspirin four times a day for 8 months to alleviate her chronic symptoms of pain and inflammation associated with arthritis. Four weeks ago, a peptic ulcer developed.

1. Explain the process in which PQ could have a peptic ulcer. How could this have been prevented?
2. Compare the similarities and differences in the side effects of salicylates with those of acetic acid agents, propionic acid agents, COX-2 inhibitors, and phenylacetic acid.
3. What patient teaching points should PQ receive before and during the time she takes aspirin?
4. How would COX-2 inhibitors prevent the development of a peptic ulcer?
5. Would DMARDs be more helpful in alleviating PQ's symptoms? Explain your answer.
6. Compare the differences in the various types of DMARDs.

NCLEX STUDY QUESTIONS

1. A patient is taking ibuprofen. The nurse understands that COX-1 and COX-2 inhibitors are different in that ibuprofen is more likely than celecoxib to cause which adverse effect?
   a. Fever
   b. Constipation
   c. Peptic ulcer disease
   d. Metallic taste when eating
2. When teaching a patient who is receiving allopurinol, what should the nurse encourage the patient to do?
   a. Eat more meat.
   b. Increase vitamin C intake.
   c. Have annual eye examinations.
   d. Take medication 2 hours before meals.
3. A patient is admitted to the hospital with an acute gout attack. The nurse expects that which medication will be ordered to treat acute gout?
   a. colchicine
   b. allopurinol
   c. probenecid
   d. sulfinpyrazone
4. A patient is taking aspirin for arthritis. Which adverse reaction should the nurse teach the patient to report to the health care provider?
   a. Tinnitus
   b. Seizures
   c. Sinusitis
   d. Palpitations
5. The nurse is teaching a patient about taking aspirin. Which are important points for the nurse to include? (Select all that apply.)
   a. Advise the patient to avoid alcohol while taking aspirin.
   b. Instruct the patient to take aspirin before meals on an empty stomach.
   c. Instruct the patient to inform the dentist of the aspirin dosage before having dental work.
   d. Instruct the patient to inform the surgeon of the aspirin dosage before having surgery.
   e. Suggest that aspirin may be given to children for flu symptoms.
6. A patient is taking infliximab (Remicade) and asks the nurse what side effects/adverse reactions to expect from this drug. The nurse lists which side effects? (Select all that apply.)
   a. Fatigue
   b. Headache
   c. Chest pain
   d. Renal damage
   e. Severe infections

Answers: 1, c; 2, c; 3, a; 4, a; 5, a, c, d; 6, a, b, c, e.

CHAPTER

26

Nonopioid and Opioid Analgesics

evolve WEBSITE

http://evolve.elsevier.com/KeeHayes/pharmacology/

- Animations
- Content Updates
- Key Points
- Review Questions for the NCLEX® Examination
- References from the Textbook
- Unfolding Case Studies

OBJECTIVES

- Differentiate between acute and chronic pain.
- Compare indications for nonopioid and opioid analgesics.
- Describe the serum therapeutic ranges of acetaminophen and aspirin.
- Contrast the side effects of aspirin and opioids.
- Explain the methadone treatment program.
- Discuss nursing interventions and patient teaching related to nonopioid and opioid analgesics.
- Apply the nursing process to the patient with patient-controlled analgesia.

OUTLINE

Pathophysiology
- Undertreatment of Pain

Nonopioid Analgesics
- Nonsteroidal Antiinflammatory Drugs
- Acetaminophen
- Nursing Process: Patient-Centered Collaborative Care: Analgesic: Acetaminophen

Opioid Analgesics
- Morphine
- Nursing Process: Patient-Centered Collaborative Care: Opioid Analgesic: Morphine Sulfate
- Meperidine
- Hydromorphone
- Combination Drugs
- Patient-Controlled Analgesia
- Transdermal Opioid Analgesics
- Analgesic Titration
- Opioid Use in Special Populations

Adjuvant Therapy

Treatment for Opioid-Addicted Individuals

Opioid Agonist-Antagonists
- Nursing Process: Patient-Centered Collaborative Care: Opioid Agonist-Antagonist Analgesic: Nalbuphine (Nubain)

Opioid Antagonists

Headaches: Migraine and Cluster
- Pathophysiology
- Treatment of Migraine Headaches

Key Websites

Critical Thinking Case Study

NCLEX Study Questions

KEY TERMS

addiction, p. 358
adjuvant analgesics, p. 363
analgesics, p. 353
cluster headaches, p. 366
endorphins, p. 353
migraine headaches, p. 365
neuropathic pain, p. 353
nociceptors, p. 353
nonopioid analgesics, p. 354
nonsteroidal antiinflammatory drugs, p. 353
opioid agonist, p. 356
opioid agonist-antagonist, p. 363
opioid antagonist, p. 365
orthostatic hypotension, p. 360
pain threshold, p. 353
pain tolerance, p. 353
patient-controlled analgesia, p. 362
withdrawal syndrome, p. 360

Pain is an unpleasant sensory and emotional experience related to tissue injury. Due to the subjective nature of pain, the nurse must be knowledgeable and skillful in the assessment and measurement of pain to achieve optimal pain management.

Pain management is regarded as such a significant component of nursing care that pain has become known as the "fifth vital sign." The Joint Commission (TJC) has incorporated the assessment, documentation, and management of pain into its 2003 standards, which reflects the importance of this vital sign. The nurse's role is to assess the patient's pain level, alleviate the patient's pain through nonpharmacologic and pharmacologic treatments, thoroughly document the patient's response to treatment, and teach patients and their significant others to manage pain control themselves when appropriate.

An individual's **pain threshold** reflects the level of stimulus needed to create a painful sensation. Individual genetic makeup contributes to the variations in pain threshold from person to person. The mu (μ) opioid receptor gene controls the number of μ receptors present. When an individual has a large amount of μ receptors, the pain threshold is high and pain sensitivity is reduced.

The amount of pain a person can endure without having it interfere with normal functioning is called **pain tolerance.** This psychological aspect of pain varies greatly in individuals, because it is very subjective. Pain tolerance is influenced by factors such as age, gender, culture, ethnicity, previous experience, anxiety level, and specific circumstances.

Analgesics, both nonopioid and opioid, are prescribed for the relief of pain. The choice of analgesic depends upon the severity of the pain. Mild to moderate pain is frequently relieved with the use of nonopioid (also known as nonnarcotic) analgesics. Moderate to severe pain usually requires an opioid (also known as narcotic) analgesic.

Drugs used for pain relief are presented in this chapter. Many of the same nonopioid analgesics that are taken for pain, such as the **nonsteroidal antiinflammatory drugs (NSAIDs)**, are also taken for antiinflammatory purposes. This application for these drugs is covered in Chapter 25.

The most common classification of pain is by duration. Acute pain can be mild, moderate, or severe and is usually associated with a specific tissue injury. The onset of acute pain is usually sudden and of short duration. Chronic pain usually has a vague origin and onset with a prolonged duration.

Pain may also be classified by its origin. **Nociceptors** (sensory pain receptors) are activated by noxious stimuli (mechanical, thermal, and chemical) in peripheral tissues. When tissue damage occurs, injured cells release chemical mediators that affect the exposed nerve endings of the nociceptors. Pain that originates from tissue injury is nociceptor pain, which includes somatic (structural tissues: bones, muscles) and visceral (organ) pain. **Neuropathic pain** is an unusual sensory disturbance often involving neural supersensitivity. This pain is due to injury or disease of the peripheral or central nervous system (CNS). The patient with neuropathic pain usually complains of burning, tingling, or electrical shocks in the affected area, often triggered by light touch. Diabetic neuropathy associated with diabetes mellitus is an example of peripheral neuropathic pain. Severe, intractable pain from a herniated disk or spinal cord injury is evidence of neuropathic pain in the CNS.

PATHOPHYSIOLOGY

The most common pain theory is called the gate theory, proposed by Melzack and Wall in 1965. According to this theory, tissue injury activates nociceptors and causes the release of chemical mediators such as substance P, prostaglandins, bradykinin, histamine, serotonin, acetylcholine, glutamate, adenosine triphosphate, leukotrienes, and potassium. These substances initiate an action potential along a sensory nerve fiber and sensitize pain receptors. Nociceptive action potentials are transmitted via afferent nerve fibers. One type of pain fiber that primarily transmits impulses from the periphery is the A delta (δ) fiber. Because A δ pain fibers are wrapped in a myelin sheath, they transmit impulses rapidly in acute pain. The C fiber is a type of pain fiber that is small and unmyelinated, and because C fibers are unmyelinated, they transmit impulses slowly. C fibers are more often associated with chronic, dull pain.

A pain signal begins at the nociceptors in the periphery and proceeds throughout the CNS. Knowing how and where pharmacologic agents work is essential to controlling pain. The body produces neurohormones called **endorphins** (peptides) that naturally suppress pain conduction, although the method is not completely understood. Opioids such as morphine activate the same receptors as endorphins to reduce pain. NSAIDs control pain at the peripheral level by blocking the action of cyclooxygenase (pain-sensitizing chemical) and interfering with the production of prostaglandins. Cortisone decreases pain by blocking the action of phospholipase, reducing the production of both prostaglandins and leukotrienes. In neuropathic pain, anticonvulsant drugs prevent the production of nerve impulses by stabilizing the neuronal membrane and inactivating peripheral sodium channels.

To ascertain severity of pain, the health care provider should ask the patient to rate the degree of pain on a scale of 1 to 10, with 10 being the worst or most severe pain. The patient's comfort level should also be determined. A patient who indicates a pain level of 9 may verbalize a decrease in pain to a level of 3 within 30 to 45 minutes after receiving pain medication. Table 26-1 lists the types of pain and the drug groups that may be effective in relieving each type of pain.

Undertreatment of Pain

Undertreatment of pain is a major issue in health care today. The National Pharmaceutical Council and TJC state that up to 75% of patients have unrelieved pain. Some reasons for undertreatment are sociocultural variables that mediate a patient's willingness to acknowledge being in pain, the patient's inability to describe pain, the nurse's inability to

TABLE 26-1 TYPES OF PAIN

TYPE OF PAIN	DEFINITION	DRUG TREATMENT
Acute	Pain occurs suddenly and responds to treatment; can result from trauma, tissue injury, inflammation, or surgery	Mild pain: Scheduled nonopioid (acetaminophen, NSAIDs q6h) Moderate pain: Scheduled combination of nonopioid and opioid (oxycodone 5 mg and acetaminophen 325 mg q4h) Severe pain: Scheduled potent opioid (morphine 15 mg q4h)
Chronic	Pain persists for greater than 6 months and is difficult to treat or control	Nonopioid drugs are suggested. Opioids, if used, should meet these criteria: • Oral or transdermal • Long duration of action • Include adjunct therapy • Cause minimal respiratory depression
Cancer	Pain from pressure on nerves and organs, blockage to blood supply, or metastasis to bone	NSAIDs and opioid drugs administered PO, transdermal, IM, IV, or PCA
Somatic	Pain of skeletal muscle, ligaments, and joints	Nonopioids: NSAIDs; also act as antiinflammatories and muscle relaxants
Superficial	Pain from surface areas such as skin and mucous membranes	Mild pain: Nonopioid Moderate pain: Combination of opioid and nonopioid analgesic drug
Vascular	Pain from vascular or perivascular tissues contributing to headaches or migraines	Nonopioid drugs
Visceral	Pain from smooth muscle and organs	Opioid drugs

IM, Intramuscular; *IV,* intravenous; *NSAIDs,* nonsteroidal antiinflammatory drugs; *PCA,* patient-controlled analgesia; *PO,* by mouth.

measure pain, lack of regular pain assessment rounds, attitudes of the health care team, an unwillingness to believe the patient's report of pain, inaccurate knowledge of the health care provider concerning addiction and tolerance, and prescription of an inadequate analgesic dose. Many scales and instruments are available to the nurse for assessment and measurement of the patient's pain level.

Unrelieved pain leads to a multitude of harmful effects involving almost all organs of the body. As a result of unrelieved pain, the patient may develop increased respiratory rate and heart rate, hypertension, increased stress response, urinary retention, fluid overload, electrolyte imbalance, glucose intolerance, hyperglycemia, pneumonia, atelectasis, anorexia, paralytic ileus, constipation, weakness, confusion, and infection.

In addition to psychological and physical suffering, inadequate pain management leads to high health care costs. It is estimated the cost of extended hospital stays, readmissions to the hospital, and outpatient visits due to inadequate pain management exceeds $100 billion per year.

NONOPIOID ANALGESICS

Nonopioid analgesics (aspirin, acetaminophen, ibuprofen, naproxen) are less potent than opioid analgesics. They are used to treat mild to moderate pain. Nonopioids are usually purchased over-the-counter (OTC), but COX-2 inhibitors require a prescription. Nonopioids are effective for the dull, throbbing pain of headaches, dysmenorrhea (menstrual pain), inflammation, minor abrasions, muscular aches and pain, and mild to moderate arthritis. Most analgesics also have an antipyretic effect and will lower an elevated body temperature. Some, such as aspirin, have antiinflammatory and antiplatelet effects as well.

Nonsteroidal Antiinflammatory Drugs

All NSAIDs have an analgesic effect as well as an antipyretic and antiinflammatory action. NSAIDs such as aspirin (ASA), ibuprofen (Motrin, Advil), and naproxen (Aleve) can be purchased as OTC drugs. Aspirin, a salicylate NSAID, is the oldest nonopioid analgesic drug still in use. Adolf Bayer marketed the original formulation in 1899, and currently aspirin can be purchased under many names and with added ingredients. Examples are Bufferin, Ecotrin (enteric-coated tablet), Anacin (containing caffeine), and Alka-Seltzer.

Aspirin should not be used in children younger than 12 years of age, and it is contraindicated for any elevated temperature, regardless of the cause, because of the danger of Reye's syndrome (neurologic problems associated with viral infection treated with salicylates). In these circumstances, acetaminophen (Tylenol) is recommended instead of aspirin.

In addition to its analgesic, antipyretic, and antiinflammatory properties, aspirin decreases platelet aggregation (clotting). Some health care providers may therefore prescribe one 81-mg, 162-mg, or 325-mg aspirin tablet every day or one 325-mg tablet every other day as a preventive measure against transient ischemic attacks (TIAs, or "small strokes"), heart attacks, or any thromboembolic episode. Aspirin is discussed in depth in Chapter 25 along with other NSAIDs.

Aspirin and other NSAIDs relieve pain by inhibiting biosynthesis of prostaglandin by different forms of the enzyme cyclooxygenase (COX). Inhibition of COX-2 decreases inflammation and pain, but inhibition of COX-1 decreases protection of the stomach lining. As a result of an NSAID's inhibition of COX-1, stomach ulcers and bleeding may occur. Aspirin is the drug of choice for alleviating pain and inflammation in arthritic conditions, but when given in high doses, severe GI problems develop in approximately 20% of patients.

Some pharmaceutical companies have developed antiinflammatory and analgesic drugs that inhibit only COX-2. The COX-2 inhibitors were developed to eliminate the GI side effects associated with aspirin and other NSAIDs. COX-2 inhibitors are discussed in depth in Chapter 25.

Side Effects and Adverse Reactions

A common side effect of NSAIDs is gastric irritation. These drugs should be taken with food, at mealtime, or with a full glass of fluid to help reduce this problem.

If an NSAID is taken for dysmenorrhea during the first 2 days of menstruation, excess bleeding might occur (more so with aspirin than with ibuprofen).

Some patients are hypersensitive to aspirin. Tinnitus, vertigo, bronchospasm, and urticaria are some of the symptoms that indicate hypersensitivity or overdose of the salicylate product. Certain foods also contain salicylates: prunes, raisins, paprika, and licorice. Those with a hypersensitivity to aspirin and salicylate products may be sensitive to other NSAIDs. This hypersensitivity may be related to inhibition of the enzyme cyclooxygenase by the salicylate product.

Acetaminophen

The analgesic acetaminophen (paraaminophenol derivative) is a popular nonprescription drug for the relief of pain, discomfort, and fever in infants, children, adults, and older adults. Acetaminophen is a nonopioid drug, but it is not an NSAID. Acetaminophen does not have the antiinflammatory properties of aspirin, so it is not the drug of choice for any inflammatory process. It constitutes 25% of all OTC drugs sold. Examples of OTC products that contain acetaminophen include Anacin; Excedrin; Midol: Maximum Strength Menstrual Formula; and Vicks: Cold & Flu Relief. Examples of prescription products on the market that contain acetaminophen include Lortab, Percocet, and Vicodin. Acetaminophen (Tylenol), first marketed in the mid-1950s, is an analgesic and antipyretic drug used for muscular aches and pains and for fever caused by viral infections. It is a safe, effective drug when used at therapeutic doses. It causes little to no gastric distress and does not interfere with platelet aggregation. An IV formulation was FDA approved in 2010 for treating pain and fever. There is no link between acetaminophen and Reye's syndrome, and it does not increase the potential for excessive bleeding if taken for dysmenorrhea, as do aspirin and NSAIDs (Prototype Drug Chart 26-1).

Pharmacokinetics Acetaminophen is well absorbed from the gastrointestinal (GI) tract. Rectal absorption may be erratic because of the presence of fecal material or a decrease in blood flow to the colon. Because of acetaminophen's short half-life, it can be administered every 4 hours as needed with a maximum dose of 4 g/day. However, it is suggested that a patient who frequently takes acetaminophen limit the dose to 2000 mg/day (2 g/day) to avoid the possibility of hepatic or renal dysfunction. More than 85% of acetaminophen is metabolized to drug metabolites by the liver.

PROTOTYPE DRUG CHART 26-1

Acetaminophen

Drug Class Analgesic Trade Names: Anacin-AF, Ofirmev Pregnancy Category: B	**Dosage** A: PO: 325-650 mg q4-6h PRN; *max:* 4000 mg/d; rectal supp: 650 mg q.i.d. A: IV: 1 g q6h or 650 mg q4h PRN; *max:* 4 g/d C >2 y: PO: 15 mg/kg q6h; *max:* 75 mg/kg/d
Contraindications Acetaminophen hypersensitivity, severe hepatic or renal disease, alcoholism	**Drug-Lab-Food Interactions** Increase effect with caffeine, diflunisal Decrease effect with oral contraceptives, antacids, anticholinergics, cholestyramine, charcoal
Pharmacokinetics Absorption: PO: Rapidly absorbed; rectal: erratic Distribution: PB: 10%-25%; crosses the placenta, excreted in breast milk Metabolism: t½: 2-4 h Excretion: In urine as metabolites	**Pharmacodynamics** PO: Onset: 10-30 min Peak: 30-60 min Duration: 3-5 h Rectal: Onset: UK Peak: UK Duration: 4-6 h
Therapeutic Effects/Uses To decrease pain and fever Mode of Action: Inhibition (weak) of prostaglandin synthesis, inhibition of hypothalamic heat-regulator center	
Side Effects Anorexia, nausea, vomiting, rash, insomnia	**Adverse Reactions** Oliguria, urticaria, elevated liver enzymes Life-threatening: Hemorrhage, hepatotoxicity, hemolytic anemia, agranulocytosis, leukopenia, thrombocytopenia

A, Adult; *C,* child; *d,* day; *h,* hour; *min,* minute; *PB,* protein-binding; *PO,* by mouth; *q.i.d.,* four times a day; *t ½,* half-life; *UK,* unknown; *y,* year; <, less than; >, greater than.

Large doses or overdoses can be toxic to the hepatic cells, so when large doses are administered over a long period, the serum level of acetaminophen should be monitored. The therapeutic serum range is 10 to 25 mcg/mL. Liver enzyme levels (aspartate aminotransferase [AST], alanine aminotransferase [ALT], alkaline phosphatase [ALP]) and serum bilirubin should also be monitored. Large doses of acetaminophen with regular alcohol intake may lead to liver injury. When acetaminophen toxicity occurs, acetylcysteine (Mucomyst) is the antidote, which reduces liver injury by converting toxic metabolites to a nontoxic form.

Pharmacodynamics Acetaminophen weakly inhibits prostaglandin synthesis, which decreases pain sensation. It is effective in eliminating mild to moderate pain and headaches and is useful for its antipyretic effect. Acetaminophen does not possess antiinflammatory action. Its onset of action is rapid, and the duration of action is 5 hours or less. Severe adverse reactions may occur with an overdose, so acetaminophen in liquid or chewable form should be kept out of children's reach.

Side Effects and Adverse Reactions

An overdose of acetaminophen can be extremely toxic to liver cells, causing hepatotoxicity. Death could occur in 1 to 4 days from hepatic necrosis. If a child or adult ingests excessive amounts of acetaminophen tablets or liquid, a poison control center should be contacted immediately and the child or adult should be taken to the emergency department. Early symptoms of hepatic damage include nausea, vomiting, diarrhea, and abdominal pain.

Table 26-2 lists the commonly used nonopioid analgesics and their dosages, uses, and considerations.

Nursing Process
Patient-Centered Collaborative Care

Analgesic: Acetaminophen

Assessment

- Obtain a medical history of liver dysfunction. Overdosing or extremely high doses of acetaminophen can cause hepatotoxicity.
- Ascertain the severity of pain. Nonopioid NSAIDs such as ibuprofen or an opioid may be necessary to relieve pain.

Nursing Diagnoses

- Risk for injury related to analgesic effect on sensorium
- Acute pain related to edema from surgical incision

Planning

- Patient's pain will be relieved or diminished.

Nursing Interventions

- Check liver enzyme tests such as alanine aminotransferase, alkaline phosphatase, gamma-glutamyl transferase, 5′ nucleotidase, and bilirubin for elevations in patients taking high doses or overdoses of acetaminophen.

Patient Teaching

General

- Teach patient to keep acetaminophen out of children's reach. Acetaminophen for children is available in flavored tablets and liquid. High doses can cause hepatotoxicity.
- Advise patient not to self-medicate with acetaminophen longer than 10 days. Teach adult caregiver not to medicate child longer than 5 days without health care provider's approval.
- Direct parent to call poison control center immediately if a child has taken a large or unknown amount of acetaminophen.
- Teach patient to check acetaminophen dosage on package label of OTC drugs. Do not exceed the recommended dosage. Suggested safe adult acetaminophen dose is 2000 mg/d (2 g/day), not to exceed 4 g/day to avoid liver damage (see Prototype Drug Chart 26-1).

Side Effects

- Encourage patient to report side effects. Overdosing can cause severe liver damage and death.
- Inform patient that liver damage may occur with excess use of acetaminophen.
- Check serum acetaminophen level if toxicity is suspected. Normal serum level is 5 to 20 mcg/mL; toxic level is >50 mcg/mL. Levels of >200 mcg/mL could indicate hepatotoxicity. The antidote for acetaminophen is acetylcysteine (Mucomyst). Dosage is based on serum acetaminophen level.

Cultural Considerations

- Involving the extended family may be important for teaching health strategies and providing support.

Evaluation

- Evaluate the effectiveness of acetaminophen in relieving pain. If pain persists, another analgesic may be needed.
- Determine if patient is taking dose as recommended. Observe and report any side effects.

HERBAL ALERT 26-1

Capsaicin

Capsaicin, which is found naturally in cayenne pepper, is selective for C fiber nociceptors and relieves some arthritis pain in topical cream or gel form.

OPIOID ANALGESICS

Opioid analgesics, called **opioid agonists,** are prescribed for moderate and severe pain. In the United States, the Harrison Opioid Act of 1914 required that all forms of opium be sold with a prescription and that it no longer be used as a nonprescription drug. The Controlled Substances Act of 1970

TABLE 26-2 ANALGESICS

GENERIC (BRAND)	ROUTE AND DOSAGE	USES AND CONSIDERATIONS
Paraaminophenol		
acetaminophen	See Prototype Drug Chart 26-1.	
NSAIDs		
aspirin (Bayer, Ecotrin)	Analgesic: A: PO/PR: 325 to 650 mg, q4h; *max:* 4 g/d C: PO/PR: 10-15 mg/kg/d q4-6h; *max:* 4 g/d	Effective in relieving headaches, muscle pain, inflammation and pain from arthritis; mild anticoagulant. Can displace other highly protein-bound drugs. If taken with acetaminophen, GI bleeding could result. Side effects: gastric discomfort, tinnitus, vertigo, deafness (reversible), increased bleeding. Should be taken with foods or at mealtime. Should not be taken with alcohol. Pregnancy category: D; PB: 80%-90%; t½: 15-20 min
diflunisal (Dolobid)	A: PO: Initially 1000 mg; *maint:* 500 mg q12h; *max:* 1500 mg/d Older adults: PO: Initially 500 mg; *maint:* 250 q8-12h; *max:* 1500 mg/d	Used for mild to moderate pain. Considered to be less toxic than aspirin. Pregnancy category: C; PB: 99%, t½: 8-12 h
Propionic Acid		
ibuprofen (Motrin, Advil) ibuprofen: IV injection (Caldolor)	Pain: A: PO: 400 mg q4-6h; *max:* 3200 mg/d A: IV: 400-800 mg over 30 min q6h Fever: A: IV: 400 mg over 30 min q4-6h PRN	For mild to moderate muscle aches and pains. Causes some gastric distress but less than aspirin. Should be taken with food, at mealtime, or with plenty of fluids. Pregnancy category: C (D, third trimester); PB: 90%-99%; t½: 2-4 h
naproxen (Naprosyn)	Mild to moderate pain: A: PO: initially 500 mg, then 250 mg q6-8h; *max:* 1250 mg/d	Treatment of inflammation and pain from osteoarthritis, rheumatoid arthritis, ankylosing spondylitis, gout, and dysmenorrhea. Pregnancy category: C; PB: 99%; t½: 12-17 h
ketorolac (Toradol)	A: PO: 10 mg q6h PRN; *max:* 40 mg/d Older adults: PO: 10 mg q4-6h PRN; *max:* 40 mg/d A: IM/IV: 30-60 mg q6h PRN; *max:* 120 mg/d Older adults: IM/IV: 15 mg q6h PRN; *max:* 60 mg/d	For short-term pain management (5 days or less). Pregnancy category: C; PB: 99%; t½: 2.5-9 h
Oxicams		
meloxicam (Mobic)	A: PO: Initially 7.5-15 mg/d; *max:* 15 mg/d	Treatment of pain from osteoarthritis. Pregnancy category: C (first and second trimester), D (third trimester); PB: 99%; t½: 15-20 h
Naphthylalkanones		
nabumetone (Relafen)	A: PO: 1000 mg/d or 500 mg b.i.d.; *max:* 2000 mg/d	Treatment of pain from osteoarthritis, rheumatoid arthritis. Pregnancy category: C (D, third trimester); PB: 99%; t½: 24 h
COX-2 Inhibitors		
celecoxib (Celebrex)	A: PO: 100-400 mg b.i.d.; *max:* 800 mg/d Older adults: 100-200 mg b.i.d.; *max:* 400 mg/d	Treatment of osteoarthritis and rheumatoid arthritis. Not indicated for patients <18 y. Use caution for patients with severe renal or liver disorders and for those allergic to sulfonamides. Pregnancy category: C (D, third trimester); PB: 97%; t½: 11.2 h
Miscellaneous		
tramadol (Ultram) tramadol ER (Ultram ER, Ryzolt)	A: PO: Initially: 25 mg/d, *maint:* 50-100 mg q4-6h PRN; *max:* 400 mg/d A >75 y: *max:* 300 mg/d A: PO: ER: 100 mg/d; *max:* 300 mg/d	Used for moderate to severe pain. Contraindicated in severe alcoholism or with use of opioids. Nausea, vomiting, dizziness, constipation, headache, anxiety, and seizures may occur. Pregnancy category: C; PB: 20%; t½: 6.3 h for immediate release, 7.9 h for ER

A, Adult; *b.i.d.,* twice a day; *C,* child; *d,* day; *ER,* extended-release; *GI,* gastrointestinal; *h,* hour; *IM,* intramuscular; *IV,* intravenous; *maint,* maintenance; *max,* maximum; *min,* minute; *NSAIDs,* nonsteroidal antiinflammatory drugs; *PB,* protein-binding; *PO,* by mouth; *PRN,* as needed; *t½,* half-life; *UK,* unknown; *y,* year; >, greater than; <, less than.

classified addicting drugs, opioids among them, in five schedule categories according to their potential for drug abuse (see Chapter 9). **Addiction** is defined as a psychological and physical dependence upon a substance beyond normal voluntary control, usually after prolonged use of a substance.

HERBAL ALERT 26-2

Opioids

Opioids taken with kava kava, valerian, and St. John's wort may increase sedation.

Morphine, a prototype opioid, is obtained from the sap of seed pods of the opium poppy plant. Codeine is another drug obtained from opium. In the past decades, many synthetic and semisynthetic opioids have been developed.

While nonopioid analgesics act on the peripheral nervous system at the pain receptor sites, opioid analgesics act mostly on the CNS. Opioids act primarily by activating the μ receptors, while also exerting a weak activation of the kappa (κ) receptors. Analgesia, respiratory depression, euphoria, and sedation are effects of μ activation. Activation of κ receptors leads to analgesia and sedation, having no effect on respiratory depression and euphoria.

Opioids not only suppress pain impulses but also respiration and coughing by acting on the respiratory and cough centers in the medulla of the brainstem. One example of such an opioid is morphine, a potent analgesic that can readily depress respirations. Codeine is not as potent as morphine (1/15 to 1/20 as potent), but it also relieves mild to moderate pain and suppresses cough, which allows it also to be classified as an antitussive. Most opioids, with the exception of meperidine (Demerol), have an antitussive (cough suppression) effect. The opioids have two isomers, levo and dextro. The levo-isomers of opioids produce an analgesic effect only; however, both levo- and dextro-isomers possess an antitussive response. The dextro-isomers do not cause physical dependence, but the levo-isomers do. Synthetic cough suppressants are discussed in Chapter 40.

In addition to pain relief and antitussive effects, many opioids possess antidiarrheal effects. Common side effects with high doses of most opioids include nausea and vomiting (particularly in ambulatory patients), constipation, a moderate decrease in blood pressure, and orthostatic hypotension. High doses of opioids may also cause respiratory depression, urinary retention (usually in older adults), and antitussive effects.

Morphine

Morphine, an extraction from opium, is a potent opioid analgesic (Prototype Drug Chart 26-2). Morphine is effective against acute pain resulting from acute myocardial infarction (AMI), cancer, and dyspnea resulting from pulmonary edema. It may be used as a preoperative medication. Although it is effective in relieving severe pain, it can cause respiratory depression, orthostatic hypotension, miosis, urinary retention, constipation resulting from reduced bowel motility, and cough suppression. An antidote for morphine excess or overdose is the opioid antagonist naloxone (Narcan).

Pharmacokinetics Morphine may be taken orally, although GI absorption can be somewhat erratic. For severe pain, such as with AMI, it is given intravenously (IV). Morphine is 30% protein-bound and may also be administered rectally and epidurally. Oral morphine undergoes first hepatic pass, meaning the liver metabolizes the drug before bioavailability to the rest of the body occurs. Only a small amount of morphine crosses the blood-brain barrier to produce an analgesic effect. It has a short half-life, and 90% is excreted in the urine. Morphine crosses the placenta and is excreted in breast milk.

Pharmacodynamics Morphine binds with the opiate receptor in the CNS. Parenterally the onset of action is rapid, especially IV. Onset of action is slower for subcutaneous (subQ) and intramuscular (IM) injections. Duration of action with most types of drug administration is 3 to 5 hours; with controlled-release morphine sulfate tablets (MS Contin), duration is 8 to 12 hours.

Nursing Process

Patient-Centered Collaborative Care

Opioid Analgesic: Morphine Sulfate

Assessment

- Obtain a medical history. Contraindications for morphine include severe respiratory disorders, increased intracranial pressure, and severe renal disease. Morphine may cause seizures.
- Determine a drug history. Report if a drug-drug interaction is probable. Morphine increases the effects of alcohol, sedatives or hypnotics, antipsychotic drugs, and muscle relaxants and might cause respiratory depression.
- Assess vital signs, noting rate and depth of respirations for future comparisons; opioids commonly decrease respirations and systolic blood pressure.
- Monitor urinary output; morphine can cause urinary retention.
- Assess type of pain, location, and duration before giving opioids.

Nursing Diagnoses

- Acute pain related to surgical tissue injury
- Ineffective breathing patterns related to excess morphine dosage
- Risk for falls related to sedative effects secondary to morphine
- Constipation related to morphine

Planning

- Patient's pain will be diminished or alleviated.

Nursing Interventions

- Administer morphine before pain reaches its peak to maximize effectiveness of the drug.

PROTOTYPE DRUG CHART 26-2

Morphine Sulfate

Drug Class Opioid Trade Names: MS Contin, Roxanol CSS II Pregnancy Category: C/D	**Dosage** A: PO: 10-30 mg q4h PRN C >6 mo: PO: 0.2-0.5 mg/kg q4-6h PRN Infants <6 mo/neonates: PO: 0.1 mg/kg q3-4h A: SR: 15-30 mg, q12h PRN A: IV/IM/subQ: 2.5-15 mg q2-6h PRN C >6 mo: IM/subQ: 0.05-0.2 mg/kg q2-4h PRN; *max:* <15 mg/dose Neonate: subQ/IM/IV: 0.05 mg/kg q4-8h
Contraindications Hypersensitivity, CNS or respiratory depression, status asthmaticus, increased intracranial pressure, shock, alcoholism, ileus, hypovolemia Caution: Respiratory, renal, or hepatic diseases; urinary retention, sleep apnea; older adults; very young	**Drug-Lab-Food Interactions** Drug: Increase effects of alcohol, sedative-hypnotics, antipsychotic drugs, muscle relaxants Lab: Increase AST, ALT
Pharmacokinetics Absorption: PO: varies; IV: rapid Distribution: PB: UK; crosses placenta, excreted in breast milk Metabolism: t½: 1.5-2 h Excretion: 90% in urine	**Pharmacodynamics** PO: Onset: Variable Peak: 1 h Duration: 4-5 h; SR: 8-12 h subQ/IM: Onset: 15-30 min Peak: 50-90 min Duration: UK IV: Onset: rapid Peak: 20 min Duration: 3-5 h
Therapeutic Effects/Uses To relieve severe pain Mode of Action: Depression of the CNS; depression of pain impulses by binding with the opiate receptor in the CNS	
Side Effects Anorexia, nausea, vomiting, constipation, drowsiness, dizziness, sedation, confusion, urinary retention, rash, blurred vision, bradycardia, flushing, euphoria, pruritus	**Adverse Reactions** Hypotension, urticaria, seizures, ileus Life-threatening: Respiratory depression, increased intracranial pressure

A, Adult; *ALT,* alanine aminotransferase; *AST,* aspartate aminotransferase; *C,* child; *CNS,* central nervous system; *CSS,* Controlled Substances Schedule; *h,* hour; *IM,* intramuscular; *IV,* intravenous; *min,* minute; *PB,* protein binding; *PO,* by mouth; *PRN,* as necessary; *subQ,* subcutaneous; *SR,* sustained-release; *t ½,* half-life; *UK,* unknown; <, less than.

- Monitor vital signs at frequent intervals to detect respiratory changes. Respirations of <10/min can indicate respiratory distress.
- Record patient's urine output because urinary retention is a side effect of morphine. Urine output should be at least 600 mL/day.
- Check bowel sounds for decreased peristalsis; constipation is a side effect of morphine. Dietary change or mild laxative might be needed.
- Check for pupil changes and reaction. Pinpoint pupils can indicate morphine overdose.
- Have naloxone (Narcan) available as an antidote to reverse respiratory depression if morphine overdose occurs.
- Validate dose of morphine before its administration. Check older adults for alertness and orientation because confusion is a side effect of morphine. Use side rails, and take other safety precautions as necessary.

Patient Teaching

General

- Encourage patient not to use alcohol or CNS depressants with any opioid analgesics such as morphine. Respiratory depression can result.
- Suggest nonpharmacologic measures to relieve pain as patient recuperates from surgery. As recovery progresses, a nonopioid analgesic may be prescribed.

Side Effects

- Alert patient that with continuous use, opioids such as morphine can become addicting. If addiction occurs, inform patient about methadone treatment programs and other resources in the area.
- Encourage patient to report dizziness while taking morphine. Dizziness could be due to orthostatic hypotension. Advise patient to ambulate with caution or only with assistance.

- Teach patient to report difficulty in breathing, blurred vision, and headaches.

Cultural Considerations

- Identify conflicts in values and beliefs about pain and its management.
- Respect cultural and religious differences concerning refusal of opioid analgesics.
- Incorporate traditional practices into Western medicine when possible.

Evaluation

- Evaluate the effectiveness of morphine in lessening or alleviating pain. If pain persists after several days, dose should be increased or opioid changed.
- Determine stability of vital signs. Any decrease in respiration and blood pressure should be reported.

Meperidine

One of the first synthetic opioids, meperidine (Demerol) became available in the mid-1950s. It is classified as a schedule II drug according to the Controlled Substances Act. Meperidine has a shorter duration of action than morphine, and its potency varies according to the dosage. Meperidine, which can be given orally, IM, and IV, is primarily effective in GI procedures. It does not have the antitussive property of opium preparations.

During pregnancy, meperidine is preferred to morphine because it does not diminish uterine contractions and causes less neonatal respiratory depression. Meperidine causes less constipation and urinary retention than morphine. Meperidine is not indicated for patients with chronic pain, severe liver dysfunction, sickle cell disease, a history of seizures, severe coronary artery disease (CAD), or cardiac dysrhythmias. When older adults and patients with advanced cancer receive large doses of meperidine, neurotoxicity (e.g., nervousness, tremors, agitation, irritability, seizures) have been reported. Meperidine should not be prescribed for long-term use; the dose is frequently limited to 600 mg in a 24-hour period for no longer than 48 to 72 hours.

Meperidine is metabolized in the liver to an active metabolite; therefore the dose should be decreased for patients with hepatic or renal insufficiency. It is excreted in the urine in a metabolite form called normeperidine. Meperidine should not be taken with alcohol or sedative-hypnotics, because the combination of these drugs causes an additive CNS depression. A major side effect of meperidine is a decrease in blood pressure, which should be monitored, especially if the patient is an older adult.

Table 26-3 lists opioids and their dosages, uses, and considerations.

SAFETY: Preventing Medication Errors

Do not confuse...

- **Meperidine** with **morphine**, **meprobamate**, or **hydromorphone**
- **Demerol** with **Desyrel**, **Dilaudid**, or **Temaril**

Hydromorphone

Hydromorphone (Dilaudid) is a semisynthetic opioid similar to morphine. The analgesic effect is approximately six times more potent than morphine with fewer hypnotic effects and less GI distress. This opioid has a faster onset and shorter duration of action than morphine. Hydromorphone is classified as a schedule II drug according to the Controlled Substances Act. Tolerance to hydromorphone increases gradually.

This drug is given orally, rectally, subQ, IM, and IV for the relief of moderate to severe pain. When given IV, dilution of each dose with 5 mL of sterile water or normal saline is preferred. Direct IV administration of 2 mg or less should be given over 2 to 5 minutes. Hydromorphone is readily absorbed in the body and excreted in the urine. Respirations should be monitored closely, and adequate hydration should be provided.

Side Effects and Adverse Reactions

Many side effects are known to accompany the use of opioids. Of particular importance are signs of respiratory depression (respiration <10/min). Other side effects include **orthostatic hypotension** (decrease in blood pressure when rising from a sitting or lying position), tachycardia, drowsiness and mental clouding, constipation, and urinary retention. In addition, pupillary constriction (a sign of toxicity), tolerance, and psychological and physical dependence may occur with prolonged use.

Increased metabolism of opioids contributes to tolerance, which causes an increased need for higher doses of the opioid. If chronic use of the opioid is discontinued, withdrawal (cessation of drug administration) symptoms usually occur within 24 to 48 hours after the last opioid dose. **Withdrawal syndrome** is caused by physical dependence. Symptoms of withdrawal syndrome include irritability, diaphoresis (sweating), restlessness, muscle twitching, and an increase in pulse rate and blood pressure. Withdrawal symptoms from opioids are unpleasant but not as severe or life-threatening as those that accompany withdrawal from sedative-hypnotics—a process that may lead to convulsions.

Contraindications

Use of opioid analgesics is contraindicated for patients with head injuries. Opioids decrease respiration, thus causing an accumulation of carbon dioxide (CO_2). With an increase in carbon dioxide retention, blood vessels dilate (vasodilation), especially cerebral vessels, which causes increased intracranial pressure.

Opioid analgesics given to a patient with a respiratory disorder only intensify the respiratory distress. In the patient with asthma, opiates decrease respiratory drive while simultaneously increasing airway resistance.

Opioids may cause hypotension and are not indicated for patients in shock or for those who have very low blood pressure. If an opioid is necessary, the dosage needs to be adjusted accordingly; otherwise, the hypotensive state may worsen. For an older adult or a person who is debilitated, the opioid dose usually needs to be decreased.

TABLE 26-3 OPIOIDS: OPIUM AND SYNTHETICS

GENERIC (BRAND)	ROUTE AND DOSAGE	USES AND CONSIDERATIONS
codeine sulfate, codeine phosphate) CSS II	A: PO/subQ/IM: 15-60 mg q4-6h PRN; *max:* 360 mg/d C: PO/subQ/IM: 0.5-1 mg/kg q4-6h, *max:* 60 mg/dose	Effective for mild to moderate pain and as an antitussive. Can be used with nonopioids (acetaminophen) for pain relief. Can cause decreased respirations, constipation, and physical dependence. Pregnancy category: C/D; PB: 7%, t½: 2.5-4 h
hydrocodone bitartrate (Hycodan) CSS II combination with acetaminophen (Lortab, Vicodin), aspirin (Lortab ASA), ibuprofen (Vicoprofin), and chlorpheniramine (Tussionex)	Analgesic: A: PO: 5 mg q4-6h PRN; *max:* 30 mg/d C >6 y: PO: 2.5 mg q4-6h PRN; *max:* 15 mg/d	For moderate to moderately severe pain. Used for antitussive purposes. Pregnancy category: C/D; PB: UK; t½: 4 h
hydromorphone HCl (Dilaudid) CSS II	A: PO: 2.5-10 mg q4-6h PRN A: IV: 0.2-1 mg q2-3h PRN Rectal: 3 mg q6-8h	For moderate to severe pain. Can be prescribed for analgesic and antitussive purposes. Pregnancy category: C; PB: 8%-19%; t½: 2-3 h
levorphanol tartrate (Levo-Dromoran) CSS II	A: PO/IV: 1 mg q3-6h A: IM/subQ: 1-2 mg q6-8h PRN	For moderate to severe pain. Has side effects similar to morphine. Pregnancy category: B; PB: 40%; t½: 11-16 h
meperidine (Demerol) CSS II	A: PO/subQ/IM/IV: 50-150 mg q3-4h PRN C: PO/subQ/IM/IV: 1-1.5 mg/kg q3-4h PRN; *max:* 150 mg q4h	For moderate to severe pain, GI procedures, and preoperative sedation. Pregnancy category: C/D; PB: 60%-80%; t½: 3-5 h
morphine sulfate CSS II	See Prototype Drug Chart 26-2.	
oxycodone HCl (OxyContin) CSS II	A: PO: 5-10 mg q6h PRN C >12 y: PO: 2.5 mg q6h PRN C 6-12 y: PO: 1.25 mg q6h PRN	For moderate to moderately severe pain, including postoperative and postpartum pain. Avoid taking drug over an extended period of time. As potent as morphine. Take with food to avoid GI distress. Pregnancy category: B (D in third trimester); PB: 40%; t½: 3-5 h
oxycodone HCl with acetaminophen (Percocet) and oxycodone terephthalate with aspirin (Percodan) CSS II	A: PO: 2.5-10 mg q4-6h PRN or 5-10 mg q6h PRN	For moderate to severe pain. Percocet contains acetaminophen. Percodan contains aspirin and can cause gastric irritation, so it should be taken with food or plenty of liquid. Pregnancy category: C; PB: UK; t½: 4 h
alfentanil (Alfenta) CSS II	A: IV: 3-8 mcg/kg for surgery Continuous infusion: 0.25-1 mcg/kg/min Total dose: 3-40 mcg/kg	Opioid analgesic with rapid onset of action. May be used to induce anesthesia. Pregnancy category: C; PB: 92%; t½: 90-111 min
fentanyl (Duragesic, Sublimaze) CSS II	A: IM: 50-100 mcg q1-2h PRN A: Sublimaze IM: 50-100 mcg q1-2h PRN A: Duragesic transdermal patch: Initially 25 mcg/h patch q3d	Short-acting potent opioid analgesic. May be used with short-term surgery. Drug available as a lozenge and transdermal patch for controlling chronic pain. Pregnancy category: C; PB: 80%-89%; t½: 7 h IV; 17 h transdermal
sufentanil citrate (Sufenta) CSS II	Primary anesthetic: A: IV: 8-30 mcg/kg with 100% oxygen and muscle relaxant Adjunct to anesthesia: IV: 1-8 mcg/kg	Potent synthetic opioid; used as part of the balanced anesthesia group. May be used as a primary anesthetic. Pregnancy category: C; PB: 93%; t½: 1-3 h
remifentanil (Ultiva) CSS II	A: IV: Postop: 0.025-0.2 mcg/min	Newest opioid analgesic. Rapid onset of action, short-acting duration (5-10 min). Can cause respiratory depression, hypotension, and bradycardia. Pregnancy category: C; PB: 70%; t½: 3-10 min
methadone (Dolophine) CSS II	Pain: A: PO/subQ/IM: 2.5-10 mg q8-12h PRN	For moderate to severe acute pain. Similar to morphine but longer duration of action. Used in drug abuse programs. Helps alleviate craving for opioids. Peak action 30-60 min. Pregnancy category: C; PB: 85%-90%; t½: 2-3 h

A, Adult; *C,* child; *CSS,* Controlled Substances Schedule; *GI,* Gastrointestinal; *h,* hour; *IM,* intramuscular; *IV,* intravenous; *maint;* maintenance; *max,* maximum; *min,* minute; *PB,* protein-binding; *PO,* by mouth; *PRN,* as necessary; *subQ,* subcutaneous; *t½,* half-life; *UK,* unknown; *y,* year.

Morphine is the opioid analgesic prototype, and all other opioids are measured in comparison to morphine.

Combination Drugs

To treat moderate to severe pain, combination drugs of an NSAID and an opioid analgesic may be used. Examples are hydrocodone and ibuprofen (Vicoprofen), which is a combination of an NSAID and an opioid. Another combination for the treatment of mild to moderate pain is acetaminophen and codeine. Using a combination of drugs for pain helps to decrease drug dependency that may result from possible long-term use of an opioid agent.

Patient-Controlled Analgesia

Patient-controlled analgesia (PCA) is an alternative route for opioid administration for self-administered pain relief as needed. Usually a loading dose (e.g., 2 to 10 mg of morphine) is given initially to achieve pain relief. Then within predetermined safety limits, the patient controls administration of the opioid analgesic, depending on the amount of pain. To receive the opioid, the patient pushes a button on the PCA device, releasing a specific dose of analgesic (e.g., 1 mg morphine) into the IV line. The nurse titrates the opioid analgesic dose by regulating the time intervals (every several minutes) at which the drug can be received. A lockout mechanism on the electronically controlled infusion pump prevents the patient from constantly pushing the button and causing a drug overdose. The PCA device maintains a near-constant analgesic level, avoiding episodes of severe pain and oversedation. Morphine is used most often for PCA, but fentanyl (Sublimaze) and hydromorphone (Dilaudid) may also be given.

Transdermal Opioid Analgesics

Transdermal opioid analgesics provide a continuous "around-the-clock" pain control that is helpful to patients who suffer from chronic pain. The transdermal method is not useful for acute or postoperative pain. An example of a transdermal opioid analgesic is fentanyl (Duragesic), which is administered via a transdermal patch. This patch comes in various strengths—12.5, 25, 50, 75, and 100 mcg/h. Maximum serum fentanyl levels occur within 24 hours of when the patch is first applied. Fentanyl is also available for IM and IV use. Fentanyl is more potent than morphine. For older adults, the use of a lower fentanyl transdermal dose is usually suggested. The health care provider must exercise caution when prescribing fentanyl for patients who weigh less than 110 pounds.

Analgesic Titration

Analgesics may be titrated to increase or decrease the dosage. Usually postoperative pain will decrease over time, and analgesics will be titrated downward. However, the patient with cancer-related pain usually has a continual increase in pain and will require an upward titration. Titration can be accomplished by changing the dose, the interval between doses, the route of administration, or the drug. When titrating analgesics, the dosage is decided after assessing the patient's respiratory rate and pain level.

Opioid Use in Special Populations

Children

Pain management in children is complex, because it is more difficult to assess their pain. Some children will not verbalize discomfort when they are in severe pain, and some are fearful of treatments like injections that relieve pain. Nurses should use age-appropriate communication skills to ascertain a child's need for pain relief. The "ouch scale" illustrated in Figure 26-1 can be helpful in determining a child's level of pain. Also, the parent may help identify the presence and degree of the child's pain. Crying and whining may be indicators of a need for pain relief or may represent other needs.

A child, like an adult, should be given medication before the pain becomes severe. The use of oral liquid medication

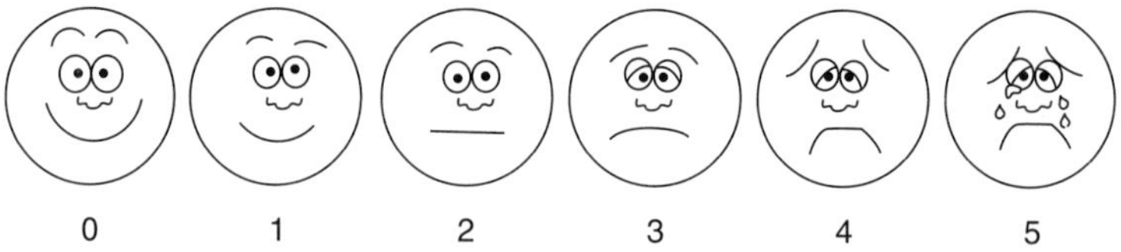

1. Explain to the child that each face is for a person who feels happy because he has no pain (hurt, or whatever word the child uses) or feels sad because he has some or a lot of pain.

2. Point to the appropriate face and state, "This face is ..."
   0-"very happy because he doesn't hurt at all."
   1-"hurts just a little bit."
   2-"hurts a little more."
   3-"hurts even more."
   4-"hurts a whole lot."
   5-"hurts as much as you can imagine, although you don't have to be crying to feel this bad."

3. Ask the child to choose the face that best describes how he feels. Be specific about which pain (e.g., "shot" or incision) and what time (e.g., now? earlier? before lunch?).

FIGURE 26–1 A scale used to rate the intensity of pain in children. From Hockenberry M: *Wong's essentials of pediatric nursing,* ed. 9, St. Louis, 2013, Mosby.

for pain relief, if appropriate, is generally more acceptable to the child. The nurse may alleviate the child's fear and help with drug compliance by using drawings and pictures related to areas of pain in the body and pain relief with smiling faces.

Older Adults

Usually, adults who are 65 years of age or older require adjustment to drug doses to avoid severe side effects. Merely decreasing the usual adult dosage of opioid analgesic is not always the answer for older adults. Many take an array of medications for their health problems, increasing the possibility of drug interactions and drug side effects. In older adults, side effects from the use of opioids become more pronounced. The nurse needs to closely monitor for adverse reactions in older adults who take opioid analgesics. As a person ages, liver and renal functions decrease, causing the rate of metabolism and excretion of the drug to decrease. As a result, drug accumulation may occur.

Older adults tend to have different beliefs and fears than younger generations regarding opioids. They may believe that pain is inevitable due to aging or fear addiction. Older adults may not want to report pain, because they do not want to be a burden. The nurse must perform pain assessment with a supportive approach in an unhurried manner and teach the patient accurate drug information.

Pain assessment may be more difficult with older adults due to the decrease in cognitive and sensory-perceptual abilities. Dementia or hearing and visual deficits may interfere with communication. The nurse may need to rely on a more thorough physical assessment to discover the presence of pain, because self-reporting may not be reliable.

In the presence of decreased renal and hepatic function, drugs that tend to be more toxic in older adults include meperidine (Demerol), pentazocine (Talwin), and propoxyphene (Darvon). Analgesics are usually metabolized in the liver and excreted in the urine. Usual doses of analgesics in older adults may result in excessive sedation and prolonged duration of action. Chronologic age is one of several factors that influence medication use and dosage. Comorbidity must also be considered.

Cognitively Impaired Individuals

Any cognitively impaired individual may be unable to report pain adequately. The nurse should use a measurement scale that is appropriate for the patient. Some physical signs of pain include moans, grimacing, clenched teeth, noisy respirations, and restlessness.

Oncology Patients

Cancer pain is managed according to three levels of analgesia based on the World Health Organization (WHO) Ladder as follows:

Step 1—Mild Pain: Nonopioids with or without an adjuvant medication

Step 2—Moderate Pain: Nonopioids and mild opioid with or without an adjuvant medication

Step 3—Severe Pain: Stronger opioid at higher dosage levels with or without an adjuvant medication

Opioids are titrated for oncology patients until pain relief is achieved or the side effects become intolerable. For effective pain management in patients with cancer, extremely high doses may be required. There are no set dosage limits for oncology patients.

Individuals with a History of Substance Abuse

Often patients with a history of substance abuse require pain medication. A thorough pain assessment is necessary to find out the cause of pain. The nurse needs to know that opioids are effective and safe in this population, even though larger doses in greater frequency may be required. Studies have shown that withholding opioids in this population has not increased recovery from addiction. However, opioid agonist-antagonists such as pentazocine (Talwin) should be avoided in chemically dependent patients, because these drugs may precipitate withdrawal syndrome.

ADJUVANT THERAPY

Medications used as **adjuvant analgesics** have been developed for other purposes and later found to be effective for pain relief in neuropathy. Adjuvant therapy is usually used along with a nonopioid and opioid. Examples of adjuvant analgesics include anticonvulsants, antidepressants, corticosteroids, antidysrhythmics, and local anesthetics.

Anticonvulsant medications (gabapentin [Neurontin]) act on the peripheral nerves and CNS by inhibiting spontaneous neuronal firing. They are used for neuropathic pain and the prevention of migraine headaches. Tricyclic antidepressants (amitriptyline [Elavil]) prevent the reuptake of serotonin and norepinephrine in the cells. Lower doses of tricyclic antidepressants than those usually prescribed for depression are effective in treating peripheral neuropathy. Corticosteroids serve as effective analgesics by reducing nociceptive stimuli. Antidysrhythmics (mexiletine [Mexitil]) block sodium channels to reduce pain. Local anesthetics (lidocaine patch) can be effective analgesics by interrupting the transmission of pain signals to the brain.

Adjuvant medications potentiate opioid analgesia for severe persistent pain in diabetic neuropathy, cancer, migraine headaches, and rheumatoid arthritis. When any of the adjuvant medications are used in conjunction with an NSAID and opioid, dosages may be kept lower to reduce adverse effects.

TREATMENT FOR OPIOID-ADDICTED INDIVIDUALS

Refer to Chapter 5 for a discussion of therapies for addiction.

OPIOID AGONIST-ANTAGONISTS

Opioid agonist-antagonists, medications in which an opioid antagonist (e.g., naloxone [Narcan]) is added to an opioid agonist, were developed in hopes of decreasing opioid abuse. Pentazocine (Talwin), the first opioid analgesic, can be given orally (tablet) and by injection (subQ, IM, and IV). Pentazocine is classified as a schedule IV drug. Butorphanol tartrate (Stadol), buprenorphine (Buprenex), and nalbuphine hydrochloride (Nubain) are examples of other opioid agonist-antagonist analgesics. Reports say that pentazocine and butorphanol can cause dependence. Opioid agonist-antagonist drugs are not given for cancer pain, because of the risk of potential CNS toxicity from the high doses required. These analgesics are considered safe for use during labor, but their safety during early pregnancy has not been established.

Prototype Drug Chart 26-3 details the pharmacologic behavior of nalbuphine, and Table 26-4 lists the various opioid agonist-antagonists.

PROTOTYPE DRUG CHART 26-3

Nalbuphine

Drug Class Opioid: agonist-antagonist Trade Name: Nubain Pregnancy Category: B/D	**Dosage** A: IV/IM/subQ: 10-20 mg q3-6h; *max:* 160 mg/d
Contraindications Hypersensitivity Caution: History of drug abuse or emotional instability, impaired respirations, head injury, increased intracranial pressure, MI, biliary tract surgery, renal or hepatic dysfunction	**Drug-Lab-Food Interactions** Drug: CNS depression is potentiated with alcohol or other CNS depressants
Pharmacokinetics Absorption: readily occurs parenterally Distribution: PB: <30%; crosses placenta, excreted in breast milk Metabolism: t½: 3-6 h Excretion: In urine, bile, feces	**Pharmacodynamics** Onset: 2-3 min IV; 15 minutes IM Peak: 30 min IV; 30 min IM Duration: 3-4 h IV; 3-6 h IM
Therapeutic Effects/Uses To relieve moderate to severe pain Mode of Action: Inhibition of pain impulses transmitted in the CNS by binding with opiate receptor and increasing pain threshold	
Side Effects Dizziness, confusion, hallucinations, blurred vision, headache, flushing, sedation, nervousness, restlessness, euphoria, depression, crying, dysphoria, unusual dreams, dry mouth, bitter taste, nausea, vomiting, abdominal cramps, clammy skin, urinary urgency	**Adverse Reactions** Bradycardia, tachycardia, hypotension, hypertension, dyspnea Life-threatening: Respiratory depression

CNS, Central nervous system; *d,* day; *h,* hour; *IM,* intramuscular; *IV,* intravenous; *max,* maximum; *MI,* myocardial infarction; *min,* minute; *PB,* protein-binding; *subQ,* subcutaneous; *t½,* half- life.

TABLE 26-4 OPIOIDS: AGONIST-ANTAGONISTS

GENERIC (BRAND)	ROUTE AND DOSAGE	USES AND CONSIDERATIONS
buprenorphine HCl (Buprenex) CSS V	Pain: A: IM/IV: Initially: 0.3 mg q4h PRN	For moderate to severe pain associated with surgery, cancer, urinary calculi, myocardial infarction, and trauma. Avoid alcohol and CNS depressants. Pregnancy category: C; PB: 96%; t½: 2-37 h
butorphanol tartrate (Stadol) CSS IV	A: IM: 1-4 mg q3-4h PRN A: IV: 0.5-2 mg q3-4h PRN Nasal spray: 1 mg (1 spray) q3-4h	Management of moderate to severe pain associated with cancer, urinary calculi, labor, musculoskeletal, and burns. Pregnancy category: C; PB: 80%; t½: 5 h
nalbuphine HCl (Nubain) CSS IV	See Prototype Drug Chart 26-3.	
pentazocine lactate (Talwin) CSS IV	A: PO: 50-100 mg q3-4h PRN; *max:* 600 mg/d A: subQ/IM/IV: 30 mg q3-4 h PRN; *max:* 360 mg/d	To control moderate to severe pain. Pregnancy category: C; PB: 60%; t½: 1.5-10 h

A, Adult; *CNS,* central nervous system; *CSS,* Controlled Substances Schedule; *d,* day; *h,* hour; *IM,* intramuscular; *IV,* intravenous; *max,* maximum; *PB,* protein-binding; *PO,* by mouth; *PRN,* as needed; *subQ,* subcutaneous; *t½,* half-life; *UK,* unknown; >, greater than.

Pharmacokinetics Nalbuphine can be administered orally, IM, subQ, or IV. It is rapidly absorbed parenterally. Nalbuphine has a short half-life. It is metabolized in the liver and excreted in the urine.

Pharmacodynamics Nalbuphine is effective in alleviating moderate to severe pain. Onset of action is rapid, and peak time occurs within 30 minutes with IV administration. Duration of action is the same for all routes of administration: approximately 5 hours.

SAFETY: Preventing Medication Errors

Do not confuse...

- **Nubain** (narcotic agonist-antagonist analgesic for moderate to severe pain) with **Nebcin** (aminoglycoside antibiotic) or **Nuprin** (OTC analgesic, antipyretic, NSAID).

Nursing Process
Patient-Centered Collaborative Care

Opioid Agonist-Antagonist Analgesic: Nalbuphine (Nubain)

Assessment

- Obtain a drug history from patient. Report if a drug-drug interaction is probable. When taken with nalbuphine, CNS depressants can cause respiratory depression.
- Note baseline vital signs for future comparison.
- Assess the type of pain, duration, and location before giving the drug.

Nursing Diagnosis

- Acute pain related to trauma
- Knowledge deficit related to unfamiliarity of drug

Planning

- Patient's intensity of pain will be lessened.

Nursing Interventions

- Monitor vital signs. Note any changes in respirations.
- Check bowel sounds and date of last bowel movement to identify constipation. Decreased peristalsis may result in constipation. A mild laxative may be necessary.
- Determine urine output. Report if urine output is <30 mL/h or <600 mL/day.
- Administer IV nalbuphine undiluted. Do not mix with barbiturates.

Patient Teaching

General

- Warn patient not to use alcohol or CNS depressants while taking nalbuphine. Respiratory depression can occur.
- Suggest nonpharmacologic methods for lessening pain like changing position or ambulation.

Side Effects

- Advise patient to report side effects of nalbuphine: dizziness, headaches, constipation, dysuria, rash, or blurred vision. Hallucinations, tachycardia, and respiratory depression are adverse reactions that might occur.

Cultural Considerations

- Accept various cultural groups' use of alternative methods in relief of pain.

Evaluation

- Evaluate effectiveness of nalbuphine in relieving pain. If ineffective, another opioid analgesic may need to be ordered.
- Determine stability of vital signs. Note if there is a change in respirations, pulse rate, or blood pressure. Report abnormal findings.

OPIOID ANTAGONISTS

Opioid antagonists are antidotes for overdoses of natural and synthetic opioid analgesics. The opioid antagonists have a higher affinity to the opiate receptor site than the opioid being taken. An **opioid antagonist** blocks the receptor and displaces any opioid that would normally be at the receptor, inhibiting the opioid action. Indications for opioid antagonists include reversal of postoperative opioid depression and opioid overdose.

Naloxone (Narcan), administered IM or IV; naltrexone hydrochloride (ReVia), administered orally by tablet or liquid; and nalmefene are opioid antagonists. These drugs are perfect examples of pharmacologic antagonists because they reverse the respiratory and CNS depression (sedation and hypotension) caused by opioids. Table 26-5 lists the opioid antagonists.

When receiving opioid antagonists, the patient should be monitored continuously. The opioid action may exceed that of opioid antagonists, and further analgesia may be needed. For example, fentanyl and a combination of drugs given during surgery may lead to excessive respiratory depression. Naloxone may be given as an opioid antidote. The patient's respiratory and CNS status should be monitored closely for indications of analgesic reversal (tachycardia, nausea, vomiting, and sweating) and possible need of further analgesia. The patient receiving naloxone should also be observed for bleeding, because this drug may cause an elevated partial thromboplastin time.

HEADACHES: MIGRAINE AND CLUSTER

Migraine headaches are characterized by a unilateral throbbing head pain accompanied by nausea, vomiting, and photophobia. These symptoms frequently persist for 4 to 24 hours and for several days in some cases. Two thirds of migraine headaches are experienced by women in their twenties and thirties. Symptoms usually decrease or are absent during pregnancy and menopause. The intensity of migraine pain can disrupt daily activities.

Pathophysiology

Migraine headaches are caused by inflammation and dilation of the blood vessels in the cranium. The etiology is unknown, but some theories suggest an imbalance in the neurotransmitter serotonin (5-hydroxytryptamine [5-HT]) that causes vasoconstriction and suppresses migraine headaches. The tendency of calcitonin gene-related peptide (CGRP) is to promote a migraine attack. Serum CGRP levels are elevated during a migraine attack. Foods such as cheese, chocolate, and red wine can trigger an attack.

The two types of migraine are (1) classic migraines, which are associated with an aura that occurs minutes to 1 hour before onset, and (2) common migraines, which are not associated with an aura.

Cluster headaches are characterized by a severe unilateral nonthrobbing pain usually located around the eye. They occur in a series of cluster attacks—one or more attacks every day for several weeks. They are not associated with an aura and do not cause nausea and vomiting. Men are more commonly affected by cluster headaches than women.

Treatment of Migraine Headaches

Preventive treatment for migraines includes (1) beta-adrenergic blockers such as propranolol (Inderal) and atenolol (Tenormin); (2) anticonvulsants such as valproic acid (Depakote) and gabapentin (Neurontin); and (3) tricyclic antidepressants such as amitriptyline (Elavil) and imipramine (Tofranil).

Treatment or cessation of a migraine attack depends on the intensity of pain. Drugs used to treat migraines include analgesics, opioid analgesics, ergot alkaloids, and selective serotonin$_1$ (5-HT) receptor agonists, also known as *triptans.* For mild migraine attacks, aspirin, acetaminophen, or NSAIDs, such as ibuprofen or naproxen (Aleve), may be prescribed. Aspirin may be used in combination with caffeine. Meperidine (Demerol) and butorphanol nasal spray (Stadol NS) are opioid analgesics that are occasionally used.

Antimigraine medication should be taken early during a migraine attack. Nausea and vomiting might occur; antiemetics decrease these symptoms. Dihydroergotamine, an ergot alkaloid, can be administered subcutaneously, intramuscularly, intravenously, and by means of a nasal spray.

The triptans (5-HT$_1$ receptor agonists) are the most recently developed group of drugs for the treatment of migraine headaches. Sumatriptan (Imitrex), a selective serotonin receptor agonist with a short duration of action, was the first triptan drug. It is considered more effective than ergot alkaloids in treating acute migraine attacks. Table 26-6 lists the ergot alkaloids and the selective serotonin$_1$ (5-HT) receptor agonists and their dosages, uses, and considerations. Do not confuse sumatriptan with zolmitriptan. Both drugs are triptans but have different dosages. Also, do not confuse Amerge (triptan used for migraines) with Amaryl (sulfonylurea used for diabetes mellitus) or Altace (angiotensin-converting enzyme inhibitor) used for hypertension and heart failure. Prototype Drug Chart 26-4 provides further pharmacology of sumatriptan.

TABLE 26-5 OPIOID ANTAGONISTS

GENERIC (BRAND)	ROUTE AND DOSAGE	USES AND CONSIDERATIONS
naloxone HCl (Narcan)	Opiate overdose or opioid-induced respiratory distress: A: IV: 0.4-2 mg; may repeat q2-3 min; *max:* 10 mg C: IV: 0.01-0.1 mg/kg; may repeat q2-3 min; *max:* 10 mg	To treat opioid overdose. Approved for use in neonates to reverse respiratory depression induced by maternal opioid use. Pregnancy category: B; PB: UK; t½: 0.5-1.5 h
naltrexone HCl (Vivitrol, ReVia)	A: PO: 25 mg/d; repeat 25 mg in 1 h if no withdrawal response; *max:* 150 mg/d A: IM: 380 mg/dose q4wk; *max:* 380 mg/dose	To treat opioid and alcohol abuse. Three to five times more potent than naloxone. Decreases but does not prevent craving for opioids. Use after patient is off opioids for 7 days or more. Do not give if patient is in opiate withdrawal; can precipitate a withdrawal reaction. High doses can cause hepatotoxicity. Pregnancy category: C; PB: 21%-28%; t½: 5-10 h

A, Adult; *C,* child; *h,* hour; *IM,* intramuscular; *IV,* intravenous; *max,* maximum; *min,* minute; *PB,* protein-binding; *PO,* by mouth; *PRN,* as needed; *t½,* half-life; *UK,* unknown.

TABLE 26-6 DRUGS USED TO TREAT SEVERE MIGRAINE HEADACHES

DRUG	ROUTE AND DOSAGE	USES AND CONSIDERATIONS
Ergot Alkaloids		
dihydroergotamine mesylate (Migranal)	A: Intranasal: 1 spray in each nostril; may repeat in 15 min; *max:* 4 sprays (2 mg)/attack, 8 sprays/d, 24 sprays/wk A: IM/IV: 1 mg; may repeat in 1 h; *max:* 6 mg/wk	To prevent or abort migraine attack. Pregnancy category: X; PB: 90%-93%; t½: 21-32 h

TABLE 26-6 DRUGS USED TO TREAT SEVERE MIGRAINE HEADACHES—cont'd

DRUG	ROUTE AND DOSAGE	USES AND CONSIDERATIONS
Selective Serotonin$_1$ Receptor Agonists (Triptans)		
sumatriptan (Imitrex)	See Prototype Drug Chart 26-4.	
naratriptan (Amerge)	A: PO: 1-2.5 mg; may repeat in 4 h; *max:* 5 mg/d	For acute migraines. Has a longer half-life, thus duration of action is longer. Causes vasoconstriction of cranial arteries. Avoid if patient has uncontrolled hypertension, IHD, prior MI. Pregnancy category: C; PB: 28%-31%; t½: 6 h
rizatriptan benzoate (Maxalt)	A: PO: 5-10 mg; may repeat in 2 h; *max:* 30 mg/d	For acute migraines. Two types of tablets: regular and melt-in-mouth. Avoid if patient has uncontrolled hypertension, IHD, prior MI. Pregnancy category: C; PB: 14%; t½: 2-3 h
zolmitriptan (Zomig)	A: PO: 2.5-5 mg; may repeat in 2 h; *max:* 10 mg/d	For acute migraines. 65% of patients respond in 2 h. Avoid if patient has uncontrolled hypertension, IHD, prior MI. Pregnancy category: C; PB: 25%; t½: 3 h
almotriptan (Axert)	A: PO: 6.25-12.5 mg; may repeat in 2 h; *max:* 25 mg/d	For acute migraines. Pregnancy category: C; PB: 35%; t½: 3-4 h
frovatriptan (Frova)	A: PO: 2.5 mg; may repeat in 2 h; *max:* 7.5 mg/d	For acute migraines. Pregnancy category: C; PB: 15%; t½: 26 h
eletriptan (Relpax)	A: PO: 20-40 mg; may repeat in 2 h; *max:* 80 mg/d	For acute migraines. Pregnancy category: C; PB: 85%; t½: 4-5 h

A, Adult; *h,* hour; *IHD,* ischemic heart disease; *IM,* intramuscular; *IV,* intravenous; *max,* maximum; *MI,* myocardial infarction; *min,* minute; *PB,* protein-binding; *PO,* by mouth; *SL,* sublingual; *subQ,* subcutaneous; *t½,* half-life; *UK,* unknown, *wk,* week.

PROTOTYPE DRUG CHART 26-4

Sumatriptan

Drug Class
5-HT$_1$ receptor agonist: antimigraine
Trade Name: Imitrex
Pregnancy Category: C

Dosage
A: PO: 25-50 mg for 1 dose, may repeat once after 2 h, *max:* 200 mg/d
A: subQ: 6 mg, may repeat with 6 mg at least 1 h after first injection, *max:* 12 mg/d
A: Intranasal: 5-20 mg in one nostril, may repeat after 2 h, *max:* 40 mg/d

Contraindications
Hypersensitivity, coronary artery disease, peripheral vascular disease, hypertension, obesity, diabetes mellitus, smoking, hepatic disease, cerebrovascular disease, older adults
Caution: Renal dysfunction, seizures

Drug-Lab-Food Interactions
Drug: Risk of vasospasm and blood pressure elevation with dihydroergotamine and other ergot alkaloids; increased levels and toxicity within 2 weeks of MAOIs; increased risk of serotonin syndrome or neuroleptic malignant syndrome with SSRIs

Pharmacokinetics
Absorption: Rapidly absorbed following subQ injection
Distribution: PB: 14%-21%
Metabolism: t½: 2 h
Excretion: Urine and feces

Pharmacodynamics
PO: Onset: 60 min
Peak: 2 h
Duration: 24-48 h
subQ: Onset: 10 min
Peak: 1 h
Duration: 24-48 h
Intranasal: Onset: 15 min
Peak: 1-1.5 h
Duration: 24-48 h

Therapeutic Effects/Uses
To treat migraine and cluster headaches
Mode of Action: Causes vasoconstriction of cranial arteries to relieve migraine attacks

Side Effects
Dizziness, fainting, tingling, numbness, warm sensation, drowsiness, muscle cramps, nausea, vomiting, dry mouth, diarrhea, abdominal cramping

Adverse Reactions
Hypotension, hypertension, heart block, angina, dysrhythmias, thromboembolism, seizures, central nervous system hemorrhage, stroke
Life-threatening: Coronary artery vasospasm, myocardial infarction, cardiac arrest

A, Adult; *h,* hour; *MAOI,* monoamine oxidase inhibitor; *max,* maximum; *min,* minute; *PB,* protein-binding; *PO,* by mouth; *subQ,* subcutaneous; *t½,* half-life; *UK,* unknown.

KEY WEBSITES

Information on Duragesic (fentanyl transdermal patch): *www.rxlist.com/cgi/generic/fentanyl.htm*

Information on acetaminophen: *www.nlm.nih.gov/medlineplus/druginfo/meds/a681004.html*

Information on zolmitriptan (Zomig): *www.zomig.com/index.aspx?ce5set*

CRITICAL THINKING CASE STUDY

RJ, a 79-year-old man, underwent abdominal surgery for resection of his colon. His physician prescribed morphine 10 mg every 3 to 4 hours PRN after the surgery. RJ did not ask for "pain medication," because he worried he might become addicted. A day after the surgery, his nurse noted that he was restless and grimaced whenever he moved in bed. He refused to breathe deeply or cough when instructed to do so. The nurse compared RJ's vital signs to his baseline findings and noted an increased pulse rate and a drop in systolic blood pressure of 6 mm Hg.

1. Should the nurse give morphine? Explain your answer.
2. What would your reaction be to RJ in regard to his restlessness, grimacing, and refusal to deep breathe and cough?
3. What is the significance of the change in vital signs?
4. What classic side effects of opioid analgesics should the nurse assess?
5. What are some possible nonpharmacologic measures that might be helpful in alleviating RJ's pain?

The second postoperative day, RJ began asking for morphine every 3 hours. On the fifth day, the physician discontinued RJ's morphine and prescribed acetaminophen with codeine.

6. Why was the opioid analgesic order changed?
7. RJ does not want to ambulate. What is an appropriate nursing response?

NCLEX STUDY QUESTIONS

1. A patient requires a nonopioid medication. The nurse knows that which medication will cause the least gastrointestinal distress?
   a. aspirin
   b. ketorolac
   c. celecoxib
   d. ibuprofen
2. A patient states during a medical history that he takes several acetaminophen tablets throughout the day. The nurse teaches the patient that the dosage should not exceed which amount?
   a. 1 g/day
   b. 2 g/day
   c. 4 g/day
   d. 6 g/day
3. For the patient receiving periodic morphine IV push, which is the most critical finding for the nurse to discover?
   a. Increased temperature
   b. Decreased bowel sounds
   c. Decreased respirations
   d. Increased red blood cell count
4. A patient is admitted to the emergency department in respiratory depression following self-injection with hydromorphone. The admitting nurse knows that which drug will reverse respiratory depression caused by opioid overdose?
   a. fentanyl
   b. naloxone
   c. butorphanol
   d. sufenta
5. Assessing a patient following IV morphine administration, the nurse notes cold, clammy skin; a pulse of 40 beats/min; respirations of 10 breaths/min; and constricted pupils. Which medication will the patient likely need next?
   a. naloxone (Narcan)
   b. meloxicam (Mobic)
   c. pentazocine (Talwin)
   d. propoxyphene (Darvon)
6. For the patient who is taking acetaminophen (Tylenol), what should the nurse do? (Select all that apply.)
   a. Monitor routine liver enzyme tests.
   b. Encourage the patient to check package labels of OTC drugs to avoid overdosing.
   c. Teach the diabetic patient taking acetaminophen to check blood glucose more frequently.
   d. Teach the female patient that oral contraceptives can increase the effect of acetaminophen.
   e. Teach the patient that caffeine decreases the effects of acetaminophen.
7. For the patient who is taking nalbuphine (Nubain), what should the nurse do? (Select all that apply.)
   a. Monitor any changes in respirations.
   b. Instruct the patient to report bradycardia.
   c. Administer IV nalbuphine undiluted.
   d. Explain to the patient to expect an excessive amount of urine output.
   e. Instruct the patient to avoid alcohol when taking nalbuphine to avoid respiratory depression.
8. A patient is having a migraine attack. The nurse should know that which drugs are used to treat migraine attacks?
   a. Triptans
   b. Anticonvulsants
   c. Tricyclic antidepressants
   d. Beta-adrenergic blockers

Answers: 1, c; 2, c; 3, c; 4, b; 5, a; 6, a, b, c; 7, a, c, e; 8, a.

UNIT VIII

Psychiatric Agents

From moods and emotions flow the various thoughts and actions of individuals, which are communicated throughout the central nervous system (CNS) by chemical neurotransmitters. An impulse is communicated by traveling through the presynaptic neuron across the synaptic cleft and binding to a receptor on the postsynaptic neuron, as illustrated in Figure VIII-1.

Neurotransmitters are synthesized in the cytoplasm in the presynaptic neuron and stored in vesicles. Vesicles safeguard neurotransmitters from being destroyed by enzymes. When an impulse arrives by way of an action potential at a presynaptic neuron, vesicles are triggered to move to the cell membrane wall and release the transmitter into the synaptic cleft.

Neurotransmitters function with the help of receptors, which are embedded in the membrane of the postsynaptic neuron. Receptors are configured in size and shape to interlock with specific transmitters. Immediately upon connection of neurotransmitters to receptors, an action is exerted and the transmitter is removed. Once released, transmitters can be broken down into inactive substances by enzymes, diffused away from the synapse into intracellular fluid, or returned to the presynaptic neuron in a process called *reuptake*.

The major neurotransmitters affecting psychopathology include gamma-aminobutyric acid (GABA), serotonin, dopamine, norepinephrine, and acetylcholine. The GABA neurotransmitter is associated with the regulation of anxiety. When the level of GABA neurotransmitters is reduced, anxiety disorders may result.

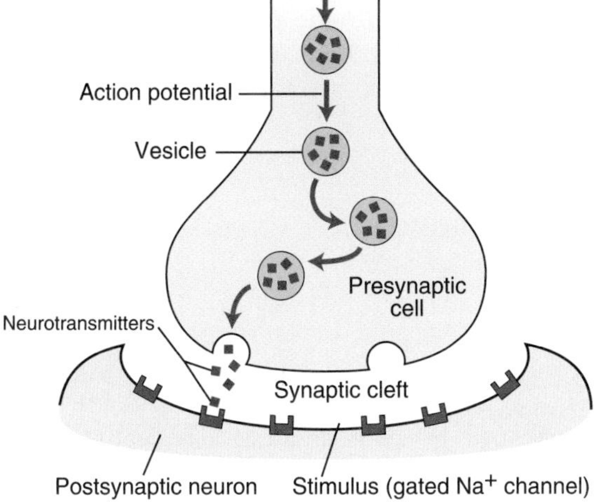

FIGURE VIII–1 Chemical neurotransmitters.

Benzodiazepines (antianxiety drugs) act by binding to a GABA receptor site, making the postsynaptic receptor more sensitive to GABA and its neurotransmission. This connection decreases the signs and symptoms of anxiety.

Serotonin neurotransmission is associated with arousal and general activity levels of the CNS. Serotonin functions to regulate sleep, wakefulness, and mood, as well as the delusions, hallucinations, and withdrawal of schizophrenia. Antidepressants block the reuptake of serotonin into the presynaptic neuron. A structurally specific drug is more likely to affect only the specific receptors for which it is intended and not the receptors specific for other neurochemicals, which would produce unintended effects. Selective serotonin reuptake inhibitor (SSRI) drugs are specific and generally produce fewer side effects in the treatment of depression than older antidepressants such as monoamine oxidase inhibitors (MAOIs).

Dopamine-containing neurons are thought to be involved in the regulation of cognition, emotional responses, and motivation, and dopamine neurotransmitters are associated with schizophrenia and other psychoses. Antipsychotic drugs block dopamine receptors in the postsynaptic neuron.

Norepinephrine is associated with control of arousal, attention, vigilance, mood, affect, and anxiety. This transmitter is involved with thinking, planning, and interpreting. Tricyclic antidepressants block the reuptake of norepinephrine into the presynaptic neuron and effectively treat depressive disorders. MAOIs inactivate norepinephrine, dopamine, and serotonin by inhibiting the monoamine oxidase enzyme to relieve signs and symptoms of depression.

Faulty release, reuptake, or elimination of neurotransmitters may lead to an imbalance of neurotransmission and pathology. Disorders can then develop that affect an individual's thoughts, feelings, and behaviors.

Knowledge of psychopharmacology is essential to psychiatric mental health nursing. A basic understanding of the actions of psychotropic drugs will help nurses rapidly comprehend and apply information and enhance the effectiveness of pharmacologic treatment. Essential responsibilities of the nurse in administering psychotropic medications are to assess behavior, monitor for side effects, and educate the patient and family. These actions are crucial to successful psychopharmacologic therapy.

Drugs used to treat psychoses and anxiety are discussed in Chapter 27. Antidepressants and mood stabilizers are discussed in Chapter 28.

CHAPTER 27

Antipsychotics and Anxiolytics

evolve WEBSITE

http://evolve.elsevier.com/KeeHayes/pharmacology/

- Animations
- Content Updates
- Key Points
- Review Questions for the NCLEX® Examination
- References from the Textbook
- Unfolding Case Studies

OBJECTIVES

- Differentiate between the two groups of drugs: antipsychotics and anxiolytics.
- Contrast the action, uses, side effects, and adverse effects of traditional/typical and atypical antipsychotics.
- Plan nursing interventions, including patient teaching, for the patient taking antipsychotics and anxiolytics.
- Apply the nursing process to the patient taking an atypical antipsychotic, a typical antipsychotic, and an anxiolytic.

OUTLINE

KEY TERMS

Antipsychotics and anxiolytics are CNS depressants used to manage symptoms of psychosis and anxiety disorders. Antipsychotics are also known as *neuroleptics* or *psychotropics,* but the preferred name for this group is either *antipsychotics* or *neuroleptics.* **Neuroleptic** refers to any drug that modifies psychotic behavior and exerts an antipsychotic effect. Anxiolytics are also called *antianxiety drugs* or *sedative-hypnotics.* Certain anxiolytics are used to treat sleep disorders, seizures, and withdrawal symptoms from alcohol or other abuse substances. Some of these drugs are also used for conscious sedation and anesthesia supplementation. However, the anxiolytics described in this chapter are used specifically to treat anxiety.

PSYCHOSIS

Psychosis, or losing contact with reality, is manifested in a variety of mental or psychiatric disorders. Psychosis is usually characterized by more than one symptom, but these may include difficulty in processing information and coming to a conclusion, delusions, hallucinations, incoherence, catatonia, and aggressive or violent behavior. **Schizophrenia,** a chronic psychotic disorder, is the major category of psychosis in which many of these symptoms are manifested.

The symptoms of schizophrenia usually develop in adolescence or early adulthood. The symptoms of this psychotic disorder are divided into two groups: "positive" symptoms and "negative" symptoms. Positive symptoms may be characterized by exaggeration of normal function (e.g., agitation), incoherent speech, hallucinations, delusions, and paranoia. Negative symptoms are characterized by a decrease or loss in function and motivation. There is a poverty of speech content, poor self-care, and social withdrawal. Negative symptoms tend to be more chronic and persistent. The typical or traditional group of antipsychotics is more helpful for managing positive symptoms than negative symptoms. A group of antipsychotics called *atypical* have been found to be more useful in treating both the positive and negative symptoms of schizophrenia. *Antipsychotics* compose the largest group of drugs used to treat mental illness. Specifically, these drugs improve the thought processes and behavior of patients with psychotic symptoms, especially those with schizophrenia and other psychotic disorders. They are not used to treat anxiety or depression. The theory is that psychotic symptoms result from an imbalance in the neurotransmitter **dopamine** in the brain. Sometimes these antipsychotics are called *dopamine antagonists.* Antipsychotics block D_2 dopamine receptors in the brain, reducing psychotic symptoms. Many antipsychotics block the chemoreceptor trigger zone and vomiting (emetic) center in the brain, producing an **antiemetic** (prevents or relieves nausea and vomiting) effect. When dopamine is blocked, however, **extrapyramidal symptoms (EPS)** of **parkinsonism** (Parkinson's disease, a chronic neurologic disorder that affects the extrapyramidal motor tract) such as tremors, masklike facies, rigidity, and shuffling gait may develop. Many patients who take high-potency antipsychotic drugs may require long-term medication for parkinsonian symptoms.

ANTIPSYCHOTIC AGENTS

Antipsychotics are divided into two major categories: *typical* (or *traditional*) and *atypical.* The **typical antipsychotics,** introduced in 1952, are subdivided into phenothiazines and nonphenothiazines. Nonphenothiazines include butyrophenones, dibenzoxazepines, dihydroindolones, and thioxanthenes. The phenothiazines and thioxanthenes block norepinephrine, causing sedative and hypotensive effects early in treatment. The butyrophenones block only the neurotransmitter dopamine.

Atypical antipsychotics make up the second category of antipsychotics. Clozapine, discovered in the 1960s and made available in Europe in 1971, was the first atypical antipsychotic agent. It was not marketed in the United States until 1990 because of adverse hematologic reactions. Atypical antipsychotics are effective for treating schizophrenia and other psychotic disorders in patients who do not respond to or are intolerant of typical antipsychotics. Because of their decreased side effects, atypical antipsychotics are often used instead of traditional typical antipsychotics as first-line therapy.

Pharmacophysiologic Mechanisms of Action

Antipsychotics block the actions of dopamine and thus may be classified as dopaminergic antagonists. There are five subtypes of dopamine receptors: D_1 through D_5. All antipsychotics block the D_2 (dopaminergic) receptor, which in turn promotes the presence of EPS, resulting in drug-induced pseudoparkinsonism in varying degrees. Atypical antipsychotics have a weak affinity to D_2 receptors, a stronger affinity to D_4 receptors, and they block the serotonin receptor. These agents cause fewer EPS than the typical (phenothiazines) antipsychotic agents, which have a strong affinity to D_2 receptors.

Adverse Reactions

Extrapyramidal Syndrome

Pseudoparkinsonism, which resembles symptoms of Parkinson's disease, is a major side effect of typical antipsychotic drugs. Symptoms of pseudoparkinsonism, or EPS, include stooped posture, masklike facies, rigidity, tremors at rest, shuffling gait, pill-rolling motion of the hand, and bradykinesia. When patients take high-potency typical antipsychotic drugs, these symptoms are more pronounced. Patients who take low-strength antipsychotics such as chlorpromazine (Thorazine) are not as likely to have symptoms of pseudoparkinsonism as those who take fluphenazine (Prolixin).

During early treatment with typical antipsychotic agents for schizophrenia and other psychotic disorders, two adverse extrapyramidal reactions that may occur are acute dystonia and akathisia. Tardive dyskinesia is a later phase of extrapyramidal reaction to antipsychotics. Use of anticholinergic drugs helps decrease pseudoparkinsonism symptoms, acute dystonia, and akathisia, but has little effect on alleviating tardive dyskinesia.

HERBAL ALERT 27-1

Antipsychotic Agents

- Kava kava may increase the risk and severity of dystonic reactions when taken with phenothiazines.
- Kava kava may increase the risk and severity of dystonia when taken concurrently with fluphenazine.

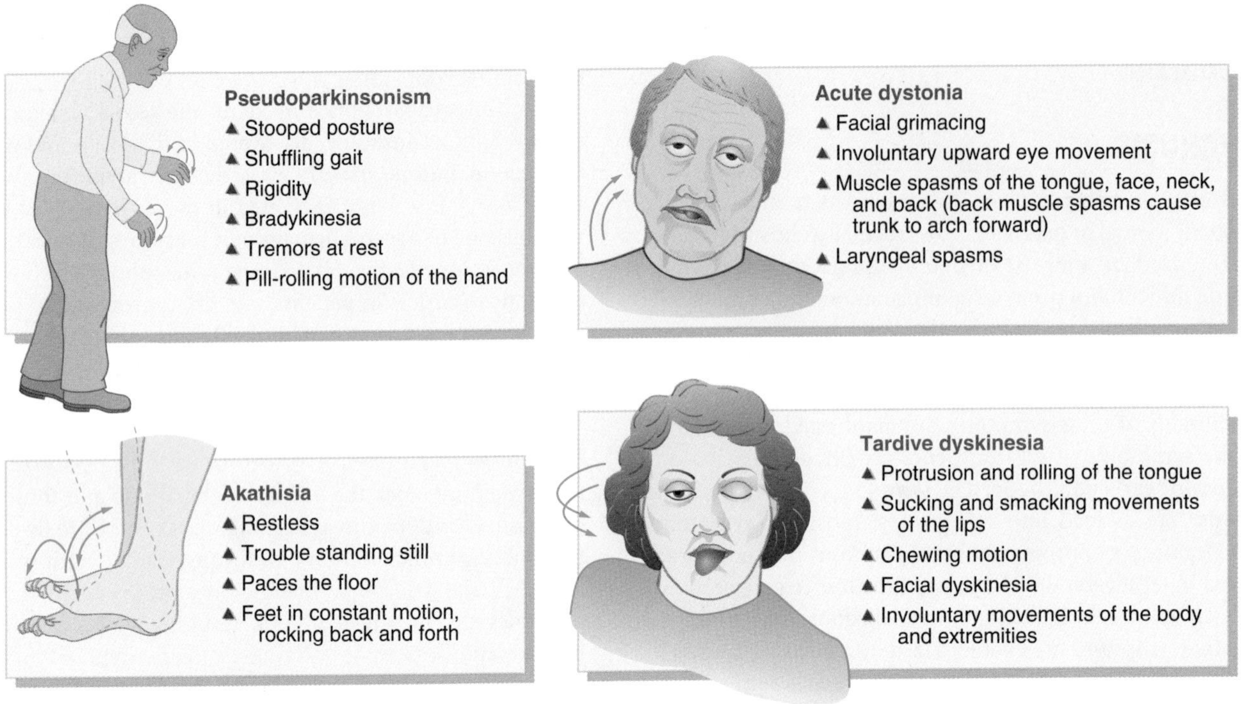

FIGURE 27–1 Characteristics of pseudoparkinsonism, acute dystonia, akathisia, and tardive dyskinesia.

The symptoms of **acute dystonia** usually occur in 5% of patients within days of taking typical antipsychotics. Characteristics of the reaction include muscle spasms of the face, tongue, neck, and back; facial grimacing; abnormal or involuntary upward eye movement; and laryngeal spasms that can impair respiration. This condition is treated with anticholinergic/antiparkinsonism drugs such as benztropine (Cogentin). The benzodiazepine lorazepam (Ativan) may also be prescribed.

Akathisia occurs in approximately 20% of patients who take a typical antipsychotic drug. With this reaction, the patient has trouble standing still, is restless, paces the floor, and is in constant motion (e.g., rocks back and forth). Akathisia is best treated with a benzodiazepine (e.g., lorazepam) or a beta blocker (e.g., propranolol).

Tardive dyskinesia is a serious adverse reaction occurring in approximately 20% to 30% of patients who have taken a typical antipsychotic drug for more than 1 year. The prevalence is higher in cigarette smokers. The likelihood of developing tardive dyskinesia depends on the dose and duration of the antipsychotic factor. Characteristics of tardive dyskinesia include protrusion and rolling of the tongue, sucking and smacking movements of the lips, chewing motion, and involuntary movement of the body and extremities. In older adults, these reactions are more frequent and severe. The antipsychotic drug should be stopped in all who experience tardive dyskinesia and another antipsychotic agent substituted. Benzodiazepines, calcium channel blockers, or beta blockers are helpful in some cases in decreasing tardive dyskinesia. No one agent is effective for all patients. High doses of vitamin E may be helpful, and its use to treat tardive dyskinesia is currently under investigation. Clozapine (Clozaril) has also been effective for treating tardive dyskinesia. Tetrabenazine (Xenazine), used to improve symptoms of Huntington's disease, seems to be effective in treating tardive dyskinesia. Tetrabenazine reduces dopamine, norepinephrine, and serotonin levels. Amantadine has also been helpful in reducing drug-induced involuntary movements. Figure 27-1 shows the characteristics of pseudoparkinsonism, acute dystonia, akathisia, and tardive dyskinesia.

Neuroleptic Malignant Syndrome

Neuroleptic malignant syndrome (NMS) is a rare but potentially fatal condition associated with antipsychotic drugs. Predisposing factors include excess agitation, exhaustion, and dehydration. NMS symptoms involve muscle rigidity, sudden high fever, altered mental status, blood pressure fluctuations, tachycardia, dysrhythmias, seizures, rhabdomyolysis, acute renal failure, respiratory failure, and coma. Treatment of NMS involves immediate withdrawal of antipsychotics, adequate hydration, hypothermic blankets, and administration of antipyretics, benzodiazepines, and muscle relaxants such as dantrolene (Dantrium).

Phenothiazines

Chlorpromazine hydrochloride (Thorazine) was the first phenothiazine introduced for treating psychotic behavior in patients in psychiatric hospitals. The **phenothiazines** are subdivided into three groups: aliphatic, piperazine, and piperidine, which differ mostly in their side effects.

TABLE 27-1 EFFECTS OF PHENOTHIAZINES (VARIES WITHIN CLASS)

GROUP	SEDATION	HYPOTENSION	EPS	ANTIEMETIC
aliphatic	+++	+++	++	++
chlorpromazine and triflupromazinec				+++
piperazine	++	+	+++	+++
piperidine	+++	+++	+	—
Nonphenothiazines				
haloperidol	+	+	+++	+++
loxapine	++	++	+++	—
molindone	+/++	+	+++	—
thiothixene	+	+	+++	—
Atypical Antipsychotics				
risperidone	+	+	+/0	—

—, No effect; *+*, mild effect; *++*, moderate effect; *+++*, severe effect; *EPS*, extrapyramidal symptoms.

The *aliphatic phenothiazines* produce a strong sedative effect, decreased blood pressure, and may cause moderate EPS (pseudoparkinsonism). Chlorpromazine hydrochloride is in the aliphatic group and may produce pronounced **orthostatic hypotension** (low blood pressure that occurs when an individual assumes an upright position from a supine position).

The *piperazine phenothiazines* produce more EPS than other phenothiazines. They cause dry mouth, urinary retention, and agranulocytosis. Examples of piperazine phenothiazines are fluphenazine (Prolixin) and perphenazine (Trilafon).

The *piperidine phenothiazines* have a strong sedative effect, cause few EPS, have a low to moderate effect on blood pressure, and have no antiemetic effect. Thioridazine (Mellaril) is an example of piperidine phenothiazines. Table 27-1 summarizes the effects of the phenothiazines.

Most antipsychotics can be given orally (tablet or liquid), intramuscularly (IM), or intravenously (IV). For oral use, the liquid form might be preferred, because some patients hide tablets to avoid taking them. In addition, the absorption rate is faster with the liquid form. Peak serum drug level occurs in 2 to 3 hours. The antipsychotics are highly protein bound (>90%), and excretion of the drugs and their metabolites is slow. Phenothiazines are metabolized by liver enzymes into phenothiazine metabolites. Metabolites can be detected in the urine several months after the medication has been discontinued. Phenothiazine metabolites may cause a harmless pinkish to red-brown urine color. The *full* therapeutic effects of antipsychotics may not be evident for 3 to 6 weeks following initiation of therapy, but an observable therapeutic response may be apparent after 7 to 10 days.

Noncompliance with antipsychotics is common. Encourage the patient to take the medication as prescribed. Explain and emphasize essential information to compensate for patients' knowledge deficit, and provide an interpreter for patients whose first language is not English.

Prototype Drug Chart 27-1 shows the drug characteristics of fluphenazine (Prolixin), a phenothiazine antipsychotic used to manage psychosis. Box 27-1 shows the symptoms and suggested treatment for overdose of phenothiazines.

BOX 27-1 SYMPTOMS AND SUGGESTED TREATMENT FOR OVERDOSE OF PHENOTHIAZINES

Symptoms

- Unable to arouse; blood pressure fluctuations; tachycardia; agitation; delirium; convulsions; dysrhythmias; neuroleptic malignant syndrome; extrapyramidal symptoms; and renal, cardiac, and respiratory failure.

Treatment

- Maintain airway, gastric lavage, activated charcoal administration, adequate hydration, anticholinergics, and norepinephrine.

Pharmacokinetics Oral absorption of fluphenazine is rapid and not affected by food. This drug is strongly protein-bound and has a long half-life; therefore, the drug may accumulate. Fluphenazine is metabolized by the liver, crosses the blood-brain barrier and placenta, and is excreted as metabolites primarily in the urine. With hepatic dysfunction, the phenothiazine dose may need to be decreased. Lack of drug metabolism in the liver will cause an elevation in serum drug level.

Pharmacodynamics Fluphenazine is prescribed primarily for psychotic disorders. This drug has anticholinergic properties and should be cautiously administered to patients with glaucoma, especially narrow-angle glaucoma. Because hypotension is a side effect of these phenothiazines, any antihypertensives simultaneously administered can cause an additive hypotensive effect. Narcotics and sedative-hypnotics administered simultaneously with these phenothiazines can cause an additive CNS depression. Antacids decrease the absorption rate of both drugs and all phenothiazines, so they should be given 1 hour before or 2 hours after an oral phenothiazine.

The onset of action for fluphenazine hydrochloride is 1 hour, with a duration rate of 6 to 8 hours. Fluphenazine decanoate has delayed absorption, with an onset of action of 24 to 72 hours and a duration of 1 to 6 weeks.

Nonphenothiazines

The many groups of nonphenothiazine antipsychotics include butyrophenone, dibenzoxazepines, dihydroindolone, and thioxanthene.

PROTOTYPE DRUG CHART 27-1

Fluphenazine

Drug Class Antipsychotic: neuroleptic piperazine phenothiazine Trade Names: Prolixin, Decanoate Pregnancy Category: C	**Dosage** Psychoses: A: PO: 0.5-10 mg/d; *max:* 40 mg/d IM/subQ: HCl 2.5-10 mg/d; *max:* 100 mg/d Older adults: PO: 1-2.5 mg/d; *max:* 40 mg/d Decanoate: 12.5-25 mg q1-4wk
Contraindications Hypersensitivity, subcortical brain damage, blood dyscrasias, renal or liver damage, coma	**Drug-Lab-Food Interactions** Drug: Increase depressive effects when taken with alcohol or other CNS depressants Herbal: Kava kava may increase dystonia
Pharmacokinetics Absorption: Rapidly absorbed Distribution: PB 91%-99% Metabolism: t½: HCl—15 h; Decanoate—7-10 d Excretion: In urine	**Pharmacodynamics** PO: HCl: Onset: HCl—1 h; Decanoate—24-72 h Peak: HCl—0.5 h Duration: HCl—6-8 h; Decanoate—1-6 wk IM: Peak: HCl—1.5-2 h
Therapeutic Effects/Uses To manage symptoms of psychosis including schizophrenia Mode of Action: Blocks dopamine receptors in the brain and controls psychotic symptoms	
Side Effects Sedation, dizziness, headache, dry mouth, nasal congestion, blurred vision, photosensitivity, nausea, constipation, urinary retention, polyuria, peripheral edema	**Adverse Reactions** Hypertension, hypotension, tachycardia, extrapyramidal symptoms (tardive dyskinesia), impaired thermoregulation, convulsions Life-threatening: agranulocytosis

A, Adult; *CNS,* central nervous system; *d,* day; *h,* hour; *IM,* intramuscular; *max,* maximum; *PB,* protein-binding; *PO,* by mouth; *t½,* half-life; *wk,* week.

In the *butyrophenone* group, a frequently prescribed nonphenothiazine is haloperidol (Haldol). Haloperidol's pharmacologic behavior is similar to that of the phenothiazines. It is a potent antipsychotic drug in which the equivalent prescribed dose is smaller than drugs of lower potency (e.g., chlorpromazine). The drug dose for haloperidol is 0.5 to 5 mg, whereas the drug dose for chlorpromazine is 10 to 25 mg. Long-acting preparations (haloperidol decanoate [Haldol] and fluphenazine decanoate [Prolixin]) are given for slow release via injection every 2 to 4 weeks. Administration precautions should be taken to prevent soreness and inflammation at the injection site. Because the medication is a viscous liquid, a large-gauge needle (e.g., 21-gauge) should be used with the Z-track method for administration in a deep muscle. See Chapter 4 for further explanation of the Z-track method of injection. The injection site should not be massaged, and sites should be rotated. These medications should not remain in a plastic syringe longer than 15 minutes. Prototype Drug Chart 27-2 provides the drug data related to haloperidol.

Pharmacokinetics Haloperidol is absorbed well through the gastrointestinal (GI) mucosa. It has a long half-life and is highly protein-bound, so the drug may accumulate. Haloperidol is metabolized in the liver and excreted in urine and feces.

Pharmacodynamics Haloperidol alters the effects of dopamine by blocking dopamine receptors; thus sedation and EPS may occur. The drug is used to control psychoses and decrease agitation in adults and children. Dosages need to be decreased in older adults because of decreased liver function and potential side effects. It may be prescribed for children with hyperactive behavior. Haloperidol has anticholinergic activity, so care should be taken when administering it to patients with a history of glaucoma.

Haloperidol has a similar onset of action, peak time of concentration, and duration of action as phenothiazines. It has strong EPS effects. Skin protection is necessary for prolonged use because of the possible side effect of photosensitivity.

From the *dibenzoxazepine* group, loxapine (Loxitane) is a moderately potent agent. It has moderate sedative and orthostatic hypotensive effects and a strong EPS effect.

The typical antipsychotic molindone hydrochloric acid (Moban) from the *dihydroindolone* group is a moderately potent agent. It has low sedative and orthostatic hypotensive effects and a strong EPS effect.

In the nonphenothiazine group known as *thioxanthenes* is thiothixene (Navane), a highly potent typical antipsychotic drug. It has side effects similar to those of molindone with low sedative and orthostatic hypotensive effects and a strong EPS effect.

Side Effects and Adverse Reactions

Several side effects are associated with antipsychotics. The most common side effect for all antipsychotics is drowsiness. Many of the antipsychotics have some anticholinergic effects: dry mouth, increased heart rate, urinary retention,

PROTOTYPE DRUG CHART 27-2

Haloperidol and Haloperidol Decanoate

Drug Class Antipsychotic: neuroleptic (nonphenothiazine) Trade Names: Haldol Pregnancy Category: C	**Dosage** A: PO: 0.2-0.5 mg q.d./b.i.d., increase to 4 mg/d PRN IM: 2-10 mg; may repeat q1h PRN; Deconoate: 50-100 mg q4wk C: PO: 0.05-0.15 mg/kg/d in divided doses; (not for child <3 y) Older adults: Decreased doses PO: 0.25-2 mg b.i.d./t.i.d.; *max:* 4 mg/d
Contraindications Narrow-angle glaucoma; severe hepatic, renal, and cardiovascular diseases; bone marrow depression; Parkinson's disease; blood dyscrasias; CNS depression; subcortical brain damage	**Drug-Lab-Food Interactions** Drug: Increase sedation with alcohol, CNS depressants; increase toxicity with anticholinergics, CNS depressants, lithium; decrease effects with phenobarbital, carbamazepine; decrease effects with caffeine
Pharmacokinetics Absorption: PO: 60% absorbed Distribution: PB: 92% Metabolism: t½: 24 h Excretion: In urine and feces	**Pharmacodynamics** PO: Onset: erratic Peak: 2-6 h Duration: 24-72 h IM: Onset: 15-30 min Peak: 30-45 min Duration: 4-8 h IM: Decanoate: Onset: UK Peak: 6-7 d Duration: 3-4 wk
Therapeutic Effects/Uses To treat acute and chronic psychoses, to treat children with severe behavior problems who are combative, to suppress narcotic withdrawal symptoms, to treat schizophrenia resistant to other drugs, to treat Tourette syndrome, to treat symptoms of dementia in older adults Mode of Action: Alters the effect of dopamine on CNS; mechanism for antipsychotic effects are unknown	
Side Effects Sedation, extrapyramidal symptoms, orthostatic hypotension, headache, photosensitivity, dry mouth and eyes, blurred vision	**Adverse Reactions** Tachycardia, seizures, urinary retention Life-threatening: Laryngospasm, respiratory depression, cardiac dysrhythmias, NMS, agranulocytosis

A, Adult; *b.i.d.,* twice a day; *C,* child; *CNS,* central nervous system; *d,* day; *h,* hour; *IM,* intramuscular; *min,* minute; *NMS,* neuroleptic malignant syndrome; *PB,* protein-binding; *PO,* by mouth; *PRN,* as needed; *t ½,* half-life; *t.i.d.,* three times a day; *UK,* unknown; *wk,* week; *y,* year; <, less than.

and constipation. Blood pressure decreases with the use of antipsychotics; aliphatics and piperidines cause a greater decrease in blood pressure than the others.

EPS can begin within 5 to 30 days after initiation of antipsychotic therapy and are most prevalent with the phenothiazines, butyrophenones, and thioxanthenes. These symptoms include pseudoparkinsonism, akathisia, **dystonia** (prolonged muscle contractions with twisting, repetitive movements), and tardive dyskinesia. Tardive dyskinesia may develop in 20% of patients taking antipsychotics for long-term therapy. Antiparkinsonian anticholinergic drugs may be given to control EPS, but they are not always effective in treating tardive dyskinesia.

High dosing or long-term use of some antipsychotics can cause **blood dyscrasias** (blood cell disorders) such as agranulocytosis. White blood cell (WBC) count should be closely monitored and reported to the health care provider if there is an extreme decrease in leukocytes.

Dermatologic side effects seen early in drug therapy are pruritus and marked photosensitivity. Patients are urged to use sunscreen, hats, and protective clothing and to stay out of the sun.

Drug Interactions

Because phenothiazine lowers the seizure threshold, dosage adjustment of an anticonvulsant may be necessary. If either aliphatic phenothiazine or the thioxanthene group is administered, a higher dose of anticonvulsant might be necessary to prevent seizures.

Antipsychotics interact with alcohol, hypnotics, sedatives, narcotics, and benzodiazepines to potentiate the sedative effects of antipsychotics. Atropine counteracts EPS and potentiates antipsychotic effects. Use of antihypertensives can cause an additive hypotensive effect.

Antipsychotics should *not* be given with other antipsychotic or antidepressant drugs except to control psychotic behavior for selected individuals who are refractory to drug therapy. Under ordinary circumstances, if one antipsychotic drug is ineffective, a different one is prescribed. Individuals should *not* take alcohol or other CNS depressants (e.g., narcotic analgesics, barbiturates) with antipsychotics, because additive depression is likely to occur.

When discontinuing antipsychotics, the drug dosage should be reduced gradually to avoid sudden recurrence of psychotic symptoms. Table 27-2 lists common antipsychotic

TABLE 27-2 PHENOTHIAZINES AND NONPHENOTHIAZINES

GENERIC (BRAND)	DRUG POTENCY	ROUTE AND DOSAGE	USES AND CONSIDERATIONS
Phenothiazines			
Aliphatics			
chlorpromazine HCl (Thorazine)	Low	A: PO: 25-100 mg t.i.d./q.i.d. A: IM/IV: 25-50 mg q4-6h C >6 mo: PO: 0.55 mg/kg q4-6h C >6 mo: IM/IV: 0.5-1 mg/kg q6-8h	For psychosis, schizophrenia, intractable hiccups, preoperative sedation, behavioral problems in children, nausea, and vomiting. Pregnancy category: C; PB: 95%; t½: 24 h
Piperazines			
fluphenazine HCl (Prolixin)	High	See Prototype Drug Chart 27-1.	
perphenazine (Trilafon)	Moderate	A: PO: 4-16 mg b.i.d./t.i.d./q.i.d.; *max:* 64 mg/d	For psychotic disorders; to control severe nausea and vomiting; to treat intractable hiccups. Used also before chemotherapy to prevent nausea. Pregnancy category: C; PB: 91%-97%; t½: 9-12 h
Piperidines			
thioridazine HCl (Mellaril)*	Low	A: PO: 50-100 mg t.i.d.; *max:* 300 mg/d Older adults: 10 mg t.i.d.; *max:* 300 mg/d C 2-12 y: PO: 0.5-3 mg/kg/d in 2-3 divided doses; *max:* 3 mg/kg/d	For psychosis only when unresponsive to other medications. Higher doses for severe psychosis. Lower doses (10-50 mg t.i.d.) for marked depression, alcohol withdrawal, intractable pain. Few EPS. Little antiemetic effect. Can cause life-threatening dysrhythmias. Pregnancy category: C; PB: 91%-99%; t½: 24-34 h
Nonphenothiazines			
Butyrophenone			
haloperidol (Haldol)	High	See Prototype Drug Chart 27-2.	
Dibenzoxazepine			
loxapine (Loxitane)	Moderate	A: PO: Initially 10-25 mg q12h; maintenance 60-100 mg/d in divided doses; *max:* 250 mg/d Older adults: 5-10 mg daily/b.i.d.; maintenance 40-50 mg/d; *max:* 250 mg/d	For acute psychosis and schizophrenia. Likely to cause EPS. Overdose can cause cardiac toxicity or neurotoxicity. Pregnancy category: C; PB: 95%; t½: 8 h
Dihydroindolone			
molindone HCl (Moban)	Moderate	A: PO: Initial: 50-75 mg in 3-4 divided doses, then 15-50 mg t.i.d./q.i.d.; *max:* 225 mg/d Older adults: ⅓-½ adult dose	Management of schizophrenia. Can cause EPS. Has less sedative effect. Pregnancy category: C; PB: UK; t½: 1.5 h
Thioxanthenes			
thiothixene HCl (Navane)	High	A: PO: 2 mg t.i.d.; *max:* 60 mg/d	Management of psychotic disorders, especially acute and chronic schizophrenia. Can cause EPS. Pregnancy category: C; PB: 90%; t½: 34 h
Atypical Antipsychotics			
clozapine (Clozaril)	Low	A: PO: Initially: 12.5 mg/d or b.i.d.; if tolerated, gradually increase to 300-450 mg/d in 3 divided doses; *max:* 900 mg/d	For severely ill schizophrenic patients, especially those who do not respond to other antipsychotics. With long-term use, monitor white blood cell count. Pregnancy category: B; PB: 95%; t½: 8-12 h

TABLE 27-2 PHENOTHIAZINES AND NONPHENOTHIAZINES—cont'd

GENERIC (BRAND)	DRUG POTENCY	ROUTE AND DOSAGE	USES AND CONSIDERATIONS
olanzapine (Zyprexa Zydis) Extended-release injectable (Zyprexa Relprevv)	UK	A: IM: 5-10 mg/d; *max:* 20 mg/d Older adults: PO: 5 mg q.d.; *max:* 20 mg/d A: IM: IR: 5-10 mg/d Older adults: IM: 2.5-5 mg/d A: IM: ER: 150-300 mg q2wk or 405 mg q4wk Older adults: IM: ER: 150 q4wk	Treatment of schizophrenia. Does not cause EPS. May cause headaches, dizziness, excess weight gain, agitation, insomnia, and somnolence. Pregnancy category: C; PB: 93%; t½: 21-54 h
quetiapine (Seroquel)	UK	A: PO: Initially 25 mg/b.i.d.; increase 25-50 mg b.i.d./t.i.d. first week up to 300-400 mg/d in 2-3 divided doses; *max:* 800 mg/d Older adults: PO: 25 mg b.i.d.; increase q.d.; *max:* 400 mg/d A: XR: 300 mg h.s.; *max:* 800 mg/d Older adults: XR: 50 mg/d, increase 50 mg/d; *max:* 200-800 mg/d	Treatment of schizophrenia, bipolar disorder, and major depression. Not likely to cause EPS. May cause dizziness, headache, sedation. Pregnancy category: C; PB: 83%; t½: 6 h
asenapine (Saphris)	UK	A: SL: 5-10 mg b.i.d.; *max:* 20 mg/d	For treatment of schizophrenia and manic bipolar disorder. Adverse effects include dizziness, appetite stimulation, dysrhythmias, and pseudoparkinsonism. Pregnancy category: C; PB: UK; t½: 24 h
risperidone (Risperdal)	Low	Psychosis: A: PO: Initially 2 mg/d, increase to 4-8 mg/d Older adults: PO: Initially 0.5-1.5 mg b.i.d.; *max:* 4 mg/d Adol: PO: Initially 0.5 mg q.d., increase up to 3 mg/d	For management of schizophrenia. May cause sedation, headaches, sexual dysfunction, hyperglycemia, EPS, and NMS. Pregnancy category: C; PB: 90%; t½: 24 h
ziprasidone (Geodon)	UK	A: PO: 20 mg b.i.d. may increase q2d; *max:* 160 mg/d A: IM: 10 mg q2h or 20 mg q4h; *max:* 40 mg/d	For management of schizophrenia. Pregnancy category: C; PB: 99%; t½: 7 h
iloperidone (Fanapt)	UK	A: PO: Initially 1 mg b.i.d., then 6-12 mg b.i.d.; *max:* 24 mg/d	For treatment of schizophrenia. Adverse effects include GI distress, blurred vision, confusion, dehydration, dysrhythmias, and pseudoparkinsonism. Pregnancy category: C; PB: 95%; t½: 18-33 h
aripiprazole (Abilify)	UK	See Prototype Drug Chart 27-3.	
paliperidone (Invega, Invega Sustenna)	UK	A: PO: 6-12 mg/d in the AM; *max:* 12 mg/d A: IM: ER: 39-234 mg/mo	Treatment of schizophrenia. Extended-release injectable is given once a month. Pregnancy category: C; PB: 74%; t½: 23 h

A, Adult; *b.i.d.*, twice a day; *C*, child; *d*, day; *EPS*, extrapyramidal symptoms; *ER*, extended-release; *h*, hour; *IM*, intramuscular; *IR*, immediate-release; *IV*, intravenous; *max*, maximum; *mo*, month; *NMS*, neuroleptic malignant syndrome; *PB*, protein-binding; *PO*, by mouth; *PR*, rectally; *q.i.d.*, four times a day; *t½*, half-life; *t.i.d.*, three times a day; *UK*, unknown; >, greater than; *SL*, sublingual; *XR*, extended release.
*Avoid spilling liquid on skin. Contact dermatitis could result.

drugs (phenothiazines and nonphenothiazines) and their dosages, uses, and considerations.

Antipsychotic Dosage for Older Adults

Older adults usually require smaller doses of antipsychotics—from 25% to 50% less than young and middle-aged adults. Regular to high doses of antipsychotics increase the risk of severe side effects. Dosage amounts need to be individualized according to the patient's age and physical status. In addition, dosage changes may be necessary during antipsychotic therapy. Antipsychotics have a black box warning that states: Increased mortality in elderly patients with dementia-related psychosis.

Atypical (Serotonin/Dopamine Antagonists) Antipsychotics

Atypical antipsychotics differ from typical/traditional antipsychotics in that the atypical agents are effective in treating both positive and negative symptoms of schizophrenia. The typical antipsychotics have not been effective in the treatment of negative symptoms. Two advantages of the atypical agents are that (1) they are effective in treating negative symptoms, and (2) they are not likely to cause EPS, including tardive dyskinesia. Atypical drugs available include clozapine, risperidone, olanzapine, ziprasidone, and aripiprazol. These agents have a greater affinity for blocking serotonin and dopaminergic D_4 receptors than primarily blocking the dopaminergic D_2 receptor responsible for mild and severe EPS. Weight gain, drowsiness, unsteady gait, headache, insomnia, depression, diabetes mellitus, and dyslipidemia are common side effects of atypical antipsychotics.

Clozapine (Clozaril) was the first atypical antipsychotic agent used to treat schizophrenia and other psychoses. It is not as likely to cause EPS, although they may occur. Tremors and occasional rigidity have been reported. Serious adverse reactions of clozapine are seizures and agranulocytosis, a decrease in the production of granulocytes that involves the body's immune defenses. Currently clozapine is only indicated for the treatment of severely ill schizophrenic patients who have not responded to traditional antipsychotic drugs. The WBC count needs to be closely monitored for leukopenia; if the WBC (leukocyte) level falls below 3000 mm^3, clozapine should be discontinued. Seizures have been reported in 3% of patients taking the drug. Dizziness, sedation, tachycardia, orthostatic hypotension, and constipation are common side effects.

Another atypical agent used to treat positive and negative symptoms of schizophrenia is risperidone (Risperdal). Its action is similar to that of clozapine, and the occurrence of EPS and tardive dyskinesia is low. It does not cause agranulocytosis. Paliperidone (Invega) is the major active metabolite of risperidone and is an extended-release tablet with once-a-day dosing. Paliperidone should be swallowed whole and not chewed, divided, or crushed. The most common adverse effects include EPS, insomnia, headache, and akathisia.

The atypical antipsychotic olanzapine (Zyprexa), like clozapine and risperidone, is effective for treating positive and negative symptoms of schizophrenia. It does not cause agranulocytosis.

Quetiapine (Seroquel), like all the other atypical antipsychotics, is less likely to cause EPS. Tardive dyskinesia for long-term use has not been determined.

For individuals with cardiac dysrhythmias, ziprasidone (Geodon) must be prescribed with caution, because its use may lead to prolonged Q-T interval; ECGs should be monitored. Ziprasidone is contraindicated in patients with a history of prolonged Q-T interval or with other concurrent drugs known to prolong Q-T interval. Patients taking quetiapine, clozapine, risperidone, olanzapine, ziprasidone, and aripiprazole should be monitored for hyperglycemia and other symptoms of diabetes mellitus.

Prototype Drug Chart 27-3 illustrates drug characteristics of aripiprazole (Abilify), an atypical antipsychotic. When anxiety, hallucinations, agitation, mania, confusion, or depression and other symptoms are noted, the health care provider should check the medications that the patient is taking.

Nursing Process
Patient-Centered Collaborative Care

Phenothiazines and Nonphenothiazines

Assessment

- Assess baseline vital signs for use in future comparison.
- Obtain a health history from patient of present drug therapy. If patient is taking an anticonvulsant, drug dose might need to be increased, because antipsychotics tend to lower seizure threshold.
- Assess mental status, cardiac, eye, and respiratory disorders before start of drug therapy, and continue daily assessment.

Nursing Diagnoses

- Disturbed sleep pattern related to medication adverse effects
- Activity intolerance related to sedation
- Acute confusion related to psychosis
- Self-care deficit related to loss of motivation

Planning

- Patient's psychotic behavior will improve with medication(s) and psychotherapy.

Nursing Interventions

- Monitor vital signs. Orthostatic hypotension is likely to occur.
- Remain with patient while medication is taken and swallowed; some patients hide antipsychotics in the mouth to avoid taking them.
- Avoid skin contact with liquid concentrates to prevent contact dermatitis. Liquid must be protected from light and should be diluted with fruit juice.
- Administer oral doses with food or milk to decrease gastric irritation.
- Dilute oral solution of fluphenazine in fruit juice, water, or milk. Avoid apple juice and caffeinated drinks.
- Administer by IM route deep into muscle, because drug irritates fatty tissue. Do not administer intravenously.
- Check blood pressure for marked decrease or increase 30 minutes after drug is injected.
- Do *not* mix in same syringe with heparin, pentobarbital, cimetidine, or dimenhydrinate.
- Chill suppository in refrigerator for 30 minutes before removing foil wrapper.
- Observe for EPS: acute dystonia, akathisia, pseudoparkinsonism, and tardive dyskinesia (see Figure 27-1). Report these promptly to the health care provider.

PROTOTYPE DRUG CHART 27-3

Aripiprazole

Drug Class	Dosage
Nonphenothiazine: atypical antipsychotic Trade Name: Abilify Pregnancy Category: C	Psychosis: A: PO: 10-15 mg/d, may increase q2wk; *max:* 30 mg/d Adol: PO: 2 mg/d, may increase q2d; *max:* 30 mg/d
Contraindications	**Drug-Lab-Food Interactions**
Hypersensitivity, dehydration, alcohol intoxication, hypovolemia, agranulocytosis, neutropenia, leucopenia, heart failure, suicidal ideation, myocardial infarction, diabetes mellitus, hyperglycemia, hypotension, seizures, parkinsonism	Drug: Antidiabetic agents decrease Abilify drug levels and increase risk of hyperglycemia; alpha blockers and antihypertensives increase risk of hypotension; other antipsychotics enhance risk of NMS, EPS, tardive dyskinesia, anticholinergic effects, hypotension, and seizures; CNS depressants may increase sedation and orthostatic hypotension; SSRIs may increase risk of serotonin syndrome; calcium channel blockers may increase blood levels Food: Grapefruit juice may increase blood levels Herbal: St. John's wort may decrease blood levels Lab: Increased blood glucose
Pharmacokinetics	**Pharmacodynamics**
Absorption: Well absorbed, not affected by food Distribution: PB: 99% Metabolism: $t\frac{1}{2}$: 75 h Excretion: In urine and feces	PO: Onset: UK Peak: 3-5 h Duration: 24 h IM: Onset: 1-3 h Peak: UK Duration: 24 h
Therapeutic Effects/Uses	
To manage symptoms of psychosis, including schizophrenia Mode of Action: Interferes with the binding of dopamine to dopamine (D_2) and serotonin 5-hydroxytryptamine (5-HT_2) receptors	
Side Effects	**Adverse Reactions**
Sedation, drowsiness, weight gain, weight loss, headaches, fatigue, blurred vision, photosensitivity, alopecia, peripheral edema, amenorrhea, hyperglycemia, hypoglycemia, insomnia, anxiety, agitation, dizziness, constipation, nausea, vomiting, arthralgia, dizziness, sexual dysfunction	Orthostatic hypotension, hypertension, tachycardia, bradycardia, EPS, dysrhythmias, seizures, angina, angioedema, diabetes mellitus Life-threatening: Suicidal ideation, NMS, agranulocytosis, neutropenia, leukopenia

A, Adult; *adol,* adolescent; *b.i.d.,* twice a day; *C,* child; *CNS,* central nervous system; *d,* day; *EPS,* extrapyramidal symptoms; *h,* hour; *IM,* intramuscular; *min,* minute; *NMS,* neuroleptic malignant syndrome; *PB,* protein-binding; *PO,* by mouth; *PRN,* as needed; *$t\frac{1}{2}$,* half-life; *t.i.d.,* three times a day; *UK,* unknown; *wk,* week; *y,* year; <, less than.

- Assess for symptoms of NMS: increased fever, pulse, and blood pressure; muscle rigidity; increased creatine phosphokinase and WBC count; altered mental status; acute renal failure; varying levels of consciousness; pallor; diaphoresis; tachycardia; and dysrhythmias.
- Record urine output as urinary retention may result.
- Monitor serum glucose level.

Patient Teaching

General

- Encourage patient to take the drug exactly as ordered. In schizophrenia and other psychotic disorders, antipsychotics do not cure the mental illness but do alleviate symptoms. Many patients on medication can function outside of the institution setting. Adherence to drug regimen is extremely important.
- Inform patient that medication may take 6 weeks or longer to achieve full clinical effect.
- Caution patient not to consume alcohol or other CNS depressants such as narcotics; these drugs intensify the depressant effect on the body.
- Recommend patient not to abruptly discontinue the drug. Seek advice from health care provider before making any changes in dosage.
- Encourage patient to read labels on OTC preparations. Some are contraindicated when taking antipsychotics.
- Teach smoking cessation, because smoking increases metabolism of some antipsychotics.
- Guide patient to maintain good oral hygiene by frequently brushing and flossing teeth.
- Encourage patient to talk with health care provider regarding family planning. The effect of antipsychotics on the fetus is not fully known; however, there may be teratogenic effects.

- Explain to the breastfeeding patient that phenothiazine passes into breast milk, possibly causing drowsiness and unusual muscle movement in the infant.
- Warn patient about importance of routine follow-up examinations.
- Encourage patient to obtain laboratory tests on schedule. WBCs are monitored for 3 months, especially during the start of drug therapy. Leukopenia, or decreased WBCs, may occur. Be alert to symptoms of malaise, fever, and sore throat, which may be an indication of agranulocytosis, a serious blood dyscrasia.
- Teach patient to report symptoms of infection promptly to the health care provider, especially when patient is taking clozapine.
- Advise patient to wear an identification bracelet indicating the medication taken.
- Inform patient that tolerance to sedative effect develops over a period of days or weeks.

Side Effects

- Direct patient to avoid potentially dangerous situations, such as driving, until drug dosing has been stabilized.
- Inform patient about EPS; instruct patient to promptly report symptoms to health care provider.
- Encourage patient to wear sunglasses for photosensitivity, to limit exposure to direct sunlight, and to use sunscreen and protective clothing to prevent a skin rash.
- Warn patient about orthostatic hypotension and possible dizziness.
- Teach patient who is taking aliphatic phenothiazines such as chlorpromazine that the urine might be pink or red-brown; this discoloration is harmless.
- Inform patient that changes may occur related to sexual functioning and menstruating. Women could have irregular menstrual periods or amenorrhea, and men might experience impotence and gynecomastia (enlargement of breast tissue).
- Suggest lozenges or hard candy if mouth dryness occurs. Advise patient to consult health care provider if dry mouth persists for more than 2 weeks.
- Encourage patient to avoid extremes in environmental temperatures and exercise.
- Advise patient to rise slowly from sitting or lying to standing to prevent a sudden decrease in blood pressure.

Cultural Considerations

- Recognize that some cultural groups may have difficulty in accepting the patient's disorder and need for medication.

Evaluation

- Evaluate the effectiveness of the drug and whether the patient has acceptably reduced psychotic symptoms at the *lowest* dose possible.
- Ascertain whether patient can cope with everyday living situations and attend to activities of daily living.
- Determine if any side effects of or adverse reactions to the drug have occurred.

SAFETY: Preventing Medication Errors

Do not confuse ...

- **Seroquel** with **Serzone** (an antidepressant) or **sertindole** (Serlect)

ANXIOLYTICS

Anxiolytics, or *antianxiety drugs,* are primarily used to treat anxiety and insomnia. The major anxiolytic group is benzodiazepines (a minor tranquilizer group). Long before benzodiazepines were prescribed for anxiety and insomnia, barbiturates were used. Benzodiazepines are considered more effective than barbiturates, because they enhance the action of gamma-aminobutyric acid (GABA), an inhibitory neurotransmitter within the CNS. Benzodiazepines have fewer side effects and may be less dangerous in overdosing. Long-term use of barbiturates causes drug tolerance and dependence and may cause respiratory distress. Currently barbiturates are not drugs of choice for treating anxiety. Benzodiazepine-like drugs are used to treat insomnia. Selective serotonin reuptake inhibitors, serotonin norepinephrine reuptake inhibitors, tricyclic antidepressants, and monamine oxidase inhibitors are used to treat various anxiety disorders. These drugs are discussed in Chapter 28.

Table 27-3 lists approved uses for benzodiazepines. Drugs used to treat insomnia, including benzodiazepines, are discussed in Chapter 21.

A certain amount of anxiety may make one more alert and energetic, but when anxiety is excessive, it can be disabling, and anxiolytics may be prescribed. The action of anxiolytics resembles that of the sedative-hypnotics but *not* that of the antipsychotics.

There are two types of anxiety—primary and secondary. *Primary anxiety* is not caused by a medical condition or by drug use; *secondary anxiety* is related to selected drug use or medical or psychiatric disorders. Anxiolytics are not usually given for secondary anxiety unless the medical problem is untreatable, severe, and causes disability. In this case, an anxiolytic could be given for a short period to alleviate any acute anxiety attacks. These agents treat the symptoms but do not cure them. Long-term use of anxiolytics is discouraged, because tolerance develops within weeks or months, depending on the agent. Drug tolerance can occur in less than 2 to 3 months in patients who take phenobarbital.

Nonpharmacologic Measures

Some of the symptoms of a severe attack of anxiety, or panic attack, include dyspnea (difficulty in breathing), choking sensation, chest pain, heart palpitations, dizziness, faintness, sweating, trembling and shaking, and fear of losing control.

TABLE 27-3 APPROVED USES FOR BENZODIAZEPINES

PRESCRIBED USES	DRUGS
Anxiety	alprazolam (Xanax) chlordiazepoxide (Librium) chlorazepate (Tranxene) diazepam (Valium) lorazepam (Ativan)
Anxiety associated with depression	alprazolam (Xanax) clonazepam (Klonopin) lorazepam (Ativan)
Insomnia: short-term use	estazolam (Prosom) flurazepam (Somnol) quazepam (Doral) temazepam (Restoril) triazolam (Halcion)
Seizures and status epilepticus	clonazepam (Klonopin) clorazepate (Tranxene) diazepam (Valium)—status epilepticus lorazepam (Ativan)—status epilepticus
Alcohol withdrawal	clorazepate (Tranxene) chlordiazepoxide (Librium) diazepam (Valium) lorazepam (Ativan)
Skeletal muscle spasms	diazepam (Valium)
Preoperative medications	chlordiazepoxide (Librium) diazepam (Valium) lorazepam (Ativan) midazolam (Versed)

Before giving anxiolytics, nonpharmacologic measures should be used for decreasing anxiety. These measures might include using a relaxation technique, psychotherapy, or support groups.

Benzodiazepines

Benzodiazepines have multiple uses as anticonvulsants, sedative-hypnotics, preoperative drugs, substance abuse withdrawal agents, and anxiolytics. Most of the benzodiazepines are used mainly for severe or prolonged anxiety. Examples include chlordiazepoxide (Librium), diazepam (Valium), clorazepate dipotassium (Tranxene), lorazepam (Ativan), and alprazolam (Xanax). The most frequently prescribed benzodiazepine is lorazepam. Many of the benzodiazepines are used for more than one purpose.

Benzodiazepines are lipid-soluble and are absorbed readily from the GI tract. They are highly protein-bound (80% to 98%). Benzodiazepines are primarily metabolized by the liver and excreted in urine, so the drug dosage for patients with liver or renal disease should be lowered accordingly to avoid possible cumulative effects. Traces of benzodiazepine metabolites could be present in the urine for weeks or months after the person has stopped taking the drug. These are controlled substance schedule IV (CSS IV) drugs.

The first benzodiazepine, chlordiazepoxide, became widely used for its sedative effect in 1962. Diazepam was the most frequently prescribed drug in the early 1970s. Lorazepam is the prototype drug of benzodiazepine and is described in Prototype Drug Chart 27-4.

HERBAL ALERT 27-2

Benzodiazepines

Kava kava should not be combined with benzodiazepines, because it increases the sedative effect.

Pharmacokinetics Lorazepam is highly lipid-soluble, and the drug is rapidly absorbed from the GI tract. The drug is highly protein-bound, and the half-life is 10 to 20 hours. Lorazepam is excreted primarily in the urine.

Pharmacodynamics Lorazepam acts on the limbic, thalamic, and hypothalamic levels of the CNS. The onset of action is 15 to 30 minutes by mouth and 1 to 5 minutes by IV. The serum levels of most oral doses of benzodiazepines peak in 2 hours. Oxazepam levels peak in 3 hours. Duration of action varies. The average is 2 to 3 hours when given orally; when given IV, the longest duration of action is 1 hour.

It is recommended that benzodiazepines be prescribed for no longer than 3 to 4 months. Beyond 4 months, the effectiveness of the drug lessens. Table 27-4 lists the anxiolytics and their dosages, uses, and considerations.

Miscellaneous Anxiolytics

The anxiolytic buspirone hydrochloride (BuSpar) binds to serotonin and dopamine receptors. It may not be effective until 1 to 2 weeks after continuous use. It has fewer side effects of sedation and physical and psychological dependency associated with many benzodiazepines. The most common side effects of buspirone include drowsiness, dizziness, headache, nausea, nervousness, and excitement. Note: Buspirone has an interaction with grapefruit juice that can lead to toxicity. To avoid this interaction, buspirone users should be advised to limit intake of grapefruit juice to 8 ounces daily or half of a grapefruit.

Nursing Process
Patient-Centered Collaborative Care

Benzodiazepines

Assessment
- Assess for suicidal ideation.
- Obtain a history of patient's anxiety reaction.
- Determine patient's support system (family, friends, groups), if any.
- Obtain patient's drug history. Report possible drug-drug interaction.

Nursing Diagnoses
- Anxiety related to situational crisis
- Impaired physical mobility related to drowsiness and weakness

PROTOTYPE DRUG CHART 27-4

Lorazepam

Drug Class Anxiolytic: benzodiazepine Trade Name: Ativan Pregnancy Category: D	**Dosage** Anxiety: A: PO: 2-6 mg/d; *max:* 10 mg/d Older adults: PO: 1-2 mg/d; *max:* 10 mg/d
Contraindications Hypersensitivity, CNS depression, shock, coma, narrow-angle glaucoma, seizures, alcohol intoxication, liver impairment, pregnancy, lactation Caution: Hepatic or renal dysfunction, suicidal ideation	**Drug-Lab-Food Interactions** Drug: Increases CNS depression when taken with alcohol, CNS depressants, and anticonvulsants; cimetidine increases lorazepam plasma levels, increases phenytoin levels, decreases levodopa effects; smoking decreases antianxiety effects
Pharmacokinetics Absorption: Rapid from GI tract Distribution: PB: 91% Metabolism: $t\frac{1}{2}$: 12-14 h Excretion: In urine	**Pharmacodynamics** PO: Onset: UK Peak: 2 h Duration: 12-24 h IM: Onset: 15-30 min Peak: 60-90 min Duration: UK IV: Onset: 1-5 min Peak: UK Duration: UK
Therapeutic Effects/Uses To control anxiety and to treat status epilepticus; for preoperative sedation; for substance withdrawal Mode of Action: Potentiate gamma-aminobutyric (GABA) effects by binding to specific benzodiazepine receptors and inhibiting GABA neurotransmission	
Side Effects Drowsiness, dizziness, weakness, confusion, blurred vision, nausea, vomiting, anorexia, restlessness, hallucinations, anterograde amnesia, sleep-related behaviors	**Adverse Reactions** Hypertension, hypotension, bradycardia, respiratory depression

A, Adult; *C,* child; *CNS,* central nervous system; *d,* day; *GI,* gastrointestinal; *h,* hour; *IM,* intramuscular; *IV,* intravenous; *max,* maximum; *min,* minute; *PB,* protein-binding; *PO,* by mouth; $t\frac{1}{2}$, half-life; *UK,* unknown.

Planning

- Patient's anxiety and stress will be reduced through nonpharmacologic methods, anxiolytic drugs, or support/group therapy.

Nursing Interventions

- Observe patient for side effects of anxiolytics. Recognize that drug tolerance and physical and psychological dependency can occur with most anxiolytics.
- Recognize that anxiolytic dosages should be lower for older adults, children, and debilitated persons than for middle-aged adults.
- Monitor vital signs, especially blood pressure and pulse; orthostatic hypotension may occur.
- Encourage family to be supportive of patient.

Patient Teaching

General

- Advise patient not to drive a motor vehicle or operate dangerous equipment when taking anxiolytics, because sedation is a common side effect.
- Warn patient not to consume alcohol or CNS depressants such as narcotics while taking an anxiolytic.
- Teach patient ways to control excess stress and anxiety (relaxation techniques, long walks).
- Inform patient that effective response may take 1 to 2 weeks.
- Encourage patient to follow drug regimen and not to abruptly stop taking the drug after prolonged use because withdrawal symptoms can occur. Drug dose is usually tapered when drug is discontinued.

Side Effects

- Encourage patient to rise slowly from sitting to standing position to avoid dizziness from orthostatic hypotension.

Cultural Considerations

- Use simple and clear instructions, modifying methods and materials to meet patient and family needs. Ask family members to assist with translation only if an

TABLE 27-4 **ANXIOLYTICS**

GENERIC (BRAND)	ROUTE AND DOSAGE	USES AND CONSIDERATIONS
Benzodiazepines		
alprazolam (Xanax) CSS IV	IR tablet, Orally disintegrating form: A: PO: 0.25-0.5 mg t.i.d.; *max:* 4 mg/d Older adults: 0.125-0.25 mg b.i.d.; *max:* 4 mg/d ER tablet: A: PO: 0.5-1 mg q.d. in morning Older adults: 0.5 mg/d; *max:* 10 mg/d	Management of anxiety and panic disorders and anxiety associated with depression. Side effects include drowsiness, dry mouth, and lightheadedness. Pregnancy category: D; PB: 90%; t½: 11-16 h
chlordiazepoxide HCl (Librium) CSS IV	Anxiety disorders: A: PO: 5-10 mg t.i.d./q.i.d. C: PO: 5 mg b.i.d./q.i.d. Acute alcohol withdrawal: A: PO: 50-100 mg q4h until agitation controlled; *max:* 300 mg/d	Effective for alcohol withdrawal syndrome (DTs), anxiety, and tension. Dose should be less for the older adult. Pregnancy category: D; PB: 96%; t½: 5-30 h
clorazepate dipotassium (Tranxene) CSS IV	A: PO: 15-60 mg/d in divided doses; *max:* 60 mg/d Older adults: 7.5-15 mg/d in divided doses; *max:* 60 mg/d	For anxiety, alcohol withdrawal syndrome, and partial seizures. Avoid taking alcohol or CNS depressants with clorazepate. Drowsiness and dizziness may occur. Pregnancy category: D; PB: 98%; t½: 40-50 h
diazepam (Valium) CSS IV	Anxiety, muscle spasm, and alcohol withdrawal: A: PO: 2-10 mg b.i.d./q.i.d. Older adults: PO: 2-2.5 mg q.d./b.i.d. C <6 mo: PO: 1-2.5 mg b.i.d./t.i.d. A: IM/IV: 2-5 mg; repeat in 3-4 h PRN Preoperative sedation: A: IV: 5-15 mg 15 min before procedure	Management of anxiety, muscle spasms, alcohol withdrawal, status epilepticus, and preoperative sedation. Pregnancy category: D; PB: 99%; t½: 25-50 h
lorazepam (Ativan) CSS IV	See Prototype Drug Chart 27-4.	
oxazepam (Serax) CSS IV	A: PO: 10-30 mg t.i.d./q.i.d; *max:* 120 mg/d Older adults: PO: 10 mg t.i.d.; *max:* 60 mg/d	For anxiety and acute alcohol withdrawal. Pregnancy category: D; PB: 85%-95%; t½: 5-15 h
Azapirones		
buspirone HCl (BuSpar)	A: PO: Initial: 7.5 mg b.i.d.; then 15-30 mg/d in divided doses; *max:* 60 mg/d Older adults: PO: 5 mg b.i.d.; then 15-30 mg/d in divided doses; *max:* 60 mg/d	For anxiety and anxiety-related depression. Takes several weeks before anxiolytic effects occur. Common side effects include drowsiness, dizziness, headache, and nausea. Pregnancy category: B; PB: 86%; t½: 2-4 h
Benzodiazepine Antagonists		
flumazenil (Romazicon)	A: IV: 0.2 mg over 15-30 sec; repeat 0.2 mg at 1-min intervals; *max:* 3 mg/h	Used to partially or completely reverse benzodiazepine dose from sedation, anesthesia, and overdose. Should not be used with antipsychotics or antidepressants. Pregnancy category: C; PB: 50%; t½: 40-80 min

A, Adult; *b.i.d.,* twice a day; *C,* child; *CNS,* central nervous system; *CSS,* Controlled Substances Schedule; *d,* day; *ER,* extended-release; *h,* hour; *IM,* intramuscular; *IR,* immediate-release; *IV,* intravenous; *max,* maximum; *min,* minute; *PB,* protein-binding; *PO,* by mouth; *q.i.d.,* four times a day; *t½,* half-life; *t.i.d.,* three times a day; *UK,* unknown.

interpreter is not available, and do not ask private questions in public.

Evaluation

- Evaluate the effectiveness of drug therapy by determining if patient is less anxious and more able to cope with stresses and anxieties.
- Determine if patient is taking the anxiolytic drug as prescribed and adhering to patient teaching instructions.

Side Effects and Adverse Reactions

The side effects associated with benzodiazepines are sedation, dizziness, headaches, dry mouth, blurred vision, rare urinary incontinence, and constipation. Adverse reactions include leukopenia (decreased WBC count) with symptoms of fever, malaise, and sore throat; tolerance to the drug dosage with continuous use; and physical dependency. Box 27-2 lists guidelines for treating benzodiazepine overdose.

Benzodiazepines should not be abruptly discontinued, because withdrawal symptoms are likely to occur. Withdrawal

BOX 27-2 SUGGESTED TREATMENT FOR OVERDOSE OF BENZODIAZEPINES

1. Administer an emetic, and follow with activated charcoal if the patient is conscious; use gastric lavage if the patient is unconscious.
2. Administer the benzodiazepine antagonist flumazenil (Romazicon) IV if required.
3. Maintain an airway, give oxygen as needed for decreased respirations, and monitor vital signs.
4. Give IV vasopressors for severe hypotension.
5. Request a mental health consultation for the patient.

IV, intravenous.

symptoms caused by short-term benzodiazepine use are similar to those from the sedative-hypnotics (agitation, nervousness, insomnia, tremor, anorexia, muscular cramps, sweating). However, they are slow to develop, taking 2 to 10 days, and can last several weeks, depending on the benzodiazepine's half-life. When discontinuing a benzodiazepine, the drug dosage should be gradually decreased over a period of days, depending on dose or length of time on the drug. Withdrawal symptoms from long-term, high-dose benzodiazepine therapy include paranoia, delirium, panic, hypertension, and status epilepticus. Convulsions during withdrawal may be prevented with simultaneous substitution of an anticonvulsant. Alcohol and other CNS depressants should *not* be taken with benzodiazepines, because respiratory depression could result. Tobacco, caffeine, and sympathomimetics decrease the effectiveness of benzodiazepines. Benzodiazepines are contraindicated during pregnancy because of possible teratogenic effects.

KEY WEBSITES

Information on risperidone: *http://psyweb.com/drughtm/jsp/risper.jsp*

Information on lorazepam: *www.drugs.com/lorazepam.html*

CRITICAL THINKING CASE STUDY

FS, a 35-year-old woman, is receiving risperidone, 3 mg b.i.d., to control a psychotic disorder. She has taken the drug for 6 months but has recently become agitated and is complaining of insomnia.

1. What is the relation between FS's drug dose and her complaints? Explain your answer.
2. What further assessment should be made concerning FS and the drug regimen?
3. How does risperidone compare with other antipsychotics such as chlorpromazine, fluphenazine, olanzapine, and haloperidol regarding actions and adverse effects?

NCLEX STUDY QUESTIONS

1. The nurse suspects that a patient who is experiencing facial grimacing, involuntary upward eye movement, and muscle spasms of the tongue and face may have which condition?
   a. Akathisia
   b. Acute dystonia
   c. Tardive dyskinesia
   d. Pseudoparkinsonism
2. A patient asks the nurse to explain how antipsychotic drugs work to make him feel better. The nurse understands that antipsychotics act in which way?
   a. Blocking actions of dopamine
   b. Blocking actions of epinephrine
   c. Promoting prostaglandin synthesis
   d. Enhancing the action of gamma-aminobutyric acid
3. An antipsychotic agent, fluphenazine (Prolixin), is ordered for a patient with psychosis. The nurse understands that this agent can lead to extrapyramidal symptoms that may be treated with which medication?
   a. quetiapine (Seroquel)
   b. aripiprazole (Abilify)
   c. benztropine (Cogentin)
   d. chlorpromazine (Thorazine)
4. An atypical antipsychotic is prescribed for a patient with psychosis. The nurse understands that this category of medications includes which drugs? (Select all that apply.)
   a. clozapine (Clozaril)
   b. fluphenazine (Prolixin)
   c. haloperidol (Haldol)
   d. olanzapine (Zyprexa)
   e. aripiprazole (Abilify)
5. A patient is prescribed lorazepam (Ativan). What does the nurse know to be true regarding lorazepam?
   a. It may cause anterograde amnesia and sleep-related behaviors.
   b. It has a maximum adult dose of 25 mg/day.
   c. When combined with cimetidine, it causes plasma levels to be decreased.
   d. It interferes with the binding of dopamine receptors.

6. A patient is receiving aripiprazole (Abilify). Which nursing intervention(s) will the nurse include in the patient's care plan? (Select all that apply.)
   a. Administer before meals on an empty stomach to facilitate absorption.
   b. Remain with the patient until medication is swallowed.
   c. Monitor vital signs to detect orthostatic hypotension.
   d. Assess the patient for evidence of neuroleptic malignant syndrome.
   e. Observe the patient for acute dystonia, akathisia, and tardive dyskinesia.
7. A patient appears to have had an overdose of phenothiazines. The nurse anticipates that which intervention(s) may be used to treat phenothiazine overdose? (Select all that apply.)
   a. Gastric lavage
   b. Adequate hydration
   c. Maintaining an airway
   d. Fluphenazine (Prolixin)
   e. Risperidone (Risperdal)
   f. Activated charcoal administration

Answers: 1, b; 2, a; 3, c; 4, a, d, e; 5, a; 6, b, c, d, e; 7, a, b, c, f.

CHAPTER

28

Antidepressants and Mood Stabilizers

evolve WEBSITE

http://evolve.elsevier.com/KeeHayes/pharmacology/

- Animations
- Content Updates
- Key Points
- Review Questions for the NCLEX® Examination
- References from the Textbook
- Unfolding Case Studies

OBJECTIVES

- Contrast the various categories of different antidepressants, giving an example of one drug for each category.
- Describe the side effects and adverse reactions of antidepressants.
- Plan nursing interventions, including patient teaching, for antidepressants (tricyclic antidepressants, monoamine oxidase inhibitors, selective serotonin reuptake inhibitors, selective norepinephrine reuptake inhibitors, and atypical antidepressants).
- Explain the uses of lithium and its serum/plasma therapeutic ranges, side effects and adverse reactions, and nursing interventions.
- Apply the nursing process to the patient taking lithium, carbamazepine, and valproic acid.

OUTLINE

KEY TERMS

Antidepressants are used for depressive episodes that are accompanied by feelings of hopelessness and helplessness. They can be prescribed for 1 month to 12 months or perhaps longer.

Mood-stabilizer agents such as lithium are effective for bipolar affective disorder. Drug therapy for treating bipolar disorder is discussed in this chapter.

DEPRESSION

Depression is the most common psychiatric problem, affecting approximately 10% to 20% of the population. Only 33% of depressed persons receive medical or psychiatric help. Women between the ages of 25 and 45 years are two to three times more likely to experience major depression than men. Depression is characterized primarily by mood changes and loss of interest in normal activities. It is second only to hypertension as the most common chronic clinical condition.

Contributing causes of depression include genetic predisposition, social and environmental factors, and biologic conditions. Some signs of major depression include loss of interest in most activities, depressed mood, weight loss or gain, insomnia or hypersomnia, loss of energy, fatigue, feelings of despair, decreased ability to think or concentrate, and suicidal thoughts. Approximately 66% of all suicides are related to depression. Depressed men, especially older white men, are more likely to commit suicide successfully than depressed women. Antidepressants can mask suicidal tendencies.

The three types of depression are (1) *reactive,* (2) *major,* and (3) *bipolar affective disorder* (previously referred to as *manic depression*). **Reactive depression** usually has a sudden onset after a precipitating event (e.g., depression resulting from a loss, such as death of a loved one). The patient knows why he or she is depressed and may call this "the blues." Usually this type of depression lasts for months. A benzodiazepine agent may be prescribed. *Major depression* is characterized by loss of interest in work and home, inability to complete tasks, and deep depression **(dysphoria).** Major depression can be either primary (i.e., not related to other health problems) or secondary to a health problem (e.g., physical or psychiatric disorder or drug use). Antidepressants have been effective in treating major depression. **Bipolar affective disorder** involves swings between two moods, the manic (euphoric) and the depressive (dysphoria). Lithium (Lithobid) was originally the drug of choice for treating this type of disorder. Other mood stabilizers, such as carbamazepine (Tegretol), valproic acid or divalproex (Depakote, Valproate), and lamotrigine (Lamictal) are also currently first-line drugs of choice for bipolar disorder.

Pathophysiology

There are many theories about the cause of major depression. A common one suggests an insufficient amount of brain monoamine neurotransmitters (norepinephrine, serotonin, perhaps dopamine). It is thought that decreased levels of serotonin permit depression to occur, and decreased levels of norepinephrine cause depression. However, there can be other physiologic causes of depression as well as social and environmental factors.

Herbal Supplements for Depression

St. John's wort and gingko biloba have been suggested for the management of mild depression. St. John's wort can decrease reuptake of the neurotransmitters serotonin, norepinephrine, and dopamine. The use of these and many herbal products should be discontinued 1 to 2 weeks before surgery. The patient should check with the health care provider regarding herbal treatments (Herbal Alert 28-1).

HERBAL ALERT 28-1

Selective Serotonin Reuptake Inhibitors

- Feverfew may interfere with SSRI antidepressants such as fluoxetine (Prozac).
- St. John's wort interacts with SSRIs, which may cause serotonin syndrome (dizziness, headache, sweating, and agitation).

ANTIDEPRESSANT AGENTS

Antidepressants are divided into five groups: (1) **tricyclic antidepressants** (TCAs), or tricyclics; (2) **selective serotonin reuptake inhibitors** (SSRIs); (3) **serotonin norepinephrine reuptake inhibitors** (SNRIs); (4) **atypical antidepressants** that affect various neurotransmitters; and (5) **monoamine oxidase inhibitors** (MAOIs). TCAs and MAOIs were marketed in the late 1950s, and many of the SSRIs and atypical antidepressants were available in the 1980s. The SSRIs and SNRIs are popular antidepressants because they do not cause sedation, hypotension, anticholinergic effects, or cardiotoxicity as do many of the TCAs. Users of SSRIs can experience sexual dysfunction, which can be managed. With unpleasant side effects or lack of improvement, the patient is usually changed to another category.

Tricyclic Antidepressants

TCAs are used to treat major depression because they are effective and less expensive than SSRIs and other drugs. Imipramine was the first TCA marketed in the 1950s.

The action of TCAs is to block the uptake of the neurotransmitters norepinephrine and serotonin in the brain. The clinical response of TCAs occurs after 2 to 4 weeks of drug therapy. If there is no improvement after 2 to 4 weeks, the antidepressant is slowly withdrawn and another antidepressant is prescribed. *Polydrug therapy,* the practice of giving several antidepressants or antipsychotics together, should be avoided if possible because of potential serious side effects.

The effectiveness of TCAs in treating major depression is well documented. This group of drugs elevates mood, increases interest in daily living and activity, and decreases insomnia. For agitated depressed persons, amitriptyline (Elavil), doxepin (Silenor), or trimipramine (Surmontil) may be prescribed, because of their highly sedative effect. Frequently TCAs are given at night to minimize problems caused by their sedative action. When discontinuing TCAs, the drugs should be gradually decreased to avoid withdrawal symptoms such as nausea, vomiting, anxiety, and akathisia. Imipramine hydrochloride (Tofranil) is used for the treatment of enuresis (involuntary discharge of urine during sleep in children).

The TCA drugs include amitriptyline, imipramine, trimipramine, doxepin, desipramine, nortriptyline, and protriptyline. The TCA drugs desipramine and nortriptyline are major metabolites of imipramine and amitriptyline.

Pharmacokinetics Amitriptyline is strongly protein-bound. The half-life is 10 to 50 hours, and a cumulative drug effect may result. Amitriptyline is primarily excreted in urine.

Pharmacodynamics Amitriptyline is well absorbed, but antidepressant effects develop slowly over several weeks. The onset of the antidepressant effect of amitriptyline is 1 to 4 weeks, and the peak concentration is 2 to 12 hours. Drug doses are decreased for older patients to reduce side effects.

Side Effects and Adverse Reactions

The TCAs have many side effects: orthostatic hypotension, sedation, anticholinergic effects, cardiotoxicity, and seizures. Rising from a sitting position too rapidly can cause dizziness and lightheadedness, so the patient should be instructed to rise slowly to an upright position to avoid *orthostatic hypotension.* This group of antidepressants blocks the histamine receptors; thus, sedation is likely to occur initially but decreases with continuous use of the drug. Because TCAs block the cholinergic receptors, they can cause anticholinergic effects such as tachycardia, urinary retention, constipation, dry mouth, and blurred vision. Other side effects of TCAs include allergic reactions (skin rash, pruritus, and petechiae) and sexual dysfunction (impotence and amenorrhea). Most TCAs can cause blood dyscrasias (leukopenia, thrombocytopenia, and agranulocytosis) requiring close monitoring of blood cell counts. Amitriptyline may lead to extrapyramidal symptoms (EPS). Clomipramine may cause neuroleptic malignant syndrome (NMS). Seizure threshold is decreased by TCAs; therefore, patients with seizure disorders may need to have the TCA dose adjusted. The most serious adverse reaction to TCAs is cardiotoxicity, such as dysrhythmias that may result from high doses of the drug. The therapeutic serum range is 100 to 200 ng/mL.

Drug Interactions

Alcohol, hypnotics, sedatives, and barbiturates potentiate central nervous system (CNS) depression when taken with TCAs. Concurrent use of MAOIs with amitriptyline may lead to cardiovascular instability and toxic psychosis. Antithyroid medications taken with amitriptyline may increase the risk of dysrhythmias.

Selective Serotonin Reuptake Inhibitors

SSRIs block the reuptake of serotonin into the nerve terminal of the CNS, thereby enhancing its transmission at the serotonergic synapse. These drugs do not block the uptake of dopamine or norepinephrine, and they do not block cholinergic and alpha$_1$-adrenergic receptors. SSRIs are more commonly used to treat depression than are TCAs. They have fewer side effects than TCAs.

The primary use of SSRIs is for major depressive disorders. They are also effective for treating anxiety disorders such as obsessive-compulsive disorder, panic, phobias, posttraumatic stress disorder, and other forms of anxiety. Fluvoxamine (Luvox) is useful for treating obsessive-compulsive disorder in children and adults. SSRIs have also been used to treat eating disorders and selected drug abuses. Miscellaneous uses for SSRIs include decreasing premenstrual tension syndrome, preventing migraine headaches, and preventing or minimizing aggressive behavior in patients with borderline personality disorder.

The SSRIs include fluoxetine (Prozac), fluvoxamine (Luvox), sertraline (Zoloft), paroxetine (Paxil), citalopram (Celexa), and escitalopram (Lexapro). Fluoxetine (Prozac) has been effective in 50% to 60% of patients who fail to respond to TCA therapy (TCA-refractory depression). Of all of the SSRIs, sertraline (Zoloft) is the most commonly prescribed antidepressant. The U.S. Food and Drug Administration (FDA) approved a weekly fluoxetine dose of 90 mg. However, before taking the weekly dose, the patient should respond to a daily maintenance dose of 20 mg/d without serious effects. It has been reported that there are some side effects to the weekly 90 mg fluoxetine dose.

Note: Many SSRIs have an interaction with grapefruit juice that can lead to possible toxicity. It is recommended that daily intake be limited to 8 ounces of grapefruit juice or one half of a grapefruit.

Prototype Drug Chart 28-1 describes the drug characteristics of the SSRI fluoxetine (Prozac). Table 28-1 lists the side effects of the various antidepressants.

Pharmacokinetics Fluoxetine is strongly protein-bound. The half-life is 2 to 3 days; therefore a cumulative drug effect may result from long-term use. Fluoxetine is metabolized and excreted by the kidneys.

Pharmacodynamics Fluoxetine is well absorbed; however, its antidepressant effect develops slowly over several weeks. The onset of fluoxetine's antidepressant effect is between 1 and 4 weeks, and peak concentration is at 6 to 8 hours after ingestion. The drug dose for older adults should be decreased to reduce side effects.

Side Effects and Adverse Reactions

Fluoxetine produces common side effects such as dry mouth, blurred vision, insomnia, headache, nervousness, anorexia, nausea, diarrhea, and suicidal ideation. Fluoxetine has fewer side effects than amitriptyline (see Table 28-1).

Some patients may experience sexual dysfunction when taking SSRIs. Men have discontinued taking fluoxetine (Prozac) after experiencing a decrease in sexual arousal. Some women have become anorgasmic when taking paroxetine HCl (Paxil). The side effects often decrease or cease over the 2- to 4-week period of waiting for the therapeutic effect to emerge.

Serotonin Norepinephrine Reuptake Inhibitors

Venlafaxine (Effexor) was the first SNRI approved for major depression in 1993. SNRIs inhibit the reuptake of serotonin and norepinephrine, increasing availability in the synapse. SNRIs are used for major depression. Other approved uses are for generalized anxiety disorder and social anxiety disorder. Other SNRIs include duloxetine (Cymbalta) and desvenlafaxine (Pristiq). The concurrent interaction of venlafaxine and St. John's wort may increase the risk of serotonin syndrome and neuroleptic malignant syndrome. Prototype Drug Chart 28-2 describes the drug characteristics of venlafaxine.

Pharmacokinetics Venlafaxine is well absorbed. The protein binding capacity of venlafaxine is 27%, and the half-life is 5 hours. It is mostly excreted in the urine.

PROTOTYPE DRUG CHART 28-1

Fluoxetine

Drug Class Antidepressant: selective serotonin reuptake inhibitor Trade Name: Prozac Pregnancy Category: C	**Dosage** A: PO: Initially 20 mg/d in AM; *max:* 80 mg/d C >7 y: PO: Initially 10 mg/d; *max:* 40 mg/d Therapeutic range: 90-300 ng/mL
Contraindications Hypersensitivity, acute myocardial infarction, taking MAOIs, dehydration, breastfeeding Caution: Severe depression with suicidal tendency, severe liver or kidney disease, glaucoma, seizure disorder, diabetes mellitus, underweight adult	**Drug-Lab-Food Interactions** Drug: Increase effects of CNS and respiratory depression, and hypotensive effect with alcohol and CNS depressants Herb: St. John's wort increases risk for serotonin syndrome Increase effect of hypoglycemics
Pharmacokinetics Absorption: PO: well absorbed Distribution: PB: 95% Metabolism: fluoxetine: $t\frac{1}{2}$: 4-6 d Excretion: Excreted primarily in urine	**Pharmacodynamics** PO: Onset: 2-4 wk Peak: 6-8 wk Duration: UK
Therapeutic Effects/Uses To treat depression with or without melancholia; bulimia disorder; obsessive-compulsive disorder; panic disorder; and premenstrual dysphoric disorder Mode of Action: Serotonin is increased in nerve cells because of blockage from nerve fibers.	
Side Effects Headache, nervousness, restlessness, insomnia, blurred vision, mydriasis, tremors, dry mouth, anorexia, nausea, diarrhea, weight loss, menstrual irregularities, sexual dysfunction	**Adverse Reactions** Seizures, hyponatremia, dehydration, bleeding, osteopenia, suicidal ideation

A, Adult; *CNS,* central nervous system; *d,* day; *ECG,* electrocardiogram; *GI,* gastrointestinal; *MAOI,* monoamine oxidase inhibitor; *max,* maximum; *PB,* protein-binding; *PO,* by mouth; $t\frac{1}{2}$, half-life; *UK,* unknown; *wk,* week.

Pharmacodynamics The onset and duration of venlafaxine are unknown. The peak action is 2 to 4 hours for immediate-release tablets and 5.5 to 9 hours for extended-release tablets.

Side Effects and Adverse Effects

Side effects for venlafaxine include drowsiness, dizziness, insomnia, headache, euphoria, amnesia, blurred vision, photosensitivity, and ejaculation dysfunction. Adverse effects of this drug are hyponatremia, bleeding, hypertension, angioedema, blood dyscrasias, suicidal ideation, and Stevens-Johnson syndrome.

Atypical Antidepressants

Atypical antidepressants, or *second-generation antidepressants,* became available in the 1980s and have been used for major depression, reactive depression, and anxiety. They affect one or two of the three neurotransmitters: serotonin, norepinephrine, and dopamine. One of the first atypical antidepressants marketed was amoxapine (Asendin); others are maprotiline, nefazodone, and trazodone.

Amoxapine and maprotiline are sometimes considered to be TCAs because of their pharmacologic similarities. Atypical antidepressants should not be taken with MAOIs and should not be used within 14 days after discontinuing MAOIs. Trazodone may have a potential drug interaction with ketoconazole, ritonavir, and indinavir that may lead to increased trazodone levels and adverse effects. Table 28-2 lists the antidepressants and how each affects the various neurotransmitters.

Monoamine Oxidase Inhibitors

Another group of antidepressants is the MAOIs. The enzyme monoamine oxidase (MAO) inactivates norepinephrine, dopamine, epinephrine, and serotonin. By inhibiting MAO, the levels of these neurotransmitters rise. In the body, there are two forms of MAO enzyme: MAO-A and MAO-B. These enzymes are found primarily in the liver and brain. MAO-A inactivates dopamine in the brain, whereas MAO-B inactivates norepinephrine and serotonin. The MAOIs are nonselective, inhibiting both MAO-A and MAO-B. Inhibition of MAO by MAOIs is thought to relieve the symptoms of depression. Four MAOIs are currently prescribed: tranylcypromine sulfate (Parnate), isocarboxazid (Marplan), selegiline HCl (Emsam, Eldepryl), and phenelzine sulfate (Nardil). These MAOIs are detailed in Table 28-2.

For the treatment of depression, MAOIs are as effective as TCAs, but because of adverse reactions such as the risk of hypertensive crisis resulting from food and drug interactions, only 1% of patients taking antidepressants take an MAOI. Currently, MAOIs are not the antidepressants of choice and are usually prescribed when the patient does not respond to TCAs or second-generation antidepressants. However, MAOIs

TABLE 28-1 SIDE EFFECTS OF ANTIDEPRESSANTS

ANTIDEPRESSANT CATEGORY	ANTICHOLINERGIC EFFECT	SEDATION	HYPOTENSION	GI DISTRESS	CARDIOTOXICITY	SEIZURES	INSOMNIA/ AGITATION
Tricyclic Antidepressants							
amitriptyline (Elavil)	++++	++++	+++	—	++++	+++	—
clomipramine (Anafranil)	++++	++++	++	—	++++	++	—
desipramine (Norpramin)	+	++	++	—	++	++	+
doxepin (Sinequan)	+++	++++	++	—	++	++	—
imipramine (Tofranil)	+++	+++	+++	+	++++	++	+
nortriptyline (Aventyl)	+	+++	+	—	+++	++	—
protriptyline (Vivactil)	+++	+	++	—	+++	++	+
trimipramine (Surmontil)	+++	++++	+++	—	++++	++	—
Selective Serotonin Reuptake Inhibitors							
citalopram (Celexa)	+	0	0	++	—	—	+
fluoxetine (Prozac)	—	+	—	+++	—	0/+	++
fluvoxamine (Luvox)	—	++	—	+++	—	—	++
paroxetine (Paxil)	—	+	—	+++	—	—	++
sertraline (Zoloft)	—	+	—	+++	—	—	++
Atypical (Heterocyclic) Antidepressants							
amoxapine (Asendin)	+++	++	+	—	+	+++	++
bupropion (Wellbutrin)	++	—	0/+	+	+	++++	++
trazodone (Desyrel)	—	+++	++	+	+	+	—
maprotiline (Ludiomil)	+++	+++	+	—	++	+++	—
venlafaxine (Effexor)	0	0	0	0	0/+	+	—
Monoamine oxidase inhibitors	—	+	++	+	—	—	++

—, No effect; +, mild effect; ++, moderate effect; +++, strong effect; ++++, severe effect; *0*, no data available.

PROTOTYPE DRUG CHART 28-2

Venlafaxine

Drug Class Antidepressant: serotonin and norepinephrine reuptake inhibitor Trade name: Effexor Pregnancy Category: C	**Dosage** Immediate-release: A: PO: 75 mg/d in 2-3 divided doses; *max:* 225 mg/d in 3 divided doses Extended-release: A: PO: Initially 75 mg once daily or 37.5 once daily for 4-7 days to allow patient to adjust, then increase to 75 mg/d; *max:* 225 mg/d Therapeutic serum range: 100-200 ng/mL
Contraindications Hypersensitivity, taking MAOIs, CNS depression, SIADH, anticoagulant therapy, pregnancy, breastfeeding, children Caution: Suicidal tendency, kidney dysfunction, narrow-angle glaucoma, seizures, underweight, hypovolemia, hyperthyroidism, recent MI, heart failure	**Drug-Lab-Food Interactions** Drug: Increase effects of CNS, respiratory depression, and hypotensive effect with alcohol and CNS depressants Hypertensive crisis and death may occur with MAOIs. Increase drug levels and toxicity with cimetidine, haloperidol Increase bleeding with anticoagulants, aspirin Increase risk of serotonin syndrome and neuroleptic malignant syndrome with other SNRIs, SSRIs, serotonin receptor agonists (triptans), and amphetamines Herb: St. John's wort may cause serotonin syndrome (potentially life-threatening state with tachycardia, hypertension, confusion, twitching, hyperreflexia, hyperthermia)
Pharmacokinetics Absorption: PO: Well absorbed Distribution: PB: 27% Metabolism: $t\frac{1}{2}$: 5 h Excretion: Excreted primarily in urine	**Pharmacodynamics** Immediate-release: PO: Onset: UK Peak: 2-4 h Duration: UK Extended-release: PO: UK Peak: 5.5-9 h Duration: UK
Therapeutic Effects/Uses To treat depression with or without melancholia; generalized anxiety disorder; social anxiety disorder; panic disorder; and posttraumatic stress disorder Mode of Action: Serotonin and norepinephrine are increased in nerve cells because of blockage from nerve fibers.	
Side Effects Drowsiness, dizziness, nervousness, insomnia, headache, euphoria, confusion, amnesia, blurred vision, cataracts, mydriasis, dry mouth and eyes, gingivitis, hirsutism, alopecia, sweating, photosensitivity, urinary retention, constipation, diarrhea, weight loss, nausea, anorexia, increased intraocular pressure, ejaculation dysfunction	**Adverse Reactions** Bradycardia, tachycardia, hyponatremia, bleeding, hypertension, serotonin syndrome, neuroleptic malignant syndrome, angioedema Life-threatening: Agranulocytosis, thrombocytopenia, leukopenia, seizures, suicidal ideation, myocardial infarction, heart failure, Stevens-Johnson syndrome

A, Adult; *b.i.d.,* twice a day; *C,* child; *CNS,* central nervous system; *d,* day; *ECG,* electrocardiogram; *h,* hour; *IM,* intramuscular; *MAOI,* monoamine oxidase inhibitor; *PB,* protein-binding; *PO,* by mouth; *q.i.d.,* four times a day; SIADH, syndrome of inappropriate antidiuretic hormone secretion; $t\frac{1}{2}$, half-life; *t.i.d.,* three times a day; *UK,* unknown; *wk,* week; >, greater than.

are still used for mild, reactive, and atypical depression (chronic anxiety, hypersomnia, fear). MAOIs and TCAs should not be taken together when treating depression.

Drug and Food Interactions

Certain drug and food interactions with MAOIs can be fatal. Any drugs that are CNS stimulants or sympathomimetics (e.g., vasoconstrictors and cold medications containing phenylephrine and pseudoephedrine) can cause a hypertensive crisis when taken with an MAOI. In addition, foods that contain tyramine (cheese [cheddar, Swiss, bleu], cream, yogurt, coffee, chocolate, bananas, raisins, Italian green beans, liver, pickled foods, sausage, soy sauce, yeast, beer, and red wines) have sympathomimetic-like effects and can cause a hypertensive crisis. MAOI users *must avoid* these types of food and drugs. Frequent blood pressure monitoring is essential, and patient teaching regarding foods and over-the-counter (OTC) drugs to avoid is an important nursing responsibility. Because of the danger associated with hypertensive crisis, many psychiatrists will not prescribe MAOIs for depression unless other drugs have failed to be effective for the patient. However, this group of drugs is effective for treating depression if properly taken.

TABLE 28-2 ANTIDEPRESSANTS

GENERIC (BRAND)	ROUTE AND DOSAGE	USES AND CONSIDERATIONS
Tricyclic Antidepressants		
amitriptyline HCl (Elavil, Tryptanol)	A: PO: 25-75 mg/d; *max:* 300 mg/d for inpatients, 200 mg/d for outpatients Older adults: PO: 10-25 mg h.s.; *max:* 150 mg/d Therapeutic serum range: 100-200 ng/mL	For depression with or without melancholia. Common side effects include drowsiness, dizziness, orthostatic hypotension, dry mouth, constipation, and urinary retention. Pregnancy category: C; PB: 95%; $t\frac{1}{2}$: 10-50 h
clomipramine HCl (Anafranil)	A: PO: 25-100 mg/d; *max:* 250 mg/d; after titration, entire dose may be given at bedtime C >10 y: PO: initially 25 mg/d, then 3 mg/kg/d; *max:* 200 mg/d	For depression and obsessive-compulsive disorder. Given at bedtime to reduce daytime sedation. Common side effects include tremor, dizziness, weight gain, and dry mouth. Pregnancy category: C; PB: 97%; $t\frac{1}{2}$: 20-30 h
desipramine HCl (Norpramin)	A: PO: Initially 50-75 mg/d; increase to 200 mg/d for outpatients; *max:* 300 mg/d for inpatients Adol/Older adults: Initially 25 mg/d h.s.; increase to 100 mg/d in divided doses; *max:* 150 mg/d Therapeutic serum range: 150-250 ng/mL	For depression. Has been used for attention deficit/hyperactivity disorder (ADHD). Take with food if GI distress occurs. Common side effects include drowsiness, dry mouth, urinary retention, and postural hypotension. Pregnancy category: C; PB: 90%; $t\frac{1}{2}$: 12-60 h
doxepin HCl (Sinequan)	A: PO: Initially 75 mg/d h.s. or in 2-3 divided doses; *max:* 300 mg/d Older adults/PO: Initially 10-25 mg/d; *max:* 300 mg/d C >12 y: PO: Initially 25-50 mg/d; *max:* 100 mg/d Therapeutic serum range: 30-50 ng/mL	For depression and anxiety related to involutional depression or bipolar disorder. Has less effect on cardiac status than other drugs in this group. Pregnancy category: C; PB: 80%-85%; $t\frac{1}{2}$: 6-8 h
imipramine HCl (Tofranil)	A: PO: 75-200 mg/d; *max:* 200 mg/d for outpatients, 300 mg/d for inpatients Older adults: 25-100 mg/d; *max:* 200 mg/d for outpatients, 300 mg/d for inpatients Therapeutic serum range: 150-250 ng/mL	For depression. Can be taken at bedtime to lessen dangers from sedative effect. Take with food if GI distress occurs. Avoid taking with alcohol or CNS depressants. Common side effects include drowsiness, dry mouth, hypotension, delayed micturition. Pregnancy category: UK; PB: 85%-95%; $t\frac{1}{2}$: 8-15 h
nortriptyline HCl (Pamelor, Aventyl)	A: PO: Initially 25-50 mg t.i.d./q.i.d.; *max:* 150 mg/d Older adults: PO: Initially 10-25 mg/d h.s.; *max:* 150 mg/d Adol: PO: 1-3 mg/kg/d in 3-4 divided doses or h.s.; *max:* 150 mg/d Therapeutic serum range: 50-150 ng/mL	For depression. Similar to imipramine HCl. Pregnancy category: C; PB: 90%-95%; $t\frac{1}{2}$: 16-90 h
protriptyline HCl (Vivactil)	A: PO: Initially 5-10 mg t.i.d.; *max:* 60 mg/d Older adults: Initially 5 mg t.i.d.; *max:* 30 mg/d Therapeutic serum range: 70-250 ng/mL	For depression. Has little sedative effect. May increase suicidal ideation. Effects are similar to imipramine HCl. Pregnancy category: C; PB: 90%; $t\frac{1}{2}$: 60-98 h
trimipramine maleate (Surmontil)	A: Initially 75 mg/d in divided doses or h.s.; *max:* 200 mg/d for outpatients, 300 mg/d for inpatients Adol/older adults: Initially 50 mg/d in divided doses or h.s.; *max:* 100 mg/d	For depression. Similar to imipramine HCl. Pregnancy category: C; PB: 95%; $t\frac{1}{2}$: 20-26 h
Selective Serotonin Reuptake Inhibitors (SSRIs)		
citalopram (Celexa)	A: PO: 20-40 mg/d; *max:* 40 mg/d Older adults >60 y: PO: 20 mg/d; *max:* 20 mg/d	For depression, panic disorder, obsessive-compulsive disorder. Wait 14 days after stopping MAOIs. May cause sexual dysfunction, insomnia, nausea, and dry mouth. Pregnancy category: C; PB: 80%; $t\frac{1}{2}$: 35 h
fluoxetine HCl (Prozac)	See Prototype Drug Chart 28-1.	
paroxetine HCl (Paxil)	Depression: Regular-release tablets A: PO: Initially 20 mg/d; *max:* 50 mg/d Older adults: PO: Initially: 10 mg/d; *max:* 40 mg/d Controlled-release tablets A: PO: Initially 25 mg/d AM; *max:* 62.5 mg/d Older adults: PO: Initially 12.5 mg/d; *max:* 50 mg/d	For depression and obsessive-compulsive disorder. Lower dose for older adults and those with renal and hepatic disorders. Side effects include dizziness, insomnia, headache, nausea, dry mouth, tremors, and postural hypotension. Pregnancy category: D; PB: 95%; $t\frac{1}{2}$: 24 h
sertraline HCl (Zoloft)	A: PO: 50 mg/d; *max:* 200 mg/d	For major depressive disorders. Do not take with MAOIs or TCAs. Take with food if GI distress occurs. Urine may be pink-red-brown color. Pregnancy category: C; PB: 98%; $t\frac{1}{2}$: 24 h

TABLE 28-2 **ANTIDEPRESSANTS—cont'd**

GENERIC (BRAND)	ROUTE AND DOSAGE	USES AND CONSIDERATIONS
fluvoxamine (Luvox)	A: PO: 50-200 mg/d; *max:* 300 mg/d C >8 y: PO: 25 mg/d; *max:* 300 mg/d	For obsessive-compulsive disorder and social anxiety disorder. Caution: Do not use with renal or hepatic disorder. Pregnancy category: C; PB: 77%; t½: 15 h
escitalopram (Lexapro)	A: PO: 10 mg/d, may increase to 20 mg/d after 1 wk; *max:* 20 mg/d Older adults: PO: 10 mg/d; *max:* 10 mg/d for depression Adol: PO: 10 mg/d; *max:* 20 mg/d	For depression and generalized anxiety disorder. Pregnancy category: C; PB: 80%; t½: 25-35 h
vilazodone (Viibryd)	A: PO: 10 mg/d for 7 d; then 20 mg/d for 7 d; then 40 mg/d	For major depression. Common adverse effects include dizziness, insomnia, diarrhea, nausea, dry mouth, decreased libido. Pregnancy category: C; PB: 96%-97%; t½: 25 h
Atypical (Heterocyclic or Second-Generation) Antidepressants		
amoxapine (Asendin)	A: PO: 50 mg b.i.d./q.i.d.; *max:* 400 for outpatients, 600 for inpatients Older adults: PO: 25 mg b.i.d./q.i.d.; *max:* 300 mg/d	For depression with anxiety and for reactive depression. Do not take with MAOIs. Side effects include drowsiness, dizziness, EPS, postural hypotension, increased appetite, urinary retention. Pregnancy category: C; PB: >90%; t½: 8 h
maprotiline HCl (Ludiomil)	A: PO: 75 mg h.s. or in divided doses; *max:* 150-225 mg/d Older adults: 25 mg h.s.; *max:* 150-225 mg/d	Same as amoxapine. Can be taken at bedtime. Pregnancy category: B; PB: 88%; t½: 27-58 h
trazodone HCl (Desyrel)	A: PO: 150 mg/d in divided doses; *max:* 400 mg/d for outpatients, 600 mg/d for inpatients	For depression. Can be taken at bedtime to lessen dangers from sedative effect. Drowsiness, lightheadedness, postural hypotension, and dry mouth might occur. Take with food to decrease GI distress. Pregnancy category: C; PB: 85%-95%; t½: 5-10 h
Norepinephrine and Dopamine Reuptake Inhibitors (NDRIs)		
bupropion HCl (Wellbutrin)	A: PO: 75-100 mg b.i.d.; *max:* 300 mg/d	For depression, seasonal affective disorder, and nicotine withdrawal. May cause increased risk of seizures. Avoid with a history of seizures. Many side effects. Pregnancy category: B; PB: 84%; t½: 8-24 h
Miscellaneous Antidepressants		
mirtazapine (Remeron)	A: PO: Initially 15 mg h.s., then 15-30 mg/d; *max:* 45 mg/d Older adults: PO: Initially 7.5 mg h.s., then 15-30 mg/d; *max:* 45 mg/d	For depression, anxiety, and insomnia. Increases both norepinephrine and serotonin neurotransmitters. Has low anticholinergic activity. Pregnancy category: C; PB: 85%; t½: 20-40 h
Serotonin and Norepinephrine Reuptake Inhibitors		
desvenlafaxine (Pristiq)—extended-release tablet	A: Extended-release tablet PO: 50 mg/d; *max:* 400 mg/d	For depression, feelings of guilt and worthlessness, and anxiety. Decrease dose with renal and hepatic disorders and for anxiety. Does not cause cardiovascular problems or sedation. Pregnancy category: C; PB: 30%; t½: 11 h
duloxetine (Cymbalta)	A: PO: 40-60 mg/d in single or divided doses; *max:* 60 mg/d	For major depression, diabetic neuropathy, fibromyalgia, generalized affective disorder, musculoskeletal pain, and osteoarthritis. Wait 14 days after stopping MAOIs. Pregnancy category: C; PB: 90%; t½: 12 h
venlafaxine (Effexor)	See Prototype Drug Chart 28-2.	
Monoamine Oxidase Inhibitors (MAOIs)		
isocarboxazid (Marplan)	A: PO: 10-20 mg/d; *max:* 40 mg/d	For depression that is refractory to TCAs. Avoid certain foods such as cheese, sour cream, wine, beer, figs, anchovies, shrimp, bananas, and chocolate, and avoid drugs (e.g., TCAs). Pregnancy category: C; PB: UK; t½: 2.5 h
phenelzine sulfate (Nardil)	A: PO: 15 to 60 mg/d in divided doses; *max:* 90 mg/d	For depression. Avoid certain foods and drugs (see isocarboxazid). Pregnancy category: C; PB: UK; t½: 12 h
tranylcypromine sulfate (Parnate)	A: PO: 30 mg/d in 2 divided doses; *max:* 60 mg/d	For depression. Avoid certain foods and drugs (see isocarboxazid). Pregnancy category: C; PB: 90%; t½: 2.5 h

Continued

TABLE 28-2 ANTIDEPRESSANTS—cont'd

GENERIC (BRAND)	ROUTE AND DOSAGE	USES AND CONSIDERATIONS
selegiline HCl (Emsam, Eldepryl)	A: PO: Regular-release: 10 mg/d A: Orally disintegrating tablet: 2.5 mg/d A: Transdermal: 6 mg/d; *max:* 12 mg/d	For major depression. No dietary restrictions are necessary at low doses. Pregnancy category: C; PB: 85%-90%; t½: PO: 10 h; transdermal 2-20.5 h
Mood Stabilizers		
lithium citrate (Eskalith, Lithobid)	See Prototype Drug Chart 28-3.	
carbamazepine (Tegretol)	A: PO: 200 mg b.i.d.; increase to 200 mg/d as needed; *max:* 1600 mg/d Therapeutic serum level: 4-12 mcg/mL	For acute manic and mixed episodes associated with bipolar disorder. Contraindicated in bone marrow depression. Pregnancy category: D; PB: 76%; t½: 25-65 h
divalproex (Valproate, Depakote)	750 mg/d in divided doses b.i.d.; *max:* 3000 mg/d or 60 mg/kg/d	For major depression, bipolar disorder, mania, tonic-clonic seizures, and migraine prophylaxis. Pregnancy category: C; PB: 90%; t½ 6-16 h
lamotrigine (Lamictal)	25 mg/d for 2 weeks, then 50 mg/d for 2 weeks, then 100 mg/d for 3 weeks; thereafter give 200 mg/d	For major depression; partial seizures, and tonic-clonic seizures Pregnancy category: C; PB: 55%; t½ 25-30 h

A, Adult; *adol,* adolescent; *b.i.d.,* twice a day; *C,* child; *CNS,* central nervous system; *d,* day; *EPS,* extrapyramidal symptoms; *GI,* gastrointestinal; *h,* hour; *h.s.,* at bedtime; *IM,* intramuscular; *maint,* maintenance; *MAOIs,* monoamine oxidase inhibitors; *max,* maximum; *PB,* protein-binding; *PO,* by mouth; *q.i.d.,* four times a day; *t½,* half-life; *t.i.d.,* three times a day; *TCAs,* tricyclic antidepressants; *UK,* unknown; *y,* year; <, less than; >, greater than.

HERBAL ALERT 28-2

Monoamine Oxidase Inhibitors

- Ginseng, ephedra, ma-huang, and St. John's wort may lead to palpitations, heart attack, and hypertensive crisis when taken with antidepressant MAOIs.
- Ginseng may lead to manic episodes when taken in combination with MAOIs such as tranylcypromine sulfate.
- An excessive dose of anise may interfere with MAOIs.
- An increased use of brewer's yeast with MAOIs can increase blood pressure.

In teaching patients about the foods and drugs to avoid when taking MAOIs, some individuals respond better to verbal instructions and education with reinforcement from videos than to printed communications. Herbal Alert 28-2 details herb interactions with MAOIs.

Side Effects and Adverse Reactions

Side effects of MAOIs include CNS stimulation (agitation, restlessness, and insomnia), orthostatic hypotension, and anticholinergic effects.

Nursing Process

Patient-Centered Collaborative Care

Antidepressants

Assessment

- Assess patient's baseline vital signs and weight for future comparison. TCAs should be avoided in patients with cardiovascular disease and hypertension.
- Note patient's liver and renal function by assessing urine output (>1500 mL/d), blood urea nitrogen (BUN), and serum creatinine and liver enzyme levels.
- Obtain a health history of episodes of depression; assess mental status, and assess for suicidal tendencies.
- Secure a drug history of the current drugs, alcohol, and herbs patient is taking. CNS depressants can cause an additive effect. Antidepressants that cause anticholinergic-like symptoms are contraindicated if patient has glaucoma.
- Assess for tardive dyskinesia and neuroleptic malignant syndrome (NMS), including hyperpyrexia, muscle rigidity, tachycardia, and cardiac dysrhythmias.

Nursing Diagnoses

- Risk for self-directed violence and injury related to feelings of despair
- Anxiety related to situational crises
- Social isolation related to feelings of sadness
- Ineffective coping related to negative thought patterns
- Hopelessness related to feelings of despair
- Deficient knowledge related to inexperience with medication
- Ineffective health maintenance related to lack of interest

Planning

- Patient's depression or bipolar behavior will be decreased.

Nursing Interventions

- Observe patient for signs and symptoms of depression: mood changes, insomnia, apathy, or lack of interest in activities.

- Monitor patient's vital signs. Orthostatic hypotension is common. Check for anticholinergic-like symptoms: dry mouth, increased heart rate, urinary retention, or constipation. Check weight two to three times per week.
- Monitor patient for suicidal tendencies when marked depression is present.
- Observe patient for seizures when patient is taking an anticonvulsant; antidepressants lower the seizure threshold. The anticonvulsant dose might need to be increased.
- Monitor for drug-drug and food-drug interactions. Sympathomimetic-like drugs and foods containing tyramine may cause a hypertensive crisis if taken with MAOIs.
- Check patient for extremely high blood pressure when taking MAOIs.
- Provide patient with a list of foods to avoid when taking MAOIs to avoid hypertensive crisis. These foods include cheese, red wine, beer, liver, bananas, yogurt, and sausage.

Patient Teaching

General

- Teach patient to take the medication as prescribed. Compliance is important.
- Inform patient that full effectiveness of drug may not be evident until 1 to 2 weeks after start of therapy.
- Encourage patient to keep medical appointments.
- Caution patient not to consume alcohol or any CNS depressants because of their addictive effect.
- Inform patient that many herbal products interact with antidepressants, especially MAOIs and SSRIs. Herbs may need to be discontinued, or the antidepressant drug dosage may need to be modified (see Herbal Alerts 28-1 and 28-2).
- Warn patient not to drive or be involved in potentially dangerous mechanical activity until stabilization of drug dose has been established.
- Advise patient not to abruptly stop taking the drug. Drug dose should be gradually decreased by health care provider.
- Encourage patient who is planning pregnancy to consult with health care provider about possible teratogenic effects of the drug on the fetus.
- Take with food if gastrointestinal (GI) distress occurs.

Side Effects

- Advise patient that antidepressants may be taken at bedtime to decrease dangers from the sedative effect. Have patient check with health care provider. Transient side effects include nausea, drowsiness, headaches, and nervousness.

Cultural Considerations

- Explain to Asian patients taking an antipsychotic (such as TCA or lithium) that the dose may need to be decreased. Explain to Hispanic patients that the dose for the antidepressant may be lower than is required for other cultural groups.

Evaluation

- Evaluate the effectiveness of the drug therapy regarding whether patient's depression is controlled or has ceased.

MOOD STABILIZERS

Mood stabilizers are used to treat bipolar affective disorder. Lithium was the first drug used to manage this disorder. Some refer to lithium as an *antimania drug* that is effective in controlling manic behavior that arises from underlying bipolar disorder. Lithium has a calming effect but may cause some memory loss and confusion. It controls any evidence of flight of ideas and hyperactivity. If the person stops taking lithium, manic behavior may return. Lithium (Lithobid), carbamazepine (Tegretol), valproic acid or divalproex (Depakote, Valproate), and lamotrigine (Lamictal) are currently first-line drugs for bipolar disorder.

Lithium is an inexpensive drug that must be closely monitored. Lithium has a narrow therapeutic serum range: 0.5 to 1.5 mEq/L. Serum lithium levels greater than 1.5 to 2 mEq/L are toxic. The serum lithium level should be monitored biweekly until the therapeutic level has been obtained and then monitored monthly on the maintenance dose. Serum sodium levels also need to be monitored because lithium tends to deplete sodium. Lithium must be used with caution, if at all, by patients taking diuretics. Prototype Drug Chart 28-3 lists the pharmacologic behavior of lithium.

Pharmacokinetics More than 95% of lithium is absorbed through the GI tract. The average half-life of lithium is 24 hours; however, in older adults the half-life can be up to 36 hours. Because of its long half-life, cumulative drug action may result. Lithium is metabolized by the liver, and most of the drug is excreted unchanged in the urine.

Pharmacodynamics Lithium is prescribed mostly for the stabilization of bipolar affective disorder. The onset of action is fast, but the patient may not achieve the desired effect for 5 to 6 days. Increased sodium intake increases renal excretion, so the sodium intake needs to be closely monitored. Increased urine output can result in body fluid loss and dehydration. Adequate fluid intake of 1 to 2 L should be maintained daily.

Anticonvulsants, such as carbamazepine (Tegretol), lamotrigine (Lamictal), and divalproex/valproic acid (Depakote) have been used in place of lithium for some patients. These agents are further discussed in Chapter 22. The antipsychotic drugs olanzapine (Zyprexa), ziprasidone (Geodon), and aripiprazole (Abilify) are approved to treat acute mania and mixed episodes of bipolar disorder. Antipsychotic drugs are discussed further in Chapter 27.

Side Effects and Adverse Reactions

The many side effects of lithium—dry mouth, thirst, increased urination (loss of water and sodium), weight gain, bloated feeling, metallic taste, and edema of the hands and ankles—can be annoying to the patient. If taken during pregnancy, lithium may have teratogenic effects.

Lithium and nonsteroidal antiinflammatory drugs (NSAIDs) should *not* be given together on a continuous basis

PROTOTYPE DRUG CHART 28-3

Lithium

Drug Class Mood stabilizer Trade Names: Eskalith, Lithane, Lithonate, Lithobid, ✤ Carbolith, Lithizine Pregnancy Category: D	**Dosage** A: PO: initially 600 mg t.i.d.; maint: 300 mg t.i.d./q.i.d.; *max:* 2.4 g/d C: PO: 15 to 20 mg/kg/d in 3-4 divided doses Therapeutic drug range: 0.5-1.5 mEq/L
Contraindications Liver and renal disease, pregnancy, lactation, severe cardiovascular disease, severe dehydration, hyponatremia, children <12 y Caution: Thyroid disease, seizure disorder	**Drug-Lab-Food Interactions** Drug: May increase lithium level with thiazide diuretics, methyldopa, haloperidol, NSAIDs, antidepressants, carbamazepine, calcium channel blockers, spironolactone, ACE inhibitors, sodium bicarbonate, phenothiazines May increase lithium excretion with theophylline, aminophylline May increase risk of serotonin syndrome with SSRIs and SNRIs May increase hyperglycemia with antidiabetics Caffeine may decrease lithium levels Amphetamines may increase risk of mania Lab: Increase urine and blood glucose, protein; decrease serum sodium level Food: Increase sodium intake; lithium may cause sodium depletion Herbs: Use of St. John's wort, kava kava, and valerian may lead to neurotoxicity
Pharmacokinetics Absorption: PO: well absorbed Distribution: PB: UK Metabolism: t½: 21-30 h Excretion: 98% in urine, mostly unchanged	**Pharmacodynamics** PO: Onset: UK Peak: 2-4 h Duration: 24 h
Therapeutic Effects/Uses To treat bipolar psychosis, manic episodes Mode of Action: Alteration of ion transport in muscle and nerve cells; increased receptor sensitivity to serotonin	
Side Effects Headache, memory impairment, blurred vision, metallic taste, dental caries, lethargy, drowsiness, dizziness, tremors, slurred speech, dry mouth, anorexia, vomiting, diarrhea, polyuria, dehydration, hypotension, abdominal pain, muscle weakness, restlessness	**Adverse Reactions** Urinary and fecal incontinence, hyperglycemia, hyponatremia, proteinurea, polyurea, leukocytosis, nephrotoxicity Life-threatening: Cardiac dysrhythmias, seizures, cardiac arrest, serotonin syndrome, neuroleptic malignant syndrome

A, Adult; *C*, child; *d*, day; *h*, hour; *max*, maximum; *NSAIDs*, nonsteroidal antiinflammatory drugs; *PB*, protein-binding; *PO*, by mouth; *q.i.d.*, four times a day; *SR*, sustained-release; *t.i.d.*, three times a day; *t ½*, half-life; *UK*, unknown; <, less than; >, greater than; ✤, Canadian drug name.

and should not be prescribed for patients who have a cardiac "sick sinus syndrome." If the patient has taken lithium for a long period, laboratory tests to determine thyroid function should be closely monitored.

Nursing Process
Patient-Centered Collaborative Care

Mood Stabilizer: Lithium

Assessment

- Assess for suicidal ideation.
- Assess patient's baseline vital signs for future comparison.
- Evaluate patient's neurologic status, including gait, level of consciousness, reflexes, and tremors.
- Note patient's hepatic and renal function by assessing urine output (>600 mL/d) and whether BUN and serum creatinine and liver enzyme levels are within normal range. Assess for toxicity. Draw weekly blood levels initially and then every 1 to 2 months. Therapeutic serum levels for acute mania are 1 to 1.5 mEq/L; for maintenance, levels are 0.5 to 1.5 mEq/L. Signs and symptoms of toxicity at serum levels of 1.5 to 2 mEq/L are persistent nausea and vomiting, severe diarrhea, ataxia, blurred vision, and tinnitus. At 2 to 3.5 mEq/L, signs and symptoms of toxicity are excessive output of dilute urine, increasing tremors, muscular irritability, psychomotor retardation, mental confusion, and giddiness. At 3.5 mEq/L or higher, levels are life-threatening and may result in impaired consciousness, nystagmus, seizures, coma, oliguria/anuria, cardiac dysrhythmias, myocardial infarction, and cardiovascular collapse.

Withhold medication and notify health care provider immediately if any of these occur.
- Obtain a health history of episodes of depression or manic-depressive behavior.
- Obtain patient's drug history. Diuretics, NSAIDs (e.g., ibuprofen), tetracyclines, methyldopa, and probenecid decrease renal clearance of lithium, causing drug accumulation.

Nursing Diagnoses
- Risk for injury or violence related to impulsiveness
- Ineffective coping related to manic behavior
- Noncompliance related to lack of adequate education regarding lithium

Planning
- Patient's manic-depressive behavior will be decreased.

Nursing Interventions
- Observe patient for signs and symptoms of depression: mood changes, insomnia, apathy, or lack of interest in activities.
- Monitor patient's vital signs. Orthostatic hypotension is common.
- Draw blood samples for lithium levels immediately before the next dose (8 to 12 hours after the previous dose).
- Monitor for signs of lithium toxicity. Report high (greater than 1.5 mEq/L) and toxic (greater than 2.0 mEq/L) serum lithium levels immediately to health care provider.
- Monitor patient for suicidal tendencies when marked depression is present.
- Evaluate patient's urine output and body weight. Fluid volume deficit may occur as a result of polyuria.
- Observe patient for fine- and gross-motor tremors and presence of slurred speech, which are signs of adverse reaction.
- Check patient's cardiac status. Loss of fluids and electrolytes may cause cardiac dysrhythmias.
- Monitor patient's serum electrolytes. Report abnormal findings.

Patient Teaching
General
- Teach patient to take lithium as prescribed. Emphasize importance of adherence to the therapy, laboratory tests, and follow-up visits with health care provider. If lithium is stopped, manic symptoms will reappear.
- Encourage patient to keep medical appointments. Have patient check with health care provider before taking OTC preparations.
- Warn patient not to drive a motor vehicle or be involved in potentially dangerous mechanical activity until stable lithium level is established.
- Advise patient to maintain adequate fluid intake: 2 to 3 L/d initially and 1 to 2 L/d maintenance. Fluid intake should increase in hot weather.
- Teach patient to take lithium with meals to decrease gastric irritation.
- Inform patient that effectiveness of drug may not be evident until 1 to 2 weeks after the start of therapy. Compliance in taking the prescribed lithium doses on a daily basis is a major problem with bipolar patients. When patient has a period of emotional stability, he or she does not believe that the drug is needed; thus, patient stops taking the lithium.
- Advise patient who is planning pregnancy to consult with health care provider about possible teratogenic effects of the drug on the fetus, especially during the first 3 months.
- Encourage patient to wear or carry an identification tag or bracelet indicating the drug taken.

Diet
- Inform patient to avoid caffeine products (coffee, tea, cola), because they can aggravate the manic phase of bipolar disorder.
- Advise patient to maintain adequate sodium intake and to avoid crash diets that affect physical and mental health.

Side Effects
- Advise patient to contact health care provider if experiencing symptoms of toxicity. Early symptoms include diarrhea, drowsiness, loss of appetite, muscle weakness, nausea, vomiting, slurred speech, trembling. Late symptoms include blurred vision, confusion, increased urination, convulsions, severe trembling, and unsteadiness.

Cultural Considerations
- Obtain an interpreter when necessary; do not rely on family members, who may not fully disclose because of honor, shame, or lack of understanding of medical terminology.

Evaluation
- Evaluate the effectiveness of the drug therapy. Patient is free of bipolar behavior.
- Allow patient to verbalize understanding of symptoms of toxicity.
- Determine if patient demonstrates a subsiding or resolution of symptoms.

KEY WEBSITES

Information on antidepressants: *www.nlm.nih.gov/medlineplus/antidepressants.html*

Information on depression: *www.nlm.nih.gov/medlineplus/depression.html*

Information on sertraline (Zoloft): *www.rxlist.com/zoloft-drug.htm*

Information on St. John's wort for treatment of depression: *http://nccam.nih.gov/health/stjohnswort/index.htm*

CRITICAL THINKING CASE STUDY

ST, a 37-year-old woman, is receiving fluoxetine (Prozac) 20 mg in the evening for depression. ST complains of insomnia and GI upset.

1. What could you suggest to ST to help her avoid insomnia? Explain your answer.
2. How might ST avoid GI upset when taking fluoxetine?

ST states that she does not think the fluoxetine is helping. She states that she has heard about herbal supplements that may be taken for depression. She has also heard that fluoxetine can be taken weekly.

3. Is ST's fluoxetine dose within normal dosage range? Explain your answer.
4. How would you respond to ST about the use of certain herbal supplements for depression?
5. What would your response be concerning the use of fluoxetine in a weekly dose?

NCLEX STUDY QUESTIONS

1. A patient is admitted with bipolar affective disorder. The nurse acknowledges that which medication is used to treat this disorder for some patients in place of lithium?
   a. thiopental
   b. gingko biloba
   c. fluvoxamine (Luvox)
   d. divalproex (Depakote)
2. The nurse realizes that some herbs interact with selective serotonin reuptake inhibitors. Which herb interaction may cause serotonin syndrome?
   a. feverfew
   b. ma-huang
   c. St. John's wort
   d. gingko biloba
3. A selective serotonin reuptake inhibitor (SSRI) is prescribed for a patient. The nurse knows that which drug is an SSRI?
   a. paroxetine (Paxil)
   b. amitriptyline (Elavil)
   c. divalproex sodium (Depakote)
   d. bupropion HCl (Wellbutrin)
4. A patient is taking tranylcypromine sulfate (Parnate) for depression. What advice should the nurse include in the teaching plan for this medication?
   a. Warn the patient about severe hypotension.
   b. Instruct the patient to avoid beer and cheddar cheese.
   c. Encourage the patient to take ginseng and ephedra.
   d. Encourage the patient to eat fruit such as bananas.
5. Which statement is true concerning lithium?
   a. The maximum dose is 3.4 g/d.
   b. The therapeutic drug range is 2.5 to 3.5 mEq/L.
   c. Lithium increases receptor sensitivity to GABA.
   d. Concurrent NSAIDs may increase lithium levels.
6. When a patient is taking an antidepressant, what should the nurse do? (Select all that apply.)
   a. Monitor the patient for suicidal tendencies.
   b. Observe the patient for orthostatic hypotension.
   c. Teach the patient to take the drug with food if GI distress occurs.
   d. Tell the patient that the drug may not have full effectiveness for 1 to 2 weeks.
   e. Advise the patient to maintain adequate fluid intake of 2 L/d.
7. A patient is taking lithium. The nurse should be aware of the importance of which nursing intervention(s)? (Select all that apply.)
   a. Observe the patient for motor tremors.
   b. Monitor the patient for orthostatic hypotension.
   c. Draw lithium blood levels immediately after a dose.
   d. Advise the patient to drink 750 mL/d of fluid in hot weather.
   e. Advise the patient to avoid caffeinated foods and beverages.
   f. Teach the patient to take lithium with meals to decrease gastric irritation.

Answers: 1, d; 2, c; 3, a; 4, b; 5, d; 6, a, b, c, d; 7, a, b, e, f.

UNIT IX

Antibacterial and Antiinfective Agents

Disease-producing microorganisms may be gram-positive or gram-negative bacteria, viruses, or fungi. The degree to which they are pathogenic depends on the microorganism and its virulence. The cell walls of bacteria differ in their structure: bacilli are elongated, cocci are spherical, and spirilla are helical.

This unit discusses agents prescribed to combat disease-producing microorganisms. Included are antibacterials-antibiotics (penicillins, cephalosporins, macrolides, tetracyclines, aminoglycosides, fluoroquinolones) and sulfonamides.

Chapter 29 discusses penicillins and cephalosporins; Chapter 30 addresses macrolides, tetracyclines, aminoglycosides, and fluoroquinolones; and Chapter 31 focuses on the sulfonamides.

CHAPTER

29

Penicillins and Cephalosporins

evolve WEBSITE

http://evolve.elsevier.com/KeeHayes/pharmacology/

- Animations
- Content Updates
- Key Points
- Review Questions for the NCLEX® Examination
- References from the Textbook
- Unfolding Case Studies

OBJECTIVES

- Explain the mechanisms of action of antibacterial drugs.
- Differentiate between bacteria that are naturally resistant and those that have acquired resistance to an antibiotic.
- Summarize the three general adverse effects associated with antibacterial drugs.
- Differentiate between narrow-spectrum and broad-spectrum antibiotics.
- Compare the effects of the natural, broad-spectrum (extended), penicillinase-resistant, and antipseudomonal penicillins.
- Contrast the effects of first-, second-, third-, and fourth-generation cephalosporins.
- Apply the nursing process for patients receiving penicillins and cephalosporins.

OUTLINE

KEY TERMS

This chapter discusses the antibacterials and their effects, which include mechanisms of antibacterial action, body defenses, resistance to antibacterials, use of antibacterial combinations, general adverse reactions to antibacterials, and narrow- and broad-spectrum antibiotics. This chapter also discusses two antibacterials in detail: penicillin and cephalosporin.

PATHOPHYSIOLOGY

Bacteria, known as *prokaryotes,* are single-celled organisms lacking a true nucleus and nuclear membrane. Most bacteria have a rigid cell wall, and the structure of the cell wall determines the shape of the bacteria. One classification of bacteria involves the appearance or shape under a microscope. A *bacillus* is a rod-shaped organism. *Cocci* are spherical. When cocci appear in clusters, they are called *staphylococci;* when cocci are arranged in chains, they are called *streptococci.* Bacteria reproduce by cell division about every 20 minutes.

Another classification of bacteria involves staining properties of the cell. The Gram staining method was devised in 1882 by Hans Christian Gram, a Danish bacteriologist. Gram staining is determined by the ability of the bacterial cell wall to retain a purple stain by a basic dye. Crystal violet is normally used in the staining process but may be substituted with methylene blue. If bacteria retain a purple stain, they are classified as *gram-positive* microorganisms. Those bacteria not stained are known as *gram-negative* microorganisms. Examples of gram-positive bacteria include *Staphylococcus aureus, Streptococcus pneumoniae, Group B streptococcus,* and *Clostridium perfringens.* Examples of gram-negative bacteria include *Neisseria meningitides, Escherichia coli,* and *Haemophilus influenzae.*

Bacteria produce toxins that cause cell lysis (cell death). Many bacteria produce the enzyme beta-lactamase, which destroys beta-lactam antibiotics such as penicillins and cephalosporins.

ANTIBACTERIAL DRUGS

Antibacterials/Antibiotics

Although the terms *antibacterial, antimicrobial,* and *antibiotic* are frequently used interchangeably, there are some subtle differences in meaning. **Antibacterials** and **antimicrobials** are substances that inhibit bacterial growth or kill bacteria and other **microorganisms** (microscopic organisms including viruses, fungi, protozoa, and rickettsiae). Technically, the term *antibiotic* refers to chemicals produced by one kind of microorganism that inhibits the growth of or kills another. For practical purposes, however, these terms may be used interchangeably. Several drugs, including antiinfective and chemotherapeutic agents, have actions similar to those of antibacterial and antimicrobial agents. Antibacterial drugs do not act alone in destroying bacteria. Natural body defenses, surgical procedures to excise infected tissues, and dressing changes may be needed along with antibacterial drugs to eliminate the infecting bacteria.

Antibacterial drugs are either obtained from natural sources or manufactured. The use of moldy bread on wounds to fight infection dates back 3500 years. In 1928, a British bacteriologist named Alexander Fleming noted that "mold" was contaminating his bacterial cultures and inhibiting bacterial growth. The mold was called *Penicillium notatum;* thus Fleming called the substance *penicillin.* In 1939 Howard Florey expanded on Fleming's findings and purified the penicillin so it could be used commercially. Penicillin was used during World War II and marketed in 1945. Sulfonamide, a synthetic antibacterial, was introduced in 1935. Sulfonamides are discussed in greater detail in Chapter 31.

Bacteriostatic drugs inhibit the growth of bacteria, whereas **bactericidal** drugs kill bacteria. Some antibacterial drugs (tetracycline and sulfonamides) have a bacteriostatic effect, whereas other antibacterials (penicillins and cephalosporins) have a bactericidal effect. Depending on the drug dose and serum level, certain drugs can have both bacteriostatic and bactericidal effects.

For drugs with a narrow therapeutic index (e.g., aminoglycosides), peaks and troughs of serum antibiotic levels are monitored to determine if the drug is within the therapeutic range for its desired effect. If the serum *peak* level is too high, drug toxicity could occur. If the serum *trough* level (drawn minutes before administration of the next drug dose) is below the therapeutic range, the patient is not receiving an adequate antibiotic dose to kill the targeted microorganism.

Mechanisms of Antibacterial Action

Five mechanisms of antibacterial action are responsible for the inhibition of growth or destruction of microorganisms: (1) inhibition of bacterial cell-wall synthesis, (2) alteration of membrane permeability, (3) inhibition of protein synthesis, (4) inhibition of the synthesis of bacterial ribonucleic acid (RNA) and deoxyribonucleic acid (DNA), and (5) interference with metabolism within the cell (Table 29-1).

Pharmacokinetics Antibacterial drugs must not only penetrate the bacterial cell wall in sufficient concentration, but also must have an affinity (attraction) to the binding sites on the bacterial cell. The time the drug remains at the binding sites increases the effect of the antibacterial action. This time factor is controlled by the pharmacokinetics (distribution, half-life, and elimination) of the drug.

Antibacterials that have a longer half-life usually maintain a greater concentration at the binding site; therefore, frequent dosing is not required. Most antibacterials are not highly protein-bound, with a few exceptions (e.g., oxacillin, ceftriaxone, cefoperazone, cefprozil, cloxacillin, nafcillin, clindamycin). Protein binding does not have a major influence on the effectiveness of most antibacterial drugs. The steady state of the antibacterial drug occurs after the fourth to fifth half-lives, and the drug is eliminated from the body, mainly through urine, after the seventh half-life.

Pharmacodynamics The drug concentration at the site or the exposure time for the drug plays an important role in bacterial eradication. Antibacterial drugs are used to achieve the minimum effective concentration (MEC) necessary to halt the growth of a microorganism. Many antibacterials have a bactericidal effect against the pathogen when the drug concentration remains constantly above the MEC during the dosing interval. Duration of time for use of the antibacterial varies according to the type of pathogen, site of infection, and immunocompetence of the host. With some severe infections, a continuous infusion regimen is more effective than intermittent dosing because of constant drug concentration and time exposure. Once-daily antibacterial dosing (e.g., aminoglycosides, macrolides, fluoroquinolones) has been effective in eradicating pathogens and has not caused severe adverse reactions (ototoxicity, nephrotoxicity) in most cases. The ease of compliance with once- or twice-daily drug dosing also increases the patient's adherence to the drug regimen.

Figure 29-1 illustrates the effect of three methods of drug dosing. The drug dose is effective when it remains above the MEC.

Body Defenses

Body defenses and antibacterial drugs work together to stop the infectious process. The effect that antibacterial drugs have on an infection depends not only on the drug but also on the host's defense mechanisms. Factors such as age, nutrition, immunoglobulins, white blood cells (WBCs), organ function, and circulation influence the body's ability to fight infection.

TABLE 29-1 MECHANISMS OF ACTIONS OF ANTIBACTERIAL DRUGS

ACTION	EFFECT	DRUGS
Inhibition of cell wall synthesis	Bactericidal effect Enzyme breakdown of cell wall Inhibition of enzyme in synthesis of cell wall.	penicillin cephalosporins bacitracin vancomycin
Alteration in membrane permeability	Bacteriostatic or bactericidal effect Increases membrane permeability. Loss of cellular substances causes lysis of the cell.	amphotericin B nystatin polymyxin colistin
Inhibition of protein synthesis	Bacteriostatic or bactericidal effect Interferes with protein synthesis without affecting normal cell. Inhibits steps of protein synthesis.	aminoglycosides tetracyclines erythromycin lincomycin
Inhibition of synthesis of bacterial RNA and DNA	Inhibits synthesis of RNA and DNA in bacteria. Binds to nucleic acid and enzymes needed for nucleic acid synthesis.	fluoroquinolones
Interference with cellular metabolism	Bacteriostatic effect Interferes with steps of metabolism within cells.	sulfonamides trimethoprim isoniazid (INH) nalidixic acid rifampin

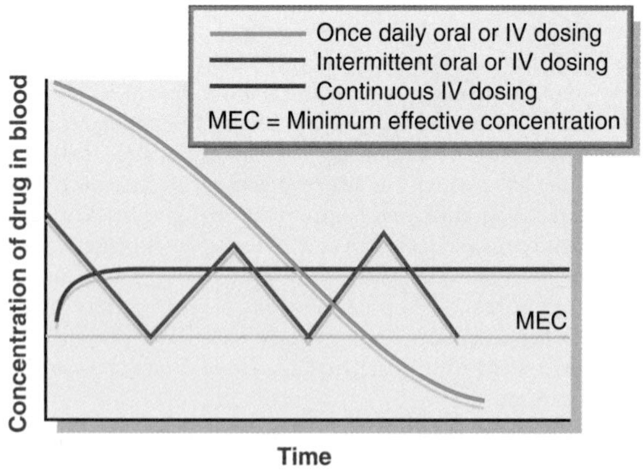

FIGURE 29–1 Effects of concentrated drug dosing.

Older adults and undernourished individuals have less resistance to infection than younger, well-nourished populations. If the host's natural body defense mechanisms are inadequate, drug therapy might not be as effective. As a result, drug therapy may need to be closely monitored or revised. When circulation is impeded, an antibacterial drug may not be distributed properly to the infected area. In addition, **immunoglobulins** (antibody proteins such as IgG and IgM) and other elements of the immune response system (WBCs) needed to combat infections may be depleted in individuals with poor nutritional status.

Resistance to Antibacterials

Bacteria may be sensitive or resistant to certain antibacterials. When bacteria are sensitive to a drug, the pathogen is inhibited or destroyed. If bacteria are resistant to an antibacterial, the pathogen continues to grow, despite administration of that antibacterial drug.

Bacterial resistance may result naturally (**inherent resistance**) or it may be acquired. A natural, or inherent, resistance occurs without previous exposure to the antibacterial drug. For example, the gram-negative (non–gram-staining) bacterium *Pseudomonas aeruginosa* is inherently resistant to penicillin G. An **acquired resistance** is caused by prior exposure to the antibacterial. Although *Staphylococcus aureus* was once sensitive to penicillin G, repeated exposures have caused this organism to evolve and become resistant to it. Penicillinase, an enzyme produced by the microorganism, is responsible for causing its penicillin resistance. Penicillinase metabolizes penicillin G, causing the drug to be ineffective. Penicillinase-resistant penicillins that are effective against *S. aureus* are available.

Antibiotic resistance is a major problem. In the early 1980s, pharmaceutical companies thought that enough antibiotics were on the market, so these companies concentrated on developing antiviral and antifungal drugs. As a result, fewer new antibiotics were developed during the 1980s. Now pharmaceutical companies have developed many new antibiotics, but antibiotic resistance continues to develop, especially when antibiotics are used frequently. As bacteria reproduce, some mutation occurs, and eventually the mutant bacteria survive the effects of the drug. One explanation is that the mutant bacteria strain may have grown a thicker cell wall.

In large health care institutions, there is a tendency toward drug resistance in bacteria. Mutant strains of organisms have developed, thus increasing their resistance to antibiotics that were once effective against them. Infections acquired while patients are hospitalized are called **nosocomial infections.** Many of these infections are caused by drug-resistant bacteria and can prolong hospitalization, which is costly to both the patient and third-party health care insurers.

Another problem related to antibiotic resistance is that bacteria can transfer their genetic instruction to another bacterial species. The other bacterial species becomes resistant to that antibiotic as well. Bacteria can pass along high resistance to a more virulent and aggressive bacterium (e.g., *S. aureus*, enterococci).

Methicillin (Staphcillin) was the first penicillinase-resistant penicillin developed in 1959 in response to a resistance of *S. aureus*. In 1968, strains of *S. aureus* were beginning to become resistant to methicillin. Highly resistant bacteria, known as methicillin-resistant *Staphylococcus aureus* (MRSA), became resistant not only to methicillin, but to all penicillins and cephalosporins as well. Resistance that was once found only in hospitals began to emerge in 1981 in the community as well. Methicillin is now off the market. The treatment of choice for MRSA is vancomycin (Vancocin). Other effective drugs used to treat MRSA include linezolid (Zyvox), daptomycin (Cubicin), trimethoprim/sulfamethoxazole (Bactrim), doxycycline (Vibramycin), and clindamycin (Cleocin). Telavancin (Vibativ), a glycopeptides antiinfective, was approved in September 2009 to treat gram-negative bacteria, including MRSA.

Many enterococcal strains are resistant to penicillin, ampicillin, gentamicin, streptomycin, and vancomycin. Another big resistance problem is vancomycin-resistant *Enterococcus faecium* (VREF), which can cause death in many persons with weakened immune systems. The incidence of VREF in hospitals has increased. A strain of MRSA has been reported to be resistant to vancomycin (vancomycin-resistant *Staphylococcus aureus,* or VRSA). Major medical problems result. One antibiotic after another is ineffective against new resistant strains of bacteria. As new drugs are developed, drug resistance will probably develop as well. Pharmaceutic companies and biotechnical firms are working on new classes of drugs to overcome the problem of bacterial resistance to antibiotics. A class of antibiotics, oxazolidinones, was discovered by a pharmaceutical company in 1988, but the company could not overcome toxicity problems in this class of drug. Another pharmaceutical company has taken the compound and made it less toxic. This antibiotic, linezolid, is effective against MRSA, VREF, and penicillin-resistant *Streptococci.* Quinupristin/dalfopristin (Synercid), which consists of two streptogramin antibacterials, is marketed in a combination of 30:70 for intravenous (IV) use against life-threatening infection caused by VREF and for treatment of bacteremia, *S. aureus,* and *Streptococcus pyogenes.*

Another way to attack antimicrobial resistance is to develop drugs that disable the antibiotic-resistant mechanism in the bacteria. Patients would take the antibiotic-resistance disabler along with the antibiotic already on the market, making the drug effective again. Developing a bacterial vaccine is another way to combat bacteria and lessen the need for antibiotics. The bacterial vaccine against pneumococcus has been effective in decreasing the occurrence of pneumonia and meningitis among various age groups.

Antibiotic misuse, a major problem today, increases antibiotic resistance. Studies reveal that 23% to 37.8% of patients in hospitals receive antibiotics and 50% of this population is receiving antibiotics inappropriately. When antibiotics are taken unnecessarily (e.g., for viral infections, when no infection is present) or incorrectly (e.g., skipping doses, not taking the full antibiotic regimen), one may develop resistance to antibacterials. Consumer education is important because many patients "demand" antibiotics for viral conditions. Antibiotics are ineffective against viruses. However, viral infections that persist could decrease the body's immune system, thus promoting a bacterial infection. The nurse should teach patients about the proper use of antibiotics to prevent situations that promote drug resistance to bacteria.

Cross-resistance can also occur between antibacterial drugs that have similar actions, such as the penicillins and cephalosporins. To ascertain the effect antibacterial drugs have on a specific microorganism, culture and sensitivity or antibiotic susceptibility laboratory testing is performed. A *culture and sensitivity* test (C&S) can detect the infective microorganism present in a sample (e.g., blood, sputum, swab) and what drug can kill it. The organism causing the infection is determined by culture, and the antibiotics the organism is sensitive to are determined by sensitivity. The susceptibility or resistance of one microorganism to several antibacterials can be determined by this method. Multiantibiotic therapy (daily use of several antibacterials) delays the development of microorganism resistance.

Use of Antibiotic Combinations

Combination antibiotics should not be routinely prescribed or administered except for specific uncontrollable infections. Usually a single antibiotic will successfully treat a bacterial infection. When there is a severe infection that persists and is of unknown origin or has been unsuccessfully treated with several single antibiotics, a combination of two or three antibiotics may be suggested. Before beginning antibiotic therapy, a culture or cultures should be taken to identify the bacteria.

When two antibiotics are combined, the result is additive, potentiative, or antagonistic. The *additive* effect is equal to the sum of the effects of two antibiotics. The *potentiative* effect occurs when one antibiotic potentiates the effect of the second antibiotic, increasing their effectiveness. The *antagonistic* result is a combination of a drug that is bactericidal, such as penicillin, and a drug that is bacteriostatic, such as tetracycline. When these two drugs are used together, the desired effect may be greatly reduced.

General Adverse Reactions to Antibacterials

Three major adverse reactions associated with the administration of antibacterial drugs are allergic (hypersensitivity) reactions, superinfection, and organ toxicity. Table 29-2 describes these adverse reactions, all of which require close monitoring of the patient.

Narrow-Spectrum and Broad-Spectrum Antibiotics

Antibacterial drugs are either narrow spectrum or broad spectrum. The **narrow-spectrum antibiotics** are primarily effective against one type of organism. For example, penicillin and erythromycin are used to treat infections caused by gram-positive bacteria. Certain **broad-spectrum antibiotics** (tetracycline and cephalosporins) can be effective against both gram-positive and gram-negative organisms. Because narrow-spectrum antibiotics are selective, they are more active against those single organisms than the broad-spectrum antibiotics. Broad-spectrum antibiotics are frequently used to treat infections when the offending microorganism has not been identified by C&S.

TABLE 29-2 GENERAL ADVERSE REACTIONS TO ANTIBACTERIAL DRUGS

TYPE	CONSIDERATIONS
Allergy or hypersensitivity	Allergic reactions to drugs may be mild or severe. Examples of mild reactions are rash, pruritus, and hives. An example of a severe response is anaphylactic shock. Anaphylaxis results in vascular collapse, laryngeal edema, bronchospasm, and cardiac arrest. Shortness of breath is frequently the first symptom of anaphylaxis. Severe allergic reaction generally occurs within 20 minutes. Mild allergic reaction is treated with an antihistamine; anaphylaxis requires treatment with epinephrine, bronchodilators, and antihistamines.
Superinfection	Superinfection is a secondary infection that occurs when the normal microbial flora of the body are disturbed during antibiotic therapy. Superinfections can occur in the mouth, respiratory tract, intestine, genitourinary tract, or skin. Fungal infections frequently result in superinfections, although bacterial organisms (e.g., *Proteus, Pseudomonas,* staphylococci) may be the offending microorganisms. Superinfections rarely develop when the drug is administered for less than 1 week. They occur more commonly with the use of broad-spectrum antibiotics. For fungal infection of the mouth, nystatin is frequently used.
Organ toxicity	The liver and kidneys are involved in drug metabolism and excretion. Antibacterials may result in damage to these organs. For example, aminoglycosides can be *nephrotoxic* (as well as ototoxic).

PENICILLINS AND CEPHALOSPORINS

Penicillins

Penicillin, a natural antibacterial agent obtained from the mold genus *Penicillium,* was introduced to the military during World War II and is considered to have saved many soldiers' lives. It became widely used in 1945 and was labeled a "miracle" drug. With the advent of penicillin, many patients survived who would have normally died from wound and severe respiratory infections.

Penicillin's beta-lactam structure (beta-lactam ring) interferes with bacterial cell-wall synthesis by inhibiting the bacterial enzyme that is necessary for cell division and cellular synthesis. The bacteria die of cell lysis (cell breakdown). The penicillins can be both bacteriostatic and bactericidal, depending on the drug and dosage. Penicillin G is primarily bactericidal.

Penicillins are mainly referred to as *beta-lactam antibiotics.* Bacteria can produce a variety of enzymes, such as beta-lactamases, that can inactivate penicillin and other beta-lactam antibiotics such as the cephalosporins. The beta-lactamases, which attack penicillins, are called *penicillinases.*

Penicillin G was the first penicillin administered orally and by injection. With oral administration, only about one third of the dose is absorbed. Because of its poor absorption, penicillin G given by injection (intramuscular [IM] and intravenous [IV]) is more effective in achieving a therapeutic serum penicillin level. Aqueous penicillin G has a short duration of action, and the IM injection is very painful, because it is an aqueous drug solution. As a result, a longer-acting form of penicillin, procaine penicillin (milky color), was produced to extend the activity of the drug. Procaine in the penicillin decreases the pain related to injection.

Penicillin V was the next type of penicillin produced. Although two thirds of the oral dose is absorbed by the gastrointestinal (GI) tract, it is a less potent antibacterial drug than penicillin G. Penicillin V is effective against mild to moderate infections, including anthrax as a biologic weapon of bioterrorism.

Initially penicillin was overused. It was first introduced for the treatment of staphylococcal infections, but after a few years mutant strains of *Staphylococcus* developed that were resistant to penicillins G and V because of the bacterial enzyme penicillinase, which destroys penicillin. This led to the development of new broad-spectrum antibiotics with structures similar to penicillin to combat infections resistant to penicillins G and V.

Food in the stomach does not significantly alter absorption of penicillin V, so it should be taken after meals. Amoxicillins are penicillins that are unaffected by food.

Broad-Spectrum Penicillins (Aminopenicillins)

Broad-spectrum penicillins are used to treat both gram-positive and gram-negative bacteria. They are not, however, as "broadly" effective against all microorganisms as they were once considered to be. This group of drugs is costlier than penicillin and therefore should not be used when ordinary penicillins, such as penicillin G, are effective. The broad-spectrum penicillins are effective against some gram-negative organisms: *Escherichia coli, Haemophilus influenzae, Shigella dysenteriae, Proteus mirabilis,* and *Salmonella.* However, these drugs are not penicillinase resistant. They are readily inactivated by beta-lactamases, thus ineffective against *S. aureus.* Examples of this group are ampicillin (Omnipen), and amoxicillin (Amoxil) (Table 29-3). Amoxicillin is the most prescribed penicillin derivative for adults and children.

Penicillinase-Resistant Penicillins (Antistaphylococcal Penicillins)

Penicillinase-resistant penicillins (antistaphylococcal penicillins) are used to treat penicillinase-producing *S. aureus.* Dicloxacillin is an oral preparation of these antibiotics; nafcillin and oxacillin are IM and IV preparations. This group of drugs is not effective against gram-negative organisms and is less effective than penicillin G against gram-positive organisms. Prototype Drug Chart 29-1 compares the similarities and differences in the broad-spectrum

PROTOTYPE DRUG CHART 29-1

Amoxicillin and Dicloxacillin

Drug Class	Dosage
amoxicillin: Broad-spectrum penicillin dicloxacillin: Penicillinase-resistant penicillin Trade Names: amoxicillin: Amoxil dicloxacillin: Dynapen Pregnancy Category: B	amoxicillin: A: PO: 250 q8h or 500 mg q12h C: PO: 20-40 mg/kg/d in 3 divided doses dicloxacillin: A: PO: 125-500 mg q6h C: PO: 12.5-25 mg/kg/d q6h
Contraindications	**Drug-Lab-Food Interactions**
amoxicillin/dicloxacillin: Allergic to penicillin, asthma, inflammatory bowel disease, pseudomembranous colitis, ulcerative colitis amoxicillin: mononucleosis Caution: amoxicillin/dicloxacillin: Hypersensitivity to cephalosporins amoxicillin: renal impairment	Drug: amoxicillin/dicloxacillin: Increase effect with aspirin, allopurinol, probenecid; increase bleeding with oral anticoagulants; increase effect of methotrexate; decrease effect with tetracycline, erythromycin Lab: Increase serum AST, ALT, BUN, and creatinine; increase PT, INR Food: Decrease effect with acidic fruits or juices
Pharmacokinetics	**Pharmacodynamics**
Absorption: PO: amoxicillin: >80% in GI tract dicloxacillin: 35%-76% in GI tract Distribution: PB: amoxicillin: 20% dicloxacillin: 95%-99% Metabolism: t½: amoxicillin: 1-1.5 h dicloxacillin: 0.5-1 h Excretion: amoxicillin: 70% in urine; clavulanate: 30%-40% in urine dicloxacillin: Excreted in bile and urine	amoxicillin: PO: Onset: 0.5 h Peak: 1-2 h Duration: 6-8 h dicloxacillin: PO: Onset: 0.5 h Peak: 1 h Duration: 4-6 h
Therapeutic Effects/Uses	
amoxicillin: To treat respiratory tract infection, urinary tract infection, otitis media, and sinusitis dicloxacillin: To treat *Staphylococcus aureus* infection Mode of Action: amoxicillin/dicloxacillin: Inhibition of the enzyme in cell wall synthesis; bactericidal effect	
Side Effects	**Adverse Reactions**
amoxicillin/dicloxacillin: Nausea, vomiting, diarrhea, rash, stomatitis, seizures, pseudomembranous colitis amoxicillin: Edema, insomnia, dysphagia dicloxacillin: Abdominal pain, flatulence	amoxicillin/dicloxacillin: Superinfections (vaginitis) Life-threatening: amoxicillin/dicloxacillin: Blood dyscrasias, thrombocytopenia, neutropenia, hemolytic anemia, bone marrow depression, Stevens-Johnson syndrome amoxicillin: Respiratory distress dicloxacillin: Eosinophilia, agranulocytosis, angioedema, liver toxicity

A, Adult; *ALT*, alanine aminotransferase; *AST*, aspartate aminotransferase; *BUN*, blood urea nitrogen; *C*, child; *d*, day; *GI*, gastrointestinal; *h*, hour; *PB*, protein-binding; *PO*, by mouth; *t ½*, half-life; >, greater than.

penicillin amoxicillin and the penicillinase-resistant penicillin dicloxacillin.

Extended-Spectrum Penicillins (Antipseudomonal Penicillins)

The antipseudomonal penicillins are a group of broad-spectrum penicillins. This group of drugs is effective against *Pseudomonas aeruginosa*, a gram-negative bacillus that is difficult to eradicate. These drugs are also useful against many gram-negative organisms such as *Proteus* spp., *Serratia* spp., *Klebsiella pneumoniae*, *Enterobacter* spp., and *Acinetobacter* spp. The antipseudomonal penicillins are not penicillinase-resistant. Their pharmacologic action is similar to that of aminoglycosides, but they are less toxic.

Table 29-3 lists the drugs in the four categories of penicillin-type antibacterials. The administration route of various types of penicillins (oral, IM, IV), along with the cephalosporins, are available on the Evolve website.

TABLE 29-3 **ANTIBACTERIALS: PENICILLINS**

GENERIC (BRAND)	ROUTE AND DOSAGE	USES AND CONSIDERATIONS
Basic Penicillins		
penicillin G procaine (Crysticillin, Wycillin)	A: IM: 600,000-1 million units/d in 1-2 divided doses C: IM: 300,000 units/d in 1-2 divided doses	For moderately serious infections. Slow IM absorption with prolonged action. Solution is milky. Pregnancy category: B; PB: 60%; t½: 0.5-1 h
penicillin G benzathine (Bicillin L-A)	A: IM: 1.2 million units as a single dose C >27 kg: IM: 900,000 units/dose C <27 kg: IM: 300,000-600,000 units/dose	Long-acting penicillin when given by injection. Used as prophylaxis for rheumatic fever. Pregnancy category: B; PB: 60%; t½: 0.5-1 h
penicillin G sodium/ potassium (Pfizerpen)	A: IM/IV: 5-24 million units/d in divided doses q4-6 h; *max:* 80 million units/d C: IM/IV: 150,000-300,000 units/d in divided doses q4-6h; *max:* 24 million units/d Neonates: IM/IV: 50,000- 75,000 units/kg/d in divided doses q6-12h; *max:* 100,000/kg/d	Treatment of lower respiratory infections. Monitor electrolyte levels with high doses. Injectable solution is clear. Pregnancy category: B; PB: 45%-68%; t½: 20-30 min
penicillin V potassium (Veetids)	A/C >12 y: PO: 125-500 mg q6h	Treatment of upper respiratory infections. Acid-stable and less active than penicillin G against some bacteria. Not recommended in renal failure. Take drug after meals. Pregnancy category: B; PB: 75%-89%; t½: 0.5 h
Broad-Spectrum Penicillins		
amoxicillin (Amoxil)	See Prototype Drug Chart 29-1.	
amoxicillin-clavulanate (Augmentin)	A/C >40 kg: PO: 250-500/125 mg q8-12h for 10 d	Treatment of lower respiratory infections, otitis media, sinusitis, skin infections, and UTIs. Pregnancy category: B; PB: 17%-30%; t½: 1-1.5 h
ampicillin (Principen)	A: PO/IM/IV: 250-500 mg q6h C: PO/IM/IV: 25-50 mg/kg/d in 4 divided doses	Treatment of lower respiratory tract infections. First broad-spectrum penicillin. Effective against gram-negative and gram-positive bacteria. Individuals with penicillin allergies may also be allergic to ampicillin. Pregnancy category: B; PB: 15%-28%; t½: 1-1.5 h
ampicillin-sulbactam (Unasyn)	A: IM/IV: 1.5-3 g q6h; *max:* 4 g sulbactam/d C: IV: 100-300 mg/kg/d, in divided doses q6h	Same as ampicillin. Treatment of streptococcus pneumonia, nosocomial pneumonia, skin infections, and *Neisseria gonorrhoeae.* Sulbactam inhibits beta-lactamase thus extending the spectrum. Pregnancy category: B; PB; 28%-38%; t½: 1-2 h
Penicillinase-Resistant Penicillins		
dicloxacillin sodium (Dynapen)	See Prototype Drug Chart 29-1.	
nafcillin (Nallpen)	A: IM/IV: 500 mg-2 g q4-6h; *max:* 12 g/d	Highly effective against penicillin G–resistant *Staphylococcus aureus.* Not recommended orally due to instability in gastric juices. Pregnancy category: B; PB: 70%-90%; t½: 0.5-1.5 h
oxacillin sodium	A/C >40 kg: IM/IV: 250 mg-1 g q4-6h; *max:* 6 g C <40 kg: IM/IV: 50-100 mg/kg/d in divided doses q4-6h; *max:* 6 g/d Neonates: IM/IV: 25 mg/kg/d in divided doses q6h	For penicillin-resistant staphylococci in bone, joint, and skin infections. Pregnancy category: B; PB: 89%-94%; t½: 0.5 h
Extended-Spectrum Penicillins		
carbenicillin indanyl (Geocillin)	A: PO: 382-764 mg q6h	The first penicillin-like drug developed to treat infections caused by *Pseudomonas aeruginosa* and *Proteus* spp. Contains large amounts of sodium. Use with caution when administering to patients with hypertension or heart failure. Pregnancy category: B; PB: 30%-60%; t½: 1 h
piperacillin-tazobactam (Zosyn)	A: IV: 3.375 g, q6h over 30 min, 7-10 d	To treat severe appendicitis, skin infections, pneumonia, and beta-lactamase–producing bacteria. Tazobactam is a beta-lactamase inhibitor. Pregnancy category: B; PB: 30%; t½: 0.7-1.5 h
ticarcillin-clavulanate (Timentin)	A: IV: 3.1 g q6h C >3 mo: IV: 50 mg/kg/d in 4-6 divided doses	Clavulanic acid protects ticarcillin from degradation by beta-lactamase enzymes. Effective for treating septicemia and lower respiratory tract, urinary tract, skin, bone, and joint infections. Pregnancy category: B; PB: 45%-65%; t½: 1 h

A, Adult; *C,* child; *d,* day; *GI,* gastrointestinal; *h,* hour; *IM,* intramuscular; *IV,* intravenous; *max,* maximum; *NB,* newborn; *NSS,* normal saline solution; *PB,* protein-binding; *PO,* by mouth; *t½,* half-life; *UK,* unknown; *UTI,* urinary tract infection; *y,* year; >, greater than; <, less than.

Beta-Lactamase Inhibitors

When a broad-spectrum antibiotic (e.g., amoxicillin) is combined with a beta-lactamase (enzyme) inhibitor (e.g., clavulanic acid), the resulting antibiotic (e.g., amoxicillin-clavulanic acid [Augmentin]) inhibits the bacterial beta-lactamases, making the antibiotic effective and extending its antimicrobial effect. There are three beta-lactamase inhibitors: clavulanic acid, sulbactam, and tazobactam. These inhibitors are not given alone but combined with a penicillinase-sensitive penicillin such as amoxicillin, ampicillin, piperacillin, or ticarcillin. The combined drugs currently marketed include the following:

- *Oral use:* amoxicillin-clavulanic acid
- *Parenteral use:* ampicillin-sulbactam (Unasyn), piperacillin-tazobactam (Zosyn), and ticarcillin-clavulanic acid (Timentin)

Pharmacokinetics Amoxicillin is well absorbed from the GI tract, whereas dicloxacillin is only partially absorbed. Protein-binding power differs between the two drugs—amoxicillin is 20% protein-bound and dicloxacillin is highly protein-bound (95%). Drug toxicity may result when other highly protein-bound drugs are used with dicloxacillin. Both drugs have short half-lives. Sixty percent of amoxicillin is excreted in the urine; dicloxacillin is excreted in bile and urine.

Pharmacodynamics Both amoxicillin and dicloxacillin are penicillin derivatives and are bactericidal. These drugs interfere with bacterial cell-wall synthesis, causing cell lysis. Amoxicillin may be produced with or without clavulanic acid, an agent that prevents the breakdown of amoxicillin by decreasing resistance to the antibacterial drug. The addition of clavulanic acid intensifies the effect of amoxicillin. The amoxicillin-clavulanic acid preparation (Augmentin) and amoxicillin trihydrate (Amoxil) have similar pharmacokinetics and pharmacodynamics, as well as similar side effects and adverse reactions. When probenecid is taken with amoxicillin or dicloxacillin, the serum antibacterial levels may be increased. The effects of amoxicillin are decreased when taken with erythromycin and tetracycline. The onset of action, serum peak concentration time, and duration of action for amoxicillin and dicloxacillin are very similar.

Geriatrics

Most beta-lactam antibiotics are excreted via the kidneys. With older adults, assessment of renal function is most important. Serum blood urea nitrogen (BUN) and serum creatinine should be monitored. With a decrease in renal function, the antibiotic dose should be decreased.

Side Effects and Adverse Reactions

Common adverse reactions to penicillin administration are hypersensitivity and **superinfection** (occurrence of a secondary infection when the flora of the body is disturbed) (see Table 29-2). Nausea, vomiting, and diarrhea are common GI disturbances. Rash is an indicator of a mild to moderate allergic reaction. Severe allergic reaction leads to anaphylactic shock. Clinical manifestations of a severe allergic reaction include laryngeal edema, severe bronchoconstriction with stridor, and hypotension. Allergic effects occur in 5% to 10% of persons receiving penicillin compounds; therefore close monitoring during the first dose and subsequent doses of penicillin is essential.

Drug Interactions

The broad-spectrum penicillins—amoxicillin and ampicillin—may decrease the effectiveness of oral contraceptives. Potassium supplements can increase serum potassium levels when taken with potassium penicillin G or V. When penicillin is mixed with an aminoglycoside in IV solution, the actions of both drugs are inactivated.

Cephalosporins

In 1948, a fungus called *Cephalosporium acremonium* was discovered in seawater at a sewer outlet off the coast of Sardinia. This fungus was found to be active against gram-positive and gram-negative bacteria and resistant to beta-lactamase (an enzyme that acts against the beta-lactam structure of penicillin). In the early 1960s, cephalosporins were used with clinical effectiveness. For cephalosporins to be effective against numerous organisms, their molecules were chemically altered, and semisynthetic cephalosporins were produced. Like penicillin, the cephalosporins have a beta-lactam structure and act by inhibiting the bacterial enzyme necessary for cell wall synthesis. Lysis to the cell occurs, and the bacterial cell dies.

First-, Second-, Third-, and Fourth-Generation Cephalosporins

Cephalosporins are a major antibiotic group used in hospitals and in health care offices. These drugs are bactericidal with actions similar to penicillin. For antibacterial activity, the beta-lactam ring of cephalosporins is necessary.

Nursing Process
Patient-Centered Collaborative Care

Antibacterials: Penicillins

Assessment

- Assess for allergy to penicillin or cephalosporins. The patient who is hypersensitive to amoxicillin should not take any type of penicillin products. Severe allergic reaction could occur. A small percentage of patients who are allergic to penicillin could also be allergic to a cephalosporin product.
- Evaluate laboratory results, especially liver enzymes. Report elevated alkaline phosphatase, alanine aminotransferase, or aspartate aminotransferase.
- Record urine output. If amount is inadequate (<30 mL/h or <600 mL/d), drug or drug dosage may need to be changed.

Nursing Diagnoses

- Risk for infection related to invasion of bacteria through surgical incision
- Risk for impaired skin integrity related to rash

- Noncompliance with drug regimen related to decreased finances
- Imbalanced nutrition, less than body requirements, related to nausea and vomiting

Planning

- Patient's infection will be controlled and later eliminated.

Nursing Interventions

- Obtain sample (e.g., swab, blood, sputum) for laboratory culture and antibiotic sensitivity testing of infective organism (also known as C&S) before antibiotic therapy is started.
- Monitor for signs and symptoms of superinfection, especially in patients taking high doses of an antibiotic for a prolonged time. Signs and symptoms include stomatitis (mouth ulcers), genital discharge (vaginitis), and anal or genital itching.
- Examine patient for allergic reaction to the penicillin product, especially after the first and second doses. This may be a mild reaction, such as a rash, or a severe reaction, such as respiratory distress or anaphylaxis.
- Have epinephrine available to counteract a severe allergic reaction.
- Do not mix aminoglycosides with a high-dose or extended-spectrum penicillin G, because this combination may inactivate the aminoglycoside.
- Assess patient for bleeding if high doses of penicillin are being given; a decrease in platelet aggregation (clotting) may result.
- Monitor body temperature and infected area.
- Dilute antibiotic for IV use in an appropriate amount of solution as indicated in the drug pamphlet.

Patient Teaching

General

- Teach patient to take *entire* prescribed penicillin product, such as amoxicillin, until the bottle is empty. If only a portion of the penicillin is taken, drug resistance to that antibacterial agent may develop in the future.
- Advise patient who is allergic to penicillin to wear a medical alert bracelet or necklace and carry a card that indicates the allergy. Patient should notify health care provider of any allergy to penicillin when reporting health history.
- Keep drugs out of reach of small children. Request childproof containers.
- Inform patient to report any side effects or adverse reaction that may occur while taking the drug.
- Encourage patient to increase fluid intake; fluids aid in decreasing the body temperature and in excreting the drug.
- Warn patient or child's parent that chewable tablets must be chewed or crushed before swallowing.
- Advise female patients of childbearing years to use an additional form of birth control while taking penicillins.

Diet

- Advise patient to take medication with food to avoid gastric irritation.

Cultural Considerations

- Recognize that patients and family members from various cultural backgrounds may have alternative practices for alleviating infections. Accept adjunctive alternative methods if not harmful to patient.
- Request a translator to obtain a history of symptoms related to infection and any allergies to antibiotics if patient does not speak English.

Evaluation

- Evaluate effectiveness of antibacterial agent by determining whether infection has ceased and whether any side effects, including superinfection, have occurred.

Four groups of cephalosporins have been developed, identified as *generations.* Each generation is effective against a broader spectrum of bacteria (Table 29-4).

Not all cephalosporins are affected by the beta-lactamases. First-generation cephalosporins are destroyed by beta-lactamases, but not all second-generation cephalosporins are affected by beta-lactamases. Third-generation cephalosporins are resistant to beta-lactamases. Most third- and fourth-generation cephalosporins (e.g., aztreonam, imipenem-cilastatin) are effective in treating sepsis and many strains of gram-negative bacilli. The cephalosporins ceftazidime and cefepime, along with aztreonam and imipenem-cilastatin, are effective against most strains of *Pseudomonas aeruginosa.* Table 29-5 lists the other unclassified beta-lactam antibiotics.

Approximately 10% of persons allergic to penicillin are also allergic to cephalosporins, because both groups of antibacterials have similar molecular structures. If a patient is allergic to penicillin and taking a cephalosporin, the nurse should watch for a possible allergic reaction to the cephalosporin, although the likelihood of a reaction is small.

Only a few cephalosporins are administered orally. These include cephalexin (Keflex), cefadroxil (Duricef), cefaclor (Ceclor), cefuroxime axetil (Ceftin), cefuroxime sodium (Zinacef), cefdinir (Omnicef), and cef-tibuten (Cedax). The rest of the cephalosporins are administered IM and IV. Prototype Drug Chart 29-2 describes the drug data related to ceftriaxone (Rocephin).

Pharmacokinetics Cefazolin is administered IM and IV, and cefaclor is given orally. The protein-binding power of cefazolin is greater than that of cefaclor. The half-life of each drug is short, and the drugs are excreted 60% to 80% unchanged in the urine.

TABLE 29-4 ACTIVITY OF THE FOUR GENERATIONS OF CEPHALOSPORINS

GENERATION	ACTIVITY
First	Effective against gram-positive bacteria (streptococci and most staphylococci). Effective against most gram-negative bacteria (*Escherichia coli* and species of *Klebsiella, Proteus, Salmonella,* and *Shigella*).
Second	Same effectiveness as first generation. Possess a broader spectrum against other gram-negative bacteria (*Haemophilus influenzae, Neisseria gonorrhoeae, Neisseria meningitidis, Enterobacter* spp., and several anaerobic organisms).
Third	Same effectiveness as first and second generations. Also effective against gram-negative bacteria (*Pseudomonas aeruginosa, Serratia* spp., and *Acinetobacter* spp). Less effective against gram-positive bacteria.
Fourth	Similar to third generation. Resistant to most beta-lactamase bacteria. Broader gram-positive coverage than third generation. Effective against *E. coli, Klebsiella, Proteus,* streptococci, certain staphylococci, and *P. aeruginosa.*

TABLE 29-5 OTHER BETA-LACTAM ANTIBIOTICS

GENERIC (BRAND)	ROUTE AND DOSAGE	USES AND CONSIDERATIONS
aztreonam (Azactam)	Severe infections: A: IM/IV: 1.0-2.0 g q6-8h; *max:* 8 g/d C >9 mo: IV: 30 mg/kg q6-8h; max: 120 mg/kg/d	For treatment of gram-negative infections of the lower respiratory tract, urinary tract, skin, and vagina. Not effective against gram-positive organisms. May be used in combination with other antibiotics. Pregnancy category: B; PB: 56%-60%; t½: 1.7-2.1 h
imipenem-cilastatin (Primaxin)	A/C: IM: 500-750 mg q12h A: IV: 250 mg q6-8h; max 1 g/d C: IV: 15-25 mg/kg q6h	For treatment of septicemia and severe infections of the lower respiratory tract, urinary tract, skin, bones, and joints. Effective against most gram-negative organisms, including *Pseudomonas aeruginosa.* Pregnancy category: C; PB: 20%-40%; t½: 1 h
meropenem (Merrem)	A: IV: 1-2 g q8h C >3 mo: IV: 20-40 mg/kg q8h	A carbapenem antibiotic, similar to cephalosporins. Effective against most strains of gram-negative organisms, including *Pseudomonas aeruginosa,* and effective for complicated appendicitis, peritonitis, meningitis, and soft-tissue infections. Pregnancy category: B; PB: 2%: t½: 1.2 h

A, Adult; *C,* child; *d,* day; *h,* hour; *IM,* intramuscular; *IV,* intravenous; *max,* maximum; *min,* minute; *PB,* protein-binding; *PO,* by mouth; *t½,* half-life; *UK,* unknown; *y,* year; >, greater than.

Pharmacodynamics Cefazolin and cefaclor inhibit bacterial cell-wall synthesis and produce a bactericidal action. For IM and IV use of cefazolin, the onset of action is almost immediate, and peak concentration time is 5 to 15 minutes for IV use. The peak concentration time for an oral dose of cefaclor is 30 to 60 minutes.

When probenecid is administered with either of these drugs, urine excretion of cefazolin or cefaclor is decreased, which increases the action of the drug. The effects of cefazolin and cefaclor can be decreased if the drug is given with tetracyclines or erythromycin. These drugs can cause false-positive laboratory results for proteinuria and glucosuria, especially when they are taken in large doses.

Table 29-6 lists the cephalosporins in their designated generation, dosages, and considerations.

Side Effects and Adverse Reactions

The side effects and adverse reactions to cephalosporins include GI disturbances (nausea, vomiting, diarrhea), alteration in blood clotting time (increased bleeding) with administration of large doses, and **nephrotoxicity** (toxicity to the kidney) in individuals with a preexisting renal disorder.

Drug Interactions

Drug interactions can occur with certain cephalosporins and alcohol. For example, alcohol consumption may cause flushing, dizziness, headache, nausea, vomiting, and muscular cramps while taking cefamandole, or cefoperazone. Taking uricosuric drugs concurrently can decrease the excretion of cephalosporins, thereby greatly increasing serum levels. Uricosurics increase the excretion rate of uric acid by inhibiting its reabsorption.

Nursing Process
Patient-Centered Collaborative Care

Antibacterials: Cephalosporins

Assessment

- Assess for allergy to cephalosporins or penicillins. If allergic to one type or class of cephalosporin, patient should not receive any other type of cephalosporin or penicillin.
- Record vital signs and urine output. Report abnormal findings, which may include elevated temperature or decreased urine output.
- Evaluate laboratory results, especially those that indicate renal and liver function (blood urea nitrogen, serum creatinine, aspartate aminotransferase, alanine aminotransferase, alkaline phosphatase, and bilirubin). Report abnormal findings. Use these laboratory results for baseline values.

PROTOTYPE DRUG CHART 29-2

Ceftriaxone

Drug Class ceftriaxone: third-generation cephalosporin Trade Name: Rocephin Pregnancy Category: B	**Dosage** ceftriaxone: A: IM/IV: 1-2/d; *max:* 4 g/d C: IM/IV: 50-75 mg/kg/d in 2 divided doses; *max:* 100 mg/kg/d
Contraindications Hypersensitivity to cephalosporins, gallbladder disease, pseudomembranous colitis, bleeding, receiving calcium salts IV Caution: Hypersensitivity to penicillins; vitamin K deficiency, anticoagulants	**Drug-Lab-Food Interactions** Drug: increase nephrotoxicity with loop diuretics, aminoglycosides, calcium salts, vancomycin; increase bleeding with anticoagulants Lab: May increase AST, ALT, ALP, LDH. May increase PT and INR
Pharmacokinetics Absorption: IM, IV Distribution: PB: 85%-95% Metabolism: t½: 6-9 h Excretion: Urine	**Pharmacodynamics** IM: Onset: UK Peak: 1.5-4 h Duration: UK IV: Onset: immediate Peak: 30 min Duration: UK
Therapeutic Effects/Uses For respiratory, urinary, bone, joint, and skin infections; otitis media; surgical infection prophylaxis, septicemia, gonorrhea, *Klebsiella pneumoniae, E. coli, Streptococcus pneumoniae,* and *S. aureus* Mode of Action: Inhibition of bacterial cell wall synthesis, causing cell death; bactericidal effect	
Side Effects Anorexia, nausea, vomiting, diarrhea, flatulence, rash, flushing, diaphoresis, dyspepsia, abdominal cramps, fever, pruritus, headaches, dizziness, vertigo, weakness, edema	**Adverse Reactions** Superinfections, bleeding, epistaxis, angioedema, palpitations, biliary obstruction, cholelithiasis, jaundice, hematuria Life-threatening: Seizures, anaphylaxis, agranulocytosis, aplastic anemia, hemolytic anemia, leukopenia, thrombocytopenia, neutropenia, pancytopenia, pseudomembranous colitis, Stevens-Johnson syndrome

A, Adult; *ALP,* alkaline phosphatase; *ALT,* alanine aminotransferase; *AST,* aspartate aminotransferase; *BUN,* blood urea nitrogen; *C,* child; *d,* day; *h,* hour; *IM,* intramuscular; *IV,* intravenous; *LDH,* lactic dehydrogenase; *max,* maximum; *min,* minute; *PB,* protein-binding; *PO,* by mouth; *t ½,* half-life; *UK,* unknown.

TABLE 29-6 ANTIBACTERIALS: CEPHALOSPORINS

GENERIC (BRAND)	ROUTE AND DOSAGE	USES AND CONSIDERATIONS
First-Generation		
cefadroxil (Duricef)	A: PO: 1-2 g/d in 1-2 divided doses C: PO: 30 mg/kg/d in 2 divided doses	For urinary tract infections, beta-hemolytic streptococcal infections, and staphylococcal skin infections. Well absorbed by GI tract and not affected by food. Pregnancy category: B; PB: 20%; t½: 1-2 h
cefazolin sodium (Ancef)	A: IM/IV: 250 mg-1 g q6-8h; *max:* 12 g/d C: IM/IV: 25-100 mg/kg/d in 3 divided doses; *max:* 6 g/d	For infections including otitis media, skin, bone, and respiratory or urinary tract. Pregnancy category: B; PB: 85%; t½: 1.5-2.5 h
cephalexin (Keflex)	A: PO: 250-500 mg q6h; *max:* 4 g/d C: PO: 25-100 mg/kg/d in 4 divided doses	First acid-stable cephalosporin sufficiently absorbed from the GI tract. For infections including otitis media, skin, bone, and respiratory or urinary tract. Pregnancy category: B; PB: 5%-15%; t½: 1 h
Second-Generation		
cefaclor (Ceclor, Raniclor)	See Prototype Drug Chart 29-2.	
cefotetan (Cefotan)	A: IM/IV: 500 mg-1 g q12h or 1-2 g q24h; *max:* 6 g/d	Effective against some gram-negative organisms, except *Pseudomonas aeruginosa.* Pregnancy category: B; PB: 75%-90%; t½: 3-4.5 h

TABLE 29-6 **ANTIBACTERIALS: CEPHALOSPORINS—cont'd**

GENERIC (BRAND)	ROUTE AND DOSAGE	USES AND CONSIDERATIONS
cefoxitin sodium (Mefoxin)	A: IM/IV: 1-2 g q6-8h; *max:* 12 g/d C: IM/IV: 80-100 mg/kg/d in divided doses q6-8h; *max:* 160 mg/kg/d	For severe infections and septicemia. Pregnancy category: B; PB: 65%-95%; t½: 45 min-1 h
cefprozil monohydrate (Cefzil)	A: PO: 250-500 mg/d or q12h × 10 d; *max:* 1 g/d C: PO: 7.5-15 mg/kg q12h × 10 d; *max:* 30 mg/kg/d	Effective against gram-positive bacilli including *Staphylococcus aureus.* With impaired renal function, dose is usually decreased by 50%. Pregnancy category: B; PB: 36%; t½: 1-1.3 h
cefuroxime (Ceftin, Zinacef)	A: PO: 250-500 mg q12h IM/IV: 750 mg-1.5 g q8h C: PO: 125-250 mg q12h IM/IV: 50-100 mg/kg/d in divided doses q6-8h	Similar to cefamandole. Effective in treating meningitis and septicemia and for cardiothoracic procedures and surgical prophylaxis. Pregnancy category: B; PB: 33%-50%; t½: 1.5 h
Third-Generation		
cefdinir (Omnicef)	A/C >43 kg: PO: 300 mg q12h C <43 kg: PO: 7 mg/kg q12h	New third-generation cephalosporin. For otitis media, acute sinusitis, chronic bronchitis, pharyngitis and tonsillitis, pneumonia, and skin infections. Active for *Haemophilus influenzae, Streptococcus pyogenes, Neisseria gonorrhoeae,* and many strains of enteric gram-negative bacilli. Pregnancy category: B; PB: 60%-70%; t½: 1.7 h
cefixime (Suprax)	A/C >50 kg: PO: 400 mg/d in divided doses q12-24h C <50 kg: PO: 8 mg/kg/d in divided doses q12-24h	For UTI, otitis media, and bronchitis. Effective against *Streptococcus pyogenes,* Streptococcus pneumonia, and gram-negative bacilli including *Haemophilus influenzae* and *Neisseria gonorrhoeae.* Pregnancy category: B; PB: 65%-70%; t½: 3-4 h
cefoperazone (Cefobid)	A: IM/IV: 1-2 g q12h	To treat respiratory, urinary tract, and female genital tract infections. Most effective against *Pseudomonas.* Pregnancy category: B; PB: 80%-90%; t½: 2 h
cefotaxime (Claforan)	A/C >50 kg: IM/IV: 1-2 g q8-12h; *max:* 12 g/d C <50 kg: IM/IV: 50-180 mg/kg/d in 4-6 divided doses; *max:* 12 g/d	First of the third generation. Effective against *P. aeruginosa.* Also used in treating gram-negative meningitis. Pregnancy category: B; PB: 13%-38%; t½: 1-2 h
cefpodoxime (Vantin)	A: PO: 200 mg q12h for 10 d C: 6 mo-12 y: PO: 10 mg/kg/d	To treat otitis media and respiratory and urinary tract infections. Food enhances drug absorption. Pregnancy category: B; PB: 22%-33%; t½: 3 h
ceftazidime (Fortaz)	A: IM/IV: 1-2 g q8-12h; *max:* 6 g/d C: IV: 30-50 mg/kg q8h; *max:* 150 mg/kg/d	Most effective against *Pseudomonas spp.* Pregnancy category: B; PB: <10%; t½: 1.5-2 h
ceftriaxone (Rocephin)	See Prototype Drug Chart 29-2.	
ceftizoxime sodium (Cefizox)	A: IM/IV: 500 mg-2 g q8-12h; *max:* 12 g/d C: IV: 50 mg/kg q6-8h; *max:* 200 mg/kg/d	For respiratory, urinary tract, skin, bone, and joint infections. For surgical prophylaxis. Pregnancy category: B; PB: 30%; t½: 1.7 h
ceftibuten (Cedax)	A: PO: 400 mg/d × 10 d C: 6 mo-12 y: PO: 9 mg/kg/d × 10 d; *max:* 400 mg/d	For chronic bronchitis, pharyngitis, and tonsillitis. Active against gram-positive and gram-negative bacteria, *H. influenzae, Streptococcus pneumoniae,* and *Streptococcus pyogenes.* Poor activity against staphylococci and pneumococci. Pregnancy category: B; PB: 65%; t½: 2-2.5 h
cefditoren pivoxil (Spectracef)	A/C: PO: 200-400 mg b.i.d. for 10 d; *max:* 800 mg/d	For chronic bronchitis, pharyngitis, tonsillitis, skin infections, and other mild to moderate bacterial infections. Pregnancy category: B; PB: 88%; t½: 1.6 h
Fourth-Generation		
cefepime (Maxipime)	Mild to moderate infection: A: IV: 0.5-2g q12h; *max:* 6 g/d C: IV: 50 mg/kg q12h; *max:* 50 mg/kg/dose	Similar to third-generation cephalosporins. Resistant to most beta-lactamase bacteria. Effective against pneumonia, *E. coli, Klebsiella, Proteus, streptococci,* certain staphylococci, and *P. aeruginosa.* Has a broader gram-positive coverage than the third-generation cephalosporins. Pregnancy category: B; PB: 16%-19%; t½: 2-2.3 h

A, Adult; *b.i.d.,* two times a day; *C,* child; *d,* day; *GI,* gastrointestinal; *h,* hour; *IM,* intramuscularly; *IV,* intravenously; *max,* maximum; *mo,* month; *PB,* protein-binding; *PO,* by mouth; *t½,* half-life; *UK,* unknown.

Nursing Diagnoses

- Risk for impaired skin integrity related to rash
- Risk for infection related to invasive procedure
- Noncompliance with drug regimen related to lack of knowledge relevant to regimen behavior
- Imbalanced nutrition, less than body requirements, related to nausea and vomiting.

Planning

- Patient's infection will be controlled and later eliminated.

Nursing Interventions

- Culture the infected area before cephalosporin therapy is started. The organism causing the infection can be determined by culture, and the antibiotics the organism is sensitive to are determined by sensitivity (C&S). (Antibiotic therapy may be started before culture result is reported. The antibiotic may need to be changed after C&S test results are received.)

Patient Teaching

General

- Keep drugs out of reach of children. Request childproof containers.
- Tell patient to report signs of superinfection, such as mouth ulcers or discharge from the anal or genital area.
- Advise patient to ingest buttermilk, yogurt, or acidophilus supplement to prevent superinfection of the intestinal flora with long-term use of a cephalosporin.
- Instruct patient to take the complete course of medication, even when symptoms of infection have ceased.
- Infuse all IV cephalosporins over 30 minutes or as ordered to prevent pain and irritation.
- Observe for hypersensitivity reactions.

Side Effects

- Warn patient to report any side effects from use of oral cephalosporin drugs; these may include anorexia, nausea, vomiting, headache, dizziness, itching, and rash.

Diet

- Advise patient to take medication with food if gastric irritation occurs.
- Encourage patient to take an adequate amount of fluids to avoid dehydration from diarrhea.

Cultural Considerations

- Allow adequate time for information processing for patient whose first language is not English. Failing to do so may result in an inaccurate response or no response.
- Provide time for patients to respond to questions, especially when there is a language barrier.
- Speak clearly and slowly, giving time for translation. Obtain an interpreter if necessary.

Evaluation

- Evaluate the effectiveness of the cephalosporin by determining whether the infection has ceased and that no side effects, including superinfection, have occurred.

KEY WEBSITES

Information on oral ampicillin: *www.nlm.nih.gov/medlineplus/druginfo/meds/a685015.html*

Information on cephalosporins: *www.emedexpert.com/compare/cephalosporins.shtml*

CRITICAL THINKING CASE STUDY

SA, age 6 years, has otitis media. The health care provider ordered amoxicillin 250 mg every 8 hours. The nurse asks SA's parent if SA is allergic to any drugs, and the parent says that SA is allergic to penicillin.

1. What are the similarities and differences in penicillin and amoxicillin? Explain your answer.
2. What nursing action should the nurse take? Why?

The health care provider changed the amoxicillin order to cefaclor (Ceclor) 250 mg every 8 hours. The therapeutic dosage for children is 20 to 40 mg/kg/d in three divided doses. The child weighs 40 pounds.

3. What are the similarities and differences in amoxicillin and cefaclor? Explain your answer.
4. Is the prescribed cefaclor dosage for SA within safe parameters? Explain your answer.
5. Explain the significance of the nurse asking about allergies to antibiotics such as penicillin. What is the relationship of penicillin and cefaclor in regard to allergies?
6. What should the nurse include in patient teaching for SA and her parents?

NCLEX STUDY QUESTIONS

1. A patient is receiving amoxicillin (Amoxil). The nurse understands that the action of this drug is by which process?
   a. Inhibition of protein synthesis
   b. Alteration of membrane permeability
   c. Inhibition of bacterial cell-wall synthesis
   d. Alteration of bacterial ribonucleic acid synthesis
2. Amoxicillin (Amoxil) is prescribed for a patient who has a respiratory infection. The nurse is teaching the patient about this medication and realizes that more teaching is needed when the patient makes which statement?
   a. "This medication should not be taken with food."
   b. "I will take my entire prescription of medication."
   c. "I should report to the physician any genital itching."
   d. "If I experience any excess bleeding, I will contact the health care provider."
3. A patient is prescribed dicloxacillin (Dynapen). For which adverse effect should the nurse monitor the patient?
   a. Constipation
   b. Renal failure
   c. Hypertension
   d. Hemolytic anemia
4. A patient is taking cefoperazone (Cefobid). The nurse anticipates which appropriate nursing intervention(s) for this medication? (Select all that apply.)
   a. Monitoring renal function studies
   b. Monitoring liver function studies
   c. Infusing IV medication over 30 minutes
   d. Monitoring the patient for mouth ulcers
   e. Advising the patient to take the medication with food
5. A patient has been prescribed amoxicillin (Amoxil). What does the nurse know is true about this medication?
   a. It has a normal adult dose of 2 grams q6h.
   b. It has a common side effect of hypotension.
   c. It has an intramuscular administration route.
   d. It is used to treat respiratory infections.
6. Penicillin G has been prescribed for a patient. Which nursing intervention(s) should the nurse perform for this patient? (Select all that apply.)
   a. Collect culture and sensitivity (C&S) before the first dose.
   b. Monitor the patient for mouth ulcers.
   c. Instruct the patient to limit fluid intake to 1000 mL/day.
   d. Have epinephrine on hand for a potential severe allergic reaction.
   e. No particular interventions are required for this patient.
7. A patient is prescribed cephradine (Velosef). Which actions should the nurse implement? (Select all that apply.)
   a. Report seizures to the health care provider.
   b. Advise the patient to eat yogurt to prevent superinfection.
   c. Monitor the patient for allergic reaction, especially after the first and second dose.
   d. Advise the patient to take medication on an empty stomach, even if GI distress occurs.
   e. Culture the infected area before administering the first dose.

Answers: 1, c; 2, a; 3, d; 4, a, b, c, d; 5, d; 6, a, b, d; 7, a, b, c, e.

CHAPTER

30

Macrolides, Tetracyclines, Aminoglycosides, and Fluoroquinolones

evolve WEBSITE

http://evolve.elsevier.com/KeeHayes/pharmacology/

- Animations
- Content Updates
- Key Points
- Review Questions for the NCLEX® Examination
- References from the Textbook
- Unfolding Case Studies

OUTLINE

OBJECTIVES

- Describe the pharmacokinetics and pharmacodynamics of erythromycin.
- Apply the nursing process for tetracyclines, including patient teaching.
- Summarize the nurse's role in detecting ototoxicity and nephrotoxicity associated with the administration of aminoglycosides.
- Explain the importance for ordering peak and trough concentration levels for aminoglycosides.
- Develop a teaching plan for a patient prescribed a fluoroquinolone (quinolone).
- Contrast the nursing interventions for each of the drug categories: macrolides, tetracyclines, aminoglycosides, and fluoroquinolones.

KEY TERMS

bactericidal, p. 414
bacteriostatic, p. 414
hepatotoxicity, p. 415
nephrotoxicity, p. 419
ototoxicity, p. 418
pathogen, p. 414
photosensitivity, p. 419
superinfection, p. 419

The groups of antibacterials discussed in this chapter include macrolides (erythromycin, clarithromycin, azithromycin, and dirithromycin), lincosamides, glycopeptides, ketolides, tetracyclines, glycylcyclines, aminoglycosides, fluoroquinolones (quinolones), and lipopeptides. The macrolides, lincosamides, and tetracyclines are primarily **bacteriostatic** (inhibit bacterial growth) drugs and may be **bactericidal** (kill bacteria), depending on the drug dose or **pathogen** (microorganism capable of producing disease). Glycopeptides, aminoglycosides, and fluoroquinolones are bactericidal drugs.

MACROLIDES, LINCOSAMIDES, GLYCOPEPTIDES, AND KETOLIDES

These four groups of drugs are discussed together, because they have spectrums of antibiotic effectiveness similar to penicillin, although they differ in structure. Drugs from these groups are used as penicillin substitutes, especially in individuals who are allergic to penicillin. Erythromycin is the drug frequently prescribed if the patient has a hypersensitivity to penicillin.

Macrolides

Macrolides, including azithromycin (Zithromax), clarithromycin (Biaxin), and erythromycin (E-Mycin), are called *broad-spectrum antibiotics*. Erythromycin, the first macrolide, was derived from the funguslike bacteria *Streptomyces erythreus* and was first introduced in the early 1950s. Macrolides bind to the 50S ribosomal subunits and inhibit protein synthesis. At low to moderate drug doses, macrolides have a bacteriostatic effect, and with high drug doses, their effect is bactericidal. Macrolides can be administered orally or intravenously (IV) but not intramuscularly (IM), because it is too painful. Administration of IV macrolides should be infused slowly to avoid unnecessary pain (phlebitis).

Gastric acid destroys erythromycin in the stomach; therefore, acid-resistant salts are added to erythromycin (e.g., ethylsuccinate, stearate, estolate) to decrease dissolution (breakdown in small particles) in the stomach. This allows the drug to be absorbed in the intestine. Normally, food does not hamper the absorption of acid-resistant macrolides. Table 30-1 lists the dosages, uses, and considerations of macrolides.

Macrolides are active against most gram-positive bacteria and moderately active against some gram-negative bacteria. Resistant organisms may emerge during treatment. Macrolides are used to treat mild to moderate infections of the respiratory tract, sinuses, gastrointestinal (GI) tract, skin and soft tissue, and diphtheria, impetigo contagiosa, and sexually transmitted infections (STIs).

Erythromycin is the drug of choice for the treatment of mycoplasmal pneumonia and Legionnaire's disease. Biaxin XL is clarithromycin in a once-a-day extended-release tablet to be taken for 7 days. Azithromycin is frequently prescribed for upper and lower respiratory infections, STIs, and uncomplicated skin infections. Table 30-1 lists the drugs developed from the derivatives of erythromycin. Prototype Drug Chart 30-1 details the pharmacologic behavior of azithromycin.

Pharmacokinetics Clarithromycin and erythromycin are readily absorbed from the GI tract, mainly by the duodenum. Azithromycin is incompletely absorbed from the GI tract, and only 37% reaches systemic circulation. Azithromycin and erythromycin are available IV, but intermittent infusions should be diluted in normal saline (NS) or in 5% dextrose in water (D_5W) to prevent phlebitis or burning sensations at the injection site. Azithromycin 500 mg should be diluted in 250 to 500 mL of fluid, and erythromycin lactobionate 1 g should be diluted in 200 to 1000 mL. Macrolides are excreted in bile, feces, and urine. Because only a small amount is excreted in urine, renal insufficiency is not a contraindication for macrolide use.

Pharmacodynamics Macrolides suppress bacterial protein synthesis. The onset of action of oral preparations of erythromycin is 1 hour, peak concentration time is 4 hours, and duration of action is 6 hours. Newer macrolides have a longer half-life and are administered less frequently. Clarithromycin (Biaxin) is administered twice a day, and Biaxin XL is administered once a day. Azithromycin (Zithromax) has up to a 40- to 68-hour half-life and is prescribed to be taken only once a day for 5 days.

Side Effects and Adverse Reactions

Side effects and adverse reactions to macrolides include GI disturbances such as nausea, vomiting, diarrhea, and abdominal cramping. Conjunctivitis may develop as a side effect of azithromycin. The patient should avoid wearing contact lenses if this occurs. Allergic reactions to erythromycin are rare. **Hepatotoxicity** (liver toxicity) can occur when erythromycin and azithromycin are taken in high doses with other hepatotoxic drugs, such as acetaminophen (high doses), phenothiazines, and sulfonamides. Liver damage is usually reversible when the drug is discontinued. Erythromycin should not be taken with clindamycin or lincomycin because they compete for receptor sites.

Drug Interactions

Macrolides can increase serum levels of theophylline (bronchodilator), carbamazepine (anticonvulsant), and warfarin (anticoagulant). If these drugs are given with macrolides, their drug serum levels should be closely monitored. To avoid severe toxic effects, erythromycin should not be used with other macrolides. Antacids may reduce zithromycin peak levels when taken at the same time.

Extended Macrolide Group

Derivatives of erythromycin have been effective in the treatment of numerous organisms. Like erythromycin, they inhibit protein synthesis. Many of these macrolides have a longer half-life and are administered once a day. The first extended macrolide group developed after the introduction of erythromycin was clarithromycin (Biaxin), which has been effective against many bacterial infections. Clarithromycin is administered twice a day and the XL formulation is given once a day. Another extended macrolide is azithromycin (Zithromax). This drug has a long half-life of up to 40 to 68 hours; therefore it is only prescribed once a day for 5 days.

Elimination of these drugs is via bile and feces. Azithromycin is frequently prescribed for upper and lower respiratory tract infections, STIs, and uncomplicated skin infections.

When erythromycin is given concurrently with verapamil (Calan), diltiazem (Cardizem), clarithromycin (Biaxin), fluconazole (Diflucan), ketoconazole (Nizoral), and itraconazole (Sporanox), erythromycin blood concentration and the risk of sudden cardiac death increase. Table 30-1 lists the drugs developed from the derivatives of erythromycin.

Common side effects of clarithromycin are nausea, diarrhea, and abdominal discomfort. With azithromycin, the side effects of nausea, diarrhea, and abdominal pain are common.

TABLE 30-1 ANTIBACTERIALS: MACROLIDES, LINCOSAMIDES, GLYCOPEPTIDES, KETOLIDES, AND LIPOPEPTIDES

GENERIC (BRAND)	ROUTE AND DOSAGE	USES AND CONSIDERATIONS
Macrolides		
azithromycin (Zithromax)	See Prototype Drug Chart 30-1.	
clarithromycin (Biaxin)	A: PO: 250-500 mg q12h × 7-14 d or XL 1 g/d; *max:* 1 g/d C: PO: 7.5 mg/kg b.i.d.; *max:* 15 mg/kg/d	For upper and lower respiratory tract infections, skin and soft-tissue infections, *Helicobacter pylori* and mycobacterial species, and gram-positive and gram-negative organisms. Report persistent diarrhea. Pregnancy category: C; PB: 65%-75%; t½: 3-6 h
erythromycin base (E-Mycin); erythromycin ethylsuccinate (E.E.S., Pediamycin) erythromycin stearate (Erythrocin Stearate)	A: PO: 250-500 mg q6h; *max:* 4 g/d C: PO: 20-50 mg/kg q6h; *max:* 2 g/d	For moderate to severe infections (e.g., pneumococcal pneumonia, acute pelvic inflammatory disease, intestinal amebiasis, Legionnaires' disease, chlamydial infections). Report persistent diarrhea. Pregnancy category: B; PB: 73%-81%; t½: PO: 1-2 h; IV: 3-5 h
erythromycin IV (Erythrocin lactobionate)	A/C/older adults: IV: 15-20 mg/kg/d in 4 divided doses; *max:* 4 g/d	For IV administration. Drug should not be dissolved in solution that contains preservative. Same as erythromycin base.
Fidaxomicin (Dificid)	A: PO: 200 mg b.i.d. for 10 d; *max:* 400 mg/d	For treatment of *Clostridium difficile*–associated diarrhea. May cause GI bleeding, GI obstruction, and elevated liver enzymes. Pregnancy category: B; PB: UK; t½: UK
Lincosamides		
clindamycin HCl (Cleocin) clindamycin palmitate (Cleocin Pediatric) clindamycin phosphate (Cleocin Phosphate)	A: PO: 150-600 mg q6-8h; *max:* 2700 mg/d C: PO: 8-20 mg/kg/d in 3-4 divided doses; *max:* 20 mg/kg/d A: IM/IV: 600-1200 mg/d in divided doses; *max:* 2700 mg/d po, 4800 mg/d IV for severe infections C: IM/IV: 20-40 mg/kg/d in 3-4 divided doses; *max:* 40 mg/kg/d	For serious infections. Available in capsule form. Should be taken with full glass of water. Not affected by food. May cause fatal colitis. Pregnancy category: B; PB: 92%-94%; t½: 2-3 h
lincomycin (Lincocin)	A: IM: 600 mg q12-24h IV: 600 mg-1 g q8-12h; *max:* 8 g/d C: IM: 10 mg/kg q12-24h IV: 10-20 mg/kg/d q8-12h	In most situations, this drug has been replaced by clindamycin. May cause fatal colitis. When IV, dilute in 100 mL of IV fluids. Pregnancy category: B; PB: 72%; t½: 4-6 h
Glycopeptides		
vancomycin HCl (Vancocin)	A: IV: 500 mg q6h or 1 g q12h C: IV: 40 mg/kg/d in 4 divided doses; dilute in IV fluids; infuse over 60-90 min	For *S. aureus*–resistant infections and cardiac surgical prophylaxis in patients with penicillin allergy. Adverse reactions include vascular collapse, ototoxicity, nephrotoxicity, and red neck syndrome. Pregnancy category: B (oral)/C (IV); PB: 55%; t½: 4-8 h
telavancin (Vibativ)	A: IV: 10 mg/kg/d over 60 min for 7-14 d; *max:* 10 mg/kg/d	For treating complicated skin and skin structure infections, as well as MRSA. Adverse reactions include hearing loss, red neck syndrome, and blood dyscrasias. Pregnancy category: C; PB: UK; t½: 4-8 h
Ketolides		
telithromycin (Ketek)	A: PO: 800 mg/d for 7-10 d	For treating community-acquired pneumonia. May cause serious hepatotoxicity and worsen myasthenia gravis. Pregnancy category: C; PB: 60%-70%; t½: 10 h
Lipopeptides		
daptomycin (Cubicin)	A: IV: 4-6 mg/kg/d	To treat complicated skin and skin structure infections. Effective against a broad spectrum of gram-positive bacteria and *S. aureus*–resistant infections. Pregnancy category: B; PB: 92%; t½: 8 h

A, Adult; *C,* child; *d,* day; *h,* hour; *IM,* intramuscular; *IV,* intravenous; *maint,* maintenance; *max,* maximum; *mo,* month; *PB,* protein-binding; *PO,* by mouth; *t½,* half-life; *UK,* unknown; *y,* year.

PROTOTYPE DRUG CHART 30-1

Azithromycin

Drug Class Antibacterial macrolide Trade Names: Zithromax, AzaSite Pregnancy Category: B	**Dosage** A: PO: 250-500 mg/d IV: 500 mg/d C >6 mo: PO: 10 mg/kg/d on day 1; then 5 mg/kg/d on days 2-5; *max:* 500 mg/d
Contraindications Hypersensitivity, bradycardia, hypokalemia, hypomagnesemia Caution: Hepatic dysfunction, lactation, renal dysfunction	**Drug-Lab-Food Interactions** Drug: Increase effect of digoxin, cyclosporine, warfarin; decrease effect of penicillins, clindamycin
Pharmacokinetics Absorption: PO: 37% absorbed Distribution: PB: 51% Metabolism: $t_{1/2}$: 68 h Excretion: In bile and small amount in urine	**Pharmacodynamics** PO: Onset: 1 h Peak: 2.5-5 h Duration: 24 h IV: Onset: UK Peak: UK Duration: UK
Therapeutic Effects/Uses To treat gram-positive and some gram-negative organisms; for patients who are allergic to penicillin; to treat upper respiratory tract infections, gonorrhea, and skin infections. AzaSite is given for bacterial conjunctivitis. Mode of Action: Inhibits the steps of protein synthesis; bacteriostatic or bactericidal effect	
Side Effects Blurred vision, headache, drowsiness, dizziness, fatigue, anorexia, nausea, vomiting, diarrhea, tinnitus, abdominal cramps, pruritus, rash	**Adverse Reactions** Superinfections, vaginitis, urticaria, stomatitis; hearing loss, dehydration, angioedema, seizures Life-threatening: Hepatotoxicity, anaphylaxis, Stevens-Johnson syndrome

A, Adult; *C*, child; *d*, day; *h*, hour; *IV*, intravenous; *PB*, protein-binding; *PO*, by mouth; $t_{1/2}$, half-life; *UK*, unknown.

Nursing Process
Patient-Centered Collaborative Care

Antibacterials: Macrolides

Assessment
- Assess vital signs and urine output. Report abnormal findings.
- Check laboratory tests (liver enzyme values) to determine liver function. Order liver enzyme tests periodically for patients taking large doses of azithromycin for a continuous period.
- Obtain a history of drugs patient currently takes. The peak level of azithromycin may be decreased by antacids.

Nursing Diagnoses
- Risk for infection related to invasion of bacteria through broken skin
- Risk for impaired tissue integrity related to azithromycin side effects

Planning
- Patient's infection will be controlled and later eliminated.

Nursing Interventions
- Obtain a sample from infected area and send to laboratory for culture and sensitivity (C&S) test before starting azithromycin therapy. Antibiotic can be initiated after obtaining culture sample.
- Monitor vital signs, urine output, and laboratory values, especially liver enzymes: alkaline phosphatase, alanine aminotransferase, aspartate aminotransferase, and bilirubin.
- Monitor patient for liver damage resulting from prolonged use and high dosage of macrolides such as azithromycin. Signs of liver dysfunction include elevated liver enzyme levels and jaundice.
- Administer oral azithromycin 1 hour before or 2 hours after meals. Give with a full glass of water, *not* fruit juice. Give the drug with food if GI upset occurs. Chewable tablets should be chewed, *not* swallowed whole.
- Dilute in an appropriate amount of solution as indicated in the drug circular for IV azithromycin.
- Administer antacids either 2 hours before or 2 hours after azithromycin.

Patient Teaching
General
- Instruct patient to take full course of antibacterial agent as prescribed. Drug compliance is most important for all antibacterials (antibiotics).

Side Effects

- Encourage patient to report side effects, including adverse reactions (nausea, vomiting, diarrhea, abdominal cramps, itching).
- Teach patient to report any evidence of superinfection. **Superinfection** (a secondary infection resulting from drug therapy) such as stomatitis or vaginitis may occur.
- Tell patient to report onset of loose stools or diarrhea. Pseudomembranous colitis should be ruled out.

Cultural Considerations

- Recognize that patient and family members from various cultural backgrounds may need a written drug schedule as to when the drug should be taken. Have instructions available in the language patient speaks or reads most easily, and emphasize reporting possible side effects to health care provider.

Evaluation

- Evaluate the effectiveness of azithromycin by determining if the infection has been controlled or has ceased and that no side effects, including superinfection, have occurred.

Lincosamides

Like erythromycin, lincosamides inhibit bacterial protein synthesis and have both bacteriostatic and bactericidal actions, depending on drug dosage. Clindamycin (Cleocin) and lincomycin (Lincocin) are examples of lincosamides. Clindamycin is more widely prescribed than lincomycin, because it is active against most gram-positive organisms, including *Staphylococcus aureus* and anaerobic organisms. It is not effective against gram-negative bacteria (e.g., *Escherichia coli, Proteus, Pseudomonas*). Clindamycin is absorbed better than lincomycin through the GI tract and maintains a higher serum drug concentration. Clindamycin is considered more effective than lincomycin and has fewer toxic effects. Table 30-1 lists the lincosamides.

Side Effects and Adverse Reactions

Side effects and adverse reactions to clindamycin and lincomycin include GI irritation, which may manifest as nausea, vomiting, and stomatitis. Rash may also occur. Severe adverse reactions include colitis and anaphylactic shock.

Drug Interactions

Clindamycin and lincomycin are incompatible with aminophylline, phenytoin (Dilantin), barbiturates, and ampicillin.

Glycopeptides

Vancomycin (Vancocin), a glycopeptide bactericidal antibiotic, was widely used in the 1950s to treat staphylococcal infections. Vancomycin is used against drug-resistant *S. aureus* and in cardiac surgical prophylaxis for individuals with penicillin allergies. Serum vancomycin levels should be monitored.

Vancomycin has become ineffective for treating enterococci. Quinupristin/dalfopristin is a combined antibacterial used to treat life-threatening vancomycin-resistant enterococci (VREF) infections. Antibiotic-resistant enterococci can cause staphylococcal endocarditis.

Telavancin (Vibativ), a glycopeptide, treats selected gram-positive bacteria and skin infections. This drug is a semisynthetic derivative of vancomycin, with bactericidal action against MRSA. Telavancin has an advantage of once-daily dosing.

Pharmacokinetics Vancomycin is given orally for treatment of staphylococcal enterocolitis and antibiotic-associated pseudomembranous colitis due to *Clostridium difficile.* When vancomycin is given orally, it is not absorbed systemically and is excreted in the feces. Vancomycin is given IV for severe infections due to MRSA; septicemia; and bone, skin, and lower respiratory tract infections that do not respond or are resistant to other antibiotics. Intermittent vancomycin doses should be diluted in 100 mL for 500 mg and 200 mL for 1 g of D_5W, NS, or LR and administered at a rate of 10 mg/min or a minimum of 60 minutes. Vancomycin is excreted in the urine when given IV. It is 30% protein-bound, and the half-life is 6 hours.

Pharmacodynamics Vancomycin inhibits bacterial cell wall synthesis and is active against several gram-positive microorganisms. The peak action is 30 minutes after the end of the infusion.

Side Effects and Adverse Reactions

Vancomycin may cause nephrotoxicity and ototoxicity. **Ototoxicity** results in damage to the auditory or vestibular branch of cranial nerve VIII. Such damage can result in permanent hearing loss (auditory branch) or temporary or permanent loss of balance (vestibular branch). Side effects may include chills, dizziness, fever, rashes, nausea, vomiting, and thrombophlebitis at the injection site. Too rapid an IV injection of vancomycin can cause a condition known as *"red man" syndrome* or *red neck syndrome.* Characterized by red blotching of the face, neck, and chest, this is a toxic effect rather than an allergic reaction. Other adverse effects include eosinophilia, neutropenia, and Stevens-Johnson syndrome. Severe hypotension, tachycardia, generalized tingling, and, rarely, cardiac arrest are also adverse reactions.

Drug Interactions

Dimenhydrinate (Dramamine) can mask ototoxicity when taken with vancomycin. The risk of nephrotoxicity and ototoxicity may be potentiated when vancomycin is taken with furosemide, aminoglycosides, amphotericin B, colistin, cisplatin, and cyclosporine. Vancomycin may inhibit methotrexate excretion and increase methotrexate toxicity. The absorption of oral vancomycin may be decreased when given with cholestyramine and colestipol.

Ketolides

Ketolides are structurally related to macrolides. The first drug in this class is telithromycin (Ketek), which is used for adults 18 years of age and older to treat mild to moderate community-acquired pneumonia. This disorder is usually caused by *Streptococcus pneumoniae* and *Haemophilus influenza.*

Pharmacokinetics Telithromycin is given orally and is well absorbed by the GI tract and not affected by food intake. Telithromycin is excreted in the feces and urine. It is 60% to 70% protein bound, and the half-life is 10 hours.

Pharmacodynamics Telithromycin inhibits protein synthesis in microorganisms by binding to the bacterial ribosomal RNA site of the 50S subunit, resulting in bacterial cell death. The peak action is 1 hour.

Side Effects and Adverse Reactions

Side effects and adverse reactions to telithromycin include visual disturbances (blurred vision and diplopia), headache, dizziness, altered taste, nausea, vomiting, diarrhea, and liver failure. Telithromycin may also lead to an exacerbation of myasthenia gravis.

Drug Interactions

Telithromycin levels are increased when taken concurrently with antilipidemics (simvastatin, lovastatin, and atorvastatin), itraconazole, ketoconazole, and benzodiazepines. Class 1A or class III antidysrhythmics may lead to life-threatening dysrhythmias. Blood levels of telithromycin are decreased when taken with rifampin, phenytoin, carbamazepine, or phenobarbital, producing a subtherapeutic level. Telithromycin can increase levels of cisapride and pimozide, leading to toxicity; therefore, these two drugs are contraindicated for the patient taking telithromycin. Digoxin, metoprolol, midazolam, ritonavir, sirolimus, and tacrolimus levels are increased when taken concurrently with telithromycin. Concurrent use of telithromycin with ergot alkaloid derivatives leads to ergot toxicity (severe peripheral vasospasm and impaired sensation).

TETRACYCLINES

Tetracyclines, isolated from *Streptomyces aureofaciens* in 1948, were the first broad-spectrum antibiotics effective against gram-positive and gram-negative bacteria and many other organisms—mycobacteria, rickettsiae, spirochetes, and chlamydiae, to name a few. Tetracyclines act by inhibiting bacterial protein synthesis and have a bacteriostatic effect.

Tetracyclines are not effective against *S. aureus* (except for the newer tetracyclines), *Pseudomonas,* or *Proteus.* They can be used against *Mycoplasma pneumoniae.* Tetracycline in combination with metronidazole and bismuth subsalicylate is useful in treating *Helicobacter pylori,* a bacterium in the stomach that can cause a peptic ulcer. For years, oral and topical tetracycline has been used to treat severe acne vulgaris. Low doses are usually prescribed to minimize the toxic effect of the drug.

Continuous use of tetracyclines has resulted in bacterial resistance to the drugs. Tetracycline resistance has increased in the treatment of pneumococcal and gonococcal infections; therefore tetracyclines are not as useful in treating these infections.

The tetracyclines are frequently prescribed for oral use, although they are also available for IM and IV use (Prototype Drug Chart 30-2). Because IM administration of tetracycline causes pain on injection and tissue irritation, this route of administration is seldom used. The IV route is used to treat severe infections. The newer oral preparations of tetracyclines (i.e., doxycycline, minocycline) are more rapidly and completely absorbed. Tetracyclines should not be taken with magnesium and aluminum antacid preparations, milk products containing calcium, or iron-containing drugs, because these substances bind with tetracycline and prevent absorption of the drug. It is suggested that tetracyclines, except for doxycycline and minocycline, be taken on an empty stomach 1 hour before or 2 hours after mealtime. The absorption of doxycycline and minocycline is improved with food ingestion. Table 30-2 describes the tetracycline preparations and their dosages, uses, and considerations. The tetracyclines are listed according to short-acting, intermediate-acting, and long-acting.

Although tetracyclines are widely used, they have numerous side effects, adverse reactions, toxicities, and drug interactions.

Side Effects and Adverse Reactions

GI disturbances such as nausea, vomiting, and diarrhea are side effects of tetracyclines. **Photosensitivity** (sunburn reaction) may occur in persons taking tetracyclines, especially demeclocycline (Declomycin). Pregnant patients should not take tetracycline during the first trimester of pregnancy because of possible teratogenic effects. Women in the last trimester of pregnancy and children younger than 8 years of age should *not* take tetracycline because it irreversibly discolors the permanent teeth. Minocycline (Minocin) can cause damage to the vestibular part of the inner ear, which may result in difficulty maintaining balance. Outdated tetracyclines should always be discarded, because the drug breaks down into a toxic by-product. **Nephrotoxicity** (kidney toxicity) results when tetracycline is given in high doses with other nephrotoxic drugs. Because tetracycline can disrupt the microbial flora of the body, **superinfection** (secondary infection resulting from drug therapy) is another adverse reaction that might result.

Drug Interactions

Antacids (Maalox and others) and iron-containing drugs can prevent absorption of tetracycline from the GI tract. Milk and drugs high in calcium can inhibit tetracycline absorption. To avoid drug interaction, these drugs should be taken at least 2 hours apart from tetracycline. Lipid-soluble tetracyclines (doxycycline and minocycline) are actually better absorbed from the GI tract when taken with milk products and food.

The desired action of oral contraceptives can be lessened when taken with tetracyclines. The activity of penicillins given with a tetracycline can be decreased. Tetracyclines could cause a bacterial resistance to the action of penicillin. Administering tetracycline with an aminoglycoside may increase the risk of nephrotoxicity.

PROTOTYPE DRUG CHART 30-2

Doxycycline

Drug Class	Dosage
Antibacterial: tetracycline Trade Names: Vibramycin, Vibra-Tabs Pregnancy Category: D	Systemic infection: A: PO: 100 mg q12h on day 1, then 100/d C >8 y & <45 kg: PO: 2.2 mg/kg q12h on day 1, then 2.2 mg/kg/d A/C >45 kg: IV: 200 mg on day 1, then 100-200 mg/d C >8 y and <45 kg: 4.4 mg/kg on day 1, then 2.2-4.4 mg/kg/d in 1-2 divided doses
Contraindications	**Drug-Lab-Food Interactions**
Hypersensitivity, sulfite hypersensitivity, pregnancy, severe hepatic or renal disease Caution: Renal and hepatic dysfunction, hypokalemia, bradycardia, proton pump inhibitor therapy, breastfeeding	Drug: May increase effects of digoxin and warfarin; decrease doxycycline absorption with sucralfate, antacids, iron, calcium, magnesium, and zinc; decrease effects of oral contraceptives, ciprofloxacin; may alter lithium levels Lab: Decrease serum potassium level Food: Dairy products decrease effect
Pharmacokinetics	**Pharmacodynamics**
Absorption: PO: 100% absorbed Distribution: PB: 23%-93% Metabolism: t½: 14-24 h Excretion: Urine and bile	PO: Onset: 1-2 h Peak: 2-4 h Duration: 12 h IV: Onset: Rapid Peak: 0.5-1 h Duration: 12 h
Therapeutic Effects/Uses	
To treat infections caused by uncommon gram-positive and gram-negative organisms, respiratory and skin infections or disorders, chlamydial infection, gonorrhea, syphilis, rickettsial infection, and inflammatory papules and pustules associated with rosacea in adults Mode of Action: Inhibits the steps of protein synthesis; bacteriostatic or bactericidal	
Side Effects	**Adverse Reactions**
Nausea, vomiting, diarrhea, rash, flatulence, abdominal discomfort, headache, photosensitivity, pruritus, heartburn, color vision changes, teeth discoloration	Superinfections, severe photosensitivity, angioedema, hyperglycemia, hypertension Life-threatening: Blood dyscrasias, hepatotoxicity, intracranial hypertension, pseudomembranous colitis, Stevens-Johnson syndrome

A, Adult; *b.i.d.*, twice a day; *C*, child; *CNS*, central nervous system; *d*, day; *h*, hour; *IV*, intravenous; *PB*, protein binding; *PO*, by mouth; *t ½*, half life; *y*, year.

GLYCYLCYCLINES

Tigecycline (Tygacil) is an antibiotic in a category called *glycylcycline*, a synthetic analogue of the tetracyclines. This drug acts by blocking protein synthesis in bacterial cells, resulting in a bacteriostatic action. Indications for use are complicated skin infections and intraabdominal infections, including *Staphylococcus aureus, Escherichia coli, Streptococcus pyogenes, Klebsiella pneumoniae,* and *Clostridium perfringens.*

Pharmacokinetics Tigecycline is administered IV at an initial loading dose of 100 mg over 30 to 60 minutes, followed by 50 mg q12h. The protein-binding capacity of tigecycline ranges from 71% to 89%, and the half-life is 42 hours. The drug is eliminated from the body in bile, feces, and urine, with biliary excretion being the primary route. The pregnancy category is D.

Pharmacodynamics Tigecycline binds to the 30S ribosomal subunit and causes cell death. It has broad-spectrum activity against gram-positive and gram-negative bacterial pathogens.

Side Effects and Adverse Reactions

Because of their related structural formulas, many side effects of tigecycline are similar to those of tetracycline. The most common side effects of tigecycline involve the GI tract and include nausea, vomiting, abdominal pain, and diarrhea. Pseudomembranous colitis may occur but is rare. Other side effects are photosensitivity, headache, dizziness, insomnia, hypertension, hypotension, anemia, leukocytosis, and thrombocythemia. Hyperglycemia, hypokalemia, elevated BUN, and elevated liver enzymes may occur.

Nursing Process
Patient-Centered Collaborative Care

Antibacterials: Tetracyclines

Assessment

- Assess vital signs and urine output. Report abnormal findings.
- Check laboratory results, especially those that indicate renal and liver function (blood urea nitrogen, serum

TABLE 30-2 ANTIBACTERIALS: TETRACYCLINES AND GLYCYLCYCLINES

GENERIC (BRAND)	ROUTE AND DOSAGE	USES AND CONSIDERATIONS
Short-Acting Tetracycline		
tetracycline (Sumycin)	A: PO: 250 mg q6h or 500 mg q12h; *max:* 4 g/d C >8y: PO: 25-50 mg/kg/d in 4 divided doses; *max:* 3 g/d	For infections caused by gram-positive and gram-negative microorganisms, respiratory and skin disorders, chlamydial infection, gonorrhea, syphilis, and rickettsial infections. Pregnancy category: D; PB: 65%; $t_{1/2}$: 6-12 h
Intermediate-Acting Tetracycline		
demeclocycline HCl (Declomycin)	A: PO: 150 mg q6h or 300 mg q12h C >8 y: PO: 8-12 mg/kg/d in 2-3 divided doses	For gram-positive and gram-negative bacteria. Severe photosensitivity may occur. Pregnancy category: D; PB: 65%-91%; $t_{1/2}$: 10-15 h
Long-Acting Tetracyclines		
doxycycline hyclate (Vibramycin)	See Prototype Drug Chart 30-2.	
minocycline HCl (Minocin)	A: PO/IV: Initially: 200 mg; 100 mg q12h C >8 y: PO/IV: Initially: 4 mg/kg/d; 2 mg/kg q12h	For bacterial infections and acne. Should take with food. Pregnancy category: D; PB: 55%-88%; $t_{1/2}$: 11-26 h
Glycylcyclines		
tigecycline (Tygacil)	A: IV: Initially: 100 mg; then 50 mg q12h for 5-14 days	For complicated skin and intraabdominal infections. Pregnancy category: D; PB: 71%-89%; $t_{1/2}$: 42 h

A, Adult; *C,* child; *d,* day; *h,* hour; *IM,* intramuscular; *IV,* intravenous; *max,* maximum; *PB,* protein-binding; *PO,* by mouth; $t_{1/2}$, half-life; *UK,* unknown; *y,* year; >, greater than.

creatinine, aspartate aminotransferase, alanine aminotransferase, bilirubin).

- Obtain a history of dietary intake and drugs patient currently takes. Dairy products, antacids, iron, calcium, and magnesium decrease drug absorption. Digoxin absorption is increased, which may lead to digitalis toxicity.

Nursing Diagnoses

- Risk for infection related to invasion of bacteria into respiratory tract
- Noncompliance with drug regimen related to denial of illness
- Risk for impaired skin integrity related to adverse effect of tetracycline (sunburn)
- Imbalanced nutrition: less than body requirements, related to nausea and vomiting.

Planning

- Patient's infection will be controlled and later eliminated.

Nursing Interventions

- Obtain a sample for culture from the infected area, and send to laboratory for culture and sensitivity test. Antibiotic therapy can be started after the culture sample has been taken.
- Administer tetracycline 1 hour before or 2 hours after meals for optimum absorption.
- Monitor laboratory values for liver and kidney functions (in particular, liver enzymes, blood urea nitrogen, serum creatinine).
- Record vital signs and urine output.

Patient Teaching

General

- Tell patient to store tetracycline away from light and extreme heat. Tetracycline decomposes in light and heat, causing the drug to become toxic.
- Advise patient to check expiration date on bottle of tetracycline; out-of-date tetracycline can be toxic.
- Inform female patients who are contemplating pregnancy to avoid taking tetracycline because of possible teratogenic effect.
- Warn parents that children younger than 8 years of age should not take tetracycline because it can cause discoloration of permanent teeth.
- Encourage patient to take complete course of tetracycline as prescribed.

Side Effects

- Advise patient to use sun block and protective clothing during sun exposure. Photosensitivity is associated with tetracycline.
- Encourage patient to report signs of a superinfection (mouth ulcers, anal or genital discharge).
- Advise patient to use additional contraceptive techniques and *not* to rely on oral contraceptives when taking the drug, because effectiveness may decrease.
- Teach patient to use effective oral hygiene several times a day to prevent or alleviate mouth ulcers (stomatitis).

Diet

- Educate patient to avoid milk products, iron, and antacids. Tetracycline should be taken 1 hour before or 2 hours after meals with a full glass of water. If GI upset occurs, the drug can be taken with nondairy foods.

Cultural Considerations

- Recognize that patient and family members from various cultural backgrounds may need a written drug schedule as to when the drug should be taken. Explain how dairy products should not be taken with specific tetracyclines, but that food helps with the absorption of minocycline and doxycycline.
- Provide a detailed explanation orally or in written form of the possible side effects that should be reported to the health care provider.

Evaluation

- Evaluate the effectiveness of tetracycline by determining whether the infection has been controlled or has ceased and that there are no side effects.

Drug Interactions

Oral contraceptives may be less effective when given concurrently with tigecycline. Warfarin levels may be increased and may lead to bleeding when taken with tigecycline.

AMINOGLYCOSIDES

Aminoglycosides act by inhibiting bacterial protein synthesis. The aminoglycoside antibiotics are used against gram-negative bacteria such as *E. coli, Proteus* spp., and *Pseudomonas* spp. Some gram-positive cocci are resistant to aminoglycosides, so penicillins or cephalosporins may be used.

Streptomycin sulfate, derived from the bacterium *Streptomyces griseus* in 1944, was the first aminoglycoside available for clinical use and was used to treat tuberculosis. Because of its ototoxicity and the bacterial resistance that can develop, it is infrequently used today. Despite its toxicity, streptomycin is the drug of choice to treat tularemia and bubonic pneumonic forms of plague.

Aminoglycosides are for serious infections. Aminoglycosides cannot be absorbed from the GI tract and cannot cross into the cerebrospinal fluid. They cross the blood-brain barrier in children but not in adults. These agents are primarily administered IM and IV, except for a few aminoglycosides (e.g., neomycin, paromomycin) that may be given orally to decrease bacteria and other organisms in the bowel. Neomycin is frequently used as a preoperative bowel antiseptic. Paromomycin is useful in treating intestinal amebiasis and tapeworm infestation.

The aminoglycosides currently used to treat *Pseudomonas aeruginosa* infection include gentamicin, tobramycin, and amikacin. *P. aeruginosa* is sensitive to gentamicin. Amikacin may be used when there is bacterial resistance to gentamicin and tobramycin. Prototype Drug Chart 30-3 lists the drug data related to the aminoglycoside gentamicin.

Pharmacokinetics Gentamicin is administered IM and IV. This drug has a short half-life, and the drug dose can be given three to four times a day. Excretion of this drug is primarily unchanged in the urine.

Pharmacodynamics Gentamicin inhibits bacterial protein synthesis and has a bactericidal effect. Gentamicin has a pregnancy category of C. The onset of action is rapid or immediate. The peak action for gentamicin is 1 to 2 hours.

To ensure a desired blood level, aminoglycosides are usually administered IV. The patient's blood levels are drawn periodically to determine the drug's peak blood level (highest concentration) and trough level (lowest concentration). A therapeutic drug level can be maintained by monitoring the trough level, and peak levels are useful to monitor for toxicity. Many other antibiotics should be monitored as well to maintain effective blood levels.

IV aminoglycosides can be given with penicillins and cephalosporins but should not be mixed together in the same container. When combinations of antibiotics are given IV, the IV line is flushed after each antibiotic has been administered to ensure that the antibiotic was completely delivered.

Side Effects and Adverse Reactions

Serious adverse reactions to aminoglycosides include ototoxicity and nephrotoxicity. Renal function, drug dose, and age are all factors that determine whether a patient will develop nephrotoxicity from aminoglycoside therapy. Careful drug dosing is especially important with younger and older patients. The nurse must assess changes in patients' hearing, balance, and urinary output. Prolonged use of aminoglycosides could result in a superinfection. Specific serum aminoglycoside levels should be closely monitored to avoid adverse reactions. Table 30-3 lists the aminoglycosides and their dosages, uses, and considerations.

Nursing Process
Patient-Centered Collaborative Care

Antibacterials: Aminoglycosides

Assessment

- Record vital signs and urine output. Compare these results with future vital signs and urine output. An adverse reaction to most aminoglycosides is nephrotoxicity.
- Assess laboratory results to determine renal and liver functions, including blood urea nitrogen, serum creatinine, alkaline phosphatase, alanine aminotransferase, aspartate aminotransferase, and bilirubin. Serum electrolytes should also be checked. Aminoglycosides may decrease serum potassium and magnesium levels.
- Obtain a medical history related to renal or hearing disorders. Large doses of aminoglycosides could cause nephrotoxicity or ototoxicity.

Nursing Diagnoses

- Risk for infection related to invasion of bacteria
- Risk for impaired tissue integrity related to aminoglycoside side effect of rash
- Imbalanced nutrition, less than body requirements, related to inability to ingest food
- Risk for ineffective peripheral tissue perfusion: renal related to an aminoglycoside adverse effect of nephrotoxicity

PROTOTYPE DRUG CHART 30-3

Gentamicin Sulfate

Drug Class Antibacterial: aminoglycoside Pregnancy Category: D	**Dosage** A: IM/IV: 3-5 mg/kg/d in 3-4 divided doses C: IM/IV: 2-2.5 mg/kg q8h TDM: Peak: 5-8 mcg/mL; trough: 0.5-2 mcg/mL
Contraindications Hypersensitivity, severe renal disease, pregnancy, and pseudomembranous colitis Caution: Renal disease, neuromuscular disorders (myasthenia gravis, parkinsonism), heart failure, older adults, neonates	**Drug-Lab-Food Interactions** Drug: Increase risk of ototoxicity with loop diuretics, methoxyflurane; increase risk of nephrotoxicity with amphotericin B, polymyxin, cisplatin, furosemide, vancomycin Lab: Increase BUN, serum AST, ALT, LDH, bilirubin, creatinine; decrease serum potassium and magnesium
Pharmacokinetics Absorption: IM, IV Distribution: PB: 0%-30% Metabolism: t½: 2 h Excretion: Unchanged in urine	**Pharmacodynamics** IM/IV: Onset: rapid Peak: 1-2 h Duration: 6-8 h
Therapeutic Effects/Uses To treat serious infections caused by gram-negative organisms (e.g., *Pseudomonas aeruginosa, Proteus*); to treat pelvic inflammatory disease; effective against methicillin-resistant *Staphylococcus aureus* infections Mode of Action: Inhibits bacterial protein synthesis; bactericidal effect	
Side Effects Anorexia, nausea, vomiting, rash, numbness, visual disturbances, headache, confusion, depression, tremors, tinnitus, hearing loss, pruritus, muscle cramps or weakness, photosensitivity, alopecia, arthralgia	**Adverse Reactions** Oliguria, urticaria, palpitations, superinfection, peripheral neuropathy, laryngeal edema, hypokalemia, hypomagnesemia, hyponatremia Life-threatening: Ototoxicity, nephrotoxicity, thrombocytopenia, agranulocytosis, neuromuscular blockade, liver damage

A, Adult; *ALT,* alanine aminotransferase; *AST,* aspartate aminotransferase; *BUN,* blood urea nitrogen; *C,* child; *d,* day; *h,* hour; *IM,* intramuscular; *IV,* intravenous; *LDH,* lactic dehydrogenase; *PB,* protein-binding; *t ½,* half-life; *TDM,* therapeutic drug monitoring; *UK,* unknown.

TABLE 30-3 ANTIBACTERIALS: AMINOGLYCOSIDES

GENERIC (BRAND)	ROUTE AND DOSAGE	USES AND CONSIDERATIONS
amikacin sulfate (Amikin)	A: IM/IV: 10-15 mg/kg/d q8-12h; *max:* 15 mg/kg/d C: IM/IV: 7.5-22.5 mg/kg/d in divided doses; *max:* 15 mg/kg/d TDM: Peak: 25-35 mcg/mL; trough: <5 mg/mL	Effective against gram-negative bacteria, including those resistant to other aminoglycosides. Used for respiratory tract, bone, joint, skin, and soft-tissue infections. Monitor for hearing loss, hepatotoxicity, and nephrotoxicity. Pregnancy category: C; PB: 0%-10%; t½: 2-4 h
gentamicin sulfate	See Prototype Drug Chart 30-3.	
kanamycin sulfate (Kantrex)	A/C: IM/IV: 10-15 mg/kg/d in divided doses	Used orally for hepatic coma. Effective against gram-negative bacteria with the exception of *Pseudomonas aeruginosa.* Monitor for hearing loss and nephrotoxicity. Pregnancy category: D; PB: 10%; t½: 2 h
neomycin sulfate (Myciguent, Neo-Fradin)	Bowel prep: A: PO: 1 g q1h for 4 doses; then 1 g q4h for 5 doses Hepatic coma: A: PO: 1-3 g q6h for 5-6 d; *max:* 12 g/d	Decreases bacteria in the bowel and is used as a preoperative bowel antiseptic. Treats skin infections and diarrhea caused by *E. coli.* Pregnancy category: C; PB: 0%-30%; t½: 3 h
streptomycin sulfate (Streptomycin)	A: IM: 1-2 g/d C: IM: 20-40 mg/kg/d TDM: Peak: 40-50 mcg/mL; trough: <10 mcg/mL	For tuberculosis. Ototoxicity is a major problem. Pregnancy category: D; PB: 35%; t½: 2-3 h
tobramycin sulfate (Nebcin)	A: IM/IV: 3-5 mg/kg/d in divided doses C: IM/IV: 2.5 mg/kg/d in divided doses TDM: Peak: 4-8 mcg/mL; trough: 0.5-2 mcg/mL	Very effective against *P. aeruginosa.* Monitor for hearing loss and nephrotoxicity. Fewer toxic effects than other aminoglycosides. Pregnancy category: D; PB: 10%; t½: 2-3 h

A, Adult; *C,* child; *d,* day; *GI,* gastrointestinal; *h,* hour; *IM,* intramuscular; *IV,* intravenous; *max,* maximum; *PB,* protein-binding; *PO,* by mouth; *t½,* half-life; *TDM,* therapeutic drug monitoring; *UK,* unknown; *wk,* week.

Planning

- Patient's infection will be controlled and later eliminated.

Nursing Interventions

- Send sample from infected area to laboratory for culture to determine organism and antibiotic sensitivity before aminoglycoside is started.
- Monitor intake and output. Urine output should be at least 600 mL/d. Immediately report if urine output is decreased. Urinalysis may be ordered daily. Check results for proteinuria, casts, blood cells, or appearance.
- Check for hearing loss. Aminoglycosides can cause ototoxicity.
- Evaluate laboratory results, and compare with baseline values. Report abnormal results.
- Monitor vital signs. Note if body temperature has decreased.
- For IV use, dilute gentamicin in 50 to 200 mL of normal saline solution or 5% dextrose in water (D_5W) solution, and administer over 30 to 60 minutes.
- Check that therapeutic drug monitoring has been ordered for peak and trough drug levels. Blood should be drawn 45 to 60 minutes after drug has been administered for peak levels and minutes before next drug dosing for trough levels. Gentamicin peak values should be 5 to 8 mcg/mL, and trough values should be 0.5 to 2 mcg/mL.
- Monitor for signs and symptoms of superinfection: stomatitis (mouth ulcers), genital discharge (vaginitis), and anal or genital itching.

Patient Teaching

General

- Unless fluids are restricted, encourage patient to increase fluid intake.

Side Effects

- Inform patient to report aminoglycoside side effects: nausea, vomiting, tremors, tinnitus, pruritus, and muscle cramps.
- Direct patient to use sun block and protective clothing during sun exposure. Aminoglycosides can cause photosensitivity.

Cultural Considerations

- Do not give directions such as "Take one blue pill" at a specified time. Instead, provide the name and dosage of the medication in the language patient speaks and reads most easily.

Evaluation

- Evaluate the effectiveness of the aminoglycoside by determining whether or not the infection has ceased and no side effects have occurred.

Drug Interactions

When aminoglycosides are administered concurrently with penicillins, the desired effects of aminoglycosides are greatly decreased. Preferably these drugs should be given several hours apart. The drug action of oral anticoagulants such as warfarin (Coumadin) can increase when taken simultaneously with aminoglycoside administration. The risk of ototoxicity increases when ethacrynic acid and aminoglycoside are given.

FLUOROQUINOLONES (QUINOLONES)

The mechanism of action of fluoroquinolones is to interfere with the enzyme DNA gyrase, which is needed to synthesize bacterial deoxyribonucleic acid (DNA). Their antibacterial spectrum includes bactericidal action on both gram-positive and gram-negative organisms. Nalidixic acid (NegGram) and cinoxacin (Cinobac) are the earliest derivatives of the fluoroquinolone group, prescribed primarily for urinary tract infection caused by common gram-negative organisms such as *E. coli.* These two drugs are no longer available on the market in the United States. The fluoroquinolones are effective against some gram-positive organisms, such as *Streptococcus pneumoniae,* and against *Haemophilus influenzae, P. aeruginosa, Salmonella,* and *Shigella.* This group of antibiotics is useful in the treatment of urinary tract, bone, and joint infections; bronchitis; pneumonia; gastroenteritis; and gonorrhea. Table 30-4 lists the various fluoroquinolones.

Ciprofloxacin (Cipro) and norfloxacin (Noroxin) are synthetic antibacterials related to nalidixic acid. These two fluoroquinolones have a broad spectrum of action on gram-positive and gram-negative organisms, including *P. aeruginosa.* Norfloxacin is indicated for urinary tract infections. Ciprofloxacin is approved for use for urinary tract infections; lower respiratory tract infections; and skin, soft-tissue, bone, and joint infections.

The use of fluoroquinolones as urinary antibiotics is discussed in Chapter 34. Prototype Drug Chart 30-4 lists the drug data related to levofloxacin. Levofloxacin's use is not limited to urinary tract infections.

Levofloxacin (Levaquin) is used primarily to treat respiratory problems, such as community-acquired pneumonia, chronic bronchitis, acute sinusitis, urinary tract infections, and uncomplicated skin infections.

Moxifloxacin (Avelox) is available for once-a-day oral and parenteral dosing. This drug is prescribed to treat the same infections other fluoroquinolones are effective against.

Nursing Process
Patient-Centered Collaborative Care

Antibacterials: Fluoroquinolones

Assessment

- Record vital signs and intake and urine output. Compare these results with future vital signs and urine output. Fluid intake should be at least 2000 mL/d.

TABLE 30-4 ANTIBACTERIALS: FLUOROQUINOLONES (QUINOLONES) AND UNCLASSIFIED DRUGS

GENERIC (BRAND)	ROUTE AND DOSAGE	USES AND CONSIDERATIONS
Fluoroquinolones		
ciprofloxacin HCl (Cipro)	A: PO: 250-500 mg q12h A: IV: 400 mg q12h C: PO: 10-20 mg/kg q12h C: IV: 6-10 mg/kg q8h	For lower respiratory tract, renal, bone, joint, and skin infections. Pregnancy category: C: PB: 20%-40%; $t\frac{1}{2}$: 4 h
levofloxacin (Levaquin)	See Prototype Drug Chart 30-4.	
moxifloxacin (Avelox)	A: PO/IV: 400 mg/d for 10 days	For sinusitis, bronchitis, community-acquired pneumonia, and skin infections. It is 4 to 8 times more active than levofloxacin against *Streptococcus pneumoniae.* Side effects similar to other fluoroquinolones. Pregnancy category: C; PB: 30%-50%; $t\frac{1}{2}$: 12 h
norfloxacin (Noroxin)	A: PO: 400 mg b.i.d. for 1-3 wk	For acute and chronic UTIs. Most potent drug of fluoroquinolone group. Food may inhibit drug absorption. Pregnancy category: C; PB: 10%-15%; $t\frac{1}{2}$: 3-4 h
ofloxacin (Floxin)	A: PO: 200-400 mg q12h for 7-10 days	For respiratory tract infections, UTIs, prostatitis, skin infections. Not to be taken with meals. Superinfection may result. Avoid excessive sunlight. Pregnancy category: C; PB: 32%; $t\frac{1}{2}$: 4-8 h
Unclassified Drugs		
chloramphenicol	A/C: IV: 50 mg/kg/d in 4 divided doses NB: 25 mg/kg/d in 4 divided doses	For severe infections. Drug can be toxic; may cause aplastic anemia. Pregnancy category: C; PB: 50%-60%; $t\frac{1}{2}$: 4.5 h
quinupristin/dalfopristin (Synercid)	A: IV: 7.5 mg/kg given over 1 h, q8h × 10 days	For vancomycin-resistant *Enterococcus faecium.* Also effective against skin infected by *Staphylococcus aureus* and *Streptococcus pyogenes.* May have thrombophlebitis at infusion site. Pregnancy category: B; PB: UK; $t\frac{1}{2}$: 1-3 h

A, Adult; *b.i.d.,* twice a day; *C,* child; *d,* day; *GI,* gastrointestinal; *h,* hour; *IM,* intramuscular; *IV,* intravenous; *max,* maximum; *NB,* newborn; *PB,* protein-binding; *PO,* by mouth; *q.i.d.,* four times a day; $t\frac{1}{2}$, half-life; *UK,* unknown; *UTI,* urinary tract infection; *wk,* week; *y,* year.

- Assess laboratory results to determine renal function: blood urea nitrogen and serum creatinine.
- Obtain a drug and diet history. Antacids and iron preparations decrease absorption of fluoroquinolones such as levofloxacin (Levaquin). Levofloxacin can increase the effects of theophylline and caffeine. Levofloxacin can increase the effects of oral hypoglycemics. When levofloxacin is taken with NSAIDs, CNS reactions including seizures may occur.

Nursing Diagnoses

- Risk for infection related to an invasion of bacteria
- Risk for impaired tissue integrity related to a fluoroquinolone adverse effect of Stevens-Johnson syndrome
- Noncompliance with drug regimen related to lack of understanding of importance of drug regimen

Planning

- Patient's infection will be controlled and later eliminated.

Nursing Interventions

- Obtain specimen from infected site, and send to laboratory for culture and sensitivity before initiating antibacterial drug therapy.
- Monitor intake and output. Urine output should be at least 750 mL/d. Patient should be well hydrated, and fluid intake should be >2000 mL/d to prevent crystalluria. Urine pH should be <6.7.
- Record vital signs. Report abnormal findings.
- Check laboratory results, especially blood urea nitrogen and serum creatinine. Elevated values may indicate renal dysfunction.
- Administer levofloxacin 2 hours before or after antacids and iron products for absorption. Give with a full glass of water. If GI distress occurs, drug may be taken with food.
- For IV levofloxacin, dilute antibiotic in an appropriate amount of solution as indicated in drug circular. Infuse over 60 minutes.
- Check for signs and symptoms of superinfection: stomatitis (mouth ulcers), furry black tongue, anal or genital discharge and itching.
- Monitor serum theophylline levels when taken concurrently. Levofloxacin can increase theophylline levels. Check for symptoms of central nervous system stimulation: nervousness, insomnia, anxiety, and tachycardia.
- Monitor blood sugar. Levofloxacin can increase effects of oral hypoglycemics.

Patient Teaching

General

- Teach patient to drink at least 6 to 8 glasses (8 oz) of fluid daily.
- Encourage patient to avoid caffeinated products.

PROTOTYPE DRUG CHART 30-4

Levofloxacin

Drug Class Antibacterials: quinolone, fluoroquinolone Trade Name: Levaquin Pregnancy Category: C	**Dosage** A: PO: 500-750 mg/d for 7-14 days IV: 500 mg/d infused over 60 min
Contraindications Severe renal disease, hypersensitivity to other quinolones, myasthenia gravis, pregnancy, and breastfeeding Caution: Seizure disorders, renal dysfunction, children <14 y, older adults, theophylline therapy, dehydration, cardiac dysrhythmias	**Drug-Lab-Food Interactions** Drug: Increase effect of oral hypoglycemics and theophylline, caffeine; decrease drug absorption with antacids, iron; may increase warfarin effects Lab: Increase AST, ALT, prolonged bleeding time
Pharmacokinetics Absorption: PO: well absorbed Distribution: PB: 24%-38% Metabolism: t½: 6-8 h Excretion: Unchanged in urine	**Pharmacodynamics** PO: Onset: 0.5-1 h Peak: 1-2 h Duration: UK
Therapeutic Effects/Uses To treat moderate to severe lower respiratory tract, renal, skin, bone, and joint infections, anthrax, cellulitis, bronchitis, pneumonia, UTI, PID, gonorrhea, *Staphalococcus aureus,* streptococcus Mode of Action: Interferes with the enzyme DNA gyrase, which is needed for bacterial DNA synthesis; bactericidal effect	
Side Effects Nausea, vomiting, diarrhea, abdominal cramps, flatulence, headache, blurred vision, dizziness, fatigue, restlessness, confusion, depression, insomnia, weakness, nightmares, tremors, rash, flushing, tinnitus, photosensitivity, tendonitis, rare possible tendon rupture	**Adverse Reactions** Palpitations, superinfection, edema, blood dyscrasias, anaphylaxis, hyperkalemia, hypotension, angioedema, peripheral neuropathy Life-threatening: Stevens-Johnson syndrome, hepatotoxicity, nephrotoxicity, encephalopathy, seizures, pseudomembranous colitis, dysrhythmias, suicidal ideation

A, Adult; *ALT,* alanine aminotransferase; *AST,* aspartate aminotransferase; *DNA,* deoxyribonucleic acid; *h,* hour; *IV,* intravenous; *min,* minute; *PB,* protein binding; *PO,* by mouth; *t ½,* half-life; *UK,* unknown; *y,* year; <, less than.

Side Effects

- Direct patient to avoid operating hazardous machinery or operating a motor vehicle while taking drug or until drug stability has occurred, because of possible drug-related dizziness.
- Inform patient that photosensitivity is a side effect of most fluoroquinolones. Patient should use sunglasses, sun block, and protective clothing when in the sun.
- Encourage patient to report side effects, such as dizziness, nausea, vomiting, diarrhea, flatulence, abdominal cramps, tinnitus, rash, and very rare tendon rupture. Older adults are more likely to develop side effects.

Cultural Considerations

- Demonstrate an interest in the patient's family and in other personal matters to establish trust among some Hispanic and Appalachian patients.
- Solicit the patient's opinions and advice.

Evaluation

- Evaluate the effectiveness of the fluoroquinolone by determining if the infection has ceased and the body temperature has returned within normal range.

Moxifloxacin is more active than levofloxacin against *S. pneumoniae.* It is also effective against some strains of *S. aureus* and enterococci, but not VREF. The fluoroquinolones are included in Table 30-4.

Pharmacokinetics Levofloxacin (Levaquin) is well absorbed from the GI tract. It has a low protein-binding effect of 50% and a moderately short half-life of 6 to 8 hours. Levofloxacin is excreted unchanged in the urine.

Pharmacodynamics Levofloxacin inhibits bacterial DNA synthesis by inhibiting the enzyme DNA gyrase. The drug has a high tissue distribution. If possible, it should be taken before meals, because food slows the absorption rate. Antacids also decrease absorption rate. Levofloxacin increases the effect of oral hypoglycemics, theophylline, and caffeine.

Levofloxacin has an average onset of action of 0.5 to 1 hour, and the peak concentration time is 1 to 2 hours. The duration of action is unknown.

LIPOPEPTIDES

Daptomycin (Cubicin) is an FDA-approved antibiotic in the category of *lipopeptides*. Daptomycin acts by binding to the bacterial membrane and causing rapid depolarization of its membrane potential, inhibiting protein, DNA, and RNA synthesis. This action results in bacterial cell death.

Indications for daptomycin include complicated skin infections due to gram-positive microorganisms, septicemia due to *Staphylococcus aureus* infections, and infective endocarditis due to MRSA.

Pharmacokinetics Daptomycin is administered IV at a dose of 4 mg/kg/day. Each 500 mg vial of the medication is diluted in 10 mL of NS 0.9% and allowed to stand for 10 minutes. After gentle rotation of vial to ensure dilution, further dilute in 50 to 100 mL of NS and administer over 30 minutes. However, it should *not* be mixed with dextrose-containing diluents. The protein-binding capacity is 92%, with a half-life of 8 hours. Daptomycin is primarily excreted by the kidneys. The pregnancy category is B.

Pharmacodynamics Daptomycin binds to the bacterial membrane and causes cell death. An effective trough concentration of 5.9 mcg/mL is usually achieved by the third dose.

Side Effects and Adverse Reactions

Side effects that may occur when taking daptomycin include hypertension, hypotension, anemia, numbness, tingling, dizziness, insomnia, pain or burning on urination, nausea, vomiting, diarrhea, constipation, and pallor. More serious adverse effects that have occurred with daptomycin are chest pain, hypokalemia, hyperkalemia, hyperglycemia, hypoglycemia, bleeding, rhabdomyolysis, and pleural effusion.

Drug Interactions

When daptomycin is given with HMG-CoA reductase inhibitors, the risk of rhabdomyolysis is increased. Daptomycin toxicity may be increased when given concurrently with tobramycin. Warfarin may lead to increased bleeding when taken with daptomycin.

UNCLASSIFIED ANTIBACTERIAL DRUGS

Several antibacterials, such as chloramphenicol, spectinomycin, and quinupristin/dalfopristin, do not belong to any major drug group. Chloramphenicol (Chloromycetin) was discovered in 1947 and has a bacteriostatic action by inhibiting bacterial protein synthesis. Because of the toxic effects of chloramphenicol, including blood dyscrasias related to bone marrow suppression, it is used only to treat serious infections. It is effective against gram-negative and gram-positive bacteria and many other microorganisms, such as rickettsiae, *Mycoplasma,* and *H. influenzae.*

Quinupristin/dalfopristin (Synercid) is effective for treating vancomycin-resistant *Enterococcus faecium* (VREF) bacteremia and skin infected by *S. aureus* and *S. pyogenes.* It acts by disrupting the protein synthesis of the organism. When administering the drug through a peripheral IV line, pain, edema, and phlebitis may occur.

KEY WEBSITES

Information on aminoglycosides: *www.merck.com/mmpe/sec14/ch170/ch170b.html*

Information on fluoroquinolones: *www.merck.com/mmpe/sec14/ch170/ch170f.html*

Information on antibiotics: *www.nlm.nih.gov/medlineplus/druginfo/meds/a682098.html*

CRITICAL THINKING CASE STUDY

JN, a 46-year-old woman, has a wound infection. The culture report stated that the infection was caused by *Pseudomonas aeruginosa* and that JN's temperature was 104° F (40° C). Amikacin sulfate (Amikin) is to be administered IV in 100 mL of D_5W over 45 minutes every 8 hours. The dosage is 15 mg/kg/day in three divided doses. JN weighs 165 pounds.

1. What is the drug classification of amikacin? How many milligrams of amikacin should JN receive every 8 hours?
2. What type of IV infusion should be used? What would be the IV flow rate?
3. When would a wound culture be obtained to determine the appropriate antibacterial agent? Explain your answer.
4. What are the similarities of amikacin to other aminoglycosides such as gentamicin? Would one aminoglycoside be preferred over another? Explain your answer.

   The nurse assesses JN for hearing and urinary function before and during amikacin therapy.
5. What should a hearing assessment include?
6. JN's urine output in the last 8 hours was 125 mL. Explain the possible cause for the amount of urine output. What nursing action should be taken?
7. What laboratory tests monitor renal function?
8. The health care provider requests peak and trough serum amikacin levels. When should the blood samples to determine peak serum level and trough serum level be drawn?

NCLEX STUDY QUESTIONS

1. A patient is taking azithromycin (Zithromax). Which nursing interventions would the nurse plan to implement for this patient? (Select all that apply.)
   a. Monitor periodic liver function tests.
   b. Dilute with 50 mL of D_5W for IV administration.
   c. Instruct the patient to report any hearing loss.
   d. Instruct the patient to report evidence of superinfection.
   e. Teach the patient to take oral drug 1 hour a.c. or 2 hours p.c.
   f. Advise the patient to avoid antacids from 2 hours prior to 2 hours after administration.
2. For which serious adverse effect should the nurse closely monitor a patient who is taking lincosamides?
   a. Seizures
   b. Ototoxicity
   c. Hepatotoxicity
   d. Pseudomembranous colitis
3. The nurse enters a patient's room to find that his heart rate is 120, his blood pressure is 70/50, and he has red blotching of his face and neck. Vancomycin (Vancocin) is running IVPB. The nurse believes that this patient is experiencing a severe adverse effect called "red man syndrome." What action will the nurse take?
   a. Stop the infusion and call the laboratory.
   b. Reduce the infusion to 10 mg/min.
   c. Encourage the patient to drink more oral fluids up to 2 L/day.
   d. Report onset of Stevens-Johnson syndrome to the health care provider.
4. A patient is receiving tetracycline (Vibramycin). Which advice should the nurse include when teaching this patient about tetracycline?
   a. Take sunscreen precautions when at the beach.
   b. Take an antacid with the drug to prevent severe GI distress.
   c. Obtain frequent hearing tests for early detection of hearing loss.
   d. Obtain frequent eye checkups for early detection of retinal damage.
5. A patient is taking levofloxacin (Levaquin). What does the nurse know to be true regarding this drug?
   a. Administered IV only
   b. May cause hypertension
   c. Classified as an aminoglycoside
   d. An adverse effect is dysrhythmia
6. Which instructions will the nurse include when teaching a patient about gentamicin? (Select all that apply.)
   a. Patient should report any hearing loss.
   b. Patient should use sunscreen.
   c. IV gentamicin will be given over 20 minutes.
   d. Patient will be monitored for mouth ulcers and vaginitis.
   e. Peak levels will be drawn 30 minutes before IV dose.
   f. Patient should increase fluid intake.
7. Which nursing intervention(s) should the nurse consider for the patient taking ciprofloxacin (Cipro)? (Select all that apply.)
   a. Obtain culture before drug administration.
   b. Tell patient to avoid taking Cipro with antacids.
   c. Monitor patient for tinnitus.
   d. Encourage fluids to prevent crystalluria.
   e. Infuse IV Cipro over 60 minutes.
   f. Monitor blood glucose, because Cipro can decrease effects of oral hypoglycemic.

Answers: 1, a, c, d, e, f; 2, d; 3, a; 4, a; 5, d; 6, a, b, d, f; 7, a, b, c, d, e.

CHAPTER

31

Sulfonamides

evolve WEBSITE

http://evolve.elsevier.com/KeeHayes/pharmacology/

- Animations
- Content Updates
- Key Points
- Review Questions for the NCLEX® Examination
- References from the Textbook
- Unfolding Case Studies

OBJECTIVES

- Differentiate between short-acting and intermediate-acting sulfonamides.
- Compare the similarities and differences between the sulfonamides and sulfadiazine.
- Explain the pharmacokinetics of the sulfonamides.
- Apply the nursing process to the patient taking trimethoprim-sulfamethoxazole.

OUTLINE

KEY TERMS

Sulfonamides are one of the oldest antibacterial agents used to combat infection. When penicillin was initially marketed, the sulfonamide drugs were not widely prescribed, because penicillin was considered the "miracle drug." However, use of sulfonamides has increased as a result of new sulfonamides and the combination drug of sulfonamide with an antibacterial agent in preparations such as trimethoprim-sulfamethoxazole (Bactrim, Septra).

SULFONAMIDES

Sulfonamides were first isolated from a coal tar derivative compound in the early 1900s and were produced for clinical use against coccal infections in 1935. It was the first group of drugs used against bacteria. Sulfonamides are not classified as an antibiotic, because they were not obtained from biologic substances. The sulfonamides are **bacteriostatic** because they inhibit bacterial synthesis of folic acid, which is essential for bacterial growth. Humans do not synthesize folic acid but acquire it through the diet; therefore, sulfonamides selectively inhibit bacterial growth without affecting normal cells. Folic acid (folate) is required by cells for biosynthesis of ribonucleic acid (RNA), deoxyribonucleic acid (DNA), and proteins.

The clinical usefulness of sulfonamides alone, not in combination, has decreased for several reasons. The availability and effectiveness of penicillin and other antibiotics has increased, and bacterial resistance to some sulfonamides can develop. Sulfonamides may be used as an alternative drug for patients who are allergic to penicillin. They are still used to treat urinary tract and ear infections and may be used for newborn eye prophylaxis. Sulfonamides are approximately 90% effective against *Escherichia coli;* therefore they are frequently a preferred treatment for urinary tract infections, which are often caused by *E. coli.* They are also useful in the treatment of meningococcal meningitis and against the organisms *Chlamydia* and *Toxoplasma gondii*. Sulfonamides are not effective against viruses and fungi.

Pharmacokinetics Sulfonamide drugs are well absorbed by the gastrointestinal (GI) tract and are well distributed to body tissues and the brain. The liver metabolizes the sulfonamide drug, and the kidneys excrete it.

Pharmacodynamics Many sulfonamides are for oral administration, because they are absorbed readily by the GI tract. They are also available in solution and ointment for ophthalmic use and in cream form (silver sulfadiazine [Silvadene] and mafenide acetate [Sulfamylon]) for burns. Most of the early sulfonamides were highly protein-bound and displaced other drugs by competing for protein sites. The following are two categories of sulfonamides, classified according to their duration of action: (1) short-acting sulfonamides (rapid absorption and excretion rate) and (2) intermediate-acting sulfonamides (moderate to slow absorption and slow excretion rate).

Sulfadiazine is useful in prophylactic treatment of streptococcal infections in patients with rheumatic fever who are hypersensitive to penicillin. Sulfadiazine is poorly soluble in urine and can cause crystallization, which could damage the kidneys if there is insufficient fluid and water intake. Table 31-1 lists the protein-binding, half-life, and solubility in urine of most drugs in the sulfonamide group.

TABLE 31-1 PHARMACOKINETICS OF SELECTED SULFONAMIDES

DRUG	PROTEIN-BINDING (%)	HALF-LIFE (HOURS)	SOLUBILITY IN URINE
Short-Acting			
sulfadiazine (Microsulfon)	20-60	17	+1
Intermediate-Acting			
sulfasalazine (Azulfidine)	99	5-10	+1
trimethoprim-sulfamethoxazole (Bactrim)	50-65	8-12	+1-2

Older sulfonamides (e.g., sulfadiazine) have low solubility and may cause crystallization in the urine. The current sulfonamides have greater water solubility; therefore, crystal formations in the urine and renal damage are unlikely. Table 31-2 describes the sulfonamides.

Side Effects and Adverse Reactions

Side effects of sulfonamides may include an allergic response such as skin rash and itching. Anaphylaxis is not common. Blood disorders such as hemolytic anemia, aplastic anemia, and low white blood cell and platelet counts could result from prolonged use and high dosages. GI disturbances (anorexia, nausea, vomiting) may also occur. The early sulfonamides were insoluble in acid urine, and **crystalluria** (crystals in urine) and hematuria were common problems. Increasing fluid intake dilutes the drug, helping prevent crystalluria from occurring. **Photosensitivity** (excessive reaction to direct sunlight or ultraviolet light leading to redness and burning of skin) can occur, so the patient should avoid sunbathing and excess ultraviolet light. **Cross-sensitivity** (a sensitivity or allergy to one sulfonamide may lead to sensitivity to another sulfonamide) might occur with the different sulfonamides but does not occur with other antibacterial drugs. Sulfonamides should be avoided during the third trimester of pregnancy.

SAFETY: Preventing Medication Errors

Do not confuse...

- **Septra** (an antibacterial-sulfonamide) with **Sectral** (a beta-adrenergic antagonist that is used to manage dysrhythmias).
- **Sulfadiazine** (a short-acting antibacterial-sulfonamide) with **sulfasalazine** (an intermediate acting antibacterial-sulfonamide)

Trimethoprim and Sulfamethoxazole

Trimethoprim is an antibacterial agent that interferes with bacterial folic acid synthesis just as sulfonamides do.

TABLE 31-2 ANTIBACTERIALS: SULFONAMIDES

GENERIC (BRAND)	ROUTE AND DOSAGE	USES AND CONSIDERATIONS
Short-Acting		
sulfadiazine (Microsulfon)	A: PO: LD: 2-4 g; then 2-4 g/d in 4-6 divided doses C >2 mo: PO: LD: 75 mg/kg; then 150 mg/kg/d in 4-6 divided doses; *max:* 6 g/d	For systemic infections. Could be classified as a short- to immediate-acting sulfonamide. When taking this drug, increase fluid intake to >2000 mL/d. Pregnancy category: C; PB: 38%-48%; $t\frac{1}{2}$: 17 h
Intermediate-Acting		
sulfasalazine (Azulfidine)	A: PO: Initially: 1 g q6-8h; *maint:* 500 mg q6h C >6 y: PO: Initially: 40-60 mg/kg/d in 4-6 divided doses; *maint:* 30 mg/kg/d in 4 divided doses; *max:* 2 g/d	For ulcerative colitis, Crohn's disease, rheumatoid arthritis (some cases), and reduces *Clostridium* and *E. coli* in stools. Take after eating. Side effects include nausea, vomiting, bloody diarrhea. Pregnancy category: B (near term: D); PB: 99%; $t\frac{1}{2}$: 6 h
trimethoprim-sulfamethoxazole (Bactrim, Septra)	See Prototype Drug Chart 31-1.	

A, Adult; *C*, child; *d*, day; *h*, hour; *LD*, loading dose; *maint*, maintenance; *max*, maximum; *mo*, month; *PB*, protein-binding; *PO*, by mouth; $t\frac{1}{2}$, half- life; *y*, year; >, greater than; ≥, greater than or equal to.

Trimethoprim is classified as a urinary tract antiinfective that may be used alone for uncomplicated urinary tract infections. This drug is effective against the gram-negative bacteria *Proteus* spp., *Klebsiella* spp., and *E. coli.* In the 1970s it was combined with the sulfonamide sulfamethoxazole (an intermediate-acting sulfonamide) to prevent bacterial resistance to sulfonamide drugs and to obtain a better response against many organisms. Giving both drugs together in one compound form causes bacterial resistance to develop much more slowly than if only one of the drugs is used alone. This combination drug, trimethoprim-sulfamethoxazole (TMP-SMZ [Bactrim, Septra]) is commonly used. The drug ratio is one part trimethoprim to five parts sulfamethoxazole (1:5). The two drugs have a **synergistic effect,** increasing the desired drug response.

TMP-SMZ is effective in treating urinary, intestinal, and lower respiratory tract infections; otitis media; prostatitis; and gonorrhea. It is also used to prevent *Pneumocystis carinii* in patients with acquired immunodeficiency syndrome (AIDS). Increased fluid intake is highly recommended to avoid complications such as crystallization in the urine. Prototype Drug Chart 31-1 describes the pharmacologic behavior of TMP-SMZ.

Pharmacokinetics TMP-SMZ is well absorbed from the GI tract and is moderately protein-bound. Its half-life is 8 to 12 hours; thus it is administered twice a day. It is excreted as unchanged metabolites in the urine.

Pharmacodynamics TMP-SMZ is known generically as *co-trimoxazole* in many countries. Trimethoprim, a nonsulfonamide antibiotic, enhances the activity of the drug combination. TMP-SMZ blocks steps in bacterial synthesis of protein and nucleic acid, producing a bactericidal effect.

TMP-SMZ can be administered orally or intravenously (IV). Orally the drug has a moderately rapid onset of action; drug action is immediate via the IV route. Serum peak concentration time for oral use is 2 to 4 hours and 0.5 to 1 hour for IV use. TMP-SMZ increases the hypoglycemic response when taken with sulfonylureas (oral hypoglycemic agents). It can also increase the activity of oral anticoagulants.

Side Effects and Adverse Reactions

Side effects of TMP-SMZ may include mild to moderate rashes, anorexia, nausea, vomiting and diarrhea, stomatitis, crystalluria, and photosensitivity. Serious adverse reactions are rare; however, agranulocytosis, aplastic anemia, and allergic myocarditis have been reported as possible life-threatening conditions.

PROTOTYPE DRUG CHART 31-1

Trimethoprim-Sulfamethoxazole (TMP-SMZ)

Drug Class Antibacterial: sulfonamide Trade Names: Bactrim, Septra Pregnancy Category: C (D near term)	**Dosage** A: PO: 160 mg TMP/800 mg SMZ q12-24h A/C: IV: 8-10 mg/kg/d in 2-4 divided doses; infuse over 1-1.5 h C <40 kg: PO: 8/40 mg/kg/d in 2 divided doses
Contraindications Severe renal or hepatic disease, hypersensitivity to sulfonamides, megaloblastic or folate-deficiency anemia, pregnancy, breastfeeding, infants Caution: Malnutrition, hypothyroidism, older adults	**Drug-Lab-Food Interactions** Drug: Increase anticoagulant effect with warfarin; increase hypoglycemic effect with an oral hypoglycemic drug, increase potassium with ACE inhibitors and potassium-sparing diuretics, increase digoxin levels, increase phenytoin and methotrexate toxicity Lab: May increase BUN, serum creatinine, AST, ALT, ALP
Pharmacokinetics Absorption: PO: Well absorbed Distribution: PB: 44% for TMP; 70% for SMZ; crosses placenta Metabolism: t½: 8-10 h for TMP; 6-12 h for SMZ Excretion: In urine as metabolites	**Pharmacodynamics** PO: Onset: 0.5-1 h Peak: 1-4 h Duration: UK IV: Onset: Immediate Peak: 0.5-1 h Duration: UK
Therapeutic Effects/Uses To treat urinary tract infection, otitis media, bronchitis, *Streptococcus pneumoniae, Pneumocystis carinii, Klebsiella, Escherichia coli,* cystitis Mode of Action: Inhibits folic acid synthesis and protein synthesis of nucleic acids; bactericidal effect	
Side Effects Anorexia, nausea, vomiting, diarrhea, abdominal pain, rash, stomatitis, fatigue, depression, headache, vertigo, insomnia, photosensitivity	**Adverse Reactions** Life-threatening: Seizures, leukopenia, thrombocytopenia, increased bone marrow depression, hemolytic anemia, aplastic anemia, agranulocytosis, angioedema, hyperkalemia, hyponatremia, hypoglycemia, crystalluria, pseudomembranous colitis, Stevens-Johnson syndrome, renal failure

A, Adult; *AIDS,* acquired immunodeficiency syndrome; *ALP,* alkaline phosphatase; *ALT,* alanine aminotransferase; *AST,* aspartate aminotransferase; *BUN,* blood urea nitrogen; *C,* child; *d,* day; *h,* hour; *IV,* intravenous; *PB,* protein-binding; *PO,* by mouth; *SMZ,* sulfamethoxazole; *TMP,* trimethoprim; *t½,* half-life; *UK,* unknown; >, greater than; <, less than.

Topical and Ophthalmic Sulfonamides

Sulfonamides can be administered for topical and ophthalmic uses, but because topical use of sulfonamides can cause hypersensitivity reactions, they are not frequently used. Mafenide acetate (Sulfamylon) is a sulfonamide derivative prescribed to prevent sepsis in cases of second- and third-degree burns. Silver sulfadiazine (Silvadene) is another topical sulfonamide used to treat burns. Both of these drugs are discussed in more detail in Chapter 50.

Nursing Process

Patient-Centered Collaborative Care

Antibacterials: Sulfonamides

Assessment

- Assess patient's renal function by checking urinary output (>600 mL/d), blood urea nitrogen (normal, 8 to 25 mg/dL), and serum creatinine (normal, 0.5 to 1.5 mg/dL).
- Obtain a medical history from patient. Sulfonamides such as co-trimoxazole (trimethoprim-sulfamethoxazole [Bactrim, Septra]) are contraindicated for patients with severe renal or liver disease.
- Determine if patient is hypersensitive to sulfonamides. An allergic reaction can include rash, skin eruptions, and itching. A severe hypersensitivity reaction includes **erythema multiforme** (erythematous macular, papular, or vesicular eruption; if severe, can cover the entire body) or **exfoliative dermatitis** (desquamation, scaling, and itching of skin).
- Obtain a history of drugs patient currently takes. Oral antidiabetic drugs (sulfonylureas) with sulfonamides increase hypoglycemic effect; use of warfarin with sulfonamides increases anticoagulant effect.
- Assess baseline laboratory results, especially complete blood count (CBC). Blood dyscrasias may occur as a result of high doses of sulfonamides over a continuous period, causing life-threatening conditions.

Nursing Diagnoses

- Risk for infection related to indwelling catheter
- Ineffective protection as evidenced by photosensitivity related to sulfonamides
- Impaired urinary elimination related to prolonged high doses of sulfonamides

Planning

- Patient's infection will be controlled and later alleviated.

Nursing Interventions

- Administer sulfonamides with a full glass of water. Extra fluid intake can prevent crystalluria and kidney stone formation.
- Record patient's intake and output. Urine output should be at least 1200 mL/d to decrease the risk of crystalluria. The sulfonamide sulfadiazine is more likely to cause crystalluria than combination drugs. Fluid intake should be at least 2000 mL/d.
- Monitor vital signs. Note if patient's temperature has decreased.
- Observe patient for hematologic reaction that may lead to life-threatening anemias. Early signs are sore throat, purpura, and decreasing white blood cell and platelet counts. Check patient's CBC, and compare with baseline findings.
- Check for signs and symptoms of superinfection (secondary infection caused by a different organism than the primary infection). Symptoms include stomatitis (mouth ulcers), furry black tongue, anal or genital discharge, and itching.

Patient Teaching

General

- Encourage patient to drink several quarts of fluid daily while taking sulfonamides to avoid the complication of crystalluria.
- Advise pregnant patients to avoid sulfonamides during the last 3 months of pregnancy.
- Inform patient not to take antacids with sulfonamides, because antacids decrease the absorption rate.
- Warn patient who has an allergy to one sulfonamide that all sulfonamide preparations should be avoided, with health care provider's approval, because of the possibility of cross-sensitivity. Observe patient for rash or any skin eruptions.

Self-Administration

- Teach patient to take the sulfonamide 1 hour before or 2 hours after meals with a full glass of water.

Side Effects

- Direct patient to report bruising or bleeding that could be a result of drug-induced blood disorder. Advise patient to have blood cell count monitored on a regular basis.
- Warn patient to wear sunglasses, avoid direct sunlight, and use sun block and protective clothing to decrease the risk of photosensitive reactions.

Cultural Considerations

- Respect cultural beliefs and values regarding alternative methods for treating infections. Explain the purpose of the drug therapy and how often the drug should be taken.
- Communicate that patient should increase fluid intake to 10 to 12 glasses per day. Written instructions in patient's own language may be necessary if patient's cultural background prevents understanding of the health problem and drug regimen.

Evaluation

- Evaluate effectiveness of sulfonamide by determining if infection has been alleviated and if blood cell count is within normal range.

Sulfacetamide sodium (AK-Sulf, Cetamide, Sodium Sulamyd, Sulf-10) is a sulfonamide for ophthalmic and topical uses. In ophthalmic preparations (liquid/drop and ointment), sulfacetamide sodium is used to treat conjunctivitis and corneal ulcers. It is often used as prophylactic treatment after an eye injury or the removal of a foreign body. Note: Do not use ointment for the eye unless it has "ophthalmic" printed on the drug label. Sulfacetamide sodium is discussed in more detail in Chapter 49.

Topical sulfacetamide sodium for the skin is an ointment and is used to treat seborrheic dermatitis and secondary bacterial skin infections. This dermatologic form is not used for the eye.

KEY WEBSITE

Information on Bactrim (trimethoprim-sulfamethoxazole [TMP/SMZ]): *www.healthsquare.com/newrx/bac1046.htm*

CRITICAL THINKING CASE STUDY

RM, a 46-year-old woman, has a severe urinary tract infection (UTI). She takes trimethoprim-sulfamethoxazole (Bactrim), 160 mg/800 mg every 6 hours.

1. Is the dose within the recommended drug dose and dosing interval? What is the nurse's responsibility?
2. What are the similarities and differences between trimethoprim-sulfamethoxazole (Bactrim) and sulfadiazine?
3. What are the signs of thrombocytopenia, hemolytic anemia, and agranulocytosis for patients who take high doses of sulfonamides? Explain the assessment and nursing interventions regarding these severe adverse reactions to sulfonamides.

Patient teaching is an important part of nursing interventions. Explain the nurse's role regarding patient teaching concerning the following:

4. What is the required amount of daily fluid intake?
5. What are the cross-sensitive effects if a patient is allergic to other sulfonamide preparations? What allergic reactions may occur?
6. What time of day should sulfonamides be taken?
7. Why should bruising and bleeding be reported?
8. What protective measures should be taken to prevent a possible photosensitive reaction? RM takes the anticoagulant Coumadin, 7.5 mg/day.
9. What effect does Bactrim have on warfarin (Coumadin), and what is the nurse's responsibility? Should RM's Coumadin dosage be increased or decreased? Explain your answer.

NCLEX STUDY QUESTIONS

1. Sulfasalazine (Azulfidine) has been ordered for a patient. The nurse knows that this drug is most effective against which organisms?
   a. *Escherichia coli* and *Clostridium*
   b. *Neisseria gonorrhoeae* and *H. Influenzae*
   c. *Pseudomonas aeruginosa* and *Helicobacter pylori*
   d. *Enterococcus faecium* and *Staphylococcus aureus*
2. A patient is taking sulfasalazine (Azulfidine). What should the nurse teach the patient to do?
   a. Drink at least 10 glasses of fluid per day.
   b. Monitor blood glucose carefully to avoid hyperglycemia.
   c. Avoid operating a motor vehicle because this drug may cause drowsiness.
   d. Take this drug with an antacid to decrease the risk of gastrointestinal distress.

3. The nurse is teaching a patient about sulfadiazine (Microsulfon). Which instructions will the nurse include in the teaching?
   a. Avoid caffeine during sulfonamide treatment.
   b. Administer in 50 mL of fluid over 30 minutes.
   c. Avoid sulfonamides during the third trimester of pregnancy.
   d. Use an ultraviolet light to enhance drug effectiveness.
4. A patient is ordered to take trimethoprim-sulfamethoxazole (Bactrim). The nurse knows to be aware of which adverse effect?
   a. Bronchospasm
   b. Dysrhythmias
   c. Pseudomembranous colitis
   d. Stevens-Johnson syndrome
5. A patient is taking a sulfonamide for an acute urinary tract infection. Which medication does the nurse realize is a short-acting sulfonamide?
   a. sulfasalazine (Azulfidine)
   b. sulfadiazine (Microsulfon)
   c. sulfamethoxazole (Gantanol)
   d. co-trimoxazole/TMP-SMZ (Bactrim)
6. The nurse is teaching a patient about trimethoprim-sulfamethoxazole (Bactrim). Which instructions will the nurse plan to include? (Select all that apply.)
   a. Report any bruising or bleeding.
   b. Report any diarrhea or bloody stools.
   c. Report any fever, rash, or sore throat.
   d. Avoid unprotected exposure to sunlight.
   e. Report thirst and polyuria.

Answers: 1, a; 2, a; 3, c; 4, d; 5, b; 6, a, b, c, d.

UNIT X

Additional Antiinfective Agents

Unit 10 discusses agents prescribed to combat disease-producing microorganisms. Included in this unit are antitubercular, antifungal, antiviral, antimalarial, and anthelmintic drugs. Urinary antiseptics and other drugs for urinary tract disorders are also presented.

Disease-producing organisms may be gram-positive or gram-negative bacteria, viruses, or fungi. The degree to which they are pathogenic depends on the microorganism and its virulence.

Viruses are very small organisms that do not have an organized cellular structure. There are numerous families of virus, including herpesviruses, cytomegalovirus, adenovirus, and papovavirus.

The fungi are divided into yeasts and molds. The few fungi that produce disease usually affect the skin and subcutaneous tissues in conditions such as athlete's foot and ringworm. Serious fungal infections are systemic and usually need aggressive drug therapy. Opportunistic fungal infections commonly result from prolonged antibiotic and steroidal therapies and debilitating diseases such as cancer. The yeast *Candida albicans* is a cause of common infections of the mucous membranes of the mouth, gastrointestinal tract, vagina, and skin. *Candida,* like most fungi, is resistant to penicillin-type antibiotics because of its rigid cell wall structure.

Chapter 32 describes the variety of topical and systemic drugs used to treat yeast and mold infections. Chapter 33 discusses antivirals, antimalarials, and anthelmintics, and Chapter 34 addresses drugs for urinary tract disorders.

CHAPTER 32

Antituberculars, Antifungals, Peptides, and Metronidazole

evolve WEBSITE

http://evolve.elsevier.com/KeeHayes/pharmacology/

- Animations
- Content Updates
- Key Points
- Review Questions for the NCLEX® Examination
- References from the Textbook
- Unfolding Case Studies

OBJECTIVES

- Compare first-line and second-line antitubercular drugs, and give examples of each.
- Differentiate between the five groups of antifungal drugs.
- Explain the uses of polyenes.
- Differentiate the adverse reactions of antitubercular, antifungal, and peptide drugs.
- Apply the nursing process for patients taking antitubercular, antifungal, and peptide drugs.
- Describe the side effects/adverse effects for metronidazole.

OUTLINE

KEY TERMS

This chapter covers antitubercular drugs, antifungal drugs, peptide drugs, and metronidazole. Although these drug categories differ from each other, they each contain drugs that inhibit or kill organisms that cause disease.

TUBERCULOSIS

Tuberculosis (TB) is caused by the acid-fast bacillus *Mycobacterium tuberculosis.* This pathogen is frequently called the *tubercle bacillus.* Tuberculosis is one of the world's major health problems, killing more persons than any other infectious disease, including **acquired immunodeficiency syndrome** (AIDS) (immune disorder characterized by opportunistic diseases). More than 1.5 billion people in the world have TB, and many are unaware of their infection. Each year more than 8 million new cases of TB are diagnosed. Until the 1980s, the incidence of TB had decreased in the United States. The later increase in TB can be attributed, in part, to the increase in people with AIDS in whom active TB has developed because of compromised immune systems. In addition, the increased incidence is partly a result of increasingly crowded living conditions in urban areas. Patients more susceptible to TB are those with alcohol addiction, AIDS, and debilitative conditions.

Pathophysiology

TB is transmitted from one person to another by droplets dispersed in the air through coughing and sneezing. The organisms are inhaled into the alveoli (air sacs) of the lung. If the body's immune system is strong and intact, phagocytes stop the multiplication of the tubercle bacilli. When the immune system is compromised, however, tubercle bacilli can spread from the lungs to other organs of the body via the blood and lymphatic system. Dissemination of TB bacilli can be found in the liver, kidneys, spleen, and other organs. Symptoms of TB include anorexia, cough and sputum production, increased fever, night sweats, weight loss, and positive acid-fast bacilli in the sputum.

ANTITUBERCULAR DRUGS

Before 1944, many people died from TB because of the absence of drug therapy. Streptomycin, a parenteral antibiotic, was the first drug used to treat TB. Isoniazid (INH), discovered in 1952, was the first oral drug preparation effective against the tubercle bacillus. Isoniazid is a bactericidal drug that inhibits tubercle cell wall synthesis and blocks pyridoxine (vitamin B_6), which is used for intracellular enzyme production. When isoniazid is prescribed, pyridoxine may also be prescribed to avoid deficiency and possible occurrence of peripheral neuropathy. Group names for drugs used to treat TB include *antimycobacterial agents* and **antitubercular drugs** (agents that treat tuberculosis).

Prophylactic antitubercular therapy is suggested for individuals who have been in close contact with persons with TB. Prophylaxis is also recommended for those who test positive for **human immunodeficiency virus** (HIV) (virus causing an infection characterized by profound immunosuppression) and also have a positive TB skin test or are in close contact with someone who has TB. Patients who have converted from a negative to a positive TB skin test should be considered candidates for prophylactic isoniazid therapy. Young children who have been in contact with persons with active TB are at high risk and should receive prophylactic antitubercular therapy. When a person is diagnosed with TB, family members are usually given prophylactic doses of isoniazid for 6 months to 1 year. For HIV-positive patients with positive TB skin tests, a 2-month prophylactic treatment with rifampin and pyrazinamide may be recommended.

Prophylactic therapy is contraindicated for persons with liver disease. Isoniazid is the primary antitubercular drug used and may cause isoniazid-induced liver damage. Other antitubercular drugs may also cause liver damage if given in high doses over an extended period.

Single-drug therapy with isoniazid proved ineffective in treating TB, because resistance to the drug developed in a short time. It was discovered that when a combination of antitubercular drugs was used, bacterial resistance did not occur, and the duration of treatment was reduced from 2 years to 6 to 9 months. Different combinations of drugs can be used: (1) isoniazid and rifampin; (2) isoniazid, rifampin, and ethambutol; or (3) isoniazid, rifampin, and pyrazinamide. Rifampin and ethambutol were discovered in the early 1960s; neither drug is effective against the tubercle bacillus when given alone. In fact, if rifampin is taken alone, bacterial resistance occurs quickly. Prototype Drug Chart 32-1 lists the drug data for isoniazid.

Multidrug therapy against TB is more effective. The treatment regimen is divided into two phases: the first, or initial, phase lasts 2 months, and the second phase covers the next 4 to 7 months. The total treatment plan is for 6 to 9 months and depends on the response to the antitubercular therapy. Table 32-1 gives examples of various drug regimens to treat TB.

If multidrug resistance to the tubercle bacilli persists, other antibacterial drugs such as the aminoglycosides (streptomycin, kanamycin, amikacin) or the fluoroquinolones (ciprofloxacin, ofloxacin) may be given as part of multidrug therapy. Susceptibility testing to determine drug resistance should be performed before drug therapy. At times, susceptibility testing of the sputum and antitubercular drugs is performed, but only if the patient has not responded to the drug therapy regimen.

Mycobacterium tuberculosis strains that are resistant to streptomycin can be sensitive to kanamycin. An aminoglycoside should not be taken if renal dysfunction is present. When antibacterial agents are used continuously or at high doses, the serum drug level should be closely monitored to avoid drug toxicity.

Pharmacokinetics Isoniazid is well absorbed from the gastrointestinal (GI) tract. It can also be administered intramuscularly (IM). It has a very low protein-binding rate (10%), and its half-life is 1 to 4 hours. Isoniazid is metabolized by the liver, and 75% of the drug is excreted in the urine.

Pharmacodynamics Isoniazid inhibits cell-wall synthesis of the tubercle bacillus. It is usually prescribed with other antitubercular

PROTOTYPE DRUG CHART 32-1

Isoniazid

Drug Class Antitubercular Trade names: INH, Nydrazid, ♣ Isotamine Pregnancy Category: C	**Dosage** Prophylaxis: A: PO/IM: 300 mg/d; or 900 mg/d when 2×/wk for 9 mo C: PO/IM: 10-15 mg/kg/d 2-3×/wk; *max:* 900 mg/d Active tuberculosis: A: PO/IM: 5 mg/kg/d for 2 mo; then 15 mg/kg/d or 2-3×/wk; *max:* 900 mg/d C: PO/IM: 10-15 mg/kg/d for 6 mo
Contraindications Severe renal or hepatic disease, alcoholism, diabetic retinopathy	**Drug-Lab-Food Interactions** Drug: Increase effect with alcohol, rifampin, cycloserine, and phenytoin; decrease GI absorption while taking aluminum antacids Lab: Increase AST, ALT, bilirubin
Pharmacokinetics Absorption: PO: Well absorbed Distribution: PB: 10% Metabolism: t½: 1-4 h Excretion: 75% in urine	**Pharmacodynamics** PO: Onset: 0.5 h Peak: 1-2 h Duration: 6-8 h IM: Peak: 1-2 h Duration: 6 h
Therapeutic Effects/Uses To treat tuberculosis; prophylactic measure against tuberculosis Mode of Action: Inhibition of bacterial cell-wall synthesis	
Side Effects Drowsiness, tremors, rash, blurred vision, photosensitivity, tinnitus, dizziness, nausea, vomiting, dry mouth, constipation	**Adverse Reactions** Psychotic behavior, peripheral neuropathy, vitamin B_6 deficiency, hyperglycemia Life-threatening: Blood dyscrasias, seizures, thrombocytopenia, agranulocytosis, hepatotoxicity

A, Adult; *ALT,* alanine aminotransferase; *AST,* aspartate aminotransferase; *C,* child; *d,* day; *GI,* gastrointestinal; *h,* hour; *IM,* intramuscular; *max,* maximum; *mo,* month; *PB,* protein-binding; *PO,* by mouth; *t ½,* half-life; *wk,* week; ♣, Canadian drug name.

TABLE 32-1 POSSIBLE DRUG REGIMENS FOR TUBERCULOSIS

PHASE	EXAMPLE I	EXAMPLE II	EXAMPLE III	EXAMPLE IV
First phase (2 mo)*	isoniazid, rifampin	isoniazid, rifampin, pyrazinamide	isoniazid, rifampin, streptomycin	isoniazid, rifampin, pyrazinamide, kanamycin or ciprofloxacin
Second phase (4-7 mo)	isoniazid, rifampin	isoniazid, rifampin, ethambutol	isoniazid, rifampin, capreomycin or cycloserine	isoniazid, rifampin, ethambutol, streptomycin or kanamycin or ciprofloxacin or clarithromycin or capreomycin

mo, Month.

*If there is bacterial resistance to isoniazid, the first phase of the drug regimen may be rifampin, ethambutol, and pyrazinamide. Adjust drug regimen according to drug susceptibility. The health care provider determines which antitubercular drug and how many combinations to use. Symptoms for drug toxicity should be closely monitored. Examples III and IV may be used in various combinations for multidrug resistance.

agents. The onset of action and peak concentration time for oral and IM routes of isoniazid are the same. Peripheral neuropathy is an adverse reaction to isoniazid, so pyridoxine (vitamin B_6) is usually taken with isoniazid to decrease the probability of neuropathy. Alcohol ingestion with the drug can increase the incidence of peripheral neuropathy. If phenytoin is taken with isoniazid, the effect of phenytoin may be decreased. Antacids decrease isoniazid absorption.

Antitubercular drugs are divided into two categories: first-line and second-line. **First-line drugs** (drugs chosen first) (i.e., isoniazid, rifampin, rifabutin, rifapentine, pyrazinamide, ethambutol, streptomycin) are considered more effective and less toxic than second-line drugs in treating TB. Rifapentine, an analog of rifampin, is the newest first-line drug for treating TB. The patient takes it only twice a week, unlike rifampin, which is given daily. To avoid resistance, rifapentine should be combined with another antitubercular drug. **Second-line drugs** (second-choice drugs) (i.e., para-aminosalicylic acid, kanamycin, cycloserine, ethionamide, capreomycin, pyrazinamide, others) are not as effective as first-line drugs; some can be more toxic. Second-line drugs may be used in combination with first-line drugs, especially to treat disseminated TB. First-line and some second-line drugs are described in Table 32-2.

Side Effects and Adverse Reactions

Side effects and adverse reactions differ according to the drug prescribed. For isoniazid, peripheral neuropathy can be a problem, especially for those who are malnourished, have diabetes mellitus, or are alcoholics. This condition can be prevented if pyridoxine (vitamin B_6) is administered. **Hepatotoxicity** (liver toxicity) is an adverse reaction to isoniazid, rifampin, and streptomycin. Patients with liver disorders should not take these drugs unless liver enzymes are closely monitored, because liver enzymes may become elevated. The patient taking isoniazid, rifampin, and streptomycin may develop headaches, blood dyscrasias, paresthesias, GI distress, and ocular toxicity. Isoniazid may cause hyperglycemia,

TABLE 32-2 ANTITUBERCULAR DRUGS

GENERIC (BRAND)	ROUTE AND DOSAGE	USES AND CONSIDERATIONS
First-Line Drugs		
ethambutol HCl (Myambutol)	A: PO: 15-25 mg/kg/d; or 50 mg/kg 2×/wk; or 25-30 mg/kg 3×/wk for 2 mo	Used as a combination drug for active TB. Decrease dose if renal insufficiency is present. May cause leucopenia and thrombocytopenia. Pregnancy category: B; PB: 20%-30%; $t\frac{1}{2}$: 3-4 h
isoniazid (INH, Nydrazid)	See Prototype Drug Chart 32-1.	
pyrazinamide PZA	A/C: PO: 15-30 mg/kg/d or 50-70 mg/kg 2×/wk; *max:* 30 mg/kg/d	Used in combination with other antitubercular drugs for short-term and initial phase of therapy. Promote fluid intake. May cause photosensitivity, angioedema, hepatic failure, thrombocytopenia. Pregnancy category: C; PB: 5%-10%; $t\frac{1}{2}$: 9-10 h
rifabutin (Mycobutin)	A: PO: 300 mg/d in 1 or 2 divided doses	For *Mycobacterium tuberculosis* infection; to prevent disseminated *Mycobacterium avium* complex disease in patients with advanced HIV infection. Pregnancy category: B; PB: 85%; $t\frac{1}{2}$: average 45 h
rifampin (Rifadin)	A: PO: 600 mg/d C: PO: 10-20 mg/kg/d as a single dose for 9-12 mo; *max:* 600 mg/d	Used as a combination drug for active TB. For selective gram-positive and gram-negative bacteria, including *Neisseria meningitidis.* Monitor liver enzymes. Pregnancy category: C; PB: 80%; $t\frac{1}{2}$: 3-5 h
rifapentine (Priftin)	A: PO: 600 mg 2×/wk for 2 mo, then 600 mg 1×/wk for 4 mo	For TB. Interval between doses should be at least 72 h. Monitor for toxicity if drug is taken with an anticoagulant, anticonvulsant, or digoxin. Contraindicated with oral contraceptives. Pregnancy category: C; PB: 95%; $t\frac{1}{2}$: 13 h
streptomycin sulfate	A: IM: 15 mg/kg/d; *max:* 1 g/d C: IM: 20-40 mg/kg/d	Used against TB as the third drug with isoniazid and rifampin or with isoniazid and ethambutol. First drug used to treat TB. Pregnancy category: D; PB: 35%; $t\frac{1}{2}$: 2-3 h
Second-Line Drugs		
aminosalicylate sodium	A: PO: 14-16 g/d in 2-3 divided doses C: PO: 275-420 mg/kg/d in 3-4 divided doses; take with food	Second-line antitubercular drug. To treat pulmonary and extrapulmonary TB. Used in combination with other antitubercular drugs. Take after meals to reduce GI irritation. Pregnancy category: C; PB: 15%; $t\frac{1}{2}$: 1 h
capreomycin (Capastat)	A: IM: 15 mg/kg/d for 2-4 mo, then 2-3 ×/wk	Effective against *Mycobacterium tuberculosis,* but should be used in combination with other antitubercular drugs; not effective when used alone. Useful when bacillus is resistant to first-line drug. Hearing loss is an adverse reaction. Patient should take supplemental pyridoxine (vitamin B_6) to avoid peripheral neuropathy. Pregnancy category: C; PB: UK; $t\frac{1}{2}$: 4-6 h
ethionamide (Trecator SC)	A/C >12 y: PO: 15-20 mg/kg/q8h; *max:* 1 g/d	Effective against tubercle bacilli. Used when first-line drugs fail. Patient should take pyridoxine (vitamin B_6) to avoid peripheral neuropathy. Side effects include GI discomfort. *Caution:* Patients with diabetes mellitus, alcoholism, and hepatic disorder should be closely monitored when taking this drug. Pregnancy category: C; PB: 30%; $t\frac{1}{2}$: 2-3 h
Other Second-Line Drugs		
Kanamycin, amikacin, ciprofloxacin, and ofloxacin are effective against tubercle bacilli in combination with antitubercular drugs. Chapter 29 includes more information about aminoglycosides, fluoroquinolones, and other antibacterial drugs.		

A, Adult; *C,* child; *d,* day; *GI,* gastrointestinal; *h,* hour; *HIV,* human immunodeficiency virus; *IM,* intramuscular; *max,* maximum; *mo,* month; *PB,* protein-binding; *PO,* by mouth; $t\frac{1}{2}$, half-life; *TB,* tuberculosis; *UK,* unknown; *wk,* week; *y,* year; >, greater than.

hyperkalemia, hypophosphatemia, and hypocalcemia. Rifampin turns body fluids orange, and soft contact lenses may be permanently discolored. The patient taking ethambutol may develop dizziness, confusion, hallucinations, and joint pain. Streptomycin may lead to many adverse effects, such as ototoxicity, optic nerve toxicity, encephalopathy, angioedema, CNS and respiratory depression, nephrotoxicity, and hepatotoxicity.

SAFETY: Preventing Medication Errors

Do not confuse...

- **rifampin** with other antituberculars, such as **rifabutin** and **rifapentine**, or an antibiotic called **rifaximin,** used to treat diarrhea due to contaminated food or drinking water.

Nursing Process
Patient-Centered Collaborative Care

Antitubercular Drugs

Assessment

- Determine patient history of any past instances of tuberculosis, last purified protein derivative (PPD) tuberculin test and reaction, last chest radiograph and result, and any allergies to antitubercular drugs if taken previously.
- Obtain a general medical history from patient. Most antitubercular drugs are contraindicated if the patient has severe hepatic disease.

- Check laboratory tests for liver enzyme values, bilirubin, blood urea nitrogen (BUN), and serum creatinine. These baseline values can be compared with future laboratory test results.
- Evaluate patient for signs and symptoms of peripheral neuropathy (numbness or tingling of extremities).
- Assess patient for hearing changes if antitubercular drug regimen includes streptomycin. Ototoxicity is an adverse reaction to streptomycin.

Nursing Diagnoses

- Risk for infection related to inadequate primary defenses
- Disturbed sensory perception related to adverse effects of antituberculars
- Risk for impaired skin integrity related to side effects of antituberculars
- Risk for injury related to peripheral neuropathy secondary to side effects of antituberculars
- Knowledge deficit related to unfamiliarity with medications

Planning

- Patient's sputum test for acid-fast bacilli will be negative 2 to 3 months after the prescribed antitubercular therapy.

Nursing Interventions

- Administer the commonly ordered antitubercular drug isoniazid (INH) 1 hour before or 2 hours after meals. Food decreases absorption rate.
- Give pyridoxine (vitamin B_6) as prescribed with isoniazid to prevent peripheral neuropathy.
- Monitor serum liver enzyme levels, especially if patient takes isoniazid, rifampin, or streptomycin. Elevated levels may indicate liver toxicity.
- Collect sputum specimens for acid-fast bacilli early in the morning. Usually three consecutive morning sputum specimens are sent to the laboratory, and the routine is repeated several weeks later.
- Encourage eye examinations for patients taking isoniazid and ethambutol, because these antitubercular drugs may cause visual disturbances.
- Emphasize the importance of complying with the drug regimen.

Patient Teaching

General

- Tell patient to take antitubercular drug such as isoniazid 1 hour before meals or 2 hours after meals for better absorption.
- Direct patient to take antitubercular drugs as prescribed. Ineffective treatment of tuberculosis might occur if drugs are taken intermittently or discontinued when symptoms are decreased or patient is feeling better. *Compliance with the drug regimen is essential.*
- Teach patient not to take antacids while taking antitubercular drugs, because they decrease drug absorption. Patient should also avoid alcohol, because it may increase risk of hepatotoxicity.
- Advise patient to keep medical appointments and participate in sputum testing. Sputum testing is important in evaluating effectiveness of drug regimen.
- Warn patients contemplating pregnancy to first check with health care provider about taking the antitubercular drugs ethambutol and rifampin.

Side Effects

- Guide patient to report any numbness, tingling, or burning of hands and feet. Peripheral neuritis is a common side effect of isoniazid. Vitamin B_6 prevents peripheral neuropathy. Neuritis may not occur if patient eats a balanced diet daily.
- Encourage patient to avoid direct sunlight to decrease risk of photosensitivity. Patient should use sun block while in the sun.
- Inform patient taking rifampin that urine, feces, saliva, sputum, sweat, and tears may turn a harmless red-orange color. Soft contact lenses may be permanently stained.
- Alert patient receiving ethambutol to take daily single doses to avoid visual problems. Divided doses of ethambutol may cause visual disturbances.

Cultural Considerations

- Increase access to health care. Community involvement and culturally sensitive patient education are important. Explain to patients who have active tuberculosis that family members should get a TB skin test and may receive a prophylactic drug for 6 months to 1 year. Emphasize the importance of family members seeking medical care.
- Provide a written sheet for drug and treatment regimens in the language patient speaks or reads most easily. Explain importance of good hygiene (e.g., discarding tissues that contain sputum, separating dishes, using a dishwasher to clean dishes if possible).
- Understand significance of community if multiple individuals in the same community are treated for latent tuberculosis infection. Make all attempts to place community members on a treatment plan to increase compliance through social support.

Evaluation

- Evaluate effectiveness of the antitubercular drugs. Sputum specimen for acid-fast bacilli should be negative after taking antitubercular drugs for several weeks or months.

ANTIFUNGAL DRUGS

An infection caused by a fungus is also called *mycosis.* A fungal or mycotic infection may be superficial or systemic. Superficial fungal infections are acquired via contact with an infected person. Fungi, known as *dermatophytes,* cause superficial fungal infections involving the integumentary system, including mucous membranes, hair, nails, and moist skin areas. An overgrowth of nonsusceptible microorganisms in normal flora following antibiotic treatment may also cause a superficial fungal infection. When *Candida albicans* affects the mouth, it is called *oral candidiasis* or *thrush.* Vaginal candidiasis is common in women who are pregnant, diabetic, or taking antibiotics or oral contraceptives. Systemic fungal infections may involve the lungs, CNS, or abdomen. They are usually transmitted to an individual through inhalation into the lungs from dust, soil, or animal droppings. Fungal infections may be mild, such as tinea pedis (athlete's foot), or severe, such as pulmonary conditions or meningitis.

Fungal infections are also classified as *opportunistic* or *nonopportunistic infections.* **Opportunistic infections** usually occur in the immunocompromised or debilitated population (e.g., patients who have cancer or AIDS) or those taking antibiotics, corticosteroids, chemotherapy, or other immunosuppressives. Fungi such as the *Candida* spp. (yeast) are part of the normal flora of the mouth, skin, intestine, and vagina. An opportunistic infection such as *candidiasis* may occur when the body's defense mechanisms are impaired, allowing overgrowth of the fungus. Other opportunistic infections are *aspergillosis, cryptococcosis,* and *mucormycosis.* Nonopportunistic infections, such as *sporotrichosis, blastomycosis, histoplasmosis,* and *coccidioidomycosis,* can occur in any individual.

Antifungal drugs, also called **antimycotic drugs,** are used to treat fungal infections. Typically, antifungals are fungistatic or fungicidal depending upon the susceptibility of the fungus and the dosage. The antifungal drugs are classified into the following groups (Table 32-3):

- Polyenes (e.g., amphotericin B, nystatin)
- Azoles (e.g., ketoconazole)
- Antimetabolites (e.g., flucytosine)
- Echinocandins (e.g., caspofungin)
- Antiprotozoals (e.g., atovaquone)

Polyenes

Amphotericin B

The polyene antifungal drug of choice for severe systemic infection is amphotericin B. Introduced in 1956 and used currently with close supervision because of its toxicity, amphotericin B is effective against numerous fungal diseases, including *histoplasmosis, cryptococcosis, coccidioidomycosis, aspergillosis, blastomycosis,* and *candidiasis* (systemic infection).

TABLE 32-3 ANTIFUNGAL DRUGS

GENERIC (BRAND)	ROUTE AND DOSAGE	USES AND CONSIDERATIONS
Polyenes		
amphotericin B (Fungizone)	A: IV: 0.3-1 mg/kg/d diluted in 500 mL D_5W over 2-6 h for 7-14 days using an inline filter and protection from light; *max:* 1.5 mg/kg/d	For a variety of systemic fungal (mycotic) infections, such as aspergillosis, blastomycosis, coccidioidomycosis, cryptococcosis, and histoplasmosis. Requires pretreatment with diphenhydramine, acetaminophen or ibuprofen, hydrocortisone. Nephrotoxicity may occur when given in high doses. Hypokalemia may occur. Pregnancy category: B; PB: 90%; t½: 24 h
nystatin (Mycostatin)	Intestinal infections: A: PO: 500,000-1,000,000 units t.i.d.	For *Candida* infections. Pregnancy category: C; PB: UK; t½: UK
Azoles		
fluconazole (Diflucan)	See Prototype Drug Chart 32-2.	
itraconazole (Sporanox)	A: PO: 200-400 mg/d	For various systemic fungal infections, particularly blastomycosis and histoplasmosis. Pregnancy category: C; PB: 99%; t½: 34-42 h
ketoconazole (Nizoral)	A: PO: 200-400 mg/d as single dose C >2 y: PO: 3.3-6.6 mg/kg/d as single dose	For *Candida* spp., histoplasmosis, blastomycosis, and other infections. Treatment may last 1 to 6 months for systemic infections. Take with food to avoid GI discomfort. Pregnancy category: C; PB: 84%-99%; t½: 2-8 h
miconazole nitrate (Monistat)	A/C >12 y: Intravaginal supp: 100 mg vaginal h.s. for 7 d; 200 mg for 3 d; 1200 mg single dose	For fungal meningitis and fungal bladder infections. Also for vaginal fungal infections. Pregnancy category: C; PB: 92%; t½: 24 h
voriconazole (Vfend)	A/C >40 kg: PO: 400 mg q12h on day 1, then 200 mg q12h C <40 kg: PO: 200 mg q12h on day 1, then 100 mg q12h A/C: IV: 6 mg/kg q12h on day 1, then 3-4 mg/kg q12h	For *Aspergillus* infection. Pregnancy category: D; PB: 58%; t½: 6 h
posaconazole (Noxafil)	A: PO: 100 mg/d up to-200 mg t.i.d. for 14-21 d	For prophylactic treatment of invasive *Aspergillus* and *Candida* infections in immunosuppressed patients. Pregnancy category: C; PB: 98%; t½: 35 h

Continued

TABLE 32-3 ANTIFUNGAL DRUGS—cont'd

GENERIC (BRAND)	ROUTE AND DOSAGE	USES AND CONSIDERATIONS
Antimetabolites		
flucytosine (Ancobon)	A: PO: 25 mg/kg q.i.d. for 7-10 d; *max:* 150 mg/kg/d TDM: 50-150 mcg/mL	Use with amphotericin B may increase therapeutic action as well as toxicity. Fungal resistance occurs if drug is given alone. Pregnancy category: C; PB: 2%-4%; $t\frac{1}{2}$: 3-6 h
Echinocandins		
caspofungin (Cancidas)	Loading dose: A: IV: 70 mg on day 1 Maintenance dose: A: IV: 50 mg/d over 1 h for 7-14 d	For *Aspergillus* infection. Pregnancy category: C; PB: 97%; $t\frac{1}{2}$: 9-11 h
micafungin (Mycamine)	A: IV: 100-150 mg/d over 1 h for 14-21 d	For esophageal candidiasis and prevention of *Candida* infection in patients having bone marrow transplantation. May cause GI distress, headache, and elevated liver enzymes. Pregnancy category: C; PB: 99%; $t\frac{1}{2}$: 14-17 h
anidulafungin (Eraxis)	Esophageal candidiasis: A: IV: 100 mg loading dose on day 1, then 50 mg/d IV for 7-14 days after last positive culture Other candidiasis infections: A: IV: 200 mg loading dose on day 1, then 100 mg/d IV for 14 days after last positive culture	For esophageal candidiasis, candidemia, and other *Candida* infections. Pregnancy category: C; PB: 99%; $t\frac{1}{2}$: 30-60 min
Antiprotozoals		
atovaquone (Mepron)	A: PO: 750 mg b.i.d. with food × 21 d	For mild to moderate *Pneumocystis carinii* pneumonia. Pregnancy category: C; PB: 99%; $t\frac{1}{2}$: 2-3 d
tinidazole (Tindamax)	A: PO: 2 g as a single dose for 3 days with food C >3 y: PO: 50 mg/kg as single dose for 3 days with food; *max:* 2 g	For giardiasis, intestinal amebiasis, trichomoniasis, and bacterial vaginosis. Pregnancy category: D (first trimester) and C (second and third trimesters); PB: 12%; $t\frac{1}{2}$: 12-14 h
Miscellaneous Antifungals		
griseofulvin (Fulvicin)	A: PO: 300-500; *max:* 750 mg microsize/d	For tinea capitis, tinea corporis, and tinea cruris. Pregnancy category: C; PB: UK; $t\frac{1}{2}$: 9-24 h

A, Adult; *b.i.d.,* twice a day; *C,* child; *d,* day; D_5W, 5% dextrose in water; *GI,* gastrointestinal; *h,* hour; *h.s.,* at bedtime; *inf,* infusion; *IV,* intravenous; *maint,* maintenance; *max,* maximum; *min,* minute; *mo,* month; *PB,* protein-binding; *PO,* by mouth; *supp,* suppository; $t\frac{1}{2}$, half-life; *TDM,* therapeutic drug monitoring; *t.i.d.,* three times a day; *UK,* unknown; *y,* year; >, greater than; <, less than.

Polyene antifungals act by binding to the fungal cell membrane and forming open channels that increase cell permeability and leakage of intracellular components, especially potassium.

Pharmacokinetics Amphotericin B is highly protein-bound and has a long half-life. Only 5% of the drug is excreted in the urine. Renal disease does not affect the excretion of amphotericin B.

Pharmacodynamics Amphotericin B is not absorbed from the GI tract; therefore it is administered IV in low doses for treating systemic fungal infections. Peak effect occurs 1 to 2 hours after IV infusion, and the duration is 20 hours.

Side Effects and Adverse Reactions

Side effects and adverse reactions for amphotericin B include flush, fever, chills, nausea, vomiting, hypotension, paresthesias, and thrombophlebitis. Amphotericin B is considered *highly toxic* and can cause nephrotoxicity and electrolyte imbalance, especially hypokalemia and hypomagnesemia (low serum potassium and magnesium levels). Urinary output, blood urea nitrogen, and serum creatinine levels need to be closely monitored.

Nystatin

Nystatin (Mycostatin), another polyene antifungal drug, is administered orally or topically to treat *Candida* infection. It is available in suspensions, cream, ointment, and vaginal tablets. Nystatin is poorly absorbed via the GI tract; however, the oral tablet form is used for intestinal candidiasis. The more common use of nystatin is in oral suspension for *Candida* infection in the mouth. The patient is instructed to swish the liquid within the mouth, making contact with the mucous membrane, and then to swallow the liquid after a few minutes. If the throat area is involved, instruct the patient to gargle with nystatin after swishing and before swallowing.

Pharmacokinetics Nystatin is poorly absorbed. Its protein-binding power and half-life are unknown. The drug is excreted unchanged in the feces.

Pharmacodynamics Nystatin increases permeability of the fungal cell membrane, thus causing the fungal cell to become unstable and to discharge its content. This drug has a fungistatic and fungicidal action. The onset of action for both the suspension and tablet is rapid. The onset of action for vaginal tablet or cream is approximately 24 or more hours.

Azole Group

The azole group is effective against candidiasis (superficial and systemic), coccidioidomycosis, cryptococcosis, histoplasmosis, and paracoccidioidomycosis. Ketoconazole was the first effective antifungal drug that was orally absorbed. Fluconazole and itraconazole are also azole drugs used to treat systemic fungal infection. These antifungals can be taken orally, unlike amphotericin B and caspofungin, which are by IV route only. Fluconazole, a systemic azole antifungal agent, is described in Prototype Drug Chart 32-2.

Azoles inhibit cytochrome P450 in fungal cells, interfering with the formation of ergosterol. Because ergosterol is a major sterol in the fungal cell membrane, cell permeability and leakage are increased. Numerous azoles are used in topical preparations to treat candidiasis and the tinea infections. These drugs are available in forms of vaginal tablet, cream, ointment, and solution. Topical antifungal agents (azoles and others) are presented in Table 32-4.

HERBAL ALERT 32-1

Ketoconazole

When ketoconazole is taken with the herb echinacea, hepatotoxicity may develop.

Antimetabolite

The antimetabolite flucytosine acts by selectively penetrating the fungal cell, which converts it into fluorouracil, an antimetabolite that disrupts fungal DNA and RNA synthesis. It is well absorbed from the GI tract. Flucytosine is used in combination with other antifungal drugs, such as amphotericin B (see Table 32-3).

Echinocandins

The action of echinocandins is to inhibit biosynthesis of essential components of the fungal cell wall, which interferes with growth and reproduction. Caspofungin (Cancidas) is used to treat *Candida* and *Aspergillus* infections. This drug is only administered IV because it is not absorbed in the GI tract. Phlebitis at the IV site and increased AST and ALT are common adverse effects.

Antiprotozoal

Atovaquone (Mepron) is an antiprotozoal agent used to treat mild to moderate *Pneumocystis carinii* pneumonia. This drug acts by disrupting mitochondrial electron transport and inhibiting DNA synthesis.

PROTOTYPE DRUG CHART 32-2

Fluconazole

Drug Class Antifungal Trade Name: Diflucan Pregnancy Category: C	**Dosage** A: PO/IV: 400 mg/d × 1, then 200-400 mg/d for 4 wk C: PO/IV: 12 mg/kg on day 1, then 6-12 mg/kg q72h
Contraindications Hypersensitivity Caution: Pregnancy	**Drug-Lab-Food Interactions** Drug: Increases PT when taking warfarin; increases hypoglycemia when taken with oral sulfonylureas; increases phenytoin, cyclosporine, and haloperidol levels; decreases fluconazole level with cimetidine and rifampin
Pharmacokinetics Absorption: PO: Well absorbed in GI tract Distribution: PB: 12% Metabolism: t½: 20-50 h Excretion: In urine	**Pharmacodynamics** PO: Onset: UK Peak: 1-2 h Duration: UK Vag: Onset: UK Peak: UK Duration: UK
Therapeutic Effects/Uses To treat *Candida* infections and cryptococcal meningitis Mode of Action: Increase permeability of the fungal cell membrane	
Side Effects PO: Anorexia, nausea, vomiting, diarrhea (large doses), stomach cramps, rash, headache Vaginal: Rash, burning sensation	**Adverse Reactions** None known

A, Adult; *C*, child; *d*, day; *GI*, gastrointestinal; *h*, hour; *IV*, intravenous; *PB*, protein-binding; *PO*, by mouth; *PT*, prothrombin time; *t ½*, half-life; *UK*, unknown; *wk*, week.

TABLE 32-4 TOPICAL ANTIFUNGAL AGENTS FOR FUNGAL INFECTIONS

DRUG	DRUG FORM	CANDIDIASIS	TINEA INFECTIONS: TINEA PEDIS	TINEA CRURIS	TINEA CORPORIS
Azoles					
butoconazole nitrate (Femstat)	2% vaginal cream	X			
clotrimazole (Femcare, Mycelex, Gyne-Lotrimin)	1% topical cream; vaginal tablet; PO: 1 troche (lozenge)	X	X	X	X
econazole (Spectazole)	1% topical cream	X	X	X	X
miconazole nitrate (Monistat, Micatin)	Vaginal suppository; 2% vaginal cream	X			
oxiconazole (Oxistat)	Cream		X	X	X
sulconazole (Exelderm)	Cream; solution		X	X	X
terconazole (Terazol-3)	Vaginal suppository; 0.4% and 0.8% vaginal cream	X			
Other Topical Antifungals					
ciclopirox olamine (Loprox)	Cream; lotion	X	X	X	X
haloprogin (Halotex)	1% cream; solution		X	X	X
naftifine (Naftin)	1% cream; gel		X	X	X
terbinafine HCl (Lamisil)	1% cream		X	X	X
tolnaftate (Aftate)	1% cream, gel, solution		X	X	X
sertaconazole (Ertaczo)	2% cream		X		

PO, By mouth.

Nursing Process
Patient-Centered Collaborative Care

Antifungals

Assessment
- Obtain a medical history from patient of any serious renal or hepatic disorder. Antifungal agents such as amphotericin B, fluconazole (Diflucan), flucytosine (Ancobon), and ketoconazole (Nizoral) are contraindicated if patient has a serious renal or liver disease.
- Check laboratory tests for liver enzyme values (alkaline phosphatase [ALP], alanine aminotransferase [ALT], aspartate aminotransferase [AST], gamma-glutamyl transferase [GGT]), blood urea nitrogen (BUN), bilirubin, and serum creatinine. Elevated levels can indicate liver or renal dysfunction. Use these test results for future comparison.
- Assess prior use of antifungals.
- Record baseline vital signs for future comparison.

Nursing Diagnoses
- Risk for infection related to poor health practices
- Impaired urinary elimination related to adverse effects of antifungals
- Deficient fluid volume related to side effects of antifungals

Planning
- Patient's fungal infection will be resolved.

Nursing Interventions
- Obtain a culture to determine fungus type (e.g., *Candida*).
- Monitor patient's urinary output; many antifungal drugs may cause nephrotoxicity.
- Check laboratory results, and compare with baseline findings (BUN, serum creatinine, ALP, ALT, AST, bilirubin, electrolytes). Certain antifungals could cause hepatotoxicity as well as nephrotoxicity when taking high doses over a prolonged period.
- Record vital signs. Compare with baseline findings.
- Observe for side effects and adverse reactions to antifungal drugs (antimycotics): nausea, vomiting, headache, phlebitis, signs and symptoms of electrolyte imbalance (hypokalemia with amphotericin B).

Patient Teaching

General
- Advise patient to take drug as prescribed. Compliance is of utmost importance, because discontinuing drug too soon may result in relapse.
- Monitor laboratory testing of serum liver enzymes, BUN, creatinine, and electrolytes.
- Inform patient taking ketoconazole not to consume alcohol.

Self-Administration
- Educate patient on administration of nystatin (Mycostatin) suspension: Place nystatin dose, usually 1 to 2 teaspoons, in the mouth. Swish solution in the mouth, and swallow afterward (swish and swallow).

Side Effects

- Teach patient to avoid operating hazardous equipment or a motor vehicle when taking amphotericin B, ketoconazole, or flucytosine, because these drugs may cause visual changes, sleepiness, dizziness, or lethargy.
- Encourage patient to report side effects (e.g., nausea, vomiting, diarrhea, dermatitis, rash, dizziness, tinnitus, edema, flatulence). These symptoms may occur when taking certain antifungal drugs.

Cultural Considerations

- Some cultures may not understand the purpose and procedure for the use of vaginal tablets or creams. A detailed explanation may be needed.
- Respect patient's apprehension and fear concerning the use of topical antifungal drugs and the desire to use alternative methods. Evaluate patient's method of topical administration in regard to safe practice. If the method is considered unsafe, explain why and suggest modifications. If appropriate, involve other persons for clarification.

Evaluation

- Evaluate the effectiveness of the antifungal (antimycotic) drug by noting the absence of the fungal infection (e.g., decrease in itching, redness, and rawness).

PEPTIDES

The two groups of **peptides** used as antibiotics are the polymyxins and bacitracin. Peptides are derived from cultures of *Bacillus subtilis,* and this group appears to interfere with bacterial cell membrane function.

Polymyxins

Polymyxins were one of the early groups of antibacterials, but many of the early drugs were discontinued because they caused nephrotoxicity. Polymyxin B is approved for pharmaceutical use. Polymyxins produce a bactericidal effect by interfering with the cell membrane of the bacterium, thereby causing cell death. They affect most gram-negative bacteria, such as *Pseudomonas aeruginosa, Escherichia coli, Klebsiella* spp., and *Shigella* spp.

Except for colistin, which exerts action on the colon and is excreted in the feces, the polymyxins are not absorbed through the oral route. Intramuscular injection of polymyxins produces marked pain at the injection site; therefore IV administration of polymyxins at a slow infusion rate is the suggested method. Table 32-5 lists the polymyxins with their dosage and uses.

Severe Adverse Effects

High serum levels of polymyxins can cause nephrotoxicity and neurotoxicity. With nephrotoxicity, the blood urea nitrogen and serum creatinine levels are elevated; however, when the serum drug level decreases, renal toxicity is usually reversed. Signs and symptoms of **neurotoxicity** (toxicity of the nerves) include **paresthesias** (abnormal sensations such as numbness, tingling, burning, and prickling) and dizziness. Neurotoxicity is usually reversible when the drug is discontinued.

Bacitracin

Bacitracin has a polypeptide structure and acts by inhibiting bacterial cell-wall synthesis and damaging the cell-wall membrane. The drug action can be bacteriostatic or bactericidal. Bacitracin is not absorbed by the GI tract and, if given orally, is excreted in the feces. Bacitracin is effective against most gram-positive bacteria and some gram-negative bacteria. Over-the-counter (OTC) bacitracin ointment is available for application to the skin.

Side Effects and Adverse Reactions

The side effects of bacitracin include redness, rash, nausea, and vomiting. Severe adverse reactions are renal damage and

TABLE 32-5 ANTIBACTERIALS: PEPTIDES

GENERIC (BRAND)	ROUTE AND DOSAGE	USES AND CONSIDERATIONS
Peptides		
Bacitracin (BaciiM, Baci-RX)	A/C: topical: Apply thin layer b.i.d. or t.i.d. A/C: ophthalmic ointment: Apply thin film to affected eye q3-4 h for 7-10 days	Topical ointment for skin infections; ophthalmic ointment for eye infections. Pregnancy category: C; PB: <20%; $t\frac{1}{2}$: UK
colistimethate sodium (Coly-Mycin M)	A/C: IM/IV: 2.5-5 mg/kg/d in divided doses; *max:* 5 mg/kg/d	For *Pseudomonas aeruginosa* infection. Pregnancy category: C; PB: UK; $t\frac{1}{2}$: 2-3 h
Additional Antibacterial Agents		
metronidazole (Flagyl, MetroGel)	A: PO: 250 mg t.i.d. or 500 mg b.i.d. for 7 days A: topical: Apply thin film to cleansed affected area	For serious gram-negative infections (e.g., UTI, septicemia, bacteremia, meningitis, *Pseudomonas aeruginosa,* skin infections) when other antibiotics are ineffective or contraindicated. Side effects may include GI discomfort, headache, and depression. Pregnancy category: B; PB: 10%; $t\frac{1}{2}$: 6-8 h

A, Adult; *C,* child; *d,* day; *h,* hour; *IM,* intramuscular; *IV,* intravenous; *PB,* protein-binding; *sol,* solution; $t\frac{1}{2}$, half-life; *UK,* unknown; *y,* year; >, greater than; <, less than.

ototoxicity. Mild to severe allergic reactions ranging from hives to anaphylaxis may occur.

METRONIDAZOLE

Metronidazole (Flagyl) acts by impairing DNA function of susceptible bacteria. This drug is used primarily to treat various disorders associated with organisms in the GI tract. It is prescribed to treat intestinal amebiasis, trichomoniasis, inflammatory bowel disease, anaerobic infections, and bacterial vaginosis and is used as perioperative **prophylaxis** (prevention of infection) in colorectal surgery. Metronidazole is commonly used with other agents to treat *Helicobacter pylori*, which is associated with frequent recurrent peptic ulcers. Table 32-5 includes data related to metronidazole. The patient taking metronidazole should avoid alcohol and alcohol-containing medications for at least 48 hours after treatment is completed. Drug interaction with alcohol may produce a *disulfiram reaction* (facial flushing, severe headache, tachycardia, palpitations, hypotension, dyspnea, sweating, slurred speech, abdominal cramps, nausea, and vomiting).

Side Effects and Adverse Reactions

The side effects and adverse reactions of metronidazole include dizziness, headache, confusion, depression, irritability, weakness, and insomnia. The patient taking high doses of metronidazole may develop dark or reddish-brown urine. Dry mouth, metallic or bitter taste, and GI distress may occur. Paresthesias, nasal congestion, decreased libido, dysuria, incontinence, and ECG changes may develop.

KEY WEBSITES

Information on isoniazid: *www.nlm.nih.gov/medlineplus/druginfo/meds/a682401.html*

Information on fluconazole: *www.nlm.nih.gov/medlineplus/druginfo/meds/a690002.html*

CRITICAL THINKING CASE STUDY

CJ, a 41-year-old man, has had a constant cough and night sweats for several months. He consumes 1 pint of whiskey per day. Sputum is positive for acid-fast (tubercle) bacillus. The health care provider orders a 6- to 9-month antitubercular drug regimen (time of therapy to be determined according to sputum and radiograph test results). For 2 months, CJ takes isoniazid, rifampin, and pyrazinamide daily. The next 4 to 7 months, CJ takes isoniazid and rifampin biweekly.

1. What could be contributing causes for CJ's contracting tuberculosis? Give other contributing causes for contracting tuberculosis.
2. CJ received first-line antitubercular drugs for treatment of tuberculosis. How can the health professional determine whether the drugs are effective in eradicating the tubercle bacilli? Explain your answer.
3. What is the nurse's role in patient teaching concerning the drug regimen?
4. Name at least two serious adverse reactions that can occur when antitubercular drugs are given over an extended period.
5. What laboratory tests should be monitored while CJ takes isoniazid and rifampin? Why?

The health care provider orders pyridoxine to be given daily.

6. Give the rationale for the use of pyridoxine. What type of drug is it? What is its purpose, and when should it be administered?
7. What health agencies may the nurse suggest that could be helpful to CJ during and after therapy?

NCLEX STUDY QUESTIONS

1. A patient is beginning isoniazid and rifampin treatment for tuberculosis. The nurse gives the patient which instruction?
   a. Do not skip doses.
   b. Take the drugs t.i.d. with food.
   c. Take an antacid with the drugs to decrease GI distress.
   d. Take rifampin initially, and then begin isoniazid after 2 months.
2. A patient is taking isoniazid and is worried about the side effects. Which of the following does the nurse realize is an adverse effect of isoniazid?
   a. Ototoxicity
   b. Hepatotoxicity
   c. Nephrotoxicity
   d. Optic nerve toxicity

3. The nurse teaches a patient taking amphotericin B to report which signs and symptoms to the health care provider?
   a. Change in sight
   b. Decrease in hearing
   c. Decrease in urine
   d. Painful red rash and blisters
4. A patient with a diagnosis of intestinal amebiasis develops severe nausea, vomiting, fever, facial flushing, slurred speech, tachycardia, hypotension, and palpitations. An assessment reveals that the patient has just had several alcoholic beverages. The nurse should obtain a drug history for which drug?
   a. bacitracin (Baci-IM)
   b. fluconazole (Diflucan)
   c. metronidazole (Flagyl)
   d. ethambutol (Myambutol)
5. A patient has developed vaginal candidiasis. The nurse knows that which medication is appropriate treatment for this condition?
   a. terconazole (Terazol-3)
   b. haloprogin (Halotex)
   c. terbinafine (Lamisil)
   d. tolnaftate (Aftate)
6. A patient has been diagnosed with tuberculosis and is to begin the antitubercular medications isoniazid, rifampin, and ethambutol. What should the nurse do? (Select all that apply.)
   a. Encourage periodic eye examinations.
   b. Instruct the patient to take medications with meals.
   c. Suggest that the patient take antacids with medications to prevent GI distress.
   d. Advise the patient to report numbness and tingling of the hands or feet.
   e. Alert the patient that body fluids may develop a red-orange color.
   f. Teach the patient to avoid direct sunlight and to use sun block.

Answers: 1, a; 2, b; 3, c; 4, c; 5, a; 6, a, d, e, f.

CHAPTER

33

Antivirals, Antimalarials, and Anthelmintics

evolve WEBSITE

http://evolve.elsevier.com/KeeHayes/pharmacology/

- Animations
- Content Updates
- Key Points
- Review Questions for the NCLEX® Examination
- References from the Textbook
- Unfolding Case Studies

OBJECTIVES

- Explain the uses of antiviral and antimalarial drugs.
- Describe the various helminths and the human body sites used for their infestation.
- Differentiate the action of antivirals, antimalarials, and anthelmintics.
- Compare the side effects and adverse reactions of antiviral, antimalarial, and anthelmintic drugs.
- Apply the nursing process for the patient taking antimalarial and anthelmintic drug therapy.

OUTLINE

KEY TERMS

VIRUSES

Viruses are more difficult to eradicate than most types of bacteria. A **virus** is an obligate intracellular organism that must reside within a living host cell to survive and reproduce. Viruses enter healthy cells and use their deoxyribonucleic acid (DNA) and ribonucleic acid (RNA) to generate more viruses. The growth cycle of viruses depends on the host cell enzymes and cell substrates for viral replication. Viruses live and reproduce when they are within living cells. Examples of common viral infections include influenza, herpes virus infections, and viral hepatitis infections.

Viral Infections

Influenza, also called *the flu,* is a highly contagious viral infection that affects the nose, throat, and lungs. This virus is seasonal and more prevalent from fall to spring. Influenza has three antigen types: A, B, and C. Influenza A causes a moderate to severe infection. Influenza B usually causes mild illness in children. Influenza C is very rare in humans. This viral infection is transmitted easily via contaminated droplets during coughing, sneezing, or talking. Droplets enter into the respiratory tract of the unaffected person and begin replication 24 hours before the appearance of symptoms. Usually influenza has an abrupt onset with the first symptoms being high fever, headache, fatigue, and myalgia (muscle aches). A sore throat, nonproductive cough, watery nasal discharge, weakness, red watery eyes, chills, and photophobia may also occur.

Herpesviruses are large viruses that cause infections. Among the most familiar are herpes simplex virus type 1 (HSV-1) and type 2 (HSV-2); varicella-zoster viruses (HSV-3 or VZV), more commonly known as *chickenpox* and *shingles*; Epstein-Barr virus (HSV-4 or EBV); and cytomegalovirus (HHV-5 or CMV). HSV-1 is usually associated with cold sores (vesicular lesions), which grow in neurons. The HSV-1 virus is capable of latency (ability to maintain disease potential without signs and symptoms). HSV-2 is usually associated with vesicular lesions and small ulcerations on the genitalia (genital herpes). The HSV-2 virus remains dormant by traveling through the peripheral nerves to the sacral dorsal root ganglia. The virus can be transported back the nerve root to the skin for reactivation at any time. While dormant, the virus continues to replicate. Both HSV-1 and HSV-2 are capable of causing recurrent infections. Both viruses can replicate in the mucous membranes and skin of the oropharynx or genitalia. The virus is transmitted by contact with infectious lesions or secretions. HSV-1 is spread by oral secretions from one individual to another. From the mouth, this virus can spread to the genital area by oral intercourse or poor hand washing. HSV-2 is usually spread by intimate sexual contact, or an infected mother can transmit the virus to her infant during childbirth. When signs and symptoms are present, they usually include eruption of small pustules and vesicles; fever; headache; malaise; myalgia; as well as tingling, itching, and pain in the genital area.

The varicella zoster virus (VZV or HSV-3) causes chickenpox and shingles. Chickenpox is a highly contagious viral infection that causes generalized pruritic vesicles and fever. It has become less common since a vaccine was developed; however, some outbreaks still occur. Shingles is a painful vesicular rash that can remain dormant in nerve cells. When a person who has previously been infected with chickenpox becomes older or develops a weakened immune system, the VZV can reactivate causing an outbreak along the region of skin innervated by the nerve where the virus resides. In addition to the rash, the patient may also develop fever, malaise, and myalgia.

Epstein-Barr virus (EBV or HSV-4) most commonly causes infectious mononucleosis, a condition manifested by fever, tonsillitis, and enlarged lymph nodes in the neck. EBV resides in lymphocytes, epithelial cells, and muscle cells and has a latency period.

Cytomegalovirus (CMV or HHV-5) is a very common infectious disease worldwide. It is thought that most adults have had this viral infection at one time and are unaware. Most individuals do not require treatment for CMV unless they are immunocompromised (e.g., babies or individuals who have had organ transplantations). CMV is transmitted via body fluids, especially saliva or urine; by kissing, sexual contact, or sharing food; or by a pregnant patient to the fetus. In susceptible individuals, CMV infection can lead to fatal pneumonia or blindness (due to an infected retina).

Hepatitis B (HBV) is a serious liver infection caused by the hepatitis B virus. The transmission of HBV is usually via a needlestick, intimate sexual contact, or childbirth. HBV is found in all body fluids, including blood, semen, and vaginal fluid. The signs and symptoms of HBV include anorexia, vomiting, diarrhea, jaundice, malaise, and myalgia.

A viral infection usually can be detected only after the virus has replicated itself. Viruses can cause mild to severe infections. General signs and symptoms of an acute viral infection include headache, low-grade fever (with a mild viral infection), nausea, vomiting, diarrhea, muscular pain, fatigue, and cough.

VACCINES

Vaccines are pharmacologic preparations that have been developed to provide immunity against and prevent diseases, such as smallpox, chickenpox, mumps, rabies, and influenza (see Chapter 36). The influenza virus vaccine may change annually because influenza (flu) virus changes its genetic structure each year. However, the influenza vaccine still promotes the production of antibodies by the immune system, despite the viruses' varying genetic structures. After influenza vaccination (flu shot), most individuals develop high antibody titer levels providing protection against similar circulating viral strains. Eggs are used to produce the flu vaccine; therefore any allergies to eggs should be determined before flu vaccine is administered to the patient. The success rate of vaccine use to prevent influenza in healthy children and adults is 65% to 90%. In older adults, vaccines are effective 60% of the time, but less than 60% if an older adult has multiple health problems.

DIAGNOSTIC TESTS FOR INFLUENZA

Several office laboratory tests can be used to diagnose influenza. The diagnostic test Directigen Flu A has been available for many years to detect influenza A; however, it does not detect influenza B. Flu OIA, QuickVue Influenza Test, and ZstatFlu are diagnostic tests that identify both influenza A and B. These tests use throat swabs, nasal swabs, or nasal aspiration. Results are available within 10 to 20 minutes. QuickVue tends to be easy and fast for a rapid diagnosis of influenza A and B.

ANTIVIRAL NON-HIV DRUGS

Antiviral drugs are used to prevent or delay the spread of a viral infection. They inhibit viral replication by interfering with viral nucleic acid synthesis in the cell. There are groups of antiviral drugs effective against various viruses, such as influenza A and B, herpes species, cytomegalovirus (CMV), and human immunodeficiency virus (HIV). Drugs for HIV are discussed in Chapter 35. The non-HIV antiviral drugs are listed in Table 33-1. Interferon alfa-2a and 2b are used to treat hepatitis B and C viruses (see Chapter 39).

Nonclassified Antivirals

The first two related antivirals, amantidine hydrochloride and rimantadine hydrochloride (Flumadine), were used to treat type A influenza. Both these antivirals are *nonclassified antivirals.* Originally, amantidine was used to treat parkinsonism and only later was found to be effective against influenza A. Neither amantidine nor rimantadine are effective against type B influenza. Three other nonclassified antivirals are (1) cidofovir, which is used to treat CMV retinitis; (2) foscarnet (Foscavir), which is used to treat HIV retinitis and herpes simplex infection in patients with **acquired immunodeficiency syndrome** (AIDS) (immune disorder characterized by opportunistic diseases); and (3) vidarabine (Vira-A), which is used to treat herpesvirus. In the late 1990s, the U.S. Food and Drug Administration (FDA) approved zanamivir (Relenza) and oseltamivir phosphate (Tamiflu), two drugs that inhibit the replication and spread of the influenza virus if given within 48 hours of symptoms; thus, early diagnosis of influenza is important.

Side Effects and Adverse Reactions

The side effects and adverse reactions to amantadine include central nervous system (CNS) effects, such as insomnia, depression, anxiety, confusion, and ataxia; orthostatic hypotension; neurologic problems, such as weakness, dizziness, and slurred speech; and gastrointestinal (GI) disturbances, such as anorexia, nausea, vomiting, and diarrhea. The CNS side effects of rimantadine occur less often than with amantadine.

Topical Antivirals

There are three topical antiviral drugs: idoxuridine (Herplex Liquifilm), penciclovir (Denavir), and trifluridine (Viroptic). These topical agents are used to treat herpes simplex viruses.

Neuraminidase Inhibitors

Neuraminidase inhibitors are a group of drugs that decrease the release of the virus from infected cells, thus decreasing viral spread and shortening the duration of flu symptoms. Zanamivir (Relenza) and oseltamivir phosphate (Tamiflu) are two neuraminidase inhibitors that should be taken within 48 hours of flu symptoms. These drugs inhibit the activity of neuraminidase, a viral glycoprotein, and are effective against type A and B influenza viruses. Zanamivir and oseltamivir phosphate are not substitutes for the "flu shot."

Gamma Globulin (Immune Globulin)

Gamma globulin (IgG) is rich in antibodies found in the blood. It provides a passive form of immunity to a virus by blocking the penetration of the virus into the host cell. It is administered during the early infectious stage of an illness to prevent a viral invasion in the body.

Human immune globulin (Gamastan) is administered intramuscularly (IM). A single-dose injection protects for approximately 2 to 3 weeks; it may be repeated 2 to 3 weeks following the first dose. For patients who need an immediate increase in immune globulin levels, intravenous (IV) immune globulin (Gamimune N) may be administered.

Purine Nucleosides

The synthetic purine nucleoside antiviral group is effective in interfering with the steps of viral nucleic acid (DNA) synthesis. Drugs in this group of nucleoside analogs include ribavirin (Virazole), acyclovir (Zovirax), famciclovir (Famvir), ganciclovir sodium (Cytovene), and valacyclovir (Valtrex). These drugs are effective in combating herpes simplex viruses (HSV-1, HSV-2), herpes zoster (shingles), varicella-zoster virus (chickenpox), and CMV. Valganciclovir (Valcyte) is a prodrug of ganciclovir and is effective for treating CMV retinitis in patients with AIDS.

The antiviral drug ribavirin was first marketed in 1986. It is used to treat respiratory syncytial virus (RSV) in children and respiratory infections caused by the influenza A and B viruses in older adults. Ribavirin is administered by aerosol.

Acyclovir

Acyclovir was introduced as an antineoplastic drug and later was found to be effective against herpesvirus, especially HSV-2, but also against HSV-1, herpes zoster (shingles), and CMV (which can cause congenital defects). There has been reported resistance to acyclovir as a result of the lack of viral-producing enzyme (thymidine kinase) needed to convert the drug to an effective antiviral compound. Prototype Drug Chart 33-1 lists the drug data for acyclovir sodium.

Pharmacokinetics Acyclovir is slowly absorbed, depending on the dose, and is widely distributed to body and organ tissues. Half the drug passes into the cerebrospinal fluid. The drug is 10% to 30% protein-bound. Its half-life is 2 to 3 hours with normal renal function. Acyclovir is excreted unchanged in the urine.

Pharmacodynamics Acyclovir interferes with the viral synthesis of DNA, thereby short-circuiting its replication. The onset of action for the oral preparation is unknown; for the intravenous (IV) route, the onset is rapid. Peak concentration time is within 2 hours for both routes of administration, and the duration of action for both is similar.

Probenecid can increase the effect of acyclovir. If an aminoglycoside or amphotericin B is taken with acyclovir, the incidence of nephrotoxicity is increased.

TABLE 33-1 NON-HIV ANTIVIRALS

GENERIC (BRAND)	ROUTE AND DOSAGE	USES AND CONSIDERATIONS
Systemic Non-HIV Antivirals		
Nonclassified Antivirals		
amantadine HCl	Influenza A: A <65 y/C >9 y: PO: 200 mg/d in 1-2 divided doses Older adults >65 y: 100 mg/d C 1-8 y: PO: 5 mg/kg/d in 2 divided doses	Primary use is prophylaxis against influenza A. Well absorbed by GI tract. Pregnancy category: C; PB: UK; t½: 11-15 h
cidofovir (Vistide)	A: IV: 5 mg/kg in 100 mL NS over 60 minutes once/wk for 2 wk, then 3-5 mg/kg every other week. Take probenecid 2 g, 3 h before infusion, and take 1 g, 8 h after infusion.	For CMV retinitis, especially in patients with AIDS. Kidney damage may occur; monitor kidney function. Pregnancy category: C; PB: UK; t½: 17-65 h
foscarnet (Foscavir)	CMV retinitis: A: IV: 60 mg/kg infused over 1 h, q8h, for 2-3 wk or 90 mg/kg/d infused over 2 h, q12h	For herpesviruses (HSV-1 and HSV-2, VZV) and CMV retinitis. Can cause kidney damage and hyperphosphatemia. Closely monitor kidney function. Does not cause granulocytopenia or thrombocytopenia. Pregnancy category: C; PB: UK; t½: 3-7 h
rimantadine HCl (Flumadine)	A/C >10 y: PO: 100 mg b.i.d. Older adults: PO: 100 mg/d	For prophylaxis and treatment against influenza A virus. Drug dose is usually reduced for patients with severe hepatic or renal impairment. Pregnancy category: C; PB: 40%; t½: 13-65 h
Influenza virus vaccine (FLUCELVAX, Flublok)	Flublok: A: IM: 0.5 mL as single dose at beginning of influenza season	Flublok is for prophylaxis against influenza subtypes A and type B. Given IM only in deltoid muscle of upper arm at the beginning of influenza season. FLUCELVAX is for treatment of influenza subtypes A and B. Given IM only in deltoid muscle of upper arm. Pregnancy category: C; PB: UK; t½: UK
telbivudine (Tyzeka)	A: PO: 600 mg/d	For chronic HBV. Pregnancy category: B; PB: 3.3%; t½: 40-49 h.
adefovir dipivoxil (Hepsera)	A/C >12 y: PO: 10 mg/d	For chronic HBV. Pregnancy category: C; PB: <4%; t½: 7.5 h.
entecavir (Baraclude)	A: PO: 0.5-1 mg/d 2 h a.c. or p.c.	For chronic HBV. Pregnancy category: C; PB: 13%; t½: 128-149 h.
Purine Nucleosides		
acyclovir (Zovirax)	See Prototype Drug Chart 33-1.	
famciclovir (Famvir)	Herpes zoster: A: PO: 500 mg q8h × 7 d Herpes simplex: A: PO: 125 mg b.i.d. × 5 d or 1000 mg b.i.d. for 1 d	For herpes zoster and HSV-1. Pregnancy category: B; PB: <20%; t½: 2-3 h
Varicella-zoster immune globulin (VariZIG)	A/Adol >40 kg: IM: 625 international units/dose within 96 h of exposure C 10-20 kg: 250 international units/dose IM within 96 h of exposure	For postexposure prophylaxis of varicella zoster. Pregnancy category: C; PB: UK; t½: 22-30 d
ganciclovir sodium (Cytovene)	A/C: IV: Initially: 5 mg/kg over 1 h q12h × 14-21 d; *maint:* 5 mg/kg/d over 1 h for 7 d, or 6 mg/kg/d over 1 h for 5 d	For CMV systemic infection in immunocompromised patients. Pregnancy category: C; PB: 1%-2%; t½: 2.5-6 h
ribavirin (Virazole)	RSV: C: Aerosol inhalation: 20 mg over 12-18 h/d for 3-7 d Hepatitis C: A >75 kg: PO: 600 mg b.i.d. for 24-48 wk A <75 kg: PO: 400 mg in morning and 600 mg in evening C: PO: 15 mg/kg/d	For respiratory syncytial viral infection in infants and children and for hepatitis C. Pregnancy category: X; PB: NA; t½: 44 h
valacyclovir HCl (Valtrex)	Herpes zoster: A: PO: 1 g t.i.d. for 7 d Recurrent genital herpes: A: PO: 500 mg b.i.d. for 3 d	Effective against VZV causing herpes zoster (shingles) and recurrent genital herpes. Monitor kidney function. Encourage patient to increase water intake. GI disturbances and headaches are common side effects. Pregnancy category: B; PB: 14%-18%; t½: 2.5-3.5 h
valganciclovir (Valcyte)	A: PO: 900 mg b.i.d. with food for 21 d	To treat CMV-infected cells of retinitis in AIDS patients. Inhibits viral DNA synthesis. May cause leukopenia, thrombocytopenia, bone marrow depression, and aplastic anemia. Pregnancy category: C; PB: 1%-2%; t½: 18 h

Continued

TABLE 33-1 NON-HIV ANTIVIRALS—cont'd

GENERIC (BRAND)	ROUTE AND DOSAGE	USES AND CONSIDERATIONS
Neuraminidase Inhibitors		
oseltamivir phosphate (Tamiflu)	A/C >40 kg: PO: 75 mg b.i.d. for 5d C 23-40 kg: PO: 60 mg b.i.d. for 5d C 15-23 kg: PO: 45 mg b.i.d. for 5d C <15 kg: PO: 30 mg b.i.d. for 5d	For uncomplicated acute influenza A and B. Treatment should begin within 48 h of flu symptoms. May be taken with or without food. Side effects include transient nausea and vomiting. Pregnancy category: C; PB: 3%, t½: 1-3 h
zanamivir (Relenza)	A: inhaler: 2 oral inhalations (one 5-mg blister/inhalation) b.i.d. for 5 d	For influenza A and B and H1N1 influenza. Treatment should begin within 48 h of flu symptoms. Less than 20% absorbed systemically. Pregnancy category: C; PB: <10%; t½: 2.5-5 h
Topical Non-HIV Antivirals		
penciclovir (Denavir)	A: topical: Apply cream q2h during the day for 4 d	For recurrent herpes labialis (cold sores). Pregnancy category: B; PB: UK; t½: UK
trifluridine (Viroptic)	A: ophthalmic solution: 1 gt q2h during the day; *max:* 9 gtt/d	Used primarily for keratoconjunctivitis due to herpes simplex virus. Pregnancy category: C; PB: UK; t½: 12 min

A, Adult; a.c., before meals; *AIDS,* acquired immunodeficiency syndrome; *b.i.d.,* twice a day; *C,* child; *CMV,* cytomegalovirus; *d,* day; *DNA,* deoxyribonucleic acid; *GI,* gastrointestinal; *gt,* drop; *gtt,* drops; *h,* hour; *HIV,* human immunodeficiency virus; HSV, herpes simplex virus; *IV,* intravenous; *maint,* maintenance; *max,* maximum; *PB,* protein-binding; p.c. after meals; *PO,* by mouth; *t½,* half-life; *t.i.d.,* three times a day; *UK,* unknown; *VZV,* varicella-zoster virus; *wk,* week; *y,* year; *>,* greater than; *<,* less than.

PROTOTYPE DRUG CHART 33-1

Acyclovir Sodium

Drug Class Antiviral Trade Name: Zovirax Pregnancy Category: B	**Dosage** Herpes simplex virus: A: PO: 400 mg t.i.d. for 5-10 d A: IV: 5 mg/kg q8h for 10-21 d Herpes zoster virus: A: PO: 800 mg q4h 5 ×/d for 7-10 d Herpes simplex encephalitis: A: IV: 10 mg/kg q8h for 10 d
Contraindications Hypersensitivity, severe renal or hepatic disease Caution: Electrolyte imbalance, dehydration, seizure disorder, nursing mothers, young children	**Drug-Lab-Food Interactions** Drug: Increase nephro-neurotoxicity with aminoglycosides, probenecid, interferon; decreases effect of phenytoin Lab: May increase AST, ALT, BUN
Pharmacokinetics Absorption: PO: Slowly absorbed Distribution: PB: 10%-30% Metabolism: t½: PO: 2.5-3 h Excretion: Urine and breast milk	**Pharmacodynamics** PO: Onset: UK Peak: 1.5-2 h Duration: 4-8 h IV: Onset: Rapid Peak: 1-2 h Duration: 4-8 h
Therapeutic Effects/Uses To treat HSV-1, HSV-2 (genital) Mode of Action: Interference with viral synthesis of DNA	
Side Effects Nausea, anorexia, vomiting, diarrhea, headache, tremors, agitation, lethargy, rash, pruritus, increased bleeding time, phlebitis at IV site	**Adverse Reactions** Urticaria, anemia, crystalluria, paresthesias Life-threatening: Neuropathy, seizures, nephrotoxicity (large doses), thrombocytopenia, leukopenia,

A, Adult; *ALT,* alanine aminotransferase; *AST,* aspartate aminotransferase; *BUN,* blood urea nitrogen; *C,* child; *d,* day; *DNA,* deoxyribonucleic acid; *h,* hour; *HSV,* herpes simplex virus; *IV,* intravenous; *PB,* protein-binding; *PO,* by mouth; *t½,* half-life; *t.i.d.,* three times a day; *UK,* unknown.

Valacyclovir (Valtrex) is converted to acyclovir, which has inhibitory activity against HSV-1, HSV-2, and varicella-zoster or herpes zoster viruses. With herpes zoster, valacyclovir offers a greater decrease in pain and an increase in healing time (40 to 43 days) than with acyclovir (59 days).

Famciclovir (Famvir), an antiviral drug developed before valacyclovir, is equally effective as acyclovir for treating acute herpes zoster.

Nursing Process
Patient-Centered Collaborative Care

Antiviral: Acyclovir

Assessment
- Obtain a medical history from patient of any serious renal or hepatic disease.
- Determine baseline vital signs and a complete blood count (CBC). Use these findings for comparison with future results.
- Assess baseline laboratory results, particularly blood urea nitrogen (BUN), serum creatinine, liver enzymes, bilirubin, and electrolytes. Use these results for future comparison.
- Evaluate baseline vital signs and urine output. Report abnormal findings.

Nursing Diagnoses
- Risk for infection related to insufficient knowledge about avoiding exposure to pathogens
- Risk for injury related to adverse effects of antivirals as evidenced by gingival hyperplasia and bone marrow depression
- Risk for impaired skin integrity related to adverse effects of antivirals as evidenced by rash and pruritus
- Deficient knowledge related to inexperience with antiviral medications.

Planning
- Patient's symptoms of viral infections will be eliminated or diminished.

Nursing Interventions
- Check patient's CBC. Report abnormal results (leukopenia, thrombocytopenia, low hemoglobin and hematocrit).
- Monitor other laboratory tests (BUN, serum creatinine, liver enzymes); compare with baseline values.
- Record patient's urinary output. An antiviral drug such as acyclovir can affect renal function.
- Monitor vital signs, especially blood pressure. Acyclovir and amantadine may cause orthostatic hypotension.
- Observe for signs and symptoms of side effects. Most antiviral drugs have many side effects (see Prototype Drug Chart 33-1).
- Check for superimposed infection (superinfection) caused by high dose and prolonged use of an antiviral drug such as acyclovir.
- Administer oral acyclovir as prescribed. Oral dose can be taken at mealtime.
- Dilute the antiviral drug in an appropriate amount of solution as indicated in the drug circular when giving IV. Administer IV drug over 60 minutes. Never give acyclovir as a bolus (IV push).

Patient Teaching
General
- Advise patient to maintain adequate fluid intake to ensure sufficient hydration for drug therapy and increase urine output.
- Instruct patient with genital herpes to avoid spreading infection by practicing sexual abstinence or by using condoms. Teach women with genital herpes to have a Pap test done as indicated by health care provider. Cervical cancer is more prevalent in those with genital herpes simplex.
- Direct patients taking zidovudine to have blood cell count monitored.

Side Effects
- Encourage patient to perform oral hygiene several times a day. Gingival hyperplasia (red, swollen gums) can occur with prolonged use of antiviral drugs.
- Guide patient to report adverse reactions, including decrease in urine output and central nervous system changes such as dizziness, anxiety, or confusion.
- Warn patient with dizziness resulting from orthostatic hypotension to arise slowly from a sitting to a standing position.
- Tell patient to report any side effects associated with the antiviral drug: nausea, vomiting, diarrhea, increased bleeding time, rash, urticaria, menstrual abnormalities.

Cultural Considerations
- Teach non–English-speaking patients and family members how to use ophthalmic preparations by using materials in the patients' first language. Pictures may be helpful.

Evaluation
- Evaluate the effectiveness of the antiviral drug in eliminating the virus or in decreasing symptoms.
- Determine whether or not side effects are absent.

Ganciclovir (Cytovene, Vitrasert) is effective in treating the herpesviruses and CMV. Its primary use is to treat CMV infections. It has serious adverse reactions.

Side Effects and Adverse Reactions. Side effects and adverse reactions to acyclovir and ganciclovir include GI disturbances (e.g., nausea, vomiting, diarrhea).

Acyclovir may cause headache, dizziness, and hematuria. Insomnia, depression, and hypotension, although infrequent, can also occur. Elevated blood urea nitrogen (BUN) and serum creatinine levels can result from renal involvement; such involvement is usually transient.

Ganciclovir can cause thrombocytopenia and granulocytopenia. Because of the possible serious adverse reactions, this drug should be prescribed primarily for severe systemic CMV infections for immunocompromised patients.

ANTIVIRAL HIV DRUGS

The microbe of the human immunodeficiency virus (HIV) is the cause of AIDS. HIV is a retrovirus. There are two classes of antiretroviral drugs: (1) reverse transcriptase inhibitors and (2) protease inhibitors. Antiviral drugs classified as reverse transcriptase inhibitors include delavirdine (Rescriptor), didanosine (Videx), lamivudine (Epivir), nevirapine (Viramune), stavudine (Zerit), and zidovudine (Retrovir, AZT). These drugs aid in inhibiting viral replication. Zidovudine was one of the first retroviral drugs approved by the FDA. It inhibits the action of viral reverse transcriptase, thus preventing the synthesis of DNA and allowing the T_4 lymphocytes to increase initially.

The protease inhibitor group includes indinavir (Crixivan), nelfinavir (Viracept), ritonavir (Norvir), and saquinavir (Invirase). This group of antivirals inhibits the replication of retroviruses (HIV-1 and HIV-2). When a protease inhibitor is used in combination with a reverse transcriptase inhibitor, these drugs may greatly reduce the viral level to the point that it is undetectable. The combination of drugs helps decrease HIV drug resistance. Antiviral drugs for suppressing HIV are discussed in Chapter 35.

ANTIMALARIAL DRUGS

Malaria, caused by the protozoan parasites *Plasmodium* spp. carried by infected *Anopheles* mosquitoes, is still one of the most prevalent protozoan diseases. After the mosquito infects the human, the protozoan parasite passes through two phases: the tissue phase and the erythrocytic phase. The **tissue phase** (invasion of body tissue) produces no clinical symptoms in the human, but the **erythrocytic phase** (invasion of the red blood cells) causes symptoms of chills, fever, and sweating. The incubation period is 10 to 35 days, followed by flulike symptoms.

There are approximately 50 species of *Plasmodium,* and 4 types of the species cause malaria: *P. malariae, P. ovale, P. vivax,* and *P. falciparum. P. vivax* is the most prevalent; *P. falciparum* is the most severe. Throughout the world there are about 200 million cases of malaria, but in the United States malaria is confined mainly to persons who enter the country from elsewhere. The incidence of malaria has increased since 1960, primarily because of travel to regions in the world where malaria is endemic, and drug-resistant malaria parasites.

Treatment of malaria depends on the type of *Plasmodium* and the organism's life cycle. Quinine was the only antimalarial drug available from 1820 until the early 1940s. Synthetic **antimalarial drugs** have since been developed that are as effective as quinine and cause fewer toxic effects. When drug-resistant malaria occurs, combinations of antimalarials are used to facilitate effective treatment. Chloroquine is a commonly prescribed drug for malaria. If drug resistance to chloroquine occurs, another antimalarial (e.g., mefloquine HCl, or combinations of antimalarials with or without antibiotics (e.g., tetracycline, doxycycline, clindamycin) may be prescribed.

Three methods used to eradicate malaria are **prophylaxis** (prevention) of malaria, treatment for the acute attack, and prevention of relapse. Many synthetic antimalarials (chloroquine, primaquine) are used prophylactically. Chloroquine and mefloquine are frequently used to treat an acute malarial attack. Mefloquine HCl and the combination drug atovaquone/proguanil (Malarone) are used to treat chloroquine-resistant *P. falciparum.* Chloroquine and hydroxychloroquine can be toxic to children and may even cause death; therefore the drug dose should be closely monitored. Prototype Drug Chart 33-2 lists the drug data for chloroquine HCl.

Pharmacokinetics Chloroquine HCl is well absorbed from the GI tract. It is moderately protein-binding, and the drug has a long half-life. The first two doses have a loading dose effect. Because of its long half-life, the next dose is given in 6 hours, the third and fourth doses are given at 24 and 48 hours, and then a dose is given once a day for 2 days. Chloroquine is metabolized in the liver to active metabolites and excreted in the urine.

Pharmacodynamics Chloroquine HCl inhibits the malaria parasite's growth by interfering with its protein synthesis. Whether the drug is given orally or IM, the onset of action is rapid. The peak effect is slower when given orally. The duration of effect of the drug is very long—days to weeks.

Side Effects and Adverse Reactions

General side effects and adverse reactions to antimalarials include GI upset, cranial nerve VIII involvement (quinine and chloroquine), renal impairment (quinine), and cardiovascular effects (quinine).

Table 33-2 lists commonly ordered antimalarial drugs and their dosage, uses, and considerations. Note: Quinine is an antimalarial drug, and quinidine is an antidysrhythmic drug. A medication guideline developed by the FDA accompanies mefloquine each time it is dispensed. This type of guideline is used only for drugs that require monitoring for serious adverse effects. Adverse effects that may occur after mefloquine use include severe anxiety, restlessness, disorientation, depression, hallucinations, paranoia, and suicidal thoughts.

SAFETY: Preventing Medication Errors

Do not confuse...

- **quinine** (antimalarial) with **quinidine** (antidysrhythmic)

PROTOTYPE DRUG CHART 33-2

Chloroquine HCl

Drug Class Antimalarial Trade Name: Aralen HCl Pregnancy Category: C	**Dosage** Acute malaria: A: PO: 1000 mg/dose; then 500 mg/dose in 6 h; then 500 mg/d at 24 h and 48 h C/Adol: PO: 16.5 mg/kg, then 8.3 mg/kg in 6 h, 24 h, and 36 h Prophylaxis: 2 wk before and for 6-8 wk after exposure A: PO: 500 mg/wk C: PO: 8.3 mg/kg/wk
Contraindications Hypersensitivity, renal disease, psoriasis Caution: Alcoholism; liver dysfunction; G-6-PD deficiency; GI, neurologic (seizures, hearing impairment), and hematologic disorders	**Drug-Lab-Food Interactions** Drug: Increase effects of digoxin, neuromuscular blocker; decrease absorption with antacids and laxatives Lab: Elevated liver enzymes; decreased red blood cell count, hemoglobin, hematocrit Food: Lemon juice decreases effects
Pharmacokinetics Absorption: Well absorbed from GI tract Distribution: PB: 50%-65% Metabolism: t½: 1-2 months Excretion: Excreted slowly in urine	**Pharmacodynamics** PO: Onset: Rapid Peak: 1-2 h Duration: Days to weeks
Therapeutic Effects/Uses To treat acute malaria; prophylaxis for malaria Mode of Action: Increased pH in the malaria parasite inhibits parasitic growth	
Side Effects Anorexia, nausea, vomiting, diarrhea, abdominal cramps, fatigue, pruritus, headache, nervousness, visual impairment, insomnia, photosensitivity, hair discoloration	**Adverse Reactions** ECG changes, hypotension, psychosis, seizures Life-threatening: Agranulocytosis, aplastic anemia, thrombocytopenia, ototoxicity, cardiovascular collapse

A, Adult; *Adol,* adolescent; *C,* child; *d,* day; *ECG,* electrocardiogram; *G-6-PD,* glucose-6-phosphate dehydrogenase; *GI,* gastrointestinal; *h,* hour; *IM,* intramuscular; *IV,* intravenous; *max,* maximum; *PB,* protein-binding; *PO,* by mouth; *PRN,* as needed; *t ½,* half-life; *wk,* week.

Nursing Process
Patient-Centered Collaborative Care

Antimalarials

Assessment
- Assess patient's hearing, especially if receiving quinine or chloroquine. These drugs may affect cranial nerve VIII.
- Check patient for visual changes. Patients who take chloroquine and hydroxychloroquine should have frequent ophthalmic examinations.

Nursing Diagnoses
- Risk for infection related to insufficient knowledge about avoiding exposure to malarial pathogens
- Risk for impaired skin integrity related to fever and excessive sweating
- Risk for imbalanced nutrition: less than body requirements related to side effects of vomiting and diarrhea
- Risk for visual injury related to side effects of blurred vision
- Deficient knowledge related to inexperience with antimalarial medications.

Planning
- Patient will be free of malarial symptoms.

Nursing Interventions
- Monitor patient's renal and liver function by checking urine output (>600 mL/d) and liver enzymes. Antimalarial drugs concentrate first in the liver; if patient drinks considerable amounts of alcohol or has a liver disorder, liver enzymes require closer monitoring. Renal impairment may occur as an adverse effect of antimalarials.
- Report if patient's serum liver enzymes are elevated or renal function tests are abnormal.

TABLE 33-2 ANTIMALARIALS

GENERIC (BRAND)	ROUTE AND DOSAGE	USES AND CONSIDERATIONS
chloroquine HCl (Aralen HCl)	See Prototype Drug Chart 33-2.	
hydroxychloroquine sulfate (Plaquenil sulfate)	Acute malaria: A: PO: 800 mg, then 400 mg at 6, 18, 24, and 36 h C: PO: 13 mg/kg/dose, then 6.5 mg/kg in 6, 18, and 24 h	Alternative to chloroquine. Dosage varies for treating malaria. Can be used adjunctively with primaquine. Give with meals to reduce GI distress. Pregnancy category: C; PB: 45%; t½: 32-50 d
mefloquine HCl	Malaria treatment: A: PO: Single dose: 1250 mg Malaria prophylaxis: A: PO: 250 mg/wk for 1-2 wk before travel and 4 wk after; take with plenty of water	Prophylaxis and treatment of acute malaria. Treatment of choice in U.S. for malaria. Pregnancy category: C; PB: 98%; t½: 10-21 d
primaquine phosphate (Primaquine)	Malaria treatment: A: PO: 15-mg base/d for 14 d Malaria prophylaxis: A: PO: 30-mg base/d for 14 d	For malaria caused by *Plasmodium vivax, P. ovale,* and *P. falciparum,* as well as *Pneumocystis carinii* pneumonia. Can affect WBC production (granulocytopenia) and cause acute hemolytic anemia in patients with G-6-PD deficiency. Pregnancy category: C; PB: UK; t½: 3.7-9.6 h
pyrimethamine (Daraprim)	Malaria prophylaxis: A/C >10 y: PO: 25 mg/wk for 2 wk before exposure and continue for 10 wk after C 4-10 y: PO: 12.5 mg/wk C <4 y: PO: 6.25 mg/wk Malaria treatment: A/C >10 y: PO: 25 mg/d for 2 d with a sulfonamide C 4-10 y: PO: 25 mg/d for 2 d	Prophylaxis use for malaria. For chloroquine-resistant *P. falciparum* infections. May be used with quinacrine, quinine, or chloroquine. Pregnancy category: C; PB: 80%-87%; t½: 80-123 h
quinine sulfate (Qualaquin)	Acute malaria: A: PO: 650 mg q8h for 3-7 d	Used in combination drug therapy or for chloroquine-resistant malaria. Pregnancy category: C; PB: 70%; t½: 8-21 h
Combination Antimalarial Drugs		
atovaquone/proguanil (Malarone)	A/C >40 kg: PO: 250/100-mg tabs: 3 tabs/d for 3 d C 31-40 kg: PO: 250/100-mg tabs: 2 tabs/d for 3 d C 11-20 kg: PO: 250/100-mg tabs: 1 tab/d for 3 d	For oral prophylaxis and treatment of malaria. Effective for chloroquine-resistant strains. Pregnancy category: C; PB: 99%/75%; t½: 2-3 d/12-20 h
artemether/lumefantrine (Coartem)	A/C >35 kg: PO: 4 tabs of artemether 80 mg/ lumefantrine 480 mg upon diagnosis, then 4 tabs in 8 h, then 4 tabs b.i.d. for 2 d A/C 25-35 kg: PO: 3 tabs artemether 60 mg with lumefantrine 360 mg in same regimen C 15-25 kg: PO: 2 tabs artemether 40 mg with lumefantrine 240 mg in same regimen C 5-15 kg: PO: 1 tab artemether 20 mg with lumefantrine 120 mg in same regimen	For malaria infections that are both drug-sensitive and drug-resistant to *Plasmodium falciparum.* Acts by inhibiting nucleic acid and protein synthesis. Rapid onset allows drug to control fever quickly. Has a high cure rate. Adverse effects include nystagmus, wheezing, hypokalemia, blood dyscrasias, and hepatomegaly. Pregnancy category: C; PB: 95%/99%; t½: 2-3 h/3-6 d

A, Adult; *C,* child; *d,* day; *G-6-PD,* glucose-6-phosphate dehydrogenase; *GI,* gastrointestinal; *h,* hour; *max,* maximum; *PB,* protein-binding; *PO,* by mouth; *t½,* half-life; *tab,* tablet; *UK,* unknown; *wk,* week; *y,* year; >, greater than; <, less than.

Patient Teaching

General

- Advise patients traveling to malaria-infested countries to receive prophylactic doses of antimalarial drug before leaving, during the visit, and upon return.
- Teach patient to take oral antimalarial drugs with food or at mealtime if GI upset occurs.
- Monitor patient returning from a malaria-infested area for malarial symptoms.
- Inform patient who takes chloroquine or hydroxychloroquine to report vision changes immediately.
- Warn patient to avoid consuming large quantities of alcohol.

Side Effects

- Direct patient to report signs and symptoms of anorexia, nausea, vomiting, diarrhea, abdominal cramps, pruritus, visual disturbances, and dizziness.

Cultural Considerations

- Advise patient from a malaria-infested country to be tested for malaria if patient complains of chills, high fever, and profuse sweating.
- Patient may receive an antimalarial drug as a prophylactic measure or for treatment of an acute attack. Explanation is necessary so patient complies with the drug regimen.

Evaluation

- Evaluate the effectiveness of the antimalarial drug by determining that patient is free of symptoms.
- Evaluate patient's understanding of medication regimen.

ANTHELMINTIC DRUGS

Helminths are large organisms (parasitic worms) that feed on host tissue. The most common site for **helminthiasis** (worm infestation) is the intestine. Other sites for parasitic infestation are the lymphatic system, blood vessels, and liver.

Groups of helminthes include (1) cestodes (tapeworms), (2) trematodes (flukes), (3) intestinal nematodes (roundworms), and (4) tissue-invading nematodes (tissue roundworms and filariae). They enter the human host via contaminated food, bites of carrier insects, or direct penetration of the skin. The cestodes (tapeworms) are segmented and enter the intestine via contaminated food. There are four species of cestodes: *Taenia solium* (pork tapeworm), *Taenia saginata* (beef tapeworm), *Diphyllobothrium latum* (fish tapeworm), and *Hymenolepis nana* (dwarf tapeworm). The segmented cestodes have heads and hooks or suckers that attach to the tissue.

The trematodes (flukes) are flat, nonsegmented parasites that feed on the host. Four types of trematodes exist: *Fasciola hepatica* (liver fluke), *Fasciolopsis buski* (intestinal fluke), *Paragonimus westermani* (lung fluke), and *Schistosoma species* (blood fluke).

Five types of nematodes may feed on intestinal tissue: *Ascaris lumbricoides* (giant roundworm), *Necator americanus* (hookworm), *Enterobius vermicularis* (pinworm), *Strongyloides stercoralis* (threadworm), and *Trichuris trichiura* (whipworm).

Two types of nematodes are tissue-invading: *Trichinella spiralis* (pork roundworm) and *Wuchereria bancrofti* (filariae). The pork roundworm, or *T. spiralis,* can cause **trichinosis** (disease caused by ingestion of raw or inadequately cooked pork that contains larvae of the *T. spiralis* parasite), which can be diagnosed by muscle biopsy. By thoroughly cooking pork, the roundworm, if present, is destroyed.

Side Effects and Adverse Reactions

The common side effects of **anthelmintics** (agents that destroy worms) include GI distress, which may manifest as anorexia, nausea, vomiting, and occasionally diarrhea and stomach cramps. The neurologic problems associated with anthelmintics are dizziness, weakness, headache, and drowsiness. Adverse reactions do not occur frequently, because the drugs usually are given for a short period (1 to 3 days), with the following exception: thiabendazole for treatment of threadworms and pork worms. Thiabendazole should be avoided if the patient has liver disease.

Table 33-3 lists eight anthelmintic drugs prescribed to treat various types of parasitic worms.

Nursing Process
Patient-Centered Collaborative Care

Anthelmintics

Assessment

- Obtain a history of foods patient has eaten, especially meat and fish, and how food was prepared.

TABLE 33-3 ANTHELMINTIC DRUGS

GENERIC (BRAND)	ROUTE AND DOSAGE	USES AND CONSIDERATIONS
bithionol (Bitin, Lorothidol))	A: PO: 30-50 mg/kg in 2 daily doses given every other day with food for 10-15 doses	Effective against flukes. For *Paragonimus* or *Fasciola* species when patient cannot receive praziquantel due to resistance or adverse effect.
diethylcarbamazine (Hetrazan)	A/C >15 kg: PO: 6 mg/kg, single dose	For treatment of tropical pulmonary eosinophilia or loiasis. Only available from CDC as investigational drug.
ivermectin (Stromectol)	A/C >15 kg: PO: 150-200 mcg/kg, single dose	Broad-spectrum antiparasitic drug. Causes paralysis to the parasite. Highly active against various mites. Pregnancy category: C; PB: UK; $t\frac{1}{2}$: 16-28 h
praziquantel (Biltricide)	A/C >4 y: PO: 20-25 mg/kg t.i.d. × 1-2 d	For beef, pork, and fish tapeworms; blood flukes; and liver, lung, and intestinal flukes. Pregnancy category: B; PB: 80%-85%; $t\frac{1}{2}$: 0.8-1.5 h
pyrantel pamoate (Pin-X)	A/C >2 y: PO: 10 mg/kg, single dose; *max:* 1 g	For giant roundworm, hookworm, and pinworm. Pregnancy category: C; PB: UK; $t\frac{1}{2}$: UK

A, Adult; *b.i.d.*, two times a day; *C*, child; *d*, day; *h*, hour; *max*, maximum; *PB*, protein-binding; *PO*, by mouth; *PRN*, as needed; $t\frac{1}{2}$, half-life; *t.i.d.*, three times a day; *UK*, unknown; *wk*, week; *y*, year; >, greater than; <, less than.

- Note if any other person in the household has been checked for helminths (worms).
- Assess patient for anal itching.
- Assess baseline vital signs, and collect a stool specimen.

Nursing Diagnoses
- Defensive coping related to invasion of helminth
- Activity intolerance related to dizziness, headache, drowsiness
- Disturbed body image related to fear of rejection by others
- Deficient knowledge related to inexperience with anthelmintic regime

Planning
- Patient will be free of helminths.
- Patient will explain how to prepare foods properly to avoid recurrence.
- Patient will describe methods of infection control.

Nursing Interventions
- Collect stool specimen in a clean container. Avoid having stool come in contact with water, urine, or chemicals, which could destroy parasitic worms.
- Administer prescribed anthelmintics after meals to prevent or minimize occurrence of GI distress.
- Report to health care provider if patient has any side effects.

Patient Teaching
- Explain to patient the importance of washing hands before eating and after going to the toilet. The parasite can be transferred within the family if proper hygiene is not used.
- Advise patient to take daily showers and not baths.
- Encourage patient to change sheets, bedclothes, towels, and underwear daily.
- Advise patient that a second course of anthelmintics may be necessary if helminthiasis persists after therapy.
- Emphasize importance of taking prescribed drug at designated times and keeping health care appointments.
- Teach patient to read all directions regarding over-the-counter drugs before use.
- Warn patient that drowsiness may occur, and operating a car or machinery should be avoided if this should happen.
- Teach patient to report any side effects/adverse reactions to health care provider.

Cultural Considerations
- Obtain an interpreter when necessary; do not rely on family members, who may not fully disclose because of honor or shame or because of lack of understanding of medical terminology.

Evaluation
- Evaluate effectiveness of anthelmintic therapy and absence of side effects.
- Determine if patient is using proper hygiene to avoid spread of parasitic worms.
- Evaluate patient's knowledge of preventative measures for helminthiasis.

KEY WEBSITES

Information on acyclovir: *www.nlm.nih.gov/medlineplus/druginfo/meds/a681045.html*

Seasonal Influenza: The Disease: *www.cdc.gov/flu/about/disease.htm*

Information on malaria: *www.cdc.gov/malaria*

CRITICAL THINKING CASE STUDY

TP, a 75-year-old woman, has shingles. She complains of pain and blisters (vesicular eruptions), which partially surround her waist. The health care provider prescribed acyclovir, 800 mg, every 4 hours, five times a day for 7 days.

1. When taking the health history, what should the nurse ask TP?
2. How does herpes zoster differ from varicella-zoster virus (VZV)? Explain who would be more susceptible to contracting herpes zoster virus infection.
3. How is acyclovir effective for relieving TP's symptoms?
4. Is the prescribed acyclovir dose correct? Explain your answer.
5. How does acyclovir differ from famciclovir and amantadine?
6. What comfort measures should the nurse suggest to TP?
7. What should the nurse teach TP about being around other people?

NCLEX STUDY QUESTIONS

1. A patient is diagnosed with HSV-3. The nurse understands that this illness is better known by which name? (Select all that apply.)
   a. Chickenpox
   b. Hepatitis B
   c. Shingles in an adult
   d. Cytomegalovirus
2. Zanamivir (Relenza) is ordered for a patient. What does the nurse know about use of this drug?
   a. Treatment of HSV-2
   b. Oral administration for treatment of HSV-1
   c. Treatment of varicella-zoster viruses
   d. Administration within 48 hours of onset of symptoms to be effective
3. A patient who is taking acyclovir asks the nurse about the drug. Which instruction should the nurse include in patient teaching?
   a. Restrict fluids to prevent complications.
   b. Monitor blood pressure for hypertension.
   c. Stevens-Johnson syndrome is an adverse effect.
   d. Blood tests are important for checking kidney function.
4. A patient with a history of malaria, presently being treated with chloroquine, is admitted to the hospital. What should the nurse advise the patient to do?
   a. Get frequent hearing checks.
   b. Take antimalarials before meals.
   c. Get frequent testing of stool specimens.
   d. Check heart rate before taking medication.
5. A patient is taking thiabendazole for trichinosis. What does the nurse realize about this condition and its treatment?
   a. The medication is given for 7 days.
   b. The medication should be avoided if the patient has renal disease.
   c. Family members should be checked for the same disease.
   d. Proper hygiene must be taught to avoid the spread of disease.
6. Acyclovir (Zovirax) has been ordered for a patient with genital herpes. Which nursing interventions are appropriate for this patient? (Select all that apply.)
   a. Monitor patient's BUN and creatinine.
   b. Monitor patient's BP for hypertension.
   c. Administer IV acyclovir over 30 minutes.
   d. Advise patient to maintain adequate fluid intake.
   e. Teach patient to perform oral hygiene several times a day.
   f. Monitor patient's CBC for blood dyscrasias.

Answers: 1, a,c; 2, d; 3, d; 4, a; 5, d; 6, a, d, e, f.

CHAPTER

34

Drugs for Urinary Tract Disorders

evolve WEBSITE

http://evolve.elsevier.com/KeeHayes/pharmacology/

- Animations
- Content Updates
- Key Points
- Review Questions for the NCLEX® Examination
- References from the Textbook
- Unfolding Case Studies

OBJECTIVES

- Compare the groups of drugs that are urinary antiseptics and antiinfectives.
- Describe the side effects and adverse reactions to urinary antiseptics and antiinfectives.
- Differentiate the uses for a urinary analgesic, a urinary stimulant, and a urinary antispasmodic.
- Apply the nursing process, including teaching, to nursing care of the patient receiving urinary antiseptic/antiinfective drugs.

OUTLINE

KEY TERMS

The largest number of urinary tract disorders are caused by **urinary tract infections** (UTIs), microbial infections of any part of the urinary tract. UTIs may result from an upper UTI, such as pyelonephritis, or a lower UTI, such as cystitis, urethritis, or prostatitis. A group of drugs called **urinary antiseptics/antiinfectives** prevents bacterial growth in the kidneys and bladder, but is not effective for systemic infections. Urinary antiseptics/antiinfectives have a **bacteriostatic** (inhibit bacterial growth) effect when given in lower dosages. They also have a **bactericidal** (kill bacteria) effect when given in higher dosages.

Urinary antiseptics/antiinfectives, **urinary analgesics** (relieve pain and burning in the urinary tract), **urinary stimulants** (agents that increase muscle tone of urinary muscles), and urinary antispasmodics/antimuscarinics are presented in this chapter. Chapters 29, 30, and 31 present further discussions of antibiotics, fluoroquinolones, and sulfonamides used to treat UTIs. Diuretics are discussed in Chapter 43.

Acute cystitis, a lower UTI, frequently occurs in female patients because of their shorter urethra. It is more common in women of childbearing age, older women, and young girls. Acute cystitis is commonly caused by *Escherichia coli.* Other bacterial causes include the gram-positive *Staphylococcus saprophyticus* and gram-negative *Klebsiella, Proteus,* and *Pseudomonas.* Symptoms of cystitis include pain and burning on urination and urinary frequency and urgency. A urine culture is usually obtained before the start of any antiinfective/antibiotic drug therapy. In male patients, a lower UTI is most likely prostatitis with symptoms similar to cystitis.

Acute pyelonephritis, an upper UTI, is commonly seen in women of childbearing age, older women, and young girls. *E. coli* is the most common organism causing pyelonephritis. Symptoms include chills, high fever, flank pain, pain during urination, urinary frequency and urgency, and pyuria. The bacterial count in the urine is greater than 100,000 bacteria/mL. In severe cases, the patient may be hospitalized and receive intravenous (IV) antibiotics (e.g., an aminoglycoside, ticarcillin/clavulanic acid, or piperacillin/tazobactam).

The most commonly used agents for treating UTIs are nitrofurantoin (Macrodantin); trimethoprim-sulfamethoxazole (Bactrim, Septra); and fluoroquinolones such as nalidixic acid (NegGram), norfloxacin (Noroxin), and ciprofloxacin (Cipro). Treatment may consist of a single double-strength dose of the chosen drug, a 3-day course, or the traditional method of 7 to 14 days of drug dosing. Fosfomycin tromethamine (Monurol), a nitrofurantoin prototype drug, is effective for UTIs as a single-dose treatment. Other agents used to treat UTIs include oral amoxicillin/clavulanic acid (Augmentin) and oral third-generation cephalosporins (cefixime, cefpodoxime proxetil, or ceftibuten). With severe UTIs, IV drug therapy followed by oral drug therapy is usually recommended.

URINARY ANTISEPTICS/ANTIINFECTIVES AND ANTIBIOTICS

Urinary antiseptics/antiinfectives are limited to the treatment of UTIs. Drug action occurs in the renal tubule and bladder, where it is effective in reducing bacterial growth. A urinalysis, as well as a culture and sensitivity test, is usually performed before the initiation of drug therapy. The groups of urinary antiseptics/antiinfectives are nitrofurantoin, methenamine, trimethoprim, and the fluoroquinolones.

Nitrofurantoin

Nitrofurantoin (Macrodantin) was first prescribed to treat UTIs in 1953. Nitrofurantoin is bacteriostatic or bactericidal, depending on the drug dosage, and is effective against many gram-positive and gram-negative organisms, especially *E. coli.* It is used to treat acute and chronic UTIs. The drug data for nitrofurantoin are given in Prototype Drug Chart 34-1.

Pharmacokinetics Nitrofurantoin is well absorbed from the gastrointestinal (GI) tract. The drug is usually taken with food to decrease GI distress. Decreased absorption occurs when the drug is taken with

PROTOTYPE DRUG CHART 34-1

Nitrofurantoin

Drug Class Urinary antiinfective Trade Names: Macrodantin Pregnancy Category: B	**Dosage** A: PO: 50-100 mg q.i.d. (with meals and h.s.); take with food; *max:* 7 mg/kg/d C >1 mo: PO: 1.25-1.75 mg/kg/d q6h; *max:* 7 mg/kg/d
Contraindications Hypersensitivity, moderate to severe renal impairment, oliguria, anuria, infants <1 mo, term pregnancy, lactation with infant suspected of having G-6-PD deficiency Caution: Vitamin B deficiency, electrolyte imbalance, diabetes mellitus	**Drug-Lab-Food Interactions** Drug: Decreased renal clearance with probenecid leading to toxicity; decreased absorption with antacids; decreased effectiveness of fluoroquinolones; decreased effectiveness of oral contraceptives
Pharmacokinetics Absorption: Well absorbed from GI tract; enhanced with food Distribution: PB: 20%-60%, crosses placenta, excreted in breast milk Metabolism: t½: 20 min Excretion: In urine; small amounts in bile	**Pharmacodynamics** PO: Onset: UK Peak: 30 min Duration: UK
Therapeutic Effects/Uses To treat acute and chronic UTIs Mode of Action: Inhibits bacterial enzymes and metabolism, also inhibits bacterial cell wall formation	
Side Effects Anorexia, nausea, vomiting, abdominal pain, rust/brown discoloration of urine, diarrhea, rash, pruritus, chills, dizziness, headache, drowsiness, confusion, depression, alopecia, nystagmus	**Adverse Reactions** Superinfection, angioedema, peripheral neuropathy, hemolytic anemia, aplastic anemia, thrombocytopenia, agranulocytosis Life-threatening: Anaphylaxis, hepatotoxicity, Stevens-Johnson syndrome

A, Adult; *C,* child; *CLcr,* creatinine clearance; *G-6-PD,* glucose-6-phosphate dehydrogenase; *GI,* gastrointestinal; *h.s.,* at bedtime; *min,* minute; *mo,* month; *PB,* protein-binding; *PO,* by mouth; *q.i.d.,* four times a day; *t½,* half-life; *UK,* unknown; *UTI,* urinary tract infection; *y,* year; <, less than.

antacids. Nitrofurantoin is moderately protein-bound. With normal renal function, the drug is rapidly eliminated because of its short half-life of 20 minutes; however, it accumulates in the serum with urinary dysfunction.

Pharmacodynamics When nitrofurantoin is given in low doses for prophylactic use, the drug has a bacteriostatic effect. High concentration of nitrofurantoin causes a bactericidal effect. Nitrofurantoin is effective against many gram-positive and gram-negative organisms such as *E. coli, Neisseria, streptococci, Staphylococcus aureus,* and others. It is not as effective against *Pseudomonas aeruginosa, Proteus species,* and some species of *Klebsiella.* The onset and duration of action are unknown. Peak action occurs 30 minutes after absorption. If sudden onset of dyspnea, chest pain, cough, fever, and chills develops, the patient should contact the health care provider. Symptoms resolve after discontinuing the drug.

The nursing process for nitrofurantoin is applicable to the other urinary antiseptics/antiinfectives.

Methenamine

Methenamine (Hiprex) produces a bactericidal effect when the urine pH is less than 5.5. Methenamine is available as hippurate salt. It is effective against gram-positive and gram-negative organisms, especially *E. coli* and *P. aeruginosa.* It is used for chronic UTIs. Methenamine should not be taken with sulfonamides, because crystalluria is likely to occur. It is absorbed readily from the GI tract, and approximately 90% of the drug is excreted in the urine unchanged. Methenamine forms ammonia and formaldehyde in acid urine; therefore the urine needs to be acidified to exert a bactericidal action. Cranberry juice (several 8-ounce glasses per day), ascorbic acid, and ammonium chloride can be taken to decrease the urine pH.

Nursing Process
Patient-Centered Collaborative Care

Urinary Antiinfective: Nitrofurantoin

Assessment
- Obtain a history from patient of clinical problems with UTI, incontinence, or other urinary tract disorders.
- Assess patient for signs and symptoms of UTI: pain or burning sensation on urination, frequency and urgency of urination.
- Monitor complete blood count (CBC) on patients with long-term therapy; monitor regularly.
- Monitor urine culture and sensitivity results.
- Assess renal and hepatic function.
- Determine urine pH. A pH of 5.5 is desired. However, alkalinization of the urine is not recommended.

Nursing Diagnoses
- Acute pain related to inflammation in the urinary tract
- Risk for infection related to insufficient knowledge to avoid invasion of pathogens

Planning
- Patient will be free of signs and symptoms of UTI within 10 days.

Nursing Interventions
- Monitor patient's urinary output and urine specific gravity. Careful attention to output is required when administering urinary antiseptics to patients with anuria and oliguria. Report promptly any decrease in urine output.
- Obtain urine culture to identify infecting organism before initiation of drug therapy to treat UTI.
- Observe patient for side effects and adverse reactions to urinary antiseptic drugs. Peripheral neuropathy (tingling, numbness of extremities) may result from renal insufficiency (inability to excrete drug) or long-term use of nitrofurantoin. Peripheral neuropathy may be irreversible.

Patient Teaching

General
- Teach patient not to crush tablets or open capsules.
- Advise patient to rinse mouth thoroughly after taking oral nitrofurantoin. Drug can stain teeth.
- Encourage patient to avoid antacids because they interfere with drug absorption.
- Teach patient to shake suspension well before administration and protect from freezing.
- Warn patient not to drive a motor vehicle or operate dangerous machinery; drug may cause drowsiness.
- Advise female patient to immediately report pregnancy to health care provider.

Diet
- Inform patient to increase fluids and take drug with food to minimize GI upset.

Side Effects
- Alert patient that urine may turn a harmless brown color.
- Encourage patient to report any signs of secondary fungal or bacterial infection (superinfection), such as stomatitis or anogenital discharge or itching.

Methenamine
- Educate patient to drink cranberry juice, eat plums, or take vitamin C (with approval of health care provider) to keep urine acidic. Foods that are alkaline, such as milk and some vegetables, may increase urine pH. Urine pH should be less than 5.5 for the antiseptic to be effective.

Fluoroquinolones
- Warn patient to avoid operating hazardous machinery or driving a car while taking drug, especially if dizziness is present.

- Encourage patient to take drug with food and avoid antacids, because they interfere with drug absorption.
- Alert patient that drug may turn urine a harmless brown color.
- Direct patient to report any signs of superinfection or secondary fungal or bacterial infection.
- Tell patient to avoid excessive exposure to sunlight.

Cultural Considerations

- Alleviate fear or concerns of patient from a different cultural background. Use culturally consistent communication when explaining the treatment regimen for a UTI. An interpreter may be necessary. The use of pamphlets in the language patient reads or speaks most easily can facilitate patient understanding.

Evaluation

- Evaluate the effectiveness of the urinary antiinfectives in alleviating the UTI. Patient is free of side effects and adverse reactions to drug.

Trimethoprim and Trimethoprim-Sulfamethoxazole

Trimethoprim (Proloprim) can be used alone for the treatment of UTIs, although it is usually used in combination with a sulfonamide, sulfamethoxazole (the combined preparation is generically called *TMP/SMZ*), to prevent the occurrence of trimethoprim-resistant organisms. This drug combination produces slow-acting bactericidal effects against most gram-positive and gram-negative organisms. TMP/SMZ (Bactrim, Septra) is discussed in Chapter 31. Trimethoprim is used in the treatment and prevention of acute and chronic UTIs. The amount of trimethoprim in the prostatic fluid is about two to three times greater than the amount in the vascular fluid. The half-life of trimethoprim is normally 8 to 11 hours, but it is longer in patients with renal dysfunction.

Fluoroquinolones (Quinolones)

Fluoroquinolones are one of the groups of urinary antibacterials that are effective against lower UTIs; they include nalidixic acid (NegGram), norfloxacin (Noroxin), ciprofloxacin hydrochloride (Cipro), and ofloxacin ., Norfloxacin, ciprofloxacin, and ofloxacin, are effective against a wide variety of UTIs. The drug dosage must be decreased when renal dysfunction is present. The half-lives of these drugs are ordinarily 2 to 8 hours, but are prolonged in patients with renal dysfunction. Table 34-1 lists the urinary antiseptics/antiinfectives and their dosages, uses, and considerations.

Side Effects and Adverse Reactions

Nitrofurantoin. Side effects of nitrofurantoin use include (1) GI disturbances such as anorexia, nausea, vomiting, diarrhea, and abdominal pain and (2) pulmonary reactions such as dyspnea, chest pain, fever, and cough.

Methenamine. Methenamine use has GI side effects, including nausea, vomiting, and diarrhea. Allergic reactions to the dye in Hiprex have occurred. Bladder irritation and crystalluria (when taken in large doses) may occur.

Trimethoprim. GI symptoms (including nausea and vomiting) and skin problems (including rash and pruritus) can accompany trimethoprim use.

Fluoroquinolones. Nalidixic acid use can have the following side effects: headaches, dizziness, syncope (fainting), peripheral neuritis, visual disturbances, and rash. Nausea, vomiting, diarrhea, headaches, and visual disturbances can occur with cinoxacin and norfloxacin use. Photosensitivity is a common side effect associated with fluoroquinolones.

Drug-Drug Interactions

The following drug-drug interactions can occur with the use of urinary antiseptics/antiinfectives:

- Antacids decrease nitrofurantoin absorption.
- Sodium bicarbonate inhibits the action of methenamine.
- Methenamine mandelate taken with sulfonamides increases the risk of crystalluria.
- Nalidixic acid enhances the effects of warfarin (Coumadin).
- Most urinary antiseptics cause false-positive Clinitest results.

URINARY ANALGESICS

Phenazopyridine

Phenazopyridine hydrochloride (Pyridium), an azo dye, is a urinary analgesic (relieves urinary pain and burning) that has been available for almost 40 years. It is used to relieve the pain, burning sensation, and frequency and urgency of urination that are symptomatic of lower UTIs. The drug can cause GI disturbances, hemolytic anemia, nephrotoxicity, and hepatotoxicity. The urine becomes a harmless reddish orange because of the dye. Phenazopyridine can alter the glucose urine test (Clinitest); therefore, a blood test should be used to monitor glucose levels.

URINARY STIMULANTS

When bladder function is decreased or lost as a result of (1) a neurogenic bladder (a dysfunction caused by a lesion of the nervous system), (2) a spinal cord injury (paraplegia, hemiplegia), or (3) a severe head injury, a parasympathomimetic may be used to stimulate **micturition** (urination). The drug of choice, bethanechol chloride (Urecholine), is a urinary stimulant, also known as a *direct-acting parasympathomimetic* (cholinomimetic). The drug action is to increase bladder tone by increasing tone of the detrusor urinal muscle, which produces a contraction strong enough to stimulate urination. Bethanechol is discussed in detail in Chapter 19.

TABLE 34-1 ANTISEPTICS AND URINARY ANTIINFECTIVES

GENERIC (TRADE) NAME	ROUTE AND DOSAGE	USES AND CONSIDERATIONS
fosfomycin tromethamine (Monurol)	A: PO: 3-g packet dissolved in 4 oz water, as a single dose	For uncomplicated UTIs in women. Has a bactericidal effect against most gram-negative and gram-positive bacteria. Side effects include headaches and diarrhea. Pregnancy category: B; PB: 0%; t½: 3-8.5 h
methenamine hippurate (Hiprex, Urex)	Hippurate: A: PO: 1 g b.i.d. C 6-12 y: PO: 0.5-1 g q12h	For chronic UTIs. Urine pH should be acidic (<5.5). Do not use with sulfonamides. May cause crystalluria, so push fluids. May cause GI irritation, so give with meals. Pregnancy category: C; PB: UK; t½: 4 h
nitrofurantoin (Macrodantin)	See Prototype Drug Chart 34-1.	
trimethoprim (Proloprim)	A: PO: 100 mg b.i.d. or 200 mg/d for 10-14 d	For prevention and treatment of acute and chronic UTIs in both men and women. High doses can cause GI upset. Drug can be combined with sulfamethoxazole (Bactrim). Pregnancy category: C; PB: 45%; t½: 8-10 h
ertapenem (Invanz)	A/Adol: IM/IV: 1 g/d for 10-14 d C >3 mo: IM/IV: 15 mg/kg b.i.d. for 10-14 d	To prevent recurring UTIs, acute pelvic infections, and diabetic foot infections. Effective against gram-positive and gram-negative bacteria. Commonly causes diarrhea, nausea, and headache. Pregnancy category: B; PB: 95%; t½: 4.5 h
Sulfonamides		
trimethoprim-sulfamethoxazole (TMP-SMZ, Bactrim, Septra)	See Prototype Drug Chart 31-1 in Chapter 31.	Effective for serious UTIs and otitis media. Pregnancy category: C; PB: 44%-70%; t½: 6-12 h
Quinolones (Fluoroquinolones)		
ciprofloxacin (Cipro)	A: PO: Mild to moderate: 250 mg q12h for 3 d A: PO: ER: 500 mg/d for 3 d A: IV: 200 q12h A: PO: severe/complicated: 500 mg q12h for 7-14 d; 1 g/d XRfor 7-14 d C: PO: 10-20 mg/kg q12h for 10-21 d A: IV: 400 mg q12h for 7-14 d; dilute and infuse over 1 h C: IV: 6-10 mg/kg q8h for 10-21 d	Has broad-spectrum antibacterial effect. For UTI, skin and soft-tissue infections, bone and joint infections, and anthrax infection. Antacid inhibits drug absorption. Use with caution in patients with seizure disorders. Can be taken without food. Photosensitivity can occur. Avoid excessive exposure to sunlight. Pregnancy category: C; PB: 20%-40%; t½: 4 h
nalidixic acid (NegGram)	A: PO: 1 g q.i.d. for 1-2 wk; 500 mg q.i.d. for long-term use; *max:* 4 g/d C >3 mo: PO: 55 mg/kg/d in 4 divided doses for 1-2 wk; 33 mg/kg/d for long-term use	For acute and chronic UTIs. Resistance to drug may occur. Highly protein-bound. Not distributed in prostatic fluid. Give with food to avoid GI upset. Photosensitivity can occur. Have patient contact health care provider if seizures or severe headaches occur. Pregnancy category: C; PB: 93%; t½: 1-2.5 h
norfloxacin (Noroxin)	A: PO: 400 mg q12h for 3-21 d on empty stomach	For acute and chronic UTIs. Most potent drug of the quinolone group. Food may inhibit drug absorption. Pregnancy category: C; PB: 10%-15%; t½: 3-4 h
ofloxacin	A: PO: 200 mg q12h for 3-10 d	For UTIs, respiratory tract infections, and skin infections. May cause headaches, dizziness, and insomnia. Pregnancy category: C; PB: UK; t½: 4-8 h
Other		
aztreonam (Azactam)	A: IM/IV: 500 mg–1 g q8-12h C >9 mo: IM/IV: 30 mg/kg q6-8h	Treatment of UTIs caused by gram-negative organisms. Also useful for lower respiratory tract infections and septicemia. Pregnancy category: B; PB: 56%-60%; t½: 1.5-2 h
imipenem/cilastatin sodium (Primaxin)	A: IV: 250 mg q6-8h; *max:* 4 g/d or 50 mg/kg/d, whichever is less	Treatment of serious UTIs. Also useful for lower respiratory tract, bone, and joint infections; septicemia; and endocarditis. Pregnancy category: C; PB: imipenem 20%/cilastatin 40%; t½: 1 h
polymyxin B SO_4	A/C: IV: 15,000-25,000 units/kg/d in divided doses q12h	Effective for UTIs and prevention of bacteruria from Foley catheter. Can cause nephrotoxicity. Monitor renal function (BUN, serum creatinine). Pregnancy category: B; PB: UK; t½: 4-6 h

A, Adult; *Adol,* adolescent; *b.i.d.,* twice a day; *BUN,* blood urea nitrogen; *C,* child; *CLcr,* creatinine clearance; *d,* day; *ER,* extended-release; *GI,* gastrointestinal; *h,* hour; *IM,* intramuscular; *IV,* intravenous; *min,* minute; *mo,* month; *PB,* protein-binding; *p.c.,* after meals; *PO,* by mouth; *q.i.d.,* four times a day; *t½,* half-life; *t.i.d.,* three times a day; *UK,* unknown; *UTI,* urinary tract infection; *wk,* week; *y,* year; *>,* greater than; *<,* less than.

URINARY ANTISPASMODICS/ ANTIMUSCARINICS

Urinary tract spasms resulting from infection or injury can be relieved with **antispasmodics** that have a direct action on the smooth muscles of the urinary tract. This group of drugs (dimethyl sulfoxide [also called *DMSO*], oxybutynin [Ditropan], and flavoxate [Urispas]) is contraindicated for use if urinary or GI obstruction is present or if the patient has glaucoma. Antispasmodics have the same effects as **antimuscarinics** (agents that block parasympathetic nerve impulses), parasympatholytics, and anticholinergics (see Chapter 19). Side effects include dry mouth, increased heart rate, dizziness, intestinal distention, and constipation. Tolterodine tartrate (Detrol) is an antimuscarinic/anticholinergic drug used to control an overactive bladder, which causes frequency in urination. This drug also decreases urge urinary incontinence. It has the same side effects as antispasmodics/anticholinergics. The patient taking antimuscarinic/anticholinergic drugs should be taught to report urinary retention, severe dizziness, blurred vision, palpitations, and confusion. The patient should be warned to use caution in hot environments to avoid heat prostration. Table 34-2 lists drugs that are urinary analgesics, stimulants, and antispasmodics/antimuscarinics.

TABLE 34-2 URINARY ANALGESICS, STIMULANTS, AND ANTISPASMODICS

GENERIC (BRAND)	ROUTE AND DOSAGE	USES AND CONSIDERATIONS
Urinary Analgesics		
phenazopyridine HCl (Pyridium)	A: PO: 200 mg t.i.d. p.c.; *max:* 600 mg/d	For chronic cystitis to alleviate pain and burning sensation during urination. Urine will be reddish orange. Can be taken concurrently with an antibiotic. Treats only symptoms, not underlying cause. Do not use long-term for undiagnosed urinary tract pain. Pregnancy category: B; PB: UK; $t\frac{1}{2}$: UK
Urinary Stimulants		
bethanechol Cl (Urecholine)	A: PO: 10-50 mg t.i.d./q.i.d. 1 h a.c. or 2 h p.c.; *max:* 200 mg/d A: subQ: 5-mg single dose, may repeat 3-4 times PRN; *max:* 40 mg/d	For hypotonic or atonic bladder. Do not take if peptic ulcer is present. Can cause epigastric distress, abdominal cramps, nausea, vomiting, diarrhea, and flatulence. Can cause dizziness, lightheadedness, and fainting, especially when standing up from lying or sitting position. Pregnancy category: C; PB: UK; $t\frac{1}{2}$: UK
Urinary Antispasmodics		
dimethyl sulfoxide (DMSO, Rimso-50)	Bladder instillation: 50 mL of 50% sol retained for 15 min; repeat q2wk until relief	For cystitis. Administered into the bladder to remain for 15 minutes. Additional effects are antiinflammatory, anesthetic, and bacteriostatic. Can cause garlic-like taste and odor on breath and skin for up to 72 h. Pregnancy category: C; PB: UK; $t\frac{1}{2}$: UK
flavoxate HCl (Urispas)	A: PO: 100-200 mg t.i.d./q.i.d.	For urinary tract spasms. Avoid in patients with glaucoma. Cautious use by older adults. Side effects include nausea, vomiting, dry mouth, drowsiness, blurred vision. Pregnancy category: B; PB: 50%-80%; $t\frac{1}{2}$: 10-20 h
oxybutynin Cl (Ditropan)	A: PO: 5 mg b.i.d./t.i.d.; *max:* 20 mg/d Older adults: PO: 2.5-5 mg b.i.d.; *max:* 20 mg/d C >5 y: PO: 5 mg b.i.d.; *max:* 15 mg/d	For urinary tract spasms and overactive bladder. Contraindicated for patients with cardiac, renal, hepatic, and prostate problems. Side effects include drowsiness, blurred vision, and dry mouth. Pregnancy category: B; PB: UK; $t\frac{1}{2}$: 2-5 h
mirabegron (Myrbetriq)	A:PO: 25 mg qd	For treatment of overactive bladder. Pregnancy category: C; PB: 71%; $t\frac{1}{2}$: 50 h
Antimuscarinics/Anticholinergics		
tolterodine tartrate (Detrol, Detrol LA)	A: PO: 2 mg b.i.d.; *max.* 4 mg/d A: ER: 4 mg/d	To control overactive bladder by decreasing urinary frequency and urgency. Patients with narrow-angle glaucoma should not take this drug. Dry mouth is common. Pregnancy category: C; PB: 96%; $t\frac{1}{2}$: 2-4 h
trospium chloride (Sanctura, Sanctura XR)	A: PO: 20 mg b.i.d.; *max:* 60 mg/d A: ER: 60 mg/d in morning	To treat overactive bladder by action of a muscarinic-receptor antagonist. Pregnancy category: C; PB: 50%-85%; $t\frac{1}{2}$: 20-35 h
solifenacin succinate (VESIcare)	A: PO: 5 mg/d initially; then up to 10 mg/d if tolerated; *max:* 10 mg/d	To treat overactive bladder by action of a muscarinic-receptor antagonist. Pregnancy category: C; PB: 98%; $t\frac{1}{2}$: 55 h
darifenacin hydrobromide (Enablex)	A: PO: 7.5-15 mg/d; *max:* 15 mg/d	To treat overactive bladder by action of a muscarinic-receptor antagonist. Pregnancy category: C; PB: 98%; $t\frac{1}{2}$: 13-19 h

A, Adult; *a.c.,* before meals; *b.i.d.,* twice a day; *C,* child; *d,* day; *ER,* extended-release; *h,* hour; *max,* maximum; *min,* minute; *PB,* protein-binding; *p.c.,* after meals; *PO,* by mouth; *PRN,* as needed; *q.i.d.,* four times a day; *subQ,* subcutaneous; *sol,* solution; $t\frac{1}{2}$, half-life; *t.i.d.,* three times a day; *UK,* unknown; *wk,* week; *XR,* extended release; *y,* year; >, greater than.

KEY WEBSITES

Information on phenazopyridine: *www.nlm.nih.gov/medlineplus/druginfo/meds/a682231.html*

Information on urecholine: *www.rxlist.com/cgi/generic3/bethane.htm*

Information on detrol: *www.rxlist.com/detrol-drug.htm*

CRITICAL THINKING CASE STUDY

FL, a 29-year-old woman, has complained to her health care provider of painful urinary frequency and urgency. The patient has an elevated temperature. A urine specimen indicates that FL has a urinary tract infection (UTI). The health care provider prescribes co-trimoxazole D.S. tablets (double-strength, T-160 mg/S-800 mg) twice a day for 14 days.

1. What other information should the health care provider obtain from the patient?
2. What other dose of co-trimoxazole (TMP-SMZ) could be prescribed? Explain your answer.
3. What should the health care provider discuss with the patient in regard to taking the drug and its possible side effects? What other information should FL receive?
4. What is the recommended time for follow-up care for FL?
5. What other drugs might be used instead of co-trimoxazole? Would one urinary antiinfective drug be more effective than another antiinfective drug? Explain your answer.

NCLEX STUDY QUESTIONS

1. A patient is taking nitrofurantoin (Macrodantin). What will the nurse teach the patient?
   a. Expect the urine to turn blue.
   b. Keep the urine acidic by drinking milk.
   c. Rinse the mouth after taking oral nitrofurantoin to avoid teeth staining.
   d. Take an antacid with oral nitrofurantoin to avoid gastrointestinal distress.
2. A patient complains about a burning sensation and pain when urinating. Which urinary analgesic does the nurse suspect will be ordered?
   a. tolterodine (Detrol)
   b. oxybutynin (Ditropan)
   c. bethanechol (Urecholine)
   d. phenazopyridine (Pyridium)
3. A patient is taking the urinary antiseptic methenamine mandelate for a urinary tract infection. The nurse understands that this drug should not be given concurrently with which other drug to avoid potential crystalluria?
   a. ertapenem (Invanz)
   b. ciprofloxacin (Cipro)
   c. nalidixic acid (NegGram)
   d. trimethoprim-sulfamethoxazole (Bactrim)
4. A patient is receiving solifenacin succinate (VESIcare). The nurse knows that this drug is used to treat which condition?
   a. Chronic cystitis
   b. Urinary tract stones
   c. Urinary tract infection
   d. Overactive bladder
5. The patient is taking tolterodine tartrate (Detrol). The nurse plans to teach the patient to report which condition?
   a. Alkaline urine
   b. Urinary retention
   c. Excessive tearing
   d. Reddish orange urine
6. The nurse is caring for a patient who is taking nitrofurantoin (Macrodantin). Which nursing interventions are appropriate for this patient? (Select all that apply.)
   a. Monitor urinary output and urine specific gravity.
   b. Monitor the patient for peripheral neuropathy.
   c. Advise the patient to take the medication on an empty stomach to enhance absorption.
   d. Warn the patient to avoid excess exposure to sunlight.
   e. Inform the patient that urine may turn a harmless brown color.

Answers: 1, c; 2, d; 3, d; 4, d; 5, b; 6, a, b, e.

UNIT XI

Immunologic Agents

Immunity comprises functions that protect people from the effects of invasion of the body by microscopic organisms such as bacteria, viruses, molds, spores, pollens, protozoa, and cells from other persons or animals. A person remains in harmony with these organisms as long as the organisms do not enter the body's internal environment. The body has various defenses (e.g., skin) that prevent microorganisms from gaining access to its internal environment. However, these defenses are not infallible, and invasion of the body's internal environment by microorganisms occurs often. A properly functioning immune system neutralizes, eliminates, or destroys the invading microorganisms. To do this without harming the body, immune system cells use defensive actions against only nonself proteins and cells. This means that immune system cells can differentiate between the body's own healthy self cells and other nonself proteins and cells.

Nonself proteins and cells include (1) all foreign cells and microorganisms, (2) infected or debilitated body cells, and (3) self cells that have undergone malignant transformation into cancer cells. This ability to recognize self versus nonself, which is necessary to prevent healthy body cells from being destroyed along with the invaders, is called *self-tolerance.* Immune system cells are the only body cells capable of recognizing self from nonself.

Unique proteins on the surface of all body cells of each individual serve as a personal identification code for that person. The cell-surface proteins of one person are recognized as "foreign" by the immune system of another person. These are antigens—proteins capable of stimulating an immune response.

Immune function is generally most efficient when people are in their twenties and thirties; it slowly declines with increasing age. Older adults have marginal immune function, causing increased susceptibility to a variety of pathologic conditions.

IMMUNE SYSTEM STRUCTURE

The immune system is not confined to any one organ or body area. Instead, immune system cells originate in the bone marrow. Some of these cells mature in the bone marrow; others leave the bone marrow and mature in different body sites. After maturation, most immune system cells are released into the blood, where they circulate throughout the body and exert specific effects.

IMMUNE SYSTEM FUNCTION

The three processes necessary for immunity together with the cells involved in these responses can be categorized as inflammation, antibody-mediated immunity (humoral immunity), and cell-mediated immunity. Inflammation is discussed in the introduction to Unit VII. Full immunity, or *immunocompetence,* requires the adequate function and interaction of all three processes, although some functions of each overlap. Long-lasting immune actions are those generated by antibody-mediated immunity and cell-mediated immunity.

Antibody-Mediated Immunity

Antibody-mediated immunity (AMI), also called *humoral immunity,* involves antigen-antibody interactions that neutralize, eliminate, or destroy foreign proteins. Antibodies for these interactions are produced by populations of B-lymphocytes.

Antigen-Antibody Interactions

Antigen-antibody interactions occur in the body's internal environment. To make an antibody that can exert its effects on a specific antigen, the body must first be exposed to that antigen to the degree that the antigen enters the body. Even when exposure includes penetration, not all exposures result in the stimulation of antibody production. Invasion by the antigen must occur in such large numbers that some of the antigen either evades detection by the normal nonspecific defenses or overwhelms the abilities of the inflammatory response to neutralize, eliminate, or destroy the invader.

Acquiring Antibody-Mediated Immunity

The two broad categories of immunity are *innate immunity* and *acquired immunity.* Innate immunity is a genetically determined characteristic of an individual, group, or species. A person either has or does not have innate immunity. For example, humans have many innate immunities to viruses and other microorganisms that cause specific diseases in animals. As a result, humans are not susceptible to such diseases as mange, distemper, hog cholera, or any of a variety of animal afflictions. This type of immunity cannot be developed or transferred from one person to another and is not an adaptive response to exposure or invasion by foreign proteins.

Acquired immunity is the immunity that every person's body makes (or can receive) as an adaptive response to invasion by foreign proteins. Antibody-mediated immunity is an acquired immunity. Acquired immunity occurs either naturally or artificially and can be either active or passive. Active immunity occurs when antigens enter the body and the body responds by making specific antibodies against the antigen. This type of immunity is active because the body takes an active part in making the antibodies. Active immunity can occur under conditions that are either natural or artificial. Natural active immunity occurs when an antigen enters the body without human assistance, and the body responds by actively making antibodies against that antigen (e.g., chickenpox virus). Most of the time, the first invasion of the body by this antigen results in the person manifesting signs and symptoms of the disease. However, processes occurring in the body at the same time allow the person to acquire immunity to that antigen so that a second exposure to the same antigen will not cause illness. This type of immunity is the most effective and the longest lasting.

Artificial active immunity is a type of protection developed against illnesses that produce such serious side effects that total avoidance of the disease is most desirable. Small amounts of specific antigens are deliberately placed in the body (as a vaccination) so that the body responds by actively making antibodies against the antigen. Because antigens used for this procedure have been specially processed to make them less likely to proliferate within the body, this exposure does not in itself cause the disease.

Examples of diseases for which artificially acquired active immunity can be obtained include tetanus, diphtheria, measles, smallpox, mumps, and rubella. This type of immunity lasts many years, although repeated but smaller doses of the original antigen are periodically required as a "booster" to maintain complete protection against the antigen.

Passive immunity occurs when antibodies against a specific antigen are in a person's body, but the person did not actively generate these antibodies. Instead, these antibodies are made in the body of another person or animal and then transferred to the body of a specific individual. Because these antibodies are foreign to the individual, the body recognizes the antibodies as nonself and takes steps to eliminate them relatively quickly. For this reason, passive immunity can provide only immediate, short-term protection against a specific antigen.

Cell-Mediated Immunity

Cell-mediated immunity (CMI), or cellular immunity, involves many leukocyte actions, reactions, and interactions that range from the simple to the complex. This type of immunity is provided by committed lymphocyte stem cells that mature in the secondary lymphoid tissues of the thymus and pericortical areas of lymph nodes. Certain CMI responses influence and regulate the activities of antibody-mediated immunity and inflammation by producing and releasing cytokines; therefore, total immunocompetence relies on optimal CMI function.

The leukocytes playing the most important roles in CMI include several specific T-lymphocyte subsets along with a special population of cells known as *natural killer cells* (NK cells). T-lymphocytes further differentiate into a variety of subsets, each of which has a specific function. The three T-lymphocyte subsets crucial to the development and continuation of CMI are helper/inducer T-cells, suppressor T-cells, and cytotoxic/cytolytic T-cells.

Protection Provided by Cell-Mediated Immunity

Specific components of CMI assist in providing protection to the body by their highly developed abilities to differentiate self from nonself. The nonself cells most easily recognized by CMI are self cells that are infected by organisms that live within host cells and self cells that are mutated at the DNA level and are thus abnormal. CMI provides a surveillance system that rids the body of self cells that might potentially harm the body. CMI is critically important in preventing development of cancer and metastasis after exposure to carcinogens.

CHAPTER

35

HIV- and AIDS-Related Drugs

Robert J. Kizior, Janice Heinssen, and Patricia Lincoln

evolve WEBSITE

http://evolve.elsevier.com/KeeHayes/pharmacology/

- Animations
- Content Updates
- Key Points
- Review Questions for the NCLEX® Examination
- References from the Textbook
- Unfolding Case Studies

OBJECTIVES

- Describe the life cycle of the human immunodeficiency virus (HIV), and relate it to the actions of pharmacologic agents used in the treatment of HIV disease.
- Identify the risk factors for HIV transmission.
- Describe the six classifications of antiretroviral therapy, and give examples of medications in each group.
- Explain specific issues of medication adherence to antiretroviral agents.
- Discuss the nurse's role in medication management and issues of adherence.
- Explain prophylactic treatment for opportunistic infections.
- Discuss the medical management for preventing mother-to-child transmission of HIV infection during pregnancy.
- Discuss health care workers' exposure risks, and relate the risk and type of exposure to recommendations.
- Apply the nursing process, including teaching, to the care of patients with HIV infection.

OUTLINE

KEY TERMS

Acquired immunodeficiency syndrome (AIDS) was first reported in the United States in 1981 and has led to the death of more than 25 million people globally since 1981. In 2009, an estimated 1.8 million deaths occurred, including 260,000 children younger than 15 years. It is estimated that 33.3 million people worldwide were living with HIV in 2009. The annual number of new HIV infections was 2.6 million in 2009, a reduction from 3 million in 2001. In the United States, it is estimated that at the end of 2009, 1.5 million people were living with HIV/AIDS, and that 210,000 people are unaware that they are HIV infected.

Significant improvement in HIV-related morbidity and mortality and a reduction in perinatal and behaviorally associated HIV transmission have become possible with combination antiretroviral therapy. Attaining viral suppression of HIV necessitates the use of at least two and preferably three active drugs from two or more drug classes.

This is referred to as **highly active antiretroviral therapy** (HAART), **combination antiretroviral therapy** (cART), or **antiretroviral therapy** (ART). Patients who engage and are retained in HIV care and treatment can now experience HIV as a chronic illness rather than a disease of death and dying. In the United States, approximately 30% of people living with HIV/AIDS are age 50 years or older. Areas of concern in older HIV patients are as follows:

1. Older HIV-infected patients may have age-related comorbid illnesses that can complicate management of HIV infection.
2. HIV may affect the biology of aging, possibly causing premature aging.
3. Reduced mucosal and immunologic defenses (such as postmenopausal atrophic vaginitis) and behavioral changes (such as decreased condom use because of less concern about pregnancy and increased use of erectile dysfunction medication) could result in increased risk of HIV acquisition and transmission.
4. Health care providers generally perceive older adults to be at decreased risk for HIV and as a result do not screen this age group as frequently as others.

Although strides have been made in the treatment of HIV/AIDS, challenges remain. One important aspect is increased drug **resistance** to current therapies. The makeup of the HIV DNA strands allows the virus to mutate from a drug-sensitive to a drug-resistant form. The patient is encouraged to achieve >95% medication **adherence** to minimize medication resistance, but studies suggest that 6% to 16% of patients who are naïve to ART have pre-existing genotypic resistance.

Nursing and public health initiatives should incorporate harm-reduction education to further minimize transmission of resistant virus (e.g., safer sex, not sharing needles or drug works, needle exchange programs).

HIV INFECTION: PATHOPHYSIOLOGY

HIV is an RNA retrovirus. It is unable to survive and replicate unless it is inside a living human cell. HIV destroys CD4+ T cells (also called *helper T cells* or *CD4 + T lymphocytes*), which play a critical role in the human **immune response** through recognition of infectious and neoplastic processes. The destruction of CD4 cells by HIV results in immune deficiency. The CD4 cell count is an indicator for immune function in those with HIV.

Normal CD4 counts range from 800 to 1200 cells/mm^3. After initial infection, there is rapid viral replication, resulting in a high level of virus in peripheral blood (viral load). There is a corresponding drop in CD4 cells, which triggers an immune response, resulting in CD4 cell replacement and HIV antibody production. The viral load drops with establishment of immune response. Symptoms range from mild to severe (fever, fatigue, pharyngitis, myalgia or arthralgia, lymphadenopathy, headache, night sweats) in those recently infected with HIV and can be experienced 2 to 12 weeks after HIV exposure. This period is called *acute retroviral syndrome, acute seroconversion syndrome,* or *primary HIV infection.* Symptoms in this stage can often be mistaken by both patient and health care provider for a transient flulike illness. Consequently, few people are diagnosed during this time. Additionally, the time delay from infection to a positive HIV test result averages 10 to 14 days, but some do not seroconvert for 3 to 4 weeks. Almost all patients seroconvert within 6 months. This time delay between infection and positive test results is known as the *window period.* For this reason, patients who are at risk for HIV infection and test negative should be counseled to have the test repeated in 3 months (the close of the window period). If HIV is strongly suspected, an HIV RNA quantitative test can be done. A high viral load would support HIV diagnosis (>10,000 c/mL and usually >100,000 c/mL).

Over time and in the absence of treatment, HIV infection generally progresses slowly with a gradual decline in CD4 cells. AIDS is a diagnosis that indicates advanced disease. The 1993 AIDS surveillance case definition includes all patients with a CD4 count <200 cells/mm^3 or <14% of total lymphocytes, or one of the other AIDS-defining conditions listed in Table 35-1. The risk of opportunistic infection increases when CD4 counts fall below 200 cells/mm^3.

TABLE 35-1 **CLASSIFICATION SYSTEM FOR HIV INFECTION***

	CLINICAL CATEGORIES FOR ADULTS		
	(A) ASYMPTOMATIC, ACUTE (PRIMARY) HIV OR PERSISTENT GENERALIZED LYMPHADENOPATHY	(B) SYMPTOMATIC, NOT (A) OR (C) CONDITIONS	(C) AIDS-INDICATOR CONDITIONS
(1) ≥500/mcL	A1	B1	C1
(2) 200-499/mcL	A2	B2	C2
(3) <200/mcL	A3	B3	C3
AIDS-indicator T-cell count			

≥, Greater than or equal to; <, less than.

From the Department of Health and Human Services, Henry J. Kaiser Family Foundation: Panel on practices for treatment of HIV infection: guidelines for the use of antiretroviral agents in HIV-infected adults and adolescents, Dec 1, 1998.

*The revised CDC classification system for HIV-infected adolescents and adults categorizes persons on the basis of CD4 T-lymphocyte counts and clinical conditions associated with HIV infection. The system is based on three ranges of CD4 T-lymphocyte counts and three clinical categories (Categories A to C).

CD4 T-LYMPHOCYTE CATEGORIES

HIV-infected persons should be classified based on existing guidelines for the medical management of HIV-infected persons; thus, the lowest accurate CD4 T-lymphocyte count (but not necessarily the most recent) should be used for classification purposes.

Clinical Categories

Category A consists of one or more of the following conditions in an adolescent or adult (13 years of age or older) with documented HIV infection. Conditions listed in categories B and C must not have occurred.

- Asymptomatic HIV infection
- Persistent generalized lymphadenopathy
- Acute (primary) HIV infection with accompanying illness or history of acute HIV infection

Category B consists of symptomatic conditions in an HIV-infected adolescent or adult that are not included in category C and are attributed to HIV infection or are considered to have a clinical course complicated by HIV infection. Examples of conditions in category B include, but are not limited to, the following:

- Bacillary angiomatosis
- Candidiasis, oropharyngeal (thrush)
- Candidiasis, vulvovaginal; persistent, frequent, or poorly responsive to therapy
- Cervical dysplasia (moderate or severe)/cervical carcinoma in situ
- Constitutional symptoms, such as fever (101.3° F or 38.5° C) or diarrhea lasting longer than 1 month
- Hairy leukoplakia, oral
- Herpes zoster (shingles), involving at least two distinct episodes or more than one dermatome
- Idiopathic thrombocytopenic purpura
- Listeriosis
- Pelvic inflammatory disease, particularly if complicated by tubo-ovarian abscess
- Peripheral neuropathy

For classification purposes, category B conditions take precedence over category A conditions.

Category C includes the clinical conditions listed in the AIDS surveillance case definition. For classification purposes, once a category C condition occurs, the person remains in category C.

- Bacterial pneumonia, recurrent (two or more episodes in 12 months)
- Candidiasis of the bronchi, trachea, or lungs
- Candidiasis, esophageal
- Cervical carcinoma, invasive, confirmed by biopsy
- Coccidioidomycosis, disseminated or extrapulmonary
- Cryptococcosis, extrapulmonary
- Cryptosporidiosis, chronic intestinal
- Cytomegalovirus disease
- HIV-related encephalopathy
- Herpes simplex: chronic ulcers or bronchitis, pneumonitis, or esophagitis
- Histoplasmosis, disseminated or extrapulmonary
- Kaposi sarcoma
- Lymphoma, Burkitt, immunoblastic, or primary central nervous system
- *Mycobacterium avium* complex (MAC) or *M. kansasii,* disseminated or extrapulmonary
- Mycobacterium tuberculosis, pulmonary or extrapulmonary
- *Pneumocystis jiroveci* (formerly *carinii*) pneumonia (PCP)
- Progressive multifocal leukoencephalopathy (PML)
- Salmonella septicemia, recurrent

HIV LIFE CYCLE

The phases of the HIV life cycle (Figure 35-1) are (1) binding and fusion: HIV begins its life cycle when it binds to a CD4 receptor and one of two co-receptors on the surface of a CD4 T-lymphocyte. The virus then fuses with the host cell. After fusion, the virus releases RNA, its genetic material, into the host cell; (2) reverse transcription: An HIV enzyme called **reverse transcriptase** (RT) converts the single-stranded HIV RNA to a double-stranded HIV DNA; (3) integration: The newly formed HIV DNA enters the host cell's nucleus, where an HIV enzyme called **integrase** "hides" the HIV DNA within the host cell's own DNA. The integrated HIV DNA is called a provirus; (4) transcription: When the host cell receives a signal to become active, the provirus uses a host enzyme called RNA polymerase to create copies of the HIV genomic material, as well as shorter strands of RNA called messenger RNA (MRNA). The mRNA is used as a blueprint to make long chains of HIV proteins; (5) **assembly:** An HIV enzyme called **protease** cuts the long chains of HIV proteins into smaller individual proteins. As the smaller HIV proteins come together with copies of HIV's RNA genetic material, a new virus particle is assembled; (6) **budding:** The newly assembled virus pushes out ("buds") from the host cell. During budding, the new virus steals part of the cell's outer envelope. This envelope, which acts as a covering, is studded with protein/sugar combinations called HIV glycoproteins. These HIV glycoproteins are necessary for the virus to bind to CD4 and co-receptors. The immature virus breaks free of the infected cell; (7) maturation: The protease enzyme finishes cutting HIV protein chains into individual proteins that combine to make a new working virus. The new copies of HIV can now move on to infect other cells.

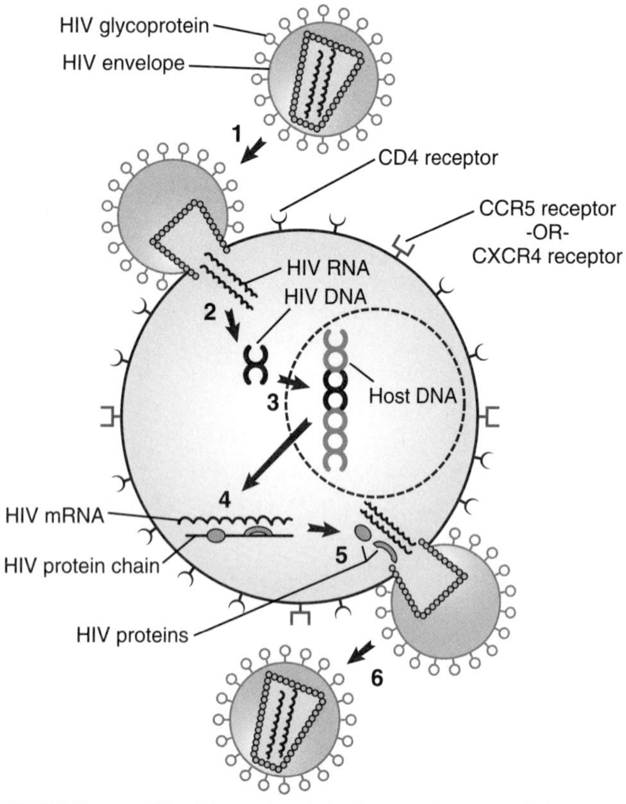

FIGURE 35–1 The life cycle of the human immunodeficiency virus. (Image courtesy of the National Institutes of Health.)

HIV TRANSMISSION

HIV is spread via intimate contact with blood, semen, vaginal fluids, and breast milk. Transmission of the virus occurs primarily by: (1) sexual contact (includes oral, vaginal, and anal sex); (2) direct blood contact (intravenous drug use with shared needles, shared drug works, shared contaminated personal care items such as razors, and blood transfusions [now extremely rare in the United States]); and (3) mother to child (through shared maternal-fetal blood circulation, by direct blood contact during delivery, or in breast milk). Included in these modes are accidental needle injury, artificial insemination with donated semen, and organ transplant. HIV is not spread by casual contact (e.g., hugging), by touching items previously touched by a person infected with the virus, or during participation in sports. Those at highest risk include persons engaging in unprotected sex, those with multiple sexual partners (either the patient themselves or partner[s] of the patient), intravenous drug users who share needles or drug works, and infants born to women with HIV. The risk of mother-to-child transmission (MTCT) is 25% without ART; the risk decreases to 1% to 2% with successful use of ART. Other factors that increase the risk of MTCT are mother with a viral load >1000 copies/mL at delivery, premature rupture of the membranes, hepatitis C virus co-infection, preterm gestation, and vaginal delivery.

LABORATORY TESTING

Several laboratory tests are important for initial patient evaluation upon entry to care, during follow-up evaluation for those not on ART, and before and after initiation or modification of ART to assess for immunologic and virologic efficacy of treatment.

The laboratory tests used to determine when to initiate medication therapy and to monitor efficacy of therapy and indications for changing therapy are **CD4 T-cell** count, plasma HIV RNA quantitative assay (or **viral load** [VL] test), and HIV resistance testing.

The count reflects the number of CD4 cells circulating in the blood. The result is listed as an absolute number and a relative percentage. The absolute count can vary in the same patient depending on laboratory used, time of day laboratory blood work is drawn, or acute illness. The CD4 percentage is a more stable reflection of the **immune system** and is used in conjunction with the absolute count to monitor health status and response to medication therapy. The patient should be encouraged to use the same laboratory at approximately the same time of day to promote consistency of results. The nurse should monitor the laboratory used, because lab value references vary from laboratory to laboratory. The HIV viral load is indicative of the level of virus circulating in the blood and is the best determinant of treatment efficacy. Two FDA-approved commercially available assays commonly used are the quantitative polymerase chain reaction assay and the branched-chain DNA. A key goal of therapy is to achieve and maintain a viral load below the limits of detection (<20 to 40 copies/mL, depending on assay used). This goal should be achieved in 16 to 24 weeks of therapy.

HIV Resistance Testing

Resistance to antiretroviral medications leads to treatment failure and to risk of transmitting drug-resistant virus. Determination of the presence of a drug-resistant strain of HIV is important to prevent ineffective medication treatment. Two types of testing are available: Genotypic resistance testing identifies mutations in the genetic code of HIV associated with drug resistance. Phenotypic testing determines if the patient's HIV is able to replicate in the presence of specific antiretroviral medications. Genotypic resistance testing is recommended upon entry into care, regardless of whether ART will be started immediately.

Additional Laboratory Evaluation

Screening for HLA-B5701 determines if the patient has a mutation associated with a hypersensitivity reaction to abacavir (Ziagen). Those with a positive HLA-B5701 result should not receive abacavir and should have it listed as a drug allergy. This test should be done and results reviewed before abacavir is considered as part of a treatment regimen.

A viral tropism assay should be done before initiation of a CCR5 antagonist medication.

CLASSIFICATION

HIV disease staging and classification systems are important tools for tracking and monitoring the HIV epidemic and providing the clinician and patient with information about HIV disease stage and clinical management.

The two major classification systems are the Centers for Disease Control and Prevention (CDC) staging system (revised in 1993 and 2008) and the World Health Organization (WHO) system (last revised in 2007). In December 2008, CDC published *Revised Surveillance Case Definitions for HIV Infection Among Adults, Adolescents, and Children Aged <18 Months and for HIV Infection and AIDS Among Children Aged 18 Months to <13 Years—United States, 2008* (*www.cdc.gov/mmwr/preview/mmwrhtml/rr5710a1.htm*).

The CDC system assesses the severity of HIV disease by CD4 cell counts and by presence of specific HIV-related conditions; the system is based on the lowest documented CD4 cell count (nadir CD4) and on previously diagnosed HIV-related conditions. The WHO system is useful in resource-constrained settings without access to CD4 cell measurements and classifies HIV disease on the basis of clinical manifestations that clinicians and those with varying levels of HIV expertise and training can recognize in diverse settings.

TREATMENT GOALS

The primary goals for initiating ART are to reduce HIV-associated morbidity and mortality and prolong the duration and quality of life; restore and preserve immunologic function; maximally and durably suppress plasma HIV viral load; and prevent HIV transmission.

INDICATIONS FOR ANTIRETROVIRAL THERAPY

Recommendations for HIV management, including initiation and ongoing treatment with **antiretroviral** medications, change rapidly based on updated clinical data and expert medical opinion. Guidelines for the Use of Antiretroviral Agents in HIV 1 Infected Adults and Adolescents have been developed by the U.S. Department of Health and Human Services (DHHS) Expert Panel on Antiretroviral Guidelines for Adults and Adolescents. This panel recommends ART for all HIV-infected individuals. The strength of this recommendation varies based on pretreatment CD4 cell count; however, regardless of CD4 count, ART is strongly recommended for HIV-infected pregnant patients; for those with a history of an AIDS-defining illness, HIV-associated nephropathy, or HIV and hepatitis B coinfection; and for serodiscordant couples. The panel posts updated information regularly at *http://aidsinfo.nih.gov.*

With increased treatment options and a better understanding of the risks of untreated HIV infection or uncontrolled viremia, there is a shift toward earlier consideration of ART. Suppression of HIV with ART may decrease inflammation and immune activation that is thought to contribute to higher rates of cardiovascular, kidney, and liver disease, neurologic complications, and malignancy in HIV-infected cohorts. If therapy is to be initiated, medications are selected based on results of genotypic resistance testing where applicable; co-morbidities (e.g., liver disease, renal dysfunction, depression); potential drug-drug interactions; pregnancy status; and assessment of patient's willingness and readiness to start therapy. Evaluation of medication readiness should include dosage regimen, pill burden, dosing frequency, food restrictions, side effects, and patient's daily routine. Tools for promoting medication adherence (e.g., alarms, pill planners) and plans for management of potential medication side effects should be reviewed before medication initiation. The patient should be instructed in the need for >95% medication adherence, the potential for development of medication resistance with less than optimal adherence, and clinical implications of resistance.

CLASSES OF ANTIRETROVIRAL MEDICATIONS

Reverse transcriptase inhibitors, protease inhibitors (PIs), **entry (fusion) inhibitors, CCR5 antagonists,** and **integrase inhibitors** make up the classification of drugs known as *antiretroviral therapy.* Reverse transcriptase inhibitors (RT inhibitors) are further divided into **nucleoside/nucleotide** (NRTI) **analogues** and **non-nucleoside** (NNRTI) **analogues.** More than 20 different antiretroviral agents are FDA approved, and various agents are available in fixed-dose combinations that contain two or more HIV medications from one or more drug classes. PIs have changed the prognosis for millions of patients infected with HIV. PIs combined with RT inhibitors can reduce viral plasma levels to undetectable levels, offering significant clinical benefits.

The most recent additions include maraviroc (Selzentry) a CCR5 antagonist; raltegravir (Isentress) and dolutegravir (Tivicay), integrase inhibitors; and etravirine (Intelence) and rilpivirine (Edurant), nucleoside reverse transcriptase inhibitors.

Antiretroviral Agents

Since the 1980s, when zidovudine monotherapy showed survival benefits in advanced HIV patients, much progress has been made. Newer agents have improved adherence (e.g., fewer pills for more convenient dosing, formulation changes that reduce dosing frequency or pill burden, combination dosage forms with two or three drugs in one pill). Other improvements include increased potency, improved side-effect profile (e.g., decreased gastrointestinal effects), and protease-inhibitor boosting with ritonavir.

ART is the standard of care in the treatment of HIV infection. The following combinations are preferred regimens for antiretroviral-naïve patients:

- Efavirenz (NNRTI)/tenofovir (NRTI)/emtricitabine (NRTI)
- Ritonavir-boosted atazanavir (PI) plus tenofovir (NRTI)/emtricitabine (NRTI)
- Ritonavir-boosted darunavir (PI) plus tenofovir (NRTI)/emtricitabine (NRTI)
- Raltegravir (integrase inhibitor) plus tenofovir (NRTI)/emtricitabine (NRTI)

Nucleoside/Nucleotide Reverse Transcriptase Inhibitors

Seven NRTIs are approved for use in the United States: zidovudine (Retrovir), didanosine (Videx), stavudine (Zerit), lamivudine (Epivir), abacavir (Ziagen), tenofovir (Viread), and emtricitabine (Emtriva). Six fixed-dose combination products are also available: Combivir (lamivudine/zidovudine), Trizivir (Abacavir/lamivudine/zidovudine), Epzicom (abacavir/lamivudine), Atripla (efavirenz/emtricitabine/tenofovir), Truvada (emtricitabine/tenofovir), and Complera (rilpivirine/emtricitabine/tenofovir). Tenofovir (Viread) is the only nucleotide analogue.

NRTIs, the foundation of ART, act by interfering with HIV viral RNA-dependent DNA polymerase, resulting in inhibition of viral replication. Two of these agents are typically included in initial ART regimens. The preferred dual NRTI is tenofovir/emtricitabine (or zidovudine/lamivudine in pregnant patients).

All NRTIs except didanosine should be taken with food for optimal tolerability. Didanosine should be taken 60 minutes before meals or 2 hours after meals for optimal absorption. With the exception of abacavir, NRTIs require dosage adjustment in persons with renal insufficiency (creatinine clearance <50 mL/min). Similarly, fixed-dose NRTI combinations should be avoided in patients with renal insufficiency. Gastrointestinal side effects (e.g., nausea, diarrhea, abdominal pain) are transient and improve within the first 2 weeks of therapy.

As a class, NRTIs are associated with changes in the body's metabolism secondary to mitochondrial toxicity. Complications include peripheral neuropathy, myopathy, pancreatitis, and lipoatrophy. Lipoatrophy, or wasting of fat on the extremities, face, and buttocks, is associated with chronic NRTI administration. Rare fatalities have occurred owing to lactic acidosis and hepatic steatosis associated with NRTIs. Drug interactions are uncommon with NRTIs. Gastrointestinal complaints and mitochondrial toxicity are less likely to occur with tenofovir. The most serious side effect with tenofovir is renal toxicity, which occurs rarely.

Adherence with NRTIs can be improved with once-daily dosing (possible with abacavir, didanosine, emtricitabine, lamivudine, and tenofovir) and with fixed-dosage combination products (e.g., Combivir and Truvada).

Prototype Drug Chart 35-1 gives pharmacologic data for zidovudine, and Prototype Drug Chart 35-2 shows the data for tenofovir.

Non-Nucleoside Reverse Transcriptase Inhibitors

Five NNRTIs are used in the United States: efavirenz (Sustiva), delavirdine (Rescriptor), nevirapine (Viramune), rilpivirine (Edurant), and etravirine (Intelence). NNRTIs prevent viral replication by competing with binding of the reverse transcriptase enzyme at the active site. The primary advantage of using NNRTIs is to reserve a protease-inhibitor–based therapy for future use. In general, an NNRTI regimen has a lower pill burden compared with most PI-based regimens. Major disadvantages are the prevalence of NNRTI-resistant viral strains and the low genetic barrier of NNRTIs for development of resistance. (Resistance testing is recommended for treatment-naïve patients before starting therapy.) NNRTIs also have the potential for drug interactions.

Efavirenz is the first-choice drug within the NNRTI class. It should be used with caution in pregnancy because neural tube defects have been reported after early human gestational exposure. Central nervous system (CNS) toxicities, including dizziness, sedation, nightmares, euphoria, or loss of concentration, may occur in up to 50% of patients. Efavirenz should be used cautiously in patients with depression or history of psychiatric or mental illness. Efavirenz is optimally administered as a component of Atripla, given once daily at bedtime on an empty stomach or with a low-fat meal to prevent excessive drug absorption.

Nevirapine may be used as an alternative in adult patients during pregnancy (especially during the first trimester) or in patients who are planning to conceive or are not using effective and consistent contraception. Nevirapine has a greater risk of severe rash and hepatotoxicity. Delavirdine appears to

PROTOTYPE DRUG CHART 35-1

Zidovudine

Drug Class Nucleoside reverse transcriptase inhibitor Trade names: ZDV, AZT, Retrovir Pregnancy category: C FDA approved: 1987 Estimated annual cost: $6700 (brand), $4350 (generic)	**Dosage** Prevention of maternal-fetal HIV transmission Maternal therapy: PO: 100 mg 5 times/d until the start of labor Intrapartum: IV: 2 mg/kg loading dose over 30-60 min followed by continuous infusion of 1 mg/kg/h until cord is clamped. For scheduled cesarean delivery, begin IV 3 h before surgery Newborn (syrup): PO: Continue dose through 6 wk of age Infant (full-term): PO: 4 mg/kg/dose b.i.d. (IV: 1.5 mg/kg/dose q6h). Infant (30-36 wk gestation at birth): PO: 2 mg/kg/dose q12h; at 2 wk of age, 3 mg/kg/dose q12h (IV: 1.5 mg/kg/dose q12h; at 2 wk of age, advance to 2.3 mg/kg/dose q12h) Infant (<30 weeks gestation at birth): PO: 2 mg/kg/dose q12h; at 4 wk of age, 3 mg/kg/dose q12h (IV: 1.5 mg/kg/dose q12h; at 4 wk of age, 2.3 mg/kg/dose q12h) Treatment: A: PO: 200 mg q8h or 300 mg q12h; IV: 1 mg/kg q4h (ATC: 5-6 doses/d) C: 4 wk to <18 y: PO: ≥30 kg: 300 mg b.i.d.; 9-29 kg: 9 mg/kg/dose b.i.d.; 4-8 kg: 12 mg/kg/dose b.i.d. C: 6 wk-11 y: IV: 120 mg/m^2/dose q6h or 20 mg/m^2/h; ≥12 y: 1 mg/kg/dose q4h ATC (5-6 doses/d)
Contraindications Life-threatening allergies to zidovudine or components of preparation Caution: Bone marrow compromise, renal and hepatic dysfunction, decreased hepatic blood flow	**Drug-Lab-Food Interactions** Drug: Ganciclovir, probenecid, valproic acid may increase concentration/adverse effects. Rifampin may decrease concentration/effects. Lab: May increase ALT, AST
Pharmacokinetics Absorption: PO: 66%-70% Distribution: PB: 25%-38%, crosses blood-brain barrier, crosses placenta, peak serum levels: 30-90 min Metabolism: t½: 0.5-3 h; extensive first-pass effect in liver Excretion: 63%-95% in urine	**Pharmacodynamics** Not applicable
Therapeutic Effects/Uses Management of patients with HIV infection; prevention of maternal-fetal HIV transmission Mode of Action: Inhibits viral enzyme reverse transcriptase, an enzyme necessary for viral HIV replication	
Side Effects Numbness, tingling, burning and pain in lower extremities, abdominal pain, rash, GI intolerance, fever, sore throat, headache, pruritus, muscle pain, difficulty swallowing, arthralgia, insomnia, confusion, mental changes, bluish-brown bands on fingernails	**Adverse Reactions** Nausea, vomiting, anemia (pale skin, unusual fatigue or weakness), neutropenia (fever, chills, sore throat), seizures

A, Adult; *b.i.d.*, twice a day; *C*, child; *d*, day; *FDA*, Food and Drug Administration; *GI*, gastrointestinal; *h*, hour; *HIV*, human immunodeficiency virus; *IV*, intravenous; *max*, maximum; *min*, minute; *PB*, protein-binding; *PO*, by mouth; *t ½*, half-life; *wk*, week; *y*, year; >, greater than; ≥, greater than or equal to; <, less than.

have the least potent antiviral activity and is not recommended as part of an initial regimen.

Etravirine is the first agent in this group to show antiviral activity in treatment-experienced patients with HIV that was resistant to an NNRTI and other antiretroviral agents. Etravirine also has many drug interactions, including combinations with fosamprenavir/ritonavir, atazanavir/ritonavir, other NNRTIs, carbamazepine, phenobarbital, and rifampin. Common side effects include rash (during the first 6 weeks of therapy), diarrhea, nausea, fatigue, abdominal pain, peripheral neuropathy, headache, and hypertension. Etravirine has been associated with potentially life-threatening and fatal skin reactions (e.g., Stevens-Johnson syndrome).

Prototype Drug Chart 35-3 presents the pharmacologic data for efavirenz.

PROTOTYPE DRUG CHART 35-2

Tenofovir

Drug Class Nucleotide reverse transcriptase inhibitor (NtRTI) Trade name: Viread Pregnancy category: B FDA approved: 2001 Estimated annual cost: $10,480	**Dosage** A/C ≥12 y: PO: 300 mg once daily with or without food (high-fat meals may increase bioavailability)
Contraindications None listed in FDA-approved labeling Caution: Renal and hepatic dysfunction	**Drug-Lab-Food Interactions** Drug: acyclovir, ganciclovir, valganciclovir may increase levels/adverse effects of tenofovir Lab: may increase triglycerides, AST, ALT, alkaline phosphatase
Pharmacokinetics Absorption: PO: 25%-40% Distribution: PB: <7% to proteins, peak serum levels: 36-84 min fasting; 96-144 min with food Metabolism: t½: converted intracellularly by hydrolysis to tenofovir, then phosphorylated to active tenofovir diphosphate Excretion: 70%-80% primarily in urine as unchanged drug	**Pharmacodynamics** Not applicable
Therapeutic Effects/Uses Management of patients with HIV infection; treatment of chronic hepatitis B Mode of Action: Inhibits viral enzyme reverse transcriptase, an enzyme necessary for viral HIV replication	
Side Effects Diarrhea, nausea, vomiting, flatulence, insomnia, dizziness, depression, fever	**Adverse Reactions** Lactic acidosis, hepatomegaly with steatosis

A, Adult; *C,* child; *d,* day; *FDA,* Food and Drug Administration; *GI,* gastrointestinal; *h,* hour; *HIV,* human immunodeficiency virus; *IV,* intravenous; *max,* maximum; *min,* minute; *PB,* protein-binding; *PO,* by mouth; *t½,* half-life; *wk,* week; *y,* year; >, greater than; ≥, greater than or equal to; <, less than.

Protease Inhibitors

PI-based regimens (one or two PIs plus two NRTIs) have revolutionized the treatment of HIV infection, leading to sustained viral suppression, improved immunologic function, and prolonged patient survival. Nine PIs are approved by the FDA: lopinavir/ritonavir (Kaletra), atazanavir (Reyataz), fosamprenavir (Lexiva), tipranavir (Aptivus), darunavir (Prezista), saquinavir (Invirase), indivavir (Crixivan), ritonavir (Norvir), and nelfinavir (Viracept). Unlike NRTIs and NNRTIs, PIs act at the end of the HIV life cycle to target viral assembly by inhibiting the activity of protease, an enzyme used to cleave nascent proteins for final assembly of new virons, resulting in formation and release of immature, defective and noninfectious virus particles. Each PI has unique characteristics based on clinical efficacy, side-effect profile, and pharmacokinetic properties. Darunavir or atazanavir (both "boosted" with ritonavir) are first-line choices of PIs in ART.

Selection of a PI-based regimen should consider dosing frequency, food and fluid requirements, pill burden, drug interaction potential, and side-effect profile. When initiating therapy with PIs, gastrointestinal side effects (nausea, vomiting, and diarrhea) can be bothersome and may negatively affect adherence. Metabolic abnormalities, including significant elevation of cholesterol and triglycerides, fat maldistribution, and insulin resistance/diabetes are associated with PI use, with each PI differing in its propensity to cause these metabolic complications. Atazanivir, a preferred PI for initial ART, has not reported insulin resistance and is less likely to elevate cholesterol and triglycerides. Metabolic abnormalities are established risk factors for cardiovascular disease, including myocardial infarction and hypertension, so lifestyle modifications, smoking cessation, exercise, and cardiac risk management are advised for those receiving chronic PI-based therapies.

Ritonavir boosting is a relatively new concept and one of the mainstays of PI therapy. The potent inhibitory effect of ritonavir on the cytochrome P450 3A4 isoenzyme allows the addition of 100 to 200 mg of ritonavir to other PIs as a pharmacokinetic booster. This helps to reduce dietary restrictions, increase drug exposure, inhibit metabolism, and maximize blood levels of the co-administered PI, thus reducing dosing frequency and pill burden and overcoming viral resistance. Because "boosted" regimens may be less complex, patients may be able to follow and tolerate them better.

Prototype Drug Chart 35-4 presents the pharmacologic data for atazanavir.

Entry Inhibitors

Enfuvirtide (Fuzeon) is the only agent approved in this class. Enfuvirtide acts by a mechanism that inhibits gp41 fusion to

PROTOTYPE DRUG CHART 35-3

Efavirenz

Drug Class
Nonnucleoside reverse transcriptase inhibitor (NNRTI)
Trade name: Sustiva
Pregnancy category: D
FDA approved: 1998
Estimated annual cost: $8275

Dosage
Note: Dose given at bedtime to minimize CNS adverse effects
A: PO: 600 mg once daily
C: PO: 10-<15 kg: 200 mg daily; 15-<20 kg: 250 mg daily; 20-<25 kg: 300 mg daily; 25-<32.5 kg: 350 mg daily; 32.5-<40 kg: 400 mg daily; ≥40 kg: 600 mg daily

Contraindications
Life-threatening allergies to efavirenz or components of preparation; concurrent use of midazolam, triazolam, ergot alkaloids
Caution: Patients with history of mental illness or drug abuse; liver impairment; seizure disorder

Drug-Lab-Food Interactions
Drug: carbamazepine, nevirapine, phenobarbital, phenytoin, rifampin; St. John's wort may decrease effect of atorvastatin, bupropion, clarithromycin, clopidrogel, methadone, and sertraline. See Contraindications.
Food: Avoid alcohol because of liver/CNS adverse effects; high-fat meals increase absorption

Pharmacokinetics
Absorption: PO: Increased following high-fat meal
Distribution: PB: >99%, widely distributed (found in CSF)
Metabolism: t½: 40-55 h; metabolized in liver Time to peak levels: 3-5 h
Excretion: 16%-41% in feces, primarily as unchanged drug; 14%-34% in urine, primarily as metabolite

Pharmacodynamics
Not applicable

Therapeutic Effects/Uses
Treatment of HIV-1 infections in combination with at least two other antiretroviral agents.
Mode of Action: Binds to reverse transcriptase, blocking RNA-dependent and DNA-dependent DNA polymerase activity including HIV-1 replication.

Side Effects
Rash; CNS effects (dizziness, insomnia, abnormal dreams/thinking, impaired concentration, amnesia, agitation, hallucinations, euphoria, anxiety); nausea, diarrhea

Adverse Reactions
Aggressive reaction, allergic reaction, convulsion, liver failure, neuropathy, suicide, abnormal vision

A, Adult; *C,* child; *CNS,* central nervous system; *CSF,* cerebrospinal fluid; *DNA,* deoxyribonucleic acid; *FDA,* U.S. Food and Drug Administration; *h,* hour; *HDL,* high-density lipoprotein; *HIV-1,* human immunodeficiency virus-1; *PB,* protein-binding; *PO,* by mouth; *RNA,* ribonucleic acid; *t½,* half-life; >, greater than; ≥, greater than or equal to; <, less than.

prevent HIV cell entry. This class of agents targets prevention of the fusion of the HIV and CD4 cell and prevents passing the viral genome to the CD4 cell. Enfuvirtide is indicated only in combination with three to five other antiretroviral agents for patients with limited treatment options requiring salvage therapy. It is expensive, and the medication must be taken by subcutaneous injection in a dose of 90 mg twice daily.

Enfuvirtide does not require dosage adjustment in patients with renal failure or hepatic impairment. It is not metabolized by CYP enzymes and is not associated with any CYP-mediated drug-drug interactions. Injection-site reactions (e.g., subcutaneous nodules, redness) occur in up to 98% of patients. Other side effects reported include rash and diarrhea. Serious allergic reactions, including anaphylaxis, fever, and hypotension, have occurred in less than 1% of patients.

CCR5 Co-Receptor Antagonists

Maraviroc, the only agent in this class, blocks the CCR5 co-receptor needed for CCR5-tropic HIV entry into immune cells, preventing viral replication. When combined with at least two other antiretroviral agents, it is effective in about 50% of patients having resistance to most classes of antiretroviral agents. For maraviroc to be effective, it is important to ensure that the HIV uses the CCR5 co-receptor rather than the CXCR4 co-receptor or a mix of both receptors for viral entry. A blood test documenting the presence of the CCR5 receptor (tropism test) must be obtained before starting the medication.

Maraviroc is indicated in combination with other antiretroviral agents for treatment-experienced adult patients with evidence of viral replication and HIV-1 strains resistant to multiple antiretroviral therapy. The most common side effects are cough, pyrexia, upper respiratory tract infection, rash, abdominal pain, and dizziness. Possible drug-induced hepatotoxicity with allergy-type features has been reported. Use caution in patients with liver or heart disease or a history of orthostatic hypotension and in those on medication that lowers blood pressure.

PROTOTYPE DRUG CHART 35-4

Atazanavir

Drug Class Protease inhibitor Trade name: Reyataz Pregnancy category: B FDA approved: 2003 Estimated annual cost: $14,115	**Dosage** ***Treatment Naïve*** A: PO: 300 mg plus ritonavir 100 mg once daily or 400 mg once daily if unable to tolerate ritonavir C: PO: 6-17 y, ≥39 kg: same as adult; 32-38 kg: 250 mg with ritonavir 100 mg once daily; 25-31 kg: 200 mg with ritonavir 100 mg once daily; 15-24 kg: 150 mg with ritonavir 80 mg once daily ***Treatment Experienced*** A: PO: 300 mg plus ritonavir 100 mg once daily C: PO: 6-17 y, 39 kg or greater: same as adult; 32-38 kg: 250 mg with ritonavir 100 mg once daily; 25-31 kg: 200 mg with ritonavir 100 mg once daily
Contraindications Hypersensitivity to atazanavir or any component, concurrent use with alfuzosin, ergot derivatives, lovastatin, midazolam (oral), rifampin, simvastatin, St. John's wort Caution: Patients with pre-existing conduction abnormalities (may prolong PR interval), hepatitis B or C, hepatic impairment, hemophilia A or B	**Drug-Lab-Food Interactions** Drug: azole antifungals, clarithromycin may increase levels/adverse effects; antacids, carbamazepine, H_2 antagonists, proton pump inhibitors, rifampin may decrease levels/effects. See Contraindications. Lab: May increase liver function tests, cholesterol, triglycerides, glucose Food: Bioavailability increased when taken with food
Pharmacokinetics Absorption: PO: Rapidly, increased with food Distribution: PB: 98%, peak levels attained in 2-3 h Metabolism: $t\frac{1}{2}$: 7-8 h (9-18 h when boosted with ritonavir). Metabolized in liver Excretion: Primarily fecal elimination (70%); urine (13%)	**Pharmacodynamics** Not applicable
Therapeutic Effects/Uses Treatment of HIV-1 infection in combination with other antiretroviral agents. Mode of Action: Inhibits HIV protease, rendering enzyme incapable of processing polyprotease precursors; production of noninfectious immature HIV particles results	
Side Effects Rash, nausea, cough	**Adverse Reactions** Hyperglycemia, diabetes mellitus, jaundice

A, Adult; *b.i.d.*, twice a day; *C*, child; *FDA*, U.S. Food and Drug Administration; *h*, hour; *HIV*, human immunodeficiency virus; *mo*, month; *PB*, protein-binding; *PO*, by mouth; *t ½*, half-life; *y*, year; >, greater than; ≥, greater than or equal to; <, less than.

Integrase Inhibitors

Raltegravir and dolutegravir exert their action by interfering with integrase, the enzyme that HIV needs to multiply, thus limiting the ability of the virus to replicate and infect new cells. They are used for the treatment of HIV-1 infections with at least two or three other antiretroviral agents in both treatment-naïve (recommended initial agent) and treatment-experienced patients. Common side effects of raltegravir include nausea, headache, diarrhea, and pyrexia. Caution is advised in patients who are at increased risk for certain types of muscle problems (e.g., myopathy and rhabdomyolysis), including patients who take medications that can increase risk, such as statins. Raltegravir is administered twice daily. Common side effects of dolutegravir include insomnia and headache. Dolutegravir is administered once daily (twice daily when given with efavirenz, fosamprenavir/ritonavir, tipranavir/ritonavir, or rifampin).

Table 35-2 shows the respective routes, dosages, and considerations of antiretroviral agents. Information on drug interactions is shown in Table 35-3.

IMMUNE RECONSTITUTION INFLAMMATORY SYNDROME

Immune reconstitution inflammatory syndrome (IRIS) is related to specific opportunistic pathogens and is experienced

TABLE 35-2 ANTIRETROVIRAL AGENTS

NAME	AVAILABILITY	DOSAGE	COMMENTS
Nucleoside Reverse Transcriptase Inhibitors (NRTIs)			
abacavir (ABC) (Ziagen) Trizivir (with ZDV + 3TC) Epzicom (with 3TC)	Ziagen: 300-mg tabs 20-mg/mL oral solution Trizivir: ABC 300 mg, ZDV 300 mg, 3TC 150 mg Epzicom: ABC 600 mg, 3TC 300 mg	Ziagen: 300 mg b.i.d. or 600 mg once daily Trizivir: 1 tab b.i.d. Epzicom: 1 tab once daily	Take without regard to meals Metabolized by alcohol dehydrogenase Excreted renally Do not use Trizivir and Epzicom for patients with CLcr <50 mL/min t½: 1.5 h Side effects: hypersensitivity reaction (avoid if HLA-B*5701 is positive due to increased risk of hypersensitivity reaction); symptoms include fever, rash, nausea, vomiting, malaise, fatigue, loss of appetite; respiratory symptoms include sore throat, cough, shortness of breath, lactic acidosis with hepatic steatosis
didanosine (DDL) (Videx EC)	Videx EC: 125 mg, 200 mg, 250 mg, 400 mg Videx 10 mg/mL powder for oral solution	Body wt >60 kg: 400 mg once daily or 200 mg b.i.d. With TDF: 250 mg/d Body wt <60 kg: 250 mg/d With TDF: 200 mg/d	Take ½ h before or 2 h after meal Excreted renally; adjust dosage in patients with renal insufficiency t½: 1.5 h Side effects: pancreatitis, peripheral neuropathy, nausea, lactic acidosis with hepatic steatosis (rare), risk of myocardial infarction, retinal changes, optic neuritis, insulin resistance, diabetes
emtricitabine (FTC) (Emtriva) Atripla (with EFV + TDF) Truvada (with TDF) Complera (with TDF and RPL)	Emtriva: 200 mg caps 10 mg/mL oral solution Atripla: EFV 600, FTC 200 mg, TDF 300 mg Truvada: FTC 200 mg, TDF 300 mg Complera: FTC 200 mg, RPL 25 mg, TDF 300 mg	Emtriva: 200-mg cap once daily or 240 mg oral solution once daily Atripla: 1 tab once daily Truvada: 1 tab once daily Complera: 1 tab once daily	Take without regard to meals Excreted renally; adjust dosage in patients with renal insufficiency Do not use Atripla/Complera for patients with CLcr <50 mL/min; Do not use Truvada for patients with CLcr <30 mL/min t½: 10 h Side effects: lactic acidosis with hepatic steatosis (rare), hyperpigmentation, skin discoloration
lamivudine (3TC) (Epivir) Combivir (with ZDV) Epizicom (with ABC) Trizivir (with ZDV + ABC)	Epivir: 150-mg, 300-mg tabs 10-mg/mL oral solution Combivir: 3TC 150 mg, ZDV 300 mg Epzicom: ABC 600 mg, 3TC 300 mg Trizivir: ABC 300 mg, ZDV 300 mg, 3TC 150 mg	Epivir: 150 mg b.i.d. or 300 mg once daily Combivir: 1 tab b.i.d. Epizicom: 1 tab once daily Trizivir: 1 tab b.i.d.	Take without regard to meals Excreted renally; adjust dosage in patients with renal insufficiency Do not use Combivir, Trizivir, Epizicom for patients with CLcr <50 mL/min t½: 5-7 h Side effects: minimal toxicity, lactic acidosis with hepatic steatosis (rare)
stavudine (d4T) (Zerit)	Zerit: 15-mg, 20-mg, 30-mg, 40-mg caps 1 mg/mL powder for oral solution	Body wt ≥60 kg: 40 mg b.i.d. Body wt <60 kg: 30 mg b.i.d.	Take without regard to meals Excreted renally; adjust dosage in patients with renal insufficiency t½: 1 h Side effects: peripheral neuropathy, lipodystrophy, pancreatitis, hyperlipidemia, rapidly progressive ascending neuromuscular weakness (rare), lactic acidosis with hepatic steatosis (rare)
tenofovir (TDF) (Viread) Atripla (with EFV+FTC) Truvada (with FTC) Complera (with FTC and RPL)	Viread: 150-mg, 200-mg, 250-mg, 300-mg tabs Atripla: EFV 600, FTC 200 mg, TDF 300 mg Truvada: FTC 200 mg, TDF 300 mg Complera: FTC 200 mg, RPL 25 mg, TDF 300 mg	Viread: 1 300-mg tab/d without regard to meals Atripla: 1 tab h.s. on empty stomach Truvada: 1 tab/d without regard to meals Complera: 1 tab/d with food	Excreted renally; adjust dosage in patients with renal insufficiency Do not use Atripla/Complera for patients with CLcr <50 mL/min; do not use Truvada for patients with CLcr <30 mL/min t½: 17 h Side effects: asthenia, headache, diarrhea, nausea, vomiting, flatulence, renal insufficiency, osteomalacia, lactic acidosis with hepatic steatosis (rare)

Continued

TABLE 35-2 ANTIRETROVIRAL AGENTS—cont'd			
NAME	**AVAILABILITY**	**DOSAGE**	**COMMENTS**
zidovudine (AZT, ZDV) (Retrovir) Combivir (with 3TC) Trizivir (with 3TC + ABC)	Retrovir: 100-mg caps 300-mg tabs 10-mg/mL IV solution 10-mg/mL oral solution Combivir: 3TC 150 mg, ZDV 300 mg Trizivir: ABC 300 mg, ZDV 300 mg, 3TC 150 mg	Retrovir: 300 mg b.i.d. or 200 mg t.i.d. Combivir: 1 tab b.i.d. Trizivir: 1 tab b.i.d.	Take without regard to meals Excreted renally; adjust dosage in patients with renal insufficiency Do not use Combivir, Trizivir for patients with CLcr <50 mL/min $t_{1/2}$: 1.1 h Side effects: bone marrow suppression, macrocytic anemia, neutropenia, GI intolerance, headache, insomnia, asthenia, lactic acidosis with hepatic steatosis (rare)
Non-Nucleoside Reverse Transcriptase Inhibitors (NNRTIs)			
delavirdine (DLV) (Rescriptor)	Rescriptor: 100-mg, 200-mg tabs	400 mg t.i.d. (100 mg may be mixed with 3 oz water; 200-mg tabs taken as intact tablets)	Take without regard to meals Metabolized by cytochrome P450, excreted in urine/feces $t_{1/2}$: 5.8 h Side effects: rash, increased transaminase levels, headaches
efavirenz (EFV) (Sustiva) Atripla (with TDF + FTC)	Sustiva: 50-mg, 200-mg caps 600-mg tabs Atripla: EFV 600, FTC 200 mg, TDF 300 mg	Sustiva: 600 mg h.s. or before on empty stomach Atripla: 1 tab/d h.s. or before	Take on empty stomach, high-fat/high-caloric meals increase concentration. Metabolized by cytochrome P450 Sustiva: no dosage adjustment in renal insufficiency Do not use Atripla for patients with CLcr <50 mL/min $t_{1/2}$: 40-55 h Side effects: rash, increased transaminase levels, CNS symptoms including dizziness, confusion, agitation, hallucinations, euphoria
etravirine (ETR) (Intelence)	25-mg, 100-mg, 200-mg tabs	200 mg b.i.d. after a meal	Caloric meals increase concentration Metabolized by cytochrome P450 No dosage adjustment in patients with renal insufficiency $t_{1/2}$: 41 +/− 20 h Side effects: rash including Stevens-Johnson syndrome, nausea
rilpivirine (RPL) (Edurant) Complera (with FTC and TDF)	Edurant: 25-mg tab Complera: FTC 200 mg, RPL 25 mg, TDF 300 mg	Edurant: 25 mg/d Complera: 1 tab once daily with food	Take with a meal $t_{1/2}$: 50 h Side effects: rash depression, headache, insomnia
nevirapine (NVP) (Viramune, Viramune XR)	Viramune: 200-mg tabs 50-mg/5-mL oral suspension Viramune ER: 100-mg, 400-mg tabs	Viramune: 200 mg/d for 14 d, then 200 mg b.i.d. Viramune ER: 400 mg once daily	Take without regard to meals Metabolized by cytochrome P450 $t_{1/2}$: 25-30 h Side effects: rash, including Stevens-Johnson syndrome, symptomatic hepatitis
Protease Inhibitors (PIs)			
atazanavir (ATV) (Reyataz)	Reyataz: 150-mg, 200-mg, 300-mg caps	Reyataz: 400 mg once daily or RTV 100 mg + ATV 300 mg once daily	Take with food; avoid taking with antacids Cytochrome P450 3A4 inhibitor and substrate Adjust dosage in patients with hepatic insufficiency $t_{1/2}$: 7 h Side effects: hyperbilirubinemia, prolonged P-R interval (use with caution in patients with underlying conduction defects or concomitant medications that prolong P-R interval), hyperglycemia, fat maldistribution, possible increased bleeding in patients with hemophilia
darunavir (DRV) (Prezista)	Prezista: 75-mg, 150-mg, 600-mg, 800-mg tabs	Prezista: (DRV 600 mg + RTV 100 mg) b.i.d.	Administer with food (increases concentration) Cytochrome P450 3A4 inhibitor and substrate Adjust dosage in patients with hepatic insufficiency $t_{1/2}$: 15 h Side effects: rash, diarrhea, nausea, headache, elevated transaminase levels, hyperglycemia, fat maldistribution, possible increased bleeding in hemophiliacs, hyperlipidemia

TABLE 35-2 **ANTIRETROVIRAL AGENTS—cont'd**

NAME	AVAILABILITY	DOSAGE	COMMENTS
fosamprenavir (fAPV) (Lexiva)	Lexiva: 700-mg tab 50-mg/mL oral suspension	Lexiva: 1400 mg b.i.d. or fAPV 1400 mg + RTV 200 mg/d or fAPV 700 mg + RTV 100 mg b.i.d.	Tablet: Take with or without food Oral suspension: Take with food Cytochrome P450 3A4 inhibitor, inducer, and substrate Adjust dosage in patients with hepatic insufficiency t½: 7.7 h Side effects: rash, diarrhea, nausea, vomiting, headache, hyperlipidemia, elevated transaminase levels, hyperglycemia, fat maldistribution, possible increased bleeding in hemophiliacs
indinavir (IDV) (Crixivan)	Crixivan: 200-mg, 400-mg caps	Crixivan: 800 mg every 8 h With RTV: IDV 800 mg + RTV 100 mg or 200 mg q12h	Unboosted: take 1 h before or 2 h after meals; with RTV: may take with or without meals Cytochrome P450 3A4 inhibitor and substrate Adjust dosage in patients with hepatic insufficiency t½: 1.5-2 h Side effects: nephrolithiasis, GI intolerance, nausea, indirect hyperbilirubinemia, headache, asthenia, blurred vision, dizziness, rash, metallic taste, thrombocytopenia, alopecia, hemolytic anemia, hyperlipidemia, elevated transaminase levels, hyperglycemia, fat maldistribution, possible increased bleeding in patients with hemophilia
lopinavir/ritonavir (LPV/r) (Kaletra)	Kaletra: Tab: LPV 200 mg and RTV 50 mg; LPV 100 mg and RTV 25 mg Oral solution: LPV 400 mg and RTV 100 mg/5 mL	Kaletra: LPV 400 mg + RTV 100 mg b.i.d. or LPV 800 mg + RTV 200 mg once daily	May take tablet with or without food; take oral solution with food Cytochrome P450 3A4 inhibitor and substrate t½: 5-6 h Side effects: GI intolerance, nausea, vomiting, diarrhea, asthenia, PR interval prolongation, pancreatitis, hyperlipidemia, elevated transaminase levels, hyperglycemia, fat maldistribution, possible increased bleeding in patients with hemophilia
nelfinavir (NFV) (Viracept)	Viracept: 250-mg, 625-mg tabs	Viracept: 1250 mg b.i.d. or 750 mg t.i.d.	Take with meal or snack Cytochrome P450 3A4 inhibitor and substrate t½: 3.5-5 h Side effects: diarrhea, hyperlipidemia, elevated transaminase levels, hyperglycemia, fat maldistribution, possible increased bleeding in hemophiliacs
ritonavir (RTV) (Norvir)	Norvir: 100-mg tabs 100-mg caps 600 mg/7.5 mL solution	Norvir: Booster: 100-400 mg in 1-2 divided doses	Take with food Cytochrome P450 3A4 potent inhibitor t½: 3-5 h Side effects: GI intolerance, nausea, vomiting, diarrhea, paresthesias, hepatitis, asthenia, taste perversion, hyperlipidemia, hyperglycemia, fat maldistribution, possible increased bleeding in patients with hemophilia
saquinavir (SQV) (Invirase)	Invirase: 200-mg caps 500-mg tabs	Invirase: SQV 1000 mg + RTV 100 mg b.i.d.	Take within 2 h of a meal Cytochrome P450 3A4 inhibitor and substrate t½: 12 h Side effects: GI intolerance, nausea, diarrhea, headache, hyperlipidemia, elevated transaminase levels, hyperglycemia, PR interval prolongation, fat maldistribution, possible increased bleeding in hemophiliacs

Continued

TABLE 35-2 ANTIRETROVIRAL AGENTS—cont'd

NAME	AVAILABILITY	DOSAGE	COMMENTS
tipranavir (TPV) (Aptivus)	Aptivus: 250-mg caps 100 mg/mL oral solution	Aptivus: TPV 500 mg + RTV 200 mg b.i.d.	Take with food Cytochrome P450 3A4 inducer and substrate t½: 6 h Side effects: hepatotoxicity, rash (has sulfonamide moiety), hyperlipidemia, hyperglycemia, fat maldistribution, possible increased bleeding in patients with hemophilia
Entry Inhibitor			
enfuvirtide (T20) (Fuzeon)	Fuzeon: Injection powder 90 mg/mL after reconstitution	Fuzeon: 90 mg subQ b.i.d.	Store vial at room temperature; following reconstitution, refrigerate and use within 24 h t½: 3.8 h Side effects: local injection site reaction (pain, erythema, induration, nodules, cysts, pruritus, ecchymosis), increased rate of bacterial pneumonia, hypersensitivity reaction (rash, fever, nausea, vomiting, chills, rigors, hypotension, elevated transaminases)
CCR5 Antagonists			
maraviroc (MRV) (Selzentry)	Selzentry: 150-mg, 300-mg tabs	300 mg b.i.d. 150 mg b.i.d. when given with strong CYP3A inhibitors (e.g., itraconazole, clarithromycin) 600 mg b.i.d. when given with strong CYP3A inducers (e.g., rifampin, carbamazepine, phenytoin)	Concentration may increase in renal dysfunction (CrCL <50); use not recommended May need to adjust dose with concomitant medications (interactions) May take without regard to food t½: 14-18 h Side effects: Fever, upper respiratory tract infection, orthostatic hypotension, hepatotoxicity, rash, cough, abdominal pain, dizziness
Integrase Inhibitors			
raltegravir (RAV) (Isentress)	Isentress: 400-mg tabs	400 mg b.i.d.	Take without regard to food No adjustment needed with renal or hepatic dysfunction Absorption increased with high-fat meal t½: 8 h Side effects: nausea, headache, diarrhea, pyrexia, increased total cholesterol, fatigue, rash including Stevens-Johnson syndrome and epidermal necrolysis
dolutagravir (Tivicay)	Tivicay: 50-mg tabs	50 mg once/d	Take without regard to meals No adjustment needed with renal or hepatic dysfunction Absorption increased with high-fat meal t½: 14 h Side effects: headache, insomnia, rash

b.i.d., Twice a day; *cap*, capsule; *d*, day; *ER*, extended-release; *GI*, gastrointestinal; *h*, hour; *h.s.*, at bedtime; *min*, minute; *subQ*, subcutaneous; *t½*, half-life; *tab*, tablet; *t.i.d.*, three times a day; *wt*, weight; >, greater than; <, less than.

by a low percentage of patients early in ART. IRIS has two distinct entities: (1) paradoxical IRIS, which is an exacerbation of treated (successful or partial) opportunistic infection (OI); and (2) unmasking IRIS, a response to undiagnosed or subclinical OI. IRIS may occur in response to many pathogens. Diagnosis is a challenge because there are no laboratory markers; it is a condition of exclusion. For example, new OI or concurrent illness must be excluded before IRIS can be diagnosed.

Risk factors for developing IRIS include a low CD4 cell count (particularly <50 cells/mcL) at time of ART initiation and a high baseline HIV RNA. Starting ART soon after

TABLE 35-3 DRUG INTERACTIONS

Drug interaction associated with HAART is a challenging issue facing providers who treat patients with HIV. Medications used as initial treatment are associated with significant drug interactions. Concurrent treatment of comorbid disease states and therapies for preventing and/or treating opportunistic infections further increase the risk of drug interactions.

Nucleoside Reverse Transcriptase Inhibitors (NRTIs)

Drug interactions associated with NRTIs are minimal because these medications are not metabolized by the CYP450 system. Nevertheless, drug interactions may still occur within the class.

Non-Nucleoside Reverse Transcriptase Inhibitors (NNRTIs)

Drugs in this class are prone to interactions because they are extensively metabolized via CYP3A4 and can act as either inducers or inhibitors of CYP3A4. Efavirenz and nevirapine are inducers of CYP3A4, and delavirdine is an inhibitor.

Protease Inhibitors (PIs)

All PIs are potent inhibitors of CYP3A4 and result in drug interactions. Levels of medications also metabolized by the same system have the potential to be markedly increased, leading to an increased incidence of adverse effects. The protease inhibitor ritonavir is the most potent inhibitor of CYP3A4 in this class.

CCR5 Antagonists

CCR5 antagonists are a substrate of CYP3A. Concentrations are significantly increased in the presence of strong CYP3A inhibitors and reduced with CYP3A inducers. Dosage adjustments are necessary when used with these agents.

Integrase Inhibitors

Integrase inhibitor raltegravir is primarily eliminated by glucouronidation mediated by UDP-glucuronosyltransferase enzymes (UGTIA1). Strong inducers of UGTIA1 enzymes can significantly decrease the concentration of raltegravir.

b.i.d., Twice a day; *d,* day; *h,* hour; *t.i.d.,* three times a day; *wk,* week.

initiation of treatment for recognized OI also increases risk for IRIS. Severity of IRIS ranges from mild to life-threatening. Treatment varies according to specific pathogen and clinical situation but typically includes continuing ART if possible, treating the OI as indicated, and adding antiinflammatory therapy (including corticosteroids) as needed.

NURSE'S ROLE IN ANTIRETROVIRAL THERAPY

Thorough assessment of the patient's physiologic and psychosocial health needs and literacy levels is required initially and for the duration of care. Follow-up assessment after ART begins should include medication side effects, adherence to regimen, and issues affecting medication adherence. Patients may confuse medication side effects with new onset of symptoms. Careful follow-up assessment can detect the need for additional medical care or medication management.

Adherence challenges are common with any medication therapy, but ART presents a greater challenge as patients are asked to achieve adherence of 95% or greater. Nonadherence can result in HIV viral replication and potential for drug resistance. Multiple strategies for adherence are available and should be discussed with patients. Medication organizers, alarms on cell phones or mobile devices, medication "maps" with pictures, and medication diaries are available tools. Friends, family members, and personal support systems can assist patients with adherence. Nurses can facilitate adherence by allowing sufficient time to educate patients about medications, developing a trusting relationship, and building a partnership with the patient.

Nursing assessment should include asking the reasons for missing medications. These commonly include stigma, forgetting, feeling ill, side effects, not having the medicine when doses are due, pill fatigue, medication costs, loss of health insurance, and lack of transportation to the pharmacy. If barriers to adherence are identified, individualized plans should be addressed with the patient and the HIV care provider.

Patient education should include purpose of each medication, dosage schedule, food and fluid restrictions, recommended food choices, and storage of medications. Additional suggestions include taking medication during a daily routine, such as brushing teeth, or using a medication calendar to track medications taken. The nurse should assess whether scheduled appointments to assist the patient with filling a medication organizer would be helpful until the patient is comfortable with completing this task. Discussion of anticipated side effects of the medications and how to manage them is necessary.

Nursing Process
Patient-Centered Collaborative Care

Antiretroviral Therapy

Assessment

- Obtain a patient history. Assess for signs and symptoms related to clinical progression of HIV disease. Assess physiologic and psychosocial needs; refer to medical care and psychological support as indicated.
- Perform medication reconciliation, including all prescription, over-the-counter (OTC), and herbal products. Assess for use of illegal drugs and other nonprescription drug use. Report potential drug-drug or drug-herbal interactions.
- Obtain a nutritional history to assess for nutritional deficits and for potential drug-food interactions. Assess for potential need for therapeutic lifestyle change if patient has or is at risk for developing a lipid disorder or diabetes.
- Assess readiness to learn and preferred method of instruction (written, verbal, pictorial).

Nursing Diagnoses

- Ineffective health self-maintenance related to knowledge deficit about HIV/AIDS
- Fear related to perceived stigma of HIV diagnosis
- Imbalanced nutrition related to loss of appetite and frequent stools
- Ineffective coping and/or compromised patient and significant other coping related to HIV diagnosis
- Risk for infection related to compromised immune system, especially if CD4 count is <200
- Ineffective health self-management related to complex medication management
- Knowledge deficit regarding drug interaction
- Readiness for enhanced health management related to expressed desire to improve knowledge about disease progression and outcomes of care
- Deficient knowledge related to medication management

Planning

- Patient's viral load will become and remain undetectable.
- Patient's CD4 count will become as high as possible.
- Patient will not experience secondary infections.
- Patient will participate in medical treatment and in spiritual and psychological support that best fits patient needs and belief system.
- Patient will promptly report new onset of symptoms and side effects.
- Patient will adhere to medication regimen and/or report difficulties related to adherence.

Nursing Interventions

- Educate patient about adherence to the therapeutic regimen by providing information on medications and timetable of dosing in the patient's preferred method of learning.
- Counsel patient about hand washing technique and methods to maintain health.
- Monitor laboratory reports for indications of decreasing CD4 counts and/or rising viral load; inform HIV health care provider.
- Refer patient for health care maintenance and appropriate health screening examinations, including PAP test, ophthalmology and dental examinations, and age- or risk-related colonoscopy.
- Refer patient for nutritional counseling as needed.
- Refer patient for spiritual support and/or for mental health or substance use counseling as needed.

Patient Teaching

General

- Explain how HIV may damage the immune system.
- Describe modes of transmission of HIV and ways to prevent transmission to others.
- Explain common emotional responses.
- Explain the need for monitoring health practices.
- Emphasize protective precautions to decrease risk for exposure to infection(s) as necessary.
- Advise patient about ways to prevent or minimize acquisition of upper respiratory infection and influenza: frequent hand washing, avoiding crowds, receiving influenza and other vaccinations as appropriate
- For patient of childbearing age, provide information about managing future pregnancies to reduce risk of HIV transmission to fetus.
- Provide personal drug therapy plan in the patient's preferred method of learning.
- Inform patient that certain medications (including OTC), foods, and herbal products may interact with antiretrovirals.
- Establish patient/family partnership in the plan.

Self-Administration

- Assist patient to develop a system for taking correct dose of correct medications at correct time.
- Counsel patient about importance of having an adequate supply of medication to avoid interruption in dosing schedule. Omission of drugs may result in deterioration of patient's condition.
- For pediatric patients unable to swallow medications, teach swallowing techniques.

Side Effects

- Advise patient about what symptoms to report promptly to health care provider.
- Discuss possible medication side effects and strategies to manage them.

Diet

- Advise patient to eat a variety of foods, to avoid raw eggs and raw fish, and to cook meats to correct temperature.
- Advise patient about how to minimize side effects (e.g., take specific drug with food).
- Discuss diet of banana, rice, applesauce, and toast for management of diarrhea.

Cultural Considerations

- Know that some cultural groups may believe the drug AZT to be harmful.
- Be aware that some cultures pressure women to reproduce regardless of health status.
- Remember that HIV remains a highly stigmatized disease in many cultures.
- Know that some religions prohibit use of contraception, especially male condom use.
- Some members of certain cultural groups may distrust health care providers and refuse treatment regimens that include research.

Evaluation
- Evaluate the effectiveness of the antiretroviral therapy.
- Determine whether the viral load is undetectable; assess for increase in CD4 count.
- Evaluate medication adherence.
- Evaluate adherence with behaviors that decrease the possibility of HIV transmission such as practicing safer sex, not sharing drug works, and participating in needle exchange programs if available and applicable.

In addition to patient assessment, education, and advocacy, nurses should identify problems that require additional investigation and research. Because of the individual needs of HIV/AIDS patients, research on strategies to promote adherence is needed. Best practices for adherence should be identified.

The nurse's role with research is also needed with clinical trials. Accurate data collection, recordkeeping, and attention to detail are necessary. Whenever medication regimens change, nurses should contribute to the ongoing evaluation of medication/regimen side effects and adverse event reporting.

OPPORTUNISTIC INFECTIONS

As HIV infection advances, patients are more vulnerable to infections and malignancies that are called **opportunistic infections** because they take advantage of the opportunity offered by a weakened immune system. Since the introduction of HAART, there has been a dramatic reduction in the incidence of OIs among HIV-positive patients receiving these medications. Although hospitalizations and deaths have decreased, OIs remain a leading cause of morbidity and mortality in HIV-infected persons. Prevention and treatment of OIs remain essential.

The most common HIV-related OIs include the following:

- Bacterial: tuberculosis, bacterial pneumonia, septicemia
- Protozoal: toxoplasmosis, cryptosporidiosis, leishmaniasis
- Fungal: *Pneumocystis jiroveci* pneumonia, candidiasis, cryptococcosis
- Viral: cytomegalovirus, herpes simplex, herpes zoster
- HIV-associated malignancies: Kaposi sarcoma, lymphoma, squamous cell carcinoma

Different conditions typically occur at different stages of HIV infection. Common with a CD4 count below 350 cells/mL are the following:

- Herpes simplex virus causes ulcers/vesicles in the mouth or genitals. Treatment includes acyclovir, famciclovir, or valacyclovir.
- Herpes zoster virus causes shingles. Shingles has a greater than 15-fold higher incidence for HIV-infected patients. Treatment includes acyclovir, famciclovir, or valacyclovir.
- Herpes simplex and herpes zoster are also capable of causing retinitis and encephalitis, which can be life-threatening.
- TB infection predominantly affects the lungs but can affect other organs, such as the bowel, brain, lining of the heart or lungs, or lining of the CNS. The CD4 cell count is not a reliable predictor of increased risk for TB disease. Treatment includes isoniazid, pyridoxine, rifampin, pyrazinamide, and ethambutol.
- Kaposi sarcoma causes dark blue lesions that can occur in a variety of locations, including the skin, mucous membranes, gastrointestinal tract, lungs, or lymph nodes; they usually appear early in the course of HIV infection. Treatment depends on the symptoms and location. For local lesions, vinblastine has been used. Radiotherapy has been used in delicate sites such as the eyes. Chemotherapy is the preferred treatment for severe widespread disease.

Common with a CD4 count below 200 cells/mL are the following:

- *Candida* esophagitis is a painful yeast infection of the esophagus. Oropharyngeal candidiasis is characterized by painless, creamy white, plaquelike lesions of the buccal or oropharyngeal mucosa or tongue surface. Fluconazole or itraconazole are effective treatments.
- Bacillary angiomatosis is skin lesions caused by *Bartonella,* usually acquired from cat scratches. Treatment includes erythromycin, clarithromycin, azithromycin, and doxycycline.
- ***Pneumocystis jiroveci* pneumonia** is caused by a fungus that shares biologic characteristics with protozoa that infects the lungs. Symptoms are mainly pneumonia, along with fever and respiratory symptoms such as dry cough, chest pain, and dyspnea. Treatment includes TMP-SMX, clindamycin, or oral primaquine.

Common with a CD4 count below 100 cells/mL are the following:

- Cryptococcal meningitis infection of the lining of the brain by a yeast
- AIDS dementia
- Toxoplasmosis encephalitis caused by a protozoan found in uncooked meat and cat feces. Infecting the brain, it can cause headache, confusion, motor weakness, and fever. If left untreated, the disease progression results in seizures, stupor, and coma. Treatment includes pyrimethamine, sulfadiazine, and clindamycin. Leucovoran is added to decrease hematologic toxicities associated with pyrimethamine therapy.
- Progressive multifocal leukoencephalopathy, a viral disease of the brain that results in a severe decline in cognitive and motor functions
- Wasting syndrome causing extreme weight loss and loss of appetite
- Cryptosporidiosis caused by protozoan parasite *cryptosporidium* infecting the small bowel mucosa, large bowel, and extraintestinal site. Symptoms include profuse, nonbloody, watery diarrhea, often with nausea, vomiting, and lower abdominal cramping.

Common with a CD4 count below 50 cells/mL are the following:

- *Mycobacterium avium* complex (MAC) is a blood infection caused by bacteria related to tuberculosis. MAC generally affects multiple organs, with symptoms including fever, night sweats, weight loss, fatigue, diarrhea, and abdominal pain. Localized syndromes include pneumonitis, osteomyelitis, skin or soft-tissue abscesses, or CNS infections. Treatment includes clarithromycin, azithromycin, ethambutol, and rifabutin.
- Cytomegalovirus infection is a virus infecting the whole body, but it most commonly appears as retinitis causing blurred vision. It can lead to blindness. Cytomegalovirus can also affect other organs, causing fever, diarrhea, nausea, pneumonia-like symptoms, and dementia. Treatment includes ganciclovir, valganciclovir, foscarnet, or cidofovir.

ANTIRETROVIRAL THERAPY IN PREGNANCY

Optimal drug therapy should be used for women of reproductive age and for those who are pregnant. When initiating ART for women of reproductive age, the criteria for starting therapy and the goals of treatment are identical to those for other adults and adolescents. Because of considerations related to the prevention of HIV transmission to the fetus during pregnancy, the timing of initiation of treatment and the selection of regimens for pregnant patients may differ from those nonpregnant adults or adolescents.

For pregnant patients, an additional goal is to prevent mother-to-child transmission, with viral suppression to at least 1000 copies/mL or less to reduce the risk of transmission of HIV to the fetus or neonate. A patient infected with HIV can transmit the virus during pregnancy, labor, and delivery, and through breastfeeding. If no preventive drugs are taken and breastfeeding is practiced, the chance of the infant becoming infected is 25%. ART medications reduce the risk of transmission to less than 2% when combined with other interventions (e.g., formula feeding).

ART is recommended in all pregnant patients who test positive for HIV infection, regardless of virologic, immunologic, or clinical parameters for the purpose of preventing mother-to-child transmission of HIV. Combination drug therapy is considered the standard of care for both treatment of maternal HIV infection and prophylaxis to reduce the risk for perinatal HIV transmission.

For the HIV-infected woman of childbearing age who is not pregnant, initiate ART per adult treatment guidelines. If the patient expresses interest in becoming pregnant and efavirenz is considered as part of the antiretroviral regimen, a risk-benefit discussion must take place regarding the risk of neural tube defects related to efavirenz in the first 5 to 6 weeks of pregnancy.

For the HIV-infected patient receiving ART who becomes pregnant, continue the current regimen if it is successfully suppressing viremia. As stated, in regimens containing efavirenz, the risk of neural tube defects is restricted to the first 5 to 6 weeks of pregnancy. Pregnancy is often not recognized during this time. Unnecessary changes in ART during pregnancy may be associated with loss of viral control and increased risk of perinatal transmission. Efavirenz can be continued in pregnant patients receiving an efavirenz-based regimen who present for antenatal care in the first trimester, provided the regimen produces virologic suppression.

For the HIV-infected pregnant patient who is not on antiretroviral agents, ART should be initiated for prophylaxis of perinatal transmission. Zidovudine (ZDV) as a component of the regimen is recommended when possible. ART may be delayed until after the first trimester.

ART is continued during the intrapartum period (ZDV is given as a continuous infusion, while other agents are given orally). For the infant, ZDV is given for 6 weeks starting 6 to 12 hours after birth (see Prototype Drug Chart 35-1 for dosage).

Clinicians treating pregnant patients infected with HIV are encouraged to report cases of prenatal exposure to antiretroviral drugs to the Antiretroviral Pregnancy Registry at *www.apregistry.com.* The registry collects data regarding antiretroviral exposure during pregnancy to assess potential teratogenicity.

OCCUPATIONAL EXPOSURE TO HIV AND POSTEXPOSURE PROPHYLAXIS

Treatment regimens after percutaneous exposure to HIV are called **postexposure prophylaxis** (PEP) regimens. Many PEP regimens are available, with varying degrees of tolerability and probability of patients completing 4 weeks of treatment. Basic and expanded PEP regimens are described in Table 35-4; HIV PEP resources and registries are shown in Box 35-1. PEP management of potential HIV exposure should be

BOX 35-1 HIV RESOURCES

AIDS Info
www.aidsinfo.nih.gov; 800-448-0440; provides information on HIV/AIDS clinical research, treatment and prevention

CDC National AIDS Hotline
800-342-AIDS, 800-344-7432 (Spanish), 800-243-7889 (TDD); provides confidential information, referrals, and general materials for the public on AIDS

National HIV/AIDS Clinicians' Consultation Center
www.nccc.ucsf.edu; 800-922-3413; provides up-to-date HIV/AIDS information to pharmacists, physicians, and nurses and is staffed by pharmacists, physicians, and nurse practitioners

National Perinatal HIV Hotline
www.nccc.ucsf.edu; 888-448-8765; offers around the clock consultation to health care providers on treating HIV-infected pregnant patients and their infants

TABLE 35-4 BASIC AND EXPANDED POSTEXPOSURE PROPHYLAXIS REGIMENS

REGIMEN	DRUG REGIMEN
Basic	zidovudine (Retrovir) + lamivudine (Epivir) available as Combivir zidovudine: 300 mg b.i.d. or 200 mg t.i.d. lamivudine: 300 mg once daily or 150 mg b.i.d. Combivir: 1 tablet b.i.d. zidovudine + emtricitabine (Emtriva) zidovudine: 300 mg b.i.d. or 200 mg t.i.d. emtricitabine: 200 mg once daily tenofovir (Viread) + lamivudine tenofovir: 300 mg once daily lamivudine: 300 mg once daily or 150 mg b.i.d. tenofovir + emtricitabine available as Truvada tenofovir: 300 mg once daily emtricitabine: 200 mg once daily Truvada: 1 tablet daily
Expanded	Basic regimen + lopinavir/ritonavir (Kaletra) Kaletra: 400/100 = 2 tablets b.i.d.

b.i.d., Twice a day.

initiated within hours of the event and continued for 4 weeks. Health care workers taking PEP have reported adverse reactions at rates of 17% to 47%, with the most common reactions being nausea, malaise, and fatigue.

HIV PREVENTION BREAKTHROUGHS

A series of HIV prevention breakthroughs cited as significant by researchers include the following: (1) Earlier initiation of ART leads to a 96% reduction in HIV transmission to uninfected partners—those who took the medication Truvada as prescribed could significantly decrease their risk of becoming infected; (2) Increased HIV testing and increased number of infected patients receiving ART help individual patients and the community by decreasing the community viral load; and (3) Medical male circumcision reduces the risk of female-to-male sexual transmission of HIV by approximately 60%, an important intervention in developing countries with limited treatment and prevention options.

KEY WEBSITES

AIDS Education and Training Center's National Evaluation Center: *www.aetcnec.ucsf.edu*

Association of Nurses in AIDS Care: *www.nursesinaidscare.org*

CDC National Prevention Information Network: *www.cdcnpin.org*

HIV/AIDS Bureau of Health Resources Services Administration: *www.hab.hrsa.gov*

CRITICAL THINKING CASE STUDY

JP is a 35-year-old patient who was recently diagnosed with HIV. Other than a recent "case of the flu" approximately 1 month ago, she has been healthy. She has been divorced for 2 years and has a 3-year-old child. JP tested HIV negative in the first trimester of her pregnancy and was not retested during the third trimester. She reports that the relationship with her husband was monogamous and that they did not use condoms. JP began a relationship with a new partner 1 year ago. He claimed to be HIV negative, and they did not use condoms (JP takes oral contraceptives for pregnancy prevention). JP denies a history of intravenous drug use and other high-risk behaviors. Her baseline labs include a CD4 of 450/20% and a viral load of 75,000 copies/mm^3. Her genotypic resistance assay shows no baseline resistance. Her preference is for a once-a-day regimen. She may want to have another child but is not certain.

1. JP asks the nurse when she may have become infected with HIV. What are some of the responses that the nurse should include in a discussion with the patient?
2. Considering JP's preference for a daily antiretroviral regimen, and in view of her history, which medication regimens could be considered for this patient? What, if any, risk-benefit discussion should occur with regard to choices?
3. JP begins ART. She takes the medication without missing any doses for 4 weeks. Her follow-up laboratory results show a CD4 count of 500/22% cells/mL and a viral load of 400 copies/mL. She schedules a follow-up appointment for 2 months later, with laboratory testing preceding her appointment. She calls after 2 weeks, complaining of a painful rash on her back. JP is diagnosed with herpes zoster. She is discouraged and thinks her HIV is worsening. What explanation can the nurse give for the occurrence of this new diagnosis?
4. At her next routine visit, JP says that she missed two doses of her medications because she had an unplanned overnight stay during a trip. What counseling and interventions should the nurse include in her discussion with the patient?

NCLEX STUDY QUESTIONS

1. During routine prenatal testing, a patient is diagnosed with HIV infection. To help prevent perinatal transmission of HIV to the fetus, what is the nurse's best action?
   a. Provide the patient with contact information for an AIDS support group.
   b. Educate the patient about the risks of HIV disease to the fetus.
   c. Notify the CDC of the patient's diagnosis.
   d. Provide written and oral education about the use of ART during pregnancy.
2. When a patient does not appear for a routine clinic visit, the nurse calls to ask about the missed visit. The patient says, "I don't need to come any longer. I'm so glad I no longer have HIV." The nurse learns that recent laboratory results indicated an "undetectable" HIV viral load and that the patient stopped his medication several weeks earlier. What is the nurse's best response?
   a. Inform the patient that he must be seen immediately because the undetectable viral load indicates that his medication stopped working.
   b. Have the patient reschedule his clinic visit.
   c. Congratulate the patient on his treatment success.
   d. Educate the patient about the continued need for his medications and ongoing laboratory monitoring.
3. The nurse advises HIV-positive patients about blood draws for CD4 count. What is the correct information to give them about when and how this laboratory blood work should be done?
   a. At the same laboratory at approximately the same time of day whenever possible
   b. After a 10-hour fast
   c. Approximately 1 hour after taking antiretroviral medications
   d. At any laboratory at any time of day
4. In collaboration with the patient on ART, the nurse formulates a plan of care. Which items are appropriate to include in planning? (Select all that apply.)
   a. Patient's viral load will become and remain undetectable.
   b. Patient will not experience secondary infection.
   c. Patient will promptly report new onset of symptoms and side effects.
   d. Patient's laboratory blood work will be within normal limits.
   e. Patient will adhere to medication regimen and/or report difficulties related to adherence.
5. A patient is to start on efavirenz (Sustiva). Which points are important for the nurse to include in health teaching for this patient? (Select all that apply.)
   a. Dose is given at bedtime to minimize CNS adverse effects.
   b. Avoid alcohol because of adverse effects to the liver.
   c. Dose is given after breakfast to minimize CNS adverse effects.
   d. High-fat meals will decrease absorption of medication.
   e. Hyperglycemia, jaundice, and diabetes mellitus are side effects.

Answers: 1, d; 2, d; 3, a; 4, a, b, c, e; 5, a, b.

CHAPTER

36

Vaccines

Lynette M. Wachholz

evolve WEBSITE

http://evolve.elsevier.com/KeeHayes/pharmacology/

- Animations
- Content Updates
- Key Points
- Review Questions for the NCLEX® Examination
- References from the Textbook
- Unfolding Case Studies

OBJECTIVES

- Compare and contrast active and passive immunity.
- Compare and contrast active natural and active acquired immunity.
- Describe infectious diseases for which vaccines are currently available.
- Outline the currently recommended childhood immunization schedule.
- Discuss vaccines routinely administered to adults.
- Discuss contraindications to the administration of recommended immunizations.
- Explain the nursing interventions, including teaching, related to the administration of vaccines.

OUTLINE

KEY TERMS

acquired immunity, p. 490
active immunity, p. 490
adjuvant, p. 490
anaphylaxis, p. 494
antibodies, p. 490
antigen, p. 490
attenuated viruses, p. 490
cocooning, p. 493
conjugate vaccines, p. 490
natural immunity, p. 490
passive immunity, p. 490
pathogen, p. 490
recombinant subunit vaccines, p. 490
seroconversion, p. 494
toxoids, p. 490
vaccination, p. 490

Timely administration of immunizations protects individuals from illness. Immunizations can also ultimately lead to the eradication of disease, as was the case with smallpox in 1977; therefore, universal immunization is a national goal. The 2009 United States National Immunization Survey estimates that 63.6% of 19- to 35-month-old children have received the recommended number of doses of DTaP, polio, hepatitis B, *Haemophilus influenzae* type B, pneumococcal, MMR, and varicella vaccines. This is down from 68.4% in 2008. Among this cohort of children, 0.6% received no immunizations at all.

Findings from the survey also found that vaccine coverage differed by ethnicity and by economic status. In general, white children had higher vaccination rates than nonwhite children. Also, poverty increased the likelihood that a child would not be fully vaccinated.

ACTIVE IMMUNITY

Active immunity occurs as a part of the human immune response, which is activated when a **pathogen** such as a bacterium or virus invades the body. The body recognizes this pathogen as a foreign substance and promptly begins producing **antibodies** (also called *immunoglobulins*) and other infection-fighting cells whose responsibility it is to rid the body of this foreign substance. On first exposure to the pathogen, the immune response is relatively slow and is typically accompanied by signs and symptoms of disease. However, the immune system retains memory of this pathogen. If this same pathogen invades the body again, the immune response, including the increased production of pathogen-specific antibodies, occurs much more rapidly and generally prevents disease. This active **natural immunity** may be present for the remaining life of the individual. Natural immunity is genetically determined in specific populations or families. Some pathogens cannot infect certain species because the environment is not suitable (e.g., measles cannot reproduce in dogs; thus, dogs have a natural immunity to measles).

Acquired immunity occurs from exposure to an antigen or from passive injection of immunoglobulins. Active protection against disease may also be provoked by immunization. **Vaccination** involves the administration of a small amount of **antigen**, which although capable of stimulating an immune response does not typically produce disease. The antigen in vaccines may be produced in several ways. Traditional vaccines contain the whole or components of an inactivated (killed) microorganism. Other vaccines are **attenuated viruses** composed of live, attenuated (weakened) microorganisms. **Toxoids** are inactivated toxins, the harmful disease-causing substance produced by some microorganisms.

Some newer vaccines are called **conjugate vaccines**. Such vaccines require a protein or toxoid from an unrelated organism to link to the outer coat of the disease-causing microorganism. This linkage creates a substance that can be recognized by the immature immune system of young infants. *Haemophilus influenzae* type B is an example of a conjugate vaccine.

Recombinant subunit vaccines involve the insertion of some of the genetic material (e.g., deoxyribonucleic acid [DNA]) of a pathogen into another cell or organism, where the antigen is then produced in massive quantities. These antigens are then used as a vaccine in place of the whole pathogen. Hepatitis B is an example of this type of vaccine.

An **adjuvant**, often an aluminum salt such as aluminum hydroxide, aluminum phosphate, or aluminum potassium sulfate, is a substance sometimes used in the production of a vaccine to increase the vaccine's immunogenicity and to prolong the immune response. Adjuvants may also be added to a vaccine to reduce the amount of antigen needed to produce a dose of vaccine. Adjuvants have been used in the production of immunizations since the 1930s and are found in many U.S. childhood vaccines.

Regardless of the composition of the vaccine, each vaccine is designed to stimulate an immune response against a specific pathogen. Booster doses are sometimes required to maintain sufficient immunity. Because the immune system retains memory, a vaccinated individual who is later exposed to the actual pathogen mounts a rapid immune response, thus preventing disease. This active artificially acquired immunity is the focus of this chapter.

PASSIVE IMMUNITY

Passive immunity occurs when an individual receives antibodies against a particular pathogen from another source. Newborn infants naturally receive passive immunity via the transfer of maternal antibodies across the placenta. Passive immunity may also be acquired through the administration of antibodies pooled from several human or animal sources that have been exposed to disease-causing pathogens. Alternatively, antibodies may be produced using recombinant DNA technology.

Whether natural or acquired, passive immunity is transient, lasting no more than several weeks to a few months. The recipient does not mount his or her own immune response. However, passive immunity is important. It helps young infants who, because of their immature immune systems, are poorly equipped to protect themselves against disease. Acquired passive immunity is important when (1) time does not permit active vaccination alone, (2) the exposed individual is at high risk for complications of the disease, or (3) the individual suffers from an immune system deficiency that renders that person unable to produce an effective immune response.

VACCINE-PREVENTABLE DISEASES

In the United States, more than 20 infectious diseases may be prevented by active vaccination. Many of these vaccines are routinely administered to healthy children and adults. Others are reserved for special populations, such as military personnel, travelers to certain foreign countries, or the chronically ill. Table 36-1 provides an overview of the disease manifestations and vaccine information, including route of administration and storage temperature. Vaccine-preventable diseases include, but are not limited to, anthrax, diphtheria, *Haemophilus influenzae* type B (Hib), hepatitis A, hepatitis B, human papillomavirus, influenza, Japanese encephalitis, measles, meningococcal disease, mumps, pertussis, pneumococcal disease, poliomyelitis, rabies, rotavirus, rubella, smallpox, tetanus, tuberculosis, typhoid, varicella, yellow fever, and herpes zoster.

TABLE 36-1 VACCINE-PREVENTABLE DISEASES

DISEASE, ROUTE OF ADMINISTRATION, AND STORAGE TEMPERATURE	MANIFESTATIONS	VACCINE
Anthrax/subQ	Spectrum involves three types of infection: Cutaneous (malignant pustule): a painless sore that develops at the site of a cut Inhalational (wool sorter's disease): severe dyspnea, cyanosis, fever, and death Gastrointestinal: abdominal pain, vomiting, bloody diarrhea, toxemia, shock, possibly death Inhalational form associated with use of bacteria in biologic warfare	Inactivated bacteria Administration limited to military personnel
Diphtheria/IM 35°-46° F (2°-8° C)	Respiratory infection May result in heart failure or paralysis if left untreated	Toxoid Contained in DTaP, Tdap, DT, Td, DTaP-Hib, DTaP-IPV, DTaP-IPV/Hib, and DTaP-IPV-hepatitis B vaccines
Haemophilus influenzae type B (Hib)/IM 35°-46° F (2°-8° C)	Causes meningitis, pneumonia, sepsis, arthritis, and skin and throat infections Most serious in children younger than 1 y	Bacterial conjugate Contained in Hib, DTaP-Hib, Hib-hepatitis B, DTaP-IPV/Hib, and Hib-MCV vaccines
Hepatitis A/IM 35°-46° F (2°-8° C)	Fever, malaise, jaundice, anorexia, and nausea Acute, self-limited illness	Inactivated viral antigen Contained in hepatitis A and hepatitis A–hepatitis B vaccines Administered to children 12-23 mo, high-risk populations, and persons traveling to certain foreign countries
Hepatitis B/IM 35°-46° F (2°-8° C)	Malaise, anorexia, arthralgias, arthritis, jaundice Chronic infection can occur, leading to liver cirrhosis, liver cancer, and death	Recombinant viral antigen Contained in hepatitis B, Hib-hepatitis B, DTaP-IPV–hepatitis B, and hepatitis A–hepatitis B vaccines
Human papillomavirus/IM 35°-46° F (2°-8° C)	Cervical, anal, and oropharyngeal cancers; genital warts	Recombinant viral antigen Administered to women 9-26 y One vaccine is also licensed for use in men 9-26 y
Influenza/IM, intradermal, intranasal *Inactivated:* 35°-46° F (2°-8° C) *Live attenuated:* ≤5° F (–15° C)	Fever, chills, headaches, malaise, myalgias, nasal congestion, and cough Occasionally causes croup and pneumonia	Inactivated viral components (IM and intradermal) or live attenuated virus (intranasal)
Japanese encephalitis/subQ 35°-46° F (2°-8° C)	Headache, fever, myalgias, encephalitis	Inactivated virus Administered to some foreign travelers
Measles/subQ 35°-46° F (2°-8° C), but may be frozen	Rash, fever, cough, nasal congestion, conjunctivitis, pneumonia Occasionally results in encephalitis	Live virus Contained in measles, MMR, and MMR-varicella vaccines
Meningococcal disease/subQ, IM 35°-46° F (2°-8° C)	Fever, sepsis, rash, meningitis	MPSV4: portions of inactivated bacterial capsule (subQ) MCV4: bacterial conjugate (IM), expected to give better, longer-lasting protection Contained in MCV4, MPSV4, and Hib-MCV vaccines
Mumps/subQ 35°-46° F (2°-8° C), but may be frozen	Swelling of salivary glands, fever, and headache Rarely causes encephalitis, inflamed testicles, and permanent hearing loss	Live attenuated virus Contained in mumps, MMR, and MMR-varicella vaccines
Pertussis ("whooping cough")/IM 35°-46° F (2°-8° C)	Severe coughing spasms Rarely causes pneumonia, seizures, encephalitis, and death Symptoms more severe in infants and young children	Antigenic components of inactivated bacteria (acellular) Contained in DTaP, Tdap, DTaP-Hib, DTaP-IPV–hepatitis B, and DTaP-IPV/Hib vaccines
Pneumococcal disease/IM, subQ 35°-46° F (2°-8° C)	Ear infections, sinus infections, pneumonia Occasionally causes sepsis and meningitis	Polysaccharide vaccine (PPV23) contains portions of 23 serotypes of pneumococcal bacterial capsules (subQ); administered to older adults and certain other high-risk populations ≥2 y Protein conjugate vaccine (PCV13) contains portions of 13 serotypes of pneumococcal bacterial capsules (IM); recommended for routine administration to children <2 y and certain older high-risk children

Continued

TABLE 36-1 VACCINE-PREVENTABLE DISEASES—cont'd

DISEASE, ROUTE OF ADMINISTRATION, AND STORAGE TEMPERATURE	MANIFESTATIONS	VACCINE
Poliomyelitis/subQ, IM 35°-46° F (2°-8° C)	Mild form causes fever, sore throat, nausea, and headaches Severe form causes paralysis and death	Inactivated virus Contained in IPV, DTaP-IPV, DTaP-IPV–hepatitis B, and DTaP-IPV/Hib vaccines
Rabies/IM 35°-46° F (2°-8° C)	Anxiety, difficulty swallowing, seizures; almost always progresses to death	Inactivated virus Administered to high-risk groups (e.g., veterinarians, animal handlers) and persons traveling to areas where rabies is common
Rotavirus/PO 35°-46° F (2°-8° C)	Vomiting and diarrhea; may be particularly severe in infants/young children	Live attenuated virus
Rubella ("German measles")/subQ 35°-46° F (2°-8° C), but may be frozen	Rash, fever Birth defects if acquired by pregnant patients	Live attenuated virus Contained in rubella, MMR, and MMR-varicella vaccines
Smallpox/skin prick 35°-46° F (2°-8° C)	High fever, severe headache, backache, abdominal pain, and lethargy lasting 2-5 days Then extensive rash that begins as macules and progresses to papules, then firm vesicles, and, finally, deep-seated, hard pustules that cause significant scarring Natural disease eradicated worldwide in 1980 May be used as a weapon of bioterrorism	Live virus Limited immunization program to include military personnel, civilian health care workers, and emergency personnel began in 2002
Tetanus ("lockjaw")/IM 35°-46° F (2°-8° C)	Headache, irritability, muscle spasms (jaw, neck, arms, legs, back, and abdomen)	Toxoid Contained in tetanus, DTaP, DTaP-Hib, DTaP-IPV, DT, DTaP-IPV–hepatitis B, DTaP-IPV/Hib, Tdap, and Td vaccines
Tuberculosis ("TB")/ID (preferred), subQ 35°-46° F (2°-8° C)	Highly contagious respiratory infection May also cause meningitis and bone, joint, and skin infections	Live attenuated bacteria Referred to as BCG vaccine Not routinely administered in the United States Prevents severe disease, but does not prevent infection with the bacterium
Typhoid/subQ, PO 35°-46° F (2°-8° C)	Fever, headache, anorexia, abdominal pain, enlarged liver and spleen, constipation, and later, diarrhea	Available as live attenuated bacteria (PO), or inactivated components of typhoid bacterial capsule (subQ) Recommended only for travelers to certain foreign countries
Varicella ("chickenpox")/subQ ≤5° F (–15° C)	Fever and rash, consisting of a few to hundreds of itchy, blisterlike lesions Symptoms more severe in older children and adults Complications may include encephalitis, bacterial skin infections, pneumonia, Reye's syndrome, and death	Live attenuated virus Contained in varicella and MMR-varicella vaccines
Yellow fever/subQ 35°-46° F (2°-8° C)	Fever, jaundice, and gastrointestinal hemorrhage	Live attenuated virus Recommended for travelers to foreign countries with high yellow fever rates Required by international regulations for travel to and from certain countries
Zoster ("shingles")/subQ ≤5° F (–15° C)	Painful, blisterlike rash in a dermatomal distribution Occurs due to reactivation of varicella virus Following resolution of rash, may have prolonged severe pain (postherpetic neuralgia)	Live attenuated virus Administered to persons ≥60 y

BCG, Bacille Calmette-Guérin; *DT,* diphtheria-tetanus; *DTaP,* diphtheria-tetanus–acellular pertussis; *Hib, Haemophilus influenzae* type B; *ID,* intradermal; *IM,* intramuscular; *IPV,* inactivated poliovirus; *MMR,* measles-mumps-rubella; *mo,* months, *PO,* by mouth; *subQ,* subcutaneous; *Td,* tetanus-diphtheria; *y,* year; >, greater than; ≥, greater than or equal to; <, less than, ≤, less than or equal to.

CHILDHOOD IMMUNIZATIONS

For the most current information on childhood immunizations, consult the Centers for Disease Control and Prevention (CDC) website at *www.cdc.gov/vaccines.* A summary of rules for childhood immunizations, updated in 2013, is also located at the Immunization Action Coalition's website at *www.immunize.org/catg.d/p2010.pdf.* Information about each vaccine includes route of administration, schedule for routine vaccine administration, minimum dosing intervals, and contraindications to use. Recommended vaccines are diphtheria-tetanus-acellular pertussis, inactivated polio, varicella, measles-mumps-rubella, *Haemophilus influenzae* type B, hepatitis A, hepatitis B, pneumococcal conjugate, influenza, meningococcal conjugate, human papillomavirus, and rotavirus. Before immunizations are administered, children and their caregivers should be questioned regarding use of prescription and over-the-counter medications, including herbal preparations, and any food or drug allergies (Herbal Alert 36-1).

HERBAL ALERT 36-1

Vaccines

Although patients should always be asked about their use of prescription and over-the-counter drugs, there are no known interactions between vaccinations and herbal preparations.

ADULT IMMUNIZATIONS

While much emphasis is placed on regularly immunizing infants and children, adult immunizations are frequently overlooked. However, immunizations are equally important to the health and well-being of adults. Routine vaccines for adults may include tetanus-diphtheria-acellular pertussis, tetanus-diphtheria, influenza, pneumococcal polysaccharide, human papillomavirus, measles-mumps-rubella, varicella, and zoster. In certain situations, adults may also be immunized with some or all of the following vaccines: hepatitis A, hepatitis B, pneumococcal polysaccharide, and meningococcal polysaccharide. The most current recommendations for adult immunization can be found at *www.cdc.gov/vaccines,* and the Immunization Action Coalition's website contains a summary of rules for adult immunization *(www.immunize.org/catg.d./p2011.pdf).* The CDC suggests review of adult immunization records on decade birthdays—ages 30, 40, and 50 years, and so on.

A strategy called **cocooning** focuses on immunizing adults in close contact with newborns and young infants to protect the babies from contracting vaccine-preventable diseases in the months before they are eligible to receive the vaccine themselves. Currently, these efforts focus on preventing pertussis in newborns and young infants by administering Tdap vaccine to parents, grandparents, and other caregivers.

SAFETY: Preventing Medication Errors

Do not confuse ...

- Hepatitis A vaccines in different doses for child/adolescent and adult
- Hepatitis B vaccines in different doses for child/adolescent and adult
- Hepatitis B vaccines and hepatitis B immunoglobulin
- DTaP and Tdap vaccines, which contain different amounts of individual vaccine components and are indicated for different age groups
- Zostavax, a vaccine administered to adults to prevent shingles, and Varivax, which prevents chickenpox and is approved for use in susceptible children and adults (both are preparations of varicella virus vaccine)

IMMUNIZATION BEFORE INTERNATIONAL TRAVEL

International travel warrants the administration of all routine vaccines indicated based on age or immunization history. It may also require consideration of additional vaccines, depending on the travel destination.

Travelers may need to consider vaccination against typhoid and yellow fever. Typhoid is caused by a bacterium, *Salmonella enterica* typhi, which is generally spread via contaminated food and water (see Table 36-1). Risk of contracting this infection is greatest for travelers to India, Pakistan, Mexico, Bangladesh, the Philippines, and Haiti. Even stays of less than 2 weeks pose significant risk. Two vaccines are available for use in the United States: The live oral vaccine can be administered to persons 6 years of age and older and consists of four capsules, one taken every 48 hours, with the series completed 1 week before potential exposure. A booster consisting of the same four-capsule regimen is recommended every 5 years. The polysaccharide vaccine may be administered to travelers 2 years of age and older. It is administered at least 2 weeks before expected exposure as a single, intramuscular (IM) injection. A booster dose is recommended every 2 years.

Yellow fever is a mosquito-borne viral illness. The disease occurs only in sub-Saharan Africa and tropical South America. The vaccine is administered as a single injection; a booster every 10 years is recommended. In the United States, the vaccine is administered only at authorized vaccine centers throughout the country.

Other vaccines needed for travel may include meningococcal, rabies, and Japanese encephalitis vaccines. Current vaccine recommendations and related travel information are available from the CDC at 1-800-CDC-INFO or *www.cdc.gov/travel.*

REPORTING OF DISEASES AND ADVERSE REACTIONS

Health care providers are responsible for reporting cases of vaccine-preventable diseases to public health officials, who make weekly reports to the CDC. These data identify whether an outbreak is occurring and the impact of immunization policies and procedures.

Vaccines are generally safe. Common mild reactions include swelling at the injection site and fever. Awareness of the contraindications for use of vaccines decreases the incidence of serious adverse reactions. Absolute contraindications include moderate or severe illness or **anaphylaxis** (a serious, potentially life-threatening allergic reaction) to a specific vaccine or vaccine component. It is important to review vaccine-specific contraindications prior to administering any vaccine. However, in general, vaccines may be given in cases of mild acute illness or convalescent phase of illness; antimicrobial therapy; exposure to infectious disease; or premature birth.

Health care providers must report adverse reactions to the Vaccine Adverse Events Reporting System. Information and forms are available at *http://vaers.hhs.gov/index.* The National Childhood Vaccine Injury Act of 1986 set forth the National Vaccine Injury Compensation Program (NVICP). This program provides compensation for injury or death caused by a vaccination. The NVICP does not require proof of negligence on the part of a health care provider. For more information, visit *www.hrsa.gov/vaccinecompensation/.*

VARICELLA VACCINE

Prototype Drug Chart 36-1 provides the pharmacologic data for varicella vaccine.

Pharmacokinetics Biologic products such as vaccines do not undergo the pharmacokinetic processes associated with other drug therapy.

Pharmacodynamics **Seroconversion** is the acquisition of detectable levels of antibodies in the bloodstream. In the case of varicella vaccine, seroconversion occurs in more than 98% of 12-month-old to 12-year-old recipients approximately 6 weeks after receiving a single dose of vaccine. Susceptible persons 13 years of age and older who receive two doses of varicella vaccine 4 to 8 weeks apart show a seroconversion rate of approximately 75% 4 weeks after the first dose and 99% 4 weeks after the second dose. Despite the high rate of initial seroconversion among children 12 months to 12 years of age, clinical trials have shown that over a 10-year period the vaccine's effectiveness in preventing disease was 94% for children receiving one dose of vaccine and 98% for those who received two doses. Therefore, beginning in 2007, a second dose of varicella vaccine was recommended for all susceptible individuals, including children.

Contraindications

Varicella vaccine should be avoided in patients with a history of previous anaphylaxis to this vaccine or to any of its

PROTOTYPE DRUG CHART 36-1

Varicella

Drug Class Vaccine Trade Name: Varivax Pregnancy Category: C	**Dosage** 0.5 mL subQ × 2 doses. First dose: 12-15 mo; second dose: 4-6 y; catch-up initiated any time after 12-15 mo <13 y: space doses at least 3 mo apart ≥13 y: space doses 4-8 wk apart **For varicella prophylaxis for outbreak control of local epidemics of wild-type varicella virus in susceptible persons following varicella exposure,** consult the current recommendations of the CDC
Contraindications Previous anaphylaxis to this vaccine or to any of its components; pregnancy or possibility of pregnancy within 1 mo; immunocompromised vaccine recipient; presence of moderate to severe acute illness; active untreated tuberculosis	**Drug-Lab-Food Interactions** Drug: Separate from other live virus vaccines (e.g., MMR, intranasal flu) by 4 wk if not given on same day; delay VV for up to 11 mo after blood transfusion or Ig; delay Ig for 2 mo after VV; high-dose immunosuppressant medications; avoid with salicylates for 6 wk after VV
Pharmacokinetics Not applicable	**Pharmacodynamics** Seroconversion rates: 12 mo–12 y: >98% at 4-6 wk after vaccination ≥13 y: ~75% 4 wk after first dose, and 99% 4 wk after second dose
Therapeutic Effects/Uses Prevention of chickenpox. When administered to susceptible individuals, vaccine results in complete protection from chickenpox for the majority. For the minority in whom breakthrough chickenpox develops after vaccination, the disease is typically very mild. The vaccine may also provide prophylaxis protection if administered within 3-5 d of exposure to chickenpox. Mode of Action: Stimulates active immunity against natural disease	
Side Effects Pain and redness at injection site, fever, chickenpox-like rash (generalized or confined to area surrounding injection site)	**Adverse Reactions** Anaphylaxis, thrombocytopenia, encephalitis, Stevens-Johnson syndrome

d, Day; *Ig,* immune globulin; *MMR,* measles-mumps-rubella; *mo,* month; *subQ,* subcutaneous; *VV,* varicella vaccine; *wk,* week; *y,* year; <, less than; ≥, greater than or equal to.

components, including gelatin and neomycin. It is also contraindicated in the presence of moderate to severe acute illness or active untreated tuberculosis.

While varicella infection can cause fetal harm, the possible effects of the vaccine on fetal development are currently unknown. Therefore, varicella vaccine is contraindicated during pregnancy. Pregnancy should also be avoided for at least 1 month after each dose of the vaccine. *Note:* This recommendation differs from the product package insert, which suggests a 3-month delay in pregnancy.

Patients who are immunocompromised because of malignancies, high-dose systemic steroids, or other immunosuppressive therapy should avoid varicella vaccine. Likewise, the vaccine is generally contraindicated in the presence of primary or acquired immunodeficiencies. However, vaccination may be considered in children with certain classes of human immunodeficiency virus (HIV) infection.

Drug Interactions

Frequently a patient is eligible for several immunizations at any given visit. A patient receiving varicella vaccine may receive all other vaccines concurrently as long as each is administered at a separate site. If the MMR or other live virus vaccine is not given the same day as the varicella vaccine, administration of the two vaccines should be separated by at least 4 weeks.

If a patient has received a transfusion of blood or blood products, including immune globulin, administration of the varicella vaccine will need to be deferred for as long as 11 months. Likewise, such blood products should be avoided for at least 2 months after vaccination if possible. Blood products and immune globulin interfere with the body's production of antibodies specific to chickenpox, thereby decreasing the likelihood that active immunity will develop.

Reye's syndrome has occasionally occurred in children following natural chickenpox infection. The majority of these children were also receiving salicylate medications (e.g., aspirin). Therefore, it is generally recommended that patients avoid salicylates for 6 weeks after vaccination.

NEWER DEVELOPMENTS AND THE FUTURE OF VACCINES

A small outbreak of anthrax cases in the United States in 2001 increased the level of awareness of the anthrax vaccine. As a biologic weapon, anthrax is highly lethal. It is easily produced, stored, and spread over large areas. Proper vaccination is an essential part of protection against this disease. Approved by the FDA in 1970, anthrax vaccine has been routinely and safely administered to laboratory and military personnel, livestock farmers, and veterinarians. The vaccine requires six injections: three given 2 weeks apart followed by three additional doses at 6, 12, and 18 months. No serious side effects have been reported, but the vaccination is contraindicated during pregnancy. Strides have been made in the development of an oral anthrax vaccine. The vaccine is derived from a genetically modified plant virus. The virus is introduced into a plant, where it then stimulates the plant to produce new proteins. These proteins are extracted and used to produce a vaccine. When the vaccine is administered to a human, the person's body reacts as if infected with anthrax and creates antibodies against the bacterium. In the event of a bioterrorism attack, large numbers of individuals can be rapidly immunized with an oral vaccine. Additional information is available at *www.anthrax.osd.mil.*

Smallpox was eradicated worldwide by 1980. The United States discontinued routine childhood immunization against smallpox in 1971. However, since the events of September 2001, concern has arisen that the smallpox (or variola) virus could be used as a bioterrorist weapon. Unlike anthrax, smallpox virus is not airborne and is transmitted through human bodily fluids or contaminated materials. A smallpox immunization plan has been implemented in the United States (*www.bt.cdc.gov/agent/smallpox/vaccination/*). However, there has been some resistance to vaccination because of a lack of perceived threat and because of the risk of significant side effects from the vaccine. The currently available vaccine is a live virus preparation. It is administered using a bifurcated needle to deliver the vaccine into the epidermis. A skin reaction occurs at the immunization site 3 to 5 days later and eventually leaves a scar. Boosters may be recommended every 10 years.

It has long been known that immunity to pertussis, or "whooping cough," wanes over time and that adolescents and adults are often responsible for transmitting this infection to vulnerable, incompletely immunized infants and young children. While a relatively benign illness in the older population, pertussis in infants is associated with significant morbidity and mortality. Two products containing tetanus and diphtheria toxoids along with acellular pertussis are licensed for use in older children and adults. Adacel is approved for use in people 11 to 64 years of age, and Boostrix is approved for use in people 10 years of age and older. Each vaccine contains the same antigens as its respective counterpart administered to young children (DTaP), but with reduced quantities of diphtheria and acellular pertussis (Tdap). It is recommended that for booster immunization, adolescents and adults receive a one-time dose of Tdap in lieu of Td vaccine.

Herpes zoster, commonly known as "shingles" or *zoster*, occurs as the result of reactivation of the varicella virus. Following a primary varicella infection ("chickenpox"), the virus persists but becomes dormant in the body, usually settling in a dorsal root ganglion. Zoster often occurs decades after the primary varicella infection. It appears that development of zoster may be related to a decline in immunity to the varicella-zoster virus (VZV). Zoster is characterized by a painful rash that presents in a dermatomal distribution. Especially in older adults, resolution of the rash may be followed by a chronic, severe, sometimes debilitating pain, referred to as *postherpetic neuralgia*. A live attenuated vaccine, Zostavax, is licensed for use as a one-time injection in adults 50 years of age and older. The vaccine has been shown to boost VZV immunity among vaccine recipients. In clinical trials,

Zostavax prevented zoster in about 50% of people who received the vaccine. Effectiveness appears to decrease with increasing age of the vaccine recipient. In those who received the vaccine yet went on to develop zoster, the duration of pain was reduced.

Rotavirus is a leading cause of severe acute gastroenteritis in infants and young children. RotaTeq, a live oral vaccine containing five strains of rotavirus, is effective in protecting against severe gastroenteritis and significantly reduces the need for hospitalization among infected children. The vaccine is administered at 2, 4, and 6 months of age. A second rotavirus vaccine, Rotarix, consists of two doses administered orally at 2 and 4 months of age.

Gardasil, the human papillomavirus (HPV) vaccine, has been called the first vaccine designed to prevent cancer. It contains four strains of human papillomavirus, which account for the vast majority of cases of cervical cancer and genital warts. HPV is also associated with several less common cancers, such as vaginal and vulvar cancers in women and anal and oropharyngeal cancers in both men and women. A recombinant vaccine, it is licensed for routine use in 9- to 26-year-old female patients and is administered as a three-shot series. The manufacturer of Gardasil has received FDA approval for use of its vaccine in male patients 9 to 26 years of age. The FDA turned down Merck's request for expanded use in women 27 to 45 years of age. A second HPV vaccine, Cervarix, is FDA approved for use in women. Because HPV is sexually transmitted, the vaccine is most effective if administered before initiation of sexual intercourse. (See Chapter 58 for more information about sexually transmitted infections and this vaccine.)

The first pneumococcal conjugate vaccine, Prevnar, provides protection against seven serotypes of pneumococci. Since its introduction, the incidence of invasive disease caused by these seven strains has dramatically decreased. However, the incidence of disease caused by nonvaccine serotypes is on the rise. One such serotype, 19A, now accounts for 42% of pneumococcal disease. In early 2010, a conjugate vaccine containing 13 serotypes, including 19A, gained FDA approval. It replaces the seven-valent vaccine.

While each vaccine as a single antigen has been available for many years, in June 2012 the FDA approved Menhibrix, a combination vaccine for infants and children 6 weeks to 18 months of age, for prevention of invasive disease cause by *Neisseria meningitides* and *Haemophilus influenza* type b. Menhibrix is given as a four-dose series at 2, 4, 6, and 12 to 15 months of age, although the first dose may be given as early as 6 weeks of age, and the fourth dose may be administered as late as 18 months of age. However, the United States Advisory Committee on Immunization Practice has not recommended routine immunization of infants against meningococcal disease, so the utility of this vaccine is currently unclear.

New delivery systems for vaccines are in development. Timed-release pills in a one-time dose have the potential to offer lifetime immunity to a targeted disease, eliminating the need for booster vaccination. In addition, skin patches may one day be used to administer tetanus and influenza vaccines.

Nursing Process
Patient-Centered Collaborative Care

Vaccines

Assessment

- Identify barriers to timely and complete immunization (e.g., belief that vaccine-preventable diseases no longer exist, misunderstanding of true contraindications to immunization, concerns regarding vaccine safety and efficacy, fear of multiple injections, cost).
- Obtain medical history, including history of malignancy or other immune deficiency.
- Determine history of pregnancy or possible pregnancy within the next month. Many vaccines are contraindicated during pregnancy.
- Obtain drug history, including high-dose immunosuppressants, blood transfusions, and immune globulin.
- Obtain a list of herbal products used by patient and mother (in case of breastfed infant).
- Determine complete allergy history, including drugs, vaccines, food, and environmental allergies.
- Assess for adverse reactions (other than allergic) to previous doses of vaccine or any vaccine component.
- Assess for symptoms of moderate to severe acute illness with or without fever.
- Screen for unvaccinated or immunocompromised household contacts at every visit.
- Obtain immunization history and history of vaccine-preventable diseases to determine current vaccine needs. For example, a person with a reliable history of chickenpox or herpes zoster ("shingles") does not need varicella vaccine; natural immunity is assumed.

Nursing Diagnoses

- Deficient knowledge related to vaccine-preventable diseases and risks and benefits of vaccination
- Risk for ineffective health maintenance related to nonadherence to recommended immunization schedule
- Risk for injury related to adverse reactions to immunizations
- Readiness for enhanced immunization status related to expressed desire to improve knowledge about vaccines

Planning

- Patient or patient's parent or guardian will possess knowledge of vaccine-preventable diseases and risks and benefits of vaccination.
- Patient or patient's parent or guardian will adhere to recommended immunization schedule for vaccine-preventable diseases unless contraindications exist.
- Patient will be free of adverse reactions.

Nursing Interventions

- Strictly adhere to individual vaccine storage requirements to ensure potency of the product.
- Upon preparation, including reconstitution of a given vaccine, administer within time limits stated in package insert to ensure potency.
- Administer at separate sites all vaccines for which patient is eligible at the time of the visit. *Do not mix vaccines in the same syringe.*
- Document in patient's record the vaccination date, route, and site of administration; vaccine type, manufacturer, lot number, and expiration date; and name, business address, and title of person administering vaccine.
- Observe patient for signs and symptoms of adverse reactions to vaccines.
- Keep epinephrine readily available for immediate use in case of anaphylactic reaction.
- Provide patient with a record of immunizations administered.

Patient Teaching

General

- Discuss vaccine-preventable diseases with patient and/or patient's family, including manifestations and risk of contracting.
- Answer all questions regarding vaccine safety and efficacy.
- Advise female patients of childbearing age to avoid pregnancy for 1 month, depending on the vaccines administered.
- Advise patients to avoid contact with immunocompromised persons, depending on vaccines to be administered.
- Provide patient or patient's family with current Vaccine Information Statements (VISs), available from the CDC, for each vaccine before its administration, as required by federal law.
- Remind patient or patient's family to bring immunization record to all visits.
- Provide patient or patient's family with return date for next vaccination(s) based on assessment of immunization history.

Side Effects

- Discuss common side effects of vaccines, such as injection site soreness, fever, and side effects specific to individual vaccines.
- Offer suggestions for management of common side effects (e.g., cold compresses for injection site soreness, acetaminophen for soreness or fever).
- Advise patient or patient's family to contact the health care provider if signs of a serious reaction are noted.

Cultural Considerations

- Modify communications to meet cultural needs of patient and family.
- Use a professional interpreter when necessary.
- Provide patient and family with VISs in preferred language (available at *www.immunize.org.*)

Evaluation

- Evaluate patient's or family's understanding of rationale for immunizations.
- Evaluate patient adherence to recommended immunization schedule.
- Evaluate if patient is free from adverse reactions.

KEY WEBSITES

CDC's National Immunization Program: *www.cdc.gov/vaccines*

CDC's Travel Health: *wwwnc.cdc.gov/travel*

Immunization Action Coalition: *www.immunize.org*

Vaccine Education Center at Children's Hospital of Philadelphia: *www.chop.edu/service/vaccine-education-center/home.html*

CRITICAL THINKING CASE STUDY

JW, 29 years of age, presents in late October to the immunization clinic, accompanied by her 2-month-old daughter and her son, who turned 6 years old in September. JW reports that they all need shots.

1. JW will soon be returning to work at a long-term care facility for developmentally disabled adults. She reports that her new employer is encouraging her to be immunized against hepatitis B. She wonders how long it will take her to complete the vaccine series. What is the nurse's best response?
2. The nurse administers JW's first dose of hepatitis B vaccine. When should JW return for the next dose?
3. The nurse asks JW about her vaccine history. JW says she does not have an immunization card but remembers receiving "a booster when I stepped on a nail at my high school graduation picnic." What "booster" did she likely

receive? At what point is another booster due? What vaccine should she receive for her next booster?

4. JW says her daughter needs her "regular shots." The infant received her first hepatitis B vaccine while in the newborn nursery. Against what vaccine-preventable illnesses should the nurse plan to vaccinate this infant today?
5. When would this infant be due for another series of immunizations?
6. JW asks the nurse about the chickenpox vaccine. She would like her daughter to be vaccinated against chickenpox as soon as possible because she does not want her to suffer through chickenpox as her son did. What is the earliest age at which her daughter can receive varicella vaccine?
7. JW says she has heard that "you can get chickenpox from the vaccination shot." How should the nurse respond to this comment?
8. JW has brought her son's immunization card. It shows he received hepatitis B vaccine at birth, at 2 months, and at 9 months of age. He received DTaP, Hib, polio (IPV), pneumococcal (PCV), and rotavirus vaccines at 2 months, 4 months, and 6 months of age. JW is worried that he will need to start his immunizations over because "he's so far behind." How should the nurse respond to her concern?
9. For what vaccines is JW's son due today?

NCLEX STUDY QUESTIONS

1. The father of a 4-month-old infant calls in to the clinic reporting that his child is having a reaction to immunizations. What is the most important piece of information the nurse should elicit?
   a. A list of the immunizations received
   b. Whether the father has given the infant any acetaminophen
   c. The signs/symptoms the infant is experiencing
   d. The sites used to administer the immunizations
2. The nurse is preparing to administer varicella vaccine to a young woman. Which factor has the greatest implication for this young woman's care?
   a. The patient tells the nurse she is "deathly afraid of needles."
   b. The medical record indicates that the patient is allergic to eggs.
   c. The medical history indicates the patient had leukemia as a young child.
   d. The patient appears to be pregnant.
3. A 38-year-old migrant farm worker presents to the clinic with a cut to his arm sustained when he reached into an old metal drum. The patient has sutures placed, and the attending provider orders "Tdap" for him. What is the nurse's most important action in carrying out this order?
   a. The nurse provides the patient with a Vaccine Information Statement about Tdap in the patient's primary language.
   b. The nurse determines the exact date of the patient's last tetanus booster.
   c. The nurse documents that the patient did not experience any side effects immediately following immunization.
   d. The nurse provides the patient with a record of the immunization administered at the visit.
4. The nurse is preparing to administer routine, recommended immunizations to a medically fragile 6-month-old child. What is the most important information to know about this infant?
   a. The infant receives all feedings via a gastrostomy tube.
   b. The infant receives inhaled steroids daily.
   c. The infant received his previous round of immunizations on time.
   d. The infant is not yet able to roll over.
5. A 61-year-old man is to receive zoster vaccine. What is the most important thing for the nurse to discuss with this patient?
   a. That the vaccine has been stored in a freezer maintained at ≤5° F
   b. The patient's medication list and allergies
   c. That an appropriate length of needle will be used to administer the vaccine subcutaneously
   d. The patient's history of shingles
6. An 18-month-old child is accompanied to the clinic by her grandmother, the child's legal guardian. The grandmother reports that the child is due for her fourth DTaP. The nurse determines that the child should not receive DTaP vaccine today for which reason?
   a. The child received varicella vaccine 2 weeks ago.
   b. The grandmother is undergoing chemotherapy for breast cancer.
   c. The third DTaP was administered 4 months ago.
   d. The child has a runny nose today.
7. The nurse is preparing to administer five immunizations to a pediatric patient. It is essential that the nurse first assess what? (Select all that apply.)
   a. Age of the child
   b. Size of the child
   c. Child's ability to understand importance of immunizations
   d. Child's current health status
   e. Ability of caregiver to protect the child from sun exposure for 24 hours
   f. Child's history of reactions to prior doses of vaccines to be administered
8. The nurse, with the help of an interpreter, has just immunized a 35-year-old woman with Tdap and MMR. It is essential that the nurse proceed with which action(s)? (Select all that apply.)
   a. Provide Vaccine Information Statements (VISs) in the patient's preferred language.

b. Document in the patient's record the date; site and route of administration; vaccine type, manufacturer, lot number, and expiration date; and the name, business address, and title of person administering the vaccine.
c. Administer a dose of ibuprofen to prevent postimmunization fever.
d. Instruct the patient to call for any injection site soreness.
e. Instruct the patient on the use of an epinephrine auto injector to administer in the event of an anaphylactic reaction.
f. Counsel the patient regarding the importance of avoiding pregnancy for 1 month.

Answers: 1, c; 2, d; 3, a; 4, a; 5, b; 6, c; 7, a, b, d, f; 8, b, f.

UNIT XII

Antineoplastic Agents

The development of cancer is a multistep process that is influenced by environmental hazards (e.g., chemicals, radiation), genetic predisposition (e.g., genetic mutations), lifestyle factors (e.g., smoking, alcohol use), diet (e.g., high in animal fats), infection (e.g., Epstein-Barr, *Helicobacter pylori*, human papillomavirus [HPV]), and immune suppression (e.g., HIV infection, immunosuppressive medications). Cancer (malignant, neoplastic) cells are characterized by unregulated growth, lack of differentiation, and spread (metastasis) to other places in the body.

CELL CYCLE

All cells progress through a distinct cycle that consists of four phases directed toward cell replication and a fifth resting stage. In this way, the cell cycles of normal and cancer cells are similar. The first phase of the cell cycle is G1, the presynthesis phase that prepares the cell for deoxyribonucleic acid (DNA) synthesis. The second phase is the S phase, whereby DNA synthesis occurs. Next is the G2 postsynthesis phase, in which the cell is prepared for mitosis. Cell division (cytokinesis) occurs in the fourth, or M (mitosis), phase. Cells may immediately progress to the G1 phase or enter the G0 or resting phase. Most cells in the human body are in the G0 stage. Exceptions include metabolically active cells (e.g., granulocytes) and epithelial cells found in the gastrointestinal tract. As each cell moves through the cell cycle, it must pass a number of checkpoints before it can continue its progression. If a cell is found to be defective at one of the checkpoints, it undergoes **apoptosis** (self-destruction). The cell cycle is illustrated in Figure XII-1.

GROWTH RATE

Growth rate (*doubling time*) is defined as the time it takes for a cancerous tumor to double in size. **Growth fraction** (the percent of actively dividing cells) decreases and doubling time increases as the tumor enlarges. Growth rate depends on several factors, including the cell-cycle activity of the proliferating cells in the tumor mass, the number of cells proliferating within the tumor (*growth fraction*), and the rate of cell loss from the tumor. In general, anticancer drugs are more effective against cancer cells that have a high growth fraction. Malignant tumors that have prolonged cell cycles and a slower growth rate are more likely to be locally confined and therefore are more amenable to surgical excision.

ANTICANCER THERAPY

Chemotherapy (chemical treatment) is the use of chemicals to kill cancer cells. Research has led to the use of new anticancer drugs and the development of standard treatment protocols (drug, dose, and schedule) to guide therapy. Nurses play a vital role in managing the treatment of those with cancer. This includes the administration of chemotherapy in health care facilities and in the homes of clients. To provide the best possible care, nurses should understand the chemotherapy regimen, contraindications, drug interactions, therapeutic effects, side effects, and adverse reactions of the chemotherapy that clients receive.

Chapter 37 discusses how selected anticancer drugs inhibit or prevent cell reproduction. The anticancer drugs are divided

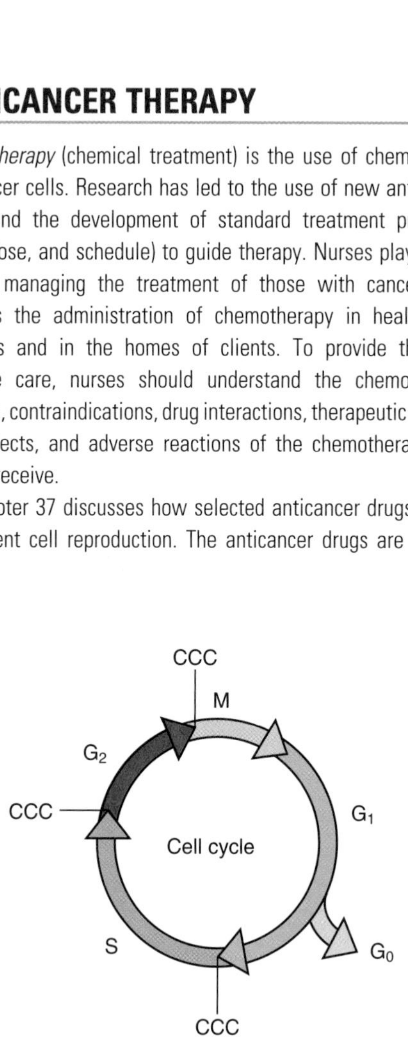

FIGURE XII–1 Cell division cycle and checkpoints. CCC, Cell cycle checkpoint. *G1 phase (postmitotic gap):* Production of enzyme for DNA synthesis. The G1 phase lasts 15 to 18 hours. *S phase (synthesis):* The DNA doubles. The S phase lasts 10 to 20 hours. G2 phase (premitotic gap): RNA synthesis for later mitosis. The G2 phase lasts approximately 3 hours. *M phase (mitosis):* Cell division produces two identical cells. The M phase lasts approximately 1 hour. *G0 phase (resting):* Cells remain in this phase or return to the cell cycle for cell replication. Cells in this phase are not as sensitive to many antineoplastic drugs. The cells must pass through a series of checkpoints to continue through the cycle. Cells that are defective undergo apoptosis (self-destruction).

into major classes that include alkylating agents, antimetabolites, antitumor antibiotics, mitotic inhibitors, and hormonal agents.

Some chemotherapy agents negatively affect cancer cells when they are actively dividing. These are called *cell cycle–specific (CCS) agents. Cell cycle–nonspecific (CCNS) drugs* work best in the G0 (resting) stage to disrupt cancer cells. Chemotherapy usually targets ribonucleic acid (RNA) or deoxyribonucleic acid (DNA) in cancer cells to prevent mitosis or induce apoptosis (self-death). The specific drugs selected are administered based on the type of tumor cells, the rate at which they divide, and the time that the drugs will be most effective. In general, chemotherapy is most effective in destroying cells that are rapidly dividing.

Chapter 38 explores targeted therapies to treat cancer. This modality targets malignant cells and is a recent development. Targeted therapies work by interfering with cancer-cell growth and division in different ways and at various points in the development, growth, and spread of cancer.

Chapter 39, describes the evolving state of biologic response modifiers that work to (1) enhance host immunologic function, (2) destroy or interfere with tumor activities, and (3) promote differentiation of stem cells.

CHAPTER

37

Anticancer Drugs

evolve WEBSITE

http://evolve.elsevier.com/KeeHayes/pharmacology/

- Animations
- Content Updates
- Key Points
- Review Questions for the NCLEX® Examination
- References from the Textbook
- Unfolding Case Studies

OBJECTIVES

- Differentiate between cell cycle–specific and cell cycle–nonspecific anticancer drugs.
- Prioritize appropriate nursing interventions to use during the treatment of patients receiving anticancer drugs.
- Compare the uses and considerations for alkylating compounds, antimetabolites, antitumor antibiotics, hormones, and biotherapy agents.
- Contrast the guidelines for administering routine parenteral medications with IV chemotherapy preparation and administration.
- Discuss ways the nurse can avoid exposure to chemotherapeutic agents.
- Apply patient-centered collaborative care, including teaching, related to anticancer drugs.
- Develop a focused teaching plan about the uses and side effects of anticancer drugs.

OUTLINE

KEY TERMS

adjuvant therapy, p. 505
alkylating agents, p. 507
antimetabolites, p. 513
antineoplastic drugs, p. 503

The authors gratefully acknowledge the work of Carolee A. Polek, who updated this chapter for the eighth edition.

antitumor antibiotics, p. 518
apoptosis, p. 503
cell cycle–nonspecific drugs, p. 504
cell cycle–specific drugs, p. 504
combination chemotherapy, p. 503
cytoprotectant (chemoprotectant), p. 510
cytotoxic therapy, p. 503
doubling time, p. 504
growth fraction, p. 504
hormones, p. 524
leucovorin rescue, p. 513
metastasis, p. 505
myelosuppression, p. 505
nadir, p. 505
neoadjuvant chemotherapy, p. 505
palliative chemotherapy, p. 505
protocol, p. 505
taxanes, p. 521
vesicant, p. 510
vesication, p. 518
vinca alkaloids, p. 521

Cancer-related deaths rank second only to heart disease in the United States. Even though cancer-related mortality has decreased since the early 1990s, 1 in 3 women and 1 in 2 men are projected to develop cancer over their lifetime. Excluding skin cancers, the highest incidence rates in men are prostate, lung, and colorectal cancer. In women, breast, lung, and colorectal cancers occur with the highest frequency. Lung cancer remains the leading cause of cancer-related death regardless of gender.

The incidence and mortality rates of cancer differ by ethnicity. African-American men have higher incidence and death rates from cancer than do white men. African-American women have a lower incidence of cancer than white women, but a higher mortality rate. Latinos have a lower incidence than non-Latinos, except for cancer of the stomach, liver, and cervix. Cancer among Asian Americans has traditionally been lower than other ethnic groups, but incidence increases as immigrants adopt a more westernized lifestyle. The incidence of liver and stomach cancer is higher among Asian immigrants, secondary to higher rates of chronic hepatitis B in this group.

Cancer is a group of diseases in which abnormal cells grow out of control and may spread to other areas of the body. Deoxyribonucleic acid (DNA) is the genetic substance in the body cells that transfers information necessary for the production of enzymes and protein synthesis. In most cases, cancer is caused by damage to the DNA within the cell. Although some cancers are inherited, most develop when genes in a normal cell become damaged or lost (mutation). More than one mutation is required before a malignancy can develop. Therefore the development of cancer is a multistep process that may take years to complete.

Pharmaceuticals are often used to destroy cancer cells and are called by different names, including *anticancer drugs, cancer chemotherapeutic agents,* **antineoplastic drugs,** or **cytotoxic therapy**. In the 1970s, the use of two or more chemotherapy agents (**combination chemotherapy**) to treat cancer was adopted and led to improved response rates and increased survival times. Chemotherapy may be used as the sole treatment of cancer or in conjunction with other modalities (e.g., radiation, surgery, biologic response modifiers). Combination chemotherapy has proved to be effective in curing some cancers. When cancer cannot be cured, anticancer drugs may be given to control the disease for a period of months to years. If cancer can no longer be controlled, chemotherapy may be used to relieve disease-related symptoms or improve quality of life. This is called *palliative treatment.*

GENETIC, INFECTIVE, ENVIRONMENTAL, AND DIETARY INFLUENCES

Cancer is a genetic disease. Genes provide the instructions for the production and function of cellular proteins that are essential for normal cellular activities. Genetic defects may occur in a variety of ways, including deletion, translocation, duplication, inversion, or insertion of genetic material. When these defects cannot be effectively repaired, cells exhibit abnormal characteristics and unregulated growth. More than 2000 genes have been causally implicated in the formation of cancer. Cancers that have a proven genetic influence include breast, ovarian, prostate, endometrial, colon, pancreatic, and lung cancers; retinoblastoma; and malignant melanoma. Many more genetic influences are expected to be found. Environment, lifestyle, viruses, and diet can influence the development of these and other types of cancers. Box 37-1 gives examples of types of environmental products, viruses, and foods that have a carcinogenic effect on cancer development in humans.

Genes can cause cells to become cancerous in several ways. *Proto-oncogenes* are normal genes that are involved in the controlled growth, division, and death (**apoptosis**) of cells. An oncogene is a mutation in a proto-oncogene. An abnormal oncogene can effect cellular growth-control proteins and trigger unregulated cell division. Tumor-suppressor (TS) genes (anti-oncogenes) signal a cell to cease multiplying and act to stop the action of oncogenes. If TS genes become lost or dysfunctional, cells could reproduce uncontrollably. Other genes repair damage to DNA. If these DNA-repair genes are damaged, mutations are not mended and are subsequently passed on to the next generation of daughter cells. It may take a long time before sufficient cell mutations take place and cause cancer to develop. As a result, cancers more commonly occur in older individuals.

A number of viruses are associated with the development of cancer. The human papillomavirus (HPV) has been found in most women with invasive cervical cancer. Individuals with human immunodeficiency virus (HIV) may develop lymphomas and anal or genital cancers. The Epstein-Barr

BOX 37-1 ENVIRONMENTAL, INFECTIVE, AND DIETARY INFLUENCES ON CANCER DEVELOPMENT

Environmental

Tobacco

Cancer of the lung, larynx, bladder, kidney, colon, cervix, stomach, pancreas, breast

Asbestos

Lung cancer

Benzene

Acute myelogenous leukemia

Formaldehyde

Nasopharyngeal cancer, leukemia

Vinyl Chloride

Sarcoma

Arsenic

Cancer of the lung, skin; sarcoma

Ionizing Radiation

Leukemia; cancer of the thyroid, breast

Ultraviolet Rays

Skin cancer

Aflatoxin

Liver cancer

Infective

Herpes Simplex 2 Virus (Genital Herpes)

Cancer of the cervix

Hepatitis B and Hepatitis C Viruses

Cancer of the liver

Epstein-Barr Virus (a cause of infectious mononucleosis)

Non-Hodgkin's lymphoma, Hodgkin's disease, nasopharyngeal cancers

Human Papilloma Virus (HPV)

Cancer of the cervix, vulva, vagina, anus, head and neck

Human Immunodeficiency Virus (HIV)

Kaposi sarcoma, Non-Hodgkin's lymphoma, cervical cancer

Human T-Cell Lymphotrophic Virus

T-cell leukemia

Helicobacter pylori

Cancer of the stomach, gastric mucosa-associated lymphoid tissue (MALT) lymphoma

Diet

Animal Fat

Cancer of the colon, rectum, breast, uterus, prostate, ovary

Heterocyclic Amines (found in some smoked meats)

Cancer of the stomach, colon, rectum, pancreas, breast

Alcohol

Cancer of the mouth, throat, esophagus, liver, breast

virus is found in almost all people with Burkitt's lymphoma in central Africa. This virus has been implicated in the development of nasopharyngeal cancer. Hepatocellular carcinoma (liver cancer) is linked to the hepatitis B or C virus. Other viruses that have a link to the development of cancer include human T-cell lymphotropic virus, type 1 (HTLV-1); human T-cell lymphotropic virus, type 2 (HTLV-2); and Kaposi sarcoma–associated herpes virus.

Bacteria can play a role in the development of cancer. The presence of *Helicobacter pylori* in the stomach is associated with an increased risk of developing gastric cancer. Some reports have indicated a link between certain bacteria and cancer of the gallbladder, colon, and lung. However, evidence that supports an association between bacterial infection and other cancers is unclear.

Environmental factors associated with the development of cancer include tobacco use, diet, infectious agents, chemicals, excessive sun exposure, and radiation. According to the American Cancer Society (ACS), the use of tobacco, an unhealthy diet, and inadequate physical activity account for 75% of cancer cases and deaths in the United States.

CELL CYCLE–NONSPECIFIC AND CELL CYCLE–SPECIFIC ANTICANCER DRUGS

The cell cycle for normal and cancer cells, growth fraction, and doubling time are discussed in Unit XII (see Figure XII-1). See the discussion at the beginning of Unit XII for clarification of the cell cycle and definitions.

Anticancer drugs cause cell death by interfering with cell replication and are classified according to their action on the cell. **Cell cycle–nonspecific (CCNS) drugs** (phase-nonspecific drugs) act during any phase of the cell cycle, including the G0 phase. **Cell cycle–specific (CCS) drugs** (phase-specific drugs) exert their influence during a specific phase or phases of the cell cycle. CCS agents are most effective against rapidly growing cancer cells. In general, the CCNS drugs include the alkylating drugs (although some alkylating agents are CCS), antitumor antibiotics, and hormones. The CCS drugs include antimetabolites and vinca alkaloids. Figure 37-1 shows selected types of anticancer drugs and the phase of the cell cycle in which they are most effective.

Growth fraction and **doubling time** are two factors that play a major role in the response of cancer cells to anticancer drugs. Anticancer drugs are more effective against neoplastic cells that have a high growth fraction (i.e., a high percentage of actively dividing cells). Leukemias and some lymphomas have high growth fractions and thus respond well to anticancer drug therapy.

Solid tumors have a large percentage of their cell mass in the G0 phase, so they generally have a low growth fraction and are less sensitive to anticancer drugs. High-dose chemotherapy results in better tumoricidal (tumor-killing) effects. Depending on the type of cancer, malignant cell growth is usually faster in the earlier stages of tumor development. As

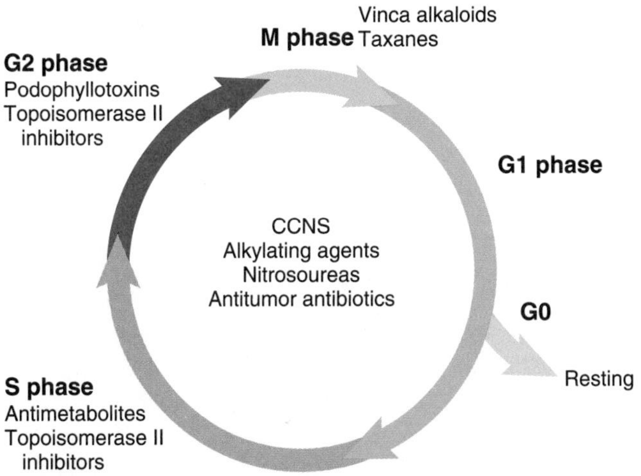

FIGURE 37–1 Selected anticancer drugs and the phases of the cell cycle in which they are most effective.

the tumor grows, the blood supply decreases, thereby slowing the growth rate. Anticancer agents are more effective against small, fast growing tumors with sufficient blood supply. As the tumor enlarges, its growth fraction decreases and its doubling time increases, reducing the effectiveness of anticancer therapy. The vascularization in solid tumors can be inconsistent. Some areas of tumor may have an adequate blood supply, while other areas are poorly perfused. This characteristic may make some large tumors resistant to anticancer drugs and therefore difficult to treat.

CANCER CHEMOTHERAPY

Anticancer drugs are not selective, so both cancer cells and normal cells are affected. The side effects of chemotherapy are largely related to the toxic effects on normal cells. Antineoplastic agents are effective because normal cells are able to repair themselves and continue to grow, whereas cancer cells are less able to do so; thus, the side effects of chemotherapy are most often temporary. Chemotherapy is usually administered systemically for cancer that has spread to other parts of the body, for tumors in multiple sites, or for tumors that are too large to be removed through other means (e.g., surgery). The most common route of chemotherapy administration is via intravenous (IV) infusion, although other routes may be used, including oral, intramuscular, subcutaneous, intraperitoneal, intraventricular (intrathecal), intrapleural, intravesicular, intra-arterial, or topical.

Some types of cancer can be cured with chemotherapy (e.g., Hodgkin's disease, Burkitt's lymphoma, testicular cancer). Other types of cancer (e.g., breast cancer, colon cancer) may be treated with surgery first, followed by chemotherapy to eliminate any residual tumor cells (microscopic metastases) that may remain in the body. This is referred to as **adjuvant therapy.** Sometimes **neoadjuvant chemotherapy** may be given first to help shrink a large tumor, so that it can be surgically removed. **Palliative chemotherapy** is used to relieve symptoms associated with advanced disease (e.g., pain, shortness of breath) and improve quality of life.

Chemotherapy administration is guided by specific **protocols** that were developed based on the results of controlled research studies. The length of treatment is determined by the type and extent of the malignancy, type of chemotherapy given, expected side effects of these drugs, and the amount of time that normal cells need to recover. Chemotherapy is usually given in cycles to improve the likelihood that cancer cells will be destroyed and that normal cells can recover. The duration, frequency, and number of cycles of chemotherapy are based on the type and size of the tumor, whether the disease has spread to other areas of the body (**metastasis**), and the condition of the patient. Chemotherapy treatment may consist of one agent or a combination of agents. Combination chemotherapy may be administered on one day or spread out over several days. The duration of each treatment varies from minutes to days and may be repeated weekly, biweekly, or monthly, based on the protocol being followed. Selected anticancer/antineoplastic drugs are listed in Box 37-2 according to classification.

Combination Chemotherapy

Single-agent drug therapy is not usually used to treat cancer, because combinations of anticancer agents have demonstrated more effective tumoricidal activity. Chemotherapy is most effective when it is able to kill cells in all phases of the cell cycle. Using two or more chemotherapy drugs at a time (combination chemotherapy) makes this more likely to occur.

To maximize cell death, CCS and CCNS drugs are often combined. Each individual chemotherapy agent used in combination therapy should have proven tumoricidal activity. Using two or more drugs together may have a synergistic effect. In addition, each drug should have a different mode of action and different dose-limiting toxicities. The use of a combination of antineoplastic agents has the advantage of decreasing drug resistance and increasing destruction of cancer cells. Some of the combinations of anticancer drugs used in cancer treatment are presented in Table 37-1.

General Side Effects and Adverse Reactions

Anticancer drugs exert adverse effects on rapidly growing normal cells (e.g., skin, hair). These drugs can also affect cells in the gastrointestinal (GI) tract, mucous membranes, bone marrow, and reproductive system. When there is a significant decrease in the cells in the bone marrow (white blood cells, platelets, red blood cells) the condition is called **myelosuppression**. Following chemotherapy administration, the time at which the blood count is at the lowest is called the **nadir** and typically occurs 7 to 10 days after treatment. Table 37-2 lists the general adverse reactions to anticancer drugs on the fast-growing cells of the body. Selected nursing measures and considerations are included.

Anticancer Therapy in Outpatient Settings and in the Home

The administration of anticancer drugs in outpatient settings is cost-effective and convenient. Although chemotherapy regimens have become increasingly aggressive, most patients

BOX 37-2 ANTICANCER DRUGS BY CLASSIFICATION*

Alkylating Agents

Mustard Gas Derivatives

nitrogen mustard (mechlorethamine hydrochloride) (Mustargen)
chlorambucil (Leukeran)
cyclophosphamide (Cytoxan)
ifosfamide (Ifex)
melphalan (Alkeran)
temozolomide (Temodar)

Nitrosoureas

carmustine (BiCNU, BCNU, Gliadel)
lomustine (CeeNU, CCNU)
streptozocin (Zanosar)

Alkylating-Like Agents

altretamine (Hexalen)
carboplatin (Paraplatin)
cisplatin (Platinol)
dacarbazine (DTIC)
oxaliplatin (Eloxatin)
thiotepa (Thioplex)

Alkyl Sulfonates

busulfan (Myleran, Busulfex))

Antimetabolites

Folic Acid Antagonists

methotrexate (MTX, amethopterin, Folex, Mexate)
pemetrexed disodium (Alimta)
trimetrexate glucuronate (Neutrexin)

Pyrimidine Analogues

azacitidine (Vidaza)
capecitabine (Xeloda)
cytarabine HCl (Cytosar-U, ARA-C)
decitabine (Dacogen)
floxuridine (FUDR)
fluorouracil (5-FU, Adrucil)
gemcitabine HCl (Gemzar)
nelarabine (Arranon)

Purine Analogues

cladribine (Leustatin)
clofarabine (Clolar)
fludarabine (Fludara)
6-mercaptopurine (6-MP, Purinethol)
thioguanine (Lanvis)

Ribonucleotide Reductase Inhibitors (Enzyme Inhibitors)

hydroxyurea (Hydrea)
2-deoxycoformycin (pentostatin [Nipent]

Plant Alkaloids

Vinca Alkaloids

vinblastine sulfate (Velban)
vincristine sulfate (Oncovin)
vincristine (liposomal) (Marqibo)
vinorelbine (Navelbine)

Antimicrotubules or Taxanes

docetaxel (Taxotere)
paclitaxel (Taxol)

Podophyllotoxins

etoposide (VP-16, Vepesid)
teniposide (VM-26, Vumon)

Camptothecan Analogs

Irinotecan (Camptosar, CPT-11)
Topotecan (Hycamtin)

Retinoids

bexarotene (Targretin)
thalidomide (Thalomid)

Antitumor Antibiotics

bleomycin sulfate (Blenoxane)
dactinomycin (Actinomycin D, Cosmegen)
daunorubicin HCl (Cerubidine)
daunorubicin (liposomal) (DaunoXome)
doxorubicin (Adriamycin, Rubex)
doxorubicin HCl (liposomal) (Doxil, Caelyx, Myocet)
epirubicin (Ellence)
idarubicin (Idamycin)
mitomycin (Mutamycin)
mitoxantrone (Novantrone)
valrubicin (Valstar)

Hormones, Hormonal Antagonists, and Enzymes

Androgens

testolactone (Teslac)
progesterone (Gesterol 50)

Hormonal Antagonists and Enzymes

aminoglutethimide (Cytadren)
anastrozole (Arimidex)
bicalutamide (Casodex)
exemestane (Aromasin)
flutamide (Eulexin)
fulvestrant (Faslodex)
goserelin acetate (Zoladex)
histrelin acetate implant (Vantas)
letrozole (Femara)
leuprolide acetate (Lupron)
megestrol acetate (Megace)
mitotane (Lysodren)
nilutamide (Nilandron)
raloxifene hydrochloride (Evista)
tamoxifen citrate (Nolvadex) (nonsteroidal antiestrogen)
toremifene (Fareston)

Miscellaneous

Enzymes

L-asparaginase (Elspar)
pegaspargase (Oncaspar)

Vaccines

Recombinant vaccines Gardasil and Cervarix

High-Alert Medications

All chemotherapeutic agents are categorized as high-alert medications for all routes of chemotherapeutic drug delivery.

*See Chapter 38 for monoclonal antibodies and targeted therapies and Chapter 39 for biologic therapies.

TABLE 37-1 SELECTED COMBINATIONS OF ANTICANCER DRUGS

GENERIC (BRAND)	ACRONYM*	SELECTED USES
doxorubicin (Adriamycin), bleomycin (Blenoxane), vinblastine (Velban), dacarbazine (DTIC)	ABVD	Hodgkin's lymphoma
fluorouracil (5-FU, Adrucil), doxorubicin/hydroxydoxorubicin (Adriamycin), cyclophosphamide (Cytoxan)	FAC*	Breast cancer, prostate cancer
cyclophosphamide (Cytoxan), doxorubicin/hydroxydoxorubicin (Adriamycin), methotrexate (Rheumatrex, Trexall)	CAM	Prostate cancer
cyclophosphamide (Cytoxan), epirubicin (Pharmorubicin), fluorouracil (5-FU, Adrucil)	CEF	Breast cancer
cyclophosphamide (Cytoxan), doxorubicin/hydroxydoxorubicin (Adriamycin), vincristine (Oncovin), prednisone, rituximab (Rituxan)	CHOP + rituximab (CHOP+R)	Non-Hodgkin's lymphoma
etoposide (VePesid, VP-16), leucovorin, fluorouracil (5-FU, Adrucil)	ELF	Esophageal cancer, stomach cancer
folinic acid (leucovorin), fluorouracil (5-FU, Adrucil), irinotecan (Camptosar)	FOLFIRI	Colorectal cancer
folinic acid (leucovorin), fluorouracil (5-FU, Adrucil), oxaliplatin (Eloxatin)	FOLFOX	Colorectal cancer
gemcitabine (Gemzar), capecitabine (Xeloda)	GEMCAP	Cancer of the pancreas
idarubicin (Idamycin), cytarabine (ARA-C, Cytosar), etoposide (VP-16, VePesid)	ICE	Acute myelogenous leukemia
mechlorethamine (Mustargen), vincristine (Oncovin), procarbazine (Matulane), prednisone	MOPP	Hodgkin's disease
melphalan (Alkeran), prednisone	MP	Multiple myeloma
mitomycin C (Mutamycin), vinblastine (Velban), cisplatin (Platinol)	MVP	Small cell lung cancer
paclitaxel (Taxol), carboplatin (Paraplatin)	PC	Non–small cell lung cancer
docetaxel (Taxotere), doxorubicin (Adriamycin), cyclophosphamide (Cytoxan)	TAC	Recurrent breast cancer
vinblastine (Velban), bleomycin (Blenoxane), cisplatin (Platinol)	VBP	Testicular cancer

*Acronyms are based on the name of the chemotherapy agents used in a specific protocol (e.g., ABVD [Adriamycin, bleomycin, vinblastine, dacarbazine], FAC [fluorouracil, Adriamycin, cyclophosphamide]). Both generic and trade names are used in acronyms.

are not hospitalized unless they require close monitoring or are very ill. Some chemotherapy agents are administered in the home. Patients receiving highly potent drugs at home may need to be closely monitored for severe adverse reactions or to assure adequate hydration. When a chemotherapy drug is given in the home, a health care provider qualified to administer anticancer agents follows the policies provided by the oncologist and the home health care agency. To reduce the nurse's exposure to chemotherapy drugs (hazardous drugs, or HD) during intravenous (IV) administration, the following precautions should be followed to minimize occupational exposure:

- Use disposable powder-free gloves (nitrile, polyurethane, neoprene) that have been tested with HD when handling chemotherapy, regardless of route of administration.
- Wear gowns (disposable, impermeable, lint-free) during the administration of IV chemotherapy.
- When there is a risk of aerosol exposure, a National Institute for Occupational Safety and Health–approved respirator is necessary. Surgical masks do not provide adequate respiratory protection.
- Use a face shield or a combination of mask and face shield if there is a danger of splashing when administering chemotherapy or disposing of body fluids.
- Change gloves after chemotherapy administration and if they become contaminated or punctured.
- Cytotoxic drugs can be accidentally absorbed by inhalation, contact with skin or mucous membranes, and ingestion. The following guidelines should be followed:
  1. Prepare chemotherapy in a separate work area. Use a plastic-backed absorbent pad to contain spills during preparation.
  2. Wash hands before and after administration of chemotherapy.
  3. Avoid hand-to-mouth or hand-to-eye contact while working with chemotherapy.
  4. Refer to agency policy for priming IV tubing and disconnecting tubing after administration.
  5. Wear gloves when disposing of body fluids (e.g., urine, feces, emesis) of patients who have received chemotherapy in the previous 48 hours.
  6. Refer to agency policy for disposal of used equipment.
  7. Refer to agency policy for chemotherapy spills or exposure.

ALKYLATING DRUGS

One of the largest groups of anticancer drugs is the alkylating compounds. **Alkylating agents** cause cross-linking of DNA strands, abnormal base pairing, or DNA strand breaks, thus preventing the cell from dividing. Drugs in this group belong to the CCNS category and kill cells in various and multiple phases of the cell cycle. However, they are most effective against cells in the G0 phase. Alkylating agents are effective against many types of cancer, including acute and chronic leukemias, lymphomas, multiple myeloma, and solid tumors (e.g., breast, ovary, uterus, lung, bladder, and stomach). Drugs in this category are classified into several groups: mustard gas derivatives (e.g., cyclophosphamide [Cytoxan]), ethylenimines (e.g., thiotepa [Thioplex]), alkylsulfonates (e.g., busulfan [Myleran]), triazines (e.g., dacarbazine [DTIC]), nitrosoureas (e.g., carmustine [BiCNU]), and metal salts (e.g., cisplatin [Platinol]). Nitrosoureas are unique because they can cross the blood-brain barrier, making them useful in the treatment of brain cancer. Table 37-3 lists the alkylating drugs, uses, and considerations.

TABLE 37-2 GENERAL ADVERSE REACTIONS TO ANTICANCER DRUGS

ADVERSE REACTIONS	NURSING MEASURES AND CONSIDERATIONS
Bone Marrow Suppression, Myelosuppression	
Low RBC count (anemia)	Assess for fatigue, shortness of breath, low blood pressure, increased heart rate, increased respiratory rate, and oliguria. Assess for cyanosis. Plan rest periods. Administer oxygen as prescribed. Elevate head of bed to facilitate breathing. Provide pain mediation if pain is increasing oxygen consumption. Provide assistance to bathroom. Monitor for mental status changes. Anemia may be treated with ferrous sulfate or infusions of RBCs. Erythropoietin may be administered to stimulate RBC production.
Low WBC count (neutropenia)	Susceptibility to infection increases as WBCs decrease. Visitors with colds or infections should take precautions (e.g., wear mask) or avoid visiting the patient. Report fever, chills, upper respiratory infections, or sore throat to health care provider. Health care providers and visitors should wash hands before and after contact with the patient. Neutrophils are the primary WBCs that fight infections. Usual signs of infection (pain, swelling, redness, warmth, pus) may be absent or greatly reduced in neutropenic patients. Monitor for increase (or decrease) in body temperature. Elevated temperature is considered a sign of infection. Avoid medications that may mask temperature. Immediately report temperatures of 101° F (38.3° C) or above to health care provider. Appropriate cultures (e.g., blood, urine, sputum) are collected, and an antibiotic regimen is initiated. Assess for localized infections. Auscultate breath sounds. Monitor WBC count. Colony-stimulating factors (e.g., filgrastim) may be administered to stimulate WBC production.
Low platelet count (thrombocytopenia)	Petechiae, bruising, bleeding of gums, and nosebleeds are signs of a low platelet count; report these signs to health care provider. Assess for bleeding, petechiae, and ecchymosis. Assess for occult bleeding in urine, feces, and emesis. Monitor platelet counts and bleeding time. Apply pressure to injection sites. Platelet transfusions may be needed. Avoid medications that may promote bleeding (e.g., aspirin). Avoid invasive procedures (e.g., injections, indwelling urinary catheters, rectal temperature).
GI Disturbances	
Anorexia	Loss of appetite may be related to anemia, pain, fatigue, or bitter taste caused by some chemotherapy agents. Provide small, frequent meals that are high in calories and protein. Plan rest periods. Address issues of pain control. Hard candy or ice chips may help relieve bitter taste.
Nausea and vomiting	Antineoplastic drugs often stimulate the chemoreceptor trigger zone (CTZ), leading to nausea and vomiting. Nausea and vomiting (N/V) may be caused by irritation of GI tract; effects of radiation to chest, abdomen, or brain; anxiety; constipation; pain; electrolyte imbalances; or other medications. Grading scales are useful to assess severity. Provide antiemetics before, during, and after chemotherapy. Assess for GI upset, and medicate appropriately. Minimize noise, stimulation, and odors. Frequent mouth care is recommended.
Diarrhea	Diarrhea may be one of three types: osmotic (absorption defects), secretory (bacterial infection, neoplasm), or exudative (secondary to chemotherapy). Chemotherapeutic agents most commonly associated with diarrhea are alkylating agents, antitumor antibiotics, and antimetabolites. Treatment (e.g., medications, diet changes) will depend on cause. Diarrhea may be caused by other medications (e.g., antibiotics); comorbid conditions (e.g., Crohn's disease); or enteral feedings (e.g., tube feeding). Assess normal bowel habits; monitor for electrolyte imbalances and dehydration. Administer appropriate antidiarrheal medications (e.g., antibiotics, anticholinergics, antispasmodics, psyllium, kaolin and pectin, octreotide acetate). Teach patient to eat small, frequent meals; follow a low-residue diet; limit spicy, fatty foods; limit intake of salty foods, whole grains, fresh fruits and vegetables; limit caffeine and carbonated drinks; and avoid very hot or very cold foods (may stimulate peristalsis). Monitor intake and output. A grading scale may be useful to assess severity.
Mucositis (stomatitis)	Many antineoplastic agents cause changes in oral mucosa; generally occur 2 to 14 days after initiation of therapy. Assess for taste changes, tissue swelling, redness, pain, dry mouth, white patches, or a white coating on the oral mucosa. Mucositis ranges from mild to severe. Symptomatic treatment may include frequent mouth rinses, topical anesthetics, antibiotics, antifungal medication, saliva substitutes, and pain medication. Patient should avoid commercial mouthwashes that contain alcohol. A soft toothbrush is recommended. Offer ice chips or ice pops to help relieve pain. Assess intake and output. Evaluate caloric needs. A grading scale may be useful to assess severity.
Other	
Alopecia	Not all chemotherapeutic agents cause hair loss. Hair thinning, patchy baldness, or complete alopecia may occur, depending on drug. Hair on all areas of the body is affected. Hair loss may be gradual (progressing with each cycle of chemotherapy) or rapid. Hair regrowth usually occurs once chemotherapy is completed; texture may be somewhat changed. Before therapy, discuss potential hair loss and ways to address problem (wigs, scarves, hats, turbans). Assess for body image changes, concerns.
Fatigue	Fatigue may be caused by chemotherapy, sleep disturbances, emotional distress, depression, bone marrow suppression, infection, pain, or electrolyte imbalances. Assess fatigue using a visual analogue scale (0 = no fatigue; 10 = worst fatigue). Address conditions that might be contributing to fatigue (e.g., lack of sleep, pain, depression). Plan ways to help patient conserve energy. Plan a well-balanced diet. Encourage patient to participate in regular (but not strenuous) exercise. Encourage stress-reduction measures (e.g., relaxation, guided imagery). A grading scale may be useful in assessing fatigue.
Infertility	If infertility occurs, it may be permanent. Pretreatment counseling is advised.

GI, Gastrointestinal; *RBC,* red blood cell; *WBC,* white blood cell.

TABLE 37-3 ANTINEOPLASTICS: ALKYLATING DRUGS

DRUG TYPE AND NAME	ROUTE AND DOSAGE	USES AND CONSIDERATIONS
Nitrogen Mustards		
chlorambucil (Leukeran)	PO: 0.1-0.2 mg/kg/d (equals 4-8 mg/m^2/d) for 3-6 wk	Lymphocytic leukemia, lymphomas, and cancer of the breast and ovaries. Side effects include nausea, vomiting, anorexia, diarrhea, abdominal upset, and leukopenia. Pregnancy category: D; PB: 99%; t½: 1.5 h
cyclophosphamide (Cytoxan)	See Prototype Drug Chart 37-1.	
ifosfamide (Ifex)	IV: 1.2-2 g/m^2/d for 5 d in combination with mesna	Testicular cancer, lymphoma, lung cancer, and sarcomas. Mesna, an uroprotective agent, is added to prevent hemorrhagic cystitis. Pregnancy category: D; PB: 69%-75%; t½: 7-15 h (high dose)
mechlorethamine HCl (Mustargen)	IV: 0.4 mg/kg, or 12-16 mg/m^2 Intracavitary: 0.2-0.4 mg/kg Topical: Dilute 10 g in 60 mL sterile water, apply with gloves (use precautions)	Hodgkin's disease, solid tumors, and pleural effusion caused by cancer of the lung. Similar side effects as chlorambucil. Pregnancy category: D; PB: UK; t½: 1 min
melphalan (Alkeran)	For multiple myeloma: 0.25 mg/kg/d; repeat every 6 wk For bone marrow transplant: IV 50-60 mg/m^2	Multiple myeloma, melanoma, and cancers of the breast, ovary, and testes. Pregnancy category: D; PB: 30%; t½: 1.5 h
temozolomide (Temodar)	PO: 150/mg/m^2/d; repeat every 28 d	Refractory anaplastic astrocytoma. Pregnancy category: D; PB: 15%, t½: UK
Nitrosoureas		
carmustine (BiCNU, BCNU)	IV: 75-100 mg/m^2/d for 2 d	Hodgkin's disease, multiple myeloma, melanoma, and brain tumors. May be used for cancer of the breast and lung. Nausea, vomiting, and stomatitis may occur. Pregnancy category: D; PB: UK; t½: 15-30 min
lomustine (CeeNu, CCNU)	PO: 130 mg/m^2 every 6 wk	Advanced Hodgkin's disease and brain tumors. Pregnancy category: D; PB: 50%; t½: 1-2 d
streptozocin (Zanosar)	IV: 500 mg/m^2/d for 5 d, repeat every 3-4 wk	Pancreatic islet cell tumor and cancer of the lung. May also be used for Hodgkin's disease and colorectal cancer. Nausea, vomiting, diarrhea, and leukopenia may occur. Pregnancy category: C; PB: UK; t½: 30-45 min
Alkyl Sulfonates		
busulfan (Myleran, Busulfex)	PO: 4-8 mg/d for 2-3 wk initially; then maintenance dose IV: 0.8 mg/kg	Myelocytic leukemia. Monitor WBCs closely. May be used as preparation agent in bone marrow transplant. Pregnancy category: D; PB: UK; t½: 2.5 h
Alkylating-Like Drugs		
altretamine (Hexalen)	PO: 260 mg/m^2/d in 4 equally divided doses for 14 d or 21 d	Ovarian cancer. Also used for breast, cervix, colon, endometrial, head/neck, and lung cancers; lymphomas. Nausea and vomiting and peripheral neuropathy may occur. Pregnancy category: D; PB: 6%; t½: 13 h
carboplatin (Paraplatin)	IV: 360 mg/m^2 every 4 wk Intraperitoneal: 200-650 mg/m^2 in 2 L For bone marrow transplant 1600 mg/m^2 IV in divided doses over 4 d	Recurrent ovarian cancer. May be used as preparation agent in bone marrow transplant. Pregnancy category: D; PB: 0%; t½: 2-6 h
cisplatin (Platinol)	IV: 50-100 mg/m^2 every 3-4 wk For ovarian cancer: intraperitoneal: 100 mg/m^2 every 3 wk	Ovarian and testicular cancer. Used as adjunctive treatment. Has been used for cancer of the bladder, head and neck, and endometrium. Nausea, vomiting, peripheral neuropathy, stomatitis, tinnitus, and blurred vision may occur. Ototoxicity occurs in 30% of patients. Pregnancy category: D; PB: >90%; t½: 58-75 h
oxaliplatin (Eloxatin)	IV: 85-130 mg/m^2 infusion in 200-250 mL 5% dextrose in water	Metastatic colorectal cancer. Used with 5-FU and leucovorin. Ovarian cancer, head and neck cancer, and malignant melanoma. Pregnancy category: D; PB: >90%; t½: 20-40 d

Continued

TABLE 37-3 ANTINEOPLASTICS: ALKYLATING DRUGS—cont'd

DRUG TYPE AND NAME	ROUTE AND DOSAGE	USES AND CONSIDERATIONS
dacarbazine (DTIC)	IV: 375 mg/m^2 every 2 wk	Metastatic malignant melanoma, sarcomas, neuroblastoma, and refractory Hodgkin's disease. May be given as an IV bolus (push) or by IV infusion. Common side effects are anorexia, nausea, and vomiting. Pregnancy category: C; PB: 5%-10%; t½: 5 h
thiotepa (Thioplex)	IV: 0.3-0.4 mg/kg IV once every 1-4 wk Intracavitary: Bladder: 60 mg in 30-60 mL of sterile water weekly for 3-4 wk Effusions: 0.6-0.8 mg/kg every 1-4 wk	Palliative therapy, especially for breast and ovarian cancer. Pregnancy category: D; PB: UK; t½: 1.5-2 h

Note: Chemotherapeutic doses and schedules will vary depending on protocol, body surface area (m^2), age, functional status, and comorbid conditions. For a full discussion of body surface area in dosage calculation, see Chapter 14.
5-FU, Fluorouracil; *d,* day; *FDA,* U.S. Food and Drug Administration; *GI,* gastrointestinal; *h,* hour; *IV,* intravenous; *min,* minute; *PB,* protein-binding; *t½,* half-life; *UK,* unknown; *WBC,* white blood cell; *wk,* week; *>,* greater than; *<,* less than.

The side effects for alkylating drugs include nausea, vomiting, hemorrhagic cystitis, alopecia, anemia, leukopenia, thrombocytopenia, bone marrow suppression (anemia, leukopenia, thrombocytopenia), secondary malignancies, and sterility. Major dose-limiting toxicities may occur in the blood cell line (red blood cell, white blood cell, platelet) and urinary systems. General adverse reactions to chemotherapeutic drugs are listed in Table 37-2.

Cyclophosphamide

Mechlorethamine (nitrogen mustard, [Mustargen]), the first alkylating drug introduced for cancer treatment, became available for clinical use during World War II. Mechlorethamine is administered as part of a chemotherapy regimen to treat Hodgkin's disease, especially if the disease is resistant to other drug combinations. This drug is a severe **vesicant** that can cause tissue necrosis if it infiltrates into the tissues. Cyclophosphamide (Cytoxan), an analogue of nitrogen mustard, may be prescribed orally, intrapleurally, or IV. The patient should be well hydrated while taking this drug to prevent hemorrhagic cystitis (bleeding as a result of severe bladder inflammation). MESNA (2-mercaptoethane sulphonate sodium [MESNEX]) is a **cytoprotectant (chemoprotectant)** drug that is often given with high-dose cyclophosphamide to inactivate urotoxic metabolites in the bladder and minimize damage to this organ.

SAFETY: Preventing Medication Errors

Do not confuse ...

- **Cytoxan** (cyclophosphamide) with **Cytosar** (cytosine arabinoside)

Pharmacokinetics Cyclophosphamide is well absorbed from the GI tract. Its half-life is moderate, and it is moderately protein-bound (<60%). The drug is metabolized by the liver, and less than 50% is excreted unchanged in the urine.

Pharmacodynamics Cyclophosphamide, an early antineoplastic drug, is still prevalent in chemotherapy protocols to treat breast cancer, leukemia, lymphoma, multiple myeloma, ovarian cancer, retinoblastoma, and neuroblastoma. The onset of action begins in 2 to 3 hours; however, therapeutic effect may take several days. It is one of the anticancer drugs that can be administered orally.

Several drug interactions may occur with cyclophosphamide. Patients should report all medications they are taking, including over-the-counter (OTC) medicines and herbal supplements. Serious drug interactions can occur when taking cyclophosphamide and aspirin, the gout medication allopurinol (Lopurin, Zyloprim), phenobarbital (Luminal), warfarin (Coumadin), thiazide diuretics, and some psychiatric medications. Herbal Alert 37-1 lists herbal supplements that may also interact with cyclophosphamide.

HERBAL ALERT 37-1

Cyclophosphamide

- Use cautiously with garlic (antiplatelet activity), ginkgo (increased antiplatelet effect), echinacea (decreased effects of immunosuppressive drugs), ginseng (altered bleeding time), St. John's wort (may interfere with chemotherapy), and kava kava (increased risk for bleeding). Toxicity and actions of both cyclophosphamide and vitamin A are altered if given together. *Do not use with mistletoe because it may promote cancer growth.*
- Astragalus (Huang-qi; milk vetch root) stimulates the immune system and may help speed recovery from immunosuppressive chemotherapy. Astragalus has blood clot–fighting properties and may increase risk of bleeding when given with cyclophosphamide.

Side Effects and Adverse Reactions

The side effects of cyclophosphamide reflect those seen in this general class of antineoplastic drugs. Hemorrhagic cystitis is a serious problem that can arise when high doses of cyclophosphamide are given. Patients who receive a high dose should be assessed for cardiomyopathy and syndrome of inappropriate antidiuretic hormone secretion (SIADH) during treatment with this drug. In addition, cyclophosphamide may cause a change (darkening) in the skin or fingernails. Prototype Drug Chart 37-1 details the pharmacologic behavior of cyclophosphamide.

PROTOTYPE DRUG CHART 37-1

Cyclophosphamide

Drug Class Alkylating drug Trade Name: Cytoxan Pregnancy Category: D	**Dosage** A: PO: Initially: 1-5 mg/kg over 2-5 d IV: Initially: 40-50 mg/kg in divided doses over 2-5 d; *max:* 100 mg/d; C: PO/IV: Initially: 1-5 mg/kg in divided doses or 50-150 mg/m^2 Many other dose regimens are used. Dose varies based on indicated use. Adjust dose if bone marrow suppression (myelosuppression) occurs.
Contraindications Hypersensitivity, severe myelosuppression Caution: Pregnancy, liver or kidney disease	**Drug-Lab-Food Interactions** Drug: Decreases digoxin level. Increases drug action of barbiturates, chloramphenicol half-life, and effects of anticoagulant drugs. Duration of leukopenia may be prolonged if given with thiazide diuretics. Potentiates doxorubicin (Adriamycin) cardiomyopathy. Actions and toxicities of allopurinol, probenicid, colchicine, phenothiazines, potassium iodide, imipramine, warfarin, and succinylcholine are altered if given with cyclophosphamide. Toxicity increased if given with corticosteroids, phenytoin, or sulfonamides. Herb: Use cautiously with garlic, ginkgo, echinacea, ginseng, St. John's wort, kava kava, grapeseed. Toxicity and actions of both cyclophosphamide and vitamin A are altered if given together. Do not use with mistletoe. Do not give with *Astragalus membranaceus* (Beg Kei, Buck Qi, Huang Chi, Milk Vetch, Yellow Leader); may decrease effects of chemotherapy Lab: Suppresses positive reaction to uric acid, purified protein derivative, mumps, Candida; Papanicolaou test (Pap smear) may cause a false-positive result
Pharmacokinetics Absorption: PO: Well absorbed Distribution: PB: <60% Metabolism: t½: 3-12 h Excretion: 25%-40% in urine unchanged; 5%-20% in feces Nadir: 7-14 d	**Pharmacodynamics** PO/IV: Onset: 7 d Peak: 10-14 d Duration: 21 d
Therapeutic Effects/Uses Breast, lung, ovarian cancers; leukemias; lymphomas, multiple myeloma. An immunosuppressant agent Mode of Action: Inhibition of protein synthesis through interference with DNA replication by alkylation of DNA	
Side Effects Nausea, vomiting, diarrhea, weight loss, hematuria, alopecia, impotence, sterility, ovarian fibrosis, headache, dizziness, dermatitis	**Adverse Reactions** Hemorrhagic cystitis, secondary neoplasm, myelosuppression Life-threatening: Leukopenia, thrombocytopenia, cardiotoxicity (very high doses), hepatotoxicity (long-term)

A, Adult; *C,* child; *d,* day; *DNA,* deoxyribonucleic acid; *h,* hour; *IV,* intravenous; *maint,* maintenance; *max,* maximum; *PB,* protein-binding; *PO,* by mouth; *t ½,* half-life.
Note: Chemotherapy drug doses are based on body weight and prescribed either as milligrams per kilogram (mg/kg) or milligrams per meter squared (mg/m^2). Doses will also vary based on drug protocol, type and stage of cancer, age, functional status, and comorbid conditions (e.g., heart disease).

Nursing Process
Patient-Centered Collaborative Care

Alkylating Drugs: Cyclophosphamide

Assessment

- Conduct a detailed medication history, including a list of all concurrent medications, including prescriptions, over-the counter medicines, antacids, dietary supplements, vitamins, and herbal supplements to avoid drug-drug interactions.
- Obtain baseline information about patient's physical status. This should include height, weight, vital signs, laboratory values (complete blood count [CBC], uric acid, electrolytes, hepatic and renal studies, cardiopulmonary assessment, intake and output, skin assessment, daily activities status (i.e., ability to perform activities of daily living [ADLs], sleep-rest cycle), nutritional status, presence or absence of underlying symptoms of disease, and the use of current or past medication and treatment.
- Assess laboratory value at the beginning of therapy and at specified time intervals (ranging from weekly to monthly) during therapy. Drug may be withheld if red blood cell, white blood cell, or platelet counts drop below predetermined levels.
- Assess results of pulmonary function tests, chest radiographs, and renal and liver function studies during therapy.
- Assess temperature; a 1- or 2-degree change in temperature may be a sign of infection.

- Monitor for adequate intake and output.
- Obtain baseline data regarding patient's psychosocial status, including educational level, ability and desire to learn, support systems, past coping strategies, presence or absence of emotional difficulties, and self-care abilities.
- Assess patient and family knowledge related to therapeutic regimen.

Nursing Diagnoses

- Risk for infection related to side effects of cancer chemotherapy treatments and disease condition
- Risk for imbalanced nutrition, less than body requirements, related to GI side effects of chemotherapy
- Impaired urinary elimination related to hemorrhagic cystitis caused by chemotherapy
- Risk for bleeding related to effects of chemotherapy on the lining of the bladder and/or bone marrow suppression
- Deficient knowledge related to chemotherapeutic protocol
- Sexual dysfunction related to interference with normal menstrual cycle (in women) or lack of sperm production (in men)
- Disturbed body image related to cancer treatment
- Anxiety related to cancer diagnosis and unknown treatment outcomes
- Risk for caregiver role strain related to cancer diagnosis, treatment, and care responsibilities

Planning

- Patient's white blood cell, red blood cell, and platelet counts will be in the desired range.
- Patient will remain free from infection.
- Patient will maintain nutritional status (adequate fluid intake and output, sufficient caloric intake, stable weight).
- Patient will maintain adequate urinary output.
- Patient will remain free from symptoms of hemorrhagic cystitis.
- Patient/family/caregiver will demonstrate understanding of chemotherapeutic protocol (e.g., dose, administration).
- Potential body image disturbances will be discussed before therapy.
- Patient/family/caregiver will verbalize an understanding of the importance of reporting chemotherapy-related side effects and adverse reactions.
- Patient and family will verbalize strategies to minimize risks related to chemotherapy
- Patient's side effects will be managed to a level that the patient can tolerate and are not life-threatening.

Nursing Interventions

- Encourage patient to drink at least 2 L of fluid per day to promote excretion of cellular breakdown products and reduce the risk of hemorrhagic cystitis. Assess need for IV hydration.
- Hydrate patient with IV and/or oral fluids before chemotherapy is administered.
- Assess for signs and symptoms of hematuria, urinary frequency, or dysuria. Teach patient to empty bladder every 2 to 3 hours.
- Monitor blood urea nitrogen (BUN) and creatinine prior to administration and throughout duration of treatment.
- Handle drug with care during preparation and administration; avoid direct skin, eye, and mucus membrane contact with anticancer drugs. Follow protocols.
- Monitor IV site frequently for irritation and phlebitis.
- Administer prescribed premedications (30 to 60 minutes before giving drug).
- Monitor fluid intake and output and nutritional intake.
- Follow institution guidelines for safe handling, preparing, administering, and dispensing of chemotherapeutic agents.
- Maintain strict medical asepsis during dressing changes and invasive procedures.

Patient Teaching

General

- Teach patient to take cyclophosphamide early in the day to prevent accumulation of drug in the bladder during the night.
- Remind patient to consult with health care provider before administration of any vaccines.
- Advise patient to promptly report signs of infection (e.g., elevated temperature, fever, chills, sore throat, frequency and/or burning on urination, redness/swelling/pain near a wound); bleeding (e.g., bleeding gums, petechiae, bruises, hematuria, blood in the stool); and anemia (e.g., increased fatigue, dyspnea, orthostatic hypotension).
- Advise patient not to visit anyone who has a respiratory infection. A decreased WBC count puts patient at high risk for acquiring an infection.
- Emphasize protective precautions as necessary (e.g., hand washing, personal hygiene).
- Explain to patient and family the rationale for chemotherapy.
- Advise breastfeeding patient that cyclophosphamide is excreted in breast milk. Advise male patient that testicular atrophy and reversible oligospermia/azoospermia may occur.
- Teach importance of using birth-control measures as appropriate. Discuss sperm banking with male patients as appropriate.
- Advise patients of childbearing age to use contraceptives during therapy and for 2 years after completion of therapy.
- Provide information on where to purchase cosmetic supplies (e.g., wigs) should hair loss occur.

Side Effects

- Advise patient about good oral hygiene with a soft toothbrush for stomatitis; have patient use a soft toothbrush when platelet count is <50,000/mm^3.
- Remind premenopausal women that they may experience amenorrhea, menstrual irregularities, or sterility; advise male patients that they may experience impotence.
- Advise patient of possible hair loss; recommend a wig, hairpiece, scarf, or turban.
- Assess for use of alternative/complementary therapy that may interact with chemotherapy agent.

Diet

- Advise patient to follow a diet low in purines (e.g., organ meats, beans, peas) to alkalize urine.
- Advise patient to avoid citric acid.
- Offer patient food and fluids that may decrease nausea (e.g., cola, crackers, ginger ale).
- Plan small, frequent meals.

Cultural Considerations

- In some cultural groups, health care decisions are made by consensus, and the family plays a key role in filtering the information given to a patient. Issues related to informed consent and full disclosure of medical information may cause distress in cultural groups who place the needs of the family above the needs of the individual. Interactions should be modified based on family structure, religious values and beliefs, time orientation, cultural health practices, and verbal and nonverbal communication.
- Cultural assessment tools can provide general guidelines for health care providers.
- Hyperpigmentation of the tongue and oral mucosa after administration has been reported in African Americans. Incidence rate of high-grade neutropenia may be higher in Asian patients.

Evaluation

- Patient is free from infection.
- Patient maintains target weight.
- Patient maintains nutritional status.
- Patient does not develop hemorrhagic cystitis.
- Patient/family/caregiver education needs are met.
- Questions related to sexuality are answered.

ANTIMETABOLITES

Antimetabolites resemble natural metabolites that synthesize, recycle, and break down organic compounds for use by the body. However, antimetabolites disrupt metabolic processes and can inhibit enzyme synthesis. They are classified as CCS and exert their effects in the S phase (DNA synthesis and metabolism) of the cell cycle. This group is classified according to the substances with which they interfere; they include folic acid (folate) antagonists (e.g., methotrexate [Rheumatrex, Trexall], pemetrexed [Altima]), pyrimidine antagonists (e.g., fluorouracil [Adrucil]), purine antagonists (e.g., 6-mercaptopurine [Purinethol]), adenosine deaminase inhibitors (e.g., fludarabine [Fludara]), and ribonucleotide reductase inhibitors (e.g., hydroxyurea (Hydrea), 2-deoxycoformycin (pentostatin [Nipent]).

Antimetabolites are used to treat acute and chronic leukemia, myelodysplastic syndrome (MDS), breast cancer, head and neck cancer, lung cancer, osteosarcoma, and lymphomas. Two drugs in this classification, fluorouracil, also known as 5-FU [Adrucil]), and floxuridine (FUDR) are considered CCNS as well as CCS.

Methotrexate, also designated as *MTX* (Rheumatrex, Trexall), a folic acid antagonist, is used for the treatment of both cancerous and noncancerous (e.g., rheumatoid arthritis, psoriasis) conditions. Methotrexate is also used to induce miscarriage in patients with ectopic pregnancies. Methotrexate acts as a substitute for folic acid, which is needed for the synthesis of proteins and DNA. Cancer patients receiving high doses of MTX must be given leucovorin calcium to "rescue" **(leucovorin rescue)** normal cells from the adverse effects of the drug.

Numerous drug interactions may occur with MTX. Protein-bound drugs (e.g., aspirin, phenytoin) increase the toxicity of MTX. Nonsteroidal antiinflammatory drugs (NSAIDs) increase and prolong MTX levels. Cotrimoxazole (Bactrim) and pyrimethamine (Daraprim) increase MTX levels. Patients who are taking penicillins, cyclooxygenase 2 (COX-2) inhibitors, and OTC herbs should share this information with their physician, because these products interact with MTX. Table 37-4 lists the antimetabolite drugs, uses, and considerations.

The general side effects of antimetabolite drugs include bone marrow suppression (anemia, leukopenia, thrombocytopenia), stomatitis (inflammation of the oral mucosa), nausea, vomiting, alopecia, and hepatic and renal dysfunction. Major dose-limiting toxicities may occur in the hematopoietic and gastrointestinal systems. General adverse reactions to chemotherapeutic drugs are listed in Table 37-2.

Fluorouracil

Fluorouracil (5-FU, Adrucil) is a mainstay of treatment for a variety of cancers, including those of the breast, stomach, liver, pancreas, and skin.

SAFETY: Preventing Medication Errors

Do not confuse ...

- **fluorouracil** with **flucytosine**

Pharmacokinetics Fluorouracil is administered IV to treat solid tumors and topically for superficial basal cell carcinoma. Less than 10% is bound to protein, and the half-life for the IV route is 10 to 20 minutes.

TABLE 37-4 ANTINEOPLASTICS: ANTIMETABOLITES

DRUG TYPE AND NAME	ROUTE AND DOSAGE	USES AND CONSIDERATIONS
Folic Acid Antagonists		
methotrexate (MTX)	IV: low dose: 10-50 mg/m^2; medium dose: 100-500 mg/m^2; high dose: 500 mg/m^2 (and higher followed by leucovorin rescue) IT: 10-15 mg/m^2 IM: 25 mg/m^2	Solid tumors, sarcomas, choriocarcinoma, leukemia. At higher doses, patients should be well hydrated; keep urine pH at 7.0 for drug solubility for excretion. Higher doses require use of leucovorin as a rescue for normal cells. Pregnancy category: D; PB: 50%; t½: 8-15 h
pemetrexed disodium (Alimta)	IV: 500 mg/m^2 day 1 of every 21-d cycle	A multitargeted antifolate to treat mesothelioma and non– small-cell lung cancer. Pregnancy category: D; PB: 81%; t½: 3.5 h
trimetrexate glucuronate (Neutrexin)	IV: 45 mg/m^2/d; infuse over 60-90 min for 21 d	Alternative drug therapy for *Pneumocystis carinii* pneumonia; treatment for patients with AIDS. May be used for colorectal cancer. Monitor CBC. Pregnancy category: D; PB: 86%-94%; t½: 11-13 h
Pyrimidine Analogues		
azacitidine (Vidaza)	SubQ: 75 mg/m^2 IV: 75-100 mg/m^2/d for 7 d, repeated every 4 wk	Treatment of chronic myelomonocytic leukemia. Pregnancy category: D; PB: UK; t½: 41 min
capecitabine (Xeloda)	PO: 2500 mg/m^2/d in two divided doses for 2 wk	Solid tumors, sarcomas, choriocarcinoma, leukemia. At higher doses, patients should be well hydrated; keep urine pH at 7.0 for drug solubility for excretion. Pregnancy category: D; PB: 50%; t½: 8-16 h
cytarabine (Cytosar-U, ARA-C, cytosine arabinoside)	For leukemia IV: 100 mg/m^2/d continuous infusion for 5-10 d For head and neck cancer: 1 mg/kg every 12 h for 5-7 d IV or subQ For bone marrow transplant 1.5 mg/m^2 continuous infusion for 48 h IT: 5-75 mg/m^2 every 2-7 d	Acute leukemias and lymphomas. Also used as an immunosuppressive drug after organ transplant. May be used in combination with other anticancer drugs. Nausea, vomiting, leukopenia, and thrombocytopenia are common side effects. Pregnancy category: D; PB: 15%; t½: 1-3 h
floxuridine (FUDR)	Intra-arterial (hepatic): 0.1-0.6 mg/kg/d for 7-14 d. Delivered by slow infusion pump	Metastatic colon cancer and hepatomas. Pregnancy category: D; PB: UK; t½: 20 h
5-fluorouracil (5-FU, Adrucil)	See Prototype Drug Chart 37-2.	
gemcitabine HCl (Gemzar)	For breast cancer: IV: 1250 mg/m^2 over 30 min days 1 and 8 of 21-d cycle For pancreatic cancer: IV: 1000 mg/m^2 over 30 min weekly for up to 7 wk For NSCL: IV: 1000 mg/m^2 over 30 min days 1 and 8 and 15 For ovarian cancer: IV: 1000 mg/m^2 over 30 min days 1 and 8 of 21-d cycle	Advanced or metastatic adenocarcinoma of the pancreas, non–small-cell lung cancer and bladder cancer. Acts at S phase of cell cycle. Monitor leukocytes and platelet count; reduce dose if values are extremely low. Pregnancy category: D; PB: UK; t½: 1-10 h
nelarabine (Arranon)	A: 1500 mg/m^2 IV over 2 hours on days 1, 3, and 5; repeat every 3 wk C: 650 mg/m^2 IV over 1 h on days 1, 2, 3, 4, 5; repeat every 3 wk	Treatment of refractory or relapsed T-cell lymphoblastic leukemia and T-cell lymphoblastic lymphoma. Pregnancy category: D; PB: <25%; t½: 30 min-3 h
Purine Analogues		
cladribine (Leustatin)	IV: 0.09 mg/kg/d as a continuous infusion for 7 d	For treatment of hairy cell leukemia and chronic lymphocytic leukemia. Adverse reactions: bone marrow suppression, fever, nausea, vomiting, diaphoresis. Pregnancy category: D; PB: 20%; t½: 5.4 h
clofarabine (Clolar)	IV: 52 mg/m^2 IV over 2 h daily for 5 d	To treat refractory or relapsed acute lymphoblastic leukemia in children. Pregnancy category: D; PB: 47%; t½: 105 min

TABLE 37-4 ANTINEOPLASTICS: ANTIMETABOLITES—cont'd

DRUG TYPE AND NAME	ROUTE AND DOSAGE	USES AND CONSIDERATIONS
fludarabine (Fludara)	PO: 40 mg/m²/d for 5 d; repeat every 28 d IV: 25 mg/m²; infuse over 30 min daily for 5 d; repeat every 28 d	Chronic lymphocytic leukemia in patients who have not responded to other alkylating drugs; low-grade non-Hodgkin's lymphoma. Anorexia, nausea, diarrhea, fever, and peripheral edema may occur. Pregnancy category: D; PB: UK; t½: 9 h
6-mercaptopurine (Purinethol)	PO: Induction dose 2.5 mg/kg/d followed by maintenance dose	First used in 1952 for treating acute lymphatic leukemia. Also used as immunosuppressive drug. Adverse reactions include hepatotoxicity, bone marrow suppression, hyperuricemia. Pregnancy category: D; PB: 19%; t½: 45 min
thioguanine (6-thioguanine, Lanvis)	PO: A: 100 mg/m² every 12 h for 5-10 d C: 100 mg/m² every 12 h for 5-10 d OR 1-3 mg/kg/d	Acute and chronic myelogenous leukemia. Long duration of action. Pregnancy category: D; PB: UK; t½: 2-11 h
Ribonucleotide Reductase Inhibitors (Enzyme Inhibitors)		
hydroxyurea (Hydrea)	PO: 20-30 mg/kg/d	Melanoma, resistant chronic myelocytic leukemia, and ovarian cancer. Long duration of action. Pregnancy category: D; PB: UK; t½: 3-4 h
pentostatin (Nipent)	IV: 4 mg/m² every other wk	Hairy cell leukemia refractory to alpha-interferon. Very long duration of action. Pregnancy category: D; PB: UK; t½: 6 h

Note: Chemotherapeutic doses and schedules will vary depending on protocol, body surface area (m²), age, functional status, and comorbid conditions. For a full discussion of body surface area in dosage calculation, see Chapter 14.

AIDS, Acquired immunodeficiency syndrome; *CBC,* complete blood cell count; *h,* hour; *min,* minute; *PB,* protein-binding; *t½,* half-life; *UK,* unknown; *wk,* week.

A small amount of the drug is excreted in the urine, and up to 80% is excreted by the lungs as carbon dioxide.

Pharmacodynamics Fluorouracil blocks the enzyme action necessary for DNA and ribonucleic acid (RNA) synthesis. The drug has a low therapeutic index and is used alone or in combination with other anticancer drugs. Fluorouracil can cross the blood-brain barrier. Its duration of action is 30 days.

HERBAL ALERT 37-2

5-Fluorouracil

- Use cautiously with ginseng and St. John's wort (may interfere with chemotherapy). *Do not use with mistletoe because it may promote cancer growth.*
- Astragalus stimulates the immune system and may help speed recovery from immunosuppressive chemotherapy. Astragalus has blood clot–fighting properties and may increase risk of bleeding when given with 5-FU.

Side Effects and Adverse Reactions

The side effects of 5-FU (Adrucil) are similar to other anticancer drugs. These include anorexia, nausea, vomiting, diarrhea, stomatitis, alopecia, photosensitivity, increased skin pigmentation, rash, and erythema. Stomatitis is an early sign of toxicity and should be reported to the physician. Myelosuppression may occur 4 to 8 days after the beginning of drug therapy.

Prototype Drug Chart 37-2 presents the pharmacologic data for 5-FU.

Nursing Process
Patient-Centered Collaborative Care

Antimetabolites: Fluorouracil

Assessment

- Conduct a detailed medication history, including a list of all concurrent medications, including prescriptions, over-the counter medicines, antacids, dietary supplements, vitamins, and herbal supplements to avoid drug-drug interactions.
- Obtain baseline information about patient's physical status. This should include height, weight, vital signs, laboratory values (CBC, uric acid, electrolytes, hepatic and renal studies, cardiopulmonary assessment, intake and output, skin assessment, daily activities status [i.e., ability to perform ADLs], sleep-rest cycle), nutritional status, presence or absence of underlying symptoms of disease, and use of current or past medication and treatment.
- Assess laboratory values at the beginning of therapy and at specified time intervals (ranging from weekly to monthly) during therapy. Drug may be withheld if red blood cell, white blood cell, or platelet counts drop below predetermined levels.
- Assess renal function studies before and during drug therapy.
- Assess temperature; fever may be an early sign of infection.
- Obtain baseline data regarding patient's psychosocial status, including educational level, ability and desire to

PROTOTYPE DRUG CHART 37-2

Fluorouracil, 5-Fluorouracil, 5-FU

Drug Class Antimetabolite Trade Names: Adrucil, 5-FU,Fluroplex, Efudex (topical) Pregnancy Category: D/X (topical)	**Dosage** A: IV: 12 mg/kg/d × 4 d; *max:* 800 mg/d; repeat with 6 mg/kg on days 6, 8, 10, and 12 or as indicated. Dose regimens are varied. Topical: 1%-2% sol/cream b.i.d. to head/neck lesions; 5% to other body areas
Contraindications Hypersensitivity, pregnancy, severe infection, myelosuppression, marginal nutritional status. Reduce dose in patients with impaired hepatic or renal function or those with malnutrition.	**Drug-Lab-Food Interactions** Drug: Bone marrow depressants increase chances of toxicity. Avoid live virus vaccines, which may potentiate virus replication. Increased 5-FU toxicity with concomitant use of leucovorin calcium. Metronidazole may increase 5-FU toxicity (clearance of 5-FU decreased). Increased pharmacologic effects of 5-FU when given with cimetidine (Tagamet). Thiazide diuretics increase myelosuppression. Lab: May decrease albumin; may increase excretion of 5-HIAA in urine Herb: Use cautiously with ginseng, St. John's wort, and gingko biloba. Do not use with mistletoe. Topical peppermint oil and eucalyptus oil may increase absorption of topical 5-FU. Avoid simultaneous use.
Pharmacokinetics Absorption: IV and topical: 5%-10% Distribution: PB: UK Metabolism: t½: 10-20 min Excretion: In urine and expired carbon dioxide Nadir: 10-14 d	**Pharmacodynamics** Effects on blood count: Peak: 10-14 d IV: Onset: 1-9 d Peak: 9-21 d Duration: 30 d Topical: Onset: 2-3 d Peak: 2-6 wk Duration: 4-8 wk
Therapeutic Effects/Uses Breast, colorectal, pancreas, stomach, esophageal, and head and neck cancers. Given in combination with levamisole after surgical resection in patients with Duke's stage C colon cancer Mode of Action: Prevention of thymidine synthetase production, thereby inhibiting DNA and RNA synthesis; not phase specific	
Side Effects Stomatitis, nausea, vomiting, diarrhea, alopecia, rash, photosensitivity. Diarrhea may be severe.	**Adverse Reactions** Bone marrow suppression Life-threatening: Thrombocytopenia, myelosuppression, hemorrhage, renal failure

5-FU, Fluorouracil; *5-HIAA,* 5-hydroxyindoleacetic acid; *A,* adult; *b.i.d.,* twice a day; *d,* day; DNA, deoxyribonucleic acid; *IV,* intravenous; *max,* maximum; *min,* minute; *PB,* protein-binding; *RNA,* ribonucleic acid; *sol,* solution; *t ½,* half-life; *UK,* unknown; *wk,* week.

learn, support systems, past coping strategies, presence or absence of emotional difficulties, and self-care abilities.

- Assess patient and family knowledge related to therapeutic regimen.

Nursing Diagnoses

- Risk for infection related to bone marrow suppression
- Risk for imbalanced nutrition, less than body requirements, related to GI side effects of chemotherapy
- Acute pain related to GI side effects (mucositis/stomatitis) of chemotherapy
- Risk for impaired skin integrity related to photosensitivity caused by chemotherapy
- Risk for impaired perianal skin integrity related to diarrhea caused by chemotherapy
- Deficient knowledge related to chemotherapeutic protocol
- Risk for caregiver role strain related to cancer diagnosis, treatment, and care responsibilities

Planning

- Patient blood counts will remain in the desired range.
- Patient will maintain nutritional status (adequate fluid intake and output, adequate caloric intake, stable weight).
- Patient will have adequate pain control.
- Patient will limit exposure to sunlight.

- Patient will not experience perianal skin breakdown.
- Patient/family/caregiver will demonstrate understanding of chemotherapeutic protocol (dose, administration, side effects, and adverse reactions).

Nursing Interventions

- Monitor IV site frequently. Extravasation produces severe pain. If this occurs, apply ice pack and notify health care provider.
- Handle drug with care during preparation and administration; avoid direct skin contact with anticancer drugs. Follow protocols.
- Administer antiemetic 30 to 60 minutes before drug to prevent vomiting.
- Monitor fluid intake and output and nutritional intake. GI effects are common.
- Assess for hyperpigmentation along the vein in which 5-FU was administered.
- Maintain strict medical asepsis during dressing changes and invasive procedures.
- Monitor blood counts and laboratory values.
- Offer patient food and fluids that may decrease nausea (e.g., crackers, cola, ginger ale).
- Encourage mouth rinses every 2 hours with normal saline.
- Plan small, frequent meals.
- Support good oral hygiene; brush teeth with soft toothbrush, and use waxed dental floss.
- Record number and consistency of stools; monitor perineal skin condition.
- Develop patient/family teaching plan on signs and symptoms of photosensitivity.

Patient Teaching

General

- Advise patient to promptly report signs of infection (e.g., fever, sore throat, chills, urinary frequency; burning on urination; redness, swelling, or pain near a wound); bleeding (e.g., bleeding gums, petechiae, bruises, hematuria, blood in the stool); or signs of anemia (e.g., increased fatigue, dyspnea, orthostatic hypotension).
- Teach patient to examine mouth daily and report signs of stomatitis (soreness, ulcerations, white patches in mouth). Oral hygiene several times a day is essential. If stomatitis occurs, rinse mouth with baking soda or normal saline. Use a soft toothbrush.
- Advise patient not to visit anyone who has a respiratory infection. A decreased white blood cell (WBC) count puts patient at risk for acquiring an infection.
- Advise patient to take year-round photosensitivity precautions. Use sunscreen when outdoors.
- Emphasize protective precautions as necessary (e.g., hand washing, personal hygiene).
- Advise patient to take pain medication as prescribed to relieve mouth pain related to mucositis/stomatitis.
- Teach importance of using birth-control measures as appropriate. Discuss sperm banking with male patients as appropriate.
- Teach patient to avoid pregnancy for 3 to 4 months after completing antineoplastic therapy in most situations. Some sources recommend that both men and women avoid conception for 2 years after completion of treatment.

Side Effects

- Advise patient about good oral hygiene with a soft toothbrush for mucositis/stomatitis; have patient use a soft toothbrush when platelet count is $\leq 50{,}000/mm^3$. Instruct patient to rinse mouth every 2 hours with normal saline and avoid use of commercial mouthwashes that contain alcohol.
- Remind premenopausal women that they may experience amenorrhea, menstrual irregularities, or sterility. Advise male patients that they may experience impotence.
- Advise patient of possible hair loss; recommend a wig, hairpiece, scarf, or turban.
- Assess for use of alternative/complementary therapy that may interact with chemotherapy.

Diet

- Encourage small frequent meals.
- Encourage use of cool, bland foods.
- Offer ice chips or ice pops to help relieve mouth pain.

Cultural Considerations

- In some cultural groups, health care decisions are made by consensus, and the family plays a key role in filtering information given to the patient. Issues related to informed consent and full disclosure of medical information may cause distress in cultural groups who place the needs of the family above the needs of the individual. Interactions should be modified based on family structure, religious values and beliefs, time orientation, cultural health practices, and verbal and nonverbal communication.
- Cultural assessment tools can provide general guidelines for health care providers.
- An increased incidence of hyperpigmentation has been reported in dark-skinned people. Hyperpigmentation may be seen on the skin, nails, hair, and oral mucosa. This usually disappears over time.

Evaluation

- Patient is free from infection.
- Oral mucosa is free from erythema and swelling.
- Pain is controlled.
- Skin integrity remains intact.
- Patient/family/caregiver education needs are met.
- Questions regarding sexuality are answered.

TABLE 37-5 ANTINEOPLASTICS: ANTITUMOR ANTIBIOTICS

DRUG TYPE AND NAME	ROUTE AND DOSAGE	USES AND CONSIDERATIONS
bleomycin (Blenoxane)	5-20 units/m^2 once a wk or 10-20 units/m^2 twice a wk IV: continuous 15 units/m^2/d for 4 d Intracavitary: Pleural space 50-60 units in 50-100 mL diluent	Squamous cell carcinomas, testicular tumor (when used with vinblastine and cisplatin), and lymphomas. Low incidence of bone marrow suppression. Lifetime dose is 400 units/m^2. A serious adverse reaction is anaphylaxis. Long duration of action. Pregnancy category: D; PB: 1%; t½: 2-5 h
dactinomycin (Actinomycin D, Cosmegen)	IV: 10-15 mcg/kg/d for 5 d (every 3-4 wk) Dose varies depending on indication	Testicular tumors, Wilms' tumor, choriocarcinoma, and rhabdomyosarcoma. Nausea and vomiting may occur during first 24 h. Long duration of action. Pregnancy category: C; PB: 80%-90%; t½: 36 h
daunorubicin HCl (Cerubidine)	IV: 30-60 mg/m^2/d for 3 d	Leukemia, Ewing's sarcoma, Wilms' tumor, neuroblastoma, and non-Hodgkin's lymphoma. Long duration of action. Pregnancy category: D; PB: 80%; t½: 19 h
doxorubicin (Adriamycin)	See Prototype Drug Chart 37-3.	
epirubicin (Ellence)	IV: 100-120 mg/m^2 every 3-4 wk	Cancers of breast, lung, lymph system, stomach, and ovaries. Metastatic node-positive breast cancer; adjuvant with anticancer therapy. May be used in combination therapy with cyclophosphamide and fluorouracil (CEF) for breast cancer; improved survival rate over cyclophosphamide, methotrexate, and fluorouracil (CMF). Adverse effects include bone marrow suppression, cardiotoxicity (less than doxorubicin), and extravasation necrosis. Less cardiotoxic than doxorubicin; similar efficacy. Pregnancy category: D; PB: 77%; t½: 33 h
idarubicin (Idamycin)	IV: Induction: 12 mg/m^2 slow IV push for 3 d	Acute monocytic leukemia and solid tumors. More potent than daunorubicin or doxorubicin. Vesicant, monitor CBC. Urine may be red. Pregnancy category: D; PB: 97%; t½: 22 h
mitomycin (Mutamycin)	IV: 10 mg/m^2 every 8 wk Intracavitary: Bladder: 20-40 mg in 20-40 mL of water	Disseminated adenocarcinoma of breast, stomach, and pancreas. Also used for cancer of the head, neck, cervix, and lung. Monitor temperature and CBC. Pregnancy category: D; PB: UK; t½: 12 min
mitoxantrone (Novantrone)	IV: For acute leukemia: Induction: 12 mg/m^2/d for 3 d	Acute nonlymphocytic leukemia; may be used for breast cancer. Rash, dyspnea, hypotension, facial swelling, blue urine, sclera, skin hue change may occur. Severe hepatic dysfunction with decreased total body clearance. Pregnancy category: D; PB: 95%; t½: 1.5-13 d
valrubicin (Valstar)	Intravesicular: Bladder: 800 mg (in 75 mL diluent) every wk for 6 wk	Bladder cancer. May cause urinary frequency and urgency, dysuria, hematuria, and bladder pain. Pregnancy category: UK; PB: >99%; t½: UK

Note: Chemotherapeutic doses and schedules will vary depending on protocol, body surface area (m^2), age, functional status, and comorbid conditions. For a full discussion of body surface area in dosage calculation, see Chapter 14.
CBC, Complete blood cell count; *d,* day; *h,* hour; *min,* minute; *PB,* protein-binding; *t½,* half-life; *UK,* unknown; *wk,* week.

ANTITUMOR ANTIBIOTICS

Antitumor antibiotics (bleomycin [Blenoxane], dactinomycin (actinomycin-D) [Cosmegen], daunorubicin [Cerubidine, Daunomycin], doxorubicin [Adriamycin], mitomycin [Mutamycin], Mitoxantrone [Novantrone]) inhibit protein and RNA synthesis and bind DNA, causing fragmentation. There are several types of antitumor antibiotics, including the anthracyclines and miscellaneous drugs. Except for bleomycin, which has its major effect on the G2 phase, they are classified as CCNS drugs. These antitumor antibiotics differ from one another and are used for various cancers, including leukemia and many solid tumors. Table 37-5 lists the antitumor antibiotics, uses, and considerations.

Adverse reactions to the antitumor antibiotics are similar to other antineoplastics and include alopecia, nausea, vomiting, stomatitis, and myelosuppression. Antitumor antibiotics are capable of causing **vesication** (blistering of tissue); exceptions to this are bleomycin (Blenoxane) and plicamycin (Mithracin). General adverse reactions to chemotherapeutic drugs are listed in Table 37-2.

Doxorubicin

Doxorubicin is used in the treatment of many types of cancer and is an important prototype drug that has led to the development of many analogs (e.g., epirubicin [Ellence], idarubicin [Idamycin]). However, it has severe cardiotoxic side effects and must be given with caution.

HERBAL ALERT 37-3

Doxorubicin

- Green tea *(Camellia sinensis)* may enhance antitumor effects of doxorubicin. Report use to the health care provider. Use cautiously with grapeseed (inhibits effects of doxorubicin), garlic (anticlotting properties, may decrease effects of chemotherapy), and St. John's wort (may decrease effectiveness of chemotherapy).
- Schisandra extract (Schisandra, gomishi, Sheng-Mai-San) may decrease the cardiotoxicity associated with doxorubicin. Schisandra stimulates hepatic metabolism and may interfere with doxorubicin, which is excreted through the liver.

Pharmacokinetics Doxorubicin is administered IV and metabolized in the liver to active and inactive metabolites. The various metabolites affect the half-life; the initial phase of doxorubicin is 12 minutes, the intermediate phase is 3.5 hours, and the final phase is 30 hours.

SAFETY: Preventing Medication Errors

Do not confuse ...
- **doxorubicin** (Adriamycin) with **idarubicin** (Idamycin)

Pharmacodynamics Doxorubicin) is prescribed in combination with other anticancer agents for the treatment of cancers of the breast, ovaries, lung, and bladder and also for leukemias and lymphomas. A major concern for clinicians is that doxorubicin can cause cardiotoxicity. Recipients of this drug are limited to a maximum lifetime dose of 550 mg/m^2. This dose may be lower for individuals who have preexisting cardiac problems, use other cardiotoxic medications, are older, or have received radiation to the chest. Prior to treatment with doxorubicin, the cardiac function of potential recipients is assessed. Dexrazoxane (Zinecard) is a cytoprotective (chemoprotective) agent that may be given to help prevent cardiotoxicity associated with doxorubicin administration.

Side Effects and Adverse Reactions

Some antitumor antibiotics can cause organ toxicities. Individuals receiving bleomycin (Blenoxane) may develop pneumonitis that progresses to pulmonary fibrosis. In addition to doxorubicin, daunorubicin (Cerubidine) and idarubicin (Idamycin) can also cause cardiotoxicity.

Prototype Drug Chart 37-3 presents the pharmacologic data for doxorubicin.

PROTOTYPE DRUG CHART 37-3

Doxorubicin

Drug Class Antitumor antibiotic Trade Name: Adriamycin Pregnancy Category: D	**Dosage** A: 40-75 mg/m^2 as a single dose every 3-4 wk or no more than 30 mg/m^2 every 2 wk with 1- wk rest IV for 3 d every 4 wk Safety and efficacy have not been established for children. Reduce dose with renal and hepatic impairment.
Contraindications Pregnancy, severe cardiac disease. Cardiac status and cardiac ejection fraction should be tested before starting doxorubicin therapy. Do not exceed a lifetime cumulative dose of 550 mg/m^2 (450 mg/m^2 if patient has had prior chest irradiation or is receiving cyclophosphamide). Dexrazoxane (Zinecard) is used to help prevent or lessen cardiac damage. Caution: Hepatic and renal impairment	**Drug-Lab-Food Interactions** Drug: Calcium channel blockers, paclitaxel (Taxol), and mitomycin increase risk of cardiotoxicity if given with doxorubicin. Doxorubicin may decrease digoxin levels. Doxorubicin decreases levels of phenytoin. Cyclophosphamide (Cytoxan) increases risk of cardiotoxicity and hemorrhage. Increased risk of hepatotoxicity when given with mercaptopurine. Increased plasma clearance of doxorubicin when given with barbiturates. Precipitate will form when doxorubicin is combined with heparin or 5-FU. Decreased metabolic clearance of 5-FU (Adrucil) and increased cytotoxicity when given with alfa interferon. Prolonged hemotoxic effects may occur if doxorubicin and cyclosporine are given together. Do not give with zidovudine (Retrovir), as it may decrease effectiveness of doxorubicin. Lab: ECG changes. Increases uric acid. Herb: Green tea may enhance antitumor effects. Report use to health care provider. Use cautiously with grapeseed, garlic, St. John's wort.
Pharmacokinetics Absorption: IV Distribution: PB: 80%-90% Metabolism: $t\frac{1}{2}$: 3-30 h Excretion: 40% in bile and 5% in urine Nadir: 10-14 d (doxorubicin)	**Pharmacodynamics** IV: Onset: 7-10 d Peak: 14 d Duration: 21 d
Therapeutic Effects/Uses Breast, bladder, ovarian, and lung cancers; leukemias; lymphomas, soft-tissue and bone sarcoma Mode of Action: Inhibits DNA and RNA synthesis; has immunosuppressant activity	
Side Effects Stomatitis, anorexia, nausea, vomiting, diarrhea, rash, alopecia. Doxorubicin is a potent vesicant. May cause a flare reaction. Nausea and vomiting are dose-related and may begin 1-3 h after administration. Causes discolored urine (pink to red) for up to 48 h. May cause "radiation recall" to previously irradiated skin.	**Adverse Reactions** Esophagitis; anemia; hyperpigmentation of nails, tongue, and oral mucosa, especially in African Americans. Teratogenic, mutagenic, and carcinogenic. Life-threatening: Thrombocytopenia, leukopenia, cardiotoxicity, congestive heart failure, electrocardiogram changes, severe myelosuppression, anaphylaxis

5-FU, Fluorouracil; *d,* day; *DNA,* deoxyribonucleic acid; *ECG,* electrocardiogram; *h,* hour; *IV,* intravenous; *PB,* protein-binding; *RNA,* ribonucleic acid; *t ½,* half-life; *wk,* week.

Nursing Process
Patient-Centered Collaborative Care
Antitumor Antibiotics: Doxorubicin

Assessment
- Conduct a detailed medication history, including a list of all concurrent medications, including prescriptions, over-the counter medicines, antacids, dietary supplements, vitamins, and herbal supplements to avoid drug-drug interactions.
- Obtain baseline information about patient's physical status. This should include height, weight, vital signs, laboratory values (CBC, uric acid, electrolytes, hepatic and renal studies, cardiopulmonary assessment, intake and output, skin assessment, daily activities status [i.e., ability to perform ADLs], sleep-rest cycle), nutritional status, presence or absence of underlying symptoms of disease, and the use of current or past medications and treatment.
- Assess laboratory tests at the beginning of therapy and at specified time intervals (ranging from weekly to monthly) during therapy. Drug may be withheld if red blood cell (RBC), white blood cell (WBC), or platelet counts drop below predetermined levels.
- Assess CBC, differential, and platelet count weekly. Drug may be withheld if RBC, WBC, or platelet counts drop below predetermined levels.
- Conduct thorough physical assessment, and document findings.
- Assess temperature; fever may be an early sign of infection.
- Obtain baseline data regarding patient's psychosocial status, including educational level, ability and desire to learn, support systems, past coping strategies, presence or absence of emotional difficulties, and self-care abilities.
- Assess patient's and family's knowledge related to therapeutic regimen.
- Assess plans for pregnancy (if appropriate).

Nursing Diagnoses
- Risk for infection related to bone marrow suppression
- Risk for decreased cardiac tissue perfusion related to cardiotoxic effects of chemotherapy
- Risk for impaired skin integrity related to vesicant properties of chemotherapy
- Deficient knowledge related to antineoplastic therapy
- Disturbed body image related to cancer treatment
- Anxiety related to cancer diagnosis and the unknown outcomes of treatment
- Risk for caregiver role strain related to cancer diagnosis, treatment, and care responsibilities

Planning
- Patient will maintain blood cell values in the desired range.
- Patient will be free from cardiac dysfunction.
- Patient's skin integrity will remain intact.
- Patient/family/caregiver will demonstrate understanding of the chemotherapy regimen, including side effects.
- Assess patient/family/caregiver knowledge related to chemotherapeutic protocol.
- Discuss potential body image disturbances prior to therapy.

Nursing Interventions
- Assess cardiac status.
- Monitor IV site frequently. Doxorubicin is a severe vesicant whose effects are not immediately apparent. Give drug through a large-bore, quickly running IV infusion. Monitor blood counts and laboratory values.
- Extravasation produces severe pain. If extravasation occurs, stop infusion immediately. Do not remove IV device from patient. Attempt to aspirate residual vesicant from IV device using a small syringe, and then remove the device. Assess the site. Notify health care provider. Apply warm packs for 15 to 20 minutes at least 4 times per day for first 24 hours. For peripheral extravasations, elevate extremity. Tissue necrosis may occur 3 to 4 weeks after infiltration into tissue.
- Handle drug with care during preparation; avoid direct skin contact with drug.
- Administer antiemetic 30 to 60 minutes before chemotherapy.
- Monitor for changes in urine color (pink to red). The drug is red and is excreted in the urine.
- Offer patient food and fluids that may decrease nausea (e.g., crackers, cola, ginger ale).
- Plan small, frequent meals.
- Administer prophylactic antibiotics to prevent infection.
- Offer analgesics for pain as prescribed.
- Maintain strict medical asepsis during dressing changes and invasive procedures.
- Support good oral hygiene. Use soft toothbrush. Use waxed dental floss.
- Monitor fluid intake and output and nutritional intake.

Patient Teaching

General
- Teach patient the signs and symptoms of cardiac dysfunction (shortness of breath, palpitations, edema in extremities) and to report these to health care provider.
- Teach patient about changes in urine color (pink or red) caused by this drug.
- Advise patient to promptly report signs of infection (e.g., fever, sore throat), bleeding (e.g., bleeding gums, petechiae, bruises, hematuria, blood in stool), and anemia (e.g., increased fatigue, dyspnea, orthostatic hypotension).

- Emphasize protective precautions (e.g., hand washing, personal hygiene).
- Teach patient that complete alopecia occurs with doses >50 mg/m^2. Teach that hair will begin to regrow within several months after therapy is completed.
- Teach patient about "radiation recall" on previously irradiated skin.
- Advise patient not to visit anyone who has a respiratory infection. A decreased WBC count puts patient at risk for acquiring an infection.
- Teach importance of using birth-control measures as appropriate. Discuss sperm banking with male patients as appropriate.
- Teach patient to avoid pregnancy for 3 to 4 months after completing antineoplastic therapy in most situations. Some sources recommend that both men and women avoid conception for 2 years after completion of treatment.
- Provide information on where to purchase cosmetic supplies (e.g., wigs) should hair loss occur.

Side Effects
- Assess for nausea/vomiting, and administer antiemetics as prescribed.
- Teach importance of using birth-control measures as appropriate. Discuss sperm banking with male patients as appropriate.
- Remind premenopausal women that they may experience amenorrhea, menstrual irregularities, or sterility; advise male patient that he may experience impotence.
- Advise patient of possible hair loss; recommend a wig, hairpiece, scarf, or turban.
- Assess for use of alternative/complementary therapies that may interact with chemotherapy agent.

Diet
- Encourage small, frequent meals.
- Encourage eating bland foods.
- Avoid foods with extreme temperatures.

Cultural Considerations
- In some cultural groups, health care decisions are made by consensus, and the family plays a key role in filtering information given to the patient. Issues related to informed consent and full disclosure of medical information may cause distress in cultural groups that place the needs of the family above the needs of the individual. Interactions should be modified based on family structure, religious values and beliefs, time orientation, cultural health practices, and verbal and nonverbal communication.
- Cultural assessment tools can provide general guidelines for health care providers.
- Hyperpigmentation of the tongue and oral mucosa has been seen after the administration of doxorubicin in African Americans. Incidence rate of high-grade neutropenia may be higher in Asian patients.

Evaluation
- Patient is free from infection.
- Cardiac function is maintained.
- Patient and family educational needs are met.
- Side effects of therapy are controlled.

PLANT ALKALOIDS

Plant alkaloids are derived from natural products that are CCS and block cell division at the M phase of the cell cycle. The **vinca alkaloids** (e.g., vinblastine [Velban], vincristine [Oncovin], and vinorelbine [Navelbine]) are obtained from the periwinkle plant. The antimicrotubules or **taxanes** group (e.g., docetaxel [Taxotere] and paclitaxel [Taxol]) were originally procured from the needles and bark of the yew tree, which only grows in the Pacific Northwest. Due to the scarcity of this natural resource, a semisynthetic form of paclitaxel was developed and then approved by the FDA. Docetaxel (Taxotere) is a semisynthetic analogue of paclitaxel. The podophyllotoxins (e.g., etoposide [VP-16, Pepesid], teniposide [VP26, Vumon]) and camptothecan analogues (e.g., Irinotecan [Camptosar, CPT-11], Topotecan [Hycamtin]) interfere with the action of topoisomerase enzymes, causing apoptosis in cancer cells. A few retinoid derivatives (e.g., bexarotene [Targretin], thalidomide [Thalomid]) play a limited role in treating cancer as well. Table 37-6 lists the plant alkaloids and their uses and considerations.

Adverse reactions to plant alkaloids include leukopenia, hypersensitivity reactions, partial-to-complete alopecia, constipation, nausea, vomiting, diarrhea, and phlebitis. The plant alkaloids damage peripheral nerve fibers and may cause reversible or irreversible neurotoxicity. Signs and symptoms of neurotoxicity include a decrease in muscular strength, numbness, tingling of fingers and toes ("stocking/glove" syndrome), constipation, and motor instability. Other adverse effects of these drugs include loss of deep tendon reflexes, muscle weakness, joint pain, and bone marrow suppression. Docetaxel may cause fluid retention. General adverse reactions to chemotherapeutic drugs are listed in Table 37-2.

Vincristine

Vincristine (Oncovin), developed from the periwinkle plant, was originally approved by the FDA in the 1960s to treat Wilms' tumor in children.

Pharmacokinetics Vincristine is given IV. Its half-life is between 19 and 155 hours, and it is primarily (~75%) protein-bound. The drug is extensively metabolized by the liver.

HERBAL ALERT 37-4

Vincristine

- Use cautiously with bromelain (an extract from the pineapple plant), which may improve the efficacy of vincristine. *Catharanthus roseus* (periwinkle) may increase risk of bone marrow suppression when given with vincristine. Schisandra extract (Schisandra, gomishi, Sheng-Mai-San) stimulates hepatic metabolism and may interfere with vincristine, which is excreted through the liver.

TABLE 37-6 ANTINEOPLASTICS: PLANT ALKALOIDS

DRUG TYPE AND NAME	ROUTE AND DOSAGE	USES AND CONSIDERATIONS
Vinca Alkaloids		
vinblastine (Velban)	IV: 1.5-2.0 $mg/m^2/d$ continuous infusion for 5 d	Cancers of the testes, breast, and kidney and treatment of lymphomas, lymphosarcomas, and neuroblastomas. Nausea, vomiting, and alopecia are common side effects. Check CBC before dosing. Pregnancy category: D; PB: 75%; t½: 25 h
vincristine (Oncovin)	IV: 0.4-1.4 $mg/m^2/wk$	Cancer of the breast, lungs, and cervix; multiple myelomas, sarcomas, lymphomas, Wilms' tumor. Assess neurologic difficulties. Used for treating Hodgkin's disease in combination therapy, MOPP (mechlorethamine, vincristine, procarbazine, and prednisone). Do not give intrathecally. Pregnancy category: D; PB: 75%; t½: triphasic 2-85 h (see Prototype Drug Chart 37-4)
vinorelbine (Navelbine)	IV: 30 $mg/m^2/wk$	First-line treatment for ambulatory patients with advanced, unresectable non–small-cell lung cancer (NSCLC). May be used alone or in combination with cisplatin for stage IV NSCLC and in combination with cisplatin for stage III NSCLC. Pregnancy category: D; PB: UK; t½: 27-43 h
Antimicrotubules/Taxanes		
docetaxel (Taxotere)	IV: 60-100 mg/m^2 over 1-h infusion every 3 wk	Advanced or metastatic breast cancer. Inhibits mitosis in cells. Greater antitumor activity with lower toxicity effect than paclitaxel (Taxol). Monitor WBC and platelet count; if low, dose may need to be decreased. Pregnancy category: D; PB: UK; t½: 11 h
paclitaxel (Taxol)	IV: For breast cancer: 175 mg/m^2 over 3-h infusion every 3 wk For ovarian cancer: 135-175 mg/m^2 over 24-h infusion	Metastatic ovarian and breast cancer. Monitor vital signs and electrocardiogram. Long duration of action (3 wk). Peak action is 11 d. Pregnancy category: D; PB: 80%-90%; t½: 5-17 h
Podophyllotoxins		
etoposide (VP-16, Vepesid)	IV: For testicular cancer: 50-100 $mg/m^2/d$ for 5 d For small-cell lung cancer 75-200 $mg/m^2/d$ for 3 d	Testicular cancer, small-cell lung cancer. Give by slow IV infusion (30-60 min), as hypotension is a side effect of rapid infusion. Bone marrow suppression is a dose-limiting toxicity; Pregnancy category: D; PB: wide variation; t½: 6-12 h
teniposide (VM-26, Vumon)	IV: 100 $mg/m^2/wk$ for 6-8 wk OR 50 mg/m^2 twice weekly for 4 wk	Acute lymphocytic leukemia, neuroblastoma, non-Hodgkin's lymphoma. Give by slow IV infusion (30-60 min), as hypotension is a side effect of rapid infusion. Pregnancy category: D; PB > 95%; t½: 5 h
Camptothecan Analogs		
irinotecan (Camptosar, CPT-11)	IV: 180 mg/m^2 over 90 min	Colon and rectal cancer. Can cause early (during administration or within 24 h) and late diarrhea. Pretreatment bowel function (without an antidiarrheal medication) should be maintained for at least 24 h before next dose of chemotherapy is given. Pregnancy category: D; PB > 90%; t½: 6 h
topotecan (Hycamtin)	IV: For ovarian cancer and SCLC: 1.5 $mg/m^2/d$ infusion over 30 min for 5 d every 21 d For relapsed SCLC: PO: 2.3 $mg/m^2/d$ for 5 d	Ovarian cancer, small-cell lung cancer. GI toxicities (nausea, vomiting, diarrhea common). Bone marrow suppression a dose-limiting toxicity. Pregnancy category: D; PB >35%; t½: 2-3 h
Retinoids		
bexarotene (Targretin)	PO: 300 $mg/m^2/d$ for 97 wk	Cutaneous T-cell lymphoma. Associated with birth defects in humans. Do *not* administer to pregnant patients. Pregnancy category: X; PB >99%; t½: 7 h
thalidomide (Thalomid)	PO: 200 mg/d	Multiple myeloma and skin lesions related to erythema nodosum leprosum. Banned by FDA in the 1960s for causing birth defects. NEVER give to pregnant patients. Pregnancy category: X; PB 55%-65%; t½: 5-7 h

Note: Chemotherapeutic doses and schedules will vary depending on protocol, body surface area (m^2), age, functional status, and comorbid conditions. For a full discussion of body surface area in dosage calculation, see Chapter 14.

CBC, Complete blood cell count; *d,* day; *h,* hour; *PB,* protein-binding; *t½,* half-life; *UK,* unknown; *WBC,* white blood cell; *wk,* week.

Pharmacodynamics Vincristine is used in chemotherapy protocols to treat acute and chronic leukemia, Hodgkin's disease, non-Hodgkin's lymphoma, neuroblastoma, sarcoma, Wilms' tumor, breast cancer, and lung cancer. The onset of action begins in a few minutes; however, the therapeutic effect may take several days. *Vincristine is an anticancer drug that is only administered IV.*

Side Effects and Adverse Reactions

Several drug interactions may occur with vincristine (Oncovin). The patient should report all medications that he or she is taking, including OTC medicines and herbal supplements. Serious drug interactions can occur when taking vincristine (Oncovin) and L-asparaginase (Elspar), the cardiac medication digoxin (Lanoxin), phenobarbital (Solfoton), calcium channel blockers, and mitomycin (Mutamycin).

Nursing Process
Patient-Centered Collaborative Care
Plant Alkaloids: Vincristine

Assessment

- Conduct a detailed medication history, including a list of all concurrent medications, including prescriptions, over-the counter medicines, antacids, dietary supplements, vitamins, and herbal supplements to avoid drug-drug interactions.
- Obtain baseline information about patient's physical status. This should include height, weight, vital signs, laboratory values (CBC, uric acid, electrolytes, hepatic and renal studies, cardiopulmonary assessment, intake and output, skin assessment, daily activities status [i.e., ability to perform ADLs], sleep-rest cycle), nutritional status, presence or absence of underlying symptoms of disease, and the use of current or past medications and treatment.
- Assess laboratory results at the beginning of therapy and at specified time intervals (ranging from weekly to monthly) during therapy. Drug may be withheld if red blood cell, white blood cell, or platelet counts drop below predetermined levels.
- Assess CBC, differential, and platelet count weekly.
- Monitor bilirubin levels. Dose may be reduced if bilirubin levels are >1.5 mg/dL.
- Conduct a thorough physical assessment, and document findings. Be especially aware of evidence of neurotoxicity, because this is a dose-limiting toxicity.
- Assess for signs of peripheral neuropathy (numbness or tingling in fingers or toes), loss of deep tendon reflexes, foot drop, slapping gait, and difficulty walking.
- Monitor bowel function. Autonomic neuropathy may lead to constipation and paralytic ileus. The use of vincristine and narcotic analgesics may increase the risk of constipation.
- Assess temperature; fever may be an early sign of infection.
- Monitor for acute bronchospasm.
- Obtain baseline data regarding patient's psychosocial status, including educational level, ability and desire to learn, support systems, past coping strategies, presence or absence of emotional difficulties, and self-care abilities.
- Assess patient and family knowledge related to therapeutic regimen.
- Assess plans for pregnancy (if appropriate).

Nursing Diagnoses

- Risk for infection related to bone marrow suppression
- Risk for constipation related to neuropathic side effects of chemotherapy
- Ineffective breathing pattern related to bronchospasm secondary to rapid infusion
- Risk for injury related to neuropathic side effects of chemotherapy
- Deficient knowledge related to antineoplastic therapy

Planning

- Patient will maintain blood cell values in the desired range.
- Patient will maintain adequate bowel function.
- Patient will be free from neuropathic dysfunction.
- Patient will be free from respiratory complications (bronchospasm).
- Patient/family/caregiver will demonstrate understanding of the chemotherapy regimen, including side effects.

Nursing Interventions

- Assess for signs of respiratory distress during and after administration.
- Monitor for signs of peripheral neuropathy (numbness and/or tingling in hands and/or feet, sensory loss, loss of deep tendon reflexes, paresthesia, foot drop, wrist drop, ataxia).
- Assess IV site carefully. Vincristine is a severe vesicant whose effects are not immediately apparent. Give drug through a large-bore, quickly running IV infusion. Monitor blood counts and laboratory values.
- Extravasation produces severe pain. If extravasation occurs, stop infusion immediately. Do not remove IV device from the patient. Attempt to aspirate residual vesicant from the IV device using a small syringe, and then remove the IV device. Assess the site. Notify health care provider. Apply warm packs for 15 to 20 minutes at least 4 times per day for first 24 hours. For peripheral extravasations, elevate extremity. Tissue necrosis may occur 3 to 4 weeks after infiltration into tissue.
- Administer antiemetic 30 to 60 minutes before chemotherapy, or as prescribed.
- Assess bowel function.
- Administer stool softener or laxative as prescribed.
- Monitor fluid intake and output, and nutritional intake.
- Maintain strict medical asepsis during dressing changes and invasive procedures.

Patient Teaching

General

- Advise patient to promptly report signs of infection (e.g., fever, sore throat), bleeding (e.g., bleeding gums, petechiae, bruises, hematuria, blood in the stool), and anemia (e.g., increased fatigue, dyspnea, orthostatic hypotension).

- Teach patient the signs and symptoms of neurotoxicity (numbness and/or tingling in hands and/or feet, sensory loss, loss of deep tendon reflexes, paresthesia, foot drop, wrist drop, ataxia). Inability to button clothes or to close zippers may be an early sign of peripheral neuropathy.
- Emphasize protective precautions (e.g., hand washing, personal hygiene) as necessary.
- Advise patient not to visit anyone who has a respiratory infection. A decreased WBC count puts patient at risk for acquiring an infection.
- Teach patient signs of "stocking/glove" syndrome (numbness/tingling of hands and feet). This may last as long as 1 year or may never completely resolve.
- Teach patient that complete alopecia may occur. Teach patient that hair will begin to regrow within several months after therapy is completed.
- Teach importance of using birth-control measures as appropriate. Discuss sperm banking with male patients as appropriate.
- Teach patient that in most situations pregnancy should be avoided for 3 to 4 months after completing antineoplastic therapy. Some sources recommend that both men and women avoid conception for 2 years after completion of treatment.

Side Effects

- Teach patient the signs of peripheral neuropathy.
- Teach patient to report constipation and abdominal pain.
- Assess for nausea and vomiting; administer antiemetics as prescribed.
- Advise patient of possible hair loss; recommend a wig, hairpiece, scarf, or turban.
- Teach importance of using birth-control measures as appropriate. Discuss sperm banking with male patients as appropriate.
- Remind premenopausal women that they may experience amenorrhea, menstrual irregularities, or sterility; advise male patient that he may experience impotence.
- Assess for use of alternative/complementary therapy that may interact with chemotherapy agent.
- Teach patient the signs of tissue extravasation, which can occur 3 to 4 weeks after administration of the drug.

Diet

- Encourage bulky high-fiber foods, adequate fluid intake, and moderate exercise to reduce risk of constipation.

Cultural Considerations

- In some cultural groups, health care decisions are made by consensus, and the family plays a key role in filtering information given to the patient. Issues related to informed consent and full disclosure of medical information may cause distress in cultural groups that place the needs of the family above the needs of the individual. Interactions should be modified based on family structure, religious values and beliefs, time orientation, cultural health practices, and verbal and nonverbal communication.
- Cultural assessment tools can provide general guidelines for health care providers.
- Asians may be at increased risk for hyponatremia and SIADH.

Evaluation

- Patient is free from infection.
- Bowel function is maintained.
- Peripheral neuropathy did not occur.
- Side effects of therapy are controlled.
- Extravasation and tissue necrosis did not occur.
- Patient/family/caregiver educational needs are met.

TARGETED THERAPIES

Chapter 38 provides in-depth information on this treatment modality.

LIPOSOMAL CHEMOTHERAPY

A more recent change in the delivery of chemotherapy involves the use of anticancer drugs that have been packaged inside synthetic fat globules called *liposomes*. The fatty coating helps the chemotherapy drug remain in the system longer, decreases side effects (e.g., hair loss, nausea, cardiotoxicity), and increases the duration of therapeutic effects. Encapsulated forms of doxorubicin (Doxil, Caelyx, Myocet), daunorubicin (DaunoXome), and Cytarabine (DepoCyt) are examples of liposomal chemotherapy.

HORMONAL AGENTS

Although **hormones** are not considered true chemotherapeutic agents, several classes of hormonal agents are used in the treatment of cancer. These include corticosteroids, sex hormones, antiestrogens, aromatase inhibitors, gonadotropin-releasing hormone analogues, and antiandrogens.

Corticosteroids

Corticosteroids (glucocorticoids) are antiinflammatory agents that suppress the inflammatory process that is associated with tumor growth. Although the exact mechanism of action is unknown, these agents may block steroid-specific receptors on the surface of cells. This blocking action slows the growth fraction of the tumor, thus retarding its growth. Prednisone (Cordrol, Deltasone), dexamethasone (Cortastat, Dalalone), and hydrocortisone (Hydrocortone, Solu-Cortef) can help decrease cerebral edema caused by a malignant brain tumor. Cortisone drugs give the patient a sense of well-being and varying degrees of euphoria. Cortisone derivatives taken internally produce many adverse side effects, including fluid retention, potassium loss, increased risk for infection, increase in blood sugar, increased fat distribution, muscle weakness, increased bleeding tendency, and euphoria.

Sex Hormones

The sex hormones (e.g., estrogen, androgen) or hormone-like agents are used to slow the growth of hormone-dependent tumors (e.g., prostate cancer, breast cancer). Estrogen therapy is a palliative treatment used to decrease the progression of prostatic cancer in men and to slow the growth of hormone-dependent breast cancer in women. Estrogen preparations suppress tumor growth and may induce remission of the cancer for up to 1 year. Examples of this group of drugs are diethylstilbestrol (Stilbestrol), ethinyl estradiol (Estinyl), chlorotrianisene (TACE), and conjugated estrogens (Premarin).

Progestins may be prescribed to treat breast cancer, endometrial carcinoma, and renal cancer. These drugs (e.g., hydroxyprogesterone caproate [Duralutin]), medroxyprogesterone acetate [Depo-Provera], and megestrol acetate [Megace]) act by shrinking the cancer tissues. Adverse reactions include fluid retention and thrombotic (clot) disorders.

Androgens are given to treat advanced breast cancer in premenopausal women. This male hormone promotes regression of tumors. If androgen therapy is used over a long period of time, masculine secondary sexual characteristics, such as body hair growth, lowering of the voice, and muscle growth, will occur. Antiestrogens such as tamoxifen (Nolvadex) and fulvestrant (Faslodex) are used to treat breast cancer tumors that are estrogen-receptor positive (ER+). Tamoxifen has shown proven efficacy in preventing tumor recurrence in both premenopausal and postmenopausal women, but it has a number of side effects associated with it. These include hot flashes, irregular menses, fatigue, headaches, nausea, and vomiting. Men who take tamoxifen may experience headaches, impotence, and a decreased interest in sexual activity. Tamoxifen increases a woman's risk for developing cancer of the uterus.

Selective estrogen receptor modulators (SERMs) act like antiestrogens to slow tumor growth, but have fewer side effects than tamoxifen. SERM drugs currently in use include raloxifene (Evista) and toremifene (Fareston). A new generation of SERM drugs is currently being evaluated to determine effects on preventing recurrent breast cancer, decreasing postmenopausal bone loss, and reducing the risk of cardiovascular disease.

Prototype Drug Chart 37-4 details the pharmacologic behavior of vincristine (Oncovin).

> **SAFETY: Preventing Medication Errors**
>
> Do not confuse …
> - **vincristine** with **vinblastine**

Gonadotropin-Releasing Hormone Analogues

Luteinizing hormone-releasing hormone (LH-RH) agonists (e.g., leuprolide [Lupron], goserelin [Zoladex]) suppress the secretion of follicle-stimulating hormone and luteinizing hormone from the pituitary gland. Initially an increase in testosterone levels is seen. However, with continued use the pituitary gland becomes insensitive to this stimulation, leading to a reduction in the production of androgens and estrogens.

Antiandrogens

Antiandrogens (e.g., flutamide [Eulexin], nilutamide [Nilandron], bicalutamide [Casodex]) are useful in treating men with hormone-responsive prostate cancer that has metastasized. These agents work by binding to androgen receptors and blocking the effects of dihydrotestosterone on the prostate cancer cells.

Aromatase Inhibitors

In postmenopausal women, the ovaries no longer produce estrogen, but androgen is converted to estrogen in this group of women. The aromatase inhibitors block the peripheral conversion of androgens to estrogens, thus suppressing the postmenopausal synthesis of estrogen and slowing tumor growth. Aromatase inhibitors are used in the treatment of hormonally sensitive breast cancer in postmenopausal women or premenopausal women who have had their ovaries removed. Anastrozole (Arimidex), letrozole (Femara), and exemestane (Aromasin) are examples of aromatase inhibitors currently in use. Increasingly these agents are being used before tamoxifen in postmenopausal women with hormonally responsive metastatic breast cancer. Table 37-7 lists hormonal agents, uses, and considerations.

MISCELLANEOUS CHEMOTHERAPY AGENTS

This category includes a number of antineoplastic agents in which the mechanism of action is unclear. Table 37-7 describes two: asparaginase (Elspar) and pegaspargase (Oncaspar).

Vaccines

Vaccines used to prevent cancer include the hepatitis B vaccine, given to prevent infection with the hepatitis B virus, which can cause liver cancer. Two recombinant vaccines, Gardasil and Cervarix, are given to girls and young women 9 to 26 years of age to prevent HPV infections that can cause cervical cancer. Cervarix is used for boys and young men 9 to 26 years of age to prevent HPV types 6 and 11, which can cause genital warts. Several experimental vaccines have shown promise in the treatment of prostate cancer.

> **SAFETY: Preventing Medication Errors**
>
> Do not confuse …
> - **busulfan** with **Buscopan**
> - **Taxotere** with **Taxol**
> - **floxuridine** with **Floxin**
> - **hydroxyurea** with **hydroxyzine hydrochloride**
> - **Oxaliplatin** with **oxaprozin**
> - **topotecan** with **Toposar**

PROTOTYPE DRUG CHART 37-4

Vincristine

Drug Class
Plant alkaloid/vinca alkaloid
Trade Name: Oncovin
Pregnancy Category: D

Dosage
A: IV: use only via free-flowing IV catheter. 0.4-1.4 mg/m^2 weekly. A 50% reduction in the dose recommended for those with a direct serum bilirubin value above 3 mg/100 mL
C: IV: use only via free-flowing IV catheter. 2 mg/m^2
For children <10 kg, starting dose is 0.05 mg/kg weekly
If peripheral neuropathies occur, reduction or discontinuance of therapy may be needed.

Contraindications
FATAL if given intrathecally
Do not give to patients receiving radiation therapy through ports into the liver.
Hypersensitivity
Do not give to patients with Charcot-Marie-Tooth syndrome.
Caution: Pregnancy, liver or kidney disease, neuromuscular disease, or infection

Drug-Lab-Food Interactions
Drug: Acute life-threatening bronchospasm may occur, especially if drug is given with mitomycin (Mutamycin).
L-asparaginase (Elspar) may reduce hepatic clearance of vincristine.
Vincristine decreases digoxin effects. Monitor digoxin levels.
Vincristine decreases phenytoin effects. Monitor patient for seizure activity.
Do not dilute in solutions that increase or decrease pH outside a range of 3.5-5.5.
Mix only with normal saline or glucose in water.
Herb: Use cautiously with bromelain (pineapple extract). *Catharanthus roseus* (periwinkle) may increase risk of bone marrow suppression when given with vincristine.
Lab: May cause hyponatremia, hyperuricemia, anemia, leukopenia, thrombocytopenia.

Pharmacokinetics
Absorption: IV
Distribution: PB: 75%
Metabolism: Liver $t_{1/2}$: first phase, 5 min; second phase, 2¼ h; terminal phase, 85 h
Excretion: 80% in feces; 10%-20% in urine
Nadir: 7-10 d

Pharmacodynamics
Effects on blood count: Decreased
IV: Onset: 7 d
Peak: 10-14 d
Duration: 21 d

Therapeutic Effects/Uses
Acute leukemia, Hodgkin's disease, non-Hodgkin's lymphoma, neuroblastoma, rhabdomyosarcoma, Ewing's sarcoma, Wilms' tumor, multiple myeloma, acute and chronic leukemia, breast and lung cancers
Mode of Action: Affects cells in the M phase of the cell cycle, and inhibits mitosis

Side Effects
Peripheral neuropathy, loss of deep tendon reflexes, phlebitis, constipation, cramps, nausea, vomiting, muscle weakness, reversible alopecia

Adverse Reactions
Sensory loss, hypotension, visual disturbances, ptosis, ileus, SIADH, hyponatremia, hyperuricemia, severe local reaction with extravasation, fever
Life-threatening: intestinal necrosis, seizures, coma, acute bronchospasm, bone marrow suppression

d, Day; *h,* hour; *IV,* intravenous; *PB,* protein-binding; *SIADH,* syndrome of inappropriate antidiuretic hormone secretion; $t_{1/2}$, half-life; ≤, less than or equal to.

TABLE 37-7 ANTINEOPLASTICS: HORMONES, HORMONE ANTAGONISTS, AND MISCELLANEOUS

DRUG TYPE AND NAME	ROUTE AND DOSAGE	USES AND CONSIDERATIONS
Androgens		
testolactone (Teslac)	PO: 250 mg 4 times/d	Palliative treatment of breast carcinoma in postmenopausal women. Monitor serum calcium levels. Voice may deepen, and facial hair may increase. Pregnancy category: D; PB: UK; $t_{1/2}$: UK
Hormonal Antagonists		
aminoglutethimide (Cytadren)	PO: 750-2000 mg/d in divided doses	Adrenal carcinoma, ectopic adrenocorticotropic hormone (ACTH)-producing tumors. Suppresses adrenal activity. May be used in breast cancer therapy. Treatment typically lasts for 3 mo. Pregnancy category: D; PB: 20%-25%; $t_{1/2}$: 7-15 h
anastrozole (Arimidex) bicalutamide (Casodex)	PO: anastrozole 1 mg/d bicalutamide 50 mg/d	Advanced breast cancer in postmenopausal women. Diarrhea, headache, hot flashes, pain, hypertension, and dyspnea might occur. Pregnancy category: D; PB: 40%; $t_{1/2}$: 50 h
exemestane (Aromasin)	PO: 25 mg/d	Advanced metastatic prostatic carcinoma. Pregnancy category: X; PB: UK; $t_{1/2}$: 5.8 d
flutamide (Eulexin)	PO: 250 mg every 8 h	Advanced breast cancer in postmenopausal women. Prostatic cancer. Pregnancy category: D; PB: UK; $t_{1/2}$: 24 h

TABLE 37-7 ANTINEOPLASTICS: HORMONES, HORMONE ANTAGONISTS, AND MISCELLANEOUS—cont'd

DRUG TYPE AND NAME	ROUTE AND DOSAGE	USES AND CONSIDERATIONS
fulvestrant (Faslodex)	IM: 500 mg as 2 5-mL injections, one in each buttock on days 1, 15, and 29 and once monthly thereafter	Metastatic prostatic carcinoma, usually in combination with other anticancer drugs. Pregnancy category: D; PB: 95%; t½: 5-10 h
goserelin acetate (Zoladex)	subQ: 3.6 mg/mo in upper abdominal wall every 28 d	Treatment of hormone-receptor positive metastatic breast cancer in postmenopausal women whose disease has progressed after antiestrogen therapy. Pregnancy category: D; PB: 99%; t½: 40 d
histrelin acetate implant (Vantas)	SubQ implant: 50 mg implanted under skin on upper, inner arm, every 12 months (remove old implant before placing new one)	Treatment of advanced prostate cancer. A small, thin implant is placed under the skin of the arm. Drug works for 12 mo, and then implant needs to be replaced. Pregnancy category: X; PB: 70%; t½: 3 h
letrozole (Femara)	PO: 2.5 mg/d	Metastatic prostatic carcinoma. Drug is a synthetic luteinizing hormone-releasing analogue. May also be used in breast cancer and endometriosis. Gynecomastia, breast swelling, and hot flashes may occur. Pregnancy category: X; PB: UK; t½: 4-6 h
leuprolide (Lupron, Viadur)	IM: Depot suspension 7.5 mg every mo Viadur implant 65 mg every 12 mo	Advanced breast cancer in postmenopausal women. Decreases estrogen biosynthesis. May be more effective than megestrol acetate and aminoglutethimide. Pregnancy category: UK; PB: UK; t½: 2 d
	subQ: 1 mg/d	Used to slow the growth of prostate cancer. Can be given daily (Lupron) or at 3- or 4-mo intervals (Lupron Depot). May be used to treat endometriosis. Hypersensitivity reactions may occur in people with allergy to benzyl alcohol. Pregnant patients should not take this drug (high risk of fetal damage). Pregnancy category: X; PB: 49%; t½: 3 h
megestrol acetate (Megace)	PO: 800 mg/d	Palliative treatment of advanced carcinoma of breast and endometrium. May Promote weight gain by increasing appetite. Pregnancy category: X; PB: UK; t½: 15-20 h
mitotane (Lysodren)	PO: 2-16 g/d	Palliative treatment of inoperable adrenal cortical carcinoma. Adverse reactions include hemorrhagic cystitis, hypouricemia, and hypercholesterolemia. Monitor vital signs. Pregnancy category: C; PB: UK; t½: 20-160 d
nilutamide (Nilandron)	PO: 300 mg/d for 30 d, then maintenance dose	Prostatic carcinoma. Loss of libido and sexual potency may occur. Monitor liver function. Pregnancy category: C: PB: UK: t½: 24-72 h
tamoxifen citrate (Nolvadex)	PO: 20 mg/d	Palliative treatment of advanced breast carcinoma with positive lymph nodes in postmenopausal women. Competes with estradiol at estrogen receptor sites. Decreases DNA synthesis. Reduces risk of breast cancer in postmenopausal women. Pregnancy category: D; PB: UK; t½: 7 d
raloxifene (Evista)	PO: 60 mg daily	Selective estrogen receptor modulator (SERM) originally approved to fight osteoporosis in postmenopausal women. Reduces risk of breast cancer with fewer side effects than tamoxifen. Pregnancy category: X; PB: 95%; t½: 27 h
toremifene citrate (Fareston)	PO: 60 mg/d	Advanced breast cancer in postmenopausal women. An antiestrogen drug. Pregnancy category: D; PB: >99%; t½: 5 d
Miscellaneous Enzymes		
asparaginase (Elspar, L-asparaginase)	IV: For leukemia induction: 200 units/kg/d for 28 d	Acute lymphocytic leukemia. Used in combination with another anticancer drug. Common side effects include nausea, vomiting, anorexia, leukopenia, and impaired pancreatic function. Pregnancy category: C; PB: 30%; t½: 8-30 h (IV)
pegaspargase (Oncaspar)	Teenagers up to 21 years of age: 2500 units/m^2 every 14 d C: BSA 0.6 m 2500 units/m every 14 d	Acute lymphoblastic leukemia. CCS agent that affects G1 phase of cell cycle. Interferes with DNA, RNA, and protein synthesis. Pregnancy category: C; PB: UK; t½: 1.4-5.2 d
Vaccines		
Hepatitis B (Engerix-B, Recombivax HB)	IM: given in a series of 3 doses: 0, 1, and 3 mo	First anticancer vaccine. Prevents hepatitis B and its serious consequences such as hepatocellular carcinoma (liver cancer).
Gardasil (quadrivalent human papillomavirus [types 6, 11, 16, 18] recombinant vaccine)	IM: 0.5 mL given in a series of 3 shots (0, 2, and 6 mo) in deltoid region of upper arm	For vaccination of women 9 to 26 years of age for prevention of diseases caused by human papillomavirus (HPV) types 6, 11 (genital warts), 16, and 18 (cervical cancer).
Cervarix	IM: 0.5 mL given in a series of 3 shots (0, 1, and 6 mo) in deltoid region of upper arm	For prevention of cervical cancer and precancerous lesions associated with most common cancer-causing HPV types.

Note: Chemotherapeutic doses and schedules will vary depending on protocol, body surface area (m^2), age, functional status, and comorbid conditions. For a full discussion of body surface area in dosage calculation, see Chapter 14.

CCS, Cell cycle–specific; *d,* day; *DNA,* deoxyribonucleic acid; *h,* hour; *IV,* intravenous; *min,* minute; *mo,* month; *PB,* protein-binding; *RNA,* ribonucleic acid; *t½,* half-life; *UK,* unknown; *wk,* week; *>,* greater than.

KEY WEBSITES

Agency for Healthcare Research and Quality: *www.ahrq.gov*
National Cancer Institute: *www.nci.nih.gov/cancertopics/chemotherapy-and-you*
Oncology Nursing Society: *www.ons.org/ClinicalResources*

CRITICAL THINKING CASE STUDY

A 63-year-old patient, recently diagnosed with breast cancer, is scheduled to receive combination chemotherapy consisting of IV fluorouracil (5-FU, Adrucil), doxorubicin (Adriamycin), and cyclophosphamide (Cytoxan). This therapy is designated by the acronym *FAC (fluorouracil, Adriamycin, cyclophosphamide)*. The patient's treatment regimen consists of the following: fluorouracil, 500 mg/m^2 IV, Day 1; doxorubicin 50 mg/m^2 IV, Day 1; cyclophosphamide, 500 mg/m^2 IV, Day 1. This cycle is to be repeated every 21 days for 6 cycles.

1. Differentiate the drug actions of fluorouracil, doxorubicin, and cyclophosphamide.
2. What side effects and adverse reactions should the nurse assess for during therapy? Why would assessment of the cardiac, GI, and genitourinary systems be important with this drug regimen?
3. What is the maximum lifetime dose for doxorubicin? Why is this so important?
4. Describe the early signs of cardiotoxicity that might be seen days to months after the administration of doxorubicin.
5. Briefly explain why hydration would be important during this drug regimen.
6. What nursing interventions would be appropriate when caring for this patient?
7. Describe the teaching that the nurse would provide to the patient and her family.
8. After two cycles of chemotherapy, the patient complains that her mouth feels sore and that it hurts to eat. Which chemotherapy agent is most likely responsible for this finding? What nursing interventions would be initiated to address this problem?
9. Analyze protective measures necessary to avoid accidental exposure to chemotherapy agents during administration.
10. The patient calls the outpatient oncology clinic and tells the nurse that she has a temperature of 101°F (38.3°C). What actions should the nurse take to address this issue?

NCLEX STUDY QUESTIONS

1. A patient is to receive a chemotherapy protocol that includes an alkylating agent, an antimetabolite, and an antitumor antibiotic. The patient asks the nurse why so much chemotherapy is needed. What is the nurse's best response?
   a. A protocol that uses a combination of chemotherapeutic agents works in the S-phase to kill cells.
   b. The rationale for using combination chemotherapy is that it increases the extent of tumor cell kill.
   c. Combination chemotherapy uses drugs that work the same way.
   d. An outcome of the use of combination chemotherapy is that it has no dose-limiting toxicities.

2. A patient is scheduled to receive chemotherapy drugs that will cause myelosuppression. Which action by the nurse will be most important?
   a. Monitor for a change in temperature.
   b. Evaluate gastrointestinal function.
   c. Assess for evidence of cardiac compromise.
   d. Question the patient about changes in sense of taste.

3. The nurse is caring for a patient with colorectal cancer who is to receive fluorouracil. Which symptom will be most important for the nurse to report to the health care provider?
   a. Nausea
   b. Decreased appetite
   c. Stomatitis
   d. Constipation

4. A patient in the outpatient oncology clinic complains of fatigue after receiving chemotherapy. Which nursing intervention will be most appropriate?
   a. Assess for other factors contributing to her fatigue (e.g., trouble sleeping).
   b. Encourage a high-protein, high-calorie diet designed with the patient.
   c. Refer the patient to a physical therapist to develop a strenuous exercise program.
   d. Encourage the patient to sleep as much as possible during the day to ease fatigue.

5. A patient in the outpatient oncology clinic has developed mucositis after receiving fluorouracil. Which statement made by the patient indicates the need for additional teaching about mucositis?
   a. "I will frequently rinse out my mouth with normal saline."
   b. "To relieve my mouth pain, I will use ice pops or ice chips."
   c. "In order to clean my mouth, I will use mouthwash with alcohol."
   d. "Using a soft toothbrush will clean my teeth and freshen my breath."

6. A patient is scheduled to receive high-dose cyclophosphamide via IV infusion as treatment for cancer. Which will be most important for the nurse to include when teaching the patient about cyclophosphamide?
   a. An indwelling urinary catheter will be placed.
   b. Drink at least 2 L of fluid per day.
   c. Empty the bladder every 4 to 6 hours.
   d. Limit fluid intake during chemotherapy.

7. A nurse is administering doxorubicin to a patient in the outpatient oncology clinic. Which information would be most important for the nurse to include in patient teaching?
   a. Blood counts will most likely remain normal.
   b. Complete alopecia rarely occurs with this drug.
   c. Report any shortness of breath, palpitations, or edema to the health care provider.
   d. Tissue necrosis usually occurs 2 to 3 days after administration.
8. A patient diagnosed with cancer is scheduled to receive vincristine. Which nursing assessment will have the highest priority when providing care for this patient?
   a. Degree of alopecia
   b. Increased digoxin (Lanoxin) levels
   c. Decreased phenytoin (Dilantin) effects
   d. Peripheral neuropathy
9. A patient is experiencing mucositis (stomatitis) secondary to receiving chemotherapy. Which symptomatic treatments will be appropriate? (Select all that apply.)
   a. Frequent mouth rinses
   b. Antiemetics
   c. Topical anesthetics
   d. Stress reduction
   e. Antibiotics
10. A nurse is teaching a patient who will receive chemotherapy that will cause thrombocytopenia. Which instructions will the nurse include in the patient's teaching plan? (Select all that apply.)
   a. Use an electric razor when shaving.
   b. Use a soft-bristled toothbrush.
   c. Use aspirin for pain or headache.
   d. Monitor oral temperature daily.
   e. Report any bleeding (gums, petechiae, bruises, hematuria, melana) to the health care provider.
11. The nurse is caring for a patient who has completed a chemotherapy protocol 10 days ago, and the drug's nadir occurs on days 7 to 14. Current laboratory values are hemoglobin 12.8 mg/dL, platelet count 162,000/mm^2, and white blood cell count 2.100/mm^2. Which action will be most appropriate for the nurse to implement?
   a. Wear a gown and mask each time you enter the patient's room.
   b. Advise the patient to avoid every person who has been vaccinated.
   c. Emphasize protective precautions (hand washing, personal hygiene).
   d. Encourage frequent periods of rest.

Answers: 1, b; 2, a; 3, c; 4, a; 5, c; 6, b; 7, c; 8, c; 9, a, c, e; 10, a, b, e; 11, c.

CHAPTER 38

Targeted Therapies to Treat Cancer

evolve WEBSITE

http://evolve.elsevier.com/KeeHayes/pharmacology/

- Animations
- Content Updates
- Key Points
- Review Questions for the NCLEX® Examination
- References from the Textbook
- Unfolding Case Studies

OBJECTIVES

- Compare the mechanisms of action of targeted therapies for cancer with those of standard chemotherapy drugs.
- Distinguish among the different types of targeted therapies for cancer treatment with regard to indications, possible side effects and adverse effects, route of administration, and nursing responsibilities.
- Incorporate the nursing process related to the needs of patients receiving targeted therapies for cancer.
- Develop and evaluate a focused teaching plan for patients/family/caregivers about the use and side effects of targeted therapy for cancer.

OUTLINE

KEY TERMS

As described in Chapter 37 and in the Unit XII opener, cancers develop from normal cells that have sustained gene damage. Cancer cells differ from normal cells in many ways, especially in their unrelenting growth and invasive spread (metastasis). This excessive growth serves no useful function and causes death when cancer cells invade normal tissues to the extent that vital organs can no longer perform their life-sustaining functions.

Traditional chemotherapy is generalized, systemic, chemical, **cytotoxic** treatment that directly kills or severely damages cells. Mechanisms of action for different categories of

The authors gratefully acknowledge the work of Carolee A. Polek, who updated this chapter for the eighth edition.

chemotherapy drugs vary, but the overall outcome is the inhibition of cell division (**mitosis**) and cell death. Often, these drugs damage the cell DNA to prevent DNA replication and formation of new cancer cells (see Chapter 37). This form of treatment has improved cancer control and increased long-term survival. Although these drugs have some selectivity for exerting cytotoxic effects on cancer cells, the drugs also have a toxic impact on many normal cells. As a result, acute side effects of traditional combination chemotherapy are uncomfortable and can be life-threatening. Thus, the cancer cell–killing effect of traditional chemotherapy is limited by the dosages and scheduling regimens needed to reduce toxic side effects on normal cells.

Targeted therapy for cancer treatment differs from traditional cancer chemotherapy by taking advantage of biologic features, such as cellular receptors, enzymes, pathways, or other molecular proteins of cancer cells that either are not present or are present in much smaller quantities in normal cells. Thus, targeted therapies are more *specific* in their mechanisms and effects than traditional cancer chemotherapy agents. The National Cancer Institute's (NCI) defines targeted therapy as drugs or other substances that block the growth and spread of cancer by interfering with specific molecules involved in tumor growth and progression. It is important to remember that, unlike traditional cytotoxic chemotherapy (which exerts its effects by damaging the DNA of nearly *any* cell), targeted therapies require a specific molecular target as the recipient of their effects. The increased specificity of targeted therapies also means that more tests are required on cancer cells to determine whether a target is present in sufficient amounts to make the targeted therapy effective. For example, not all breast cancer cells have the molecular target for trastuzumab (Herceptin), and not all leukemia cells have the molecular target for imatinib (Gleevec). *Cancers that do not have sufficient quantities of the specific molecular target will not respond to targeted therapy.*

PATHOPHYSIOLOGY

Normal Cell Growth Regulation

Genetic Control over Cell Division

As shown in Figure XII-1 at the beginning of Unit XII, which depicts the cell cycle, cell cycle checkpoints must be overcome to enter the cell cycle and continue to progress through each phase of the cycle to mitosis. Initially, general factors determine whether the cell enters the cell cycle.

Signal transduction is a method of communication that allows events, conditions, and substances outside of the cell to influence the cell's decision to divide, not to divide, or to perform its designated function. Some of the known external and internal signaling substances that promote cell division are enzymes; growth factors; adhesion proteins; steroid hormones; and cell-to-cell physical, chemical, and electrical interactions. Figure 38-1 shows a segment of a cell with one interconnecting signal transduction pathway that, when activated, leads to gene activation for those proteins that promote cell division. This pathway can be activated by growth factors binding to their receptors, the interaction of certain drugs with the cell plasma membrane, the presence of adhesion proteins, changes in ion movement (especially sodium and calcium), ligand binding, and other cell-to-cell interactions. When any of these conditions activate the signal transduction pathway, the amount of tyrosine kinases inside the cell is increased.

Tyrosine kinases (TKs) are a family of enzymes that activate other substances by adding a phosphate group (PO_4) to them, a process known as *phosphorylation*. There are many different TKs. Some are unique to the cell type; others may be present only in cancer cells that express a specific gene mutation. Regardless of how a pro–cell-division signal transduction pathway is activated, the result is an increase in TK levels that propagate the signal by activating a variety of transcription factors within the pathway.

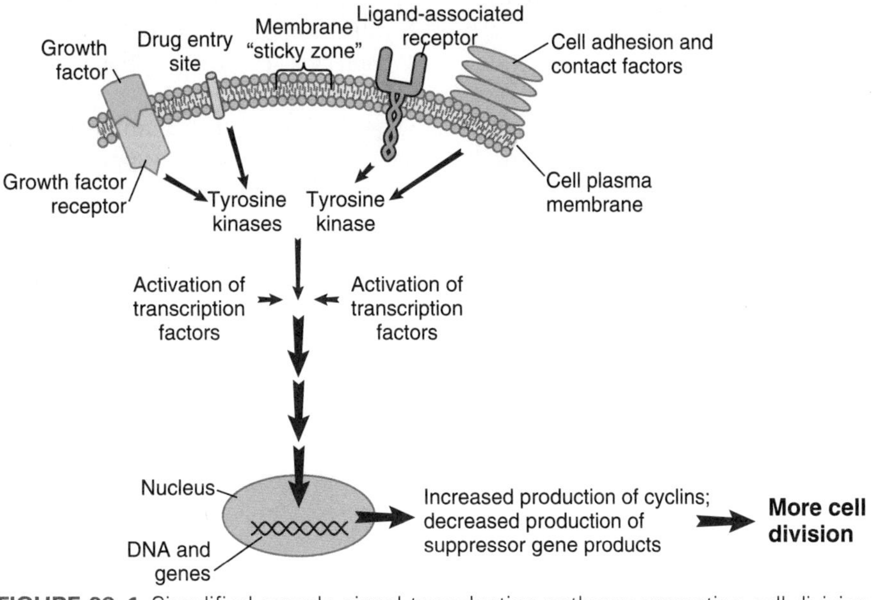

FIGURE 38–1 Simplified sample signal transduction pathway promoting cell division.

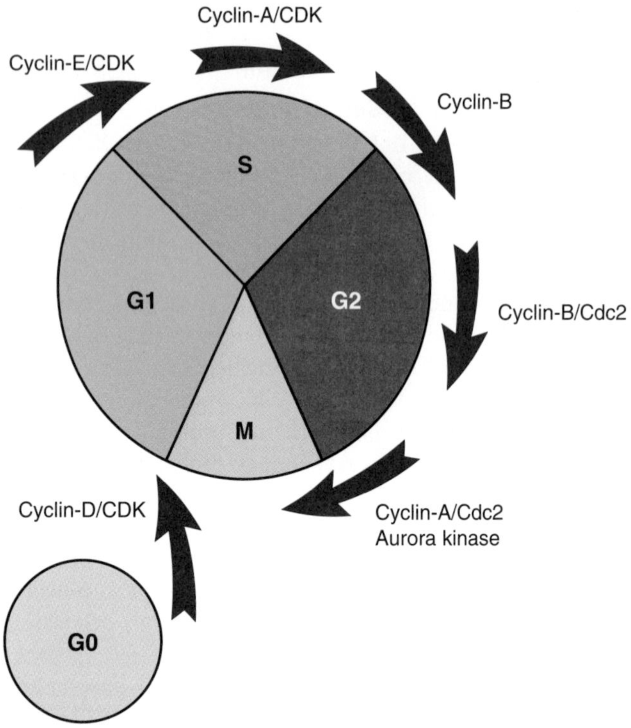

FIGURE 38–2 Cyclin activity promoting progression through the cell cycle.

Transcription factors for cell division are substances that enter the nucleus and signal the cell that mitosis is needed. Many different types of substances serve as transcription factors. The overall response is greater expression of oncogene products (cyclins) that promote cell division, and the reduced expression of **suppressor gene** products that inhibit cell division. When the cell responds to these mitotic signals indicating that cell division is needed and resources are adequate, the cell leaves the G_0 phase and enters the G_1 phase of the cell cycle. Once the cell enters the G_1 phase, the presence of specific cyclins determines whether it can progress to the next phase (Figure 38-2).

SAFETY: Preventing Medication Errors

Do not confuse...

- **trastuzumab** (Herceptin) with **tositumomab** (Bexxar)
- **bortezomib** (Velcade) with **bevacizumab** (Avastin)

Cyclins are part of a family of proteins that, when active, stimulate the cell to move through the cell cycle. They are the products of oncogenes, and most are activated when a phosphorous group is added to the cyclin chemical structure. (Removal of a phosphorous molecule from a cyclin [*dephosphorylation*] inhibits its activity.) Kinases that activate cyclins are *cyclin-dependent kinases* (CDKs). CDKs combine with cyclins to form complexes that initiate cell mechanisms to complete cell division. In normal cells, the oncogenes that produce cyclins are carefully regulated by suppressor gene products so that cell division only occurs when it is needed and to the degree that it is needed.

The amount and type of cyclins as well as which specific CDK is present in the cell during cell division vary by the phase of the cycle. These differences in types of cyclins and CDKs determine when or if a particular cell moves from one phase of the cycle to the next. Many different groups of cyclins have been identified, with the D group being most well understood.

A common signal for entering and starting the cell cycle at G_1 is the combining of a cyclin-D with the appropriate CDK to form a cyclin-D/CDK complex (see Figure 38-2). Movement of the cell from G_1 into the S, G_2, and M phases of the cell cycle is regulated by the continued presence of pro–cell-division transcription factors that promote DNA transcription and increased synthesis of specific pro–cell-division cyclins and CDKs.

Even when cell division is needed, the process is well controlled in normal cells. Proteins synthesized by suppressor genes determine how much oncogene expression is needed to allow cell division to occur but not lead to excessive cell division. Such control is exemplified by normal wound repair. For example, when a person falls and scrapes skin from the knee, the skin cells at the edge of the wound are signaled to divide and fill in the gap. When the wound area is closed, cell division normally stops. The person does not have uncontrolled cell division in this area to the extent that a large skin flap develops over and past the wound site.

When cell division is not needed, external signals, such as growth factor inhibitors and the surrounding of a cell plasma membrane with other cells, send signals that are inhibitory to the pro–cell-division signal transduction pathway (Figure 38-3). The result of this inhibition leads to low levels of TKs and reduced levels of pro–cell-division transcription factors. Instead, suppressor gene activity is increased, resulting in production of more suppressor gene products that inhibit the synthesis of cyclins and CDKs by oncogenes. There are many suppressor genes, and, although all are present in every cell type, specific suppressor genes may be more active in selected types of tissues. For example, the *BRCA1* suppressor gene appears most active in suppressing excessive cell division in breast, ovary, and genitourinary tract tissues. One of the most well-characterized suppressor genes is the *Tp53* suppressor gene. Its gene product restricts the entry of cells into the cell cycle and restricts progression through the cell cycle for many cell types. Without suppressor gene products, oncogenes would be overexpressed continually, leading to uncontrolled and unneeded cell division.

Internal cell conditions, such as poor cell nutrition and reduced energy stores, can trigger the activation of suppressor genes to disrupt the pro–cell-division signal transduction pathway, even when external conditions indicate a need for cell division (Figure 38-4). Thus, healthy and active suppressor genes guard against cell division when it is not in the body's best interest.

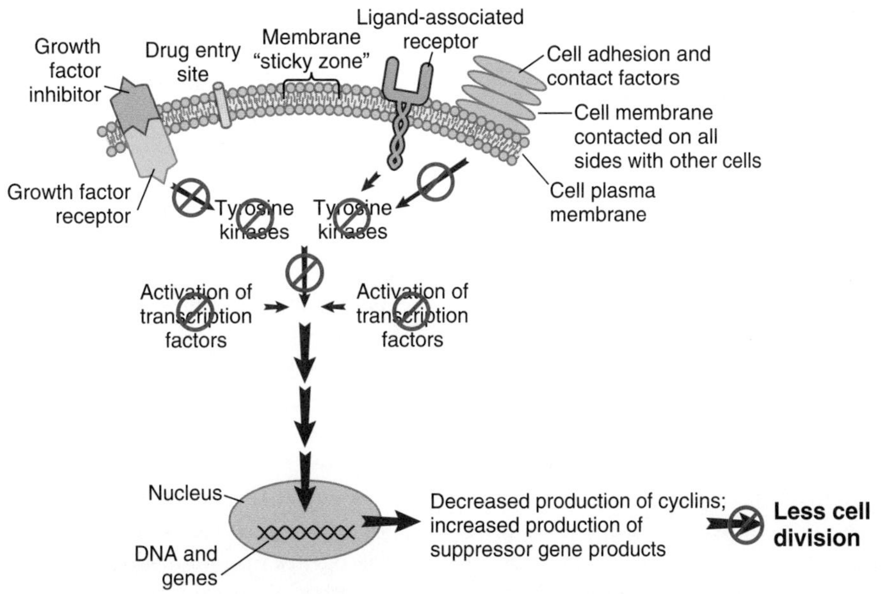

FIGURE 38–3 External signals that inhibit the sample signal transduction pathway, resulting in greatly reduced cell division.

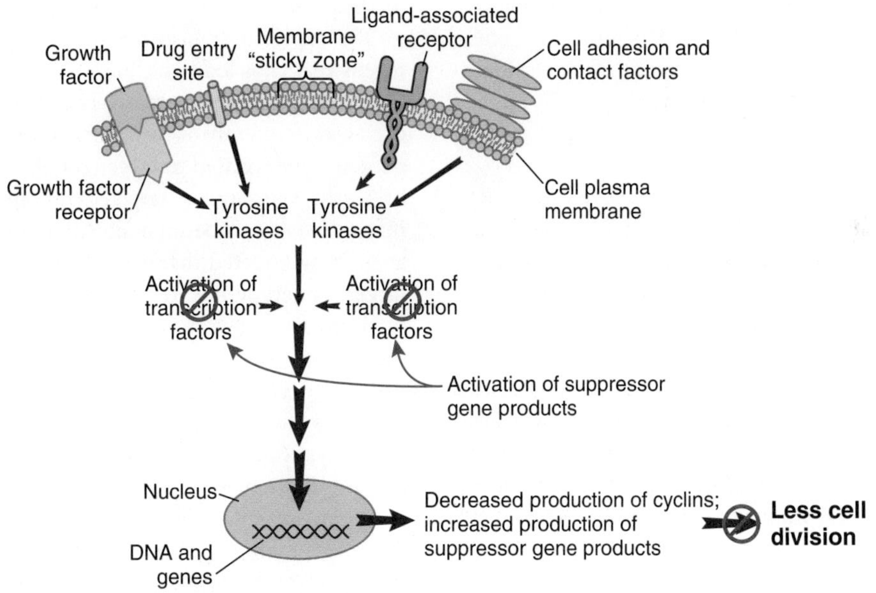

FIGURE 38–4 Suppressor gene activity inhibiting the sample signal transduction pathway, resulting in greatly reduced cell division.

Genetic Control over Cell Death

As some cells age, they begin to function less optimally. When a cell is damaged, reduced function occurs at an earlier cell age. In normal tissues that are capable of cell division, damaged cells and older cells respond to signals for **apoptosis**, which is programmed cell death, intended to ensure that tissues and organs contain only healthy and optimally functional cells. Apoptosis is under strict genetic control in normal tissues so that healthy functional cells do not self-destruct faster than they can be replaced, and that older or damaged cells unable to perform vital functions do not overpopulate a tissue and reduce organ efficiency. Maintenance of optimally functional organs depends on a balance of cell division with apoptosis.

The signals for apoptosis may come from the aging cell with the loss of telomeric DNA. **Telomeric DNA** is special DNA that caps the ends of each chromosome much like plastic tips cap the ends of a shoelace to prevent raveling (Figure 38-5). The function of telomeric DNA is to maintain the integrity of the double DNA strands within each chromosome. With each round of cell division, the telomeric DNA shortens. When the cell has undergone its lifespan's worth of cell divisions, the telomeric DNA that capped the chromosomes is gone, allowing the DNA to unravel and fragment.

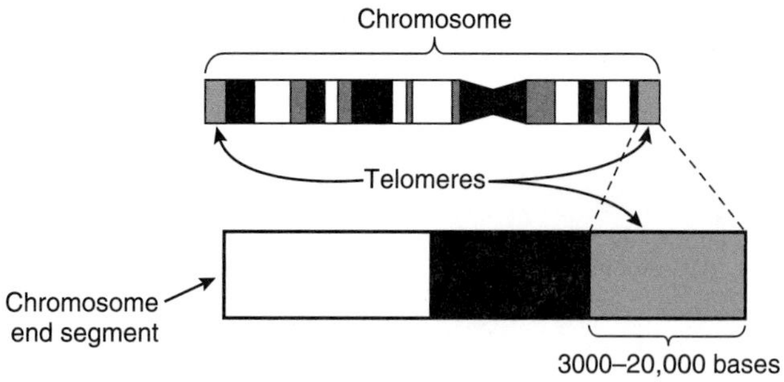

FIGURE 38–5 Chromosome with telomeric DNA and chromosome end segment with telomeric DNA.

These processes then trigger genetic and other intracellular signals for self-destruction through the action of autoenzymes, especially caspase 9. Activated caspase 9 leads to a cascade reaction for rapid activation of many more types of caspase enzymes. These enzymes degrade the cell's internal structures and cause the plasma membrane to lyse and break the cell into small fragments that are removed from the body by white blood cells.

Apoptosis is regulated by different gene products, including those of the *Tp53* (tumor protein 53) suppressor gene. When cells reach a certain age or experience DNA damage, the *Tp53* gene is expressed and older or damaged cells either undergo apoptosis or are prohibited from progression through the cell cycle.

Growth Regulation and Cancer

Loss of Genetic Control of Cell Growth. As stated earlier in the chapter, cancers develop from cells that were once normal. Normal cells become cancer cells when external or internal conditions lead to gene damage. Although cancer can develop from a normal cell that has sustained damage to its oncogenes, most commonly, one or more suppressor genes are damaged and are no longer able to control oncogene expression. As a result of excessive oncogene expression, cyclins and CDKs are overproduced and cell division occurs when it is not needed.

Excessive cell division from gene damage/mutations appears to be self-perpetuating, leading to further gene mutations that do the following:

- Allow one or more specific pro–cell-division signal transduction pathways to become more active
- Allow greater expression of cancer cell membrane receptors that trigger pro–cell-division signal transduction pathways
- Increase or amplify the production of specific TKs and transcription factors

Loss of Apoptosis. Mutations that occur in suppressor genes as a result of DNA damage inactivate the suppressor genes, preventing them from controlling oncogene activity. Some suppressor genes, such as the *Tp53* gene, also regulate apoptosis. Inactivation of suppressor genes that regulate apoptosis makes cancer cells unresponsive to apoptotic signals. These cancer cells are now resistant to natural cell death, a feature known as *cellular immortality*. The combined effects of lack of regulation for cell division and the loss of apoptosis result in cancer cells having no balance between cell division and apoptosis. This unbalanced condition favors continuous cancer cell division.

TARGETED THERAPY DRUGS

Targeted cancer therapies are a relatively new approach in cancer treatment. They work by interfering with cancer cell growth and division in different ways. These drugs are broadly known as *signal transduction inhibitors*. Targeted therapies generally inhibit cancer cell division by blocking a cancer membrane receptor, blocking tyrosine kinase activity, interfering with signal transduction, stimulating an immune system attack on cancer cells, or inducing the cell to undergo apoptosis. These agents may be used as monotherapy (a single agent), in combination with traditional chemotherapy, and with radiotherapy. Some targeted therapies are oral and are self-administered at home where it is convenient for patients; others are administered parenterally. All targeted therapies to treat cancer are categorized as high-alert medications.

The rapid identification of specific cancer-cell targets in recent years has led to an increased development of targeted therapies. Some are in relatively common use, and others are used less frequently or for rarer cancer types. Management of patient issues related to targeted therapies is an evolving area of study. With many targeted therapies being new to the market, costs can be high and may not be covered by insurance. New targeted therapies are approved frequently. Older targeted therapy drugs may be newly approved for use in a different way or with a different cancer type. Expect to see indications for use of different targeted therapies in additional cancer types in the future. Because newly approved therapies have been less widely used and their adverse effects are not yet fully characterized, this chapter focuses on therapies that have been in use for 1 year or more.

There are several major classes of targeted cancer therapies, based on their most common mechanism of action (Table 38-1). Some targeted therapies have more than one action. Those discussed in this chapter include tyrosine kinases inhibitors, multikinase inhibitors, epidermal growth factor/receptor inhibitors, vascular endothelial growth factor/receptor inhibitors, proteasome inhibitors, angiogenesis inhibitors, and monoclonal antibodies. The targeted therapies have been divided into two categories: monoclonal antibody (MoAb) and small-molecule inhibitor.

Tyrosine Kinase Inhibitors

Several types of targeted therapies have as an outcome the inhibition of tyrosine kinases using a variety of mechanisms. Specific drugs that cause this action as their main mechanisms are referred to as **tyrosine kinase inhibitors** (TKIs). The most common TKIs currently prescribed are *imatinib mesylate* (Gleevec) and *dasatinib* (Sprycel). Table 38-1 lists the TKIs and their dosages, routes, uses, and considerations.

TABLE 38-1 TARGETED THERAPIES FOR CANCER TREATMENT

DRUG TYPE AND NAME	ROUTE AND DOSAGE	USES AND CONSIDERATIONS
Tyrosine Kinase Inhibitors (TKIs)		
dasatinib (Sprycel)	A: PO: 100-140 mg once in the morning and once in the evening, with or without a meal.	Approved for chronic myelogenous leukemia (CML) and acute lymphocytic leukemia (ALL). Do not crush or cut tablets; if tablets are crushed or broken, handle with gloves. If patient on antacids, administer 2 h before and 2 h after each dose; Avoid H_2 blockers and proton pump inhibitors (PPIs) Pregnancy category: D; PB: 95%; t½: 3-5 h
imatinib mesylate (Gleevec)	For leukemia and myelodysplastic syndrome: A: PO: recommended starting dose is 400 mg/d for chronic phase and 600 mg/d for accelerated phase or blast crisis. Dose increases to max of 800 mg (given as 400 mg twice daily); can take with meal and large glass of water; drug can be dissolved in water or apple juice. For GIST: A: PO: recommended starting dose is 400 mg/d C >3 y: PO: 340 mg/m^2/d (not to exceed 600 mg/d) PO given as single daily dose, or dose may be divided and given once in morning and once in evening.	Approved for Philadelphia chromosome–positive CML, metastatic malignant GIST, ALL, and MDS. Avoid pregnancy and breastfeeding. Pregnancy category: D; PB: 95%; t½: 18-40 h
Multikinase Inhibitors (MKIs)		
sorafenib (Nexavar)	A: PO 400 mg twice daily Administer orally without food (at least 1 h before or 2 h after meal).	Approved for hepatocellular cancer and advanced renal cell carcinoma. Pregnancy category: D; PB: 99.5%: t½: 25-48 h
sunitinib (Sutent)	A: PO: 50 mg PO once daily on schedule of 4 wk on treatment followed by 2 wk off treatment. Administer orally with or without food.	Approved for GIST and advanced renal cell carcinoma (RCC). Pregnancy category: D; PB: 90%; t½ of sunitinib is 40-60 h, and that of its major metabolite is 80-110 h.
Epidermal Growth Factor/Receptor Inhibitors (EGFRIs)		
cetuximab (Erbitux)	A: IV: initial infusion dose is 400 mg/m^2 IV over 2 h. Then continue weekly infusions of 250 mg/m^2 IV over 60 min.	Colorectal cancer and head and neck cancers. Administer only as an IV infusion with an infusion controller and never as a bolus or IV push. Administer with low-protein–binding 0.22-micron filter. Do not shake or further dilute vial. Do not mix with other drugs. Premedicate patient with H_1 antagonist (e.g., diphenhydramine 50 mg IV) 30-60 minutes before first dose. Pregnancy category: C; t½: 41-214 h
erlotinib (Tarceva)	A: PO: 150 mg once daily Give drug on empty stomach, either 1 h before or 2 h after meal (administering with food increases risk for side effects). Administer at same time each day between meals	Approved for non–small-cell lung cancer (NSCLC) and pancreatic cancer. Pregnancy category: D; PB: 93%; t½: 36 h
gefitinib (Iressa)	A: PO: 250 mg once daily Administer tablet with water without regard to meals.	Approved for NSCLC. Drug may be held for up to 14 d if poorly managed diarrhea occurs. Pregnancy category: D; PB: 90%; t½: 48 h

Continued

TABLE 38-1 TARGETED THERAPIES FOR CANCER TREATMENT—cont'd

DRUG TYPE AND NAME	ROUTE AND DOSAGE	USES AND CONSIDERATIONS
panitumumab (Vectibix)	A: IV: 6 mg/kg administered over 60 min given once every 2 wk	Approved for EGFR-expressing cancers: colorectal, lung, breast, bladder, pancreas, kidney, head and neck. Administer only as an IV infusion with an infusion controller and never as a bolus or IV push. Administer with low-protein– binding 0.2-micron or 0.22-micron in-line filter. Flush line with 0.9% sodium chloride injection before and after administration. Do not mix with other drugs or infusions. Instruct patient to avoid breastfeeding. Pregnancy category: C; t½: 7.5 d
trastuzumab (Herceptin)	A: IV: 4 mg/kg infused over 90 min on week 1. If patient tolerates initial infusion, starting at week 2 administer 2 mg/kg IV over at least 30 min once weekly	Approved for breast cancer that overexpresses *EGFR2* (HER2/neureceptor). Do not administer IV push or as bolus. Monitor patient for infusion-related reactions such as fever or chills, respiratory distress, or severe hypersensitivity reactions. Interrupt infusion if patient experiences dyspnea or significant hypotension. Pregnancy category: D; t½: 25 d
Vascular Endothelial Growth Factor/Receptor (VEGFR) Inhibitors		
bevacizumab (Avastin)	For metastatic breast cancer: A: IV: 10 mg/kg every 2 wk in combination with paclitaxel For colorectal cancer: A: IV: 5 mg/kg every 2 wk in combination with 5-fluorouracil–based chemotherapy. For non–small-cell lung cancer: A: IV: 15 mg/kg every 3 wk in combination with carboplatin and paclitaxel. For metastatic renal cell carcinoma: A: IV: 10 mg/kg IV every 2 weeks in combination with interferon alfa	Approved for metastatic breast cancer, colorectal cancer, NSCLC, and RCC. Administer only as an IV infusion with an infusion controller and never as a bolus or IV push. Administer IV over 90 min as infusion; if tolerated well, may administer second dose over 60 min. Mix infusions with only 0.9% sodium chloride and never with dextrose solutions. Discard any unused portion left in the vial, as product contains no preservatives. Pregnancy category: C; t½: 11-50 d
Proteasome Inhibitors		
bortezomib (Velcade)	For mantle cell lymphoma: 1.3 mg/m^2 IV bolus on days 1, 4, 8, and 11 followed by a 10-day rest period (days 12-21). For multiple myeloma: A: IV: Treatment administered for nine 6-wk cycles. In cycles 1-4, 1.3 mg/m^2/dose IV bolus given on days 1, 4, 8, and 11 followed by 10-d rest period (days 12-21) and again on days 22, 25, 29, and 32 followed by a 10-d rest period (days 33-42) in combination with melphalan and prednisone on days 1-4; this 6-wk cycle is considered one course.	Approved for mantle cell lymphoma (MCL) and multiple myeloma. At least 72 hours should elapse between consecutive doses of bortezomib (Velcade) to give normal cells time to recover. Administered as an IV injection bolus over 3-5 sec followed by saline flush Reconstitute for injection each vial with 3.5 mL of 0.9% sodium chloride for a final concentration of 1 mg/mL. Final product should be a clear, colorless, solution. Pregnancy category: D; PB: 83%: t½: 9-15 h

TABLE 38-1 TARGETED THERAPIES FOR CANCER TREATMENT—cont'd

DRUG TYPE AND NAME	ROUTE AND DOSAGE	USES AND CONSIDERATIONS
Angiogenesis Inhibitors		
temsirolimus (Torisel)	A: IV: 25 mg IV given over 30-60 min once a wk	Approved for advanced RCC. During preparation, protect drug from excessive room light and sunlight. Premedicate with diphenhydramine (Benadryl) 25-50 mg IV, or a similar antihistamine, approximately 30 min before the start of each dose. Two dilutions are required before IV infusion. Use only supplied diluent for initial dilution. Use an in-line polyethersulfone filter with pore size of ≤5 microns and an infusion pump. Administer only through polyethylene-lined administration sets. Administer dose over 30-60 min. Pregnancy category: D; t½: 17-20 d
Monoclonal Antibodies		
alemtuzumab (Campath)	A: IV: Start at 3 mg IV over 2 h once daily. When 3-mg dose is tolerated (infusion reactions grade 2 or less), escalate daily dose to 10 mg IV once daily and continue until infusion reactions are grade 2 or less, then start the maintenance dose of 30 mg IV given 3 times weekly on alternate days (e.g., Monday, Wednesday, Friday); total therapy duration including dose escalation is 12 wk.	Approved for chronic lymphocytic leukemia (CLL). Administer as an IV infusion with an infusion controller over 2 h and never as a bolus or IV push. Monitor patient closely for serious, sometimes fatal, infusion-related reactions. Premedicate 30 min before first dose, with any dose escalation, and as needed with diphenhydramine (Benadryl) (50 mg) and acetaminophen (Tylenol) (500-1000 mg). Withhold alemtuzumab (Campath) administration if a grade 3 or 4 infusion reaction occurs Pregnancy category: C; t½: 12 d
ibritumomab tiuxetan (Zevalin)	A: IV: Step 1: Rituximab 250 mg/m² IV is administered first (see rituximab monograph). Within 4 h of completing rituximab infusion, give 5 mCi (1.6 mg total antibody dose) of In-111 ibritumomab tiuxetan IV over 10 min. Step 2: Seven to nine d following step 1, give a second dose of rituximab 250 mg/m² IV. Within 4 h of completing the rituximab infusion, give Y-90 ibritumomab tiuxetan 0.4 mCi/kg (14.8 MBq/kg) or 0.3 mCi/kg (11.1 MBq/kg) IV over 10 min.	Approved for B-cell NHL. Use appropriate precautions for handling, preparing, and administering radiopharmaceuticals. Do not administer In-111 ibritumomab tiuxetan (Zevalin) and Y-90 ibritumomab tiuxetan unless rituximab (Rituxan) predose has been administered. Do not give Y-90 ibritumomab tiuxetan if platelet count <100,000/mm³). Pregnancy category: D; t½: 30 h
rituximab (Rituxan)	A: IV: 375 mg/m² once weekly for 4 doses; may be retreated for additional 4 doses.	Relapsed or refractory, low-grade, or follicular CD20-positive B-cell NHL. Premedicate 30 min before administration with diphenhydramine (Benadryl) (50 mg), acetaminophen (Tylenol) 650-1000 mg (adults), and possibly corticosteroids. Do not administer as IV push or bolus. Administer first IV infusion at initial rate of 50 mg/h. If no hypersensitivity or infusion-related events, increase infusion rate in 50 mg/h increments every 30 min, to a maximum of 400 mg/h. Monitor patients closely during infusion for profound hypotension, dyspnea, and cardiovascular infusion–related reactions. Do not mix rituximab solution with other drugs. Pregnancy category: C; t½: 31.5-52.6 h

Continued

TABLE 38-1 TARGETED THERAPIES FOR CANCER TREATMENT—cont'd

DRUG TYPE AND NAME	ROUTE AND DOSAGE	USES AND CONSIDERATIONS
I-131 tositumomab (Bexxar) (radioimmunotherapeutic agent)	A: IV: Step 1: Dosimetric step: On day 0, give 450 mg unlabeled tositumomab IV over 1 h followed by I-131 tositumomab 5 mCi (35 mg tositumomab) IV over 20 min. Total body gamma counts using a gamma camera obtained on day 0; day 2, 3, or 4; and day 6 or 7. Using these counts, perform calculations based on standard internal radiation dosimetry methods to determine patient-specific activity (in mCi) of radiolabeled tositumomab required to deliver maximum tolerated dose of 75 cGy total-body dose. Step 2: Therapeutic step: 450 mg unlabeled tositumomab IV over 1 h followed by patient-specific activity (in millicuries) iodine I-131 labeled to 35 mg of tositumomab IV between days 7 and 14.	Refractory CD20-positive, follicular NHL. Administer thyroid protection agents at least 24 h before step 1 and step 2. Do not administer to patients with known murine (mouse) hypersensitivity. Premedicate 30 min before administration with oral diphenhydramine (Benadryl) (50 mg) and acetaminophen (Tylenol) 650-1000 mg (adults). Use appropriate precautions for handling, preparing, and administering radiopharmaceuticals. Administer through IV tubing set with 0.22-micron in-line filter. Use same IV tubing set and filter throughout entire dosimetric or therapeutic step. Administer iodine I-131 tositumomab (Bexxar) infusion over 60 min. After infusion of iodine I-131 tositumomab (Bexxar) is complete, close stopcock to syringe. Flush extension set and secondary IV infusion set with 0.9% sodium chloride for injection. Pregnancy category: X; t½: 8.5 d

d, Day; *GIST,* gastrointestinal stromal tumors; *mBq,* megabecquerels; *mCi,* millicuries; *MDS,* myelodysplastic syndrome, *h,* hour; *min,* minute; *wk,* week; ≤, less than or equal to.

Prototype Drug Chart 38-1 lists specific drug information about the TKI imatinib (Gleevec). Other approved TKIs include lapatinib (Tykerb), which is used with other drugs in the treatment of *HER2*-positive breast cancer.

TKIs exert their effects by directly inhibiting only specific types of tyrosine kinases. The types they inhibit are the SRC kinases, which are present in many cells (normal and cancerous) and a very specific type, the BCR-ABL tyrosine kinase. As shown in Figure 38-1, receptors on the cell membrane can activate tyrosine kinases, which then turn on signal transduction pathways promoting cell division. The TKIs are nonreceptor kinase inhibitors because they do not bind to the receptors on the plasma membrane. Instead they work directly on the tyrosine kinase molecule.

The SRC kinases are involved in the activation of signal transduction pathways promoting cell division in many cell types. The BCR-ABL tyrosine kinase is present only in cancer cells that have a specific gene mutation resulting from a chromosome structural rearrangement that forms a "Philadelphia chromosome." This mutation is highly present in chronic myelogenous leukemia (CML) cells and has been found in some other cancer cell types. When activated and expressed, BCR-ABL tyrosine kinase turns on a strong pro–cell-division signal transduction pathway that leads to proliferation of cancer cells. TKIs prevent activation of tyrosine kinases, which then inhibits further activation of the signal transduction pathway and stops the proliferation of cancer cells. This action can control the disease but cannot alone eradicate it.

Dasatinib

Dasatinib (Sprycel) is approved for chronic myelogenous leukemia (CML) and acute lymphocytic leukemia (ALL).

Pharmacokinetics Dasatinib is an oral drug that is readily absorbed from the gastrointestinal (GI) tract and can be taken with or without food. Antacids slow the absorption. The drug is extensively metabolized in the liver by the cytochrome P450 (CYP) 3A4 isoenzyme.

Pharmacodynamics Dasatinib most specifically targets BCR-ABL tyrosine kinase, found in CML cells. The drug blocks the ATP (adenosine triphosphase) binding site on the tyrosine kinase so that it does not become activated. This lack of BCR-ABL tyrosine kinase activation inhibits further activation of the signal transduction pathway and stops the proliferation of cancer cells. The drug has the greatest effects on cancer cells expressing the Philadelphia chromosome genetic mutation.

Side Effects and Adverse Reactions. Dasatinib often causes electrolyte imbalances, especially low serum levels of phosphorus and calcium. These imbalances may require phosphorus and calcium replacement. ECG abnormalities, especially prolonged QT interval, have been seen in patients taking dasatinib. This drug should be used cautiously in anyone at risk for long QT, such as those who have hypokalemia or hypomagnesemia and those with a family history of long QT syndrome. Fluid retention has also been seen in up to 50% of patients. Hematologic side effects of myelosuppression with anemia, thrombocytopenia, and neutropenia are relatively common.

Drug Interactions. CYP3A4 enzyme inhibitors decrease dasatinib metabolism, resulting in an increased serum concentration and increased risk for toxicity. Other drugs that

PROTOTYPE DRUG CHART 38-1

Imatinib Mesylate

Drug Class	Dosage
Tyrosine kinase inhibitor Trade Name: Gleevec Pregnancy Category: D	Leukemias; myelodysplastic syndrome; GIST: A: PO: Recommended starting dose is 400 mg/d for chronic phase and 600 mg/d for accelerated phase or blast crisis. Dose increases to max of 800 mg (given as 400 mg twice daily); C >3 y: PO: 260 mg/m^2/day PO given as a single daily dose, or the dose may be divided given once in the morning and once in the evening.
Contraindications	**Drug-Lab-Food Interactions**
Patients who may become pregnant, are pregnant, or are breastfeeding; have severe heart failure or severe kidney disease; have moderate to severe liver disease and are also taking another hepatotoxic chemotherapy drug(s); or have severe neutropenia, anemia, or thrombocytopenia	Drug: Any agent that inhibits cytochrome P450 (CYP) 3A4 may decrease the metabolism of imatinib and increase imatinib concentrations leading to an increased incidence of adverse reactions (examples include ketoconazole, amiodarone, antiretroviral protease inhibitors, dalfopristin quinupristin, and mifepristone). Any drug that induces cytochrome P450 (CYP) 3A4 may increase the metabolism of imatinib and decrease imatinib concentrations and clinical effects (examples include barbiturates, bosentan, carbamazepine, dexamethasone, phenobarbital, rifabutin, and rifapentine). Any drug that is metabolized by cytochrome P450 (CYP) 2D6 may have higher than normal blood levels of the drug (examples include amoxapine, atomoxetine, carvedilol, metoprolol, propranolol, timolol, clozapine, codeine, cyclobenzaprine, darifenacin, fenfluramine, dexfenfluramine, dextromethorphan, flecainide, haloperidol, hydrocodone, maprotiline, methadone, methamphetamine, mexiletine, morphine, oxycodone, paroxetine, perphenazine, propafenone, risperidone, thioridazine, tramadol, trazodone, tricyclic antidepressants, and venlafaxine). St. John's wort decreases imatinib blood levels and may decrease its effectiveness. Taking imatinib with acetaminophen increases the risk for acetaminophen poisoning. Taking imatinib with NSAIDs increases hypertension and disruption of platelet aggregation. Taking imatinib with warfarin increases the risk for severe bleeding. Lab: May alter liver enzyme levels and bilirubin levels. Food: Grapefruit juice increases imatinib plasma concentrations.
Pharmacokinetics	**Pharmacodynamics**
Absorption: Bioavailability is 98%. Steady-state levels achieved in 1-2 days. Distribution: 95% PB with extensive distribution Metabolism: Metabolized mainly in the liver by the cytochrome P450 (CYP) 3A4 and CYP2D6 isoenzymes; t½ of drug is 18 hours, of its major metabolite 40 hours. Excretion: Mainly in the feces	Oral absorption is fast and not affected by meal timing. Can take with meal and large glass of water; drug can be dissolved in water or apple juice.
Therapeutic Effects/Uses	
Approved for leukemia, GIST, and MDS Mode of Action: Imatinib competitively inhibits the ATP binding site on tyrosine kinases specific for Abl, PDGF, SCF, and c-Kit, preventing the activation of those specific tyrosine kinases. This action inhibits platelet-derived growth factor (PDGF) and stem cell factor (SCF) mediated cellular events. This leads to reduced cancer cell division and induction of apoptosis. This action results in blockage of downstream EGFR-TK mediated signal transduction pathways, cell cycle arrest, and inhibition of angiogenesis.	
Side Effects	**Adverse Reactions**
Edema, fluid retention, GI irritation, nausea, vomiting, neutropenia, thrombocytopenia, and hepatotoxicity	Allergic reactions, severe neutropenia increasing the risk for infection, severe thrombocytopenia increasing the risk for excessive bleeding/hemorrhage, liver impairment, kidney impairment.

A, Adult; *GIST,* gastrointestinal stromal tumors; *MDS,* myelodysplastic syndrome, *PB,* protein-binding; *PO,* by mouth; *t ½,* half-life; *y,* year; >, greater than.

strongly increase the serum concentration of dasatinib include atazanavir, clarithromycin, indinavir, itraconazole, ketoconazole, nefazodone, nelfinavir, ritonavir, saquinavir, telithromycin, triazolobenzodiazepines, and voriconazole.

Drugs that enhance the activity of the CYP3A4 enzyme decrease dasatinib serum levels and reduce its effectiveness. Such drugs include aminoglutethimide, barbiturates, carbamazepine, dexamethasone, griseofulvin, modafinil, nafcillin, phenytoin, primidone, rifabutin, and rifampin. Other drugs that appear to reduce the effectiveness of dasatinib include antacids, H_2 blockers, and proton pump inhibitors.

Dasatinib may interfere with the metabolism of other drugs that use the CYP3A4 enzyme system, such as alfentanil, astemizole, terfenadine, cisapride, cyclosporine, fentanyl, pimozide, quinidine, sirolimus, tacrolimus, and ergot alkaloids.

Multikinase Inhibitors

The **multikinase inhibitors** (MKIs) are chemicals that directly inhibit the activity of specific kinases in cancer cells and in cancer cell vasculature. (Recall that kinases are enzymes that activate other proteins, including those that activate signal transduction pathways promoting cancer cell division.) Table 38-1 lists the MKIs and their dosages, routes, uses, and considerations.

Sorafenib

Sorafenib (Nexavar) is a multikinase inhibitor that specifically targets serine/threonine and receptor tyrosine kinases, which are activated as a result of gene mutations and are most commonly found in pancreatic cancer, colon cancer, and non–small-cell lung cancer. In addition, the drug may be used in those hepatocellular carcinomas and renal cell carcinomas that overexpress the target.

Pharmacokinetics Sorafenib (Nexavar) is an oral drug whose absorption and bioavailability are inhibited when taken with a high-fat meal. The drug is metabolized in the liver, mainly by the CYP3A4 enzyme system. It is 99.5% protein-bound and reaches peak plasma level in about 3 hours. The drug is eliminated in the feces and urine, with a half-life of 25 to 48 hours.

Pharmacodynamics Sorafenib inhibits Raf kinase, vascular endothelial growth factor (VEGF) receptors VEGFR-2 and VEGFR-3, platelet-derived growth factor receptor (PDGFR), Kit receptor tyrosine kinase (KIT), fms-like tyrosine kinase 3 (FLT-3), and RET. When cytokines or growth factors activate these tyrosine kinase receptors, a protein-kinase–mediated cascade starts, leading to uncontrolled cellular proliferation. The inhibition of these signaling pathways by sorafenib results in decreased cancer cellular proliferation. In addition, sorafenib specifically inhibits two VEGF receptors (VEGFR-2 and VEGFR-3), which are key receptor tyrosine kinases involved in angiogenesis. This action results in reduced blood vessel formation in cancer cells. This anticancer activity is present only when the drug is present, and cancer growth returns when therapy is completed.

Side Effects and Adverse Reactions. Sorafenib has many common side effects. Hypertension is very common and can occur within the first 6 weeks of therapy. Skin side effects include alopecia, pruritus, dry skin, exfoliative dermatitis, acne, flushing, and palmar-plantar erythrodysesthesia (hand-foot syndrome), which also manifest within the first 6 weeks. Other side effects include weight loss, nausea/vomiting, diarrhea, anorexia, constipation, abdominal pain, mucositis, dyspepsia, dysphagia, and mild neutropenia and thrombocytopenia. More severe effects are possible, including pancreatitis, erectile dysfunction, and myocardial ischemia.

Drug Interactions. Sorafenib levels are not increased by the presence of other drugs, even those that inhibit the enzyme that metabolizes sorefenib. However, drugs that induce metabolizing enzyme activity can reduce the blood levels and effectiveness of sorafenib. These include rifampin, phenytoin, phenobarbital, carbamazepine, dexamethasone, rifabutin, and rifapenten.

Sorafenib can increase the blood levels of rapaglinide, amiodarone, ibuprofen, loperamide, irinotecan, propofol, and warfarin.

Sunitinib

Sunitinib (Sutent) inhibits more than 80 tyrosine kinases. This inhibition results in regression of tumor growth, especially in clear cell renal cell carcinoma (RCC) and gastrointestinal stromal tumors (GIST).

Pharmacokinetics Sunitinib is an oral drug that is well absorbed with or without meals. It is 90% protein-bound and reaches peak plasma levels in 6 to 12 hours. The drug is metabolized in the liver, mainly by the CYP3A4 enzyme system, and is eliminated in the feces. The half-life of sunitinib is 40 to 60 hours, and its major active metabolite has a half-life of 80 to 110 hours.

Pharmacodynamics The action of sunitinib is the inhibition of many receptor tyrosine kinases (RTKs), including those of platelet-derived growth factor receptors (PDGFR), vascular endothelial growth factor receptors (VEGFR1, VEGFR2, VEGFR3), and a variety of others. This inhibition results in decreased cancer cell proliferation and in reduced blood vessel formation in cancer cells. This drug also increases adverse effects on normal tissues, especially hair and skin.

Side Effects and Adverse Reactions. Side effects and adverse reactions are more widespread as a result of the number of different types of kinases sunitinib inhibits. Cardiovascular effects include hypertension, peripheral edema, left ventricular dysfunction, prolonged QT interval, and venous thromboembolism. GI effects include nausea/vomiting, diarrhea, stomatitis, and dyspepsia. Neuromuscular effects include fatigue, asthenia, headache, dizziness, peripheral neuropathy, mild arthralgia, limb pain, myalgia, and back pain. Liver impairment may occur with elevated liver enzyme levels and jaundice of the skin and sclera. Common integumentary changes include depigmentation of the skin, skin discoloration, rash, dry skin, and palmar-plantar erythrodysesthesia. Endocrine changes may include hypothyroidism and adrenal insufficiency. Hematologic changes may include myelosuppression. Respiratory-associated effects may include mild dyspnea and cough.

Drug Interactions. Sunitinib's blood levels and activity are increased by drugs that inhibit CYP3A4 enzyme levels, including atazanavir, clarithromycin, ketoconazole, itraconazole, indinavir, nefazodone, nelfinavir, ritonavir, saquinavir, telithromycin, voriconazole, diltiazem, and verapamil. When these drugs are used during sunitinib therapy, side effects of sunitinib are more common and more severe. Drugs that increase sunitinib elimination and reduce its effectiveness include rifampin, phenytoin, phenobarbital, carbamazepine, dexamethasone, rifabutin, and rifapentin.

Epidermal Growth Factor/Receptor Inhibitors

The epidermal growth factor/receptor inhibitors (EGFRIs) include erlotinib, gefitinib, panitumumab, and cetuximab. Most EGFRIs ultimately also inhibit tyrosine kinase, but they do it more indirectly than the TKIs. As shown in Figure 38-1, the growth factor receptors on the cell membrane can activate tyrosine kinases, which then turn on signal transduction pathways promoting cell division. The EGFRIs bind to different areas of the epidermal growth factor receptor, blocking its activity so that it cannot activate tyrosine kinase. As a result, the downstream signal transduction pathway for promotion of cell division is inhibited and cell proliferation is severely limited. Table 38-1 lists the EGFRIs and their dosages, routes, uses, and considerations. Prototype Drug Chart 38-2 lists the specific drug information for erlotinib (Tarceva).

Nursing Process
Patient-Centered Collaborative Care

Tyrosine Kinase Inhibitors and Multikinase Inhibitors for Cancer Treatment

Assessment

- Conduct a detailed medication history, including a list of all concurrent medications, including prescriptions, over-the-counter medicines, antacids, dietary supplements, vitamins, and herbal supplements to avoid drug-drug interactions.
- Obtain baseline information about patient's physical status before initiating targeted therapy regimen and during treatment period. Include height, weight, vital signs, and laboratory values (complete blood count [CBC], uric acid, electrolytes, hepatic and renal studies, cardiopulmonary assessment, intake and output).

PROTOTYPE DRUG CHART 38-2

Erlotinib

Drug Class Epidermal growth factor/receptor inhibitor Trade Name: Tarceva Pregnancy Category: D	**Dosage** For non–small-cell lung cancer and pancreatic cancer: A: PO: 150 mg once daily
Contraindications Patients who may become pregnant, are pregnant, or are breastfeeding; have preexisting respiratory problems (pulmonary fibrosis may occur); or are dehydrated or have liver impairment (risk for renal failure is high). Use cautiously in patients with history of peptic ulcer disease or diverticulitis (increases risk for GI perforation).	**Drug-Lab-Food Interactions** Drug: Drugs that increase blood levels of erlotinib and may lead to increased adverse reactions or toxicities include ketoconazole, atazanavir, clarithromycin, indinavir, itraconazole, nefazodone, nelfinavir, ritonavir, saquinavir, telithromycin, troleandomycin (TAO), and voriconazole. Drugs that reduce effectiveness of erlotinib include rifampicin, rifabutin, rifapentine, phenytoin, carbamazepine, phenobarbital, H_2 blockers, and proton pump inhibitors. Lab: Erlotinib may increase INR and lead to increased risk for bleeding. Food: Grapefruit juice increases erlotinib levels and increases the risk for adverse effects. St. John's wort decreases erlotinib levels and reduces its effectiveness. Cigarette smoking also decreases erlotinib levels.
Pharmacokinetics Absorption: Bioavailability is 60%. Distribution: 93% PB. Steady-state levels are achieved in 7-8 d. Metabolism: Liver (CYP3A4 and CYP1A2 enzymes) Excretion: Mainly in feces	**Pharmacodynamics** Give drug on an empty stomach, either 1 h before or 2 h after meal (administering with food increases risk for side effects). Administer at same time each day between meals. Oral absorption is moderately fast and is enhanced with food intake. High gastric pH levels inhibit oral absorption.
Therapeutic Effects/Uses Approved for treatment of non–small-cell lung cancer (NSCLC) and pancreatic cancer. Mode of Action: Erlotinib selectively inhibits activation of epidermal growth factor receptor-tyrosine kinase (EGFR-TK).	
Side Effects Diarrhea and skin reactions	**Adverse Reactions** Ocular changes (inflammation, corneal perforation), GI perforation, skin desquamation, renal failure, hepatic failure.

A, Adult; *d*, day; *h*, hour; *PB*, protein-binding; *PO*, by mouth.

- Assess laboratory studies, including CBC with differential, hepatic and renal studies, electrolytes, and urinalysis at the beginning of therapy and at specified time intervals (ranging from weekly to monthly) during therapy.
- Assess patient and family knowledge related to therapeutic regimen.

Nursing Diagnoses

- Deficient knowledge related to targeted therapy regimen
- Risk for impaired skin integrity related to dermatologic effects and toxicities of therapy
- Risk for infection related to bone marrow suppression
- Risk for deficient fluid volume related to GI effects of therapy
- Risk for electrolyte imbalance related to actions of targeted therapy

Planning

- Patient/family/caregiver will verbalize understanding of targeted therapy as part of an anticancer treatment regimen.
- Patient/family/caregiver will demonstrate understanding of importance of reporting targeted therapy–related side effects and adverse reactions.
- Patient/family/caregiver will verbalize strategies to minimize risks related to targeted therapy–related side effects.
- Patient's side effects will be managed to a level that the patient can tolerate and are not life threatening.
- Patient will remain infection-free.
- Patient's fluid balance and electrolytes are maintained at expected normal ranges.

Nursing Interventions

- Monitor complete blood cell count with differential and platelet count at baseline, once weekly for the first month, every other week for the second month, and at least every 2 to 3 months thereafter.
- Monitor electrolytes regularly during treatment and for 8 weeks after treatment is discontinued, especially phosphorus and calcium levels, because low levels may require replacement.
- Monitor liver function and renal function tests at baseline and at least once monthly during therapy.
- Monitor blood pressure at baseline and at least weekly during therapy.
- Monitor ejection fraction at baseline and periodically during therapy.
- Monitor thyroid function if patient experiences symptoms of hypothyroidism (cold intolerance, hair loss, decreased memory or mental alertness, constipation, bradycardia).
- Monitor adrenal function in patients receiving sunitinib who are exposed to stress (e.g., surgery, shock, trauma, infections).
- Monitor hands and feet for signs of palmar-plantar erythrodysesthesia (redness, pain, swelling or blisters).
- Follow agency policy for safe handling, preparing, administering, and dispensing of targeted therapy agents.
- Administer prescribed premedications according to established protocols for specific targeted therapies.
- Discontinue therapy before elective surgery.
- Sorafenib potentiates the activity of warfarin. Check the patient's INR weekly.

Patient Teaching

- Teach patients to take imatinib with food or with at least 240 mL of water to reduce gastric irritation.
- Teach patients to weigh themselves daily and report a weight gain of more than 2 pounds in 1 day or 4 pounds in 1 week to the health care provider.
- Teach patients to check hands and feet daily for signs of palmar-plantar erythrodysesthesia (redness, pain, swelling, or blisters) and to report these symptoms when they appear.
- Avoid alcohol and nonessential drugs that are cleared by the liver or have liver-toxic effects (e.g., acetaminophen).
- Report symptoms of adverse effects or severe side effects promptly, especially fever, chills, persistent sore throat, swelling, weight gain, or increasing shortness of breath.
- Report symptoms of bleeding immediately, including black stools, emesis that looks like coffee grounds, or easy bleeding/bruising.
- Report symptoms of liver impairment immediately, including stomach/abdominal pain, yellowing of eyes or skin, dark urine, or unusual fatigue.
- Remind women with childbearing potential to avoid pregnancy throughout treatment and for up to 12 months after treatment is completed.
- Advise breastfeeding patients to stop breastfeeding during and for 60 days after therapy.
- Teach patients that drinking grapefruit juice can increase blood levels of most targeted therapy drugs and worsen side effects or adverse effects. Encourage patient to avoid grapefruit juice while receiving targeted therapies.
- Teach patients to avoid using the herbal St. John's wort while receiving treatment with targeted therapies because this agent decreases the effectiveness of most of these drugs.
- Remind patients receiving sorafenib who also take warfarin to keep all appointments for INR testing.

Evaluation

- Patient/family/caregiver education needs are met.
- Patient/family/caregiver understands therapy-related side effects/adverse reactions.

- Patient/family/caregiver understands strategies to minimize side effects/adverse reactions.
- Side effects are managed effectively.
- Patient is free from infection.
- Patient's fluid balance and electrolytes are maintained at expected normal ranges.

Some epidermal growth factor/receptor inhibitors carry a boxed warning for adverse effects. A boxed warning indicates that the FDA has provided notice that a drug may produce serious or even life-threatening effects in some people in addition to its beneficial effects. This warning is printed on the package insert sheet and is bordered in black. Drugs with this warning can still be used, but prescribers are instructed to make certain that such drugs are prescribed only for patients who meet strict criteria and who understand the serious nature of the possible adverse effects.

Gefitinib

Gefitinib (Iressa) is a synthetic anilinoquinazoline that selectively inhibits the epidermal growth factor receptor–tyrosine kinase (EGFR-TK). It is most commonly used in the management of locally or advanced metastatic non–small-cell lung cancer.

Pharmacokinetics Gefitinib is absorbed slowly in the gastrointestinal tract, with 60% reaching systemic circulation. It is metabolized mainly in the liver by the CP3A4 enzyme and is primarily excreted in the feces. The half-life is 48 hours.

Pharmacodynamics Gefitinib selectively inhibits EGFR-TK. This action results in blockage of downstream EGFR-TK–mediated signal transduction pathways, cell cycle arrest, and inhibition of angiogenesis.

Side Effects and Adverse Reactions. Gefitinib can cause conjunctivitis and abnormal eyelash growth. Rash occurs in about 43% of patients. Some patients experience a moderate to low potential for nausea/vomiting and diarrhea. Patients can also experience acne, pruritus, anorexia, and an increase in hepatic transaminases.

Drug Interactions. Gefitinib activity is affected by CYP3A4 enzyme inhibitors, which decrease dasatinib metabolism, resulting in an increased serum concentration and increased risk for toxicity. These drugs include atazanavir, clarithromycin, indinavir, itraconazole, ketoconazole, nefazodone, nelfinavir, ritonavir, saquinavir, telithromycin, and voriconazole. Drugs that lower gefitinib serum levels and reduce its activity include carbamazepine, phenytoin, phenobarbital, rifabutin, and rifampin. Because gefitinib works best in an acid environment, its activity is reduced with the use of H_2 histamine blockers and proton pump inhibitors. When this drug is received by patients on warfarin therapy, the effectiveness of warfarin (Coumadin) is greatly increased and bleeding risks are increased. The dosage of warfarin should be adjusted based on INR results.

Panitumumab

Panitumumab (Vectibex) is a fully humanized monoclonal antibody (Table 38-2). (Refer to the Monoclonal Antibodies section later in this chapter for a more complete description of antibody types.) It is most commonly used in the management of advanced metastatic colorectal carcinomas that express or overexpress EGFR.

TABLE 38-2 SUFFIXES OF TARGETED CANCER THERAPIES

SUFFIX	MEANING
mab	A monoclonal antibody
momab	Composed of only murine (mouse) proteins
imab	Composed of more human proteins (>60%) than murine proteins (~30%)
zumab	Composed of mostly human proteins (95% or more) and only a few murine proteins (<5%)
umab	Composed of only human proteins and no murine proteins
inib	A tyrosine kinase inhibitor
zomib	A proteasome inhibitor

Pharmacokinetics Panitumumab is administered as an intravenous infusion. It is a small immunoglobulin that appears to be eliminated in the feces. The half-life is 7.5 days.

Pharmacodynamics Panitumumab binds strongly to the EGFR when it is overexpressed on malignant cells. It binds specifically to the EGFR on both normal and tumor cells, and prevents formation of a ligand (arm) that usually attaches epidermal growth factor to the receptor. As a result, EGFR-TKs are not activated and the signals are not conducted downstream. Other effects of this drug also include inhibition of cell growth, induction of apoptosis, and decreased proinflammatory cytokine and vascular growth factor production. In addition, binding of panitumumab to the EGFR causes the receptor to be taken into the cell, preventing it from binding to agonists that activate the receptor. Tumors must express EGFR for patients to be candidates for panitumumab.

Side Effects and Adverse Reactions. Panitumumab carries a boxed warning for dermatologic problems and toxicity. Manifestations usually occur within the first 2 weeks of therapy and include erythema, acneform rash, pruritus, exfoliation, rash, skin fissures, acne, dry skin, and paronychia and other nail disorders. Electrolyte imbalances (specifically hypomagnesemia and hypocalcemia) may occur and require replacement. Severe diarrhea can occur when panitumumab is given along with irinotecan. Severe infusion reactions, including angioedema and anaphylaxis, have occurred with hypotension and bronchospasm. Although this reaction is rare, patients should be monitored closely throughout the infusion.

Drug Interactions. This drug has not been shown to be associated with general drug interactions. However, when administered with other EGFRIs, side effects and toxicities are additive and more severe. Panitumumab is not recommended for use in combination with other antineoplastic drug regimens.

Cetuximab

Cetuximab (Erbitux) is a partially humanized monoclonal antibody (see Table 38-2). (Refer to the Monoclonal Antibodies section later in this chapter for a more complete description of antibody types.) It is most commonly used for the management of colorectal and head and neck cancers.

Pharmacokinetics Cetuximab is administered as an intravenous infusion. Steady-state concentration occurs by the third weekly infusion. The half-life is long, ranging from 41 to 213 hours, with a mean of 97 hours.

Pharmacodynamics Cetuximab still contains about 30% mouse proteins. It binds specifically to EGFR on both normal and tumor cells and prevents formation of a ligand that usually attaches epidermal growth factor to the receptor. This action prevents the receptor from binding to agonists that activate it. As a result, EGFR-TKs are not activated and the signals are not conducted downstream. Other effects of this drug also include inhibition of cell growth, induction of apoptosis, decreased proinflammatory cytokine and vascular growth factor production, and internalization of the EGFR. Cetuximab may make cancer cells more vulnerable to other cancer chemotherapy agents and radiation therapy. The drug is most effective in causing regression in tumors that have the wild-type *K-RAS* oncogene and overexpress EGFR.

Side Effects and Adverse Reactions. Cetuximab carries a boxed warning for infusion reactions, usually with the initial dosing, although severe reactions also have been reported during later infusions. Manifestations include rapid onset of airway obstruction, including bronchospasm, stridor, hoarseness, urticaria, and hypotension. Cetuximab is associated with dermatologic changes that typically involve the face, upper chest, and back. An acneform rash occurs in 90% of patients, usually within the first 2 weeks of therapy. Most patients continue to have the rash for at least 28 days after therapy is discontinued.

Drug Interactions. This drug has not been shown to be associated with general drug interactions. However, when administered with other EGFRIs, side effects and toxicities are additive and more severe.

Trastuzumab

Trastuzumab (Herceptin) is a monoclonal antibody that binds to the HER2 protein on the surface of cancer cells that overexpress this receptor. The HER2 receptor is structurally related to the EGFR. The HER2 receptor is overexpressed in some breast, ovarian, and colon cancers. When this receptor is overexpressed, there is increased cancer cell proliferation and increased angiogenesis. Trastuzumab is most commonly used in combination with chemotherapy agents to manage breast, ovarian, and colorectal cancers that have demonstrated overexpression of the HER2 receptor.

Pharmacokinetics Trastuzumab is administered as a weekly intravenous infusion. Its half-life averages 25 days, but it may be present in the blood for as long as 18 weeks after therapy is discontinued. Just like most monoclonal antibodies, trastuzumab appears to be eliminated slowly through the feces.

Pharmacodynamics Trastuzumab is a mostly humanized monoclonal antibody that binds to the HER2 protein on the surface of breast, ovarian, and colon cancer cells that overexpress this receptor. This drug specifically inhibits the proliferation of cancer cells that overexpress HER2 receptors. In addition, binding of trastuzumab to the cancer cell receptor increases killing of these cells through attack by immune system cells, especially natural killer cells and monocytes.

Side Effects and Adverse Reactions. Trastuzumab carries a boxed warning for cardiomyopathy manifesting as congestive heart failure when the drug is used as monotherapy. This risk is increased when the drug is given in combination with other drugs that cause cardiotoxicity, such as the anthracyclines and cyclophosphamide. Hypersensitivity reactions, including anaphylaxis, may occur but are not common. Trastuzumab is associated with headache, dizziness, hypotension, fever, chills, and nausea during the initial infusion. After the initial infusion, these symptoms typically usually do not recur. Other common side effects include headache, muscle aches, and loss of appetite.

Drug Interactions. Trastuzumab can increase the incidence and severity of cardiac dysfunction in patients who receive trastuzumab in combination with anthracyclines and cyclophosphamide. This drug may increase myelosuppressive effects of other antineoplastic agents.

Vascular Endothelial Growth Factor/Receptor Inhibitors

Bevacizumab

Bevacizumab (Avastin) is a humanized monoclonal antibody (see Table 38-1). It binds to vascular endothelial growth factor (VEGF) and prevents the binding of VEGF with its receptors, VEGFR-1 (Flt-1) and VEGFR-2 (Flk-1/KDR), which are found on the surface of endothelial cells. The role of VEGF is critical in angiogenesis, the formation of new blood vessels. In human cancers, increased VEGF expression is associated with increased microvascular density, tumor growth, metastasis, and poor prognosis. The result of bevacizumab therapy is the reduction of microvascular growth and inhibition of metastatic disease progression. Bevacizumab is approved for many types of malignancies, all in combination with chemotherapy.

Pharmacokinetics Bevacizumab is administered as an intravenous infusion, usually every 2 to 3 weeks. The half-life is about 20 days (range of 11 to 50 days) and steady-state levels are achieved in about 100 days. Clearance varies with weight, gender, and tumor burden, with men clearing the drug faster than women.

Pharmacodynamics Bevacizumab binds to the vascular endothelial growth factor receptor (VEGFR) on tumors that overexpress this receptor. The result of this binding is the competitive inhibition of vascular endothelial growth factor with the VEGFR. This action leads to reduced tumor vascularity, the development of tumor necrosis, and reduced metastatic potential.

Side Effects and Adverse Reactions. Bevacizumab carries a boxed warning for GI perforations, wound dehiscence, impaired wound healing, hemorrhage, and fistula formation after surgery. Thus, the drug should not be given within 28 days after major surgery. Hypertension is a common side effect of bevacizumab. Other side effects are associated with hematopoietic suppression, including neutropenia and thrombocytopenia. Proteinuria can be seen in about 36% of patients, and nephrotic syndrome has developed in rare situations. The risk for thromboembolism and deep vein thrombosis is increased among patients taking the drug for colon cancer and non–small-cell lung cancer.

Drug Interactions. No specific drug interactions have been reported with bevacizumab; however, coadministration of drugs with similar pharmacologic effects, especially traditional chemotherapy agents, may cause additive pharmacologic effects, including toxicity.

Nursing Process
Patient-Centered Collaborative Care

Epidermal Growth Factor/Receptor Inhibitors and Vascular Endothelial Growth Factor/Receptor Inhibitors for Cancer Treatment

Assessment
- Conduct a detailed medication history, including a list of all concurrent medications, including prescriptions, over-the counter medicines, antacids, dietary supplements, vitamins, and herbal supplements to avoid drug-drug interactions.
- Obtain baseline information about patient's physical status before initiating targeted therapy and during the treatment period. Include height, weight, vital signs, and laboratory values (CBC, uric acid, electrolytes, hepatic and renal studies, cardiopulmonary assessment, intake and output).
- Assess laboratory studies, including CBC with differential, hepatic and renal studies, electrolytes, and urinalysis at the beginning of therapy and at specified time intervals (ranging from weekly to monthly) during therapy.
- Conduct a detailed medication history, including a list of all concurrent medications, including prescriptions, over-the-counter medicines, antacids, dietary supplements, vitamins, and herbal supplements to avoid drug-drug interactions.
- Assess patient/family/caregiver knowledge related to therapeutic regimen.

Nursing Diagnoses
- Deficient knowledge related to targeted therapy regimen
- Risk for impaired skin integrity related to dermatologic effects and toxicities of therapy
- Risk for infection related to bone marrow suppression
- Risk for deficient fluid volume related to GI effects of therapy
- Risk for electrolyte imbalance related to actions of targeted therapy

Planning
- Patient and family will verbalize understanding of targeted therapy as part of an anticancer treatment regimen.
- Patient and family will demonstrate understanding of the importance of reporting targeted therapy–related side effects and adverse reactions.
- Patient and family will verbalize strategies to minimize risks related to targeted therapy–related side effects.
- Patient's side effects will be managed to a tolerable level and are not life-threatening.
- Patient will remain free from infection.
- Patient's fluid balance and electrolytes are maintained at expected normal ranges.

Nursing Interventions
- When administering monoclonal antibodies intravenously, have resuscitation equipment nearby, and stay with the patient during the first 15 minutes of the infusion. Thereafter, monitor vital signs every 15 to 30 minutes during the infusion and for 1 hour after infusion is complete.
- Examine patient's skin closely at each visit for the presence of erythema, rash, peeling, or blister formation, and rate the severity of dermatologic reactions. Also determine whether infection is present in any nonintact skin.
- Monitor electrolytes regularly during treatment and for 8 weeks after treatment is discontinued, especially phosphorus and calcium levels, because low levels may require replacement.
- Assess lower extremities for deep vein thrombosis at every visit.
- Monitor renal function tests at baseline and at least once monthly during therapy.
- Monitor complete blood cell count with differential and platelet count at baseline, and as often as recommended for specific agents.
- Administer prescribed premedications according to established protocols for specific targeted therapies.
- Follow agency policy for safe handling, preparing, administering, and dispensing targeted therapy agents.
- Gefitinib potentiates the activity of warfarin. Check the patient's INR weekly.
- Before administering trastuzumab, ask whether the patient has a known allergy to hamsters or hamster products.
- With trastuzumab therapy, monitor electrocardiogram and ejection fraction at baseline and periodically during treatment.
- Use with caution in patients older than 65 years of age because the incidence of serious adverse events is higher among older adults.
- Monitor blood pressure at least every 2 to 3 weeks during therapy. Monitor more frequently if hypertension develops.
- Monitor for proteinuria with a urine dipstick before each dose. Patients with a 2+ or greater reading should undergo further assessment, such as 24-hour urine collection.
- Initiate bevacizumab therapy at least 28 days after major surgery or when the surgical incision is completely healed, whichever occurs later. Consider discontinuing bevacizumab before elective surgery or delaying the surgery until 2 months after therapy is discontinued.

Patient Teaching

- Advise patients to seek medical help immediately if chest pain, symptoms of stroke (e.g., change in mental awareness; inability to talk or move one side of the body; sudden numbness or weakness of the face, arm, or leg; seizures), severe abdominal pain, or swelling associated with redness or pain in one leg occurs.
- Report symptoms of adverse effects or severe side effects promptly, especially fever, chills, persistent sore throat, swelling, weight gain, or increasing shortness of breath.
- Report symptoms of bleeding immediately, including black stools, vomit that looks like coffee grounds, and easy bleeding/bruising.
- Advise patients taking erlotinib to immediately report worsening of skin rash; severe or persistent diarrhea, nausea, anorexia, or vomiting; onset or worsening of unexplained shortness of breath or cough; or eye irritation.
- Teach patients to weigh themselves daily and report a weight gain of more than 2 pounds in 1 day or 4 pounds in 1 week to the health care provider.
- Advise patients to notify the health care provider if foaming of urine occurs (an indication of protein in the urine).
- Teach patients to avoid taking NSAIDs, such as aspirin (except for low-dose aspirin), celecoxib (Celebrex), ibuprofen (Advil, Motrin), and naproxen (Aleve), to prevent excessive bleeding.
- Teach patients receiving bevacizumab ways to promote venous return and avoid deep vein thrombosis (DVT), such as avoiding becoming dehydrated, not wearing clothing that restricts circulation, and avoiding smoking cigarettes.
- Remind women with childbearing potential to avoid pregnancy throughout treatment and for up to 12 months after treatment is completed.
- Advise breastfeeding women to stop breastfeeding during and for 60 days after therapy.
- Teach patients to avoid direct sunlight and tanning beds to prevent worsening of skin side effects.
- Teach patients to avoid cigarette smoking while taking erlotinib.
- Remind patients taking gefitinib who also take warfarin (Coumadin) to keep all appointments for INR testing.

Evaluation

- Patient/family/caregiver education needs are met.
- Patient/family/caregiver understands therapy-related side effects/adverse reactions.
- Patient/family/caregiver understands strategies to minimize side effects/adverse reactions.
- Side effects are managed effectively.
- Patient is free from infection.
- Patient's fluid balance and electrolytes are maintained at expected normal ranges.

Proteasome Inhibitors

Bortezomib

Bortezomib (Velcade) works by inhibiting the 26S proteasome, which is part of the most common proteasome pathway (see Table 38-1). A **proteasome** is a large complex of proteins in cell fluid (cytoplasm) and cell nucleus that regulates protein expression and the degradation of damaged or old proteins within the cell. Its activity is critical to activation or suppression of cellular functions. This system regulates the expression of substances that mediate cell cycle progression (especially oncogene products and cyclins), suppressor genes (especially the *Tp53* gene), and proteins that signal apoptosis. When proteasomes are inhibited, cells are much more likely to undergo apoptosis. Although proteasomes are present in normal and cancer cells, the cancer cells are much more sensitive to the effects of proteasome inhibition than normal cells. Thus, proteasome inhibition results in suppression of cancer cell division and enhancement of cancer cell apoptosis. Bortezomib is most commonly used to manage mantle-cell lymphoma and multiple myeloma.

Pharmacokinetics Bortezomib is administered as an intravenous bolus injection. More than 80% of the drug is protein-bound and distributed to most body tissues, including the myocardium. The half-life ranges from 9 to 15 hours. Bortezomib is metabolized by the CYP3A4, CYP2C19, and CYP1A2 enzymes in the liver. At present, elimination pathways are not known.

Pharmacodynamics Bortezomib inhibits the activity of the 26S proteasome. This inhibition causes an increase in cell cycle checkpoint activity, a decrease in cell proliferation, and a greater responsiveness to cellular signals for apoptosis. The overall results are inhibition of cancer cell growth and an increase in cancer cell apoptosis.

Side Effects and Adverse Reactions. The most common side effects of bortezomib are nausea, vomiting, anorexia, abdominal pain, bowel changes (constipation or diarrhea), and decreased taste sensation. Most patients also experience either new-onset peripheral neuropathy or worsening of existing peripheral neuropathy, including both loss of sensation and orthostatic hypotension. Other general side effects include headache, insomnia, rash, pruritus, back pain, arthralgia, bone pain, and muscle cramps. Respiratory effects include dyspnea, cough, and pneumonia. Weakness (asthenia) and low-grade fever are relatively common. Moderate to severe thrombocytopenia, anemia, and neutropenia can occur during bortezomib therapy.

Rare but serious cardiopulmonary side effects have been reported. These include new-onset congestive heart failure or worsening of preexisting heart failure, decreased left ventricular function, and pulmonary pneumonitis.

Additional neurologic side effects may include anxiety, fatigue, headaches, lethargy, dizziness, insomnia, and blurred or double vision. An uncommon adverse event is the development of reversible posterior leukoencephalopathy syndrome (RPLS) in patients receiving bortezomib. RPLS is a reversible neurologic condition that can present as seizures, hypertension, headache, lethargy, confusion, visual impairment (including blindness), or other neurologic disturbances.

Because bortezomib causes rapid killing of cancer cells, the development of tumor lysis syndrome (TLS), including hyperkalemia and hyperphosphatemia, is possible. This complication is more likely in patients with a high tumor burden at the start of bortezomib therapy.

Drug Interactions. Drugs that inhibit the CYP3A4 enzyme can lead to increased serum levels of bortezomib, which increases the risk for severe side effects. These drugs include ketoconazole (Nizoral), atazanavir (Reyataz), clarithromycin (Biaxin), indinavir (Crixivan), itraconazole (Sporanox), nefazodone (Serzone, Nefadar), nelfinavir (Viracept), ritonavir (Norvir), saquinavir (Invirase), telithromycin (Ketek), voriconazole (Vfend), amprenavir (Agenerase), aprepitant (Emend), diltiazem (Cardizem), fluconazole (Diflucan), verapamil (Isoptin, Verelan), and cimetidine (Tagamet).

Drugs that induce CYP3A4 enzyme activity may lower bortezomib blood serum levels and reduce its effectiveness. These drugs include rifampin (Rifadin), carbamazepine (Tegretol), and phenytoin (Dilantin).

Angiogenesis Inhibitors

Temsirolimus/Sirolimus

Temsirolimus (Torisel) and its active metabolite, sirolimus, is the major drug in this class. The target of this drug is a protein kinase known as the *mammalian target of rapamycin* (mTOR). When temsirolimus or sirolimus bind to an intracellular protein called FKBP-12, a protein-drug complex forms that directly inhibits the activity of mTOR. Inhibition of mTOR greatly reduces the concentration of vascular endothelial growth factor (VEGF). In addition, by its inhibition of mTOR, a variety of downstream pro–cell-division signal transduction pathways are disrupted, especially in renal cell carcinoma cells. This drug is most commonly used to manage advanced renal cell carcinoma.

Pharmacokinetics Temsirolimus is administered by intravenous infusion. It is extensively metabolized in the liver by CYP3A4 into five active metabolites, including sirolimus. The half-life or temsirolimus is 17 hours, and the half-life of sirolimus is 54 hours. The drug and its metabolites are primarily excreted in the feces.

Pharmacodynamics Temsirolimus and its metabolites bind to an intracellular protein forming a drug-protein complex that inhibits the protein kinase, mTOR, in the tumor cells of renal cell carcinoma (RCC). As a result of this inhibition RCC tumors lose vascularity. Inhibition of mTOR also reduces production of cyclin D so that progression through the cell cycle does not occur. RCC cell proliferation is inhibited, even under hypoxic kidney conditions.

Side Effects and Adverse Reactions. Hypersensitivity reactions to temsirolimus are common, and pretreatment is recommended (see the Nursing Process section). Hyperglycemia is very common (about 89%) in patients receiving temsirolimus, and it may require treatment with oral antidiabetic agents or with insulin. Hematologic side effects of anemia, neutropenia, and thrombocytopenia may be moderate to severe. Other common side effects include headache, insomnia, nausea and vomiting, back pain, arthralgia, myalgia, mucositis, and diarrhea. Integumentary problems such as rash, pruritus, nail disorders, dry skin, acne, and abnormal wound healing may occur.

Respiratory adverse effects of interstitial pneumonitis or other interstitial lung disease are possible. Liver impairment and renal impairment have been reported. Cardiovascular effects of edema formation, chest pain, hypertension, venous thromboembolism, and thrombophlebitis are possible.

Drug Interactions. Drugs that inhibit the CYP3A4 enzyme can lead to increased serum levels of temsirolimus, which increases the risk for severe side effects. These drugs include ketoconazole (Nizoral), atazanavir (Reyataz), clarithromycin (Biaxin), indinavir (Crixivan), itraconazole (Sporanox), nefazodone (Serzone, Nefadar), nelfinavir (Viracept), ritonavir (Norvir), saquinavir (Invirase), telithromycin (Ketek), voriconazole (Vfend), amprenavir (Agenerase), aprepitant (Emend), diltiazem (Cardizem), fluconazole (Diflucan), verapamil (Isoptin, Verelan), and cimetidine (Tagamet).

Drugs that induce CYP3A4 enzyme activity may lower temsirolimus blood serum levels and reduce its effectiveness. These drugs include rifampin (Rifadin), carbamazepine (Tegretol), and phenytoin (Dilantin).

Patients taking antihypertensive drugs such as angiotensin-converting enzyme (ACE) inhibitors or angiotensin II receptor antagonists during temsirolimus therapy are at increased risk for angioedema of the face and upper airways. The combination of temsirolimus and sunitinib may result in dose-limiting integumentary toxicities of erythematous maculopapular rash and gout/cellulitis that require hospitalization. The use of live vaccines such as intranasal influenza, measles, mumps, rubella, oral polio, BCG, yellow fever, varicella, and typhoid vaccines should be avoided during treatment with temsirolimus.

Monoclonal Antibodies

Monoclonal antibodies largely exert their effects on specific cell-membrane surface proteins. All FDA-approved monoclonal antibodies currently used in cancer treatment are given intravenously because their protein structure would be altered and inactivated in the GI tract.

Antigens are normal cell surface proteins or ligands that serve as targets for binding engineered monoclonal antibodies for the treatment of cancer. Ideal target antigens for cancer treatment should be specific to tumor cells; be located on the surface of the tumor cell and not shed into the bloodstream; occur in high numbers; and play a role in tumor cell survival.

Monoclonal antibody therapy is aimed specifically at tumor cells expressing the target antigen. The side effects of monoclonal antibodies are related to activation of the immune system, location of the target antigen, and type of monoclonal antibody. Some monoclonal antibodies sensitize tumor cells to chemotherapy and overcome chemotherapy resistance.

The function of an antibody or immunoglobulin is to recognize an antigen and then interact with other serum proteins to eliminate the antigen or the cell associated with that antigen. The Y shape of the antibody has two active sites (Fab and Fc) and the following two activities:

1. The Fab portion of the antibody contains the antigen-binding sites that recognize and bind to a specific antigen.

2. The Fc or constant region is the end of the antibody that signals the immune system to destroy the cell the antibody has bound.

The binding of antibody to antigen is highly selective, rather like a lock-and-key fit. When an antibody selectively binds to a specific antigen, the antibody/antigen complex acts as a flag or target, drawing other immune cells to the bound cell to destroy it.

A monoclonal antibody recognizes only a single unique antigen and is produced by cloning a single cell. Hybridoma technology, developed in 1975, allowed for mass production of monoclonal antibodies. In this technique, a mouse is inoculated with a purified antigen, and antibody-producing cells are isolated from the mouse spleen. Then antibody producing cells are mixed with myeloma cells (immortal cells that are unable to produce antibodies). When antibody-producing cells fuse with myeloma cells, the resulting cells can make large quantities of the specific monoclonal antibody.

Binding of a monoclonal antibody to its specific target antigen on the cancer cell inactivates or destroys the cancer cell by one or more of the following mechanisms:

- Causing neutralization of tumor cell growth by direct interference with normal biologic activities of the antigen, such as signal transduction of cell growth messages. This cytostatic process can slow growth of the tumor cells.
- Promoting antibody-dependent cell-mediated cytotoxicity (ADCC) in which the Fc portion of the bound monoclonal antibody recruits effector cells such as phagocytes, T-cells, and natural killer cells of the immune system to release cytokines that destroy the target cell.
- Initiating complement-dependent cytotoxicity (CDC), which activates the complement system (a cascade of naturally circulating blood proteins), thus enhancing immune system destruction of antibody-bound cells.
- Directly inducing apoptosis, or programmed cell death.
- In fully human antibodies, the entire antibody has been engineered to contain only human antibody protein sequences. Human antibodies are usually named with the suffix "umab" (see Table 38-2).

Murine monoclonal antibodies are derived from mice. Mouse antibodies have a very short half-life in the human body, are not as effective as human antibodies in eliciting a response from the CDC and ADCC systems, and can cause development of human anti-mouse antibodies (HAMA) that neutralize and render the mouse antibodies ineffective against the tumor. Mouse antibodies are usually named with the suffix "momab." Chimeric monoclonal antibodies end with the suffix "ximab" and contain both human and mouse protein sequences (typically 70% human and 30% mouse).

Humanized monoclonal antibodies ending in "zumab" contain human and gene mouse sequences; however, they are not considered chimeric because they contain more human sequences than do chimeric monoclonal antibodies, usually 90% to 95% human and 5% to 10% mouse.

When monoclonal antibodies are named, not only is the suffix a clue to the makeup, but you can tell what they target by the name. If a generic monoclonal antibody has a *u* in the name, then the target is on a tumor cell. Monoclonal antibodies can be *naked,* or *unconjugated,* with nothing attached to them. They also may be *conjugated* with other anticancer agents (e.g., chemotherapy agents, toxins, or radioisotopes) attached to the antibody. Although agents attached to conjugated antibodies are targeted specifically against tumor cells, nearby healthy cells can still be negatively affected, especially if radioisotopes are used. If the specific target antigen is found on normal cells, these antibodies also cause damage to these cells.

The four major monoclonal antibodies currently in use for cancer therapy are alemtuzumab, ibritumomab tiuxetan, rituximab, and tositumomab (see Table 38-1). Prototype Drug Chart 38-3 lists specific drug information for rituximab.

Alemtuzumab

Alemtuzumab (Campath) is an unconjugated, humanized monoclonal antibody against the cell surface antigen CD52. CD52 is found on most B- and T-lymphocytes; the majority of monocytes, macrophages, and natural killer (NK) cells; and some granulocytes, stem cells, and mature spermatozoa. Although normal cells may express this antigen, malignant cells are much more sensitive to the destructive activity of this antibody. This drug is most commonly used for management of chronic lymphocytic leukemia.

Pharmacokinetics Alemtuzumab is administered as an intravenous infusion. Its average half-life is 12 days, and steady-state levels are reached by about 6 weeks. Because all monoclonal antibodies bind to target cell surfaces and are destroyed along with the target cell, they are cleared as debris from the blood by the liver and eliminated in the feces.

Pharmacodynamics Alemtuzumab binds to leukemic cells expressing the CD52 cell surface antigen and induces antibody-dependent lysis. T-cell prolymphocytic leukemia cells are most sensitive to this drug, but monocytes and monocytic leukemias are resistant to it, despite expressing similar amounts of antigen. As an unconjugated monoclonal antibody, this drug relies on inducing apoptotic signals and the activation of mechanisms such as complement or T-cells to attack and kill the targeted cells. Alemtuzumab is also associated with the release of tumor necrosis factor (TNF), interleukin-6, and interferon gamma.

Side Effects and Adverse Reactions. Alemtuzumab therapy induces fatigue as the most common side effect that is not related to infusion reactions or pancytopenia. This drug carries a boxed warning because of profound bone marrow suppression that may require dose interruptions or reduction, based on severity. This suppression is more profound in patients who are also receiving standard cytotoxic chemotherapy. In addition, infusion reactions with fever, nausea, chills, blood pressure changes, hyperglycemia, and hypoxia are common and often require premedication with antihistamines and acetaminophen. Some patients have reduced reactions with subsequent infusions.

Drug Interactions. Specific drug interactions have not been reported with this drug; however, concomitant administration of drugs with similar pharmacologic effects may cause additive side effects, including toxicity.

PROTOTYPE DRUG CHART 38-3

Rituximab

Drug Class	Dosage
Monoclonal antibody Trade Name: Rituxan Pregnancy Category: C	A: IV: 375 mg/m^2 IV once weekly for 4 doses; may be retreated for an additional 4 doses.
Contraindications	**Drug-Lab-Food Interactions**
Patients who may become pregnant, are pregnant, or are breastfeeding; have previously had hepatitis B; have active bacterial or viral infection; have moderate to severe renal, liver, and/or cardiac disease; or have preexisting pulmonary fibrosis	Drug: Potentiation of hypotension when coadministered with antihypertensive drugs Potentiation of bone marrow suppression when coadministered with drugs that also cause bone marrow suppression, increasing risk for infection and bleeding Reduces effectiveness of vaccinations Lab: None known Food: None known
Pharmacokinetics	**Pharmacodynamics**
Absorption: 100% bioavailability after intravenous infusion Distribution: Throughout extracellular fluid, bone marrow, and secondary lymphoid tissues (primarily the spleen) Metabolism: Degraded by circulating and liver-based phagocytic cells Excretion: As cellular debris in feces	Antibody binding specifically to the CD20 cell surface antigen on B-lymphocytes
Therapeutic Effects/Uses	
CD20-positive non-Hodgkin's lymphoma (NHL) Moderate to severe rheumatoid arthritis (lower dosages) Mode of Action: Binds to CD20-positive B-lymphocytes and lymphoma cells, leading to complement-dependent cytotoxicity, antibody-dependent cellular cytotoxicity, and apoptosis.	
Side Effects	**Adverse Reactions**
Bone marrow suppression with pancytopenia, Tumor lysis syndrome, hypotension, night sweats, joint and muscle aches, headaches, soreness at injection site	Infusion reactions Reactivation of dormant viruses, pulmonary fibrosis, cardiac dysrhythmias, heart failure

A, Adult; *IV*, intravenous.

Ibritumomab Tiuxetan

Ibritumomab tiuxetan (Zevalin) is a conjugated murine monoclonal antibody. Ibritumomab is the antibody, and tiuxetan is a linker-chelater to which either Indium-111 or Yttrium-90 can be bound. Like rituximab, this drug combination binds specifically to the human B-lymphocytes that express the CD20 cell surface antigen. This drug is most commonly used for management of B-cell types of non-Hodgkin's lymphoma that express the CD20 cell surface protein.

Pharmacokinetics Ibritumomab tiuxetan is administered as an intravenous infusion. Its physical half-life is 64 hours, and its biologic half-life (determined by radioactivity detection) is 30 hours. The drug is excreted to a slight degree by the kidneys but is mostly eliminated in the feces.

Pharmacodynamics Ibritumomab tiuxetan binds to the CD20 antigen on B-lymphocytes and lymphoma cells. Following binding with the CD20 antigen, beta wave radioactive emissions from the attached radionuclide, Y-90, induce cellular damage by the formation of free radicals in the target and neighboring cells. This cellular damage prevents cells from dividing and also causes cell death.

Side Effects and Adverse Reactions. Ibritumomab tiuxetan carries a boxed warning for infusion reactions with fever, nausea, chills, and blood pressure changes. Severe infusion reactions warrant discontinuing the drug. Less severe infusion reactions may be managed using premedication with antihistamines and acetaminophen. Some patients experience reduced reactions with the second and subsequent infusions. Additional boxed warnings for this drug include severe cytopenia and severe cutaneous and mucocutaneous reactions, fetal damage if given during pregnancy, and possible second malignancies. Just as with all monoclonal antibodies, this drug causes profound bone marrow suppression that may require dose interruptions or reduction (based on severity) and are more profound in patients who are also receiving standard cytotoxic chemotherapy. Ibritumomab tiuxetan side effects and adverse effects not associated with bone marrow suppression or infusion reaction include nausea, vomiting, diarrhea, abdominal pain, cough, rash, pruritus, and urticaria.

Drug Interactions. Ibritumomab tiuxetan increases the risk for bleeding or hemorrhage when used along with anticoagulant or antiplatelet therapy. Other specific drug interactions are not associated with this drug; however, concomitant administration of drugs with similar pharmacologic effects may cause additive side effects, including toxicity.

Tositumomab

Tositumomab (Bexxar) is a murine monoclonal antibody conjugated with the radioactive isotope iodine-131 (^{131}I). Like rituximab and ibritumomab tiuxetan, the antibody portion of this drug binds specifically to the human B-lymphocytes that express the CD20 cell surface antigen. This drug is most commonly used to manage B-cell non-Hodgkin's lymphoma that does not respond to rituximab.

Pharmacokinetics Tositumomab is administered as an intravenous infusion. It has a median blood clearance of 68.2 mg/hour (with 485-mg dosage). The mean total-body effective half-life is 67 hours. The radioisotope (131I) decays over time (half-life is 8 days) and is eliminated in the urine.

Pharmacodynamics Tositumomab induces cytotoxicity by combining the immunologic effects of antibody binding with the preferential targeting of radiation therapy against CD20-positive lymphocytes and lymphoma cells. Actions of the antibody include the induction of complement-mediated cytolysis, antibody-dependent cellular cytotoxicity, and apoptosis. Radiation activity is cytotoxic not only to the cells bound by the radiolabeled antibody, but also to adjacent cells that may not have been bound by the antibody or do not express the target antigen (a process called the *cross-fire effect*). Together, these actions result in sustained depletion of circulating CD20-positive lymphocytes and lymphoma cells.

Side Effects and Adverse Reactions. Tositumomab carries a boxed warning for severe hypersensitivity reactions (anaphylaxis), severe bone marrow suppression, and fetal damage (when used during pregnancy). Specific tositumomab side effects and adverse effects include asthenia, headache, hypotension, nausea, vomiting, abdominal pain, diarrhea, hypothyroidism, cough, dyspnea, pleural effusion, and pneumonia. Toxicities associated with radioimmunotherapy can be acute, delayed, or long-term. The most common acute toxicities are fever, rigors, fatigue, headache, and nausea, whereas hypotension and allergic reactions are less common. Delayed toxicities include shortness of breath, fever, signs of infection, inflammation, pain with urination, rash, sore joints, and bone marrow suppression. Long-term toxicities are myelodysplasia or acute leukemia, secondary malignancies, and hypothyroidism. Just as with other monoclonal antibodies, this drug causes profound bone marrow suppression that may require dose interruptions or reduction, based on severity, and are more profound in patients who are also receiving standard cytotoxic chemotherapy. In addition, infusion reactions with fever, nausea, chills, blood pressure changes, hyperglycemia, and hypoxia are common and often require premedication with antihistamines and acetaminophen. Some patients have reduced reactions with subsequent infusions.

Drug Interactions. Tositumomab increases the risk for bleeding or hemorrhage when used along with anticoagulant or antiplatelet therapy. Other specific drug interactions have not been reported with this drug; however, concomitant administration of drugs with similar pharmacologic effects may cause additive side effects, including toxicity.

Nursing Process
Patient-Centered Collaborative Care

Proteosome Inhibitors, Angiogenesis Inhibitors, and Monoclonal Antibodies for Cancer Treatment

Assessment

- Conduct a detailed medication history, including a list of all concurrent medications, to avoid drug-drug interactions. Include prescriptions, over-the-counter medicines, antacids, dietary supplements, vitamins, and herbal supplements.
- Obtain baseline information about patient's physical condition before initiating targeted therapy and during the treatment period. Include height, weight, vital signs, and laboratory values (CBC, uric acid, electrolytes, hepatic and renal studies, cardiopulmonary assessment, intake and output).
- Assess laboratory studies, including CBC with differential, hepatic and renal studies, electrolytes, and urinalysis, at the beginning of therapy and at specified time intervals during therapy (ranging from weekly to monthly).
- Assess patient/family/caregiver knowledge related to therapeutic regimen.

Nursing Diagnoses

- Deficient knowledge related to targeted therapy regimen
- Risk for impaired skin integrity related to dermatologic effects and toxicity of therapy
- Risk for infection related to bone marrow suppression
- Risk for deficient fluid volume related to GI effects of therapy
- Risk for electrolyte imbalance related to actions of targeted therapy

Planning

- Patient and family will verbalize understanding of targeted therapy as part of anticancer treatment regimen.
- Patient and family will demonstrate understanding of importance of reporting targeted therapy–related side effects and adverse reactions.
- Patient and family will verbalize strategies to minimize risks related to targeted therapy–related side effects.
- Patient's side effects will be managed to a level that the patient can tolerate and are not life threatening.
- Patient will remain infection-free.
- Patient's fluid balance and electrolytes are maintained at expected normal ranges.

Nursing Interventions

- Monitor CBC count with differential and platelet count at baseline, and as often as recommended for specific agents.

- Monitor liver function tests and renal function tests at baseline and at least once monthly during therapy.
- Administer prescribed premedications according to established protocols for specific targeted therapies.
- Follow agency policy for safe handling, preparing, administering, and dispensing of targeted therapy agents.

Bortezomib

- Ensure that patient is adequately hydrated before, during, and after therapy to reduce risk for tumor lysis syndrome.
- Check for manifestations of tumor lysis syndrome (decreased urine output, hyperkalemia, and hypertension).
- Check patient's peripheral sensation and blood pressure at each visit throughout treatment.
- Discuss with health care provider the possible need for prophylactic allopurinol therapy.
- Monitor output and serum potassium levels closely.

Temsirolimus/Sirolimus

- Ensure that resuscitation equipment is nearby, and stay with patient during first 15 minutes of infusion. Thereafter, monitor vital signs every 15 to 30 minutes during infusion and for 1 hour after infusion is complete.
- Check patient's blood glucose level before, during, and after drug administration.
- Ask patient about known hypersensitivity to temsirolimus or sirolimus.
- If prescribed, premedicate patient with diphenhydramine 25 to 50 mg IV, or a similar antihistamine, approximately 30 minutes before the start of each dose.
- Monitor fasting blood glucose and serum electrolytes at baseline and at least every 2 weeks during therapy.
- Monitor chest radiograph at baseline and periodically during therapy for onset of pulmonary toxicity.
- Monitor renal and hepatic function at baseline and then periodically during therapy.

Monoclonal Antibodies

- Infusion reactions are common with intravenous infusion of monoclonal antibodies. Ensure that resuscitation equipment is nearby, and stay with the patient during the first 15 minutes of the infusion. Thereafter, monitor vital signs every 15 to 30 minutes during the infusion and for 1 hour after infusion is complete.
- Ensure that patient is adequately hydrated before, during, and after rituximab therapy to reduce risk for tumor lysis syndrome.
- Monoclonal antibodies against leukocytes can profoundly suppress bone marrow activity and increase patient's risk for infection.
- Monitor for signs and symptoms of infection.
- Patients receiving alemtuzumab are usually prescribed to start antimicrobial prophylaxis beginning on the first day of therapy to reduce the risk for serious infection. Prophylaxis is continued for 2 months after the last dose.
- Gemtuzumab ozogamicin can cause liver toxicity. Closely monitor liver function tests.
- Screen patients for hepatitis B infection before the initiation of rituximab therapy.
- Monitor output and serum potassium levels closely.
- Check for manifestations of tumor lysis syndrome (decreased urine output, hyperkalemia).

General

- Report symptoms of bleeding immediately, including black stools, vomit that looks like coffee grounds, easy bleeding/bruising.
- Report symptoms of adverse effects or severe side effects promptly, especially fever, chills, persistent sore throat, swelling, weight gain, or increasing shortness of breath.
- Report symptoms of liver impairment immediately, including stomach/abdominal pain, yellowing eyes or skin, dark urine, or unusual fatigue.
- Avoid alcohol and nonessential drugs that are cleared by the liver or have liver-toxic effects (e.g., acetaminophen).
- Remind women with childbearing potential to avoid pregnancy throughout treatment and for up to 12 months after treatment is completed.
- Advise breastfeeding patients to stop breastfeeding during and for 60 days after therapy.

Bortezomib

- Advise patient (or family member) to immediately report convulsions, persistent headache, reduced eyesight, increased blood pressure, or blurred vision.
- Teach patient to drink at least 4 liters of fluid daily on day before therapy, on days of therapy, and for 2 days following therapy. Stress importance of keeping fluid intake consistent throughout 24-hour day, and help patients draw up a schedule of fluid intake.
- Advise patient to contact health care provider or cancer clinic immediately if nausea and vomiting prevent adequate fluid intake so they can be started on parenteral fluids.
- Teach patient to avoid driving or operating dangerous machinery during periods of blurred or double vision or when fatigue is extreme.

Temsirolimus/Sirolimus

- Advise patients who develop swelling of the face, lips, or tongue to immediately go to the nearest emergency department.
- Advise nondiabetic patients to report symptoms of hyperglycemia (excessive thirst or any increase in the volume or frequency of urination).
- Advise diabetic patients to test blood glucose levels more frequently. If prescribed dosages of oral antidiabetic

drugs are not sufficient to maintain target blood glucose levels, advise patient to contact the health care provider for diabetic therapy adjustments.
- Advise the patient and live-in family members not to receive any vaccinations without consulting the oncologist.

Monoclonal Antibodies
- Teach patient the signs and symptoms of bone marrow suppression and infection.
- Advise the patient receiving alemtuzumab therapy and live-in family members not to receive any live-virus vaccinations during therapy and for 2 months after therapy is completed.
- Teach patient that monoclonal antibodies conjugated to radioisotopes (ibritumomab tiuxetan and tositumomab) will make him or her somewhat radioactive for a time after the infusion and will pose a radiation hazard to others for 4 to 7 days. Teach patient to use the following precautions for 1 week after each drug administration:
  - Sleep in a separate bed.
  - Maintain a distance of 6 feet or more from children and pregnant women.
  - Limit time spent in public places.
  - Use a separate bathroom and sit while urinating.
  - Wash hands frequently, especially after using the toilet or handling genitals.
  - Drink plenty of liquids (at least 3 L daily).
  - Keep eating utensils separate from others.
  - Wash laundry separately from those of others.
  - Avoid using disposable products.
  - Avoid sexual contact and avoid becoming pregnant.
  - Clean spilled urine, and dispose of body fluid–contaminated material so that others will not inadvertently handle it.

Evaluation
- Patient/family/caregiver education needs are met.
- Patient/family/caregiver understands therapy-related side effects/adverse reactions.
- Patient/family/caregiver understands strategies to minimize side effects/adverse reactions.
- Side effects are managed effectively.
- Patient is free from infection.
- Patient's fluid balance and electrolytes are maintained at expected normal ranges.

KEY WEBSITES

American Cancer Society: *www.cancer.org/cancer/cancerbasics/thehistoryofcancer/the-history-of-cancer-cancer-treatment-targeted-therapy*
National Cancer Institute: *www.cancer.gov/cancertopics/factsheet/Therapy/targeted*
National Comprehensive Cancer Network: *www.nccn.org*

CRITICAL THINKING CASE STUDY

MR is a 64-year-old man who is diagnosed with stage III B-cell non-Hodgkin's lymphoma (NHL). He is scheduled to receive rituximab (Rituxan) and a traditional chemotherapy regimen of cyclophosphamide (Cytoxan), doxorubicin (Adriamycin), vincristine (Oncovin), and prednisolone, a combination known as "CHOP." The dosage and schedule of rituximab for this patient is 600 mg IV on days 1 and 6 before the first CHOP chemotherapy cycle (which will be administered on day 8). The next two doses will be administered 2 days before the third and fifth cycles, and the remaining two cycles of rituximab will be administered after the sixth cycle of CHOP on days 134 and 141. MR has a friend who is taking imatinib (Gleevec) daily as an oral drug for chronic myelogenous leukemia. He asks why rituximab must be taken intravenously and, because he has an implanted port, if his spouse, who is an LPN, could administer it at home so he won't have to travel to the cancer center in addition to his standard chemotherapy appointments.

1. What is your best response about why rituximab must be administered intravenously?
2. How are rituximab and imatinib different?
3. Why can't MR's spouse administer rituximab at home?
4. What side effects are specific for rituximab?
5. What are the most common adverse effects of rituximab?
6. What should you teach this patient specifically related to rituximab therapy?

NCLEX STUDY QUESTIONS

1. A patient on chemotherapy for breast cancer asks why she is not receiving trastuzumab (Herceptin) like her sister received with breast cancer. What is the nurse's best response?
   a. "Your breast cancer cells are estrogen receptor–positive, and targeted therapy is not needed."
   b. "You are much older than your sister and would not tolerate the treatment well."
   c. "The drug is expensive, and your insurance does not cover it."
   d. "Your cancer cells do not have the target for trastuzumab."

2. Which instruction is important for the nurse to include when teaching a patient about imatinib (Gleevec) therapy?
   a. Do not drink grapefruit juice while taking this drug.
   b. Go immediately to the emergency department if you develop a headache while taking this drug.
   c. This drug will only work for about 2 months before your cancer develops resistance to it.
   d. Be sure to take this drug on an empty stomach, either 1 hour before or at least 3 hours after eating.
3. Which is the priority nursing diagnosis for patients receiving epidermal growth factor/receptor inhibitors?
   a. Risk for infection related to bone marrow suppression and neutropenia
   b. Risk for impaired skin integrity related to skin side effects
   c. Risk for injury related to reduced platelet activity
   d. Disturbed body image related to alopecia
4. The nurse should be most alert to a possible infusion reaction when administering which class of targeted therapies?
   a. Tyrosine kinase inhibitors
   b. Multikinase inhibitors
   c. Monoclonal antibodies
   d. Proteasome inhibitors
5. A patient taking sunitinib (Sutent) reports that the skin on her hands and feet is red, is painful, and has some blisters. What is the nurse's best action?
   a. The only action needed is to document the report because this is a mild side effect.
   b. Advise the patient to wear gloves and mittens when going outdoors in cold weather.
   c. Advise the patient to avoid getting her hands wet and touching food.
   d. Notify the oncologist to determine if a dosage reduction is needed.
6. Which action is most important for the nurse to teach a patient taking tositumomab (Bexxar)?
   a. Avoid drinking alcohol for 1 week after receiving this drug.
   b. Avoid smoking cigarettes for the entire treatment period.
   c. Use a separate bathroom and sit while urinating for 1 week after receiving this drug.
   d. Be sure to take this drug on an empty stomach, either 1 hour before or 2 hours after eating.
7. Which activity will the nurse advise the patient taking erlotinib (Tarceva) to avoid?
   a. Drinking alcoholic beverages
   b. Taking aspirin or aspirin-containing drugs
   c. Exposing self to crowds or persons who are ill
   d. Exposing self to direct sunlight or tanning beds
8. A patient receiving a targeted therapy asks the nurse why St. John's wort must be avoided. What is the nurse's best response?
   a. This herbal drug increases blood levels of most targeted therapies and increases the risk for severe side effects or adverse reactions.
   b. This herbal drug decreases blood levels of most targeted therapies and reduces their effectiveness.
   c. Targeted therapies increase blood levels of St. John's wort, increasing the risk of an overdose of this herbal agent.
   d. Targeted therapies bind with St. John's wort in the intestinal tract, preventing absorption of both the drug and the herbal agent.
9. A patient taking imatinib (Gleevec) has gained 5 pounds in the past week. Is this cause for concern?
   a. No, weight gain is an expected side effect of this drug because it increases the appetite.
   b. Yes, weight gain is an indication of slow metabolism and possible hypothyroidism.
   c. Yes, weight gain is an indication of water retention and possible renal impairment.
   d. Yes, weight gain is an indication of a drug interaction between imatinib and loop diuretics.

Answers: 1, d; 2, a; 3, b; 4, c; 5, d; 6, c; 7, d; 8, b; 9, c.

CHAPTER

39

Biologic Response Modifiers

evolve WEBSITE

http://evolve.elsevier.com/KeeHayes/pharmacology/

- Animations
- Content Updates
- Key Points
- Review Questions for the NCLEX® Examination
- References from the Textbook
- Unfolding Case Studies

OBJECTIVES

- Compare the mechanisms of action of drugs classified as *biologic response modifiers* with those of standard chemotherapy drugs.
- Distinguish among the different types of biologic response modifiers with regard to indications, common side effects and adverse effects, route of administration, and nursing responsibilities.
- Discuss three common side effects of interferons, colony-stimulating factors, and interleukin-2.
- Distinguish anaphylaxis reactions from the anaphylactoid reactions caused by the administration of monoclonal antibody therapy.
- Incorporate the nursing process related to the needs of patients receiving biologic response modifiers.

OUTLINE

KEY TERMS

The authors gratefully acknowledge the work of Carolee A. Polek, who updated this chapter for the eighth edition.

Biologic response modifiers (BRMs) are a class of pharmacologic agents used to enhance the body's immune system. (Another group of immunostimulants are monoclonal antibodies, considered targeted therapy agents, which are discussed in Chapter 38.) **Recombinant DNA** (the genetic engineering process that produces mass quantities of human proteins) and **hybridoma technology** (the process that uses mice to mass-produce monoclonal antibodies) are two advances that have led to commercial mass-production of BRMs (Figure 39-1). Interferons (α, β, γ), colony-stimulating factors, interleukins, and monoclonal antibodies are some currently known BRMs. With the exception of monoclonal antibodies, BRMs are complex proteins produced by the cells of the immune system (Figure 39-2). Individuals taking BRMs are immunocompromised and should be counseled on concurrent drug and herb use (Herbal Alert 39-1).

HERBAL ALERT 39-1

Biologic Response Modifiers

Herbal preparations are generally not recommended for patients receiving BRMs. Several herbs (e.g., elderberry, echinacea, ginseng, goldenseal, green tea) act to stimulate the immune system. However, patients who take BRMs are immunocompromised, and taking any herbal preparations in combination is not recommended.

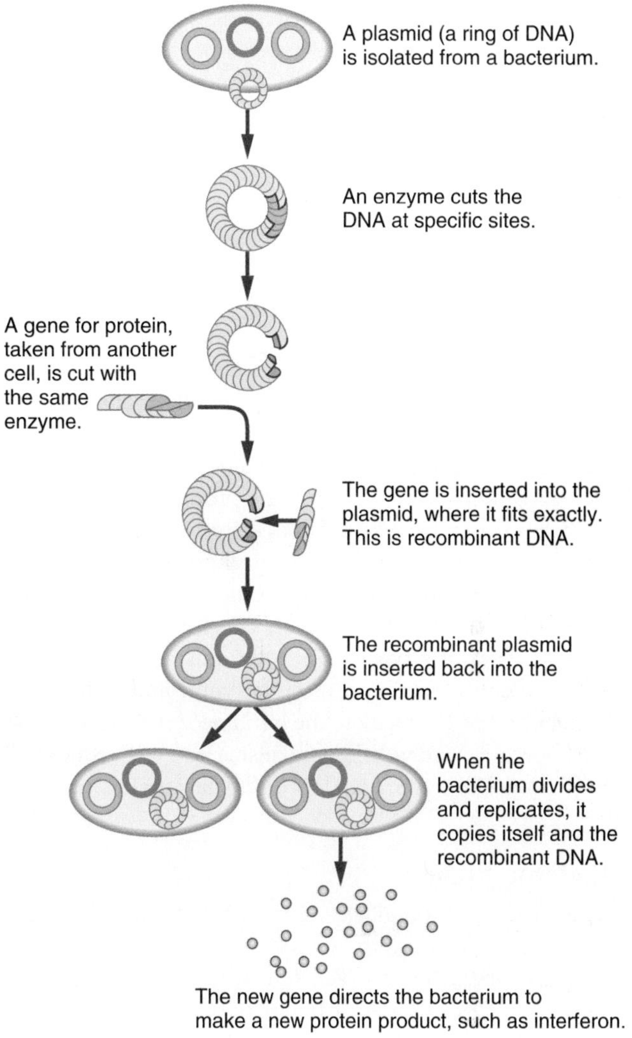

FIGURE 39–1 Recombinant DNA.

Three functions of BRM have been identified:

- Enhance host immunologic function (immunomodulation)
- Destroy or interfere with tumor activities (cytotoxic/cytostatic effects)
- Promote differentiation of stem cells (other biologic effects) (see Figure 39-2).

New BMR drugs are always under development and are being investigated for clinical effectiveness. Several categories

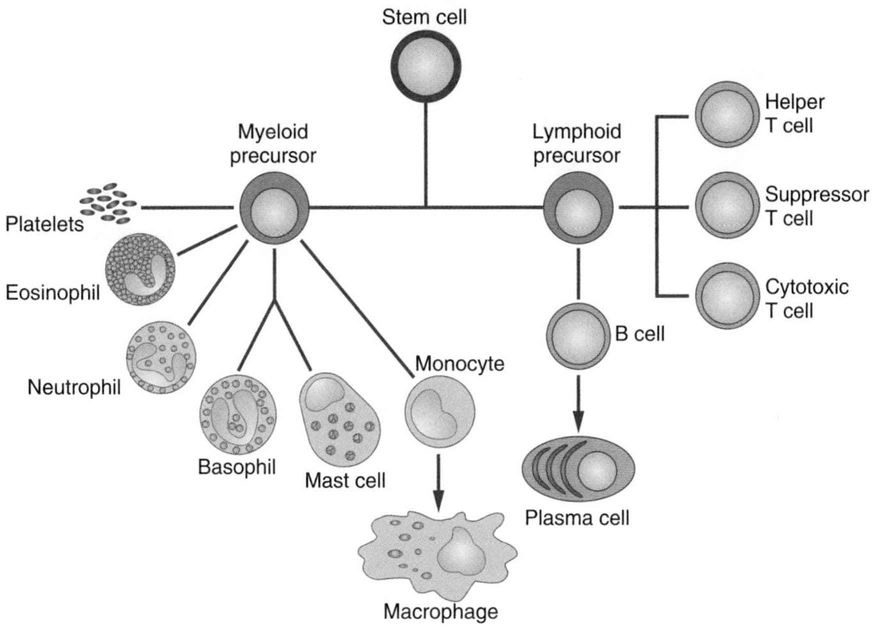

FIGURE 39–2 Cells of the immune system.

of these drugs have been approved by the U.S. Food and Drug Administration (FDA) and are commercially available: interferons, colony-stimulating factors (erythropoietin-stimulating agents, granulocyte colony-stimulating factors, granulocyte macrophage colony-stimulating factors, thrombopoietic growth factors), and interleukin-2. In addition, a number of monoclonal antibodies have been approved by the FDA (see Chapter 38). Interferons, colony-stimulating factors, and interleukin-2 are discussed in this chapter.

INTERFERONS

Interferons (IFNs) are a family of naturally occurring proteins that were first discovered in the 1950s. Three major types of IFNs have been identified: alpha (α) IFN, beta (β) IFN, and gamma (γ) IFN. Each type is produced by a different cell within the immune system. All three types can be manufactured using recombinant DNA technology. Type I IFNs include IFN-α and IFN-β, which bind selectively to either α- or β-cell surface receptors on effector cells. Interferon gamma (IFN-γ) is a type II IFN and binds to a different cell surface receptor. Common to both Type I and II IFNs are their abilities to (1) regulate the immune system to improve resistance to invading microorganisms and (2) reduce cell proliferation. However, each IFN group has specific functionality as well.

Interferon Alpha

B-cells, T-cells, **macrophages** (type of monocyte—the major phagocytic cells of the immune system), and null cells produce interferon alpha (IFN-α) (Roferon-A, Intron A) in response to the presence of viruses or tumor cells. This interferon has been shown to have antiviral, antiproliferative, and immunomodulatory effects, which means that IFN-α inhibits intracellular replication of viral DNA, interferes with tumor cell growth, and enhances natural killer (NK) cell (antitumor) activity. Recombinant IFN-α is manufactured as Roferon-A (alpha-2a) and Intron A (alpha-2b).

Roferon-A is used in the treatment of (1) hairy cell leukemia; (2) chronic myelogenous leukemia (CML), and (3) AIDS-related Kaposi's sarcoma. Intron A is used in the treatment of (1) malignant melanoma, (2) hairy cell leukemia, (3) follicular non-Hodgkin's lymphoma (NHL), (4) AIDS-related Kaposi sarcoma, and (5) nonmalignant chronic hepatitis B and C and condylomata acuminata. Clinically IFN-α has been used to treat non-Hodgkin's lymphoma (intermediate grade), cutaneous T-cell lymphoma, multiple myeloma, renal cell carcinoma, bladder cancer, and carcinoid (a type of cancer-like disease). Intravesical administration of IFN-α has proved successful for low-grade bladder tumors; intraperitoneal administration of IFN-α has been used to treat ovarian cancer; and intralesional application of IFN-α has been used to treat melanoma and basal cell carcinoma. IFN-α-n3 is a human leukocyte-derived interferon that binds to the same receptors as IFN-α-2b. It is FDA approved for intralesional treatment of refractory or recurring external condylomata acuminata.

Interferon Beta

Interferon beta (IFN-β) (Betaseron, IFN-β-1b) is indicated for the treatment of multiple sclerosis. Specifically this interferon (1) enhances the activity of suppressor T-cells (thymocyte-dependent lymphocytes that turn off an immune reaction—an active part of the cell-mediated immune system), (2) reduces the production of proinflammatory cytokines, (3) reduces antigen-presentation (recruiting members of the immune system to start an immune reaction), and (4) inhibits the movement of lymphocytes in the central nervous system.

Interferon Gamma

Interferon gamma (IFN-γ) (Actimmune, IFN-γ-1b) is indicated for (1) delaying time to disease progression in patients with severe malignant osteopetrosis, (2) reducing the frequency and severity of serious infections related to chronic granulomatous disease, and (3) treating patients with chronic myelogenous leukemia and renal cell carcinoma. IFN-γ-1b has been shown to (1) enhance oxidative metabolism of macrophages, (2) enhance antibody-dependent cell cytotoxicity (ADCC), (3) activate natural killer (NK) cells, and (4) enhance Fc receptors (on antibody) and major histocompatibility antigens (HLA). Malignant osteopetrosis is a congenital disorder hallmarked by two characteristic defects: a defect in osteoclasts that causes bone overgrowth and a defect in phagocyte oxidative metabolism, which can be improved with IFN-γ-1b. Chronic granulomatous disease (CGD) is an inherited error in leukocyte function related to enzyme defects that are responsible for killing invading microorganisms (phagocyte superoxide generation).

Pharmacokinetics IFN-α is metabolized by the liver and filtered by the kidneys. However, the body absorbs approximately 80% of the dose. Peak serum concentrations are reached 4 to 8 hours after administration. IFN-α can be administered subcutaneously (subQ), intramuscularly (IM), and intravenously (IV), although subQ and IM are the preferred routes of administration; subQ administration is recommended for patients with platelet counts below 50,000. Interferons-α-n3, -β and -γ are not discussed further because they are not used as antineoplastic agents.

Side Effects and Adverse Reactions

The major side effect of IFN-α is a flulike syndrome. Other effects occur in the gastrointestinal (GI), neurologic, cardiopulmonary, renal, hepatic, hematologic, and dermatologic systems.

The flulike syndrome is characterized by chills, fever, fatigue, malaise, and myalgias (muscle aches). Chills can occur 3 to 6 hours after IFN-α administration and may progress to rigors. A fever as high as 101° F to 104° F (39° C to 40° C) may occur within 30 to 90 minutes after the onset of chills and last 24 hours. Fatigue, malaise, and myalgias are cumulative side effects; fatigue is the **dose-limiting toxicity** (i.e., the side effect that necessitates a decrease in dose or discontinuation of the drug).

GI side effects include nausea, diarrhea, vomiting, anorexia, taste alterations, and xerostomia (dry mouth). These side effects are mild; anorexia is considered the dose-limiting toxicity for this system.

Neurologic side effects are reversible (after the drug is stopped) and occur in 70% of patients who receive IFN-α. These effects are manifested by mild confusion, somnolence (sleepiness), irritability, poor concentration, seizures, transient aphasia (temporary loss of ability to speak), hallucinations, paranoia, and psychoses. Depression, suicidal ideation, and suicide attempts have occurred in patients taking IFN-α, requiring drug discontinuance.

Cardiopulmonary side effects are dose-related and occur more frequently in older adults and patients with underlying cardiac disease. Side effects include tachycardia, pallor, cyanosis, tachypnea, nonspecific electrocardiographic changes, rare myocardial infarction, and orthostatic hypotension.

Renal and hepatic effects are dose-dependent and usually result in few or no symptoms. The effects are manifested by increased blood urea nitrogen (BUN) and creatinine levels, proteinuria, and elevated transaminases.

Hematologic effects are reversible and dose-limiting. Neutropenia (decreased number of neutrophils in the blood) and **thrombocytopenia** (decreased number of thrombocytes in the blood) are manifestations of such effects. Neutropenia is usually rare and does not predispose the patient to infection. Thrombocytopenia is more common in patients with hematopoietic (affecting the formation of blood cells) diseases than in those with solid tumors.

Maculopapular rashes of the trunk and extremities, pruritus, irritation at the injection site, desquamation (shedding of epithelial cells of the skin), and alopecia are dermatologic effects of IFN-α. Alopecia can occur after more than 4 months of therapy.

Dosing and Preparation

Roferon-A is supplied in prefilled syringes containing 3 million International Units (IU) per 0.5 mL, 6 million IU per 0.5 mL, and 9 million IU per 0.5 mL. All prefilled syringes must be refrigerated at 36° F to 46° F (2° C to 8° C). The syringes should not be frozen or shaken and must be protected from light.

Intron A is supplied as single-use vials (either powder or liquid), multidose vials, and multidose pens. The lyophilized powder is for single-dose use and is available in 10, 18, and 50 million IU. The powder is reconstituted with 1 mL of the provided diluent (sterile water for injection) and gently swirled to dissolve. Final vial concentrations are 10 million IU/mL, 18 million IU/mL, and 50 million IU/mL. The single-dose solution vial for injection is available as 10 million IU (10 million IU/mL). Multidose vials are available as 18 million IU (3 million IU/0.5 mL) and 25 million IU (5 million IU/0.5 mL). Multidose pens for injection are available containing 3 million IU (concentration 22.5 million IU/1.5 mL, delivering 3 million IU/0.2 mL, and containing 6 doses), 5 million IU (concentration 37.5 million IU/1.5 mL, delivering 5 million IU/0.2 mL, and containing 6 doses), and 10 million IU (concentration 75 million IU/1.5 mL, delivering 10 million IU/0.2 mL, and containing 6 doses). Multidose solutions and pens must be stored at 36° F to 46° F (2° C to 8° C). The IFN alphas are listed in Table 39-1 with their dosages, uses, and considerations.

Administration

The administration of IFN-α is contraindicated in patients with a known hypersensitivity to IFN-α, mouse immunoglobulin, or any component of the product. It should be used cautiously in patients with severe cardiac, renal, or hepatic disease and in those with seizure disorders or central nervous system dysfunction. Manufacturers recommend administering the agent to persons 18 years or older only under the supervision of a qualified physician. Women of childbearing age should use contraceptives while receiving IFN-α because of the agent's effects on serum estradiol and progesterone concentrations. Studies have not demonstrated fertility or teratogenic effects in men.

It is recommended that baseline and periodic complete blood counts (CBCs) and liver function tests be performed during the course of IFN therapy. Manufacturers suggest that patients undergo IFN therapy for at least 6 months before a decision is made to continue treatment in those who respond or discontinue treatment in those who do not; optimal treatment duration has not been determined. Patients should be well hydrated during IFN therapy, especially during treatment for malignant melanoma, because this minimizes severe side effects. Dose reductions of 50% or drug discontinuation should be considered if severe adverse reactions occur. Concurrent or prior treatment with chemotherapeutic agents or radiation therapy may increase the effectiveness and toxicity of IFN-α.

COLONY-STIMULATING FACTORS

Hematopoietic **colony-stimulating factors** (CSFs) are proteins that stimulate or regulate the growth, maturation, and differentiation of bone marrow stem cells. CSFs are manufactured through recombinant DNA techniques.

Although CSFs are not directly tumoricidal, they are useful in cancer treatment, because they do the following:

- Decrease the length of posttreatment neutropenia (the length of time **neutrophils,** a type of white blood cell [WBC], are decreased secondary to chemotherapy), thereby reducing the risk, incidence, and duration of infection
- Permit the delivery of higher doses of drugs. **Myelosuppression** (suppression of bone marrow activity) is often a dose-limiting toxicity of chemotherapy. Higher, possibly tumoricidal, doses of drugs cannot be administered because of potentially life-threatening side effects. Colony-stimulating factors can minimize the myelosuppressive toxicity, thus allowing the delivery of higher doses of drugs.
- Reduce bone marrow recovery time after bone marrow transplantation
- Enhance macrophage or granulocyte tumor-, virus-, and fungus-destroying ability

TABLE 39-1 BIOLOGIC RESPONSE MODIFIERS: INTERFERONS

GENERIC (BRAND)	ROUTE AND DOSAGE	USES AND CONSIDERATIONS
interferon alpha-2a (Roferon-A)	Hairy-cell leukemia: A: subQ/IM: 3 million IU daily for 16-24 wk, then maintenance dose 3 million IU subQ/IM 3 times/wk Chronic myelogenous leukemia: A: subQ: 9 million IU daily (gradually increase initial dose of 3 million IU daily for 3 days to 6 million IU for 3 days, and then increase to final 9 million IU dose daily	For hairy-cell leukemia, chronic myelogenous leukemia, condyloma acuminata, and AIDS-related Kaposi's sarcoma. Flulike symptoms such as fatigue, aches, pain, fever, chills, and headaches may occur. Pregnancy category: C; PB: UK; $t\frac{1}{2}$: 2-3 h
interferon alpha-2b (Intron A)	Hairy cell leukemia: A: Subcutaneous/IM: 2 million IU/m² 3 times/wk for up to 6 mo Kaposi's sarcoma: A: IM/subQ: Initially: 30 million IU/m² 3 times/wk until severe intolerance or maximal response at 16 wk; use only 50-million IU strength; 50% dose reduction for severe side effects Malignant melanoma: A: Induction: 20 million IU/m² IV over 20 min daily for 5 consecutive d/wk for 4 wk. Maint: 10 million IU/m² subQ 3 times/wk for 48 wk Follicular lymphoma: A: 5 million IU subQ 3 times/wk for up to 18 mo, together with anthracycline-containing chemotherapy regimen and then alone after chemotherapy is completed	For hairy-cell leukemia, adjuvant to surgical resection of malignant melanoma, follicular non-Hodgkin's lymphoma, condyloma acuminata, AIDS-related Kaposi's sarcoma, and chronic hepatitis B and non-A hepatitis. Flulike symptoms, fatigue, GI symptoms (nausea, vomiting, diarrhea) may occur. Low blood counts. Monitor CBC, AST, ALT, ALP, LDH. Pregnancy category: C; PB: UK; $t\frac{1}{2}$: 2 h
interferon gamma-1b (Actimmune)	Body surface area: >0.5 m²: A: subQ: 50 mcg/m² 3 times/wk Body surface area: <0.5 m²: A/C >1 y: subQ: 1.5 mcg/kg/dose 3 times/wk	For chronic granulomatous disease. Flulike symptoms may occur. Pregnancy category: C; PB: UK; $t\frac{1}{2}$: 0.5-6 h
interferon alpha-n3 (Alferon N)	Condylomata acuminata: A: Inject into wart: 250,000 units (0.05 mL) twice weekly; *max:* 8 wk Do not repeat for >3 mo after end of therapy	For recurring condylomata acuminata (genital venereal warts). Flulike symptoms may occur. Monitor CBC, AST, ALT, ALP, LDH. Pregnancy category: C; PB: UK; $t\frac{1}{2}$: 6-8 h
interferon beta-1b (Betaseron)	Reduce number of clinical exacerbations of multiple sclerosis: A >18 y: subQ: 0.0625 mg every other day C: Not recommended	For multiple sclerosis (MS). Flulike symptoms may occur. Pregnancy category: C; PB: UK; $t\frac{1}{2}$: 8 min–4.3 h

A, Adult; *AIDS,* acquired immunodeficiency syndrome; *ALT,* alanine aminotransferase; *ALP,* alkaline phosphatase; *AST,* aspartate aminotransferase; *C,* child; *CBC,* complete blood count; *h,* hour; *IM,* intramuscular; *IV,* intravenous; *LDH,* lactate dehydrogenase; *maint,* maintenance; *max,* maximum; *min,* minute; *mo,* month; *PB,* protein-binding; *subQ,* subcutaneous; $t\frac{1}{2}$, half-life; *UK,* unknown; *wk,* week; *y,* year; >, greater than; <, less than.

- Prevent severe thrombocytopenia after myelosuppressive chemotherapy

CSFs have been used to treat patients with neutropenia secondary to disease or treatment and can be administered both IV and subQ. The CSFs that are FDA approved for clinical use are erythropoietin-stimulating agents, granulocyte colony-stimulating factor, granulocyte macrophage colony-stimulating factor, and thrombopoietic growth factor.

Erythropoietin-Stimulating Agents

Erythropoietin-stimulating agents (ESAs) include epoetin alpha (Procrit, Epogen) and darbepoetin alpha (Aranesp). **Erythropoietin** is a glycoprotein produced by the kidney; it stimulates red blood cell (RBC) production in response to hypoxia (decreased oxygen to body tissues). Specifically, erythropoietin stimulates the division and differentiation of committed RBC progenitors (parent cells destined to become circulating RBCs) in the bone marrow. ESAs have undergone close scrutiny as data from clinical trials reveal more deaths in cancer patients receiving ESAs when compared to patients receiving RBC transfusions. Therefore ESAs must be used cautiously and only as indicated, because of the increased risk for death and serious cardiovascular events when administered to increase hemoglobin levels to >12 g/dL. Procrit is currently FDA approved for treatment of anemia secondary to chronic renal failure (CRF), zidovudine (AZT)-treated human immunodeficiency virus (HIV) infections, cancer chemotherapy, and anemia in patients who are undergoing surgery. Aranesp is FDA-approved for treatment of anemia resulting from CRF and for use with chemotherapy treatment of nonmyeloid malignancies. The use of ESAs in patients with anemia may decrease the need for and frequency of RBC transfusion.

Pharmacokinetics ESAs can be administered IV (push) or subQ. According to the manufacturer, ESAs administered by IV are eliminated at a rate consistent with first-order kinetics (process by which the drug

PROTOTYPE DRUG CHART 39-1

Epoetin Alpha (Erythropoietin)

Drug Class	**Dosage**
Biologic response modifier Trade Names: Epogen, Procrit, ♣ Eprex Pregnancy Category: C Boxed Warning: ESAs increased the risk for death when given to target Hgb or >12 g/dL in cancer patients.	A: Modify dose to keep target hemoglobin <12 g/dL CRF: 50-100 units/kg 3 times/wk, Cancer chemotherapy: 50-150 units/kg 3 times/wk or 40,000 units/wk IV: Dialysis patients (administer at end of dialysis treatment) IV/subQ: Nondialysis, CRF patients IV/subQ: 100 U/kg 3 times/wk for 8 wk in AZT-treated HIV-infected patients Initial dose to those with EPO levels <500 mU/mL and receiving <4200 mg of AZT/wk; patients with EPO level >500 mU/mL unlikely to respond to EPO therapy subQ: Cancer chemotherapy
Contraindications	**Drug-Lab-Food Interactions**
Uncontrolled hypertension, hypersensitivity to mammalian cell-derived products or human albumin	Drug: None known Lab: Increase hematocrit, decrease plasma volume Iron stores need to be monitored and replaced: Patients with serum ferritin <100 mcg/L, or serum transferring saturation <20% should receive supplemental iron therapy Food: None known Caution: Pregnancy, lactation, porphyria; safety in children not established; increased mortality and/or tumor progression, serious cardiovascular and thromboembolic events if target hemoglobin of 12 g/dL exceeded.
Pharmacokinetics	**Pharmacodynamics**
Absorption: subQ, IV Distribution: PB: UK Metabolism: $t\frac{1}{2}$: 4-13 h in patients with CRF; 20% less in those with normal renal function Excretion: In urine	IV: Onset: 7-10 d Peak: 2-4 wk Duration: UK subQ: Onset: 7-10 d Peak: 5-4 h Duration: UK
Therapeutic Effects/Uses	
To treat anemia secondary to CRF or AZT (zidovudine) treatment of HIV infections. Use in patients with anemia secondary to cancer chemotherapy Mode of Action: Increased production of RBCs triggered by hypoxia or anemia	
Side Effects	**Adverse Reactions**
Sense of well-being, hypertension, arthralgias, nausea, edema, fatigue, injection site reaction, rash, diarrhea, shortness of breath	Seizures, hyperkalemia Life-threatening: Cerebrovascular accident, myocardial infarction

A, Adult; *CRF*, chronic renal failure; *d*, day; *EPO*, erythropoietin; *h*, hour; *HIV*, human immunodeficiency virus; *IV*, intravenous; *PB*, protein-binding; *RBC*, red blood cell; *subQ*, subcutaneous; $t\frac{1}{2}$, half-life; *UK*, unknown; *wk*, week; <, less than; >, greater than; ♣, Canadian drug name.

is eliminated in part by hepatic and renal blood flow). It has a circulating half-life ranging from approximately 4 to 13 hours in patients with CRF. Plasma levels of Procrit have been detected for at least 24 hours. After subQ administration of Procrit to CRF patients, peak serum levels are achieved within 5 to 24 hours. The half-life of IV-administered Procrit is approximately 20% shorter in normal patients without CRF than in patients with CRF. Prototype Drug Chart 39-1 details the characteristics of this BRM.

Side Effects and Adverse Reactions

It is imperative that the target hemoglobin never exceed 12 g/dL, because the risks of death, serious cardiovascular events, and tumor progression increase at greater values. Close monitoring of hemoglobin response to the ESA and possible dose modification are essential to safe therapy.

The side effects of erythropoietin include hypertension, headache, arthralgias (joint pain), nausea, edema, fatigue, diarrhea, vomiting, chest pain, injection site skin reaction, asthenia (weakness), dizziness, seizures, thrombosis (clots), and allergic reactions. Studies demonstrate that ESA administration is usually well tolerated, and there have been no reports of serious allergic reactions or anaphylaxis. Rare transient skin reactions have been reported. Blood pressure may increase in patients with CRF who receive ESA during the early phase of treatment when the hematocrit (Hct) is on the rise. About 25% of patients with CRF who receive dialysis may require initiation of or increase in antihypertensive therapy. It is postulated that increases in blood pressure may relate to increases in Hct; therefore it is recommended that the dose of ESA be decreased if the Hct increase exceeds 4 points in any 2-week period. Similarly an increase in Hct may cause increased vascular access clotting (clots in the blood vessel at the connection site of the artificial kidney) in hemodialysis patients. Patients may require increased heparinization during ESA therapy to prevent clotting of the artificial kidney. Seizures occurred in patients with CRF who received ESA during clinical trials; activity was particularly evident during the first 90 days of therapy.

Dosing

Procrit should be administered at a starting dose of 50 to 100 units/kg three times a week for patients with CRF. For patients receiving cancer chemotherapy, therapy should not be initiated if the patient's hemoglobin (Hgb) level is ≥10 g/dL. The Hgb should be monitored on a weekly basis until the level becomes stable. The dose should be titrated for each patient to achieve and maintain the lowest Hgb level sufficient to avoid blood transfusions. The initial recommended dose of Procrit in adults is 150 units/kg 3 times a week or 40,000 units per week given subQ. The dose should be reduced by 25% when the Hgb reaches a level needed to avoid a transfusion or increases >1 g/dL in any 2-week period. The dose should be held if the Hgb exceeds a level needed to avoid transfusion and then restarted at 25% below the previous dose. Aranesp dose is 0.45 mcg/kg subQ every week or 500 mcg subQ every 3 weeks. If the rate of Hgb increase is >1 g/dL in 2 weeks or if the Hgb reaches a level needed to avoid transfusion, the dose should be reduced by 25% of the prior dose. If the Hgb exceeds a level needed to avoid transfusion, the dose should be held until the Hgb approaches a level where transfusion may be required. At this point, the dose should be restarted at 25% of the previous dose. ESAs should be discontinued if after 8 weeks of therapy there is no response as measured by Hgb levels or if transfusions are still required. Otherwise, discontinue ESAs at the completion of the course of chemotherapy.

The following situations must be considered and evaluated if a patient does not respond or maintain a response to an ESA:

1. Iron deficiency
2. Underlying infections, inflammatory, or malignant processes
3. Occult blood loss
4. Underlying hematologic disease
5. Folic acid or vitamin B_{12} deficiency
6. Hemolysis
7. Aluminum intoxication
8. Osteitis fibrosa cystica (fibrous degeneration with formation of cysts and nodules secondary to hyperparathyroidism)

Administration

Erythropoietin-stimulating agent administration is contraindicated in patients with (1) uncontrolled hypertension, (2) known hypersensitivity to mammalian cell–derived products, and (3) known hypersensitivity to human albumin or polysorbate. Evaluation of iron stores should occur during erythropoietin therapy. Transferrin saturation should be at least 20%, and ferritin should be at least 100 ng/mL. Iron supplements may be used to increase and maintain transferrin saturation to support erythropoietin-stimulated erythropoiesis. There are no known ESA drug interactions.

Aranesp is available in 1-mL single-dose polysorbate-preserved vials; single-dose prefilled syringes (with polysorbate) in 200-mcg/0.4 mL, 300-mcg/0.6 mL, or 500-mcg/1 mL dose with a 27-gauge ½-inch needle (SingleJect); single-dose prefilled SureClick autoinjectors (with polysorbate) in 25-mcg/0.42 mL, 40-mcg/0.4 mL, 60-mcg/0.3 mL, 100-mcg/0.5 mL, 150-mcg/0.3 mL, 200-mcg/0.4 mL, 300-mcg/0.6 mL, or 500-mcg/1 mL dose.

Preparation of ESAs

1. Do not shake, because shaking may denature the glycoprotein, rendering it biologically inactive.
2. Store the vials at 36° F to 46° F (2° C to 8° C). Do not freeze.
3. The single-dose vial of Procrit contains no preservatives, so any unused drug must be discarded immediately; the multidose vial contains preservatives and must be stored at 36° F to 46° F (2° C to 8° C) between doses; discard 21 days after initial access.
4. Protect Aranesp from light.

Granulocyte Colony-Stimulating Factor

Recombinant DNA technology can produce colony-stimulating factors for human **granulocytes** (a type of WBC responsible for fighting infection). Two commercially available forms are filgrastim (Neupogen) and pegfilgrastim (Neulasta). **Granulocyte colony-stimulating factor** (G-CSF) is a glycoprotein produced by monocytes (a type of WBC), fibroblasts (immature fiber-producing cells), and endothelial cells (cells that line the heart cavity and blood and lymph vessels). It regulates the production of neutrophils (granular leukocytes, WBCs) within the bone marrow. It is approved and available for the following indications to decrease the incidence of infections in patients: (1) receiving myelosuppressive cancer chemotherapy, (2) receiving induction or consolidation chemotherapy for acute myeloid leukemia, (3) receiving bone marrow transplantation for cancer, (4) undergoing peripheral blood progenitor cell collection and therapy (mobilization of stem cells for rescue), and (5) with severe, chronic neutropenia. G-CSF has been evaluated as an adjunct to chemotherapy for both solid tumor and hematologic malignancies and has been evaluated in studies using a number of different chemotherapy regimens. Filgrastim and pegfilgrastim are commercially available forms of G-CSF. Prototype Drug Chart 39-2 gives the drug data for filgrastim (Neupogen) and pegfilgrastim (Neulasta).

Filgrastim

Pharmacokinetics Filgrastim administration results in a two-phase neutrophil response. An early response is seen within 24 hours of

PROTOTYPE DRUG CHART 39-2

Filgrastim and Pegfilgrastim

Drug Class Granulocyte colony-stimulating factor Trade Names: Neupogen, G-CFS, Neulasta Pregnancy Category: C	**Dosage** A: IV inf/subQ: 5 mcg/kg/d Neupogen C: Neupogen: 5 mcg/kg/d; Neulasta: 6 mg subQ × 1 during chemotherapy cycle Refer to specific protocols.
Contraindications Hypersensitivity to *Escherichia coli*–derived proteins; 24 hours before or after cytotoxic chemotherapy Caution: Pregnancy, lactation; safety in children not established	**Drug-Lab-Food Interactions** Drug: None known Lab: Increase lactic acid, LDH, alkaline phosphatase; transient increase in WBC and neutrophil count Food: None known
Pharmacokinetics Absorption: subQ: Well absorbed Distribution: PB: UK Metabolism: $t\frac{1}{2}$: 2-3.5 h; Neulasta: 15-80 h Excretion: Probably in urine	**Pharmacodynamics** IV/subQ: Onset: 24 h Peak: 3-5 d Duration: 4-7 d
Therapeutic Effects/Uses To decrease incidence of infection in patients receiving myelosuppressive chemotherapeutic agents, including patients with AML undergoing induction or consolidation therapy, and patients undergoing bone marrow transplant; adjunct to chemotherapy for both solid tumor and hematologic malignancies; and for mobilization of progenitor stem cells used in autologous transplant; also for treatment of patients with severe, chronic neutropenia. Mode of Action: Increases production of neutrophils, and enhances their phagocytosis	
Side Effects Nausea, vomiting, skeletal pain, alopecia, diarrhea, fever, skin rash, anorexia, headache, cough, chest pain, sore throat, constipation	**Adverse Reactions** Neutropenia, dyspnea, splenomegaly, psoriasis, hematuria Life-threatening: Thrombocytopenia, myocardial infarction, adult respiratory distress syndrome in patients with sepsis, splenic rupture

A, Adult; *C,* child; *d,* day; *h,* hour; *inf,* infusion; *IV,* intravenous; *LDH,* lactate dehydrogenase; *PB,* protein-binding; *subQ,* subcutaneous; $t\frac{1}{2}$, half-life; *UK,* unknown.

administration, and then there is a second peak in circulating neutrophils following the chemotherapy-induced **nadir** (lowest value of formed blood cells). The proliferation-induced increase in neutrophils usually begins 4 to 5 days after administration is initiated, but timing may vary based on type and dose of myelosuppressive therapy, the patient's underlying disease, and prior treatment history. The elimination half-life of G-CSF in both normal patients and those with cancer is 3.5 hours. Clearance rates are approximately 0.5 to 0.7 mL/min/kg.

Side Effects and Adverse Reactions. The side effects of filgrastim therapy include nausea, vomiting, skeletal pain, alopecia, diarrhea, neutropenia, fever, mucositis, fatigue, anorexia, dyspnea, headache, cough, skin rash, chest pain, generalized weakness, sore throat, stomatitis, constipation, and pain of unspecified origin. Of these reactions, bone pain is the only consistently observed reaction attributed to G-CSF therapy, and this relates to the expanding bone marrow. Bone pain is of mild to moderate severity and is well controlled with nonopioid analgesia. It occurs more frequently in patients receiving higher IV doses (20 to 100 mcg/kg/day) than in patients receiving lower subcutaneous doses (3 to 10 mcg/kg/day). Rarely splenic rupture may occur, and patients who complain of left upper abdominal pain and/or shoulder tip pain should be evaluated for an enlarged spleen or splenic rupture. The drug may rarely cause adult respiratory distress syndrome in neutropenic patients who are septic and may cause sickle cell crisis in patients with sickle cell disease.

Dosing. G-CSF should not be administered during the 24-hour period before and the 24-hour period after chemotherapy agents are administered because of the potential sensitivity of rapidly dividing myeloid cells to chemotherapy. It may stimulate the proliferation of rapidly dividing cells that may be destroyed by chemotherapy drugs. G-CSF can be administered subQ and by IV infusion. The recommended starting dose of G-CSF for patients receiving myelosuppressive cancer chemotherapy is 5 mcg/kg/day subQ or IV infusion over 15 to 30 minutes. Doses may be increased in 5-mcg/kg/day increments for each chemotherapy cycle, according to the duration and severity of the absolute neutrophil count nadir. The **absolute neutrophil count (ANC)** is determined using the following equation:

$$\text{Total white blood cell count (WBC)} \times (\%\ \text{neutrophils} + \%\ \text{bands})$$

G-CSF causes a transient increase in neutrophil counts 1 to 2 days after initiation of therapy. However, to achieve a sustained therapeutic response, G-CSF therapy should continue until postchemotherapy nadir ANC is 10,000/mm^3. Premature discontinuation of G-CSF therapy before expected ANC recovery is not recommended.

The dose of G-CSF given for bone marrow transplantation is 10 mcg/kg/day IV infusion over 4 hours or as a continuous IV infusion over 24 hours. The first dose must be given at least 24 hours after cytotoxic chemotherapy and at least 24 hours after bone marrow infusion. Subsequent dosing is determined by the ANC. The dose of G-CSF for stem cell mobilization (progenitor cell collection) is 10 mcg/kg/day subQ or IV as a bolus or continuous infusion. It is given for at least 4 days prior to the first leukapheresis procedure and is continued until the last leukapheresis. Monitor the ANC closely, and modify the dose if the WBC is >100,000/mm^3.

Administration. G-CSF administration has no demonstrable effects on fertility in male and female rats. Its carcinogenic potential is not known. Caution should be used when G-CSF is given to pregnant and nursing patients. The manufacturer recommends that the benefits justify the potential risks.

Filgrastim's efficacy has not been demonstrated in children, although safety data indicate that it does not cause any greater toxicity in children than in adults.

There has been no evidence of other drug interaction with filgrastim, but its administration is contraindicated in patients with known hypersensitivity to *Escherichia coli*–derived proteins.

Preparation. Neupogen is supplied either as 1-mL vials containing 300 mcg of filgrastim; 1.6-mL vials containing 480 mcg of filgrastim; or prefilled syringes (SingleJect with UltraSafe needle guard) containing 300 mcg of filgrastim in 0.5 mL (600 mcg/mL), or 480 mcg in 0.8 mL (600 mcg/mL). Both the vials and prefilled syringes are preservative-free, therefore the manufacturer recommends that the vials and syringes be used one time only and that any vials left at room temperature for longer than 6 hours be discarded. Filgrastim should be stored in a refrigerator at 36° F to 46° F (2° C to 8° C). Do not freeze or shake the vials or syringes.

Pegfilgrastim

Pharmacokinetics Filgrastim is eliminated via the kidneys. Pegfilgrastim is a pegylated form of filgrastim (**pegylation** is the process of adding a polyethylene glycol [PEG] molecule to another molecule). Pegfilgrastim therefore becomes a larger substance and as a result is not as easily eliminated from the body via the kidneys. The decreased rate of urinary excretion keeps this G-CSF in the body longer, thereby reducing the frequency of injections. Filgrastim requires daily IV or subQ injections for up to 2 weeks to be effective, whereas pegfilgrastim only requires a once per chemotherapy cycle injection to be effective. For patients and their families, this reduction in dosing frequency alleviates the burden of daily clinic trips for injections.

Pegfilgrastim is FDA approved to decrease the incidence of infections and febrile neutropenia in patients with nonmyeloid malignancies receiving chemotherapy associated with clinically significant febrile neutropenia.

Side Effects and Adverse Reactions. Side effects are similar to those of filgrastim with the most frequently reported adverse event being bone pain. This bone pain is effectively reduced with acetaminophen 650 mg or ibuprofen 400 mg by mouth every 4 to 6 hours.

Dosing and Administration. The recommended dose is 6 mg of pegfilgrastim administered as a single subcutaneous injection given at least 24 hours after chemotherapy once per chemotherapy cycle. The drug should not be administered during the period 14 days before and 24 hours after administration of cytotoxic chemotherapy.

Preparation, Storage, and Handling. Pegfilgrastim is supplied in prefilled syringes containing 6 mg in 0.6 mL. This colorless, preservative-free medication should be protected from light and refrigerated at 36° F to 46° F (2° C to 8° C). Only one injection is to be given, and any unused pegfilgrastim must be discarded.

Granulocyte-Macrophage Colony-Stimulating Factor

Granulocyte-macrophage colony-stimulating factor (GM-CSF), or sargramostim, belongs to a group of growth factors that support survival, clonal expression, and differentiation (maturation) of hematopoietic progenitor cells. It induces partially committed progenitor (parent) cells to divide and differentiate in the granulocyte macrophage (a type of WBC responsible for recognizing and destroying bacteria through phagocytosis) pathway. GM-CSF, unlike G-CSF, is a multilineage factor that promotes proliferation of myelomonocytic, megakaryocytic, and erythroid progenitors. Activated T-cells, endothelial cells, and fibroblasts produce GM-CSF in vivo. Commercial production of GM-CSF is accomplished through recombinant DNA technology and is FDA approved for use to induce and support myeloid reconstitution (1) after induction of chemotherapy in acute myelogenous leukemia (AML), (2) in both autologous and allogeneic bone marrow transplant (BMT), (3) for mobilization of autologous peripheral blood progenitor cells, and (4) in BMT failure or delayed engraftment. Sargramostim (GM-CSF) is commercially available as Leukine. Prototype Drug Chart 39-3 presents the drug data for sargramostim.

Pharmacokinetics GM-CSF has been found to effectively accelerate myeloid engraftment (growth and development of bone marrow and subsequent circulating blood cell activity) in autologous BMT. After autologous BMT in patients with non-Hodgkin's lymphoma, acute lymphoblastic leukemia, or Hodgkin's disease, GM-CSF administration resulted in accelerated myeloid engraftment, decreased duration of antibiotic use, reduced duration of infectious episodes, and shortened hospitalizations.

Side Effects and Adverse Reactions

Side effects of GM-CSF administration include fever, mucous membrane disorder, asthenia (weakness), malaise, sepsis, nausea, diarrhea, vomiting, anorexia, liver damage, alopecia, rash, peripheral edema, dyspnea, blood dyscrasias, renal dysfunction, and central nervous system disorder. This drug should be administered with caution to patients with preexisting pleural or pericardial effusions, because it may increase fluid retention. Sequestration of granulocytes in the pulmonary circulation has been seen with GM-CSF administration. The phenomenon results in dyspnea and suggests that special attention be given to respiratory symptoms during or immediately following GM-CSF infusions, a caution that is especially important for patients with underlying pulmonary

PROTOTYPE DRUG CHART 39-3

Sargramostim

Drug Class	Dosage
Granulocyte-macrophage colony-stimulating factor Trade Name: Leukine Pregnancy Category: C	A: IV: 250 mcg/m²/d as a 2-h infusion for 21 d after autologous BMT Some protocols use subQ administration.
Contraindications	**Drug-Lab-Food Interactions**
Within 24 h of chemotherapy administration or within 12 h after last dose of radiation therapy; excessive leukemia myeloid blast cells in bone marrow; hypersensitivity to GM-CSF, yeast-derived products Caution: Pregnancy, lactation, heart failure; safety in children not established; not FDA approved for children	Drug: Lithium and steroids may increase effect Lab: Increase in WBC and platelet counts, bilirubin, creatinine, and liver enzymes Food: None known
Pharmacokinetics	**Pharmacodynamics**
Absorption: IV: Essentially complete Distribution: PB: UK Metabolism: t½: 2 h Excretion: Probably in urine	IV: Onset: 7-14 d Peak: UK Duration: Baseline WBCs by 1 wk after administration
Therapeutic Effects/Uses	
To accelerate growth and development of bone marrow and circulating blood cell activity in autologous BMT Mode of Action: Increased production and functional activity of eosinophils, macrophages, monocytes, and neutrophils	
Side Effects	**Adverse Reactions**
Generally well tolerated; diarrhea, fatigue, chills, weakness, local irritation at injection site; peripheral edema, rash	Pleural/pericardial effusion, rigors, GI hemorrhage, dyspnea

A, Adult; *BMT*, bone marrow transplant; *d*, day; *FDA*, Food and Drug Administration; *GI*, gastrointestinal; *h*, hour; *IV*, intravenous; *PB*, protein-binding; *subQ*, subcutaneous; *t ½*, half-life; *UK*, unknown; *WBC*, white blood cell; *wk*, week.

disease. The GM-CSF infusion should be reduced by half or discontinued if the patient experiences dyspnea.

Supraventricular dysrhythmia has been observed during GM-CSF infusion, suggesting cautious administration in patients with preexisting cardiac disease. Renal and hepatic dysfunction, as indicated by elevated serum creatinine, bilirubin, and liver function tests, have occurred with GM-CSF administration. If these values become elevated, GM-CSF dosage should be reduced or therapy interrupted.

GM-CSF therapy is contraindicated in patients with excessive leukemia myeloid blast cells in the bone marrow or peripheral blood (>10%) and in patients with a known hypersensitivity to GM-CSF, yeast-derived products, or any component of the product. Because of the sensitivity of rapidly dividing hematopoietic progenitor cells to cytotoxic chemotherapy or radiologic therapy, GM-CSF should not be administered within 24 hours before or after chemotherapy or within 12 hours before or after radiation therapy.

GM-CSF should be administered to pregnant or nursing patients only if clearly indicated (i.e., if benefits outweigh risks). Efficacy in the pediatric population has not been established.

Carcinogenic, mutagenic, or fertility effects have not been determined. A full evaluation of drug interactions has not been conducted, but drugs that may potentiate the myeloproliferative effects of GM-CSF, such as lithium and corticosteroids, should be used with caution.

Dosing

The recommended dose of GM-CSF is 250 mcg/m²/day for 21 days as a 2-hour infusion beginning 2 to 4 hours after autologous bone marrow infusion; or on day 11 (4 days after completion of induction chemotherapy for AML) until ANC is >1500 cells/mm³ for 3 consecutive days. When used for stem cell mobilization, the dose is given daily prior to and throughout the period of stem cell collection; when used after stem cell reinfusion, the drug is administered daily until ANC is >1500 cells/mm³. When used for bone marrow transplant graft failure or delay, the drug is given daily for 14 days as a 2-hour infusion, followed by an assessment of the response.

Administration

GM-CSF is administered IV over 2 to 4 hours or subQ. The drug should not be administered within 24 hours of chemotherapy administration or within 12 hours before or after radiation therapy. Manufacturers recommend dose reduction or discontinuation in the presence of a severe adverse reaction, appearance of blast cells (immature, possibly malignant cells), or disease progression. To avoid potential complications associated with leukocytosis, therapy should be stopped if the ANC is >20,000 cells/mm³.

Preparation

Leukine is available as lyophilized Leukine (250 mcg), a sterile, white, preservative-free powder that requires reconstitution, or as liquid Leukine (500 mcg). The powder is reconstituted with 1 mL of sterile water for injection. During reconstitution, the diluent should be directed at the side of the vial and the contents gently swirled but not shaken. Further dilution with 0.9% sodium chloride only is done in preparation for the 2-hour IV infusion. The final concentration of solution should be >10 mcg/mL. The infusion should be completed within 6 hours of preparation to ensure stability and potency. Sargramostim powder, reconstituted vials, and diluted solution should be refrigerated at 36° F to 46° F (2° C to 8° C). The liquid sargramostim vials can be stored at 36° F to 46° F (2° C to 8° C) for up to 20 days once the vial has been entered.

Thrombopoietic Growth Factor

Oprelvekin is recombinant human interleukin-11, a platelet (thrombocyte) growth factor available commercially as Neumega. This product can potentially prevent recurrent severe chemotherapy-induced thrombocytopenia. According to the manufacturer, Oprelvekin stimulates megakaryocyte and thrombocyte production. This effect results in functionally and morphologically normal circulating platelets. Neumega is indicated to prevent severe thrombocytopenia and to reduce the need for platelet transfusions following myelosuppressive chemotherapy in adult patients with nonmyeloid malignancies who are at high risk for severe thrombocytopenia. Neumega is not indicated following myeloablative (transplant) chemotherapy. It has the potential to prevent severe thrombocytopenia and to reduce the need for platelet transfusions following myelosuppressive chemotherapy. Efficacy is most evident in those who experience severe thrombocytopenia following the previous chemotherapy cycle. However, in clinical practice the potential side effect of severe fluid retention limits its use.

Pharmacokinetics Product dosing should begin 6 to 24 hours after completion of chemotherapy. Studies have shown that daily subQ dosing for 14 days increased the platelet count in a dose-dependent way. Platelet counts begin to increase between 5 and 9 days after the start of Neumega administration. After administration of the product stops, the platelet count continues to increase for up to 7 days, returning to baseline within 14 days.

Animal studies demonstrate that Neumega is cleared rapidly from the serum and distributed to highly perfused organs. The kidney is the primary route of elimination, although most of the product is metabolized before excretion. Neumega is contraindicated in patients with a history of hypersensitivity to the product or any of its components and should be used cautiously in patients with heart failure.

Side Effects and Adverse Reactions

The side effects of Neumega include serious fluid retention, cardiovascular events, ophthalmologic events, and severe hypersensitivity reactions. Fluid retention as evidenced by peripheral edema; exertional dyspnea; and worsening of preexisting pleural effusions, ascites, and pericardial effusions is reversible within several days once the product is discontinued. Transient atrial arrhythmias (fibrillation or flutter) have occurred in approximately 10% of patients, and postmarketing reports have indicated that ventricular arrhythmias occur as well. These arrhythmias may be related to fluid retention, advanced age, or underlying cardiac disease. Papilledema and transient visual blurring have been reported in about 1.5% of patients. Postmarketing reports also indicate that hypersensitivity reactions including anaphylaxis have occurred, and the drug should be discontinued if there is evidence of symptomatic bronchospasm or anaphylaxis.

Drug interactions include Neumega and diuretics, which may increase the risk of hypokalemia. Laboratory abnormalities include a decrease in hemoglobin related to increased plasma volume (fluid retention), decreased serum proteins (albumin, transferrin, gamma globulins), and elevated plasma fibrinogen. No studies have been done to assess the carcinogenic potential of the product, and no studies have determined its safety and effectiveness in children, pregnant patients, or breastfeeding patients. Use in these situations should be evaluated carefully.

Dosing

The recommended dose of Neumega in adults is 50 mcg/kg given once daily. It should be administered subQ as a single injection in the thigh, abdomen, hip, or upper arm. If the patient has severe renal impairment (creatinine clearance <30 mL/min), the dose is reduced to 25 mcg/kg. Safety and efficacy in pediatric patients has not been established. The first dose of Neumega should be given 6 to 24 hours after completion of chemotherapy. Platelet counts should be monitored to determine the duration of Neumega therapy.

Administration

Administration should continue until the postnadir count is >50,000 cells/mcL. Dosing beyond 21 days is not recommended. Neumega should be discontinued at least 2 days before chemotherapy is begun.

Preparation

Neumega is available for subQ administration in single-use vials containing 5 mg of oprelvekin as a sterile, lyophilized powder. When reconstituted with 1 mL of sterile water for injection, it has a concentration of 5 mg/mL. Reconstituted Neumega is a clear, colorless, isotonic solution with a pH of 7.0. During reconstitution, avoid excessive shaking of the vial; direct sterile water for injection at the side of the vial, and swirl contents gently. Do not reenter or reuse a single-dose vial. The parenteral drug product should be visually inspected and discarded if there is discoloration or visible particulate matter.

Neumega should be used within 3 hours of reconstitution whether it has been stored refrigerated at 36° F to 46° F (2° C to 8° C) or at room temperature up to 77° F (25° C). Do not freeze, and do not shake the reconstituted product.

Patient Information

Self-administration of Neumega should not be attempted until the patient fully understands the health care provider's instructions about its preparation, correct dose, and proper method for injection. The injection site should not be rubbed. The dose is given at the same time each day. If a dose is missed, the next scheduled dose should be taken. Note: Patients can safely receive concurrent doses of ESA, G-CSF, and Neumega. Different injection sites should be used for each agent.

INTERLEUKIN-2

Interleukins are a group of proteins produced by the body's WBCs—the lymphocytes. Because interleukins are hormone-like glycoproteins manufactured by the lymphocytes, they are sometimes called **lymphokines**. One of the most widely studied interleukins is interleukin-2 (IL-2).

First defined in 1976, this substance was found to have antitumor activities, particularly in renal cell carcinoma and malignant melanoma. IL-2 is produced commercially through recombinant DNA technology as aldesleukin (Proleukin). Proleukin is FDA approved for treatment of metastatic renal cell carcinoma and metastatic melanoma.

Pharmacokinetics Proleukin, administered either by IV infusion or subQ injection, is rapidly distributed to the extravascular extracellular space and eliminated by the kidneys. The serum half-life of IL-2 is short, and because of this rapid clearance, IL-2 is administered frequently in short infusions.

Side Effects and Adverse Reactions

Proleukin should be administered only to patients with normal cardiac and pulmonary function, because side effects may be severe. The principal serious side effects are capillary leak syndrome and infection. *Capillary leak syndrome* is characterized by loss of vascular tone with leakage of plasma fluids into the extravascular space, including the lungs. This can cause hypotension and decreased blood circulation to vital organs, resulting in angina, myocardial infarction, respiratory distress, gastrointestinal bleeding, and mental status changes. Infection may result from alteration in neutrophil function, with the most severe infection being sepsis and bacterial endocarditis. Many patients with cancer are at risk for gram-negative infections related to their indwelling central lines, and they may benefit from prophylactic antibiotic therapy. The most frequent side effects reported as a result of IL-2 use include hypotension, nausea, vomiting, diarrhea, mental status changes, oliguria/anuria, anemia, thrombocytopenia, fever, chills, sinus tachycardia, pulmonary congestion, dyspnea, pain at injection site, fatigue, weakness, malaise, and elevated liver function tests. Table 39-2 lists adverse events/effects of IL-2. According to the manufacturer, Proleukin should be discontinued permanently if certain organ system toxicities occur (Table 39-3) and should be held and restarted under specific parameters for other toxicities (Table 39-4).

Preparation

Proleukin is supplied in single-use vials, each containing 22 million (1.3 mg) units of Proleukin. Unreconstituted vials should be stored refrigerated at 36° F to 46° F (2° C to 8° C). After aseptic reconstitution with 1.2 mL of sterile water for injection (*not* bacteriostatic water), each mL contains 18 million IU (1.1 mg) of Proleukin. Inject the sterile water into the vial, and swirl gently; do not shake. The resulting solution should be a clear, colorless to pale yellow liquid. Withdraw the indicated dose of Proleukin from the vial, and dilute in a 50-mL 5% dextrose IV bag. If not used immediately, the IV bag can be stored for 48 hours in a refrigerator. Infuse over a 15-minute period through nonfiltered IV tubing. Discard any unused portion of the reconstituted drug. Table 39-5 presents route, dosage, use, and considerations information for Proleukin.

TABLE 39-2 INCIDENCE OF ADVERSE EVENTS TO INTERLEUKIN-2

EVENTS BY BODY SYSTEM	% OF PATIENTS	EVENTS BY BODY SYSTEM	% OF PATIENTS
Cardiovascular		**Gastrointestinal**	
Hypotension	85	Nausea and vomiting	87
(requiring pressors)	71	Diarrhea	76
Sinus tachycardia	70	Stomatitis	32
Arrhythmias	22	Anorexia	27
Atrial	8	Gastrointestinal bleeding	13
Supraventricular	5	(requiring surgery)	2
Ventricular	3	Dyspepsia	7
Junctional	1	Constipation	5
Bradycardia	7	Intestinal perforation/ileus	2
Premature ventricular contractions	5	Pancreatitis	1
Premature atrial contractions	4		
Myocardial ischemia	3	**Neurologic**	
Myocardial infarction	2	Mental status changes	73
Cardiac arrest	2	Dizziness	17
Congestive heart failure	1	Sensory dysfunction	10
Myocarditis	1	Special sensory disorders (vision, speech, taste)	7
Stroke	1		
Gangrene	1	Syncope	3
Pericardial effusion	1	Motor dysfunction	2
Endocarditis	1	Coma	1
Thrombosis	1	Seizure (grand mal)	1

TABLE 39-3 ORGAN SYSTEM TOXICITIES WITH INTERLEUKIN-2

ORGAN SYSTEM	PERMANENTLY DISCONTINUE TREATMENT FOR THE FOLLOWING TOXICITIES
Cardiovascular	Sustained ventricular tachycardia (5 beats)
	Cardiac rhythm disturbances not controlled or unresponsive to management
	Recurrent chest pain with electrocardiographic changes, documented angina, or myocardial infarction
	Pericardial tamponade
Pulmonary	Intubation required >72 h
Renal	Renal dysfunction requiring dialysis >72 h
Central nervous system	Coma or toxic psychosis lasting >48 h
	Repetitive or difficult-to-control seizures
Gastrointestinal	Bowel ischemia/perforation/gastrointestinal bleeding requiring surgery

h, hour; >, greater than.

KERATINOCYTE GROWTH FACTOR

Keratinocyte growth factor (palifermin) is available commercially as Kepivance and is indicated for decreasing the incidence and duration of severe oral mucositis in patients with hematologic malignancies receiving myelotoxic therapy requiring hematologic stem cell support. There is no evidence at this time as to its safety (may stimulate growth of tumors dependent upon this growth factor) or efficacy in patients receiving chemotherapy for solid tumors. The drug is contraindicated in patients with hypersensitivity to *E. coli*–derived therapy or to palifermin.

Pharmacokinetics Kepivance binds to the keratinocyte growth factor receptor on epithelial cells, such as those of the oral mucosa, and initiates proliferation, differentiation, and migration of the epithelial cells. Thicker buccal mucosa is laid down, and in clinical trials this led to a significantly reduced incidence of grade 3/4 oral mucositis, a decreased duration of oral mucositis, and less opioid use for oral mucositis in transplant patients.

TABLE 39-4 INTERLEUKIN-2 DOSE HELD AND GIVEN

ORGAN SYSTEM	HOLD DOSE IF:	SUBSEQUENT DOSES MAY BE GIVEN IF:
Cardiovascular	Patient has atrial fibrillation, supraventricular tachycardia, or bradycardia that requires treatment or is recurrent or persistent	Patient is asymptomatic with full recovery to normal sinus rhythm
	Systolic BP is <90 mm Hg with increasing requirements for pressors	Systolic BP is 90 mm Hg and stable or improving requirements for pressors
	Any ECG change consistent with MI or ischemia with or without chest pain; suspicion of cardiac ischemia	Patient is asymptomatic, MI has been ruled out, clinical suspicion of angina is low
Pulmonary	O_2 saturation <94% on room air or <90% with 2 L O_2 by nasal prongs	O_2 saturation 94% on room air or 90% with 2 L O_2 by nasal prongs
Central nervous system	Mental status changes, including moderate confusion or agitation	Mental status changes have completely resolved
Systemic	Patient has sepsis syndrome and is clinically unstable	Sepsis syndrome has resolved, patient is clinically stable, and infection is under treatment
Renal	Serum creatinine is >4.5 mg/dL, or serum creatinine is ≥4 mg/dL in presence of severe volume overload, acidosis, or hyperkalemia	Serum creatinine is <4 mg/dL, and fluid and electrolyte status is stable
	Persistent oliguria, urine output of 10 mL/h for 16-24 h with rising serum creatinine	Urine output is >10 mL/h with decrease of serum creatinine 1.5 mg/dL or normalization of serum creatinine
Hepatic	Signs of hepatic failure, including encephalopathy, increasing ascites, liver pain, and hypoglycemia	All signs of hepatic failure have resolved*
Gastrointestinal	Stool guaiac is repeatedly >3 to 4+	Stool guaiac is negative
Skin	Bullous dermatitis or marked worsening of preexisting skin condition (avoid topical steroid therapy)	All signs of bullous dermatitis have been resolved

*Discontinue all further treatment for that course. Consider starting a new course of treatment at least 7 weeks after cessation of adverse event and hospital discharge.

BP, Blood pressure; *ECG*, electrocardiographic; *h*, hour; *MI*, myocardial infarction; *O_2*, oxygen; >, greater than; <, less than.

TABLE 39-5 INTERLEUKIN*

GENERIC (BRAND)	ROUTE AND DOSAGE	USES AND CONSIDERATIONS
interleukin-2 (Proleukin)	Two 5-day treatment periods separated by a rest period A: IV: 600,000 IU/kg (0.037 mg/kg) by 15-min IV infusion q8h for maximum of 14 doses. Following 9 days of rest, repeat the schedule for another 14 doses, for a maximum of 28 doses per course	For treating metastatic renal cancer and metastatic melanoma. *Do not* give dexamethasone during treatment unless absolutely necessary; it may negate the effects of Proleukin.

*Patients receiving IL-2 by any route, in any dose, and in any setting—inpatient or outpatient—should be monitored closely for signs of toxicity.

A, Adult; *d*, day; *h*, hour; *IV*, intravenous; *min*, minute; *wk*, week.

Side Effects and Adverse Reactions

The most common side effects of Kepivance are skin toxicities (rash, erythema, edema, pruritus) and oral toxicities (tongue thickening, oral/perioral dysesthesia [distorted sensation], tongue discoloration, and taste alteration). Other side effects are hypertension and transient increases in serum lipase and serum amylase. The most concerning potential adverse reaction is the possible stimulation of tumor growth, in that some solid tumors are composed of epithelial cells, which are stimulated to grow when Kepivance stimulates keratinocyte growth receptors. For this reason, the drug is approved only in hematologic malignancies treated with myelotoxic chemotherapy requiring stem cell support.

Drug Interactions

Kepivance binds to heparin, so lines containing heparin should be flushed with normal saline prior to the infusion of Kepivance and following the infusion of Kepivance.

Dosing and Administration

Kepivance must not be administered within 24 hours of, during, or within 24 hours after the administration of myelotoxic chemotherapy. Kepivance is administered in a dose of 60 mcg/kg/day as an IV bolus for 3 consecutive days *before* and 3 consecutive days *after* myelotoxic chemotherapy, for a total of 6 doses. The third dose must be administered 24 to 48 hours before chemotherapy. The fourth dose is given on the same day as, but after, stem cell reinfusion and at least 4 days after the third dose of Kepivance. Flush central lines with normal saline before and after the administration of Kepivance if heparin has been used in the line.

Preparation, Storage, and Handling

Kepivance is available as a white lyophilized powder for IV injection, which is reconstituted with 1.2 mL Sterile Water for Injection, USP, yielding a clear, colorless solution with a Kepivance concentration of 5 mg/mL. Do not shake or vigorously agitate the vial to mix. The reconstituted solution remains stable refrigerated in its carton at 36° F to 46° F (2° C to 8° C) for up to 24 hours. Prior to administration, remove the reconstituted vial from the refrigerator and bring it to room temperature for up to 1 hour, while keeping it protected from light in its carton. Discard the vial if it is out of the refrigerator for more than 1 hour. Also discard any remaining drug after the dose is withdrawn. Do not freeze or filter the drug.

SAFETY: Preventing Medication Errors

Do not confuse...

- sargramostim (Leukine) with Leukeran
- interferon alpha-2a (Roferon-A) with interferon alpha-2b
- interferon alpha-2b (Intron-A) with interferon alpha-2a
- interferon beta-1a (Avonex, Rebif) with interferon beta-1b (Avelox)
- interferon beta-1b (Betaseron) with interferon beta-1a
- interleukin-2 (IL2, Proleukin) with interferon 2

Nursing Process
Patient-Centered Collaborative Care

Biologic Response Modifiers

Assessment

- Obtain a drug and herbal supplement history from patient.
- Obtain baseline information about patient's physical status. This should include height, weight, vital signs, laboratory values (complete blood count [CBC], uric acid, electrolytes, blood urea nitrogen [BUN], creatinine, and liver function tests), cardiopulmonary assessment, intake and output, skin assessment, daily activities status (i.e., ability to perform activities of daily living [ADLs], sleep-rest cycle), nutritional status, presence or absence of underlying symptoms of disease, and use of current or past medication and treatment.
- Assess CBC (with filgrastim, pegfilgrastim, sargramostim, and oprelvekin) before therapy and biweekly throughout therapy to avoid leukocytosis and thrombocytosis. Assess renal and hepatic function tests in patients with dysfunction (liver enzymes, BUN, serum creatinine). With erythropoietin-stimulating agents, assess hematocrit and hemoglobin, serum ferritin, and serum iron–transferrin saturation. Most patients will need supplemental iron. Desired levels are >100 ng/mL for serum ferritin and >20% for serum iron–transferrin saturation. Assess blood pressure before start of and, especially, early in therapy.
- Obtain baseline data regarding patient's psychosocial status, including educational level, ability and desire to learn, support systems, past coping strategies, presence or absence of emotional difficulties, and self-care abilities.
- Assess patient for signs and symptoms associated with BRMs, such as fatigue, chills, diarrhea, and weakness. With filgrastim, be alert to changes in patients with preexisting cardiac conditions. With oprelvekin, assess for peripheral edema and impact on cardiopulmonary system. With aldesleukin, assess for signs and symptoms of capillary leak syndrome, including hypotension and respiratory distress.
- Assess patient's/family's/caregiver's ability to administer subcutaneous BRMs.
- Determine patient's/family's/caregiver's understanding of BRMs and related side effects.

Nursing Diagnoses

- Imbalanced nutrition, less than body requirements, related to side effects of biologic response modifier therapy
- Risk for infection related to side effects of cancer chemotherapy treatments and disease condition
- Risk for deficient fluid volume related to side effects of cancer therapy

- Impaired oral mucous membrane skin integrity related to side effects of cancer chemotherapy and disease condition
- Fatigue related to side effects of biologic response modifier therapy
- Anxiety related to cancer diagnosis and unknown outcomes of treatment
- Fear related to cancer diagnosis
- Risk for caregiver role strain related to cancer diagnosis, treatment, and care responsibilities

Planning

- Patient and family will verbalize understanding of importance of reporting BRM-related side effects.
- Patient and family will demonstrate correct and safe BRM administration.
- Patient and family will identify strategies to deal with BRM-related side effects.
- Patient will remain free from infection.
- Patient will remain free from hemorrhage.

Nursing Interventions

- Monitor patient's temperature at onset of chills.
- Encourage patient to drink at least 2 L of fluid a day to promote excretion of cellular breakdown products. Assess need for IV hydration, especially during IFN-α therapy.
- Encourage patient to rest when tired and to notify health care provider if profound fatigue or anorexia occurs.
- Administer antiemetic as necessary. Premedicate patient with antiemetic, and administer it around the clock for 24 hours after BRM administration to further delay nausea or vomiting.
- Premedicate patient with acetaminophen to reduce chills and fever and with diphenhydramine to reduce nausea.
- Administer BRM at bedtime to decrease consequences of fatigue.
- Cover patient with blankets to promote warmth during chills.
- Administer prescribed meperidine 25 mg to 50 mg intravenously to decrease rigors.
- Consult dietitian, social worker, and physical or occupational therapist as necessary.
- Provide patient and family the opportunity to discuss effect of BRM therapy on quality of life.
- Refer patient and family to financial counselor if reimbursement of BRM therapy is problematic.
- Continue with same brand of BRM, and notify health care provider if considering changing brand.
- Remember that palifermin binds with heparin, so if patient has a central line, it must be flushed with normal saline before and after administration of palifermin.

Patient Teaching

General

- Explain to patient and family the rationale for BRM therapy.
- Explain the frequency and rationale for studies and procedures during BRM therapy.
- Inform patient and family that most BRM side effects disappear within 72 to 96 hours after discontinuation of therapy.
- Instruct patients of childbearing age to use contraceptives during BRM therapy and for 2 years after completion of therapy.
- Provide patient with information regarding the effect of BRM-related fatigue on ADLs, including sexuality.
- Explain to patient that concurrent use of herbal products with BRM therapy is not recommended (see Herbal Alert 39-1).

Side Effects

- Advise patient to report episodes of difficulty in concentration, confusion, or somnolence.
- Report weight loss.
- Report dyspnea, palpitations, and signs of infection or bleeding.

Self-Administration

- Demonstrate correct drug administration techniques.
- Provide patient/family/caregiver with written or video instructions regarding BRM self-administration.

Cultural Considerations

- Obtain an interpreter when necessary; do not rely on family members who may not fully disclose personal information because of cultural norms.

Evaluation

- Evaluate patient/family/caregiver education strategies by asking them to discuss the potential effect of BRM therapy on quality of life.
- Evaluate patient/family/caregiver BRM administration technique if appropriate.
- Periodically evaluate patient/family/caregiver management of BRM-related side effects.
- Patient will have a decreased incidence of infection after autologous bone marrow transplantation.
- Patient will have a decreased incidence of thrombocytopenia after chemotherapy administration.

KEY WEBSITES

Biological Response Modifier: What Is It?: *arthritis.about.com/cs/enbrel/a/biologics.htm*

National Cancer Institute: *www.cancer.gov/cancertopics/treatment/biologicaltherapy*

CRITICAL THINKING CASE STUDY

JW, a 55-year-old man, has metastatic non–small-cell cancer of the lung. His past treatment regimen included external-beam chest irradiation and combination chemotherapy. Two weeks before hospitalization, JW received a course of carboplatin and paclitaxel as an outpatient. He was admitted to the hospital with neutropenia, thrombocytopenia, and anemia. Upon assessment, he was cachectic, weak, and able to perform activities of daily living only with assistance. Admitting laboratory data were Hgb (hemoglobin) 6.9, Hct (hematocrit) 20.6, platelets 16,000, and WBC 600 with ANC 96. JW was started on filgrastim 480 mcg/day subQ; erythropoietin 40,000 units subQ once a week; and oprelvekin 50 mcg/kg/day subQ. Parenteral antibiotic therapy was also initiated. Nursing diagnoses for JW included a potential for infection related to neutropenia, bleeding related to thrombocytopenia, fatigue related to anemia, and anxiety related to hospitalization. Nursing interventions included the following:

- Maintaining scrupulous hand washing and hand hygiene before and after patient contact
- Allowing no one with cold or infection to enter patient's room
- Obtaining vital signs and pulmonary assessment every 4 hours
- Inspecting all sites associated with risk for infection (e.g., venipuncture sites, oral cavity, perirectal area) during every shift
- Protecting skin and mucosal surfaces to prevent entry of microorganisms by not using suppositories, enemas, or urinary catheters; by avoiding IM injections; and by not obtaining rectal temperatures
- Monitoring laboratory values daily
- Providing bedside range-of-motion exercises and physical therapy
- Giving emotional support to patient/family/caregiver
- Instructing patient/family/caregiver about giving subQ injections and self-assessment of the signs and symptoms of infection and bleeding

JW continued therapy with filgrastim, oprelvekin, and erythropoietin. The following laboratory data were obtained:

TESTS	DAY 1	DAY 2	DAY 3	DAY 4	DAY 5
Hgb	6.9	6.5	7.1	7.8	7.9
Hct	20.6	19.4	21.6	22.9	22.9
Platelets	16,000	15,000	16,000	20,000	30,000
WBC/ANC	600/96	1000/0	1200/168	9400/4700	31,500/18,270

Filgrastim was discontinued on day 5, and antibiotics were discontinued on day 4, but erythropoietin and oprelvekin were continued. JW's physical therapy was continued in the physical therapy department. JW refused red blood cell transfusion on the basis of religious beliefs and was discharged to home (day 5) on procrit 40,000 units subQ once a week and Neumega 50 mcg/kg/day subQ for 7 days.

1. Why were filgrastim, oprelvekin, and erythropoietin indicated?
2. What is an often overlooked side effect of erythropoietin?
3. Based on this side effect, what should be closely monitored in a patient receiving this agent?
4. Why was the patient receiving this agent on days 1 to 4, and what risk does this pose?

NCLEX STUDY QUESTIONS

1. A patient is being seen regularly for treatment of chronic leukemia. The nurse understands that this patient has been treated with interferon alpha (Roferon-A). What is the primary action of this biologic response modifier?
   a. Enhancing immune function, producing white blood cells, producing antigen/antibody reaction
   b. Causing allergic reactions, producing red blood cells, producing interferon
   c. Immunomodulation, causing cytotoxic/cytostatic effects, differentiating stem cells
   d. Producing cytokines, producing interleukin, fighting infection
2. A patient diagnosed with malignant melanoma, a skin cancer, is treated with interferon alpha-2a (Roferon-A). The nurse teaches this patient about which side effect of interferon-α that will make the patient uncomfortable?
   a. Increase in white blood cells
   b. Increase in red blood cells
   c. Flulike syndrome
   d. Gastrointestinal symptoms
3. A patient has a low platelet count (thrombocytopenia). The nurse reviews the list of medications and is aware that platelet production can be stimulated with which drug?
   a. epoetin alpha (Procrit, Epogen)
   b. filgrastim (Neupogen)
   c. interleukin-11 (Oprelvekin)
   d. sargramostim (Leukine)
4. The nurse is caring for a patient who has previously received the biologic response modifiers as a subcutaneous injection either in the outpatient office or at home. The patient will now be receiving a drug that is not often used in clinical practice because of its serious side effects and must be administered by IV infusion. Which drug meets this criterion?
   a. Epoetin alpha (Procrit or Epogen)
   b. interleukin-2 (Proleukin)
   c. G-CSF (Neupogen or Neulasta)
   d. GM-CSF (sargramostim)

5. A patient lives 120 miles from her oncologist's medical office and relies on her working son for transportation to and from the office. In developing a plan of care for the patient, the nurse understands that the order for pegfilgrastim was prescribed for what reason?
   a. Pegfilgrastim is eliminated via the kidneys.
   b. Pegfilgrastim is a pegylated filgrastim.
   c. Pegfilgrastim is not easily eliminated from the body.
   d. Pegfilgrastim requires a once per chemotherapy cycle injection.
6. The nurse is caring for a patient who arrives at the outpatient office for a scheduled dose of an erythropoietin-stimulating agent (ESA) to be administered today. The patient arrives with the following laboratory values noted on the chart: Hemoglobin 12.8 mg/dL; platelet count 148,000/mm^2; white blood cell count 4.800/mm^2. Which action is most appropriate for the nurse to implement?
   a. Discuss with the health care provider the potential need for a colony-stimulating factor such as G-CSF based on the laboratory results.
   b. Contact the health care provider to discuss the laboratory results and a possible discontinuation of the ordered ESA.
   c. After comparing the patient's laboratory results with the previous results, discuss the laboratory values with the health care provider to determine whether a colony-stimulating factor such as interleukin-2 should be given.
   d. Discuss with the health care provider the potential need for more laboratory tests prior to administration of ESA.

Answers: 1, a; 2, c; 3, c; 4, b; 5, d; 6, c.

UNIT XIII

Respiratory Agents

The respiratory tract is divided into two major parts: (1) the upper respiratory tract, which consists of the nares, nasal cavity, pharynx, and larynx, and (2) the lower respiratory tract, which consists of the trachea, bronchi, bronchioles, alveoli, and alveolar-capillary membrane. Air enters through the upper respiratory tract and travels to the lower respiratory tract, where gas exchanges occur. Figure XIII-1 illustrates these components.

Ventilation and *respiration* are distinct terms and should not be used interchangeably. Ventilation is the movement of air from the atmosphere through the upper and lower airways to the alveoli. *Respiration* is the process whereby gas exchange occurs at the alveolar-capillary membrane. Respiration has three phases: ventilation, perfusion, and diffusion.

1. *Ventilation* is the phase in which oxygen passes through the airways. With every inspiration, air is moved into the lungs, and with every expiration, air is transported out of the lungs.
2. *Perfusion* involves blood flow at the alveolar-capillary bed. Perfusion is influenced by alveolar pressure. For gas exchange to occur, the perfusion of each alveolus must be matched by adequate ventilation. Factors such as mucosal edema, secretions, and bronchospasm increase resistance to air flow and decrease ventilation and diffusion of gases.

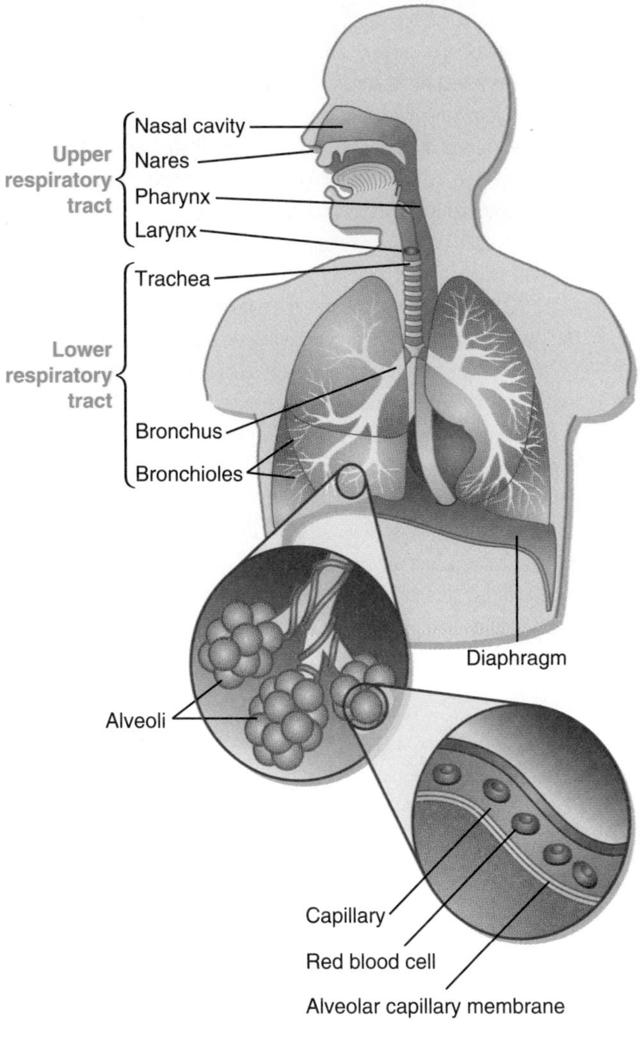

FIGURE XIII–1 Basic structures of the respiratory tract.

3. *Diffusion* (molecules move from higher to lower concentration) of gases takes place when oxygen passes into the capillary bed to be circulated, and carbon dioxide leaves the capillary bed and diffuses into the alveoli for ventilatory excretion.

The chest cavity is a closed compartment bounded by 12 ribs, the diaphragm, thoracic vertebrae, sternum, neck muscles, and intercostal muscles between the ribs. The pleura are membranes that encase the lungs. The lungs are divided into lobes; the right lung has three lobes, and the left lung has two lobes. The heart, which is not attached to the lungs, lies on the mid-left side in the chest cavity.

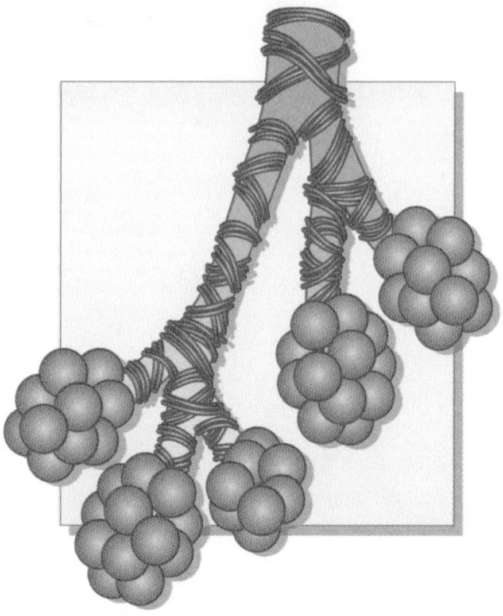

FIGURE XIII–2 Bronchial smooth muscle fibers become more closely spaced as they near the alveoli.

LUNG COMPLIANCE

Lung compliance is the lung volume based on the unit of pressure in the alveoli. This volume determines the lung's ability to stretch. Factors that influence lung compliance include (1) connective tissue (collagen and elastin) and (2) surface tension in the alveoli, which is controlled by surfactant. Surfactant lowers the surface tension in the alveoli and prevents interstitial fluid from entering. Increased lung compliance is present with chronic obstructive pulmonary disease (COPD), and decreased lung compliance occurs with restrictive pulmonary disease. With low compliance, there is decreased lung volume resulting from increased connective tissue or increased surface tension. The lungs become "stiff," and it takes greater-than-normal pressure to expand lung tissue.

CONTROL OF RESPIRATION

Oxygen (O_2), carbon dioxide (CO_2), and hydrogen (H^+) ion concentration in the blood influence respiration. *Chemoreceptors* are sensors that are stimulated by changes in these gases and ions. The central chemoreceptors, located in the medulla near the respiratory center and cerebrospinal fluid, respond to an increase in carbon dioxide and a decrease in pH by increasing ventilation. However, if the carbon dioxide level remains elevated, the stimulus to increase ventilation is lost.

Peripheral chemoreceptors, located in the carotid and aortic bodies, respond to changes in oxygen (PO_2) levels. A low blood oxygen level (PO_2 <60 mm Hg) stimulates the peripheral chemoreceptors, which in turn stimulate the respiratory center in the medulla, and ventilation is increased. If oxygen therapy increases the oxygen level in the blood, the PO_2 may be too high to stimulate the peripheral chemoreceptors, and ventilation will be depressed.

BRONCHIAL SMOOTH MUSCLE

The tracheobronchial tube is composed of smooth muscle whose fibers spiral around the tracheobronchial tube, becoming more closely spaced as they near the terminal bronchioles (Figure XIII-2). Contraction of these muscles constricts the airway. The sympathetic and parasympathetic nervous systems affect the bronchial smooth muscle in opposite ways. The vagus nerve (parasympathetic nervous system) releases acetylcholine, which causes bronchoconstriction. The sympathetic nervous system releases epinephrine, which stimulates the $beta_2$ receptor in the bronchial smooth muscle, resulting in bronchodilation. These two nervous systems counterbalance each other to maintain homeostasis.

Cyclic adenosine monophosphate (cyclic AMP) in the cytoplasm of bronchial cells increases bronchodilation by relaxing the bronchial smooth muscles. The pulmonary enzyme phosphodiesterase can inactivate cyclic AMP. Drugs of the methylxanthine group (theophylline) inactivate phosphodiesterase, thus permitting cyclic AMP to function.

This unit includes Chapter 40, Drugs for Upper Respiratory Disorders, and Chapter 41, Drugs for Lower Respiratory Disorders. Chapter 40 discusses drugs used to relieve cold symptoms, such as antihistamines, decongestants, antitussives, and expectorants. Drugs used to alleviate and control airway obstruction are presented in Chapter 41. These include the sympathomimetics (adrenergics), particularly the $beta_2$ adrenergics; methylxanthines such as theophylline; leukotriene receptor antagonists; glucocorticoids; cromolyn sodium; and mucolytics.

CHAPTER

40

Drugs for Upper Respiratory Disorders

evolve WEBSITE

http://evolve.elsevier.com/KeeHayes/pharmacology/

- Animations
- Content Updates
- Key Points
- Review Questions for the NCLEX® Examination
- References from the Textbook
- Unfolding Case Studies

OBJECTIVES

- Compare antihistamine, decongestant, antitussive, and expectorant drug groups.
- Differentiate between rhinitis, sinusitis, and pharyngitis.
- Describe the side effects of nasal decongestants and how they can be avoided.
- Apply the nursing process for drugs used to treat the common cold.

OUTLINE

KEY TERMS

acute pharyngitis, p. 581
acute rhinitis, p. 573
allergic rhinitis, p. 574
antihistamines, p. 574
antitussives, p. 578
common cold, p. 573
decongestants, p. 574
expectorants, p. 578
rebound nasal congestion, p. 575
rhinorrhea, p. 574
sinusitis, p. 581

Upper respiratory infections (URIs) include the common cold, acute rhinitis, sinusitis, and acute pharyngitis. The **common cold** is the most prevalent type of URI. Adults have an average of 2 to 4 colds per year, and children have an average of 4 to 12 colds per year. Incidence is seasonally variable, with approximately 50% of the population experiencing a winter cold and 25% experiencing a summer cold. A cold is not considered a life-threatening illness, but, it causes physical and mental discomfort and loss of time at work and school. The common cold is an expensive illness in the United States—more than $40 billion is spent each year on over-the-counter (OTC) cold and cough preparations.

COMMON COLD, ACUTE RHINITIS, AND ALLERGIC RHINITIS

The common cold is caused by the rhinovirus and affects primarily the nasopharyngeal tract. **Acute rhinitis** (acute inflammation of the mucous membranes of the nose) usually accompanies the common cold. Acute rhinitis is not the same as **allergic rhinitis,** often called *hay fever,* which is caused by pollen or a foreign substance (e.g., animal dander). Nasal secretions increase in both acute rhinitis and allergic rhinitis.

A cold is most contagious 1 to 4 days before the onset of symptoms (the incubation period) and during the first 3 days of the cold. Transmission occurs more frequently from touching contaminated surfaces and then touching the nose or mouth than it does from viral droplets released by sneezing.

The groups of drugs used to manage cold symptoms include antihistamines (H_1 blockers), decongestants (sympathomimetic amines), antitussives, and expectorants. These drugs can be used singly or in combination preparations.

Symptoms of the common cold include **rhinorrhea** (watery nasal discharge), nasal congestion, cough, and increased mucosal secretions. If a bacterial infection secondary to the cold occurs, infectious rhinitis may result, and nasal discharge becomes tenacious, mucoid, and yellow or yellow-green. The nasal secretions are discolored by white blood cells and cellular debris that are by-products of the fight against the bacterial infection. Antibiotics used to treat bacterial respiratory infections are discussed in Chapters 29, 30, and 31.

Antihistamines

Antihistamines, H_1 blockers or H_1 antagonists, compete with histamine for receptor sites, preventing a histamine response. The two types of histamine receptors, H_1 and H_2, cause different responses. When the H_1 receptor is stimulated, the extravascular smooth muscles, including those lining the nasal cavity, are constricted. With stimulation of the H_2 receptor, an increase in gastric secretions occurs, which is a cause of peptic ulcer (see Chapter 48). These two types of histamine receptors should not be confused. Antihistamines decrease nasopharyngeal secretions by blocking the H_1 receptor.

Although antihistamines are commonly used as cold remedies, these agents can also treat allergic rhinitis. However, the antihistamines are not useful in an emergency situation such as anaphylaxis. Most antihistamines are rapidly absorbed in 15 minutes, but they are not potent enough to combat anaphylaxis.

First-Generation Antihistamines

The antihistamine group can be divided into first and second generations. Most first-generation antihistamines cause drowsiness, dry mouth, and other anticholinergic symptoms, whereas second-generation antihistamines have fewer anticholinergic effects and a lower incidence of drowsiness. Many OTC cold remedies contain a first-generation antihistamine, which can cause drowsiness; therefore patients should be alerted not to drive or operate dangerous machinery when taking such medications. The anticholinergic properties of most antihistamines cause dryness of the mouth and decreased secretions, making them useful in treating rhinitis caused by the common cold. Antihistamines also decrease the nasal itching and tickling that cause sneezing.

The first-generation antihistamine diphenhydramine (Benadryl) has been available for years and is frequently combined with other ingredients in cold remedy preparations. Its primary use is to treat rhinitis. Prototype Drug Chart 40-1 lists the pharmacologic behavior of diphenhydramine.

Pharmacokinetics Diphenhydramine can be administered orally, intramuscularly (IM), or intravenously (IV). It is well absorbed from the gastrointestinal (GI) tract, but systemic absorption from topical use is minimal. It is highly protein-bound (98%) and has an average half-life of 2 to 7 hours. Diphenhydramine is metabolized by the liver and excreted as metabolites in the urine.

Pharmacodynamics Diphenhydramine blocks the effects of histamine by competing for and occupying H_1 receptor sites. It has anticholinergic effects and should not be used by patients with narrow-angle glaucoma. Drowsiness is a major side effect of the drug; in fact, it is sometimes used in sleep-aid products. Diphenhydramine is also used as an antitussive (i.e., it alleviates cough). Its onset of action can occur in as few as 15 minutes when taken orally and IM. IV administration results in an immediate onset of action. The duration of action is 4 to 6 hours.

Diphenhydramine can cause CNS depression if taken with alcohol, narcotics, hypnotics, or barbiturates.

> **SAFETY: Preventing Medication Errors**
>
> **Do not confuse:**
> - **Benadryl** (antihistamine) with **benazepril** (ACE inhibitor)

Side Effects of Most First-Generation Antihistamines. The most common side effects of first-generation antihistamines are drowsiness, dizziness, fatigue, and disturbed coordination. Skin rashes and anticholinergic symptoms (e.g., dry mouth, urine retention, blurred vision, wheezing) may also occur.

Second-Generation Antihistamines

The second-generation antihistamines are frequently called *nonsedating antihistamines* because they have little to no effect on sedation. In addition, these antihistamines cause fewer anticholinergic symptoms. Although a moderate amount of alcohol and other central nervous system (CNS) depressants may be taken with second-generation antihistamines, many clinicians advise against such use.

The second-generation antihistamines cetirizine (Zyrtec), fexofenadine (Allegra), and loratadine (Claritin) have half-lives between 7 and 15 hours. Azelastine (Astelin) is a second-generation antihistamine that has a half-life of 22 hours and is administered by nasal spray. Table 40-1 lists the first- and second-generation antihistamines used to treat allergic rhinitis.

Nasal and Systemic Decongestants

Nasal congestion results from dilation of nasal blood vessels caused by infection, inflammation, or allergy. With this dilation, there is a transudation of fluid into the tissue spaces, resulting in swelling of the nasal cavity. Nasal **decongestants** (sympathomimetic amines) stimulate the alpha-adrenergic receptors, producing vascular constriction (vasoconstriction) of the capillaries within the nasal mucosa. The result is

PROTOTYPE DRUG CHART 40-1

Diphenhydramine

Drug Class	Dosage
Antihistamine Trade Names: Benadryl, ♣ Aller-Dryl Pregnancy Category: B	A: PO: 25-50 mg q6-8h; *max:* 300 mg/d C: 6-12 y: PO: 12.5-25 mg q4-6h C: 2-6 y: PO: 6.25 q4-6h A: IM/IV: 10-50 mg as single dose, q4-6h; *max:* 400 mg/d C: IM/IV: 5 mg/kg/d in 4 divided doses; *max:* 300 mg/d
Contraindications	**Drug-Lab-Food Interactions**
Acute asthmatic attack, severe liver disease, lower respiratory disease, neonate Caution: Narrow-angle glaucoma, benign prostatic hypertrophy, pregnancy, newborn or premature infant, breastfeeding, urinary retention	Drug: Increase CNS depression with alcohol, opioids, hypnotics, barbiturates; avoid use with MAOIs
Pharmacokinetics	**Pharmacodynamics**
Absorption: PO: Well absorbed Distribution: PB: 98% Metabolism: t½: 2-7 h Excretion: In urine as metabolites	PO: Onset: 15-45 min Peak: 1-4 h Duration: 4-6 h IM: Onset: 15-30 min Peak: 1-4 h Duration: 4-7 h IV: Onset: Immediate Peak: 0.5-1 h Duration: 4-7 h
Therapeutic Effects/Uses	
To treat allergic rhinitis and itching; to prevent motion sickness; sleep aid; antitussive Mode of Action: Blocks histamine$_1$, thereby decreasing allergic response; affects respiratory system, blood vessels, and GI system	
Side Effects	**Adverse Reactions**
Drowsiness, dizziness, fatigue, nausea, vomiting, urinary retention, constipation, blurred vision, dry mouth and throat, reduced secretions, hypotension, abdominal pain, diarrhea, hearing disturbances; excitation in children; photosensitivity	Life-threatening: Agranulocytosis, hemolytic anemia, thrombocytopenia

A, Adult; *C,* child; *CNS,* central nervous system; *d,* day; *GI,* gastrointestinal; *h,* hour; *IM,* intramuscular; *IV,* intravenous; *MAOI,* monoamine oxidase inhibitor; *max,* maximum; *min,* minute; *PB,* protein-binding; *PO,* by mouth; *t ½,* half-life; ♣, Canadian drug name.

shrinking of the nasal mucous membranes and a reduction in fluid secretion (runny nose).

Nasal decongestants are administered by nasal spray or drops or in tablet, capsule, or liquid form. Frequent use of decongestants, especially nasal spray or drops, can result in tolerance and **rebound nasal congestion** (rebound vasodilation instead of vasoconstriction). Rebound nasal congestion is caused by irritation of the nasal mucosa.

Nursing Process
Patient-Centered Collaborative Care

Antihistamine: Diphenhydramine

Assessment
- Determine baseline vital signs.
- Obtain drug history; report if drug-drug interaction is probable.
- Assess for signs and symptoms of urinary dysfunction, including retention, dysuria, and frequency.
- Note complete blood count (CBC) during drug therapy.
- Assess cardiac and respiratory status.
- Obtain history of environmental exposures if patient has an allergic reaction regarding drugs, recent foods eaten, and stress.

Nursing Diagnoses
- Ineffective airway clearance related to nasal congestion
- Risk for imbalanced fluid volume related to excessive sweating and loss of fluids
- Sleep deprivation related to frequent coughing

Planning
- Patient will have decreased nasal congestion, mucosal secretions, and cough.
- Patient will sleep 6 to 8 hours per night.

TABLE 40-1 ANTIHISTAMINES FOR TREATMENT OF ALLERGIC RHINITIS

GENERIC (BRAND)	ROUTE AND DOSAGE	USES AND CONSIDERATIONS
First-Generation Antihistamines		
Alkylamine Derivatives		
brompheniramine maleate (Dimetane)	A: PO: 4-8 mg q6-8h or SR: 12-24 mg once daily; *max:* 24 mg/d A: subQ/IM/IV: 5-20 mg q6-12h; *max:* 40 mg/d C: >6 y: PO: 2-4 mg q6-8h; *max:* 12 mg/d	For allergies. Also present in various cough and decongestant formulas. Pregnancy category: C; PB: UK; t½: 12-34 h
chlorpheniramine maleate (Chlor-Trimeton)	A: PO: 2-4 mg q4-6h; *max:* 24 mg/24 h SR: 12-18 mg b.i.d.; *max:* 36 mg/d C: 6-12 y: PO: 2 mg q4-6h; *max:* 12 mg/d	For allergies including allergic rhinitis. May be used in combination with nasal decongestant. Pregnancy category: C; PB: 72%; t½: 10-24 h
dexchlorpheniramine maleate	A/C >12 y: PO: 2 mg (5 mL) q4-6h C: >6 y: PO: 1 mg (2.5 mL) q4-6h C: 2-5 y: PO: 0.5 mg (1.25 mL) q4-6h	For allergic rhinitis. May be used with epinephrine to treat anaphylactic reaction. Pregnancy category: B; PB: 72%; t½: 20-24 h
Ethanolamine Derivatives		
clemastine fumarate	A/C: >12 y: PO: 1.34-2.68 mg b.i.d./t.i.d.; *max:* 8 mg/d	For allergic rhinitis and urticaria. Pregnancy category: B; PB: UK; t½: 4-6 h
diphenhydramine (Benadryl)	See Prototype Drug Chart 40-1.	
Piperidine Derivatives		
cyproheptadine HCl	A: PO: 4-20 mg/d in divided doses; *max:* 0.5 mg/kg/d C: 7-14 y: PO: 4 mg/d in divided doses; *max:* 16 mg/d C: 2-6 y: PO: 0.25 mg/kg/d in divided doses; *max:* 12 mg/d	For allergies (rhinitis, conjunctivitis, pruritus). Common side effects include drowsiness, dry mouth, dizziness, and epigastric distress. Pregnancy category: B; PB: UK; t½: 1-4 h
Piperazine Derivatives		
levocetirizine (Xyzal)	A/C>12 y: PO: 2.5-5 mg once daily in evening C: 6-11 y: PO: 1.25-2.5 mg once daily in evening	For allergic rhinitis, chronic urticaria. Common side effects include drowsiness, fatigue, and weakness. Pregnancy category: B; PB: 91%-92%; t½: 8-9 h
Other Antihistamines		
codeine, triprolidine and pseudoephedrine (Triacin-C)	Codeine 10 mg, triprolidine 2 mg, pseudoephedrine 30 mg in 5-mL oral syrup A: PO: 10 mL q4-6h; *max:* 20 mL/d C: 6-12 y: PO: 5 mL q4-6h; Codeine 20 mg, triprolidine 4 mg, pseudoephedrine 60 mg in oral tablet A/C: >12y: PO: 1 tab q6h	For rhinitis. Combination of an antihistamine and decongestant. Pregnancy category: C; PB: UK; t½: 3 h
azelastine and fluticasone (Dymista)	A: nasal spray: 1 spray per nostril b.i.d.	For seasonal allergic rhinitis. Most common side effect is bad taste. Pregnancy category: C; PB: 88%-97%; t½: 8-25 h
Second-Generation Antihistamines		
azelastine (Astelin)	Nasal spray: A/C ≥12 y: 1-2 sprays in each nostril q12h C: <11 y: 1 spray in each nostril b.i.d.	For allergic rhinitis. May cause headaches, mild sedation, and bitter taste. Pregnancy category: C; PB: 88%; t½: 22 h
cetirizine (Zyrtec)	A/C: >6 y: PO: 5-10 mg/d Older adults: PO: 5 mg/d	For allergic rhinitis and urticaria. Has few anticholinergic effects. Pregnancy category: B; PB: 93%; t½: 8 h
fexofenadine (Allegra) with pseudoephedrine (Allegra-D)	Fexofenadine 180 mg, pseudoephedrine 240 mg (Allegra-D 24-Hour) A/C: ≥12 y: PO: 1 tab once daily	For allergic rhinitis and rhinorrhea. Has less sedative effect. Pregnancy category: C; PB: 60%-70%; t½: 14.4 h
loratadine (Claritin)	A/C: >6 y: PO: 10 mg/d	For allergic rhinitis and urticaria. Long-acting H_1-blocking effect. Pregnancy category: UK; PB: 97%; t½: 12-15 h
desloratadine (Clarinex)	A/C: >12 y: PO: 5 mg/d C: 6-12 y: PO: 2.5 mg/d C: 2-5 y: PO: 1.25 mg/d	For allergic rhinitis. Pregnancy category: C; PB: 82%-87%; t½: 27 h

A, Adult; *b.i.d.*, twice a day; *C*, child; *d*, day; *h*, hour; *h.s.*, at bedtime; *IM*, intramuscular; *IV*, intravenous; *max*, maximum; *mo*, month; *PB*, protein-binding; *PO*, by mouth; *q.i.d.*, four times a day; *subQ*, subcutaneous; *SR*, sustained-release; *t½*, half-life; *tab*, tablet; *t.i.d.*, three times a day; *UK*, unknown; *y*, year; >, greater than; <, less than.

Nursing Interventions
- Give oral form with food to decrease gastric distress.
- Administer IM form in large muscle. *Avoid subQ injection.*

Patient Teaching

General
- Warn patient to avoid driving a motor vehicle and performing other dangerous activities if drowsiness occurs or until stabilized on drug.
- Advise patient to avoid alcohol and other central nervous system depressants.
- Encourage patient to take drug as prescribed. Notify health care provider if confusion or hypotension occurs.
- Teach patient on prophylaxis for motion sickness to take drug at least 30 minutes before offending event and also before meals and at bedtime during event.
- Inform breastfeeding mothers that small amounts of drug pass into breast milk. Because children are more susceptible to side effects of antihistamines (e.g., unusual excitement or irritability), breastfeeding is not recommended while using these drugs.

Side Effects
- Advise family members or parents that children are more sensitive to effects of antihistamines. Nightmares, nervousness, and irritability are more likely to occur in children.
- Inform older adults that they are more sensitive to effects of antihistamines and are more likely to experience confusion, difficult or painful urination, dizziness, drowsiness, feeling faint, and dryness of mouth, nose, or throat.
- Suggest using sugarless candy or gum, ice chips, or a saliva substitute for temporary relief of mouth dryness.

Cultural Considerations
- Decrease language barriers by decoding jargon used in the health care environment for those with language difficulties and those who are not in the health care field.

Evaluation
- Evaluate effectiveness of drug in relieving allergic symptoms or as a sleep aid.

Systemic decongestants (alpha-adrenergic agonists) are available in tablet, capsule, and liquid form and are used primarily for allergic rhinitis, including hay fever and acute coryza (profuse nasal discharge). Examples of systemic decongestants are ephedrine (Ephedrine), phenylephrine (Neo-Synephrine), and pseudoephedrine (Sudafed). In the past, phenylpropanolamine was used in many cold remedies; however, the U.S. Food and Drug Administration (FDA) ordered its removal from OTC cold remedies and weight-loss aids because reports suggest that the drug might cause stroke, hypertension, renal failure, and cardiac dysrhythmias. Ephedrine, phenylephrine, and pseudoephedrine are frequently combined with an antihistamine, analgesic, or antitussive in oral cold remedies. The advantage of systemic decongestants is that they relieve nasal congestion for a longer period than nasal decongestants; however, currently there are long-acting nasal decongestants. Nasal decongestants usually act promptly and cause fewer side effects than systemic decongestants. Table 40-2 lists systemic and nasal decongestants and their dosages, uses, and considerations.

Side Effects and Adverse Reactions

The incidence of side effects is low with topical preparations such as nose drops. Decongestants can make a patient jittery, nervous, or restless. These side effects decrease or disappear as the body adjusts to the drug.

Use of nasal decongestants for as little as 3 days could result in rebound nasal congestion. Instead of the nasal membranes constricting, vasodilation occurs, causing increased stuffy nose and nasal congestion. The nurse should emphasize the importance of limiting the use of nasal sprays and drops.

As with any alpha-adrenergic drug (e.g., decongestants), blood pressure and blood glucose levels can increase. These drugs are contraindicated or used with extreme caution in patients with hypertension, cardiac disease, hyperthyroidism, and diabetes mellitus.

Drug Interactions

When using decongestants with other drugs, drug interactions can occur. Pseudoephedrine may decrease the effect of beta blockers. Taken together with monoamine oxidase inhibitors (MAOIs), decongestants may increase the possibility of hypertension or cardiac dysrhythmias. The patient should also avoid large amounts of caffeine (coffee, tea) because it can increase restlessness and palpitations caused by decongestants.

Intranasal Glucocorticoids

Intranasal glucocorticoids or steroids are effective for treating allergic rhinitis. Because these agents are steroids, they have an antiinflammatory action, thus decreasing the allergic rhinitis symptoms of rhinorrhea, sneezing, and congestion. The following are examples of intranasal steroids:

- Beclomethasone (Beconase)
- Budesonide (Pulmicort, Rhinocort)
- Dexamethasone (Decadron)
- Flunisolide
- Fluticasone (Flonase, Flovent)
- Triamcinolone (Nasacort AQ)

These drugs may be used alone or in combination with an H_1 antihistamine. With continuous use, dryness of the nasal mucosa may occur.

TABLE 40-2 SYSTEMIC AND NASAL DECONGESTANTS (SYMPATHOMIMETIC AMINES)

GENERIC (BRAND)	ROUTE AND DOSAGE	USES AND CONSIDERATIONS
ephedrine HCl (Primatene)	Bronchospasm: A: PO: 25-50 mg t.i.d./q.i.d. PRN; *max:* 150 mg/d A: subQ/IM/IV: 12.5-25 mg; may repeat; *max:* 150 mg once daily C: PO: 6-12 y: 2-3 mg/kg/d in 4-6 divided doses; *max:* 3 mg/kg/d Nasal spray for nasal congestion: A/C: >12 y: 2-3 sprays in each nostril q4h PRN C: 6-12 y: 1-2 sprays q4h PRN	For nasal congestion, asthma; acute bronchospasm, improves opioid-impaired respiration; corrects hypotension. Alpha- and beta-adrenergic agonist. OTC drug used alone or in combination. Pregnancy category: C; PB: UK; t½: 3-6 h
naphazoline HCl (Privine)	A/C: >12 y: 1-2 sprays 0.05% spray in each nostril q4-6h	For nasal congestion and allergic rhinitis. Can cause rebound congestion, transient hypertension, bradycardia, and cardiac dysrhythmias. Pregnancy category: C; PB: UK; t½: UK
oxymetazoline HCl (Afrin)	A/C: >6 y: 0.05% gtt or spray; 1-2 sprays in each nostril b.i.d. C: 2-5 y (0.025% solution only): 2-3 gtt b.i.d.	Long-acting decongestant. Taken twice a day (morning and evening). Can cause rebound congestion. Use only for 3-5 d. Pregnancy category: C; PB: UK; t½: UK
phenylephrine HCl (Neo-Synephrine Nasal)	A: sol (0.25%-1%): 2-3 sprays in each nostril q4h	For rhinitis. Less potent than epinephrine. Can cause transient hypertension and headaches. Use only for 3-5 d. Pregnancy category: C; PB: UK; t½: 2.5 d
pseudoephedrine (Sudafed)	A: PO: 60 mg q4-6h; SR 120 mg q12h; *max:* 240 mg/d C: 6-12 y: 30 mg q4-6h; *max:* 120 mg/d C: 2-5 y: 15 mg q4-6h; *max:* 60 mg/d	For rhinitis. Less CNS stimulation and hypertension than ephedrine. Pregnancy category: C; PB: UK; t½: 9-15 h
tetrahydrozoline (Tyzine)	A/C: >6 y: Nasal: 2-4 sprays in each nostril q3h PRN C: 2-6 y: Nasal: 2-3 sprays in each nostril q3h PRN	For nasopharyngeal congestion. Pregnancy category: C; PB: UK; t½: UK

A, Adult; *b.i.d.,* twice a day; *C,* child; *CNS,* central nervous system; *d,* day; *gtt,* drops; *h,* hour; *IM,* intramuscular; *IV,* intravenous; *max,* maximum; *OTC,* over-the-counter; *PB,* protein-binding; *PO,* by mouth; *PRN,* as necessary; *q.i.d.,* four times a day; *sol,* solution; *subQ,* subcutaneous; *t½,* half-life; *t.i.d.,* three times a day; *UK,* unknown; *y,* year; *>,* greater than; *<,* less than.

It is rare for systemic effects of steroids to occur, but they are more likely to result with the use of intranasal dexamethasone, which should not be used for longer than 30 days. The other intranasal glucocorticoids undergo rapid deactivation after absorption. Most allergic rhinitis is seasonal; therefore the drugs are for short-term use unless otherwise indicated by the health care provider. Table 40-3 lists the intranasal glucocorticoids and their dosages, uses, and considerations.

Antitussives

Antitussives act on the cough-control center in the medulla to suppress the cough reflex. The cough is a naturally protective way to clear the airway of secretions or any collected material. A sore throat may cause coughing that increases throat irritation. If the cough is nonproductive and irritating, an antitussive may be taken. Hard candy may decrease the constant, irritating cough. Dextromethorphan, a nonnarcotic antitussive, is widely used in OTC cold remedies. Prototype Drug Chart 40-2 lists the drug data related to dextromethorphan (Benylin DM).

The three types of antitussives are nonnarcotic, narcotic, or combination preparations. Antitussives are usually used in combination with other agents (Table 40-4).

Pharmacokinetics Dextromethorphan is available in numerous cold and cough remedy preparations in syrup or liquid form, chewable capsules, and lozenges. Brand name formulations include Robitussin, and Sucrets. The drug is rapidly absorbed and exerts its effects 15 to 30 minutes after oral administration. Its protein-binding percentage is unknown, and the half-life is 11 hours. Dextromethorphan is metabolized by the liver and excreted in the urine.

Pharmacodynamics Dextromethorphan, a nonnarcotic antitussive, suppresses the cough center in the medulla but does not depress respiration. It causes neither physical dependence nor tolerance. The patient should notify the health care provider and seek medical care if the cough lasts longer than 1 week and a fever or rash is present. Patients with underlying medical conditions should seek prompt medical attention.

The onset of action for dextromethorphan is relatively fast, and its duration is 3 to 6 hours. Usually preparations containing dextromethorphan can be used several times a day. CNS depression may occur if the drug is used with alcohol, opioids, sedative-hypnotics, barbiturates, or antidepressants.

Expectorants

Expectorants loosen bronchial secretions so they can be eliminated by coughing. They can be used with or without other pharmacologic agents. Expectorants are found in many OTC cold remedies along with analgesics, antihistamines, decongestants, and antitussives. The most common expectorant in such preparations is guaifenesin. Hydration is the best natural expectorant. When taking an expectorant, patients should increase fluid intake to at least 8 glasses per day to help loosen mucus. Table 40-4 lists the dosages, uses, and considerations for antitussives and expectorants.

TABLE 40-3 INTRANASAL GLUCOCORTICOIDS

GENERIC (BRAND)	ROUTE AND DOSAGE	USES AND CONSIDERATIONS
beclomethasone (Beconase AQ, Qnasl)	A: 1-2 puffs/sprays b.i.d. C: 6-12 y: 1 spray b.i.d.	For seasonal or perennial allergic and nonallergic rhinitis. Pregnancy category: C; PB: 87%; t½: 15 h
budesonide (Pulmicort, Rhinocort)	A/C: >6 y: 1-2 sprays b.i.d. or 4 sprays in the morning	For seasonal rhinitis in adults and children. Maintenance therapy for asthma. Pregnancy category: C; PB: 90%; t½: 2.5-3 h
dexamethasone (Decadron)	A/C: 6-12 y: 1-2 sprays b.i.d.	For allergic and inflammatory conditions. Administered orally, intravenously, ophthalmically, topically, and intranasally. A potent steroid used for short-term therapy. May have a systemic effect. Pregnancy category: C; PB: UK; t½: 2-3.5 h
flunisolide	A: 2 sprays b.i.d./t.i.d. C: 6-14 y: 1 spray t.i.d. or 2 sprays b.i.d.	For seasonal rhinitis in adults and children. May be used for steroid-dependent asthma. Pregnancy category: C; PB: UK; t½: 1-2 h
fluticasone (Flonase, Flovent)	A: 2 sprays once daily or 1 spray b.i.d. C: >6 y: 1 spray/d	For seasonal allergic rhinitis. When symptoms decrease, reduce dose to 1 spray daily. Pregnancy category: C: PB: 91%; t½: 8 h
mometasone furoate (Nasonex)	A: 2 sprays once daily C: 1 spray once daily	For seasonal allergic rhinitis. Pregnancy category: C; PB: UK; t½: UK Note: Direct spray away from nasal septum; gently sniff.
triamcinolone (Nasacort AQ)	A/C: 1-2 sprays once daily	For allergic rhinitis. Has many uses, such as an immunosuppressant. Pregnancy category: C; PB: UK; t½: 2-5 h

A, Adult; *b.i.d.,* twice a day; *C,* child; *h,* hour; *PB,* protein-binding; *q.i.d.,* four times a day; *t½,* half-life; *t.i.d.,* three times a day; *UK,* unknown; *y,* year; >, greater than.

PROTOTYPE DRUG CHART 40-2

Dextromethorphan Hydrobromide

Drug Class Antitussive Trade Names: Robitussin, Sucrets, Benylin DM Pregnancy Category: UK	**Dosage** A: PO: 10-20 mg q4h; *max:* 120 mg/d C: 6-12 y: PO: 5-10 mg q4h; *max:* 60 mg/d C: 2-5 y: PO: 2.5-5.0 mg q4h; *max:* 30 mg/d
Contraindications Chronic obstructive pulmonary disease, chronic productive cough, hypersensitivity; children <2 y	**Drug-Lab-Food Interactions** Drug: Increase effect/toxicity with MAOIs, SSRIs, SNRIs, opioids, sedative-hypnotics, barbiturates, antidepressants, and alcohol Food: Grapefruit juice can increase risk of toxicity.
Pharmacokinetics Absorption: PO: Rapidly absorbed Distribution: PB: UK Metabolism: t½: 11 h Excretion: In urine	**Pharmacodynamics** PO: Onset: 15-30 min Peak: UK Duration: 3-6 h
Therapeutic Effects/Uses To provide temporary suppression of nonproductive cough; to reduce viscosity of tenacious secretions Mode of Action: Inhibits cough center in the medulla	
Side Effects Nausea, dizziness, drowsiness, fatigue, sedation	**Adverse Reactions** Hallucinations (high doses)

A, Adult; *C,* child; *d,* day; *h,* hour; *MAOIs,* monoamine oxidase inhibitors; *max,* maximum; *min,* minute; *PB,* protein-binding; *PO,* by mouth; *t½,* half-life; *UK,* unknown; *y,* year.

Nursing Process
Patient-Centered Collaborative Care

Common Cold

Assessment

- Determine whether there is a history of hypertension, especially if a decongestant is an ingredient in the cold remedy.
- Note baseline vital signs. An elevated temperature of 99°F to 101°F (37.2°C to 38.3°C) may indicate a viral infection caused by a cold.
- Obtain drug history; report if drug-drug interaction is probable. Dextromethorphan HCl given with MAOIs, narcotics, sedative-hypnotics, barbiturates, antidepressants, and alcohol may increase toxicity.
- Assess cardiac and respiratory status.

TABLE 40-4 ANTITUSSIVES AND EXPECTORANTS

GENERIC (BRAND)	ROUTE AND DOSAGE	USES AND CONSIDERATIONS
Opioid Antitussives		
codeine CSS II	A: PO: 10-20 mg q4-6h; *max:* 120 mg/d	Schedule II drug. Can be Schedule V when combined in cough syrup. Usually mixed with antihistamine, decongestant, and/or expectorant. Can cause drowsiness, dizziness, nausea, constipation, and respiratory depression. Pregnancy category: C; PB: 7%; t½: 3-4 h
guaifenesin and codeine (Cheratussin AC, Tussi-Organidin NR) CSS V	Guaifenesin 300 mg, codeine 10 mg per 5 mL A: PO: 5 mL q4h; *max:* 60 mL/d (codeine 120 mg) C: 6-12 y: PO: 2.5 mL q4-6h; *max:* 20 mL/d C: 2-6 y: PO: 2.5 mL q4-6h; *max:* 6 mL/d	An expectorant combined with an opioid antitussive. Also used to control cough caused by bronchitis or common cold. Pregnancy category: C; PB: UK; t½: 1-4 h
homatropine and hydrocodone (Tussigon, Mycodone) CSS III	A: PO: 5-10 mg q4-6h; *max:* 15 mg/d C: >6y: PO: 2.5 mg q4-6h	Relief of cough and pain. Similar side effects as codeine. Pregnancy category: C; PB: UK; t½: 3-4 h
Nonopioid Antitussives		
benzonatate (Tessalon Perles)	A/C: >10 y: PO: 100 mg t.i.d. PRN; *max:* 600 mg/d	Relief of nonproductive cough without respiratory depression. Pregnancy category: C; PB: UK; t½: UK
dextromethorphan hydrobromide (Benylin DM)	See Prototype Drug Chart 40-2.	
promethazine with dextromethorphan	A: PO: 5 mL q4-6h; *max:* 30 mL/d C: 6-12 y: PO: 2.5-5 mL q4-6h; *max:* 20 mL/d C: 2-6 y: PO: 1.25-2.5 mL, q4-6h; *max:* 10 mL/d	For cough. Combination of a phenothiazine and nonnarcotic antitussive. Pregnancy category: C; PB: 80%-93%; t½: 10-14 h
Expectorants		
guaifenesin (Robitussin)	A: PO: 200-400 mg q4h; *max:* 2.4 g/d C: 6-12 y: PO: 100-200 mg q4h; *max:* 1.2 g/d C: 2-5 y: PO: 50-100 mg q4h; *max:* 600 mg/d	For dry, unproductive cough. Can cause nausea and vomiting. May be combined with other cold remedies. Take with water to loosen mucus. Pregnancy category: C; PB: UK; t½: 1 h
Antitussive/Expectorant		
guaifenesin and dextromethorphan (Robitussin-DM)	A: PO: 20-30 mL q4h PRN C: 6-12 y: PO: 10 mL q4h PRN C: 2-5 y: PO: 5 mL q4h PRN	For nonproductive cough. Pregnancy category: C; PB: UK; t½: UK

A, Adult; *C*, child; *CSS*, Controlled Substances Schedule; *d*, day; *h*, hour; *max*, maximum; *PB*, protein-binding; *PO*, by mouth; *PRN*, as necessary; *t½*, half-life; *t.i.d.*, three times a day; *UK*, unknown; *y*, year; <, less than.

Nursing Diagnoses

- Ineffective airway clearance related to nasal congestion
- Risk for imbalanced fluid volume related to excessive sweating and loss of fluids
- Sleep deprivation related to chronic coughing
- Fatigue related to sleep deprivation
- Risk for infection related to insufficient knowledge to avoid exposure to pathogens

Planning

- Patient will be free from nonproductive cough.
- Patient will be free from a secondary bacterial infection.

Nursing Interventions

- Monitor vital signs. Blood pressure can become elevated when a decongestant is taken. Dysrhythmias can also occur.
- Observe color of bronchial secretions. Yellow or green mucus is indicative of a bronchial infection. Antibiotics may be needed.
- Warn patient that codeine preparations for cough suppression can lead to tolerance and physical dependence.

Patient Teaching

General

- Tell patient that hypotension and hyperpyrexia may occur when dextromethorphan is taken with MAOIs.
- Teach patient about proper use of a nasal spray and proper use of "puff" or squeeze products.
- Caution patient not to use more than one or two puffs, four to six times a day, for 5 to 7 days. Rebound congestion can occur with overuse.
- Advise patient to read labels on OTC drugs and to check with health care provider before taking cold remedies.

This is especially important when taking other drugs or when patient has a major health problem such as hypertension or hyperthyroidism. Also, acetaminophen may be in many products, promoting an overdose.

- Inform patient that antibiotics are not helpful in treating common cold viruses. However, they may be prescribed if a secondary infection occurs.
- Encourage older patient with heart disease, asthma, emphysema, diabetes mellitus, or hypertension to contact the health care provider concerning the selection of drug, including OTC drugs.
- Direct patient not to drive during initial use of a cold remedy containing an antihistamine because drowsiness is common.
- Tell patient to maintain adequate fluid intake. Fluids liquefy bronchial secretions to ease elimination with coughing.
- Teach patient not to take a cold remedy before or at bedtime. Insomnia may occur if it contains a decongestant.
- Encourage patient to get adequate rest.
- Inform patient that common cold and flu viruses are transmitted frequently by hand-to-hand contact or by touching a contaminated surface. Cold viruses can live on the skin for several hours and on hard surfaces for several days.
- Advise patient to avoid environmental pollutants, fumes, smoking, and dust to lessen irritating cough.
- Teach patient to perform three effective coughs before bedtime to promote uninterrupted sleep.
- Direct patient and parents to store drug out of reach of children; request childproof caps.
- Advise patient to contact health care provider if cough persists for more than 1 week or is accompanied by chest pain, fever, or headache.

Self-Administration

- Teach patient to self-administer medications such as nose drops and inhalants.
- Encourage patient to cough effectively, to take deep breaths before coughing, and to be in the upright position.

Cultural Considerations

- Allow patient to incorporate traditional remedies for treating common cold into prescribed Western medical practices (if remedies are harmless). Discuss practices that could cause harm.
- Identify conflicts in values and beliefs in treatment of common cold.
- Respectfully present treatment methods to care for the common cold for patients from various cultural backgrounds, such as increasing fluid intake, getting adequate rest, and using disposable tissues to remove nasal and bronchial secretions.
- Advise patient to contact a health professional if cold persists and if body temperature is greater than 101° F (38.3° C).

Evaluation

- Evaluate effectiveness of drug therapy. Determine that patient is free from nonproductive cough, has adequate fluid intake and rest, and is afebrile.

SINUSITIS

Sinusitis is an inflammation of the mucous membranes of one or more of the maxillary, frontal, ethmoid, or sphenoid sinuses. A systemic or nasal decongestant may be indicated. Acetaminophen, fluids, and rest may also be helpful. For acute or severe sinusitis, an antibiotic may be prescribed.

ACUTE PHARYNGITIS

Acute pharyngitis (inflammation of the throat, or "sore throat") can be caused by a virus, beta-hemolytic streptococci (strep throat), or other bacteria. It can occur alone or with the common cold and rhinitis or acute sinusitis. Symptoms include elevated temperature and cough. A throat culture should be obtained to rule out beta-hemolytic streptococcal infection. If the culture is positive for beta-hemolytic streptococci, a 10-day course of antibiotics is often prescribed. Saline gargles, lozenges, and increased fluid intake are usually indicated. Acetaminophen may be taken to decrease elevated temperature. Antibiotics are not effective for viral pharyngitis.

KEY WEBSITES

Information on cetirizine: *www.nlm.nih.gov/medlineplus/druginfo/medmaster/a698026.html*

Information on loratadine: *www.medicinenet.com/loratadine/article.htm*

CRITICAL THINKING CASE STUDY

GH, a 35-year-old patient, has allergic rhinitis. Her prescriptions include loratadine (Claritin) 5 mg/day and fluticasone (Flonase, Flovent) two nasal inhalations/day. Previously she had taken OTC drugs and asked if she should continue to take the OTC drug with her prescriptions. She has never used a nasal inhaler.

1. What additional information is needed from GH concerning her health problem?
2. What is your response to GH concerning the use of OTC drugs with her prescription drugs?
3. How would you instruct GH to use a nasal inhaler? Explain your answer.
4. What are the similarities and differences between loratadine and diphenhydramine? Could one of these antihistamines be more effective than the other? Explain your answer.
5. Design a patient teaching plan for GH in regard to medications and environmental allergens.
6. What could you suggest to decrease allergens (e.g., dust mites) in the home?

NCLEX STUDY QUESTIONS

1. A patient tells the nurse that he has started to take an over-the-counter (OTC) antihistamine, diphenhydramine (Benadryl). In teaching about side effects, what is most important for the nurse to tell the patient?
   a. Do not to take this drug at bedtime to avoid insomnia.
   b. Avoid driving a motor vehicle until stabilized on the drug.
   c. Nightmares and nervousness are more likely in an adult.
   d. Medication may cause him to have excessive secretions.
2. A patient complains of a sore throat and has been told it is due to beta-hemolytic streptococcal infection. The nurse anticipates that the patient has which acute condition?
   a. Rhinitis
   b. Sinusitis
   c. Pharyngitis
   d. Rhinorrhea
3. A patient is prescribed the decongestant oxymetazoline (Afrin) nasal spray. What will the nurse teach the patient?
   a. Take this drug at bedtime because it may cause drowsiness.
   b. Directly spray the medication away from the nasal septum, and gently sniff.
   c. This drug may be used in maintenance treatment for asthma.
   d. Limit use of the drug to 5 to 7 days to prevent rebound nasal congestion.
4. A patient has been prescribed guaifenesin (Robitussin). The nurse understands that the purpose of the drug is to accomplish what?
   a. Treat allergic rhinitis and prevent motion sickness.
   b. Loosen bronchial secretions so coughing can eliminate them.
   c. Compete with histamine for receptor sites, thus preventing a histamine response.
   d. Stimulate alpha-adrenergic receptors, thus producing vascular constriction of capillaries in nasal mucosa.
5. Beclomethasone (Beconase) has been prescribed for a patient with allergic rhinitis. What should the nurse teach the patient regarding this medication?
   a. This may be used for an acute attack.
   b. An oral form is available if the patient prefers to use it.
   c. Avoid large amounts of caffeine intake because an increased heart rate may occur.
   d. With continuous use, dryness of the nasal mucosa/lining may occur.
6. The nurse is teaching a patient about diphenhydramine (Benadryl). Which instructions should the nurse include in the patient's teaching plan? (Select all that apply.)
   a. Take medication on an empty stomach to facilitate absorption.
   b. Avoid alcohol and other central nervous system depressants.
   c. Notify the health care provider if confusion or hypotension occurs.
   d. Use sugarless candy, gum, or ice chips for temporary relief of dry mouth.
   e. Avoid handling dangerous equipment or performing dangerous activities until stabilized on the medication.

Answers: 1, b; 2, c; 3, d; 4, b; 5, d; 6, b, c, d, e.

CHAPTER 41

Drugs for Lower Respiratory Disorders

evolve WEBSITE

http://evolve.elsevier.com/KeeHayes/pharmacology/

- Animations
- Content Updates
- Key Points
- Review Questions for the NCLEX® Examination
- References from the Textbook
- Unfolding Case Studies

OBJECTIVES

- Compare chronic obstructive pulmonary disease (COPD) and restrictive lung disease.
- Differentiate the drug groups used to treat COPD and asthma and the desired effects of each.
- Compare the side effects of beta$_2$-adrenergic agonists and methylxanthines.
- Describe the therapeutic serum or plasma theophylline level and the toxic level.
- Contrast the therapeutic effects of leukotriene antagonists, glucocorticoids, cromolyn, antihistamines, and mucolytics for COPD and asthma.
- Apply the nursing process for the patient taking drugs commonly used for COPD, including asthma, and restrictive lung disease.

OUTLINE

KEY TERMS

asthma, p. 584
bronchial asthma, p. 585
bronchiectasis, p. 584
bronchodilators, p. 584
bronchospasm, p. 585
chronic bronchitis, p. 584
chronic obstructive pulmonary disease, p. 584
emphysema, p. 584
glucocorticoids, p. 595
mucolytics, p. 597
restrictive lung disease, p. 584

Chronic obstructive pulmonary disease (**COPD**) and restrictive pulmonary disease are the two major categories of lower respiratory tract disorders. COPD is caused by airway obstruction with increased airway resistance of air flow to lung tissues. Four major pulmonary disorders cause COPD: chronic bronchitis, bronchiectasis, emphysema, and asthma. Chronic bronchitis, bronchiectasis, and emphysema frequently result in irreversible lung tissue damage. The lung tissue changes resulting from an acute asthmatic attack are normally reversible; however, if the attacks are frequent and asthma becomes chronic, irreversible changes in the lung tissue may result. Patients with COPD usually have a decrease in forced expiratory volume in 1 second (FEV_1) as measured by pulmonary function tests.

Restrictive lung disease is a decrease in total lung capacity as a result of fluid accumulation or loss of elasticity of the lung. Pulmonary edema, pulmonary fibrosis, pneumonitis, lung tumors, thoracic deformities (scoliosis), and disorders affecting the thoracic muscular wall (e.g., myasthenia gravis) are among the types and causes of restrictive pulmonary disease.

Drugs discussed in this chapter are primarily used to treat COPD, particularly asthma. These drugs include **bronchodilators** (sympathomimetics [primarily $beta_2$-adrenergic agonists], methylxanthines [xanthines]), leukotriene antagonists, glucocorticoids, cromolyn, anticholinergics, and mucolytics. Some of these drugs may also be used to treat restrictive pulmonary diseases.

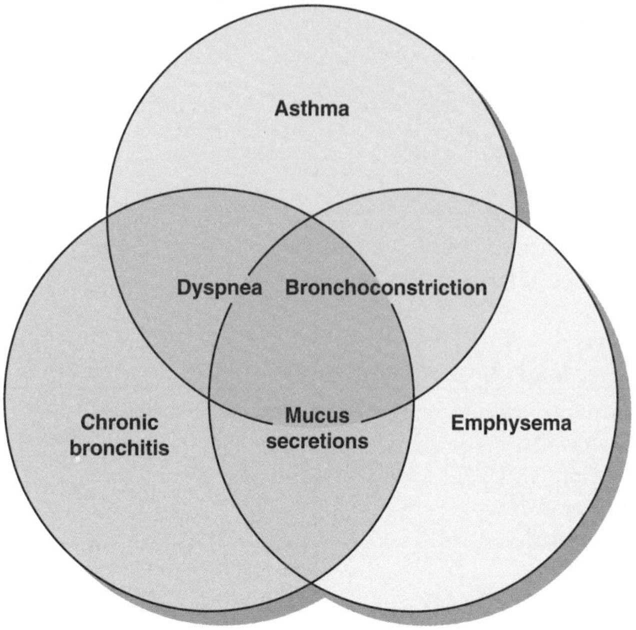

FIGURE 41–1 Overlapping signs and symptoms of chronic obstructive pulmonary disease (COPD) conditions.

CHRONIC OBSTRUCTIVE PULMONARY DISEASE

Asthma is an inflammatory disorder of the airway walls associated with a varying amount of airway obstruction. This disorder is triggered by stimuli such as stress, allergens, and pollutants. When activated by stimuli, the bronchial airways become inflamed and edematous, leading to constriction of air passages. Inflammation aggravates airway hyperresponsiveness to stimuli, causing bronchial cells to produce more mucous, which obstructs air passages. This obstruction contributes to wheezing, coughing, dyspnea (breathlessness), and tightness in the chest, particularly at night or in the early morning.

Bronchial asthma, one of the COPD lung diseases, is characterized by bronchospasm (constricted bronchioles), wheezing, mucus secretions, and dyspnea. There is resistance to air flow caused by obstruction of the airway. In acute and chronic asthma, minimal to no changes are seen in the structure and function of lung tissues when the disease process is in remission. In chronic bronchitis, emphysema, and bronchiectasis, there is permanent, irreversible damage to the physical structure of lung tissue. Symptoms are similar to those of asthma in these three pulmonary disorders, except wheezing does not occur. Figure 41-1 shows the overlapping symptoms of COPD conditions. Frequently, there is a steady deterioration over a period of years.

Chronic bronchitis is a progressive lung disease caused by smoking or chronic lung infections. Bronchial inflammation and excessive mucous secretion result in airway obstruction. Productive coughing is a response to excess mucus production and chronic bronchial irritation. Inspiratory and expiratory rhonchi may be heard on auscultation. Hypercapnia (increased carbon dioxide retention) and hypoxemia (decreased blood oxygen) lead to respiratory acidosis.

In **bronchiectasis,** there is abnormal dilation of the bronchi and bronchioles secondary to frequent infection and inflammation. The bronchioles become obstructed by the breakdown of the epithelium of the bronchial mucosa. Tissue fibrosis may result.

Emphysema is a progressive lung disease caused by cigarette smoking, atmospheric contaminants, or lack of the $alpha_1$-antitrypsin protein that inhibits proteolytic enzymes that destroy alveoli (air sacs). Proteolytic enzymes are released in the lung by bacteria or phagocytic cells. The terminal bronchioles become plugged with mucus, causing a loss in the fiber and elastin network in the alveoli. Alveoli enlarge as many of the alveolar walls are destroyed. Air becomes trapped in the overexpanded alveoli, leading to inadequate gas (oxygen and carbon dioxide) exchange.

Cigarette smoking is the most common risk factor for COPD, especially with chronic bronchitis and emphysema. There is no cure for COPD at this time; however, it remains preventable in most cases. Because cigarette smoking is the most directly related cause, not smoking significantly prevents COPD from developing. Quitting smoking will slow the disease process.

Medications frequently prescribed for COPD include the following:

- Bronchodilators such as sympathomimetics (adrenergics), parasympatholytics (anticholinergic drug, Atrovent), and

methylxanthines (caffeine, theophylline) are used to assist in opening narrowed airways.
- Glucocorticoids (steroids) are used to decrease inflammation.
- Leukotriene modifiers reduce inflammation in the lung tissue, and cromolyn and nedocromil act as antiinflammatory agents by suppressing the release of histamine and other mediators from the mast cells.
- Expectorants are used to assist in loosening mucus from the airways.
- Antibiotics may be prescribed to prevent serious complications from bacterial infections.

See the Key Websites at the end of the chapter for recommended methods for smoking cessation.

Bronchial Asthma

Bronchial asthma is a COPD characterized by periods of bronchospasm resulting in wheezing and difficulty breathing. **Bronchospasm,** or bronchoconstriction, results when the lung tissue is exposed to extrinsic or intrinsic factors that stimulate a bronchoconstrictive response. Factors that can trigger an asthmatic attack (bronchospasm) include humidity; air pressure changes; temperature changes; smoke; fumes (exhaust, perfume); stress; emotional upset; exercise; and allergies to animal dander, dust mites, food, and drugs (e.g., aspirin, ibuprofen, beta-adrenergic blockers). Reactive airway disease (RAD) is a cause of asthma resulting from sensitivity stimulation from allergens, dust, temperature changes, and cigarette smoking.

Pathophysiology

Mast cells, found in connective tissue throughout the body, are directly involved in the asthmatic response, particularly to extrinsic factors. Allergens attach themselves to mast cells and basophils, resulting in an antigen-antibody reaction on the mast cells in the lung; thus the mast cells stimulate the release of chemical mediators such as histamines, cytokines, serotonin, eosinophil chemotactic factor of anaphylaxis (ECF-A), and leukotrienes. Eosinophil counts are usually elevated during an allergic reaction, which indicates that an inflammatory process is occurring. These chemical mediators stimulate bronchial constriction, mucous secretions, inflammation, and pulmonary congestion. Histamine and ECF-A are strong bronchoconstrictors. Bronchial smooth muscles are wrapped spirally around the bronchioles and contract as they are stimulated by these mediators. Exposure to an allergen results in bronchial hyperresponsiveness, epithelial shedding of the bronchial wall, mucous gland hyperplasia and hypersecretion, leakage of plasma leading to swelling, and bronchoconstriction.

Figure 41-2 shows factors contributing to bronchoconstriction. Cyclic adenosine monophosphate (cyclic AMP, or cAMP), a cellular signaling molecule, is involved in many cellular activities and is responsible for maintaining bronchodilation. When histamine, ECF-A, and leukotrienes inhibit the action of cAMP, bronchoconstriction results. The sympathomimetic (adrenergic) bronchodilators and methylxanthines increase the amount of cAMP in bronchial tissue cells.

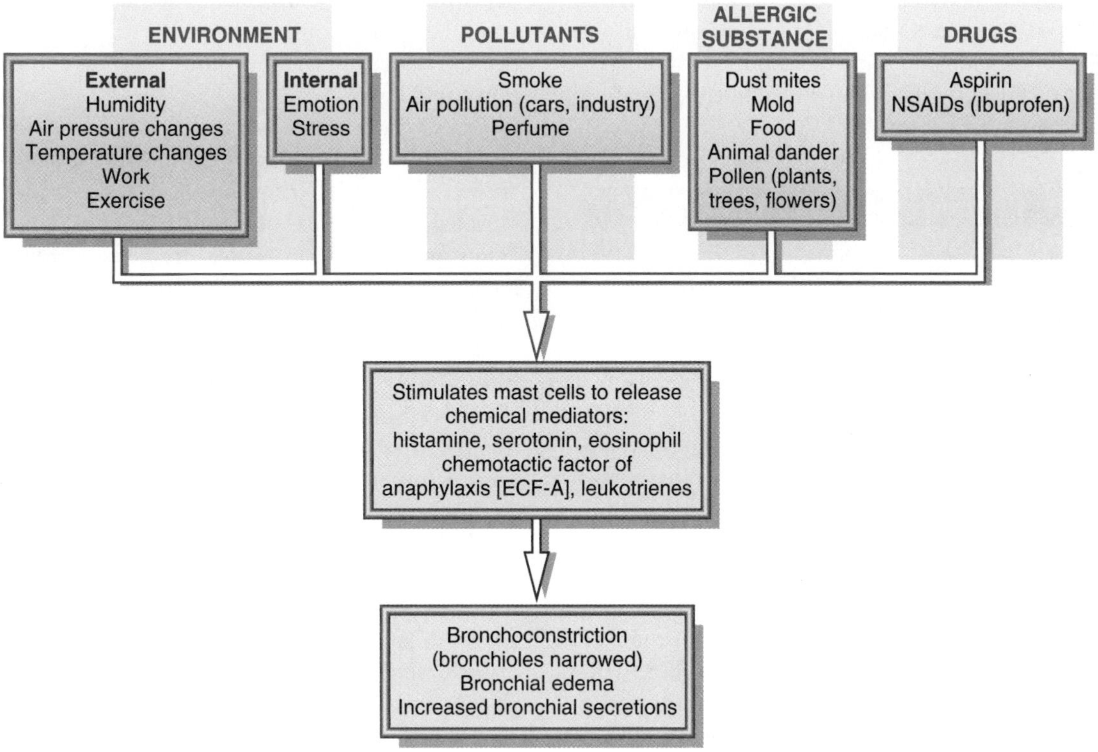

FIGURE 41–2 Factors contributing to bronchoconstriction.

In an acute asthmatic attack, the short-acting sympathomimetics ($beta_2$-adrenergic agonists) are the first line of defense. They promote cAMP production and enhance bronchodilation. Long-acting sympathomimetics are used for maintenance. Sympathomimetics (adrenergics) are also discussed in Chapter 18.

SYMPATHOMIMETICS: ALPHA- AND $BETA_2$-ADRENERGIC AGONISTS

Sympathomimetics increase cAMP, causing dilation of the bronchioles. In an acute bronchospasm caused by anaphylaxis from an allergic reaction, the nonselective sympathomimetic epinephrine (Adrenalin), which is an $alpha_1$, $beta_1$, and $beta_2$ agonist, is given subcutaneously to promote bronchodilation and elevate blood pressure. Epinephrine is administered in emergency situations to restore circulation and increase airway patency (see Chapter 59).

For bronchospasm associated with chronic asthma or COPD, selective $beta_2$-adrenergic agonists are given by aerosol or as a tablet. These drugs act primarily on the $beta_2$ receptors; therefore side effects are less severe than those of epinephrine, which acts on $alpha_1$, $beta_1$, and $beta_2$ receptors.

Albuterol

The newer beta-adrenergic drugs for asthma are more selective for $beta_2$ receptors. High doses or overuse of the $beta_2$-adrenergic agents for asthma may cause some degree of $beta_1$ response such as nervousness, tremor, and increased pulse rate. The ideal $beta_2$ agonist is one that has a rapid onset of action, longer duration of action, and few side effects. Albuterol (Proventil, Ventolin) is a selective $beta_2$ drug that is effective for treatment and control of asthma by causing bronchodilation with long duration of action. (See Prototype Drug Chart 18-2 for drug data related to albuterol.)

> **SAFETY: Preventing Medication Errors**
>
> **Do not confuse...**
> - **albuterol** ($beta_2$-adrenergic) with **Accupril** (cardiovascular agent).

Metaproterenol

The second beta-adrenergic agent is metaproterenol (Alupent), which was first marketed in 1961. It has some $beta_1$ effect but is primarily used as a $beta_2$ agent. It can be administered orally or by inhalation with a metered-dose inhaler or a nebulizer.

For long-term asthma treatment, $beta_2$-adrenergic agonists are frequently administered by inhalation. This route of administration usually delivers more of the drug directly to the constricted bronchial site. The effective inhalation drug dose is less than it would be by the oral route, and there are also fewer side effects using this route. The onset of action of the drug is more rapid by inhalation (1 minute) than orally (15 minutes).

Isoproterenol

The first beta-adrenergic agent used for bronchospasm was isoproterenol (Isuprel), introduced in 1941. It has no alpha-agonist properties, but it is considered a nonselective beta agonist because it stimulates both $beta_1$ and $beta_2$ receptors. $Beta_1$ stimulation causes heart rate increases, and tachycardia may result. $Beta_2$ stimulation promotes bronchodilation. Isoproterenol is administered by inhalation, using an aerosol inhaler or nebulizer, or intravenously (IV) for severe asthmatic attacks. Its duration of action is short. Because of its severe side effects from $beta_1$ response, it is seldom prescribed.

> **SAFETY: Preventing Medication Errors**
>
> **Do not confuse...**
> - **Isuprel** (beta-adrenergic) with **Isordil** (nitrate vasodilator).

Use of an Aerosol Inhaler

If the $beta_2$ agonist is given by metered-dose inhaler (MDI) or dry-powder inhaler (DPI), correct use of the inhaler and dosage intervals need to be explained to the patient. If the patient does not receive effective relief from the inhaler, either the technique is faulty or the canister is empty. A spacer device may be attached to the inhaler to improve drug delivery to the lung with less deposition in the mouth. If the patient does not use the inhaler properly to deliver the drug dose, the medication may be trapped in the upper airways. Because of drug inhalation, mouth dryness and throat irritation could result.

Excessive use of the aerosol drug can lead to tolerance and loss of drug effectiveness. Occasionally, severe paradoxical airway resistance (bronchoconstriction) develops with repeated, excessive use of sympathomimetic oral inhalation. Frequent dosing can cause tremors, nervousness, and increased heart rate. Table 41-1 lists the sympathomimetics used as bronchodilators.

Side Effects and Adverse Reactions

The side effects and adverse reactions of epinephrine include tremors, dizziness, hypertension, tachycardia, heart palpitations, cardiac dysrhythmias, and angina. The patient needs to be closely monitored when epinephrine is administered.

The side effects associated with $beta_2$-adrenergic drugs (e.g., albuterol) include tremors, headaches, nervousness, increased pulse rate, and palpitations (high doses). The $beta_2$ agonists may increase blood glucose levels, so patients with diabetes should be taught to closely monitor their serum glucose levels. Side effects of $beta_2$ agonists may diminish after 1 week or longer. The bronchodilating effects may decrease with continued use. It is believed that tolerance to these drugs

TABLE 41-1 ADRENERGIC BRONCHODILATORS AND ANTICHOLINERGICS

GENERIC (BRAND)	ROUTE AND DOSAGE	USES AND CONSIDERATIONS
Alpha- and Beta-Adrenergics		
ephedrine sulfate (Primatene) Alpha$_1$, beta$_1$, beta$_2$	A/C: >12 y: PO: 12.5 to 25 mg q4h; *max:* 150 mg/d; subQ/IM/IV: 25 to 50 mg	For nasal congestion, asthma, acute bronchospasm; improves respiration caused by narcotic excess; corrects hypotensive state. Nervousness, tachycardia, and insomnia could occur. Pregnancy category: C; PB: UK; t½: 3 h
epinephrine (EpiPen) Alpha$_1$, beta$_1$, beta$_2$	A: subQ: 0.2-1 mg of 1:1000 sol; may repeat q10-15min PRN C: subQ: 0.01 mg of 1:1000 sol; may repeat q15min-4h for 3-4 doses or q4h PRN	For acute bronchospasm and to combat anaphylaxis, angioedema, nasal congestion, status asthmaticus. Used frequently by nebulizer. Side effects include nervousness, tremors, dizziness, palpitations, tachycardia, and other cardiac dysrhythmias. Pregnancy category: C; PB: UK; t½: UK
Beta-Adrenergics		
albuterol (Proventil HFA, Ventolin HFA) Beta$_2$	A/C: >6 y: inhal MDI: 1 to 2 puffs q4-6h or 2 puffs 15 min before exercise A: PO immediate release: 2 to 4 mg t.i.d./q.i.d.; *max:* 32 mg/d A: PO:SR: 4 to 8 mg q12h; *max:* 32 mg/d C: 6 to 12 y: PO: immediate release: 2 mg t.i.d./q.i.d.; *max:* 24 mg/d C: 6 to 12 y: PO: SR: 4 to 8 mg q12h; *max:* 24 mg/d	For acute and chronic asthma, bronchitis, and exercise-induced bronchospasm. Onset of action orally is 30 min, and duration of action is 4 to 6 h (SR 8 to 12 h). Pregnancy category: C; PB: UK; t½: 4 to 6 h
isoproterenol (Isuprel) Beta$_1$ and beta$_2$	A/C: inhal: 1 to 2 puffs q4-6h; *max:* 12 inhal/d	For acute bronchospasm, COPD. Nonselective (beta$_1$ and beta$_2$). Beta$_1$ effect causes heart rate to increase. Monitor heart rate and blood pressure. Absorption of sublingual drug can be variable and unpredictable. Pregnancy category: C; PB: UK; t½: 2 to 5 min
levalbuterol (Xopenex HFA) Beta$_2$	Bronchospasm prophylaxis A/C: >12 y: nebulizer 0.63 to 1.25 mg q8h Acute bronchospasm A/C: >12yr: 1.25 to 2.5 mg q20min for 3 doses, then 1.25 to 5 mg q1-4h PRN; C: 6 to 11 yr: 0.75 mg/kg q20min for 3 doses, then 0.075 to 0.15 mg/kg q1-4h PRN	For acute bronchospasm and prevention of exercise-induced asthma. Product from albuterol derivative. Expensive. Rapid absorption and short acting. Side effects are nervousness and tremors. Pregnancy category: C; PB: UK; t½: 3.3 to 4 h
metaproterenol sulfate Beta$_1$ (some) and beta$_2$	A: PO: 20 mg t.i.d./q.i.d.; *max:* 80 mg/d	For acute bronchospasm, asthma, and COPD. Pregnancy category: C; PB: UK; t½: UK
formoterol fumarate (Foradil Aerolizer)	A/C: >5 y: inhal: Inhale contents of 1 capsule (12 mcg) q12h; *max:* 2 inhal/d	For asthma and prevention of exercise-induced asthma. Pregnancy category: C; PB: UK; t½: 10 h
salmeterol (Serevent Diskus) Beta$_2$	Maintenance bronchodilation A/C: > 4 y: Inhal: 1 puff q12h Prevention of exercise-induced bronchospasm A/C: >4 y: Inhal MDI: 1 puff at least 30 min before exercise	For chronic asthma and exercise-induced bronchospasm. Not effective for treating acute bronchospasm. Has a long duration of action (12 h). Pregnancy category: C; PB: 94% to 98%; t½: 5 h
terbutaline sulfate (Brethine) Beta$_2$	A: PO: 2.5 to 5 mg t.i.d.; *max:* 15 mg/d subQ: 0.25 to 0.5 mg q8h C: >12 y: PO: 2.5 mg t.i.d.; *max:* 7.5 mg/d	For reversible airway obstruction caused by asthma, bronchitis, acute bronchospasm, and emphysema. May cause nervousness, tremors, lightheadedness, palpitations, or tachycardia if taken in excess. Pregnancy category: C; PB: 25%; t½: 3 to 4 h
arformoterol tartrate (Brovana) Beta$_2$	A: inhal nebulizer: 15 mcg q12h; *max:* 30 mcg/d	For long-term maintenance treatment of COPD. Not effective for treating acute bronchospasm. Has a long duration of action. Pregnancy category: C; PB: 52% to 65%; t½: 26 h
indacaterol (Arcapta, Neohaler)	A: oral inhal: 75 mcg/d; max: 1 inhal/d	Long-acting beta$_2$ agonist to treat airflow obstruction from COPD. This maintenance bronchodilator should be administered at same time every dat. Most common adverse effects include post-inhalation cough and nasopharyngitis. Pregnancy category: C; PB: 95%; t½: 45.5 to 126 h

Continued

TABLE 41-1 ADRENERGIC BRONCHODILATORS AND ANTICHOLINERGICS—cont'd

GENERIC (BRAND)	ROUTE AND DOSAGE	USES AND CONSIDERATIONS
Anticholinergics		
ipratropium bromide (Atrovent HFA)	COPD A: inhal MDI: 2 puffs t.i.d./q.i.d., *max:* 12 inhal/d	For bronchospasm associated with COPD, including asthma. Use with caution in patients with narrow-angle glaucoma. Pregnancy category: B; PB: UK; $t\frac{1}{2}$: 1.5 to 2 h
ipratropium with albuterol (DuoNeb)	A: inhaled via nebulizer: 3 mL q6h; *max:* 3 mL q4h	Anticholinergic agent combines with $beta_2$-adrenergic agonist to increase bronchodilation. With use of this combination of drugs, duration of action is prolonged. Pregnancy category: C; PB: UK; $t\frac{1}{2}$: 2 to 4 h
aclidinium (Tudorza Pressair)	A: oral inhal: 400 mcg b.i.d.	For long-term treatment of bronchospasm associated with COPD. Most common adverse effects are headache and nasopharyngitis. Administered by MDI with dry powder. Pregnancy category: C; PB: UK; $t\frac{1}{2}$: 5 to 8 h
tiotropium (Spiriva HandiHaler)	See Prototype Drug Chart 41-1.	

A, Adult; *b.i.d.,* two times a day; *C,* child; *COPD,* chronic obstructive pulmonary disease; *d,* day; *h,* hour; *inhal,* inhalation; *IM,* intramuscular; *IV,* intravenous; *max,* maximum; *MDI,* metered-dose inhaler; *min,* minute; *PB,* protein-binding; *PO,* by mouth; *PRN,* as needed; *q.i.d.,* four times a day; *sol,* solution; *SR,* sustained-release; *subQ,* subcutaneous; $t\frac{1}{2}$, half-life; *t.i.d.,* three times a day; *UK,* unknown; *y,* year; >, greater than.

can develop; if this occurs, the dose may need to be increased. Failure to respond to a previously effective dose may indicate worsening asthma that requires reevaluation before increasing the dose.

ANTICHOLINERGICS

Tiotropium (Spiriva) is an anticholinergic drug used for maintenance treatment of bronchospasms associated with COPD. This drug is administered by inhalation only with the HandiHaler device (dry-powder capsule inhaler). Patients should discard any capsules that are opened and not used immediately. HandiHalers should be washed with warm water and dried. The most common adverse effects of tiotropium include dry mouth, constipation, vomiting, dyspepsia, abdominal pain, depression, insomnia, headache, joint pain, and peripheral edema. Chest pain has been reported following tiotropium administration. Prototype Drug Chart 41-1 lists the drug data related to tiotropium.

The anticholinergic drug ipratropium bromide (Atrovent) is used to treat asthmatic conditions by dilating the bronchioles. Unlike other anticholinergics, ipratropium bromide has few systemic effects. It is administered by aerosol.

Patients who use a beta-agonist inhalant should administer it 5 minutes before using ipratropium. When using the anticholinergic agent in conjunction with an inhaled glucocorticoid (steroid) or cromolyn, the ipratropium bromide should be used 5 minutes before the steroid or cromolyn. This causes the bronchioles to dilate so the steroid or cromolyn can be deposited in the bronchioles.

The combination of ipratropium bromide with albuterol sulfate (Combivent) is used to treat chronic bronchitis. The combination is more effective and has a longer duration of action than if either agent is used alone. These two agents combined increase the FEV_1, the index used to evaluate asthma and obstructive lung disease and the patient's response to bronchodilator therapy. Table 41-2 lists the inhalants for asthma control.

TABLE 41-2 INHALANTS FOR ASTHMA CONTROL

CATEGORIES	INHALANT AGENTS
Adrenergics	
$Beta_1$ and $beta_2$	isoproterenol (Isuprel)
$Beta_2$ and some $beta_1$	metaproterenol sulfate (Alupent, Metaprel)
$Beta_2$	albuterol (Proventil, Ventolin)
	pirbuterol acetate (Maxair)
	salmeterol (Serevent)
	terbutaline sulfate
	arformoterol tartrate (Brovana)
Anticholinergics	ipratropium bromide (Atrovent)
	ipratropium and albuterol (Combivent)
Antiinflammatory Drugs	
Cromolyn and nedocromil	cromolyn (NasalCrom)
	nedocromil
Glucocorticoids (corticosteroids)	beclomethasone (Beconase AQ)
	budesonide (Rhinocort Aqua)
	dexamethasone (Decadron)
	flunisolide
	fluticasone (Flonase)
	mometasone furoate (Nasonex)
	triamcinolone (Nasacort AQ, Kenalog IV)
	prednisone delayed release tablets (Rayos)

PROTOTYPE DRUG CHART 41-1

Tiotropium

Drug Class Anticholinergic Trade Name: Spiriva Pregnancy Category: C	**Dosage** A: Oral inhalation: 18 mcg inhalation/d at same time each day
Contraindications Hypersensitivity, children, adolescents Caution: Lactose hypersensitivity, Narrow-angle glaucoma, breastfeeding, older adults	**Drug-Lab-Food Interactions** Drug: Increase anticholinergic effects with phenothiazines; decrease action of prokinetics (cisapride, metoclopramide, parasympathomimetics)
Pharmacokinetics Absorption: PO: Well absorbed Distribution: PB: 72% Metabolism: t½: 5-6 d Excretion: In urine as metabolites	**Pharmacodynamics** Inhalation: PO: Onset: 30 min Peak: 1-4 h Duration: 4-24 h
Therapeutic Effects/Uses For maintenance treatment of bronchospasm associated with COPD Mode of Action: Relaxes smooth muscle of bronchi; dilates bronchi by inhibiting M3 receptors	
Side Effects Insomnia, dizziness, depression, headache, nausea, vomiting, abdominal pain, constipation, urinary retention, hyperglycemia, muscle cramping in extremities, peripheral edema, blurred vision, oral ulceration	**Adverse Reactions** Anaphylaxis, angioedema, dehydration, hyperglycemia Life-threatening: Cardiac dysrhythmias, cardiac arrest, paradoxical bronchoconstriction

A, Adult; *C,* child; *h,* hour; *PB,* protein-binding; *PO,* by mouth; *t ½,* half-life; *UK,* unknown; *y,* year.

METHYLXANTHINE (XANTHINE) DERIVATIVES

The second major group of bronchodilators used to treat asthma is the methylxanthine (xanthine) derivatives, which include aminophylline, theophylline, and caffeine. Xanthines also stimulate the central nervous system (CNS) and respiration, dilate coronary and pulmonary vessels, and cause diuresis. Because of their effect on respiration and pulmonary vessels, xanthines are used in the treatment of asthma.

Theophylline

The first theophylline preparation, aminophylline, was produced in 1936. Theophylline relaxes the smooth muscles of the bronchi, bronchioles, and pulmonary blood vessels by inhibiting the enzyme phosphodiesterase, resulting in an increase in cAMP, which promotes bronchodilation.

Theophylline has a low therapeutic index and a narrow therapeutic range (10 to 20 mcg/mL). The serum or plasma theophylline concentration level should be monitored frequently to avoid severe adverse effects. Toxicity is likely to occur when the serum level is greater than 20 mcg/mL. Certain theophylline preparations can be given with sympathomimetic (adrenergic) agents, but the dose may need to be adjusted.

Theophylline was once used as the first-line drug for treating patients with chronic asthma and other COPDs. However, theophylline use has declined sharply, because there is a potential danger of serious adverse effects (e.g., dysrhythmias, convulsions, cardiorespiratory collapse), and efficacy has not been found to be greater than beta agonists or glucocorticoids. Because of its numerous adverse reactions, drug-drug interactions, and narrow therapeutic drug range, it is prescribed mostly for maintenance therapy in patients with chronic stable asthma and other COPDs. Theophylline drugs are *not* prescribed for patients with seizure disorders or cardiac, renal, or liver disease. Patients who receive theophylline preparations need to be closely monitored for serious side effects and drug interactions.

Table 41-3 lists the theophylline preparations and their dosages, uses, and considerations.

Pharmacokinetics Theophylline is usually well absorbed after oral administration, but absorption may vary according to the specific dosage form. Theophylline is also well absorbed from oral liquids and uncoated plain tablets. Sustained-release dosage forms are slowly absorbed. Food and antacids may decrease the rate but not the extent of absorption; large volumes of fluid and high-protein meals may increase the rate of absorption. The dose size can also affect the rate of absorption: larger doses are absorbed more slowly. Theophylline can also be administered in IV fluids.

Theophylline drugs are metabolized by liver enzymes, and 90% of the drug is excreted by the kidneys. Tobacco smoking increases metabolism of theophylline drugs, thereby decreasing its half-life. The half-life is also shorter in children. With a short half-life, theophylline is readily excreted by the kidneys, so the dose may need to be increased to maintain therapeutic serum/plasma range. In nonsmokers and older adults,

TABLE 41-3 THEOPHYLLINE PREPARATIONS

GENERIC (BRAND)	ROUTE AND DOSAGE	USES AND CONSIDERATIONS
aminophylline—theophylline ethylenediamine (Elixophyllin, Theo-24)	Acute bronchospasm A: PO: IV: LD: 5-7 mg/kg infused over 20 min; *max:* 25 mg/min IV A: PO: maint: 300 mg q8h; *max:* 900 mg/d A: IV: maint: 0.5 mg/kg/hr infusion A/older adults: IV: maint: 0.375 mg/kg/hr infusion Caution: Individual titration based on serum theophylline levels. A: PO: LD 400 mg; then increase dose according to body weight; *max:* 24 mg/kg/d	IV for acute asthmatic attack. For IV use, drug must be diluted. Oral preparations are tablets or elixirs. For oral use, give with food to avoid GI distress. Side effects include restlessness, syncope, palpitations, tachycardia, hyperventilation, and cardiac dysrhythmias. Therapeutic range: 10-20 mcg/L. Pregnancy category: C; PB: 40%; t½: 6.5-10.5 h
dyphylline (Lufyllin, Dylix, Neothylline)	A: PO: 15 mg/kg q6h; *max:* 60 mg/kg/d Therapeutic serum theophylline range: 10-20 mcg/mL	Treatment of asthma, chronic bronchitis, and emphysema. One tenth as potent as theophylline. Structure similar to that of theophylline, but it does not convert to theophylline in the body. Pregnancy category: C; PB: UK; t½: 2 h

A, Adult; *C,* child; *COPD,* chronic obstructive pulmonary disease; *d,* day; *GI,* gastrointestinal; *h,* hour; *IM,* intramuscular; *IV,* intravenous; *LD,* loading dose; *max,* maximum; *min,* minute; *PB,* protein-binding; *PO,* by mouth; *q.i.d.,* four times a day; *t½,* half-life; *UK,* unknown; *y,* year; >, greater than; <, less than.

the average half-life of theophylline is 7 to 9 hours, and the dose requirements may be decreased. However, in smokers and children, the half-life is 4 to 5 hours, and the dose requirement may be increased. In premature infants, the half-life is 15 to 55 hours. In patients with heart failure (HF), cor pulmonale, COPD, or liver disease, the half-life is 12 hours. Kidney function may be decreased in older adults, so caution should be used regarding the theophylline dosage to avoid drug toxicity.

Pharmacodynamics Theophylline increases the level of cAMP, resulting in bronchodilation. The average onset of action is 30 minutes for oral preparations and 1 to 2 hours for sustained-release capsules. The duration of action is 8 to 24 hours for the sustained-release form and approximately 6 hours for other oral and IV theophylline preparations.

Side Effects and Adverse Reactions

Side effects and adverse reactions to theophylline include anorexia, nausea and vomiting, gastric pain caused by increased gastric acid secretion, intestinal bleeding, nervousness, dizziness, headache, irritability, cardiac dysrhythmias, tachycardia, palpitations, marked hypotension, hyperreflexia, and seizures. Adverse CNS reactions (e.g., headaches, irritability, restlessness, nervousness, insomnia, dizziness, seizures) are often more severe in children than in adults. To decrease the potential for side effects, patients should not take other xanthines while taking theophylline.

Theophylline toxicity is most likely to occur when serum concentrations exceed 20 mcg/mL. Theophylline can cause hyperglycemia, decreased clotting time, and, rarely, increased white blood cell count (leukocytosis). Because of the diuretic effect of xanthines, including theophylline, patients should avoid caffeinated products (e.g., coffee, tea, cola, chocolate) and increase fluid intake.

Rapid IV administration of aminophylline (a theophylline product) can cause dizziness, flushing, hypotension, severe bradycardia, and palpitations. To avoid severe adverse effects, IV theophylline preparations *must be administered slowly* via an infusion pump.

Drug Interactions

Beta blockers, cimetidine (Tagamet), propranolol (Inderal), and erythromycin (E-Mycin) decrease the liver metabolism rate and increase the half-life and effects of theophylline; barbiturates and carbamazepine (Tegretol) decrease its effects. In both situations, the theophylline dosage would need adjustment. Theophylline increases the risk of digitalis toxicity and decreases the effects of lithium. Phenytoin (Dilantin) decreases theophylline levels. If theophylline and a beta-adrenergic agonist are given together, a synergistic effect can occur and result in cardiac dysrhythmias.

LEUKOTRIENE RECEPTOR ANTAGONISTS AND SYNTHESIS INHIBITORS

Leukotriene (LT) is a chemical mediator that can cause inflammatory changes in the lung. The cysteinyl leukotrienes promote an increase in eosinophil migration, mucus production, and airway wall edema, which result in bronchoconstriction. LT receptor antagonists and LT synthesis inhibitors, called *leukotriene modifiers,* are effective in reducing the inflammatory symptoms of asthma triggered by allergic and environmental stimuli. These drug groups are not recommended for treatment of acute asthmatic attack. They are used for exercise-induced asthma. Three leukotriene modifiers—zafirlukast (Accolate), zileuton (Zyflo CR), and montelukast sodium (Singulair)—are available in the United States. These drugs are listed in Table 41-4.

TABLE 41-4 ANTIINFLAMMATORY DRUGS FOR CHRONIC OBSTRUCTIVE PULMONARY DISEASE

GENERIC (BRAND)	ROUTE AND DOSAGE	USES AND CONSIDERATIONS
Leukotriene Modifiers (Do Not Administer for Acute Asthmatic Attack)		
Leukotriene Receptor Antagonists		
zafirlukast (Accolate)	A: PO: 20 mg b.i.d. 1 h before or 2 h after meals; *max:* 40 mg/d C: >5 y: PO: 10 mg b.i.d.; *max:* 20 mg/d	For prophylaxis and maintenance therapy for chronic asthma. Reduces inflammation within bronchial tubes and airways. Pregnancy category: B; PB: 99%; t½: 10 h
montelukast (Singulair)	See Prototype Drug Chart 41-2.	
Leukotriene Synthesis Inhibitors		
zileuton (Zyflo CR)	ER: A: PO: 1200 mg b.i.d. within 1 h after morning and evening meal	For prophylaxis and maintenance therapy for chronic asthma. Reduces inflammation in airways and decreases bronchoconstriction. Hepatotoxicity may result; closely monitor liver enzymes. Pregnancy category: C; PB: 93%; t½: 2.5 h
Glucocorticoids (Corticosteroids)		
Intranasal Spray (see Chapter 40)		
Phosphodiesterase-4 Inhibitor		
roflumilast (Daliresp)	A: PO: 500 mcg/d	For treatment of exacerbations in severe COPD. Common adverse effects include diarrhea and weight loss. Contraindicated in moderate to severe liver impairment. Pregnancy Category: C; PB: 99%; t½: 17 h
beclomethasone (Beconase AQ, QNASL)		
budesonide (Pulmicort, Rhinocort Aqua)		
flunisolide		
fluticasone (Flonase)		
mometasone furoate (Nasonex)		
triamcinolone (Nasacort AQ)		
Aerosol Inhalation (see Chapter 51)		
beclomethasone (Qvar)		
flunisolide (Aerospan)		
budesonide (Pulmicort Flexhaler)		
fluticasone (Flovent Diskus)		
Oral and Intravenous Administration (see Chapter 51)		
betamethasone dipropinate		
cortisone acetate		
dexamethasone (Decadron)		
fludrocortisone acetate		
hydrocortisone (Cortef, Aquacort)		
methylprednisolone (Medrol, Solu-Medrol, Depo-Medrol)		
prednisolone (Flo-Pred, Orapred)		
prednisone		
triamcinolone (Kenalog IV)		
Combination Drug: Glucocorticoid and Beta$_2$ Agonist		
fluticasone propionate and salmeterol (Advair Diskus, Advair HFA)	A/C: >12 y: Inhal DPI Diskus: 1 puff q12h	For asthma; not to treat acute asthmatic attacks. If insufficient response, fluticasone dose may be increased. Pregnancy category: C; PB: 91%-98%; t½: 3-8 h
fluticasone propionate and vilanterol (Breo Ellipta)	A: Inhal: 1 inhalation qd	For long-term maintenance of COPD, including bronchitis or emphysema. Pregnancy category: C; PB: 93.7%-99.6%; t½: 21.3-24 h

Continued

TABLE 41-4 ANTIINFLAMMATORY DRUGS FOR CHRONIC OBSTRUCTIVE PULMONARY DISEASE—cont'd

GENERIC (BRAND)	ROUTE AND DOSAGE	USES AND CONSIDERATIONS
Cromolyn and Nedocromil (Do Not Use for Acute Asthmatic Attack)		
cromolyn sodium (Gastrocrom)	A/C: >6 y: Inhal MDI: 1-2 puffs 10-15 min before exercise	For chronic asthma and prophylactic use. Suppresses inflammation in bronchial tubes; does not have bronchodilating effects. Prevents release of histamine. Pregnancy category: B; PB: UK; $t\frac{1}{2}$: 80 min
nedocromil sodium	A/C: >6 y: Inhal MDI: 2 puffs q.i.d.; may decrease to b.i.d./t.i.d.	For maintenance therapy in mild to moderate asthma. Has antiinflammatory effect. Suppresses release of histamine. Pregnancy category: B; PB: UK; $t\frac{1}{2}$: 2.3 h

A, Adult; *b.i.d.,* twice a day; *C,* child; *DPI,* dry-powder inhaler; *ER,* extended-release; *h,* hour; *inhal,* inhalation; *MDI,* metered-dose inhaler; *min,* minute; *PB,* protein binding; *PO,* by mouth; *q.i.d.,* four times a day; $t\frac{1}{2}$, half-life; *t.i.d.,* three times a day; *UK,* unknown; *y,* year; >, greater than.

Nursing Process
Patient-Centered Collaborative Care

Bronchodilators

Assessment
- Obtain a medical and drug history; report probable drug-drug interactions.
- Note baseline vital signs and pulse oximetry for abnormalities and future comparisons.
- Assess for wheezing, decreased breath sounds, cough, and sputum production.
- Assess sensorium for confusion and restlessness caused by hypoxia and hypercapnia.
- Determine hydration; diuresis may result in dehydration in children and older adults.
- Assess serum theophylline levels. Toxicity occurs at a higher frequency with levels greater than 20 mcg/mL.

Nursing Diagnoses
- Ineffective breathing pattern related to fatigue
- Ineffective airway clearance related to retained secretions in the bronchi
- Impaired gas exchange related to ineffective airway clearance
- Noncompliance with drug therapy related to inadequate financial resources
- Activity intolerance related to fatigue and an imbalance between oxygen supply and demand

Planning
- Patient will be free from wheezing, and lung fields will be clear within 2 to 5 days.
- Patient will self-administer oral drugs and inhaler as prescribed.

Nursing Interventions
- Monitor vital signs. Blood pressure and heart rate can increase greatly. Check for cardiac dysrhythmias.
- Provide adequate hydration. Fluids aid in loosening secretions.
- Monitor drug therapy.
- Observe for side effects.
- Administer medication after meals to decrease gastrointestinal distress.
- Administer medication at regular intervals around the clock to have a sustained therapeutic level.
- Do *not* crush enteric-coated or sustained-released (SR) tablets or capsules.
- Check serum theophylline levels (normal level is 10 to 20 mcg/mL).

Patient Teaching

General
- Teach patient to monitor pulse rate.
- Encourage patient to monitor amount of medication remaining in the canister.
- Advise patient not to take over-the-counter (OTC) preparations without first checking with health care provider. Some OTC products may have an additive effect.
- Encourage patient contemplating pregnancy to seek medical advice before taking a theophylline preparation.
- Advise patient to avoid smoking. Avoid marked sudden changes in smoking amounts, which could affect theophylline blood levels. Smoking increases drug elimination, which may require an increased drug dose.
- Discuss ways to alleviate anxiety, such as relaxation techniques and music.
- Advise patient having asthmatic attacks to wear an ID bracelet or MedicAlert tag.
- Inform patient that certain herbal products may interact with theophylline (Herbal Alert 41-1).
- Advise patient to notify health care provider of aggressive or altered behavior and suicidal thoughts.

Self-Administration

- Teach patient to correctly use inhaler or nebulizer. Caution against overuse, because side effects and tolerance may result.
- Teach patient to monitor pulse rate and report to health care provider any irregularities in comparison with baseline.

Diet

- Advise patient that high-protein, low-carbohydrate diet increases theophylline elimination. Conversely, low-protein, high-carbohydrate diet prolongs half-life; dosage may need adjustment.

Correct Use of Metered-Dose Inhaler to Deliver Beta$_2$ Agonist

- Insert medication canister into plastic mouthpiece.
- Shake inhaler well *before* using. Remove cap from mouthpiece.
- Breathe *out* through the mouth. Open mouth wide, and hold mouthpiece 1 to 2 inches from mouth, or place inhaler mouthpiece in mouth. A spacer may be used. Discuss technique with health care provider.
- Open mouth, take a *slow deep* breath through the mouth, and at the same time push top of medication canister once.
- Hold breath for a few seconds; exhale slowly through pursed lips.
- Wait 2 minutes if a second dose is required, and then repeat the procedure by first shaking the inhaler with the mouthpiece cap in place.
- Do a "test spray" before administering the metered dose of a new inhaler or when the inhaler has not been used recently.
- Self-administer a bronchodilator first when taken at the same time as a steroid, and then *wait 5 minutes* for optimal bronchodilator effect before using the steroid.

Cultural Considerations

- Respect cultural beliefs and practices concerning alternative ways to treat asthma or other chronic obstructive pulmonary disease, and incorporate alternative treatments into patient care if they are harmless. If traditional practices/medicines are unsafe, explain in terms that can be understood.
- If patient from different cultural background does not comply with drug regimen, consult health care provider of similar background, and provide a written plan in language patient speaks and reads most easily.

Evaluation

- Evaluate effectiveness of bronchodilator. Patient is breathing without wheezing and free from side effects of the drug.
- Determine serum theophylline levels to assure therapeutic range.

HERBAL ALERT 41-1

Lower Respiratory Disorders

- Ephedra may increase the effect of the theophylline group and may cause theophylline toxicity.
- St. John's wort may decrease montelukast concentration.

Zafirlukast (Accolate) was the first drug in the class of leukotriene modifiers. It acts as an LT receptor antagonist, reducing the inflammatory process and decreasing bronchoconstriction. It is administered orally and absorbed rapidly. It has a moderate to moderately long half-life and is given twice a day. Zileuton (Zyflo CR) is an LT synthesis inhibitor. It decreases the inflammatory process and bronchoconstriction. Zileuton has a short half-life of 2.5 hours. Montelukast (Singulair) is a newer LT receptor antagonist (Prototype Drug Chart 41-2). It has a short half-life of 2.7 to 5.5 hours and is considered safe for use in children 6 years of age and older.

Nursing Process
Patient-Centered Collaborative Care

Leukotriene Receptor Antagonists

Assessment

- Obtain a medical, drug, and herbal history; report probable drug-drug or drug-herb interactions.
- Note baseline vital signs for identifying abnormalities and for future comparisons.
- Assess for wheezing, decreased breath sounds, cough, and sputum production.
- Assess sensorium for confusion and restlessness caused by hypoxia and hypercapnia.
- Assess for a history of phenylketonuria when montelukast is prescribed, because children's chewable tablets contain phenylalanine.
- Determine hydration; diuresis may result in dehydration in children and older adults.

Nursing Diagnoses

- Ineffective airway clearance related to retained secretions in bronchi
- Activity intolerance related to imbalance between oxygen supply and demand
- Deficient knowledge of OTC drug interaction related to lack of exposure to information

Planning

- Patient will be free from wheezing, or wheezing has significantly improved.
- Patient's lung fields will be clear within 2 to 5 days.
- Patient will take medications as prescribed.

PROTOTYPE DRUG CHART 41-2

Montelukast

Drug Class Bronchodilator: leukotriene receptor antagonist Trade Name: Singulair Pregnancy Category: B	**Dosage** A: PO: 10 mg/d at least 2 h before exercise C: 6-15 y: PO: 5 mg/d at least 2 h before exercise
Contraindications Hypersensitivity, severe asthmatic attack, status asthmaticus or acute bronchospasm Caution: Severe liver disease, suicidal ideation, breastfeeding, corticosteroid withdrawal	**Drug-Lab-Food Interactions** Lab: Abnormal liver function tests (ALT, AST)
Pharmacokinetics Absorption: Well absorbed Distribution: PB: 99% Metabolism: $t_{1/2}$: 2.7-5.5 h Elimination: Feces, bile	**Pharmacodynamics** PO: Onset: UK Peak: 3-4 h Duration: 24 h
Therapeutic Effects/Uses For prevention of bronchospasm and maintenance treatment of asthma Mode of Action: Binds with leukotriene receptors to inhibit smooth muscle contraction and bronchoconstriction	
Side Effects Fever, headache, drowsiness, dizziness, fatigue, restlessness, insomnia, confusion, depression, nasal congestion, cough, sore throat, dental pain, influenza, dyspepsia, nausea, vomiting, abdominal pain, weight loss, rash	**Adverse Reactions** Angioedema, bleeding, vasculitis, seizures, edema Life-threatening: anaphylaxis, suicidal ideation, Stevens-Johnson syndrome

A, Adult; *ALT,* alanine aminotransferase; *AST,* aspartate aminotransferase; *C,* child; *h,* hour; *PB,* protein-binding; *PO,* by mouth; $t_{1/2}$, half-life; *UK,* unknown; *y,* year.

Nursing Interventions

- Monitor respirations for rate, depth, rhythm, and type.
- Monitor lung sounds for rhonchi, wheezing, or rales.
- Observe lips and fingernails for cyanosis.
- Monitor drug therapy for effectiveness.
- Observe for side effects.
- Provide adequate hydration; fluids aid in loosening secretions.
- Monitor liver function tests; AST and ALT may be elevated with zafirlukast and montelukast.
- Provide pulmonary therapy by chest clapping and postural drainage, as appropriate.

Patient Teaching

General

- Advise patient that if allergic reaction occurs (i.e., rash, urticaria), drug should be discontinued and health care provider should be notified.
- Monitor periodic liver function tests.
- Direct patient not to take St. John's wort without first checking with health care provider, because this herb may decrease montelukast concentration.
- Warn patient that black or green tea and guarana with montelukast and zafirlukast may cause increased stimulation.
- Encourage patient to stop smoking.
- Discuss ways to alleviate anxiety (relaxation techniques, music).
- Advise patient having frequent or severe asthmatic attacks to wear an ID bracelet or MedicAlert tag.
- Encourage patient contemplating pregnancy to seek medical advice before taking montelukast.
- Caution patient or significant other not to open oral granule packets until ready for use. After opening packet, dose must be administered within 15 minutes. If mixed with baby formula or approved food (applesauce, carrots, rice, or ice cream), do not store for future use.
- Advise patient with known aspirin sensitivity to avoid a bronchoconstrictor response by avoiding aspirin and NSAIDs while taking montelukast.

Self-Administration

- Teach patient not to use montelukast for reversal of an acute asthmatic attack, because it is only recommended for prevention of acute attacks and treatment of chronic asthma.
- Advise patient to continue to use the usual regimen of inhaled prophylaxis and short-acting rescue medication for exercise-induced bronchospasm.

- Encourage patient to inform health care provider if short-acting inhaled bronchodilators are needed more often than usual with montelukast.
- Tell patient to comply with medication regimen even during symptom-free periods.
- Advise patient (especially children) that chewable tablets are to be chewed thoroughly because swallowing whole may alter absorption.

Diet

- Tell patient to take leukotriene receptor antagonists in the evening for maximum effectiveness.

Cultural Considerations

- Use both hands to show respect when offering a prescription, instructions, or pamphlets to Asians and Pacific Islanders.

Evaluation

- Evaluate the effectiveness of the bronchodilators. Patient is breathing without wheezing and without side effects of the drug.
- Evaluate tolerance to activity.

This category of drugs is the newest group used to control asthma. Again, LT receptor antagonists and synthesis inhibitors should *not* be used during an acute asthmatic attack. They are only for prophylactic and maintenance drug therapy for chronic asthma.

GLUCOCORTICOIDS (STEROIDS)

Glucocorticoids, members of the corticosteroid family, are used to treat respiratory disorders, particularly asthma. These drugs have an antiinflammatory action and are indicated if asthma is unresponsive to bronchodilator therapy or if the patient has an asthmatic attack while on maximum doses of theophylline or an adrenergic drug. It is thought that glucocorticoids have a synergistic effect when given with a $beta_2$ agonist.

Glucocorticoids can be given using the following methods:

- *MDI inhaler:* beclomethasone (Beconase AQ, QNASL, Qvar)
- *Tablet:* dexamethasone (Decadron), prednisone, prednisolone, and methylprednisolone
- *Intravenous:* dexamethasone (Decadron), hydrocortisone

Inhaled glucocorticoids are not helpful in treating a severe asthmatic attack, because it may take 1 to 4 weeks for an inhaled steroid to reach its full effect. When maintained on inhaled glucocorticoids, asthmatic patients demonstrate an improvement in symptoms and a decrease in asthmatic attacks. Inhaled glucocorticoids are more effective for controlling symptoms of asthma than $beta_2$ agonists, particularly in the reduction of bronchial hyperresponsiveness. The use of an oral inhaler minimizes the risk for adrenal suppression associated with oral systemic glucocorticoid therapy. Inhaled glucocorticoids are preferred over oral preparations unless they fail to control the asthma.

Patients with acute asthma exacerbations are usually given systemic glucocorticoids (i.e., IV) for rapid effectiveness in large doses (20 to 40 mg prednisone for 5 days; 1 to 2 mg/kg/day for children for 3 to 5 days). An additional week with a reduced dose may be needed. With a single dose or short-term use, glucocorticoids may be discontinued abruptly after symptoms are controlled. Suppression of adrenal function does not usually occur within 1 to 2 weeks.

When severe asthma requires prolonged glucocorticoid therapy, weaning or tapering of the dose may be necessary to prevent an exacerbation of asthma symptoms and suppression of adrenal function. Previously, alternate-day therapy (ADT) with oral prednisone was used in some asthmatic patients. Currently, inhaled glucocorticoids are thought to be preferable in the treatment of most patients with asthma. Glucocorticoid preparations are discussed in detail in Chapter 51.

Glucocorticoids can irritate the gastric mucosa and should be taken with food to avoid ulceration. A combination drug containing the glucocorticoid fluticasone propionate 100 mcg and salmeterol 50 mcg (Advair Diskus 100/50) is effective in controlling asthma symptoms. Advair is used every day, but requires only one inhalation in the morning and one at night. This drug does not replace fast-acting inhalers for sudden symptoms. The purpose of Advair is to alleviate airway constriction and inflammation.

Side Effects and Adverse Reactions

Side effects associated with orally inhaled glucocorticoids are generally local (e.g., throat irritation, hoarseness, dry mouth, coughing) rather than systemic. Oral, laryngeal, and pharyngeal fungal infections have occurred but can be reversed with discontinuation and antifungal treatment. *Candida albicans* oropharyngeal infections may be prevented by using a spacer with the inhaler to reduce drug deposits in the oral cavity, rinsing the mouth and throat with water after each dose, and washing the apparatus (cap and plastic nose or mouthpiece) daily with warm water.

Oral and injectable glucocorticoids have many side effects when used long-term, but short-term use usually causes no significant side effects. Most adverse reactions are seen within 2 weeks of glucocorticoid therapy and are usually reversible. Side effects that may occur include headache, euphoria, confusion, sweating, hyperglycemia, insomnia, nausea, vomiting, weakness, and menstrual irregularities. Adverse effects may include depression, peptic ulcer, loss of bone density and development of osteoporosis, and psychosis.

When oral and IV steroids are used for prolonged periods, electrolyte imbalance, fluid retention (puffy eyelids, edema in the lower extremities, moon face, weight gain), hypertension, thinning of the skin, purpura, abnormal subcutaneous (fat) distribution, hyperglycemia, and impaired immune response are likely to occur.

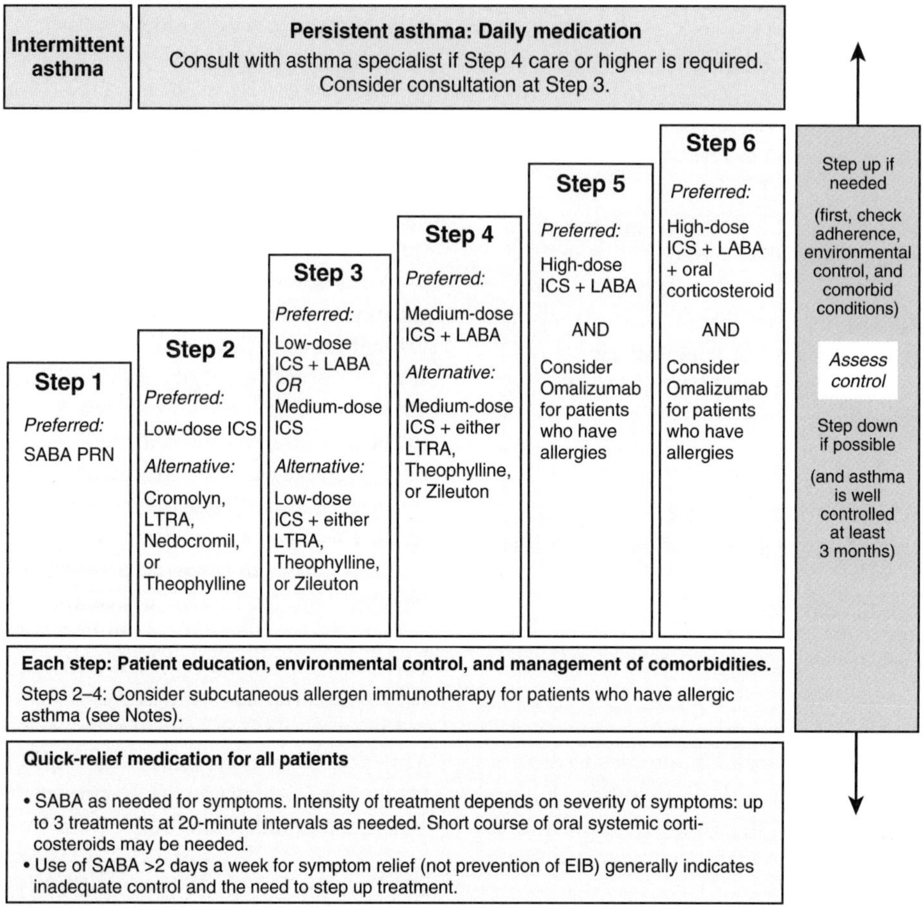

Key: **Alphabetical order is used when more than one treatment option is listed within either preferred or alternative therapy.** ICS, inhaled corticosteroid; LABA, long-acting inhaled beta$_2$-agonist; LTRA, leukotriene receptor antagonist; SABA, inhaled short-acting beta$_2$-agonist

Notes:

- The stepwise approach is meant to assist, not replace, the clinical decision making required to meet individual patient needs.
- If alternative treatment is used and response is inadequate, discontinue it and use the preferred treatment before stepping up.
- Zileuton is a less desirable alternative due to limited studies as adjunctive therapy and the need to monitor liver function. Theophylline requires monitoring of serum concentration levels.
- In Step 6, before oral corticosteroids are introduced, a trial of high-dose ICS + LABA + either LTRA, Theophylline, or Zileuton may be considered, although this approach has not been studied in clinical trials.
- Step 1, 2, and 3 preferred therapies are based on Evidence A; Step 3 alternative therapy is based on Evidence A for LTRA, Evidence B for Theophylline, and Evidence D for Zileuton. Step 4 preferred therapy is based on Evidence B, and alternative therapy is based on Evidence B for LTRA and Theophylline and Evidence D Zileuton. Step 5 preferred therapy is based on Evidence B. Step 6 preferred therapy is based on (EPR–2 1997) and Evidence B for Omalizumab.
- Immunotherapy for Steps 2–4 is based on Evidence B for house-dust mites, animal danders, and pollens; evidence is weak or lacking for molds and cockroaches. Evidence is strongest for immunotherapy with single allergens. The role of allergy in asthma is greater in children than in adults.
- Clinicians who administer immunotherapy or Omalizumab should be prepared and equipped to identify and treat anaphylaxis that may occur.

FIGURE 41–3 Stepwise approach for managing asthma in patients 12 years and older. (From the National Asthma Education and Prevention Program Expert Panel Report 3: *Guidelines for the diagnosis and management of asthma.* Washington, DC, National Heart, Lung, and Blood Institute, U.S. Department of Health and Human Services. Accessed November 14, 2012, at *www.nhlbi.nih.gov/guidelines/asthma/asthgdln.htm.*)

CROMOLYN AND NEDOCROMIL

Cromolyn sodium (NasalCrom) is used for prophylactic treatment of bronchial asthma and must be taken daily. It is not used for acute asthmatic attacks. Cromolyn does not have bronchodilator properties, but instead acts by inhibiting histamine release to prevent an asthma reaction. Its most common side effects are cough and a bad taste. These effects can be decreased by drinking water before and after using the drug.

Cromolyn is administered by inhalation. It can be used with beta adrenergics and xanthine derivatives. Rebound bronchospasm is a serious side effect of cromolyn. The drug should not be discontinued abruptly, because a rebound asthmatic attack can result.

Action and uses of nedocromil sodium are similar to those of cromolyn sodium. It has an antiinflammatory effect and suppresses the release of histamine, leukotrienes, and other mediators from the mast cells. Like cromolyn it should not be used during an acute asthmatic attack, but instead to prevent bronchospasm and acute asthmatic attack. Inhalation may cause an unpleasant taste. Nedocromil is believed to be more effective than cromolyn.

Table 41-4 lists antiinflammatory drugs for COPD, including LT receptor antagonists, LT synthesis inhibitors, glucocorticoids (intranasal spray, aerosol inhalation, combination drug, and oral, intramuscular, and intravenous form), cromolyn sodium, and nedocromil sodium.

DRUG THERAPY FOR ASTHMA ACCORDING TO SEVERITY

Chronic asthma may be controlled through a long-term drug treatment program and by a quick-relief program during an acute phase. Figure 41-3 presents a list of steps for controlling and treating chronic asthma according to severity. This treatment regimen was developed in 1997 and updated in 2007 by the National Asthma Education and Prevention Program of the National Heart, Lung, and Blood Institute in Bethesda, Maryland. The long-term drug treatment program may vary according to the symptoms of the asthma and its severity. The quick-relief drug therapy is the same for all classes of asthma.

DRUG THERAPY FOR ASTHMA ACCORDING TO AGE

Young Children

Cromolyn and nedocromil are drugs used to treat the inflammatory effects of asthma in children. Oral glucocorticoids may be prescribed for the young child to control a moderate to severe asthmatic state. An inhalation dose of a glucocorticoid should be about 1 to 2 inhalations 3 to 4 times a day or 40 to 80 mcg twice a day. If the condition is severe, selected young children may be ordered an oral beta$_2$-adrenergic agonist.

Older Adults

Drug selection and dosage need to be considered for the older adult with an asthmatic condition. Beta$_2$-adrenergic agonists and methylxanthines (e.g., theophylline) can cause tachycardia, nervousness, and tremors in older adults, especially those with cardiac conditions. Frequent use of glucocorticoids can increase the risk of the patient developing cataracts, osteoporosis, and diabetes mellitus. If a theophylline drug is ordered, dosages of glucocorticoids are normally decreased.

MUCOLYTICS

Mucolytics act like detergents to liquefy and loosen thick mucous secretions so they can be expectorated. Acetylcysteine (Mucomyst) is administered by nebulization. *The drug should not be mixed with other drugs.* When patients with asthma or hyperactive airway disease produce increased secretions that obstruct bronchial airways, acetylcysteine may be administered as an adjunct to a bronchodilator (not mixed together). The bronchodilator should be given 5 minutes before the mucolytic. Side effects include nausea and vomiting, stomatitis (oral ulcers), and "runny nose."

Acetylcysteine (Mucomyst) can be used as an antidote for acetaminophen (Tylenol) overdose if given within 12 to 24 hours after the overdose ingestion. It can be given orally, diluted in juice or soft drinks.

Dornase alfa (Pulmozyme) is an enzyme that digests deoxyribonucleic acid (DNA) in thick sputum secretions of patients with cystic fibrosis (CF). This agent helps reduce respiratory infections and improves pulmonary function. Improvement usually occurs in 3 to 7 days with its use. Side effects include chest pain, sore throat, laryngitis, and hoarseness.

ANTIMICROBIALS

Antibiotics are used only if a bacterial infection results from retained mucus secretions. Trimethoprim-sulfamethoxazole is effective for the treatment of mild to moderate acute exacerbations of chronic bronchitis (AECB) from infectious causes.

KEY WEBSITES

Metered-dose inhaler: *www.familydoctor.org/online/famdocen/home/common/asthma/medications/040.html*

Singulair: *www.singulair.com/montelukast_sodium/singulair/consumer/index.jsp*

Smoking cessation: *www.nlm.nih.gov/medlineplus/quittingsmoking.html*

CRITICAL THINKING CASE STUDY

MA, a 55-year-old patient, was recently diagnosed with bronchial asthma. Her mother and three brothers also have asthma. In the past year, MA has had three asthmatic attacks that were treated with prednisone and albuterol (Proventil) inhaler. At an office visit today, prednisone is prescribed for 4 weeks, and the order is written as follows: day 1—1 tablet 4 times a day; day 2—1 tablet 3 times a day; day 3—1 tablet 2 times a day; day 4—1 tablet in the morning; day 5—one-half tablet in the morning.

1. Explain the purpose for the use of prednisone during an asthmatic attack. Explain why the dosage is decreased (tapered) over a period of 5 days.
2. Can cromolyn sodium (NasalCrom) be substituted for prednisone during an asthmatic attack? Explain your answer.
3. MA is prescribed albuterol (Proventil, Ventolin). What effect does albuterol have on controlling asthma?
4. For each drug dose, MA is to take two puffs of albuterol administered by the inhaler. What instructions should she be given concerning use of the inhaler?

To minimize the frequency of MA's asthmatic attacks, the health care provider prescribes theophylline (Elixophyllin) 200 mg twice a day. The albuterol inhalation is to be taken as needed. Nursing interventions include patient history of asthmatic attacks and physical assessment.

5. When taking the patient's history, what should the nurse include concerning asthmatic attacks? What physical assessment would suggest an asthmatic attack?
6. What type of drug is Elixophyllin? Why should the nurse ask MA if she smokes?
7. What are the side effects, adverse reactions, and drug interactions related to Elixophyllin?
8. What nonpharmacologic measures can the nurse suggest that may decrease the frequency of asthmatic attacks?
9. Which are appropriate rescue medications used for acute asthmatic attacks? Which drugs are used as preventive medications?

NCLEX STUDY QUESTIONS

1. An Advair Diskus, fluticasone propionate (Flonase) and salmeterol (Serevent) 100 mcg/50 mcg, is ordered for a patient with COPD. What does the nurse know about this medication? (Select all that apply.)
   a. It can be used to treat an acute attack.
   b. It is delivered as a dry powdered inhaler.
   c. It contains a beta$_1$ agonist and Cromolyn.
   d. It is taken as one puff two times a day.
   e. It promotes bronchodilation.
2. A patient with COPD has an acute bronchospasm. The nurse anticipates that the health care provider will prescribe which medication?
   a. zafirlukast (Accolate)
   b. epinephrine (Adrenalin)
   c. dexamethasone (Decadron)
   d. oxtriphylline-theophyllinate
3. A patient is prescribed aminophylline–theophylline. For what adverse effect should the nurse monitor the patient?
   a. Drowsiness
   b. Hypoglycemia
   c. Increased heart rate
   d. Decreased white blood cell count
4. A patient is receiving IV aminophylline. The nurse checks the patient's lab values. The serum theophylline level is 32 mcg/mL. What action should the nurse take?
   a. Assess the patient's breath sounds for improvement.
   b. Increase the dosage per sliding scale directions.
   c. Notify the health care provider of the level.
   d. Have the laboratory collect another sample to verify the results.
5. A patient with COPD is taking a leukotriene antagonist, montelukast (Singulair). The nurse is aware that this medication is given for which purpose?
   a. Maintenance treatment of asthma
   b. Treatment of acute asthmatic attack
   c. Reversing bronchospasm associated with COPD
   d. Treatment of inflammation in chronic bronchitis

Answers: 1, b, d, e; 2, b; 3, c; 4, c; 5, a.

UNIT XIV

Cardiovascular Agents

The cardiovascular system includes the heart, blood vessels (arteries and veins), and blood flow. Blood that is abundant in oxygen (O_2), nutrients, and hormones moves through vessels called *arteries,* which narrow to arterioles and then capillaries. Capillaries transport nourished blood to body cells and absorb waste products, such as carbon dioxide (CO_2), urea, creatinine, and ammonia. The deoxygenated blood returns to the circulation by small venules and larger veins to be eliminated by the lungs and kidneys with other waste products (Figure XIV-1).

The heart's pumping action serves as the energy source that circulates blood to body cells. Blockage of vessels can inhibit blood flow.

HEART

The heart is composed of four chambers including the right and left atria and the right and left ventricles (Figure XIV-2). The right atrium receives deoxygenated blood from the circulation, and the right ventricle pumps blood through the pulmonary artery to the lungs for gas exchange (carbon dioxide for oxygen). The left atrium receives oxygenated blood, and the left ventricle pumps the blood into the aorta for systemic circulation.

The heart muscle, called the *myocardium,* surrounds the ventricles and atria. The ventricles have thick walls (especially the left ventricle) to produce the muscular force needed to pump blood to the pulmonary and systemic circulations. The atria have thin walls, have less pumping action, and receive blood from the circulation and lungs.

The heart has a fibrous covering called the *pericardium,* which protects it from injury and infection. The *endocardium* is a three-layered membrane that lines the inner part of the heart chambers. Four valves—two atrioventricular (tricuspid and mitral) and two semilunar (pulmonic and aortic)—control blood flow between the atria and ventricles and between the ventricles and the pulmonary artery and the aorta. There are two main coronary arteries. The right coronary artery divides into branches that supply blood to the right atrium and both ventricles of the heart. The left coronary artery divides near its origin to form the left circumflex artery and the anterior descending artery, which supply blood to the left atrium and both ventricles of the heart. Blockage to one of these arteries can result in a myocardial infarction (MI), or heart attack.

CONDUCTION OF ELECTRICAL IMPULSES

The myocardium is capable of generating and conducting its own electrical impulses. The cardiac impulse normally originates in the *sinoatrial (SA)* node located in the posterior wall of the right atrium. The SA node is frequently called the *pacemaker,* because it regulates the heartbeat (firing of cardiac impulses), which is approximately 60 to 80 beats/min in the normal adult. The *atrioventricular (AV) node,* located in the posterior right side of the interatrial septum, has a continuous tract of fibers called the *bundle of His,* or the AV bundle. The AV node is called the

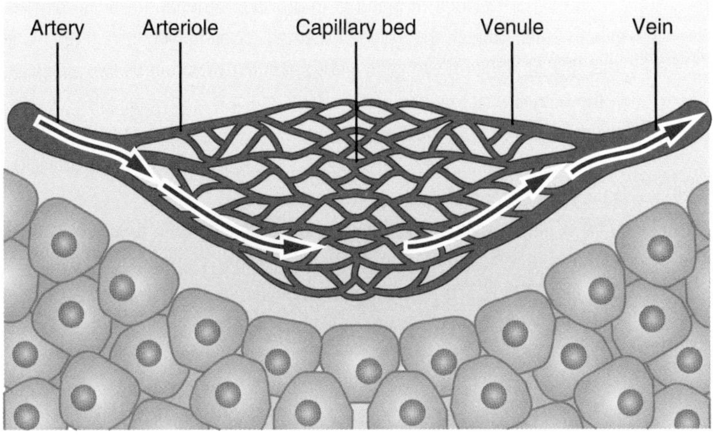

FIGURE XIV–1 Basic structures of the vascular system.

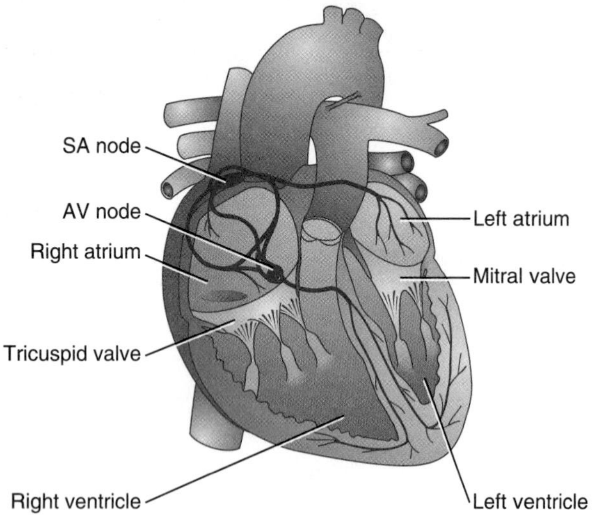

FIGURE XIV–2 Anatomy of the heart. *AV node,* Atrioventricular node; *SA node,* sinoatrial node.

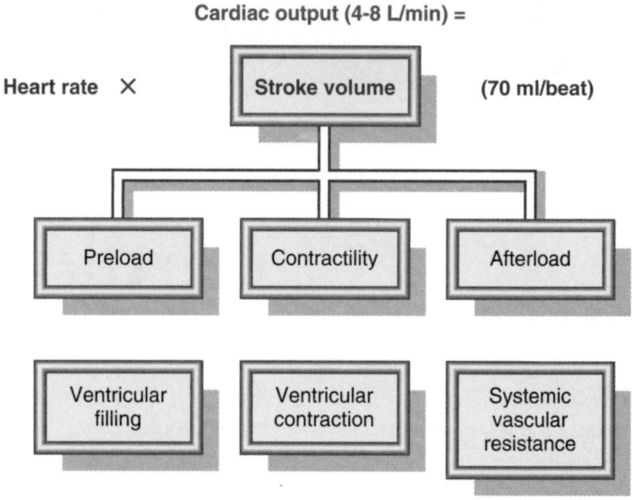

FIGURE XIV–3 Cardiac output and stroke volume.

pacemaker, having an adult rate of 40 to 60 beats/min. If the SA node fails, the AV node takes over, thus causing a slower heart rate. The AV node sends impulses to the ventricles. These two conducting systems (SA node and AV node) can act independently of each other. The ventricle can contract independently 30 to 40 times per minute.

Drugs that affect cardiac contraction include calcium, digitalis preparations, quinidine, and its related preparations. The autonomic nervous system (ANS) and drugs that stimulate or inhibit it influence heart contractions. The sympathetic nervous system and drugs that stimulate it *increase* heart rate; the parasympathetic nervous system and drugs that stimulate it *decrease* heart rate.

REGULATION OF HEART RATE AND BLOOD FLOW

The heart beats approximately 60 to 80 times per minute in an adult, pumping blood into the systemic circulation. As blood travels, resistance to blood flow develops and arterial pressure increases. The average systemic arterial pressure, known as *blood pressure,* is 120/80 mm Hg. Arterial blood pressure is determined by peripheral resistance and *cardiac output.* Cardiac output is the volume of blood expelled from the heart in 1 minute, which is calculated by multiplying the heart rate by the stroke volume. The average cardiac output is 4 to 8 L/min. *Stroke volume,* the amount of blood ejected from the left ventricle with each heartbeat, is approximately 70 mL/beat.

Three factors—preload, contractility, and afterload—determine the stroke volume (Figure XIV-3). *Preload* refers to the blood flow force that stretches the ventricle at the end of diastole. However, an increase in preload can increase stroke volume, and a decrease in preload can decrease stroke volume. *Contractility* is the force of ventricular contraction, and afterload is the resistance to ventricular ejection of blood, which is caused by opposing pressures in the aorta and systemic circulation. If afterload increases, stroke volume will decrease, and if afterload decreases, stroke volume will increase.

Specific drugs can increase or decrease preload and afterload, affecting both stroke volume and cardiac output. Most vasodilators decrease preload and afterload, thus decreasing arterial pressure and cardiac output.

CIRCULATION

There are two types of circulation—pulmonary and systemic. With pulmonary circulation, the heart pumps deoxygenated blood from the right ventricle through the pulmonary artery to the lungs. The pulmonary artery carries blood that has a high concentration of carbon dioxide. Oxygenated blood returns to the left atrium by the pulmonary vein.

With systemic circulation, also called *peripheral circulation,* the heart pumps blood from the left ventricle to the aorta and into the general circulation. Arteries and arterioles carry the blood to capillary beds. Nutrients in the capillary blood are transferred to cells in exchange for waste products. Blood returns to the heart through venules and veins.

BLOOD

Blood is composed of plasma, red blood cells (erythrocytes), white blood cells (leukocytes), and platelets. Plasma, made up of 90% water and 10% solutes, constitutes 55% of the total blood volume. The solutes in plasma include glucose, protein, lipids, amino acids, electrolytes, minerals, lactic and pyruvic acids, hormones, enzymes, oxygen, and carbon dioxide.

The major function of blood is to provide nutrients, including oxygen, to body cells. Most of the oxygen is carried on the hemoglobin of red blood cells (RBCs). White blood cells (WBCs) are the major defense mechanism of the body and act by engulfing microorganisms. They also produce antibodies. The platelets are large cells that cause blood to coagulate. RBCs have a life span of approximately 120 days, whereas the life span of a WBC is only 2 to 24 hours.

This unit is composed of five chapters dealing with drugs for cardiac disorders, diuretics and antihypertensive drugs, and drugs for circulatory disorders. Cardiac glycosides, antianginals, and antidysrhythmics are described in Chapter 42. Chapter 43 discusses the five categories of diuretics. Five major categories of antihypertensive agents are presented in Chapter 44. The five groups of drugs covered in Chapters 45 and 46 are the anticoagulants, antiplatelets, thrombolytics, antihyperlipidemics, and peripheral vasodilators.

CHAPTER

42

Cardiac Glycosides, Antianginals, and Antidysrhythmics

evolve WEBSITE

http://evolve.elsevier.com/KeeHayes/pharmacology/

- Animations
- Content Updates
- Key Points
- Review Questions for the NCLEX® Examination
- References from the Textbook
- Unfolding Case Studies

OBJECTIVES

- Differentiate the actions of cardiac glycosides, antianginal drugs, and antidysrhythmic drugs.
- Describe the signs and symptoms of digitalis toxicity.
- Compare the side effects and adverse reactions of nitrates, beta blockers, calcium channel blockers, quinidine, and procainamide.
- Apply the nursing process, including patient teaching, related to cardiac glycosides, antianginal drugs, and antidysrhythmic drugs.

OUTLINE

KEY TERMS

Three groups of drugs—cardiac glycosides, antianginals, and antidysrhythmics—are discussed in this chapter. Drugs in these groups regulate heart contraction, heart rate and rhythm, and blood flow to the myocardium (heart muscle).

CARDIAC GLYCOSIDES

Digitalis began being used as early as 1200 AD, making it one of the oldest drugs. It is still used in a purified form. Digitalis is obtained from the purple and white foxglove plant, and it can be poisonous. In 1785, William Withering of England used digitalis to alleviate "dropsy," edema of the extremities caused by kidney and cardiac insufficiency. Withering and his medical colleagues did not realize that dropsy was the result of heart failure, however. Digitalis preparations have come to be known for their effectiveness in treating heart failure (HF), also known as *cardiac failure* (CF), and previously referred to as **congestive heart failure (CHF).** When the heart muscle *(myocardium)* weakens and enlarges, it loses its ability to pump blood through the heart and into the systemic circulation. This is called **heart failure,** or pump failure. When compensatory mechanisms fail and the peripheral and lung tissues are congested, the condition is CHF. The causes of HF include chronic hypertension, myocardial infarction (MI), coronary artery disease (CAD), valvular heart disease, congenital heart disease, and arteriosclerosis.

Heart failure can be left-sided or right-sided. The patient has left-sided HF when the left ventricle does not contract sufficiently to pump the blood returned from the lungs and left atrium out through the aorta into the peripheral circulation; this causes excessive amounts of blood to back up into the lung tissue. Usually the patient has shortness of breath (SOB) and dyspnea. Right-sided HF occurs when the heart does not sufficiently pump the blood returned into the right atrium from the systemic circulation. As a result, the blood and its constituents are backed up into peripheral tissues, causing peripheral edema. Left-sided heart failure may lead to right-sided failure and vice versa. Myocardial hypertrophy resulting in *cardiomegaly* (increased heart size) can be a major problem associated with progressive HF.

In the cardiac physiology of HF, there is an increase in *preload* and *afterload.* An increased preload results from an excess of blood volume in the ventricle at the end of diastole. This occurs because of a pathologic increase in the stretching and thickening of the ventricular walls, which allows a greater filling pressure associated with a weakened heart. Increased afterload is an additional pressure or force in the ventricular wall caused by excess resistance in the aorta. This resistance must be overcome to open the aortic valve so blood can be ejected into the circulation. In 2001, the American College of Cardiology (ACC) and the American Heart Association (AHA) (ACC/AHA), classified HF in stages according to its severity. Table 42-1 lists the stages of HF according to the ACC/AHA. In the early stage of HF, there are no symptoms and no structural heart damage. Detailed information related to the staging process of HF can be found on the Internet at www.hearthope.com/about-heart-failure/nyha-scale.asp.

TABLE 42-1 ACC/AHA STAGES OF HEART FAILURE

STAGE	CHARACTERISTICS ACCORDING TO STAGES
1 (A)	High risk for HF without symptoms or structural heart disease
2 (B)	Some level of cardiac changes, e.g., decreased ejection fraction without symptoms of HF.
3 (C)	Structural heart disease with symptoms of HF, i.e., fatigue, shortness of breath, edema, and decrease in physical activity.
4 (D)	Severe structural heart disease and marked symptoms of HF at rest.

ACC, American College of Cardiology; *AHA,* American Heart Association; *HF,* heart failure.

Naturally occurring **cardiac glycosides** are found in a number of plants, including *Digitalis.* Also called *digitalis glycosides,* this group of drugs inhibits the sodium-potassium pump, resulting in an increase in intracellular sodium. This increase leads to an influx of calcium, causing the cardiac muscle fibers to contract more efficiently. Digitalis preparations have three effects on heart muscle: (1) positive **inotropic** action (*increases* myocardial contraction stroke volume), (2) negative **chronotropic** action (*decreases* heart rate), and (3) negative **dromotropic** action (*decreases* conduction of heart cells). The increase in myocardial contractility strengthens cardiac, peripheral, and kidney function by enhancing cardiac output, decreasing preload, improving blood flow to the periphery and kidneys, decreasing edema, and promoting fluid excretion. As a result, fluid retention in the lung and extremities is decreased. Digoxin does not prolong life. It acts by increasing the force and velocity of myocardial systolic contraction.

Digoxin is a secondary drug for HF. First-line drugs used to treat acute HF include intravenous inotropic agents (dopamine and dobutamine) and phosphodiesterase inhibitors, such as milrinone. Other drugs prescribed for HF include oral diuretics, beta blockers, ACE inhibitors, angiotensin-receptor blockers (ARBs), calcium channel blockers, and vasodilators, all of which are more convenient to self-administer. Oral administration allows the patient to go home on these medications.

Cardiac glycosides are also used to correct **atrial fibrillation** (cardiac dysrhythmia with rapid uncoordinated contractions of atrial myocardium) and **atrial flutter** (cardiac dysrhythmia with rapid contractions of 200 to 300 beats/min). This is accomplished by the negative chronotropic effects (decreased heart rate) and negative dromotropic effects (decreased conduction through the atrioventricular [AV] node).

When digoxin cannot convert atrial fibrillation to normal heart rhythm, the goal is to slow the heart rate by decreasing electrical impulses through the AV node. For management of atrial fibrillation, a calcium channel blocker such as verapamil (Calan) may be prescribed. To prevent thromboemboli resulting from atrial fibrillation, warfarin (Coumadin) is prescribed concurrently with other drug therapy. Warfarin is discussed in Chapter 45.

Nonpharmacologic Measures to Treat Heart Failure

Nondrug therapy is an integral part of the regimen for controlling HF. The nondrug component of the regimen should be tailored to meet the needs of each patient, but the following are some general recommendations. The patient should limit salt intake to 2 g/day, which is approximately 1 teaspoon. Alcohol intake should be either decreased to 1 drink per day or completely avoided, because excessive alcohol use can lead to cardiomyopathy. Fluid intake may be restricted. Smoking should be avoided, because it deprives the heart of oxygen (O_2). Mild exercise, such as walking or bicycling, is recommended as well as restricting fluids in severe conditions. Obesity may increase cardiovascular problems if it is associated with unhealthy behaviors; thus, obese patients should modify their behaviors as needed. Mild exercise, such as walking or bicycling, is recommended.

Laboratory Tests

Atrial Natriuretic Hormone or Peptide. Reference value: 20 to 77 pg/mL; 20 to 77 ng/L (SI units). An elevated atrial natriuretic hormone (ANH) or peptide (ANP) may confirm HF. ANH is secreted from the atria of the heart and acts as an antagonist to renin and aldosterone. It is released during expansion of the atrium, produces vasodilation, and increases glomerular filtration rate. Results of ANH secretion include a large volume of urine that decreases blood volume and blood pressure.

Brain Natriuretic Peptide. Reference values: Desired value: less than 100 pg/mL; positive value: greater than 100 pg/mL. The brain natriuretic peptide (BNP) is primarily secreted from atrial cardiac cells and, when tested, aids in the diagnoses of HF. Diagnosing HF is difficult in persons with lung disease who are experiencing dyspnea and in those who are obese or older. An elevated BNP helps differentiate that dyspnea is due to HF rather than lung dysfunction. Frequently the BNP is higher than 100 pg/mL in women who are 65 years of age or older. An 80-year-old woman may have a BNP of 160 pg/mL. However, the BNP is markedly higher (i.e., 400 pg/mL) in HF. BNP is considered a more sensitive test than ANP for diagnosing HF. Today there is a bedside/emergency department machine to measure BNP.

> **SAFETY: Preventing Medication Errors**
>
> **Do not confuse...**
>
> - **digoxin** with **digitoxin.** Both drugs are cardiac glycosides. **Digoxin** (Lanoxin) is usually the first-choice drug, because its half-life is 36 hours, whereas the half-life of **digitoxin** is 4 to 9 days. **Digitoxin** is rarely prescribed and is not available in the United States.

Digoxin

Prototype Drug Chart 42-1 gives the pharmacologic data for digoxin, a cardiac glycoside.

Pharmacokinetics The absorption rate of digoxin in oral tablet form is 70%. The rate is 90% in liquid and capsule form. The protein-binding power for digoxin is 30%. The half-life is 30 to 40 hours. Because of its long half-life, drug accumulation can occur. Side effects should be closely monitored to detect digitalis toxicity. Patients should be made aware of side effects that need to be reported to the health care provider. Serum digoxin levels are most commonly drawn when actual digitoxicity is suspected. This allows the health care provider to ascertain the extent of such toxicity and to confirm elimination of the drug after it is stopped or decreased in dosage (see the Digitalis [Digoxin] Toxicity section later in this chapter).

Thirty percent of digoxin is metabolized by the liver, and 50% to 70% is excreted by the kidneys mostly unchanged. Kidney dysfunction can affect the excretion of digoxin. Thyroid dysfunction can alter the metabolism of cardiac glycosides. For patients with hypothyroidism, the dose of digoxin should be decreased; in hyperthyroidism, the dose may need to be increased.

Pharmacodynamics In patients with a failing heart, cardiac glycosides increase myocardial contraction, which increases cardiac output and improves circulation and tissue perfusion. Because these drugs decrease conduction through the AV node, the heart rate decreases. The onset and peak actions of oral and intravenous (IV) digoxin vary. The **therapeutic serum level** is 0.8 to 2.0 ng/mL for digoxin. To treat HF, the lower serum therapeutic levels should be obtained, and for atrial fibrillation, the higher therapeutic serum levels are required.

Digoxin can be administered orally or IV. Table 42-2 lists the digitalis preparations and their dosages, uses, and considerations.

Digitalis (Digoxin) Toxicity

Overdose or accumulation of digoxin causes digitalis toxicity. Signs and symptoms include anorexia, diarrhea, nausea and vomiting, **bradycardia** (pulse rate below 60 beats/min), premature ventricular contractions, cardiac dysrhythmias, headaches, malaise, blurred vision, visual illusions (white, green, yellow halos around objects), confusion, and delirium. Older adults are more prone to toxicity.

Cardiotoxicity is a serious adverse reaction to digoxin; ventricular dysrhythmias result. Three cardiac-altered functions can contribute to digoxin-induced ventricular dysrhythmias: (1) suppression of AV conduction, (2) increased automaticity, and (3) a decreased refractory period in ventricular muscle. The antidysrhythmics phenytoin and lidocaine are effective in treating digoxin-induced ventricular dysrhythmias. Lidocaine should be limited to short-term treatment.

Antidote for Cardiac/Digitalis Glycosides

Digoxin immune Fab (ovine, Digibind) may be given to treat severe digitalis toxicity. This agent binds with digoxin to form complex molecules that can be excreted in the urine; thus, digoxin is unable to bind at the cellular site of action. Signs and symptoms of digoxin toxicity should be reported promptly to the health care provider. Serum digoxin levels

PROTOTYPE DRUG CHART 42-1

Digoxin

Drug Class Cardiac glycoside Trade Name: Lanoxin Pregnancy Category: C	**Dosage** A: PO: 0.5-1 mg initially in 2 divided doses (digitalization); maint: 0.125-0.5 mg/d IV: Same as PO dose but given over 5 min Older adults: 0.125 mg/d C: 1 mo-2y: PO: 0.01-0.02 mg/kg in 3 divided doses; maint: 0.012 mg/kg/d in 2 divided doses C: IV: Dosage varies C: 2-10y: PO: 0.012-0.04 mg/kg in divided doses Pediatric doses are usually ordered in mcg in elixir form.
Contraindications Ventricular dysrhythmias, second- or third-degree heart block Caution: AMI, renal disease, hypothyroidism, hyperthyroidism, hepatic dysfunction, bradycardia, hypokalemia	**Drug-Lab-Food Interactions** Drug: Increase digoxin serum level with quinidine, flecainide, verapamil; decrease digoxin absorption with antacids, colestipol; increase risk for digoxin toxicity with thiazide diuretics, loop diuretics Lab: Hypokalemia, hypomagnesemia, hypercalcemia can increase digitalis (digoxin) toxicity
Pharmacokinetics Absorption: PO: tablet: 60%-70%; PO: liquid: 90% PO: capsule: 90%-100% Distribution: PB: 20%-30% Metabolism: t½: 30-40 h Excretion: 70% in urine; 30% by liver metabolism	**Pharmacodynamics** PO: Onset: 30 min–2 h Peak: 2-6 h Duration: UK IV: Onset: 5-30 min Peak: UK Duration: UK
Therapeutic Effects/Uses To treat HF, atrial fibrillation Mode of Action: Inhibits sodium-potassium ATPase, promoting increased force of cardiac contraction, cardiac output, and tissue perfusion; decreases ventricular rate	
Side Effects Anorexia, nausea, vomiting, diarrhea, abdominal pain, headache, blurred vision (yellow-green halos), diplopia, photophobia, drowsiness, dizziness, fatigue, confusion	**Adverse Reactions** Bradycardia, visual disturbances Life-threatening: Atrioventricular block, cardiac dysrhythmias

A, Adult; *AMI,* acute myocardial infarction; *ATPase,* adenosine triphosphatase; *C,* child; *d,* day; *HF,* heart failure; *h,* hour; *IV,* intravenous; *maint,* maintenance; *min,* minute; *mo,* month; *PB,* protein-binding; *PO,* by mouth; *t ½,* half-life; *y,* year.

should be closely monitored. Digitalis toxicity may result in first-degree, second-degree, or complete heart block.

Drug Interactions

Drug interaction with digitalis preparations can cause digitalis toxicity. Many of the potent diuretics, such as furosemide (Lasix) and hydrochlorothiazide (Esidrix, Microzide), promote the loss of potassium from the body. The resultant **hypokalemia** (low serum potassium level) increases the effect of digoxin at its myocardial cell site of action, resulting in digitalis toxicity. Cortisone preparations taken systemically promote sodium retention and potassium excretion or loss and can also cause hypokalemia. Patients who take digoxin along with a potassium-wasting diuretic or a cortisone drug should consume foods rich in potassium or take potassium supplements to avoid hypokalemia and digitalis toxicity. Antacids can decrease digitalis absorption if taken at the same time. To prevent this problem, doses should be staggered.

Phosphodiesterase Inhibitors

Phosphodiesterase inhibitors are another positive inotropic group of drugs given to treat acute HF. This drug group inhibits the enzyme phosphodiesterase, promoting a positive inotropic response and vasodilation. A drug in this group is milrinone lactate. This drug increases stroke volume and cardiac output and promotes vasodilation. It is administered IV for no longer than 48 to 72 hours. Severe cardiac dysrhythmias might result from the use of phosphodiesterase inhibitors, so the patient's electrocardiogram (ECG) and cardiac status should be closely monitored.

TABLE 42-2 CARDIAC GLYCOSIDES AND INOTROPIC AGENTS

GENERIC (BRAND)	ROUTE AND DOSAGE	USES AND CONSIDERATIONS
Rapid-Acting Digitalis		
digoxin (Lanoxin)	See Prototype Drug Chart 42-1.	
Phosphodiesterase Inhibitors (Positive Inotropic Bipyridines)		
milrinone lactate	A: IV: Initially: 50 mcg/kg/over 10 min Continuous infusion: 0.375-0.75 mcg/kg/min with 0.45%-0.9% saline	For short-term treatment of HF. May be given before heart transplantation. Heart rate and blood pressure should be closely monitored. Pregnancy category: C; PB: 70%; t½: 1.5-2.5 h
Atrial Natriuretic Peptide Hormones		
nesiritide (Natrecor)	A: IV bolus: 2 mcg/kg, followed by 0.01 mcg/kg/min, by IV infusions; *max:* 0.03 mcg/kg/min continuous IV infusion	To treat acute HF by increasing sodium loss. Useful in managing dyspnea at rest. Causes vasodilation. Contraindicated for patients with systolic BP <90 mm Hg. Pregnancy category: C; PB: UK; t½: 18 min
Antidote for Digitalis Toxicity		
digoxin immune Fab (Digibind)	A: IV: 760-800 mg IV diluted in 50 mL NSS. Infuse over 30 min	For serious digitalis toxicity. Agent binds with digoxin to form complex molecules. (Serum digoxin level >2 ng indicative of digitalis toxicity.) Onset of action: 30 min; duration of action: 3-4 d. Pregnancy category: C; PB: UK; t½: 23 h

A, Adult; *BP,* blood pressure; *d,* day; *HF,* heart failure; *inf,* infusion; *IV,* intravenous; *LD,* loading dose; *maint,* maintenance; *min,* minute; *NSS,* normal saline solution; *PB,* protein-binding; *PO,* by mouth; *t½,* half-life; *UK,* unknown; >, greater than.

OTHER AGENTS USED TO TREAT HEART FAILURE

Vasodilators, angiotensin-converting enzyme (ACE) inhibitors, angiotensin II receptor antagonists (blockers), diuretics (thiazides, furosemide), spironolactone (Aldactone), and some beta blockers are other drug groups prescribed to treat HF.

Vasodilators can be used to treat HF. The vasodilators decrease venous blood return to the heart resulting in a decrease in cardiac filling, ventricular stretching (preload), and oxygen demand on the heart. Arteriolar dilators act in three ways: (1) to reduce cardiac afterload, which increases cardiac output; (2) to dilate the arterioles of the kidneys, which improves renal perfusion and increases fluid loss; and (3) to improve circulation to the skeletal muscles.

Nursing Process
Patient-Centered Collaborative Care

Cardiac Glycosides: Digoxin

Assessment

- Obtain a drug and herbal history. Report if drug-drug or drug-herb interaction is probable. If patient is taking digoxin and a potassium-wasting diuretic or cortisone drug, hypokalemia might result, causing digitalis toxicity. Low serum potassium level enhances action of digoxin. Patients taking a thiazide and/or cortisone with digoxin should take a potassium supplement.
- Obtain a baseline pulse rate for future comparisons. Apical pulse should be taken for a full minute and should be greater than 60 beats/min.
- Assess for signs and symptoms of digitalis toxicity. Common symptoms include anorexia, nausea, vomiting, bradycardia, cardiac dysrhythmias, and visual disturbances. Report symptoms immediately to the health care provider.

Nursing Diagnoses

- Decreased cardiac output related to decreased cardiac pumping ability
- Ineffective peripheral tissue perfusion related to decreased cardiac pumping ability
- Anxiety related to threat to cardiac health status

Planning

- Patient will check pulse rate daily before taking digoxin.
- Patient will report pulse rate when less than 60 beats/min or a marked decline in pulse rate.
- Patient will eat foods high in potassium to maintain a desired serum potassium level (see Patient Teaching and Diet sections).

Nursing Interventions

- Ascertain apical pulse rate before administering digoxin. Do *not* administer if pulse rate <60 beats/min.
- Determine signs of peripheral and pulmonary edema, which indicate HF is present.
- Monitor serum digoxin level (normal therapeutic drug range is 0.8 to 2 ng/mL). A serum digoxin level greater than 2 ng/mL is indicative of digitalis toxicity.

- Monitor serum potassium level (normal range is 3.5 to 5.3 mEq/L), and report if hypokalemia (<3.5 mEq/L) is present.

Patient Teaching

General

- Explain to patient the importance of adherence to drug therapy. A visiting nurse may ensure that medications are properly taken.
- Advise patient to avoid adverse drug interactions by not taking over-the-counter (OTC) drugs without first consulting health care provider.
- Keep drugs out of reach of small children. Request childproof bottles.
- Teach patient or child's parent to check pulse rate before administering drug.
- Inform patient of possible herb-drug interactions (Herbal Alert 42-1).

Self-Administration

- Teach patient how to check pulse rate before taking digoxin and to notify health care provider if pulse rate is <60 beats/min or irregular.

Side Effects

- Instruct patient to report side effects: pulse rate <60 beats/min, nausea, vomiting, headache, diarrhea, and visual disturbances, including diplopia.

Diet

- Advise patient to eat foods high in potassium, such as fresh and dried fruits, fruit juices, and vegetables, including potatoes.

Cultural Considerations

- Analyze conflicts in values and beliefs, and use culturally consistent communication practices. It is essential that patients taking digoxin, diuretics, and potassium supplements for HF do not miss any doses of their medication. Patient should be fully aware of adverse effects and readily report them to the health care provider.
- Validate patient's understanding of purposes for taking these drugs. Be aware of potential cultural differences related to response to authority and involvement of family members. For example, Amish people often respect authority and may follow instructions without question, but family members must be involved in decision making.

Evaluation

- Evaluate the effectiveness of digoxin by noting patient's response to drug (decreased heart rate, decreased rales) and absence of side effects. Continue monitoring pulse rate.

HERBAL ALERT 42-1

Cardiac Glycosides: Digoxin

- Ginseng may falsely elevate digoxin levels.
- St. John's wort decreases absorption of digoxin and thus decreases serum digoxin level.
- Psyllium (Metamucil) may decrease digoxin absorption.
- Hawthorn may increase the effect of digoxin.
- Licorice can potentiate the effect of digoxin. It promotes potassium loss (hypokalemia), which increases the effect of digoxin. It may cause digitalis toxicity.
- Aloe may increase the risk of digitalis toxicity. It increases potassium loss, which increases the effect of digoxin.
- Ma-huang or ephedra increases the risk of digitalis toxicity.
- Goldenseal may decrease the effects of cardiac glycosides and increase the effects of antidysrhythmics.

ACE inhibitors are usually prescribed for HF. ACE inhibitors dilate venules and arterioles, improving renal blood flow and decreasing blood fluid volume. They also moderately decrease the release of aldosterone, which in turn reduces sodium and fluid retention.

ACE inhibitors can increase potassium levels, so serum potassium levels should be monitored, especially if potassium-sparing diuretics (e.g., spironolactone [Aldactone]) are being taken concurrently. Angiotensin II receptor blockers (ARBs), such as valsartan (Diovan) and candesartan (Atacand) have been approved for HF in patients who cannot tolerate ACE inhibitors. Refer to Chapter 44 for a complete discussion of ACE inhibitors and ARBs.

Diuretics are the first-line drug treatment for reducing fluid volume. They are frequently prescribed with digoxin or other agents.

Spironolactone (Aldactone), a potassium-sparing diuretic, is used in treating moderate to severe HF. Aldosterone secretions are increased in HF. This promotes body loss of potassium and magnesium needed by the heart and increases sodium and water retention. Spironolactone blocks the production of aldosterone. This drug improves heart rate variability and decreases myocardial fibrosis by its cardioprotective effect of blocking aldosterone in the heart and blood vessels to promote cardiac remodeling. The recommended dose is 12.5 to 25 mg/day. Occurrence of hyperkalemia (excess serum potassium) is rare unless the patient is receiving 50 mg/day and has renal insufficiency. However, the serum potassium level should be closely monitored.

In the past, all beta blockers were contraindicated for patients with HF, because this drug class reduces cardiac contractility. With dosage control, beta blockers (carvedilol [Coreg], metoprolol [Lopressor, Toprol-XL], and bisoprolol [Zebeta]) have been shown to improve cardiac performance. Doses should be low initially and gradually increased. It may take 1 to 3 months for a beneficial effect to develop. Refer to Chapters 18 and 44 for more information on beta blockers.

Nesiritide (Natrecor) is an atrial natriuretic peptide hormone that inhibits antidiuretic hormone (ADH) by increasing urine sodium loss. Its effect in correcting HF is achieved by promoting vasodilation, natriuresis, and diuresis. It is useful for treating patients who have acute decompensated HF with dyspnea at rest or who have dyspnea with little physical exertion.

BiDil, a combination of hydralazine (for blood pressure) and isosorbide dinitrate (a dilator to relieve heart pain) has received FDA approval for treating HF, especially in African Americans. African Americans have more than twice the rate of HF as whites, and a research study has shown this drug to be effective in treating HF in the African-American population.

ANTIANGINAL DRUGS

Antianginal drugs are used to treat **angina pectoris.** This is a condition of acute cardiac pain caused by inadequate blood flow to the myocardium due to either plaque occlusions within or spasms of the coronary arteries. With decreased blood flow, there is a decrease in oxygen to the myocardium, which results in pain. Anginal pain is frequently described by the patient as tightness, pressure in the center of the chest, and pain radiating down the left arm. Referred pain felt in the neck and left arm commonly occurs with severe angina pectoris. Anginal attacks may lead to MI (*heart attack*). Anginal pain usually lasts for only a few minutes. Stress tests, echocardiogram, cardiac profile laboratory tests, and cardiac catheterization may be needed to determine the degree of blockage in the coronary arteries and then also to treat the condition.

Types of Angina Pectoris

The frequency of anginal pain depends on many factors, including the type of angina. There are three types of angina:

- *Classic (stable):* Occurs with predictable stress or exertion
- *Unstable (preinfarction):* Occurs frequently with progressive severity unrelated to activity; unpredictable regarding stress/exertion and intensity
- *Variant (Prinzmetal, vasospastic):* Occurs during rest

The first two types are caused by a narrowing or partial occlusion of the coronary arteries; variant angina is caused by vessel spasm (vasospasm). It is common for a patient to have both classic and variant angina. Unstable angina often indicates an impending MI. This is an emergency that needs immediate medical intervention.

Nonpharmacologic Measures to Control Angina

A combination of pharmacologic and nonpharmacologic measures is usually necessary to control and prevent anginal attacks. Nonpharmacologic methods of decreasing anginal attacks are to avoid heavy meals, smoking, extreme weather changes, strenuous exercise, and emotional upset. Proper nutrition, moderate exercise (only after consulting with a health care provider), adequate rest, and relaxation techniques are used as preventive measures.

Types of Antianginal Drugs

Antianginal drugs increase blood flow either by increasing oxygen supply or by decreasing oxygen demand by the myocardium. Three types of antianginals are nitrates, beta blockers, and calcium channel blockers. The major systemic effect of nitrates is a reduction of venous tone, which decreases the workload of the heart and promotes vasodilation. Beta blockers and calcium channel blockers decrease the workload of the heart and decrease oxygen demands.

Nitrates and calcium channel blockers are effective in treating variant (vasospastic) angina pectoris. Beta blockers are not effective for this type of angina and may aggravate it. With stable angina, beta blockers can effectively be used to prevent angina attacks. Table 42-3 lists the effects of antianginal drug groups on angina.

With unstable angina, immediate medical care is necessary. Nitrates are usually given sublingually and intravenously as needed. If the cardiac pain continues, a beta blocker is given intravenously, and if the patient is unable to tolerate beta blockers, a calcium channel blocker may be substituted.

Nitrates

Nitrates, developed in the 1840s, were the first agents used to relieve angina. They affect coronary arteries and blood vessels in the venous circulation. Nitrates cause generalized vascular and coronary vasodilation, which increases blood flow through the coronary arteries to the myocardial cells. This group of drugs reduces myocardial ischemia but can cause hypotension.

TABLE 42-3 EFFECTS OF ANTIANGINAL DRUG GROUPS ON ANGINA

DRUG GROUPS	VARIANT (VASOSPASTIC) ANGINAS	CLASSIC (STABLE) ANGINAS
Nitrates	Relaxation of coronary arteries, which decreases vasospasms and increases O_2 supply	Dilation of veins, which decreases preload and decreases O_2 demand
Beta blockers	Not effective	Decreases heart rate and contractility, which decreases O_2 demand
Calcium channel blockers	Relaxation of coronary arteries, which decreases vasospasms and increases O_2 supply	Dilation of arterioles, which decreases afterload and decreases O_2 demand. Verapamil and diltiazem decrease heart rate and contractility

O_2, Oxygen.

SAFETY: Preventing Medication Errors

Do not confuse...

- **Nitrostat** and **Nystatin.** Nitrostat is a nitroglycerin drug that promotes coronary vasodilation and thus increases blood flow to the coronary arteries. Nystatin is an antifungal antibiotic that has fungistatic and fungicidal activity against yeasts and fungi.

The sublingual (SL) nitroglycerin tablet, which is absorbed under the tongue, comes in various dosages, but the average prescribed dose is 0.4 mg following cardiac pain. If pain has not subsided or worsened, then 911 should be called. The effects of SL nitroglycerin last for 10 minutes. The SL tablets decompose when exposed to heat and light, so they must be kept in their original airtight glass containers. The tablets themselves are normally dispensed in these original glass containers, which have screw-cap tops that are not child-proof. This facilitates emergency use by older adults who may have reduced manual dexterity and are experiencing an anginal attack. After a dose of nitroglycerin, the patient may experience dizziness, faintness, or headache as a result of the peripheral vasodilation. If pain persists, the patient should immediately call for medical assistance.

Sublingual (SL) nitroglycerin is the most commonly used nitrate. It is not swallowed, because it undergoes first-pass metabolism by the liver, which decreases its effectiveness. Instead, it is readily absorbed into the circulation through the SL vessels. Nitroglycerin is also available in other forms: topical (ointment, transdermal patch), translingual, oral extended-release capsule and tablet, aerosol spray (inhalation), and IV. Prototype Drug Chart 42-2 summarizes the action of nitroglycerin (nitrates).

There are various types of organic nitrates. Isosorbide dinitrate (Isordil) can be administered in SL tablet form and is also available as chewable tablets, immediate-release tablets, and sustained-release tablets and capsules. Isosorbide mononitrate (Imdur) can be given orally in immediate-release and sustained-release tablets.

Pharmacokinetics Nitroglycerin, taken SL, is absorbed rapidly and directly into the internal jugular vein and the right atrium. Approximately 40% to 50% of nitrates absorbed through the gastrointestinal (GI) tract are inactivated by first-pass metabolism in the liver. The nitroglycerin in Nitro-Bid ointment and in the Transderm-Nitro patch is absorbed slowly through the skin. It is excreted primarily in the urine.

Pharmacodynamics Nitroglycerin acts directly on the smooth muscle of blood vessels, causing relaxation and dilation. It decreases cardiac **preload** (amount of blood in the ventricle at the end of diastole) and **afterload** (peripheral vascular resistance) and reduces myocardial O_2 demand. With dilation of the veins, there is less blood return to the heart, and with dilation of the arteries, there is less vasoconstriction and resistance.

The onset of action of nitroglycerin depends on the method of administration. With SL and IV use, the onset of action is rapid (1 to 3 minutes); it is slower with the transdermal method (30 to 60 minutes). The duration of action of the transdermal nitroglycerin patch is approximately 24 hours. Because Nitro-Bid ointment is effective for only 6 to 8 hours, it must be reapplied three to four times a day. The use of Nitro-Bid ointment has declined since the advent of the transdermal nitroglycerin patch, which is applied only once a day. It is important to note that the patch should be removed nightly to allow for an 8- to 12-hour nitrate-free interval. This is also true for most other forms of nitroglycerin. This is necessary to avoid tolerance associated with uninterrupted use or continued dosage increases of nitrate preparations. Table 42-4 lists the nitrates and their dosages, uses, and considerations.

Side Effects and Adverse Reactions

Headaches are one of the most common side effects of nitroglycerin, but they may become less frequent with continued use. Otherwise acetaminophen may provide some relief. Other side effects include hypotension, dizziness, weakness, and faintness. When nitroglycerin ointment or transdermal patches are discontinued, the dose should be tapered over several weeks to prevent the rebound effect of severe pain caused by **myocardial ischemia** (lack of blood supply to the heart muscle). In addition, *reflex tachycardia* may occur if the nitrate is given too rapidly. The heart rate increases greatly because of overcompensation of the cardiovascular system.

Drug Interactions

Beta blockers, calcium channel blockers, vasodilators, and alcohol can enhance the hypotensive effect of nitrates. IV nitroglycerin may antagonize the effects of heparin.

Beta Blockers

Beta-adrenergic blockers block the $beta_1$- and $beta_2$-receptor sites. **Beta blockers** decrease the effects of the sympathetic nervous system by blocking the action of the catecholamines (epinephrine and norepinephrine), thereby decreasing the heart rate and blood pressure. They are used as antianginal, antidysrhythmic, and antihypertensive drugs. Beta blockers are effective as antianginals because by decreasing the heart rate and myocardial contractility, they reduce the need for oxygen consumption and consequently reduce anginal pain. These drugs are most useful for classic (stable) angina.

Beta blockers should not be abruptly discontinued. The dose should be tapered over a specified number of days to avoid reflex tachycardia and recurrence of anginal pain. Patients who have decreased heart rate and blood pressure usually cannot take beta blockers. Patients who have second- or third-degree AV block should not take beta blockers.

Beta blockers, discussed in detail in Chapter 18, are subdivided into *nonselective* beta blockers (block $beta_1$ and $beta_2$) and *selective* (cardiac) beta blockers (block $beta_1$).

Examples of nonselective beta blockers are propranolol (Inderal), nadolol (Corgard), and pindolol (Visken). These drugs decrease the heart rate and can cause bronchoconstriction. The cardioselective beta blockers act more strongly on the $beta_1$ receptor, which decreases heart rate but avoids bronchoconstriction, because of their lack of activity at the $beta_2$ receptor. Examples of selective beta blockers are atenolol (Tenormin) and metoprolol (Lopressor, Toprol-XL). Selective beta blockers are the group of choice for controlling angina pectoris. Table 42-4 lists the beta blockers most frequently used for angina and their dosages, uses, and considerations.

PROTOTYPE DRUG CHART 42-2

Nitroglycerin

Drug Class Antianginal Trade Names: Nitrostat, Nitro-Bid, Transderm-Nitro patch, NTG, ♣ Nitrogard SR Pregnancy Category: C	**Dosage** A: PO/SL: 0.3, 0.4, 0.6 mg; repeat q5min × 3 as needed; SR: 2.5- 6.5 mg, 2-4 times/d IV: Initially: 5 mcg/min; dose may be increased Ointment: 2% 1-2 inches to chest or thigh area Patch: 2.5-15 mg/d to chest or thigh area
Contraindications Increased intracranial pressure, severe anemia, cardiomyopathy Caution: Severe renal or hepatic disease, acute MI, severe hypotension, hypovolemia, pregnancy, breastfeeding	**Drug-Lab-Food Interactions** Drug: Increase effect with alcohol, beta blockers, calcium channel blockers, antihypertensives, aspirin, benzodiazepines, vasodilators; decrease effects of heparin Herbs: hawthorn increases nitroglycerin levels
Pharmacokinetics Absorption: SL: Greater than 75% absorbed; ointment and patch: slow absorption	**Pharmacodynamics** SL: Onset: 1-3 min Peak: 4 min Duration: 30 min SR Cap: Onset: 20-45 min Duration: 8-12 h Ointment: Onset: 20-60 min Peak: 1-2 h Duration: 6-8 h Patch: Onset: 30-60 min Peak: 1-2 h Duration: 20-24 h Distribution: PB: 60% Metabolism: $t\frac{1}{2}$: 1-4 min Excretion: Liver and urine IV: Onset: 1-3 min Duration: 3-5 min
Therapeutic Effects/Uses To control angina pectoris (anginal pain) Mode of Action: Decreases myocardial demand for oxygen; decreases preload by dilating veins, indirectly decreasing afterload	
Side Effects Nausea, vomiting, headache, blurred vision, dizziness, syncope, weakness, diaphoresis, flushing, confusion, pallor, rash, dry mouth, palpitations, tolerance	**Adverse Reactions** Hypotension, reflex tachycardia, paradoxical bradycardia Life-threatening: Circulatory collapse

A, Adult; *AMI*, acute myocardial infarction; *cap*, capsule; *d*, day; *h*, hour; *IV*, intravenous; *MI*, myocardial infarction; *min*, minute; *NTG*, nitroglycerin; *PB*, protein-binding; *PO*, by mouth; *SL*, sublingual; *SR*, sustained-release; $t\frac{1}{2}$, half-life; ♣, Canadian drug name.

TABLE 42-4 ANTIANGINALS

GENERIC (BRAND)	ROUTE AND DOSAGES	USES AND CONSIDERATIONS
Nitrates		
Short Acting		
nitroglycerin (Nitrostat, Nitro-Bid, Transderm-Nitro)	See Prototype Drug Chart 42-2.	
Long Acting		
isosorbide dinitrate (Isordil, Sorbitrate)	A: PO: IR: Initially 5-20 mg b.i.d/t.i.d.; maint: 10-40 mg b.i.d./t.i.d. A: SL: 2.5-10 mg q2-3h PRN A: SR: 40-160 mg/d	To prevent anginal attacks. Can lower blood pressure. Tolerance builds up over time. Headaches, dizziness, lightheadedness, and flush may occur. Pregnancy category: C; PB: UK; $t\frac{1}{2}$: 1-4 h

Continued

TABLE 42-4 ANTIANGINALS—cont'd

GENERIC (BRAND)	ROUTE AND DOSAGES	USES AND CONSIDERATIONS
isosorbide mononitrate (Imdur)	A: PO: IR: 5-20 mg b.i.d.; *max:* 40 mg/d A: PO: SR: 30-60 mg in morning; *max:* 240 mg/d	To prevent anginal attacks. SR form provides controlled delivery and a 6-hour drug-free period, which helps reduce drug tolerance and increase effectiveness. Pregnancy category: C; PB: 5%; t½: 5 h
Beta-Adrenergic Blockers		
atenolol (Tenormin) ($beta_1$)	A: PO: 25-100 mg/d; *max:* 200 mg/d	To control angina pectoris. Also effective in managing hypertension. Closely monitor blood pressure and heart rate. Cardioselective drug; blocks $beta_1$. Can be used by patients with asthma. Pregnancy category: D; PB: 5%-15%; t½: 6-7 h
metoprolol tartrate (Lopressor, Toprol XL) ($beta_1$)	A: PO: 50-100 mg in 2 divided doses; may increase to 100-400 mg/d A: PO: ER: 100 mg/d; may increase to 400 mg/d A: IV: 5 mg q2min; followed in 1-2 h by PO: 25-50 mg q6h	Similar to atenolol in blocking $beta_1$. High doses of metoprolol can affect $beta_2$ and could cause bronchoconstriction. Can reduce cardiac oxygen demand, which decreases heart rate and contractility. Pregnancy category: C; PB: 12%; t½: 3-7 h
nadolol (Corgard) ($beta_1$ and $beta_2$)	A: PO: 40 mg/d; may increase dose; *max:* 240-320 mg/d in divided doses	For angina pectoris and hypertension. Pregnancy category: C; PB: 30%; t½: 10-24 h
propranolol HCl (Inderal) ($beta_1$ and $beta_2$)	A: PO: Initially: 40 mg b.i.d.; maint: 160-480 mg/d in 2-3 divided doses; *max:* 640 mg/d SR: 80-160 mg/d; may increase to 120-160 mg/d; *max:* 640 mg/d	First beta blocker; blocks $beta_1$ and $beta_2$. No longer drug of choice to prevent angina because drug poses risk for bronchospasm. Monitor heart rate, blood pressure, and respiratory status. Pregnancy category: C; PB: 90%; t½: 2-6 h
Calcium Channel Blockers		
amlodipine (Norvasc)	A: PO: Initially: 5 mg/d; maint: 5-10 mg/d; *max:* 10 mg/d Older adults: Initially: 2.5 mg/d; maint: 2.5-10 mg/d	For angina pectoris and hypertension. May be given with another antianginal or antihypertensive drug. Pregnancy category: C; PB: 93%; t½: 30-50 h
diltiazem HCl (Cardizem)	A: PO: 30-60 mg q.i.d.; may increase to 360 mg/d in 4 divided doses; *max:* 480 mg/d SR: 60 mg q12h; *max:* 360 mg/d CR: 120-180 mg/d; *max:* 360 mg/d	For angina pectoris. Hypotensive effect not as severe as with nifedipine. Monitor kidney function. Pregnancy category: C; PB: 70%-80%; t½: 3.5-9 h
felodipine (Felendil XL)	A: PO: Initially: 5 mg/d single dose; maint: 2.5-10 mg/d; *max:* 10 mg/d Older adults: Initially: 2.5 mg/d; *max:* 10 mg/d	To treat chronic angina pectoris and manage hypertension. Reduces O_2 demand by the heart. Potent peripheral vasodilator; increases heart rate and myocardial contractility. Pregnancy category: C; PB: >99%; t½: 10-16 h
isradipine (DynaCirc)	A: PO: 2.5-7.5 mg b.i.d.; *max:* 10 mg/d	Primary use is to treat hypertension. Also given for angina pectoris. Pregnancy category: C; PB: 95%; t½: 8 h
nicardipine HCl (Cardene SR, Cardene IV)	A: PO: 20 mg t.i.d.; maint: 20-40 mg t.i.d. A: PO: SR: 30 mg b.i.d.; maint: 30-60 mg b.i.d. A: IV: Initially 5 mg/h infusion; *max:* 15 mg/h	For angina pectoris. May be used alone or in combination with other antianginals. Also used for hypertension. Peripheral edema, headache, dizziness, and lightheadedness may occur. Pregnancy category: C; PB: 95%; t½: 2-4 h
nifedipine (Procardia, Adalat)	A: PO: Initially 10 mg t.i.d.; 30 mg q6-8h; *max:* 180 mg/d A: PO: ER: 30-60 mg/d; *max:* 90 mg/d	For angina pectoris. Closely monitor blood pressure, especially if patient taking nitrates or beta blockers. A potent calcium channel blocker. Pregnancy category: C; PB: 92%-98%; t½: 2-5 h
nisoldipine (Sular)	A: PO: ER: Initially 17 mg/d; maint: 17-34 mg/d Older adults: PO: Initially 8.5 mg/d; maint: 8.5-34 mg/d	For angina pectoris and hypertension. Suppresses contraction of cardiac and vascular smooth muscle. Increases heart rate and cardiac output. Decreases blood pressure. Caution: Patients with heart disease are prone to MI and HF. Pregnancy category: C; PB: 99%; t½: 7-12 h
verapamil HCl (Calan, Isoptin)	A: PO: 40-120 mg t.i.d.; *max:* 480 mg/d IV: 5-10 mg over 2 min; may repeat in 30 min if needed	For angina pectoris, cardiac dysrhythmias, and hypertension. Peripheral edema, constipation, dizziness, headache, and hypotension may occur. Pregnancy category: C; PB: 90%; t½: 3-8 h

A, Adult; *a.c.*, before meals; *b.i.d.*, twice a day; *CR*, controlled-release; *d*, day; *ER*, extended-release; *h*, hour; *h.s.*, at bedtime; *HF*, heart failure; *IR*, immediate-release; *IV*, intravenous; *maint*, maintenance; *max*, maximum; *MI*, myocardial infarction; *min*, minute; O_2, oxygen; *PB*, protein-binding; *PO*, by mouth; *PRN*, as necessary; *q.i.d.*, four times a day; *SL*, sublingual; *SR*, sustained-release; *t.i.d.*, three times a day; *t½*, half-life; *UK*, unknown; >, greater than.

Pharmacokinetics Beta blockers are well absorbed orally. Absorption of sustained-release capsules is slow. The half-life of propranolol (Inderal) is 3 to 6 hours. Of the selective beta blockers, atenolol (Tenormin) has a half-life of 6 to 7 hours, and metoprolol (Lopressor) has a half-life of 3 to 7 hours. Propranolol and metoprolol are metabolized and excreted by the liver. Half an *oral* dose of atenolol is absorbed from the GI tract, with the remainder excreted unchanged in feces. When given IV, 85% of a dose is excreted in urine within 24 hours.

Pharmacodynamics Because beta blockers decrease the force of myocardial contraction, oxygen demand by the myocardium is reduced. Therefore, the patient can tolerate increased exercise with less oxygen requirement. Beta blockers are effective for classic (stable) angina.

The onset of action of the nonselective beta blocker propranolol is 30 minutes, its peak action is reached in 1 to 1.5 hours, and its duration is 4 to 12 hours. For the cardioselective beta blockers, the onset of action of atenolol is 60 minutes, its peak action occurs in 2 to 4 hours, and its duration of action is 24 hours. The onset of action of selective metoprolol is reached in 15 minutes, and the duration of action is 6 to 12 hours.

Side Effects and Adverse Reactions. Both nonselective and selective beta blockers cause a decrease in heart rate and blood pressure. For the nonselective beta blockers, bronchospasm, behavioral or psychotic response, and impotence (with use of Inderal) are potential adverse reactions.

Vital signs need to be closely monitored in the early stages of beta blocker therapy. When discontinuing use, the dosage should be tapered for 1 or 2 weeks to prevent a rebound effect such as reflex tachycardia or life-threatening cardiac dysrhythmias.

Calcium Channel Blockers

Calcium channel blockers (CCBs), or *calcium blockers,* were introduced in 1982 for the treatment of stable and variant angina pectoris, certain dysrhythmias, and hypertension. Calcium activates myocardial contraction, increasing the workload of the heart and the need for more oxygen. CCBs relax coronary artery spasm (variant angina) and relax peripheral arterioles (stable angina), decreasing cardiac oxygen demand. They also decrease cardiac contractility (negative inotropic effect that relaxes smooth muscle), decrease afterload, decrease peripheral resistance, and reduce the workload of the heart, which decreases the need for oxygen. CCBs achieve their effect in controlling variant (vasospastic) angina by relaxing coronary arteries and in controlling classic (stable) angina by decreasing oxygen demand. Figure 42-1 shows the suggested steps for treating classic and variant angina pectoris. Table 42-4 presents the drug data for the CCBs used to treat angina and their dosages, uses, and considerations.

Pharmacokinetics Three calcium channel blockers—verapamil (Calan), nifedipine (Procardia), and diltiazem (Cardizem)—have been effectively used for the long-term treatment of angina. Eighty to ninety percent of CCBs are absorbed through the GI mucosa. However, first-pass metabolism by the liver decreases the availability of free circulating drug, and only 20% of verapamil, 45% to 65% of diltiazem, and 35% to 40% of nifedipine are bioavailable. All three drugs are highly protein-bound (80% to 90%), and their half-lives are 2 to 9 hours.

Several other CCBs are available, such as nicardipine HCl (Cardene SR), amlodipine (Norvasc), felodipine (Felendil XL), and nisoldipine (Sular). All are highly protein-bound (greater than 95%). Nicardipine has the shortest half-life at 5 hours.

Pharmacodynamics Bradycardia is a common problem with the use of verapamil, the first calcium blocker. Nifedipine, the most potent of the calcium blockers, promotes vasodilation of the coronary and peripheral vessels, and hypotension can result. The onset of action is 10 minutes for verapamil and 30 minutes for nifedipine and diltiazem. Verapamil's duration of action is 3 to 7 hours when given orally and 2 hours when given IV. The duration of action for nifedipine and diltiazem is 6 to 8 hours.

Side Effects and Adverse Reactions. The side effects of calcium blockers include headache, hypotension (more common with nifedipine and less common with diltiazem), dizziness, and flushing of the skin. Reflex tachycardia can occur as a result of hypotension. Peripheral edema may occur with several CCBs including nicardipine, nifedipine, and

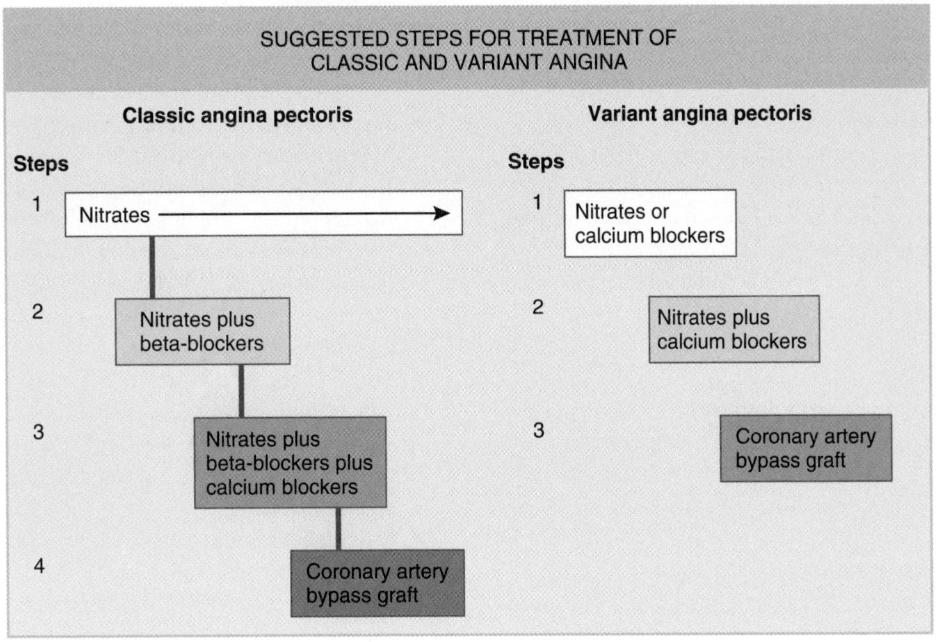

FIGURE 42–1 Suggested steps for treating classic and variant angina pectoris.

verapamil. CCBs can cause changes in liver and kidney function. Serum liver enzymes should be checked periodically. CCBs are frequently given with other antianginal drugs such as nitrates to prevent angina.

Nifedipine, in its immediate-release form (10- and 20-mg capsules), has been associated with an increased incidence of sudden cardiac death, especially when prescribed in high doses for outpatients. This is not true of the sustained-release preparations (Procardia XL, Adalat CC). For this reason, immediate-release nifedipine is usually prescribed only as needed in the hospital setting for acute increase in blood pressure.

Nursing Process
Patient-Centered Collaborative Care

Antianginals

Assessment
- Obtain baseline vital signs for future comparisons.
- Obtain health and drug histories. Nitroglycerin is contraindicated for marked hypotension or acute myocardial infarction (AMI).

Nursing Diagnoses
- Decreased cardiac output related to poor myocardial perfusion
- Anxiety related to perceived threat of death
- Acute pain related to anginal pain due to inadequate coronary perfusion and lack of oxygen
- Activity intolerance related to lack of oxygen due to poor blood perfusion to heart and lungs

Planning
- Patient's angina pain will be controlled by nitroglycerin or other antianginals.

Nursing Interventions
- Monitor vital signs. Hypotension is associated with most antianginal drugs.
- Position patient sitting or lying down when taking a nitrate for the first time. After administration, check vital signs while patient is lying down and then sitting up. Have patient rise slowly to standing position.
- Offer sips of water before giving sublingual (SL) nitrates; dryness may inhibit drug absorption.
- Monitor effects of IV nitroglycerin. Report angina that persists.
- Apply Nitro-Bid ointment to designated mark on paper. Do *not* use fingers because drug can be absorbed; use tongue blade or gloves. For Transderm-Nitro patch, do not touch medication portion.
- Do *not* apply Nitro-Bid ointment or Transderm-Nitro patch in any area on the chest in the vicinity of defibrillator-cardioverter paddle placement. Explosion and skin burns may result.

Patient Teaching
General
- Administer SL nitroglycerin tablet if chest pain occurs. If pain has not subsided or has worsened in 5 minutes, call 911.
- Advise patient not to ingest alcohol while taking nitroglycerin to avoid hypotension, weakness, and faintness.
- Advise patient to notify health care provider if chest pain is not completely alleviated. Tolerance to nitroglycerin can occur.
- Inform patient not to discontinue beta blockers and calcium blockers without health care provider's approval. Withdrawal symptoms (reflex tachycardia and pain) may be severe.

Self-Administration
- Demonstrate how (SL) nitroglycerin tablets are taken. Tablet is placed under tongue for quick absorption. Stinging or biting sensation indicates that tablet is fresh; however, with newer SL nitroglycerin tablets, biting sensation may not be present.
- Teach patient to store medication bottle away from light and to keep it dry. Keep drug in original screw-cap, amber glass bottle. Amber color of glass provides light protection, and screw-cap closure protects from moisture in the air, which can easily reduce potency of tablets.
- Teach patient about Transderm-Nitro patch. Apply once a day, usually in morning. Rotate skin sites. Patch is usually applied to chest wall, but thighs and arms may also be used. Avoid hairy areas.
- Advise patient to seek medical attention if nitroglycerin does not relieve pain.

Side Effects
- Suggest acetaminophen (Tylenol) to patient for relief of headache, which commonly occurs when first taking nitroglycerin products and lasts about 30 minutes.
- Place patient in supine position with legs elevated if hypotension results from SL nitroglycerin.
- Instruct patient how to take pulse rate.
- Advise patient taking beta blockers and calcium blockers to notify health care provider if dizziness or faintness occurs, as this may indicate hypotension.

Cultural Considerations
- Address cultural issues directly, especially in matters concerning dietary contributors to cardiac conditions. Family and community are important resources for promoting adherence to medication regimens and lifestyle changes.
- Provide printed materials in language that patient speaks and reads most easily. An interpreter may be necessary to establish sound, trusting relationship and ensure compliance with drug and diet regimens.

Evaluation

- Evaluate patient's response to nitrate product for relieving anginal pain. Note headache, dizziness, or faintness.

ANTIDYSRHYTHMIC DRUGS

Cardiac Dysrhythmias

A **cardiac dysrhythmia (arrhythmia)** is defined as any deviation from the normal rate or pattern of the heartbeat. This includes heart rates that are too slow (bradycardia), too fast (**tachycardia**), or irregular. The terms *dysrhythmia* (disturbed heart rhythm) and *arrhythmia* (absence of heart rhythm) are used interchangeably, despite the slight difference in meaning.

The ECG identifies the type of dysrhythmia. The P wave of the ECG reflects atrial activation, the QRS complex indicates ventricular depolarization, and the T wave reflects ventricular **repolarization** (return of cell membrane potential to resting after depolarization). The P-R interval indicates AV conduction time, and the Q-T interval reflects ventricular action potential duration. Atrial dysrhythmias prevent proper filling of the ventricles and decrease cardiac output by 33%. Ventricular dysrhythmias are life-threatening because ineffective filling of the ventricle and ineffective pumping results in decreased or absent cardiac output. With ventricular tachycardia, ventricular fibrillation is likely to occur, followed by death. Cardiopulmonary resuscitation (CPR) is necessary to treat these patients.

Cardiac dysrhythmias frequently follow an MI (heart attack) or can result from **hypoxia** (lack of oxygen to body tissues), **hypercapnia** (increased carbon dioxide in the blood), thyroid disease, coronary artery disease, cardiac surgery, excess catecholamines, or electrolyte imbalance.

Cardiac Action Potentials

Electrolyte transfer occurs through the cardiac muscle cell membrane. When sodium and calcium enter the cardiac cell, **depolarization** (myocardial contraction) occurs. Sodium enters rapidly to start the depolarization, and calcium enters later to maintain it. Calcium influx leads to an increased release of intracellular calcium from the sarcoplasmic reticulum, resulting in cardiac contraction. In the presence of myocardial ischemia, the contraction can be irregular.

Cardiac action potentials are transient depolarizations followed by repolarizations of myocardial cells. Figure 42-2 illustrates the action potential of a ventricular cardiac cell (myocyte) during the course of a heartbeat. There are five phases. Phase 0 is the rapid depolarization caused by an influx of sodium ions. Phase 1 is initial repolarization, which coincides with termination of sodium ion influx. Phase 2 is the plateau and is characterized by the influx of calcium ions, which prolong the action potential and promote atrial and ventricular muscle contraction. Phase 3 is rapid repolarization caused by influx of potassium ions. Phase 4 is the resting membrane potential between heartbeats. It is normally flat in

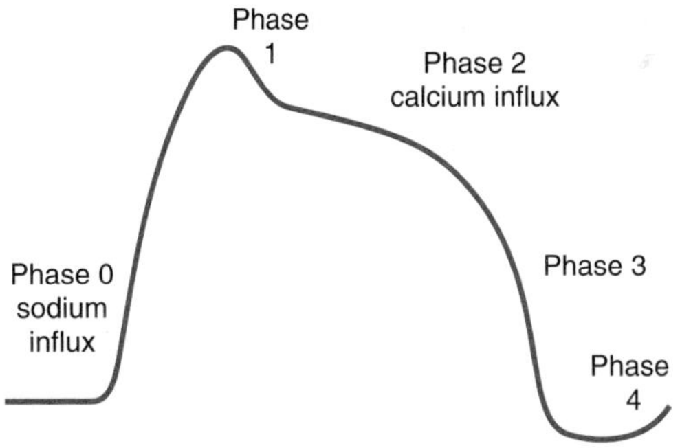

FIGURE 42–2 Action potential of a ventricular myocyte during the course of a heartbeat.

BOX 42-1 PHARMACODYNAMICS OF ANTIDYSRHYTHMICS

Mechanisms of Action

- Block adrenergic stimulation of the heart
- Depress myocardial excitability and contractility
- Decrease conduction velocity in cardiac tissue
- Increase recovery time (repolarization) of the myocardium
- Suppress automaticity (spontaneous depolarization to initiate beats)

ventricular muscle, but it begins to rise in the cells of the sinoatrial (SA) node as they slowly depolarize toward the threshold potential just before depolarization occurs, initiating the next heartbeat.

Types of Antidysrhythmic Drugs

The desired action of **antidysrhythmic (antiarrhythmic) drugs** is to restore the cardiac rhythm to normal. Box 42-1 describes the various mechanisms by which this is accomplished.

The antidysrhythmics are grouped into four classes: (1) sodium (fast) channel blockers IA, IB, and IC; (2) beta blockers; (3) drugs that prolong repolarization; and (4) calcium (slow) channel blockers. Table 42-5 lists the classes, actions, and indications for cardiac antidysrhythmic drugs. Table 42-6 lists the commonly administered antidysrhythmics and their dosages, uses, and considerations.

Class I: Sodium Channel Blockers

A sodium channel blocker decreases sodium influx into cardiac cells. Responses to the drug are decreased conduction velocity in cardiac tissues; suppression of automaticity, which decreases the likelihood of ectopic foci; and increased recovery time (repolarization or refractory period). There are three subgroups of sodium channel blockers. Class IA slows conduction and prolongs repolarization (quinidine, procainamide, disopyramide). Class IB slows conduction and shortens repolarization (lidocaine, mexiletine HCl). Class IC prolongs conduction with little to no effect on repolarization (flecainide).

Lidocaine, a Class IB sodium channel blocker, was used in the 1940s as a local anesthetic and is still used for this purpose. It was later discovered to have antidysrhythmic properties as

TABLE 42-5 CLASSES, ACTIONS, AND INDICATIONS OF ANTIDYSRHYTHMIC DRUGS

CLASSES	ACTIONS	INDICATIONS
Class I		
Sodium Channel Blockers		
IA	Slow conduction and prolong repolarization	Atrial and ventricular dysrhythmias, paroxysmal atrial tachycardia (PAT), supraventricular dysrhythmias
IB	Slow conduction and shorten repolarization	Acute ventricular dysrhythmias
IC	Prolong conduction with little to no effect on repolarization	Life-threatening ventricular dysrhythmias
Class II		
Beta blockers	Reduce calcium entry Decrease conduction velocity, automaticity, and recovery time (refractory period)	Atrial flutter and fibrillation, tachydysrhythmias, ventricular and supraventricular dysrhythmias
Class III		
Drugs that prolong repolarization	Prolong repolarization during ventricular dysrhythmias Prolong action potential duration	Life-threatening atrial and ventricular dysrhythmias resistant to other drugs
Class IV		
Calcium channel blockers	Block calcium influx Slow conduction velocity Decrease myocardial contractility (negative inotropic) Increase refraction in AV node	Supraventricular tachydysrhythmias; prevention of PSVT

AV, Atrioventricular, *PVST,* paroxysmal supraventricular tachycardia.

TABLE 42-6 ANTIDYSRHYTHMICS

GENERIC (BRAND)	ROUTE AND DOSAGE	USES AND CONSIDERATIONS
Class I		
Sodium Channel Blockers IA		
disopyramide phosphate (Norpace)	A: PO: 100-200 mg q6h; *max:* 800 mg/d C: 4-12 y: PO: 10-15 mg/kg/d in divided doses A: PO: ER: 200-300 mg q12h; *max:* 800 mg/d	Prevention and suppression of unifocal and multifocal premature ventricular contractions (PVCs). For ventricular dysrhythmias. May cause anticholinergic symptoms. Serum therapeutic level is 3-8 mcg/mL. Pregnancy category: C; PB: 90%; t½: 4-10 h
procainamide HCl	A: PO: LD: 1000-1250 mg q3-4h A: IM: 50 mg/kg/d in 4 divided doses A: IV: LD: 20-50 mg/min; maint: 1-4 mg/min continuous inf C: IV: LD: 15 mg/kg over 30-60 min TDM: 4-10 mcg/mL	Controls dysrhythmias (PVCs) and ventricular tachycardia. Depresses myocardial excitability by slowing down conductivity of cardiac tissue. Pregnancy category: C; PB: 15%, t½: 3-4 h
quinidine sulfate,	A: PO: 200-300 mg t.i.d./q.i.d. A: PO: ER: 300-600 mg q8-12h TDM: 2-6 mcg/mL	For atrial, ventricular, and supraventricular dysrhythmias. Nausea, vomiting, diarrhea, and abdominal pain or cramps are common side effects. If given with digoxin, can increase digoxin concentration. Pregnancy category: C; PB: 80%-90%; t½: 6-7 h
Sodium Channel Blockers IB		
lidocaine (Xylocaine)	A: IV: 50-100 mg bolus in 2-3 min; *max LD:* 300 mg over 1 h, then IV inf: 20-50 mcg/kg/min TDM: 1.5-6 mcg/mL	For acute ventricular dysrhythmias following MI and cardiac surgery. Pregnancy category: B; PB: 60%-80%; t½: 1.5-2 h
mexiletine HCl	A: PO: 200-300 mg q8h; *max:* 1200 mg/d TDM: 0.5-2 mcg/mL	Analogue of lidocaine. Treatment for acute and chronic ventricular dysrhythmias. Take with food to decrease GI distress. Common side effects are nausea, vomiting, heartburn, tremor, dizziness, nervousness, lightheadedness. Pregnancy category: C; PB: 50%-60%; t½: 10-12 h

TABLE 42-6 ANTIDYSRHYTHMICS—cont'd

GENERIC (BRAND)	ROUTE AND DOSAGE	USES AND CONSIDERATIONS
Sodium Channel Blockers IC		
flecainide (Tambocor)	A: PO: Initial: 50-100 mg q12h; Increase by 50 mg q12h q4d; maint: 150 mg q12h; *max:* 400 mg/d	For life-threatening ventricular dysrhythmias and prevention of PSVT and PAF. Contraindicated in cardiogenic shock, second- or third-degree heart block, or right bundle branch block. Pregnancy category: C; PB: 40%-50%; $t\frac{1}{2}$: 12-30 h
propafenone HCl (Rythmol)	A: PO: 150-300 mg q8h; *max:* 900 mg/d A: PO: ER: 225-325 mg q12h; *max:* 850 mg/d	For life-threatening ventricular dysrhythmias. Contraindicated if cardiogenic shock, uncontrolled HF, heart block, severe hypotension, bradycardia, or bronchospasm present. Pregnancy category: C; PB: 85%-97%; $t\frac{1}{2}$: 5-8 h
Class II		
Beta-Adrenergic Blockers		
acebutolol HCl (Sectral) (beta$_1$ blocker)	See Prototype Drug Chart 42-3.	
esmolol (Brevibloc) (beta$_1$ blocker)	A: IV: LD: 500 mcg/kg over 1 min; maint: 50-100 mcg/kg/min; *max:* 200 mcg/kg/min	To control atrial flutter and fibrillation. For short-term use only. Mainly for patients having dysrhythmias during surgery. May cause bradycardia, heart block, and HF. Pregnancy category: C; PB: 55%; $t\frac{1}{2}$: 9 min
propranolol HCl (Inderal, Inderal LA) (beta$_1$ and beta$_2$ blocker)	A: PO: 10-30 mg t.i.d./q.i.d. ER: 80 mg/d A: IV bolus: 0.5-3 mg at 1 mg/min	For ventricular dysrhythmias, PAT, and atrial and ventricular ectopic beats. Contraindicated for patients with asthma. Pregnancy category: C; PB: 90%; $t\frac{1}{2}$: 2-6 h
sotalol HCl (Betapace) (beta$_1$ and beta$_2$ blocker; also Class III)	A: PO: 80 mg b.i.d.; *max:* 240-320 mg/d in divided doses Increase dose interval with renal dysfunction	For sustained ventricular dysrhythmias. Contraindicated if bronchial asthma or heart block present. Correct hypokalemia and hypomagnesemia prior to initiating sotalol. Pregnancy category: B; PB: 0%; $t\frac{1}{2}$: 12 h
Class III		
Drugs That Prolong Repolarization		
adenosine (Adenocard)	A: IV: Initially, 6 mg rapid IV bolus (1-2 sec) Repeat if necessary: 12 mg rapid IV bolus × 2 doses	Treatment of PSVT, Wolff-Parkinson-White syndrome. Contraindicated if second- or third-degree AV block or atrial flutter or fibrillation present. Pregnancy category: C; PB: UK; $t\frac{1}{2}$: <10 sec
amiodarone HCl (Cordarone)	A: PO: LD: 400-1600 mg/d in divided doses; maint: 200-600 mg/d; dose may be individualized TDM: 1-2.5 mcg/mL	For life-threatening ventricular dysrhythmias. Initially dosage is greater, and then it decreases over time. Pregnancy category: D; PB: >99%; $t\frac{1}{2}$: 7-50 d
dofetilide (Tikosyn)	PO: 250-1000 mcg/d in 2 divided doses Dose usually individualized based on calculated creatinine clearance	Selective potassium channel blocker that prolongs repolarization. Prescribed for atrial flutter and fibrillation. Monitor renal function. Pregnancy category: C; PB: 60%-70%; $t\frac{1}{2}$: 10 h
ibutilide (Corvert)	A: >60 kg: IV: 0.1 mg/kg or 1 mg (1 vial) over 10 min; may repeat in 10 min. A: <60 kg: IV: 0.01 mg/kg given over 10 min	Prolongs action potential and increases atrial and ventricular refractories; prolongs Q-T interval. May be given to convert atrial flutter and fibrillation to normal sinus rhythm. Pregnancy category: C; PB: 40%; $t\frac{1}{2}$: 2-12 h
sotalol (Betapace)	A: PO: Same as Class II (see sotalol in Class II)	Beta blocker. Can be classified as Class II or III. To treat life-threatening ventricular dysrhythmias (ventricular tachycardia). Slows heart rate, decreases AV conduction, increases AV refractory period, and decreases systolic and diastolic BP. Caution: Contraindicated if second- and third-degree heart block present. (See sotalol in Class II.)
Class IV		
Calcium Channel Blockers		
verapamil HCl (Calan, Isoptin)	A: PO: 240-480 mg/d in 3-4 divided doses A: IV: 2.5-10 mg IV push over 2 min; may repeat in 30 min	For supraventricular tachydysrhythmias, prevention of PSVT, angina pectoris, and hypertension. Contraindicated if cardiogenic shock, second- or third-degree AV block, severe hypotension, or severe HF present. Serum therapeutic level: 80-300 ng/mL or 0.08-0.3 mcg/mL. Pregnancy category: C; PB: 90%; $t\frac{1}{2}$: 3-8 h
diltiazem (Cardizem)	A: IV: 0.25 mg/kg IV bolus over 2 min, or 5-10 mg/h in IV inf	For PSVT and atrial flutter or fibrillation. Contraindicated if second- or third-degree AV block or hypotension present. Pregnancy category: C; PB: 70%-80%; $t\frac{1}{2}$: 3-8 h

Continued

TABLE 42-6 ANTIDYSRHYTHMICS—cont'd

GENERIC (BRAND)	ROUTE AND DOSAGE	USES AND CONSIDERATIONS
Others		
digoxin (Lanoxin)	A: PO: LD: 10-15 mcg/kg q6-8h given in 3 divided doses A/C: >10 y: IV: LD: 8-12 mcg/kg Maintenance: 0.125-0.5 mg/d	For atrial flutter or fibrillation; to prevent recurrence of paroxysmal atrial tachycardia. Pregnancy category: C; PB: 30%; t½: >36 h
dronedarone (Multaq)	A: PO: 400 mg b.i.d. with morning and evening meal	For atrial fibrillation and atrial flutter. Has antidysrhythmic properties of all four classes. May lead to photosensitivity and severe diarrhea. Contraindicated if severe heart failure present. Avoid grapefruit and grapefruit juice. Pregnancy category: X; PB: 98%; t½: 13-19 h

A, Adult; *AV,* atrioventricular; *b.i.d.,* two times a day; *BP,* blood pressure; *C,* child; *CR,* controlled-release; *d,* day; *ER,* extended-release; *FDA,* U.S. Food and Drug Administration; *h,* hour; *HF,* heart failure; *GI,* gastrointestinal; *IM,* intramuscular; *inf,* infusion; *IV,* intravenous; *LD,* loading dose; *maint,* maintenance; *max,* maximum; *MI,* myocardial infarction; *min,* minute; *PAT,* paroxysmal atrial tachycardia; *PAF,* paroxysmal atrial fibrillation (or flutter); *PVST,* paroxysmal supraventricular tachycardia; *PB,* protein-binding; *PO,* by mouth; *q.i.d.,* four times a day; *SR,* sustained-release; *TDM,* therapeutic drug monitoring; *t½,* half-life; *t.i.d.,* three times a day; *UK,* unknown; *y,* year; >, greater than; <, less than.

well. Lidocaine is still used by some cardiologists to treat acute ventricular dysrhythmias. It slows conduction velocity and decreases action potential amplitude. Onset of action (IV) is rapid. About one third of lidocaine reaches the general circulation. A bolus of lidocaine is short-lived. Another Class IB sodium channel blocker is mexiletine.

Class II: Beta Blockers

The drugs in the second class, beta blockers, decrease conduction velocity, automaticity, and recovery time (refractory period). Examples are propranolol (Inderal), acebutolol (Sectral), esmolol (Brevibloc), and sotalol (Betapace). Beta blockers are more frequently prescribed for dysrhythmias than sodium channel blockers. Prototype Drug Chart 42-3 lists the drug data related to the beta blocker acebutolol HCL (Sectral), which can be prescribed to treat recurrent stable ventricular dysrhythmias.

Pharmacokinetics The cardioselective beta drug acebutolol (Sectral) is well absorbed in the GI tract. It is metabolized in the liver to active metabolites; 50% to 60% of the drug is eliminated in the bile via feces, and 30% to 40% is excreted in the urine. The half-life for the drug is 3 to 4 hours, but the half-life for its metabolites is 8 to 13 hours.

Pharmacodynamics Acebutolol is prescribed for ventricular dysrhythmias as well as for angina pectoris and hypertension. As an antidysrhythmic drug, the onset of action is 1 hour; peak time is 4 to 6 hours, and duration of action is 10 hours. To treat hypertension, the duration of action is 20 to 24 hours.

Class III: Drugs That Prolong Repolarization

Drugs in the third class prolong repolarization and are used in emergency treatment of ventricular dysrhythmias when other antidysrhythmics are ineffective. Amiodarone (Cordarone) increases the refractory period (recovery time) and prolongs the action potential duration (cardiac cell activity).

Class IV: Calcium Channel Blockers

The fourth class consists of the calcium channel blockers verapamil (Calan, Isoptin) and diltiazem (Cardizem). Verapamil is a slow (calcium) channel blocker that blocks calcium influx, thereby decreasing the excitability and contractility (negative inotropic) of the myocardium. It increases the refractory period of the AV node, which decreases ventricular response. Verapamil is contraindicated for patients with AV block or HF.

Side Effects and Adverse Reactions for Antidysrhythmic Drugs. Quinidine, the first drug used to treat cardiac dysrhythmias, has many side effects (e.g., nausea, vomiting, diarrhea, confusion, hypotension). It can also cause heart block and neurologic and psychiatric symptoms. Procainamide causes less cardiac depression than quinidine.

High doses of lidocaine can cause cardiovascular depression, bradycardia, hypotension, seizures, blurred vision, and double vision. Less serious side effects may include dizziness, lightheadedness, and confusion. The use of lidocaine is contraindicated in patients with advanced AV block. It should also be used with caution in patients with liver disorder and HF. Mexiletine and tocainide have side effects similar to lidocaine. They are contraindicated for use in patients with cardiogenic shock or in those with second- or third-degree heart block.

Side effects of beta blockers are bradycardia and hypotension. Bretylium and amiodarone can cause nausea, vomiting, hypotension, and neurologic problems. Side effects of calcium blockers include nausea, vomiting, hypotension, and bradycardia.

It should be noted that *all* antidysrhythmic drugs are potentially prodysrhythmic. This is because of both the pharmacologic activity of the drug on the heart and the inherently unpredictable activity of a diseased heart, with or without the use of drugs. In some cases, life-threatening ventricular dysrhythmias can result from appropriate and skillful attempts at drug therapy to treat patients with heart disease. For these reasons, antidysrhythmic drug therapy is often initiated during continuous cardiac monitoring of the patient's heart rhythm in a hospital setting.

PROTOTYPE DRUG CHART 42-3

Acebutolol HCl

Drug Class $Beta_1$ blocker: cardioselective beta-adrenergic antagonist Trade Names: Sectral Pregnancy Category: B	**Dosage** Ventricular dysrhythmia: A: PO: 200 mg q12h May increase to 600-1200 mg in 2 divided doses; *max:* 1200 mg/d Older adults: PO: 200-400 mg/d; *max:* 800 mg/d Not for children <12 y
Contraindications Second- and third-degree heart block, severe bradycardia, severe HF, cardiogenic shock Caution: Undergoing major surgery, renal and hepatic impairment, diabetes mellitus, hyperthyroidism, asthma, bronchitis, COPD	**Drug-Lab-Food Interactions** Drug: Increase effects with diuretics; prolong hypoglycemic effects of insulin and oral antidiabetics; antagonist effect with albuterol, metaproterenol, terbutaline. Lab: May increase ALT, AST, ALP, ANA titer, BUN, lipoproteins, potassium.
Pharmacokinetics Absorption: Well absorbed Distribution: PB: 26% Metabolism: $t\frac{1}{2}$: 3-4 h; metabolites: 8-13 h Excretion: 90%-100% in bile, feces, and urine	**Pharmacodynamics** Ventricular dysrhythmias: PO: Onset: 1 h Peak: 2.5-3.5 h Duration: 10 h
Therapeutic Effects/Uses To aid in treatment of recurrent stable ventricular dysrhythmias, angina pectoris, and hypertension. Mode of Action: Blocks $beta_1$-adrenergic receptors in cardiac tissues.	
Side Effects Dizziness, nausea, vomiting, anorexia, edema, headache, visual impairment, hypotension, diaphoresis, fatigue, insomnia, constipation, diarrhea, impotence	**Adverse Reactions** Palpitations with abrupt withdrawal, bradycardia, chest pain, hyperglycemia, hypoglycemia, diabetes mellitus Life-threatening: agranulocytosis, bronchospasm (high doses)

A, Adult; *ALP*, alkaline phosphatase; *ALT*, alanine aminotransferase; *ANA*, antinuclear antibodies; *AST*, aspartate aminotransferase; *b.i.d.*, twice a day; *BUN*, blood urea nitrogen; *h*, hour; *HF*, heart failure; *PB*, protein-binding; *PO*, by mouth; $t\frac{1}{2}$, half-life; *UK*, unknown; <, less than.

Nursing Process
Patient-Centered Collaborative Care

Antidysrhythmics

Assessment
- Obtain health and drug histories. History may include shortness of breath, heart palpitations, coughing, chest pain (type, duration, and severity), previous angina or cardiac dysrhythmias, and drugs patient currently takes.
- Obtain baseline vital signs and electrocardiogram (ECG) for future comparison.
- Monitor early cardiac enzyme results (aspartate aminotransferase, lactate dehydrogenase, creatine phosphokinase) and troponins (cardiac-specific) for future comparison.

Nursing Diagnoses
- Decreased cardiac output related to cardiac dysrhythmia
- Anxiety related to irregular heartbeat
- Risk for activity intolerance related to lack of oxygen due to irregular heart rate

Planning
- Patient will no longer experience abnormal sinus rhythm.
- Patient will comply with antidysrhythmic drug regimen.

Nursing Interventions
- Monitor vital signs because hypotension can occur.
- Administer drug by IV push or bolus over a period of 2 to 3 minutes or as prescribed.
- Monitor ECG for abnormal patterns, and report findings such as premature ventricular contractions (PVCs), increased P-R and Q-T intervals, and/or widening of QRS complex. Increased Q-T interval is a risk factor for *torsades de pointes*.

Patient Teaching
General
- Teach patient to take prescribed drug as ordered because drug compliance is essential.

- Provide specific instructions for each drug (e.g., photosensitivity for amiodarone).

Side Effects
- Tell patient to report side effects and adverse reactions to health care provider, including dizziness, faintness, nausea, and vomiting.
- Advise patient to avoid alcohol, caffeine, and tobacco. Alcohol can intensify hypotensive reaction; caffeine increases catecholamine level; and tobacco promotes vasoconstriction.

Cultural Considerations
- Advise patient to focus on relationship between certain dietary habits and cardiac disease. Discuss importance of drug regimen in terms that directly address cultural issues and accommodate family's values. An interpreter may be necessary to ensure patient's understanding and compliance with drug and dietary regimens.

Evaluation
- Evaluate effectiveness of prescribed antidysrhythmic by comparing heart rates with baseline heart rate and assessing patient's response to drug.
- Report side effects and adverse reactions. Drug regimen may need to be adjusted. Proarrhythmic effect may occur, which may require discontinuation of drug.

KEY WEBSITES

American Heart Association: *www.americanheart.org*

American College of Cardiology: *www.acc.org*

CRITICAL THINKING CASE STUDY

ST, a 64-year-old patient, has heart failure (HF), which is being controlled with digoxin (Lanoxin), furosemide (Lasix), and a low-sodium diet. She is taking potassium chloride (KCl) 20 mEq per day orally. Three days ago, ST had flulike symptoms such as anorexia, lethargy, and diarrhea. Her fluid and food intake was diminished. She refused to take the KCl and stated that the drug makes her sick. She has been taking the digoxin and furosemide daily.

The nurse's assessment during the home visit includes poor skin turgor, poor muscle tone, irregular pulse rate, and decreased bowel sounds. The nurse obtained a blood sample for serum electrolytes; results indicated potassium (K) 2.9 mEq/L, sodium (Na) 137 mEq/L, and chloride (Cl) 96 mEq/L.

1. List reference values for serum potassium (K), serum sodium (Na), and serum chloride (Cl). Are ST's electrolyte levels within normal range? Explain your answer.
2. Match ST's physical findings with the corresponding electrolyte imbalance.
3. What are the reasons for the electrolyte imbalance?
4. ST said she was not taking KCl because the drug makes her sick. What information can you give her concerning the administration of potassium?
5. What is the effect of furosemide on digoxin when there is a potassium deficit? Explain your answer.
6. Why should the nurse assess ST for digitalis toxicity? List the signs and symptoms of digitalis toxicity.

ST was referred to the health care provider because of her serum potassium deficit and its effect on digoxin. A repeat serum potassium determination was taken, and the result was 2.8 mEq/L. A liter of 5% dextrose in water with KCl 40 mEq/L was administered over 4 hours.

7. How many milliequivalents of KCl per hour would ST receive? Does this amount constitute an acceptable dosage?
8. Why is it important that the nurse monitor the rate of intravenous fluids containing potassium, the hourly urine output, and vital signs?
9. Because of the low serum potassium level, what other electrolyte value should be checked? Explain your answer.

After ST's serum electrolytes returned to normal, the health care provider instructed her to continue taking the prescribed KCl dosage daily with her other medications.

10. ST asks why she has to continue taking these drugs. What is the nurse's best response?
11. The nurse instructs ST to eat foods rich in potassium. Which foods are the richest sources of potassium?

NCLEX STUDY QUESTIONS

1. The patient is receiving digoxin for treatment of heart failure. Which finding would suggest to the nurse that heart failure is improving?
   a. Pale and cool extremities
   b. Absence of peripheral edema
   c. Urine output of 60 mL/4 h
   d. Complaints of increasing dyspnea
2. The patient's serum digoxin level is 3.0 ng/mL. What does the nurse know about this serum digoxin level?
   a. It is in the high (elevated) range.
   b. It is in the low (decreased) range.
   c. It is within the normal range.
   d. It is in the low average range.
3. The nurse is assessing a patient for possible evidence of digitalis toxicity. The nurse acknowledges that which is included in the signs and symptoms for digitalis toxicity?
   a. Apical pulse rate of 100 beats/min
   b. Apical pulse of 72 beats/min with an irregular rate
   c. Apical pulse of 90 beats/min and an irregular rate
   d. Apical pulse of 48 beats/min and irregular rate
4. A patient is taking a potassium-depleting diuretic and digoxin. The nurse expects that a low potassium level (hypokalemia) could have what effect on digoxin (Lanoxin)?
   a. Increase serum digoxin sensitivity level
   b. Decrease serum digoxin sensitivity level
   c. Have no effect on serum digoxin sensitivity level
   d. Cause a low average serum digoxin sensitivity level
5. A patient takes an initial dose of a nitrate. Which symptom(s) will the nurse expect to occur?
   a. Nausea and vomiting
   b. Headaches
   c. Stomach cramps
   d. Irregular pulse rate
6. A patient is prescribed a beta blocker. The nurse acknowledges that beta blockers are as effective as antianginals because they do what?
   a. Increase oxygen to the systemic circulation
   b. Maintain heart rate and blood pressure
   c. Decrease heart rate and decrease myocardial contractility
   d. Decrease heart rate and increase myocardial contractility
7. The health care provider is planning to discontinue a patient's beta blocker. Which instruction will the nurse give the patient regarding the beta blocker?
   a. The beta blocker should be abruptly stopped when another cardiac drug is prescribed.
   b. The beta blocker should not be abruptly stopped; the dose should be tapered down.
   c. The beta blocker dose should be maintained while taking another antianginal drug.
   d. Half the beta blocker dose should be taken for the next several weeks.
8. The beta blocker acebutolol (Sectral) is prescribed for dysrhythmias. The nurse knows that what is the primary purpose of the drug?
   a. Increase $beta_1$ and $beta_2$ receptors in cardiac tissues
   b. Increase the flow of oxygen to cardiac tissues
   c. Block $beta_1$-adrenergic receptors in cardiac tissues
   d. Block $beta_2$-adrenergic receptors in cardiac tissues
9. A patient who has angina is prescribed nitroglycerin. Which are appropriate nursing interventions for nitroglycerin? (Select all that apply.)
   a. Have patient sit or lie down when taking a nitroglycerin sublingual tablet.
   b. Teach patient who has taken a tablet to call 911 in 5 minutes if chest pain persists.
   c. Apply Transderm-Nitro patch to a hairy area to protect skin from burning.
   d. Call the health care provider after taking five tablets if chest pain persists.
   e. Warn patient against ingesting alcohol while taking nitroglycerin.

Answers: 1, b; 2, a; 3, d; 4, a; 5, b; 6, c; 7, b; 8, c; 9, a, b, e.

CHAPTER 43

Diuretics

evolve WEBSITE

http://evolve.elsevier.com/KeeHayes/pharmacology/

- Animations
- Content Updates
- Key Points
- Review Questions for the NCLEX® Examination
- References from the Textbook
- Unfolding Case Studies

OBJECTIVES

- Compare the action and uses of thiazide, loop, and potassium-sparing diuretics.
- Differentiate side effects and adverse reactions related to thiazide, loop, and potassium-sparing diuretics.
- Explain the nursing interventions, including patient teaching, related to thiazide, loop, and potassium-sparing diuretics.
- Apply the nursing process for the patient taking thiazide, loop, and potassium-sparing diuretics.

OUTLINE

KEY TERMS

antihypertensive, p. 621
diuresis, p. 620
diuretics, p. 620
hypercalcemia, p. 622
hyperglycemia, p. 623
hyperkalemia, p. 629
hypertension, p. 620
hyperuricemia, p. 623
hypokalemia, p. 624
natriuresis, p. 621
natriuretic, p. 625
oliguria, p. 623
osmolality, p. 626
potassium-sparing diuretics, p. 621
potassium-wasting diuretics, p. 621
saluretic, p. 625

Diuretics are used for two main purposes: to decrease hypertension (lower blood pressure) and to decrease edema (peripheral and pulmonary) in heart failure (HF) and renal or liver disorders. **Hypertension** is an elevated blood pressure. Diuretics discussed in this chapter are used either alone or in combination to decrease blood pressure and edema.

Diuretics produce increased urine flow, or **diuresis,** by inhibiting sodium and water reabsorption from the kidney tubules. Most sodium and water reabsorption occurs throughout the renal tubular segments (proximal, loop of Henle [descending loop and ascending loop], and collecting tubule). Diuretics can affect one or more segments of the renal tubules. Figure 43-1 illustrates the renal tubule along with the normal process of water and electrolyte reabsorption and diuretic effects on the tubules.

Every 1.5 hours, the total volume of the body's extracellular fluid (ECF) goes through the kidneys (glomeruli) for cleansing; this is the first process for urine formation. Small

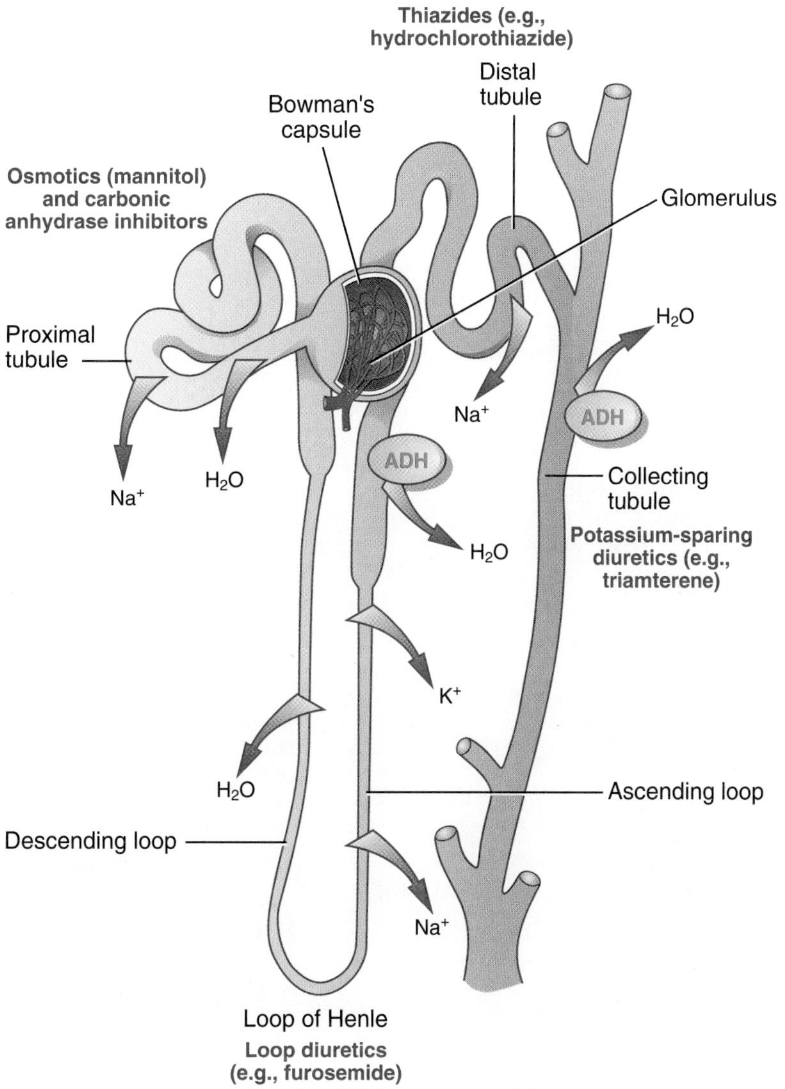

FIGURE 43–1 Diuretics act on different segments of the renal tubule. Osmotic, mercurial, and carbonic anhydrase inhibitor diuretics affect the proximal tubule; loop diuretics affect the loop of Henle; thiazides affect the distal tubule; and potassium-sparing diuretics act primarily on the collecting tubules.

particles such as electrolytes, drugs, glucose, and waste products from protein metabolism are filtered in the glomeruli. Larger products such as protein and blood cells are not filtered with normal renal function, and they remain in the circulation. Sodium and water are the largest filtrate substances.

Normally 99% of the filtered sodium that passes through the glomeruli is reabsorbed; 50% to 55% of sodium reabsorption occurs in the proximal tubules, 35% to 40% in the loop of Henle, 5% to 10% in the distal tubules, and <3% in the collecting tubules. Diuretics that act on the tubules closest to the glomeruli have the greatest effect in causing **natriuresis** (sodium loss in the urine). A classic example is the osmotic diuretic mannitol. The diuretic effect depends on the drug reaching the kidneys and its concentration in the renal tubules.

Diuretics have an **antihypertensive** effect because they promote sodium and water loss by blocking sodium and chloride reabsorption. This causes a decrease in fluid volume, lowering blood pressure. With fluid loss, edema (fluid retention in body tissues) should decrease, but if sodium is retained, water is also retained, and blood pressure increases.

Many diuretics cause the loss of other electrolytes, including potassium, magnesium, chloride, and bicarbonate. The diuretics that promote potassium excretion are classified as **potassium-wasting diuretics,** and those that promote potassium retention are called **potassium-sparing diuretics.**

The following five categories of diuretics are effective in removing water and sodium:

- Thiazide and thiazide-like
- Loop or high-ceiling
- Osmotic
- Carbonic anhydrase inhibitor
- Potassium-sparing

Thiazide, loop, and potassium-sparing diuretics are most frequently prescribed for hypertension and for edema

TABLE 43-1 DIURETICS

GENERIC (BRAND)	ROUTE AND DOSAGE	USES AND CONSIDERATIONS
Thiazides		
Short-Acting		
chlorothiazide (Diuril)	A: PO: 250-1000 mg/d in 1-2 divided doses A: IV: 500-1000 mg/d in 1-2 divided doses C: PO: 10-20 mg/kg/d in 1-2 divided doses	For hypertension and peripheral edema. Adults may be given IV chlorothiazide, but not recommended for infants and children. Pregnancy category: C; PB: 20%-80%; t½: 1-2 h
hydrochlorothiazide (Esidrix, HCTZ)	See Prototype Drug Chart 43-1.	
Intermediate-Acting		
bendroflumethiazide with Nadolol (Corzide)	A: PO: 40 mg nadolol/5 mg bendroflumethiazide; *max:* 80/5	Treatment of hypertension and edema associated with HF and cirrhosis. Has similar effects as prototype drug HCTZ. Hypokalemia, hyperglycemia, and hyperuricemia may occur. Pregnancy category: C; PB: nadolol: 95%; bendroflumethiazide: 95%; t½: nadolol: 10-24 h; bendroflumethiazide: 3 h
Long-Acting		
methyclothiazide	Hypertension/edema: A: PO: 2.5-10 mg/d; *max:* 5 mg/d for hypertension; 10 mg/d for edema	For hypertension and edema associated with HF and renal or liver dysfunction. Side effects and drug interactions similar to those of HCTZ. Long duration of action. Pregnancy category: B; PB: UK; t½: UK
Thiazide-Like Diuretics		
chlorthalidone (Hygroton, Thalitone)	Hypertension: A: PO: 12.5-50 mg/d; 50 mg/d C: PO: 2 mg/kg/d Edema: A: PO: 25-100 mg/d; *max:* 200 mg/d	For hypertension and edema associated with HF and renal or liver dysfunction. Very long duration of action (24-72 h). Pregnancy category: B; PB: 75%; t½: 40-60 h
indapamide	Hypertension/edema: A: PO: 1.25-2.5 mg/d; may increase to 5 mg/d; *max:* 5 mg/d	For hypertension and edema. Long-acting diuretic. May be classified as loop diuretic. Pregnancy category: B; PB: 71%-79%; t½: 14-18 h
metolazone (Zaroxolyn)	Hypertension: A: PO: 2.5-5.0 mg/d C: PO: 0.2-0.4 mg/kg/d in divided doses Edema: A: PO: 5-20 mg/d	For hypertension and edema. Intermediate-acting diuretic. More effective than thiazides in patients with decreased renal function. Pregnancy category: B; PB: 33%; t½: 14 h

A, Adult; *b.i.d.,* twice a day; *C,* child; *d,* day; *h,* hour; *HF,* heart failure; *IV,* intravenous; *maint,* maintenance; *max,* maximum; *mo,* month; *PO,* by mouth; *PB,* protein-binding; *t½,* half-life; *UK,* unknown; *wk,* week; *y,* year; >, greater than; <, less than.

associated with HF. Except for those in the potassium-sparing group, all diuretics are potassium-wasting.

Combination diuretics that contain both potassium-wasting and potassium-sparing drugs have been marketed primarily for the treatment of hypertension. Combinations have an additive effect in reducing blood pressure and are discussed in more detail in the Potassium-Sparing Diuretics section later in this chapter. Chapter 44 takes a closer look at the combinations of antihypertensive agents with hydrochlorothiazide (HCTZ).

THIAZIDES AND THIAZIDE-LIKE DIURETICS

The first thiazide, chlorothiazide (Diuril), was marketed in 1957 and followed a year later by hydrochlorothiazide. There are numerous thiazide and thiazide-like preparations. Thiazides act on the distal convoluted renal tubule, beyond the loop of Henle, to promote sodium, chloride, and water excretion. Thiazides are used to treat hypertension and peripheral edema. They are not effective for immediate diuresis and should not be used to promote fluid loss in patients with severe renal dysfunction. Table 43-1 lists thiazide and thiazide-like diuretics and their dosages, uses, and considerations. Drug dosages for hypertension and edema are similar.

Thiazide diuretics are used primarily for patients with normal renal function. If the patient has a renal disorder and creatinine clearance is less than 30 mL/min, the effectiveness of the thiazide diuretic is greatly decreased. Thiazides cause a loss of sodium, potassium, and magnesium, but they promote calcium reabsorption. **Hypercalcemia** (calcium excess) may result, and the condition can be hazardous to the patient who is digitalized or has cancer that causes hypercalcemia. Thiazides affect glucose tolerance, so hyperglycemia can also occur. Thiazides should be used cautiously in patients with diabetes mellitus. Laboratory test results (e.g., electrolytes, glucose) need to be monitored.

The thiazide drug hydrochlorothiazide has been combined with selected angiotensin-converting enzyme (ACE) inhibitors, beta-blockers, alpha-blockers, angiotensin II blockers, and centrally acting sympatholytics to control hypertension. Prototype Drug Chart 43-1 outlines the pharmacologic data for hydrochlorothiazide.

Pharmacokinetics Thiazides are well absorbed from the gastrointestinal (GI) tract. Hydrochlorothiazide has moderate protein-binding power. The half-life of the thiazide drugs is longer than that of the loop diuretics. For this reason, thiazides should be administered in the morning to avoid nocturia (nighttime urination) and sleep interruption.

Pharmacodynamics Thiazides act directly on arterioles to cause vasodilation, which can lower blood pressure. Other action includes the promotion of sodium chloride and water excretion, resulting in a decrease in vascular fluid volume and a concomitant decrease in cardiac output and blood pressure. The onset of action of hydrochlorothiazide occurs within 2 hours. Peak concentration times are long (3 to 6 hours). Thiazides are divided into three groups, according to their duration of action: short-acting (duration less than 12 hours), intermediate-acting (duration 12 to 24 hours), and long-acting (duration more than 24 hours).

Side Effects and Adverse Reactions. Side effects and adverse reactions of thiazides include electrolyte imbalances (hypokalemia, hypercalcemia, hypomagnesemia, and bicarbonate loss), **hyperglycemia** (elevated blood sugar), **hyperuricemia** (elevated serum uric acid level), and hyperlipidemia (elevated blood lipid level). Signs and symptoms of hypokalemia should be assessed, and serum potassium levels must be closely monitored. Potassium supplements are frequently needed. Serum calcium and uric acid levels should be checked, because thiazides block calcium and uric acid excretion. Thiazides affect the metabolism of carbohydrates, and hyperglycemia can result, especially in patients with high to high-normal blood sugar levels. Thiazides can increase serum cholesterol, low-density lipoprotein, and triglyceride levels. A drug may be ordered to lower blood lipids. Other side effects include dizziness, headache, nausea, vomiting, constipation, urticaria, or hives (rare), and blood dyscrasias (rare). Table 43-2 summarizes the serum chemistry abnormalities that can occur with thiazide use.

Contraindications. Thiazides are contraindicated for use in renal failure. Symptoms of severe kidney impairment or shutdown include **oliguria** (marked decrease in urine output), elevated blood urea nitrogen (BUN), and elevated serum creatinine.

Drug Interactions. Of the numerous thiazide drug interactions, the most serious occurs with digoxin. Thiazides can

PROTOTYPE DRUG CHART 43-1

Hydrochlorothiazide

Drug Class Thiazide diuretic Trade Names: HCT, Esidrix Pregnancy Category: B	**Dosage** Hypertension: A: PO: 12.5-50 mg/d; *max:* 50 mg/d Edema: A: PO: 25-100 mg/d in single or divided doses; *max:* 200 mg/d C: PO: 1-2 mg/kg/d in divided doses C: <6 mo: PO: 1-3 mg/kg/d in divided doses
Contraindications Renal failure with anuria, electrolyte depletion Caution: Hepatic dysfunction, renal dysfunction, diabetes mellitus, gout, systemic lupus erythematosus	**Drug-Lab-Food Interactions** Drug: Increase digitalis toxicity with digitalis if hypokalemia is present; increase renal toxicity with aspirin; increase potassium loss with steroids; decrease antidiabetic effect; decrease thiazide absorption and effects with NSAIDs, cholestyramine, and colestipol Lab: Increase serum calcium, glucose, uric acid; decrease serum potassium, sodium, magnesium
Pharmacokinetics Absorption: Readily absorbed from GI tract Distribution: PB: 65% Metabolism: t½: 6-15 h Excretion: In urine	**Pharmacodynamics** PO: Onset: 2 h Peak: 4 h Duration: 6-12 h
Therapeutic Effects/Uses To increase urine output; to treat hypertension, edema from HF, hepatic cirrhosis, renal dysfunction Mode of Action: Action is on the renal distal tubules, promoting sodium, potassium, and water excretion and decreasing preload and cardiac output; also decreases edema; acts on arterioles, causing vasodilation, thus decreasing blood pressure	
Side Effects Dizziness, vertigo, weakness, nausea, vomiting, diarrhea, abdominal pain, hyperglycemia, constipation, rash, photosensitivity, blurred vision	**Adverse Reactions** Severe dehydration, hypotension, gout Life-threatening: Severe potassium depletion, marked hypotension, aplastic anemia, hemolytic anemia, thrombocytopenia, agranulocytosis, renal failure

A, Adult; *C,* child; *d,* day; *GI,* gastrointestinal; *h,* hour; *HF,* heart failure; *maint,* maintenance; *mo,* month; *PB,* protein-binding; *PO,* by mouth; *t½,* half-life.

TABLE 43-2 SERUM CHEMISTRY ABNORMALITIES ASSOCIATED WITH THIAZIDES

SERUM CHEMISTRY PARAMETER	ABNORMAL RESULTS
Electrolytes, Normal Levels	
Potassium, 3.5-5.3 mEq/L	Hypokalemia (low serum potassium). Potassium is excreted from the distal renal tubule.
Magnesium, 1.8-3.0 mg/dL	Hypomagnesemia (low serum magnesium). Potassium and sodium loss prompt magnesium loss.
Calcium, 4.5-5.5 mEq/L	Hypercalcemia (elevated serum calcium). Thiazides may block calcium excretion.
Chloride, 95-105 mEq/L	Hypochloremia (low serum chloride). Sodium and potassium losses produce chloride loss.
Bicarbonate, 24-28 mEq/L	Minimal bicarbonate loss from proximal tubule.
Uric acid, 2.8-8.0 mg/dL	Hyperuricemia (elevated uric acid). Thiazides can block uric acid excretion.
Blood sugar, 70-110 mg/dL	Hyperglycemia (increased blood sugar). Thiazides increase fasting blood sugar levels and those of prediabetic state.
Blood Lipids	
Cholesterol: <200 mg/dL LDL: <100 mg/dL Triglyceride: 10-190 mg/dL	Can elevate cholesterol, LDLs, and triglycerides.

LDL, Low-density lipoprotein.

cause **hypokalemia,** which enhances the action of digoxin, and digitalis toxicity can occur. Potassium supplements are frequently prescribed, and serum potassium levels are monitored. Thiazides also induce hypercalcemia, which enhances the action of digoxin, resulting in possible digitalis toxicity. Signs and symptoms of digitalis toxicity (bradycardia, nausea, vomiting, visual changes) should be reported. Thiazides enhance the action of lithium, and lithium toxicity can occur. Thiazides potentiate the action of other antihypertensive drugs, which may be used to advantage in combination drug therapy for hypertension.

LOOP (HIGH CEILING) DIURETICS

The loop, or high-ceiling, diuretics act on the thick ascending loop of Henle to inhibit chloride transport of sodium into the circulation (inhibit passive reabsorption of sodium). Sodium and water are lost, together with potassium, calcium, and magnesium. Loop diuretics can affect blood sugar and increase uric acid levels. Drugs in this group are extremely potent and cause marked depletion of water and electrolytes. This high diuretic potential is the reason they are often called *high-ceiling diuretics* or *potassium-wasting diuretics.* The effects of loop diuretics are dose-related (i.e., increasing the dose increases the effect and response of the drug). More potent than thiazides for promoting diuresis (inhibiting reabsorption of sodium two to three times more effectively), loop diuretics are less effective as antihypertensive agents.

Loop diuretics should not be prescribed if a thiazide could alleviate body fluid excess. If furosemide (Lasix) alone is not effective in removing body fluid, a thiazide may be added, but furosemide should never be combined with another loop diuretic. Furosemide is usually administered as an oral dose in the morning or intravenously when the patient's condition warrants immediate removal of body fluid, for example, in cases of acute heart failure or pulmonary edema.

Nursing Process
Patient-Centered Collaborative Care

Diuretics: Thiazides

Assessment
- Assess vital signs, weight, urine output, and serum chemistry values (electrolytes, glucose, uric acid) for baseline levels.
- Check peripheral extremities for presence of edema. Note pitting edema.
- Obtain a history of drugs and herbal supplements taken daily. Review for drugs and herbals that may cause drug interaction (digoxin, corticosteroids, antidiabetics, ginkgo, licorice).

Nursing Diagnoses
- Risk for deficient fluid volume related to use or overuse of thiazides
- Impaired urinary elimination related to kidney dysfunction
- Excess fluid volume related to body fluid retention

Planning
- Patient's blood pressure will be decreased and/or return to normal value.
- Patient's edema will be decreased.
- Patient's serum chemistry levels will remain within normal ranges.

Nursing Interventions
- Monitor vital signs and serum electrolytes, especially potassium, glucose, uric acid, and cholesterol levels. Report changes. If patient is taking digoxin and hypokalemia occurs, digitalis toxicity frequently results.
- Observe for signs and symptoms of hypokalemia (e.g., muscle weakness, leg cramps, cardiac dysrhythmias).
- Monitor patient's weight daily. Weight gain of 2.2 lb is equivalent to 1 L of body fluids.
- Note urine output to determine fluid loss or retention.

Patient Teaching

General

- Emphasize the need for adherence. Patient may not "feel better" for some time or may not "feel worse" if treatment is missed or discontinued.
- Suggest that patient take hydrochlorothiazide in early morning to avoid sleep disturbance resulting from nocturia.
- Instruct patient to keep drugs out of reach of small children. Request childproof bottle.
- Inform patient that certain herbal products may interact with thiazide diuretics (Herbal Alert 43-1).

Self-Administration

- Instruct patient or family member on how to take blood pressure and record daily results.

Side Effects

- Instruct patient to slowly change positions from lying to standing, because dizziness may occur as a result of orthostatic (postural) hypotension.
- Advise patient who may be prediabetic to have blood sugar checked periodically, because large doses of hydrochlorothiazide increase blood glucose levels.
- Suggest that patient use sunblock when in direct sunlight for photosensitivity

Diet

- Teach patient to eat foods rich in potassium (fruits, fruit juices, and vegetables). Potassium supplements may be ordered.
- Instruct patient to take drugs with food to avoid gastrointestinal upset.

Cultural Considerations

- Respect cultural practices and values. If patient from a different background tells the health care provider that she or he does not eat fruits and vegetables, the nurse may have two options: to encourage patient to eat fruits and vegetables, or to contact health care provider so that an adequate potassium supplement can be prescribed to overcome potassium loss. An interpreter may be necessary.
- Emphasize importance of patient taking potassium supplement with potassium-wasting diuretic. In addition, advise patient of consequences and dangers of not taking potassium supplements or lacking appropriate nutrition while taking potassium-wasting diuretics. Monitor serum potassium levels.

Evaluation

- Evaluate the effectiveness of drug therapy. Patient's blood pressure and edema will be reduced, and blood chemistry will remain within normal range.
- Determine absence of side effects and adverse reactions to therapy.

HERBAL ALERT 43-1

Diuretics

- Aloe can decrease the serum potassium level, thereby causing hypokalemia, when taken with a potassium-wasting diuretic such as a thiazide.
- Gingko may increase blood pressure when taken with thiazide diuretics.
- Licorice can increase potassium loss, leading to hypokalemia.
- Hawthorne may potentiate hypotension.

Loop diuretics can increase renal blood flow up to 40%. Furosemide is a frequently prescribed diuretic for patients whose creatinine clearance is less than 30/min and for those with end-stage renal disease. This group of diuretics causes excretion of calcium, unlike thiazides, which inhibit calcium loss.

The first loop diuretic marketed was ethacrynic acid (Edecrin), followed by furosemide (Lasix) and then bumetanide (Bumex), which is more potent than furosemide on a milligram-for-milligram basis. Furosemide and bumetanide are derivatives of sulfonamides. Ethacrynic acid, a phenoxyacetic acid derivative, is a seldom-chosen loop diuretic. It is usually reserved for patients who are allergic to sulfa drugs. Prototype Drug Chart 43-2 lists the drug data for the loop diuretic furosemide.

Pharmacokinetics Loop diuretics are rapidly absorbed by the GI tract. These drugs are highly protein bound with half-lives that vary from 30 minutes to 1.5 hours. Loop diuretics compete for protein-binding sites with other highly protein-bound drugs.

Pharmacodynamics Loop diuretics have a great **saluretic** (sodium-chloride–losing) or **natriuretic** (sodium-losing) effect and can cause rapid diuresis, decreasing vascular fluid volume and causing a decrease in cardiac output and blood pressure. Because furosemide is a more potent diuretic than thiazide diuretics, it causes a vasodilatory effect; thus renal blood flow increases before diuresis. Furosemide is used when other conservative measures, such as sodium restriction and use of less potent diuretics, fail. The oral dose of furosemide is usually twice that of an intravenous (IV) dose.

The onset of action of loop diuretics occurs within 30 to 60 minutes. The onset of action for IV furosemide is 5 minutes. Duration of action is shorter than that of the thiazides.

Side Effects and Adverse Reactions. The most common side effects of loop diuretics are fluid and electrolyte imbalances such as hypokalemia, hyponatremia, hypocalcemia, hypomagnesemia, and hypochloremia. Hypochloremic metabolic alkalosis may result, which can worsen hypokalemia. Orthostatic hypotension can occur. Thrombocytopenia, skin disturbances, and transient deafness are rarely seen. Table 43-3 lists the physiologic and laboratory changes associated with loop diuretics.

Drug Interactions. The major drug interaction is with digitalis preparations. If the patient takes digoxin with a loop diuretic, digitalis toxicity can result. Hypokalemia enhances the action of digoxin and increases the risk for digitalis toxicity. The patient needs potassium replacement with food or supplements. Serum potassium levels should be closely monitored, especially when the patient is taking high dosages of

PROTOTYPE DRUG CHART 43-2

Furosemide

Drug Class	Dosage
Loop diuretic Trade Names: Lasix Pregnancy Category: C	A: PO: 20-80 mg single dose/d; may increase in 6-8 h, 20-40 mg; maint: 40-120 mg/d; *max:* 600 mg/d A: IM/IV: 20-40 mg over 1-2 min IV; repeat 20 mg in 2 h; *max:* 4 mg/min inf C: PO: 1-2 mg/kg single dose; repeat in 6-8 h *max:* 6 mg/kg/d C: IM/IV: 1-2 mg/kg single dose; repeat 1 mg/kg in 6-12 h; *max:* 6 mg/kg/d
Contraindications	**Drug-Lab-Food Interactions**
Presence of severe electrolyte imbalances, hypovolemia, anuria, hepatic coma, hypersensitivity to sulfonamides Caution: Heart failure, diabetes mellitus, hypotension, systemic lupus erythematosus, gout, patients with hearing impairment	Drug: Increase orthostatic hypotension with alcohol; increase ototoxicity with aminoglycosides; increase bleeding with anticoagulants; increase potassium loss with steroids, Amphotericin B, amiodarone; increase digitalis toxicity and cardiac dysrhythmias with digoxin and hypokalemia; increase lithium toxicity; increase amphotericin B ototoxicity and nephrotoxicity Food: licorice may increase potassium loss Lab: Increase BUN, blood/urine glucose, serum uric acid, ammonia; decrease potassium, sodium, calcium, magnesium, chloride serum levels Herbs: Hawthorn may potentiate hypotension, Ginseng may decrease action of loop diuretics
Pharmacokinetics	**Pharmacodynamics**
Absorption: PO: Readily absorbed from GI tract Distribution: PB: 95% Metabolism: t½: 30-60 min Excretion: In urine, some in feces; crosses placenta	PO: Onset: less than 60 min Peak: 1-4 h Duration: UK IV: Onset: 5 min Peak: 20-30 min Duration: 2 h
Therapeutic Effects/Uses	
To treat fluid retention/fluid overload caused by HF, renal dysfunction, cirrhosis; hypertension; acute pulmonary edema Mode of Action: Inhibition of sodium and water reabsorption from loop of Henle and distal renal tubules; potassium, magnesium, and calcium also may be excreted	
Side Effects	**Adverse Reactions**
Nausea, diarrhea, electrolyte imbalances, vertigo, abdominal cramping, constipation, rash, headache, weakness, ECG changes, blurred vision, photosensitivity, muscle cramping	Severe dehydration; marked hypotension, hyperglycemia, gout, hearing loss Life-threatening: Renal failure, thrombocytopenia, agranulocytosis

A, Adult; *BUN,* blood urea nitrogen; *C,* child; *d,* day; *ECG,* electrocardiogram; *GI,* gastrointestinal; *h,* hour; *HF,* heart failure; *IM,* intramuscular; *inf,* infusion; *IV,* intravenous; *max,* maximum; *min,* minute; *PB,* protein-binding; *PO,* by mouth; *t ½,* half-life.

loop diuretics. Table 43-4 lists the data for the four loop diuretics.

OSMOTIC DIURETICS

Osmotic diuretics increase the **osmolality** (concentration) and sodium reabsorption in the proximal tubule and loop of Henle. Sodium, chloride, potassium (to a lesser degree), and water are excreted. This group of drugs is used to prevent kidney failure, to decrease intracranial pressure (ICP) (e.g., in cerebral edema), and to decrease intraocular pressure (IOP) (e.g., in glaucoma). Mannitol is a potent osmotic potassium-wasting diuretic frequently used in emergency situations such as ICP and IOP. In addition, mannitol can be used with cisplatin and carboplatin in cancer chemotherapy to induce a frank diuresis and decreased side effects of treatment.

Mannitol is the most frequently prescribed osmotic diuretic, followed by urea. Diuresis occurs within 1 to 3 hours after IV administration. Table 43-4 describes Mannitol.

Side Effects and Adverse Reactions. The side effects and adverse reactions of mannitol include fluid and electrolyte imbalance, pulmonary edema from rapid shift of fluids, nausea, vomiting, tachycardia from rapid fluid loss, and acidosis. Crystallization of mannitol in the vial may occur when the drug is exposed to a low temperature. The vial should be warmed to dissolve the crystals. The mannitol solution should not be used for IV infusion if crystals are present and have not been dissolved.

TABLE 43-3 PHYSIOLOGIC AND LABORATORY CHANGES ASSOCIATED WITH LOOP DIURETICS

PHYSIOLOGIC/LABORATORY CHANGES	POSSIBLE EFFECTS OF LOOP (HIGH-CEILING) DIURETICS
Physiologic Changes	
Hypotension	Postural (orthostatic) hypotension can result because of ECFV deficit.
Ototoxicity	Hearing impairment, although rare, may occur. It is more common with use of ethacrynic acid. Diuretics in other categories are not considered ototoxic. Caution: Avoid taking a loop diuretic with a drug that can be ototoxic, such as an aminoglycoside.
Skin disturbances	Pruritus, urticaria, exfoliative dermatitis, and purpura may occur in some persons allergic to the drug or when taking the loop diuretic in high doses over a long period.
Photosensitivity	When exposed to sun or sunlamp for a prolonged time, severe sunburn could result. Patient should use sunblock and avoid long sun exposure.
Hypovolemia	Excess extracellular fluid is lost through increased urine excretion.
Laboratory Changes	
Hypokalemia, hypomagnesemia, hyponatremia, hypocalcemia, hypochloremia	Potassium, magnesium, sodium, calcium, and chloride are lost from the body from increased urine excretion. Chloride, an anion, is attached to the cations potassium and sodium; thus, chloride is lost along with potassium and sodium.
Hyperglycemia	Increased glycogenolysis may contribute to elevated blood sugar level. Patients with diabetes should closely monitor blood glucose levels when taking a loop diuretic.
Hyperuricemia	Elevated uric acid levels are common in patients susceptible to gout.
Elevated BUN and creatinine	These elevations may result from ECFV loss. Hemoconcentration can cause elevated BUN and creatinine levels, which are reversible when fluid volume returns to normal levels.
Thrombocytopenia, leukopenia	Decreases in platelet and white blood cell counts are rare, but they should be closely monitored.
Elevated lipids	Loop diuretics can decrease high-density lipoproteins (HDL) and increase low-density lipoproteins (LDL). Patients with elevated cholesterol levels should have their HDL and LDL levels checked. Regardless of the lipid effects, loop diuretics are useful for patients with serious fluid retention caused by a cardiac condition such as HF.

BUN, Blood urea nitrogen; *ECFV,* extracellular fluid volume; *HF,* heart failure.

Contraindications. Mannitol must be given with extreme caution to patients who have heart disease and HF. It should be immediately discontinued if the patient develops HF or renal failure.

Nursing Process
Patient-Centered Collaborative Care

Diuretics: Loop

Assessment

- Obtain a history of drugs that are taken daily. Note if patient is taking a drug that may interact with loop diuretic (e.g., alcohol, aminoglycosides, anticoagulants, corticosteroids, lithium, amphotericin B, digitalis). Recognize that furosemide is highly protein-bound and can displace other protein-bound drugs such as warfarin (Coumadin).
- Assess vital signs, serum electrolytes, weight, and urine output for baseline levels.
- Compare patient's drug dose with recommended dose, and report discrepancy.
- Note whether patient is hypersensitive to sulfonamides.

Nursing Diagnoses

- Risk for deficient fluid volume related to fluid loss with excessive use of loop diuretics
- Risk for electrolyte imbalance (potassium deficit related to excessive use of loop diuretics)

Planning

- Patient's edema and/or hypertension will be decreased.
- Patient's serum chemistry levels will remain within normal ranges.

Nursing Interventions

- Monitor urinary output to determine body fluid gain or loss. Urinary output should be at least 30 mL/h or 600 mL/24 h.
- Notify health care provider if urine output does not increase. Severe renal disorder may be present.
- Weigh patient to determine fluid loss or gain. A loss of 2.2 lb is equivalent to a fluid loss of 1 L.
- Monitor vital signs. Be alert for marked decrease in blood pressure.

TABLE 43-4 DIURETICS: LOOP, OSMOTICS, AND CARBONIC ANHYDRASE INHIBITORS

GENERIC (BRAND)	ROUTE AND DOSAGE	USES AND CONSIDERATIONS
Loop		
bumetanide	A: PO: 0.5-2.0 mg/d; *max:* 10 mg/d IV: 0.5-1 mg/dose slowly over 1 min; repeat in 2-4 h	Treatment of renal disease and hypertension and edema associated with HF. Similar effects as furosemide. Pregnancy category: C; PB: 96%; t½: 1-1.5 h
ethacrynic acid (Edecrin)	A: PO: 50-100 mg/d or b.i.d.; *max:* 400 mg/d C: PO: 1 mg/kg/d; *max:* 3 mg/kg/d A: IV: 0.5-1 mg/kg/dose or 50-100 mg/d C: IV: 1 mg/kg once daily	For severe edema (pulmonary and peripheral). Potent diuretic with rapid action. Also used for hypercalcemia. Moderate to high doses may cause ototoxicity. Pregnancy category: B; PB: 95%; t½: 1-1.5 h
furosemide (Lasix)	See Prototype Drug Chart 43-2.	
torsemide (Demadex)	Hypertension: A: PO: Initially: 5 mg/d; maint: PO: 5-10 mg/d; HF: A: PO/IV: 10-20 mg/d; *max:* 200 mg/d	Similar to furosemide. Pregnancy category: B; PB: 97%-99%; t½: 2-4 h
Osmotics		
mannitol	ICP/IOP: A: IV: Initially 1-2 g/kg followed by 0.25-1 g/kg; 15%-25% sol infused over 30-90 min Edema, ascites, or oliguria: A: IV: 50-100 g; 10%-20% sol infused over 90 min–6 h	For oliguria and decreasing ICP. To prevent acute renal failure. Used in narrow-angle glaucoma for reducing IOP. Patient should have effective renal function. Potent diuretic. Pregnancy category: C; PB: UK; t½: 15 min–1.5 h
Carbonic Anhydrase Inhibitors		
acetazolamide (Diamox)	Glaucoma: A: PO/IV: 250 mg once daily/q.i.d.; *max:* 1 g/d A: IV: 500 mg, may repeat in 2-4 h; *max:* 1 g/d A: SR: 500 mg q12h; *max:* 1000 mg/d Edema: A: PO: IV: 250-375 mg in morning	For edema, treating absence (petit mal) seizures, and open-angle glaucoma. May cause hyperglycemia, hyperuricemia, and hypercalcemia. Metabolic acidosis can result. Pregnancy category: C; PB: 90%; t½: 10-15 h
methazolamide (Neptazane)	A: PO: 50-100 mg b.i.d./t.i.d.; *max:* 300 mg/d	Similar to dichlorphenamide. Pregnancy category: C; PB: 50%-60%; t½: 14 h

A, Adult; *b.i.d.,* twice a day; *C,* child; *d,* day; *h,* hour; *HF,* heart failure; *ICP,* intracranial pressure; *inf,* infusion; *IOP,* intraocular pressure; *IV,* intravenous; *maint,* maintenance dose; *max,* maximum; *min,* minute; *PB,* protein-binding; *PO,* by mouth; *sol,* solution; *SR,* sustained-release; *t½,* half-life; *t.i.d.,* three times a day; *UK,* unknown; *y,* year; >, greater than.

- Administer IV furosemide slowly; hearing loss may occur if rapidly injected.
- Observe for signs and symptoms of hypokalemia (less than 3.5 mEq/L), such as muscle weakness, abdominal distention, leg cramps, and/or cardiac dysrhythmias.
- Monitor serum potassium levels, especially when patient is taking digoxin. Hypokalemia enhances action of digitalis, causing digitalis toxicity.

Patient Teaching

General

- Advise patient to take furosemide in morning and *not* in evening to prevent sleep disturbance and nocturia.

Side Effects

- Teach patient to rise slowly from lying or sitting to standing to prevent dizziness resulting from fluid loss.

Diet

- Suggest taking furosemide with food to avoid nausea.

Cultural Considerations

- Respect cultural practices and values. If patient from a different background tells health care provider that she or he does not eat fruits and vegetables, the nurse may have two options: to encourage patient to eat fruits and vegetables or to contact health care provider so that an adequate potassium supplement can be prescribed to overcome potassium loss. An interpreter may be necessary.
- Emphasize the importance of patient taking potassium supplement with potassium-wasting diuretic. In addition, advise patient of consequences and dangers of not taking potassium supplements or lacking appropriate nutrition while taking potassium-wasting diuretics.

Evaluation

- Evaluate effectiveness of drug action, such as decreased fluid retention or fluid overload, decreased respiratory distress, and increased cardiac output.
- Check for side effects and increased urine output.

CARBONIC ANHYDRASE INHIBITORS

The carbonic anhydrase inhibitors acetazolamide, dichlorphenamide, ethoxzolamide, and methazolamide block the action of the enzyme *carbonic anhydrase,* which is needed to maintain the body's acid-base balance (hydrogen and bicarbonate ion balance). Inhibition of this enzyme causes increased sodium, potassium, and bicarbonate excretion. With prolonged use, metabolic acidosis can occur.

This group of drugs is used primarily to decrease IOP in patients with open-angle (chronic) glaucoma. These drugs are not used in narrow-angle or acute glaucoma. Other uses include diuresis, management of epilepsy, and treatment of high-altitude or acute mountain sickness. Table 43-4 presents the drug data for carbonic anhydrase inhibitor diuretics. The drug may also be used for a patient in metabolic alkalosis who needs a diuretic. Carbonic anhydrase inhibitors may be alternated with a loop diuretic.

Side Effects and Adverse Reactions. Acetazolamide can cause fluid and electrolyte imbalance, metabolic acidosis, nausea, vomiting, anorexia, confusion, orthostatic hypotension, and crystalluria. Hemolytic anemia and renal calculi can also occur. These drugs are contraindicated during the first trimester of pregnancy.

POTASSIUM-SPARING DIURETICS

Potassium-sparing diuretics, which are weaker than thiazides and loop diuretics, are used as mild diuretics or in combination with another diuretic (e.g., hydrochlorothiazide, antihypertensive drugs). Continuous use of potassium-wasting diuretics requires a daily oral potassium supplement, because the kidneys excrete potassium, sodium, and body water. However, potassium supplements are *not* used when the patient takes a potassium-sparing diuretic; in fact, serum potassium excess, called **hyperkalemia,** results when a potassium supplement is taken with a potassium-sparing diuretic. The serum potassium should be periodically monitored when the patient continuously takes a potassium-sparing diuretic. If the serum potassium level is greater than 5.3 mEq/L, the patient should discontinue the potassium-sparing diuretic and restrict foods high in potassium.

Potassium-sparing diuretics act primarily in the collecting duct renal tubules and late distal tubule to promote sodium and water excretion and potassium retention. The drugs interfere with the sodium-potassium pump controlled by the mineralocorticoid hormone aldosterone (sodium retained and potassium excreted).

Spironolactone (Aldactone), an aldosterone antagonist discovered in 1958, was the first potassium-sparing diuretic. Aldosterone is a mineralocorticoid hormone that promotes sodium retention and potassium excretion. Spironolactone blocks the action of aldosterone and inhibits the sodium-potassium pump (i.e., potassium is retained and sodium is excreted). Spironolactone (Aldactone) has been prescribed by cardiologists for patients with cardiac disorders because of its potassium-retaining effect. As a result of the action of spironolactone, the heart rate is more regular, and the possibility of myocardial fibrosis is decreased. The effects of spironolactone may take 48 hours.

Amiloride (Midamor), triamterene (Dyrenium), and eplerenone (Inspra) are additional commonly prescribed potassium-sparing diuretics. Amiloride and eplerenone are effective as antihypertensive agents. Triamterene is useful in the treatment of edema caused by HF or cirrhosis of the liver. Low doses of spironolactone (Aldactone) and eplerenone are effective for chronic HF. Spironolactone, amiloride, triamterene, and eplerenone should not be taken with ACE inhibitors and angiotensin II receptor blockers (ARBs) because they can also increase serum potassium levels. Prototype Drug Chart 43-3 provides the pharmacologic data for spironolactone.

When potassium-sparing diuretics are used alone, they are less effective than when used in combination to reduce body fluid and sodium. These drugs are usually combined with a potassium-wasting diuretic, primarily hydrochlorothiazide or a loop diuretic. The combination of potassium-sparing and potassium-wasting diuretics intensifies the diuretic effect and prevents potassium loss. The common combination diuretics contain spironolactone and hydrochlorothiazide (Aldactazide), amiloride and hydrochlorothiazide (HCTZ), and triamterene and hydrochlorothiazide (Dyazide, Maxzide). Table 43-5 lists the potassium-sparing diuretics and the combination potassium-wasting and potassium-sparing diuretics.

Side Effects and Adverse Reactions. The main side effect of these drugs is hyperkalemia. Caution must be used when giving potassium-sparing diuretics to a patient with poor renal function, because the kidneys excrete 80% to 90% of potassium. Urine output should be at least 600 mL/day. Patients should *not* use potassium supplements while taking potassium-sparing diuretics, unless the serum potassium level is low. If a potassium-sparing diuretic is given with antihypertensive ACE inhibitors, hyperkalemia could become severe or life threatening, because both drugs retain potassium. Monitoring serum potassium levels is essential to safe drug therapy. GI disturbances (anorexia, nausea, vomiting, diarrhea, and numbness and tingling of the hands and feet) can occur.

Nursing Process
Patient-Centered Collaborative Care

Diuretics: Potassium-Sparing

Assessment

- Obtain a history of drugs taken daily. Note whether patient is taking a potassium supplement or using a salt substitute.
- Assess vital signs, serum electrolytes, weight, and urinary output for baseline levels.

PROTOTYPE DRUG CHART 43-3

Spironolactone

Drug Class Potassium-sparing diuretic Trade Name: Aldactone Pregnancy Category: C	**Dosage** Edema: A: PO: 25-200 mg/d in divided doses; *max:* 400 mg/d C: PO: 1.5-3.3 mg/kg/d in divided doses; *max:* 3.3 mg/kg/d Hypertension: A: PO: 50-100 mg/d; *max:* 400 mg/d
Contraindications Severe kidney or hepatic disease, anuria, severe hyperkalemia Caution: Renal or hepatic dysfunction, diabetes mellitus	**Drug-Lab-Food Interactions** Drug: Increase serum potassium level with potassium supplements; increase effects of antihypertensives and lithium; life threatening: hyperkalemia if given with ACE inhibitor Lab: Increase serum potassium level; may increase BUN, AST, alkaline phosphatase levels; decrease serum sodium, chloride
Pharmacokinetics Absorption: PO: Rapidly absorbed from GI tract Distribution: PB: 90% Metabolism: t½: 1.5-2 h Excretion: In urine, mostly as metabolites and bile	**Pharmacodynamics** PO: Onset: UK Peak: 2-3 d Duration: 2-3 days or longer
Therapeutic Effects/Uses To increase urine output; to treat fluid retention/overload associated with HF, hepatic cirrhosis, or nephrotic syndrome Mode of Action: Acts on distal renal tubules to promote sodium and water excretion and potassium retention	
Side Effects Nausea, vomiting, diarrhea, rash, dizziness, headache, weakness, dry mouth, photosensitivity	**Adverse Reactions** Life-threatening: Severe hyperkalemia, thrombocytopenia, megaloblastic anemia

A, Adult; *ACE,* angiotensin-converting enzyme; *AST,* aspartate aminotransferase; *BUN,* blood urea nitrogen; *C,* child; *d,* day; *GI,* gastrointestinal; *h,* hour; *HF,* heart failure; *PB,* protein-binding; *p.c.,* after meals; *PO,* by mouth; *t½,* half-life.

TABLE 43-5 DIURETICS: POTASSIUM-SPARING

GENERIC (BRAND)	ROUTE AND DOSAGE	USES AND CONSIDERATIONS
Single Agents		
amiloride HCl (Midamor)	A: PO: 5-10 mg/d; *max:* 20 mg/d	For diuretic-induced hypokalemia; used for hypertension, HF, and cirrhosis of the liver. Monitor serum potassium level to detect hyperkalemia. Pregnancy category: B; PB: 40%; t½: 6-9 h
eplerenone (Inspra)	A: PO: 25-50 mg/d; *max:* 100 mg/d for hypertension; 50 mg/d for HF	For hypertension or chronic HF post MI. Approved in 2002. Also classified as a selective aldosterone receptor blocker. Serum potassium should be monitored to detect hyperkalemia. Pregnancy category: B ; PB: 50%; t½: 4-6 h
spironolactone (Aldactone)	See Prototype Drug Chart 43-3.	
triamterene (Dyrenium)	A: PO: Initially 50-100 mg b.i.d.; *max:* 300 mg/d	For edema and hypokalemia. May increase excretion of magnesium. May cause severe hyperkalemia with resultant life-threatening cardiac dysrhythmias. Pregnancy category: C; PB: 67%; t½: 1-2 h
Combinations		
amiloride HCl and hydrochlorothiazide (Moduretic)	A: PO: 1-2 tab (amiloride 5 mg/ hydrochlorothiazide 50 mg)	Combinations contain potassium-wasting and potassium-sparing diuretics. Drugs are to control hypertension and edema. They are used to prevent the occurrence of hypokalemia.
spironolactone and hydrochlorothiazide (Aldactazide)	A: PO: 1 tab (25 mg spironolactone/25 mg HCTZ); *max:* 200 mg/d of each	Same as Moduretic
triamterene and hydrochlorothiazide (Dyazide, Maxzide)	A: PO: 1-2 cap p.c. (triamterene 37.5 mg/ hydrochlorothiazide 25 mg)	Same as Moduretic

A, Adult; *b.i.d.,* twice a day; *C,* child; *cap,* capsule; *d,* day; *h,* hour; *HF,* heart failure; *MI,* myocardial infarction; *PB,* protein-binding; *p.c.,* after meals; *PO,* by mouth; *t½,* half-life; *tab,* tablet; *UK,* unknown.

- Compare patient's drug dose with recommended dose, and report any discrepancy.

Nursing Diagnoses

- Risk for deficient fluid volume related to fluid loss with excessive use of potassium-sparing diuretic
- Risk for electrolyte imbalance (potassium excess related to excessive use of potassium-sparing diuretic)

Planning

- Patient's fluid retention and blood pressure will be decreased.
- Patient's serum electrolytes will remain within normal ranges.

Nursing Interventions

- Note the half-life of spironolactone. With a long half-life, drug dose is usually administered once a day, sometimes twice a day.
- Monitor urinary output. Urine output should increase. Report if urine output is <30 mL/h or <600 mL/day.
- Record vital signs. Report abnormal changes.
- Observe for signs and symptoms of hyperkalemia (serum potassium >5.3 mEq/L). Nausea, diarrhea, abdominal cramps, numbness and tingling of the hands and feet, leg cramps, tachycardia and later bradycardia, peaked narrow T wave on electrocardiogram, or oliguria may signal hyperkalemia.
- Administer spironolactone in the morning and not in the evening to avoid nocturia.

Patient Teaching

General

- Teach patient to take spironolactone with or after meals to avoid nausea.
- Encourage patient not to discontinue drug without consulting health care provider.

Side Effects

- Caution patient to avoid exposure to direct sunlight, because drug can cause photosensitivity.
- Advise patient to report possible side effects of drug (e.g., rash, dizziness, weakness, GI upset).

Diet

- Advise patients with high serum potassium levels to avoid foods rich in potassium when taking potassium-sparing diuretics.

Evaluation

- Evaluate effectiveness of potassium-sparing diuretic (e.g., triamterene). Fluid retention (edema) should be decreased or absent.
- Determine whether urine output has increased and serum potassium level is within normal range.

KEY WEBSITES

Information on hydrochlorothiazide: *www.nlm.nih.gov/medlineplus/druginfo/meds/a682571.html*

Information on spironolactone: *drugs.com/spironolactone.html*

CRITICAL THINKING CASE STUDY

JQ, a 58-year-old patient, has been recently diagnosed with hypertension. His resting blood pressure is 158/92. He is prescribed hydrochlorothiazide 50 mg/day and told to eat foods rich in potassium.

1. How does hydrochlorothiazide differ from furosemide (Lasix)? What are their similarities and differences?
2. Why is it necessary for JQ to eat foods rich in potassium when taking hydrochlorothiazide? Explain your answer.
3. What are the nursing interventions that should be considered while JQ takes hydrochlorothiazide?

   After 1 month on hydrochlorothiazide therapy, JQ becomes weak and complains of nausea and vomiting. His muscles are "soft." His serum potassium level is 3.3 mEq/L. JQ's diuretic is changed to triamterene/hydrochlorothiazide (Dyazide). Again, he is advised to eat foods rich in potassium.
4. Explain the rationale for changing JQ's diuretic.
5. Should JQ receive a potassium supplement? Explain your answer.
6. What nursing interventions should the nurse follow for JQ?
7. What care plan should the nurse develop for JQ in relation to patient teaching?
8. What medical follow-up care is needed for JQ?

NCLEX STUDY QUESTIONS

1. A patient is taking hydrochlorothiazide (HCTZ) 50 mg/day and digoxin (Lanoxin) 0.25 mg/day. The nurse plans to monitor the patient for which potential electrolyte imbalance?
   a. Hypocalcemia
   b. Hypokalemia
   c. Hyperkalemia
   d. Hypermagnesemia
2. The nurse knows that which statement is correct regarding nursing care of a patient receiving hydrochlorothiazide (HCTZ)? (Select all that apply.)
   a. Monitor patient for signs of hypoglycemia.
   b. Administer ordered potassium supplements.
   c. Monitor serum potassium and uric acid levels.
   d. Assess blood pressure before administration.
   e. Notify health care provider if patient has had oliguria for 24 hours.
   f. Assess for decreased cholesterol and triglyceride levels.
3. A patient has heart failure, and a high dose of furosemide (Lasix) is ordered. What suggests a favorable response to Lasix?
   a. Decrease in level of consciousness and sleeping more
   b. Respiratory rate decreases from 28/min to 20/min and the depth increases.
   c. Increased congestion heard in breath sounds and complains of shortness of breath
   d. Urine output of 50 mL/4 h and intake of 200 mL
4. What does the nurse know to be correct concerning the use of mannitol (Osmitrol) in patients?
   a. Decreases intracranial pressure
   b. Increases intraocular pressure
   c. Causes sodium and potassium retention
   d. Causes diuresis in several days
5. What should the nurse do when a patient is taking furosemide (Lasix)?
   a. Instruct patient to change positions quickly when getting out of bed.
   b. Assess blood pressure before administration.
   c. Administer at bedtime for maximum effectiveness
   d. Teach to avoid fruits to prevent hyperkalemia.
6. For the patient taking a diuretic, a combination such as triamterene and hydrochlorothiazide may be prescribed. The nurse realizes that this combination is ordered for which purpose?
   a. To decrease serum potassium level
   b. To increase serum potassium level
   c. To decrease glucose level
   d. To increase glucose level
7. The patient has been receiving spironolactone (Aldactone) 50 mg/day for heart failure. The nurse should closely monitor the patient for which condition?
   a. Hypokalemia
   b. Hyperkalemia
   c. Hypoglycemia
   d. Hypermagnesemia

Answers: 1, b; 2, b, c, d, e; 3, b; 4, a; 5, b; 6, b; 7, b.

CHAPTER

44

Antihypertensives

evolve WEBSITE

http://evolve.elsevier.com/KeeHayes/pharmacology/

- Animations
- Content Updates
- Key Points
- Review Questions for the NCLEX® Examination
- References from the Textbook
- Unfolding Case Studies

OBJECTIVES

- Differentiate the pharmacologic action of the various categories of antihypertensive drugs.
- Compare the side effects and adverse reactions to sympatholytics, direct-acting vasodilators, and angiotensin antagonists.
- Apply the nursing process related to antihypertensives including nursing interventions and teaching.
- Describe the blood pressure guidelines for determining hypertension.

OUTLINE

KEY TERMS

antihypertensive, p. 635
essential hypertension, p. 633
hypertension, p. 633
secondary hypertension, p. 633
sympatholytics, p. 635

HYPERTENSION

Hypertension is an increase in blood pressure such that the systolic pressure is greater than 140 mm Hg and the diastolic pressure is greater than 90 mm Hg. **Essential hypertension** is the most common type, affecting 90% of persons with high blood pressure. The exact origin of essential hypertension is unknown; however, contributing factors may include family history of hypertension, hyperlipidemia, African-American background, diabetes, aging, stress, excessive alcohol ingestion, smoking, and obesity. Ten percent of hypertension cases are related to renal and endocrine disorders and are classified as **secondary hypertension**.

Selected Regulators of Blood Pressure

The kidneys and blood vessels strive to regulate and maintain a "normal" blood pressure. The kidneys regulate blood pressure by control of fluid volume and the renin-angiotensin-aldosterone system. Kidneys control sodium and water elimination/retention, which affects cardiac output and systemic arterial blood pressure. Figure 44-1 illustrates the renin-angiotensin-aldosterone system (RAAS). Renin (from the renal cells) stimulates production of angiotensin II (a potent vasoconstrictor), which causes the release of aldosterone (adrenal hormone that promotes sodium retention and thereby water retention). Retention of sodium and water causes fluid volume to increase, elevating blood pressure.

The baroreceptors in the aorta and carotid sinus and the vasomotor center in the medulla also assist in the regulation of blood pressure. Catecholamines such as norepinephrine, released from the sympathetic nerve terminals, and epinephrine, released from the adrenal medulla, increase blood pressure through vasoconstriction activity.

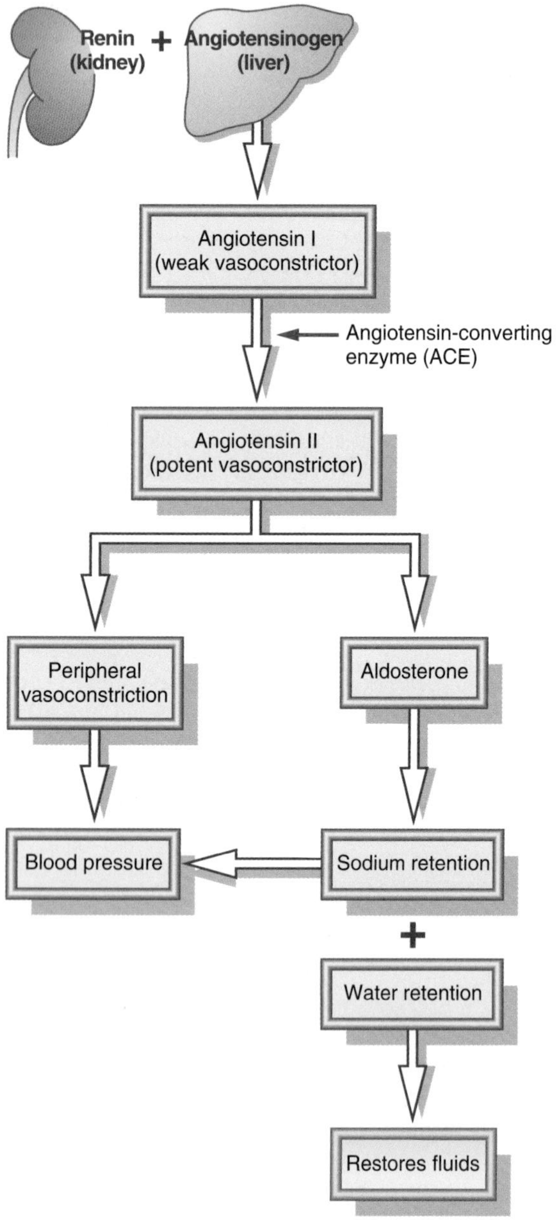

FIGURE 44–1 The renin-angiotensin-aldosterone system (RAAS). Renin, an enzyme located in the juxtaglomerular cells of the kidney, is released when blood pressure decreases. This diagram shows how the RAAS restores fluid balance and stabilizes blood pressure.

Other hormones that contribute to blood pressure regulation are antidiuretic hormone (ADH), atrial natriuretic peptide (ANP) hormone, and brain natriuretic peptide (BNP) hormone. ADH is produced by the hypothalamus and is stored and released by the posterior pituitary gland (neurohypophysis). This hormone stimulates the kidneys to conserve and retain water when there is a fluid volume deficit. When there is fluid overload, ADH secretion is inhibited, and the kidneys then excrete more water.

Physiologic Risk Factors

Certain physiologic risk factors contribute to hypertension. A diet high in saturated fat and simple carbohydrates can increase blood pressure. Carbohydrate intake can affect sympathetic nervous activity. Alcohol increases renin secretions, causing the production of angiotensin II. Obesity affects the sympathetic and cardiovascular systems by increasing cardiac output, stroke volume, and left ventricular filling. Two-thirds of hypertensive persons are obese. Normally weight loss can decrease hypertension, as can mild to moderate sodium restriction.

Cultural Responses to Antihypertensive Agents

African Americans are more likely to develop hypertension at an earlier age than white Americans. They also have a higher mortality rate from hypertension than the white population. The use of beta-adrenergic blockers (beta blockers) and angiotensin-converting enzyme (ACE) inhibitors is less effective for the control of hypertension in African Americans unless the drug is combined or given with a diuretic. This group is susceptible to low-renin hypertension; therefore, they do not respond well to beta blockers and ACE inhibitors. The antihypertensive drugs that are effective for African Americans are $alpha_1$ blockers and calcium channel blockers (calcium blockers). African-American patients do respond to diuretics as the initial monotherapy for controlling hypertension. White patients usually have high-renin hypertension and respond well to all antihypertensive agents.

Asian Americans are twice as sensitive as whites to beta blockers and other antihypertensives. A reduction in antihypertensive dosing is frequently needed. Native Americans have a reduced or lower response to beta blockers compared with whites. Monitoring blood pressure and drug dosing should be an ongoing assessment for patients in these cultural groups.

Hypertension in Older Adults

By 65 years of age, 26% of men and 30% of women are hypertensive. Between 65 and 75 years of age, 30% of men and 45% of women are hypertensive. Both systolic and diastolic hypertension are associated with increased cardiovascular morbidity and mortality. With antihypertensive therapy, the greatest decrease in cardiovascular disorders is 34% for stroke and 19% for coronary heart disease.

One of the troublesome side effects of the use of antihypertensive agents in older adults, especially frail or institutionalized persons, is orthostatic (postural) hypotension.

This episode of sudden low blood pressure presents dizziness due to blood pooling in lower extremities when an individual changes to an upright position. In older adults, the sympathetic nervous system does not respond as quickly to correct the situation, especially when potentiated by antihypertensive drug administration. If orthostatic hypotension occurs, the antihypertensive drug dose may need to be decreased or another antihypertensive drug used. Older adults with hypertension should be instructed to modify their lifestyle activities. This includes restricting dietary sodium to 2400 mg daily, avoiding tobacco, modifying diet, exercising, and decreasing stress.

NONPHARMACOLOGIC CONTROL OF HYPERTENSION

A sufficient decrease in blood pressure can be accomplished by nonpharmacologic methods. There are many nonpharmacologic ways to decrease blood pressure, but if the systolic pressure is greater than 140 mm Hg, **antihypertensive** drugs are generally ordered. Nondrug methods to decrease blood pressure include stress-reduction techniques, exercise, salt restriction, decreased alcohol ingestion, and smoking cessation.

When hypertension cannot be controlled by nonpharmacologic means, antihypertensive drugs are prescribed. However, nonpharmacologic methods should be combined with antihypertensive drugs to control hypertension.

GUIDELINES FOR HYPERTENSION

Blood pressure guidelines for determining hypertension have been revised and are contained in the Seventh Report of the Joint National Committee on Prevention, Detection, Evaluation, and Treatment of High Blood Pressure, or JNC 7. The purpose of these guidelines is to decrease the risk of cardiovascular disease (CVD) in the American population. The guideline for normal blood pressure is less than 120/80 mm Hg. *Prehypertension* is defined as systolic blood pressure (SBP) of 120 to 139 and diastolic blood pressure (DBP) of 80 to 89. Stage 1 hypertension falls between 140/90 and 159/99, and stage 2 hypertension is 160/100 or greater.

Two out of three patients with hypertension have uncontrolled blood pressure or are not optimally treated. SBP is more important than DBP as a CVD risk for patients 50 years of age or older. According to the JNC 7, if the blood pressure is greater than 20/10 mm Hg above goal, a drug regimen should be started. CVD risk doubles with each increase of 20/10 mm Hg, starting at 115/75 mm Hg.

PHARMACOLOGIC CONTROL OF HYPERTENSION

An individualized approach to the treatment of hypertension is used by many health care providers. All drugs are considered *initial agents* when first prescribed for hypertension. Reduction of other cardiovascular risk factors and the use of fewer drugs (i.e., substituting instead of adding drugs) at the lowest effective doses are emphasized. Often more than one antihypertensive is used to control blood pressure, which also may lead to less adverse effects.

Antihypertensive drugs, used either singly or in combination with other drugs, are classified into six categories: (1) diuretics, (2) sympatholytics (sympathetic depressants), (3) direct-acting arteriolar vasodilators, (4) ACE inhibitors, (5) angiotensin II receptor blockers (ARBs), and (6) calcium channel blockers.

Diuretics

Diuretics promote sodium depletion, which decreases extracellular fluid volume (ECFV). Diuretics are effective as first-line drugs for treating mild hypertension. Hydrochlorothiazide (HCTZ) is the most frequently prescribed diuretic for controlling mild hypertension by decreasing excess fluid volume. It can be used alone for recently diagnosed or mild hypertension or with other antihypertensive drugs. Many antihypertensive drugs can cause fluid retention; therefore diuretics are often administered together with antihypertensive agents. The various types of diuretics are discussed in Chapter 43.

Thiazide diuretics are not recommended for patients with renal insufficiency (creatinine clearance <30 mL/min). The loop (high-ceiling) diuretics such as furosemide (Lasix) are usually recommended, because they do not depress renal blood flow. Loop diuretics are not used if hypertension is the result of renin-angiotensin-aldosterone system involvement because they tend to elevate serum renin level immediately. Instead of a single thiazide drug, a combination of potassium-wasting and potassium-sparing diuretics may be useful; less potassium excretion would occur. In addition, thiazides can be combined with other antihypertensive drugs to increase their effectiveness. Box 44-1 lists the combinations of thiazides with other drugs. Many drug products on the market include combinations of thiazide diuretics and potassium-sparing diuretics, beta blockers, ACE inhibitors, or angiotensin II receptor blockers. ACE inhibitors tend to increase serum potassium (K) levels, so when they are combined with a thiazide diuretic, serum potassium loss is minimized.

Sympatholytics (Sympathetic Depressants)

The **sympatholytics** comprise five groups of drugs: (1) beta-adrenergic blockers, (2) centrally acting $alpha_2$ agonists, (3) alpha-adrenergic blockers, (4) adrenergic neuron blockers (peripherally acting sympatholytics), and (5) $alpha_1$- and $beta_1$-adrenergic blockers. Beta-adrenergic blockers block the beta receptors, and alpha-adrenergic blockers block the alpha receptors.

Beta-Adrenergic Blockers

Beta-adrenergic blockers, frequently called *beta blockers,* are used as antihypertensive drugs or in combination with a diuretic. Beta blockers are also used as antianginals and antidysrhythmics and are discussed in this context in Chapter 42.

BOX 44-1 COMBINATION OF THIAZIDES WITH ANTIHYPERTENSIVE DRUGS AND OTHER COMBINATIONS

Thiazide with Potassium-Sparing Diuretics
- hydrochlorothiazide with spironolactone (Aldactazide)
- hydrochlorothiazide with amiloride (Moduretic)
- hydrochlorothiazide with triamterene (Dyazide, Maxzide)

Thiazide with Beta Blockers
- hydrochlorothiazide with bisoprolol fumarate (Ziac)
- hydrochlorothiazide with metoprolol (Lopressor HCT)
- bendroflumethiazide with nadolol (Corzide)
- hydrochlorothiazide with propranolol (Inderide)
- hydrochlorothiazide with timolol (Timolide)
- chlorthalidone (thiazide-like diuretic) with atenolol (Tenoretic)

Thiazide with ACE Inhibitors
- hydrochlorothiazide with benazepril (Lotensin HCT)
- hydrochlorothiazide with captopril (Capozide)
- hydrochlorothiazide with enalapril maleate (Vaseretic)
- hydrochlorothiazide with fosinopril (Monopril HCT)
- hydrochlorothiazide with lisinopril (Prinzide, Zestoretic)
- hydrochlorothiazide with moexipril (Uniretic)
- hydrochlorothiazide with quinapril (Accuretic)

Thiazide with Angiotensin II Antagonists
- hydrochlorothiazide with candesartan (Atacand HCT)
- hydrochlorothiazide with eprosartan (Teveten HCT)
- hydrochlorothiazide with irbesartan (Avalide)
- hydrochlorothiazide with losartan (Hyzaar)
- hydrochlorothiazide with olmesartan medoxomil (Benicar HCT)
- hydrochlorothiazide with telmisartan (Micardis HCT)
- hydrochlorothiazide with valsartan (Diovan HCT)

Thiazide with Centrally Acting Alpha$_2$ Agonist
- chlorthalidone with clonidine (Combipres)
- hydrochlorothiazide with methyldopa (Aldoril)

Thiazide with Alpha Blocker
- polythiazide with prazosin (Minizide)

Combination of ACE Inhibitors with Calcium Channel Blocker
- See Table 44-3.

Combination of Calcium Channel Blocker with Statin Drug
- amlodipine with atorvastatin (Caduet)

ACE, Angiotensin-converting enzyme; *HCT,* hydrochlorothiazide.

Beta (β+ and β–)-adrenergic blockers reduce cardiac output by diminishing the sympathetic nervous system response to decrease basal sympathetic tone. With continued use of beta blockers, vascular resistance is diminished, and blood pressure is lowered. Beta blockers reduce heart rate, contractility, and renin release. There is a greater hypotensive response in patients with higher renin levels.

African-American hypertensive patients do not respond well to beta blockers alone for the control of hypertension. Instead, hypertension can be controlled by combining beta blockers with diuretics.

There are many types of beta blockers. Nonselective beta blockers, such as propranolol (Inderal) and carvedilol (Coreg) inhibit beta$_1$ (heart) and beta$_2$ (bronchial) receptors. Heart rate slows (blood pressure decreases secondary to the decrease in heart rate), and bronchoconstriction occurs because of unopposed parasympathetic tone. Cardioselective beta blockers are preferred, because they act mainly on the beta$_1$ rather than the beta$_2$ receptors and bronchoconstriction is less likely to occur. Acebutolol (Sectral), atenolol (Tenormin), betaxolol (Kerlone), bisoprolol (Zebeta), and metoprolol (Lopressor) are cardioselective beta blockers that block beta$_1$ receptors.

Cardioselectivity does not confer absolute protection from bronchoconstriction. In tests measuring forced expiratory volume in 1 second (FEV_1) as a measure of β– reactivity, only atenolol demonstrated true protection. Other cardioselective beta blockers were only partially effective. Studies also show that at the upper end of the dosage range, cardioselectivity is less effective. In patients with preexisting bronchospasm or other pulmonary disease, beta blockers, even those considered cardioselective, should be used with caution. Some experts regard this as a relative contraindication. The real value of beta selectivity is in maintaining renal blood flow and minimizing the hypoglycemic effects of beta blockade.

The combination of beta blockers with hydrochlorothiazides is packaged together in tablet form (see Box 44-1). Usually the hydrochlorothiazide dose is 12.5 to 25 mg, approximately half the average dose.

Beta blockers tend to be more effective in lowering blood pressure in patients who have an elevated serum renin level. The cardioselective prototype drug metoprolol (Lopressor) is presented in Prototype Drug Chart 44-1.

Beta blockers should not be used by patients with second- or third-degree atrioventricular (AV) block or sinus bradycardia. A noncardioselective beta blocker such as propranolol (Inderal) should not be given to a patient with chronic obstructive pulmonary disease (COPD).

Pharmacokinetics Metoprolol is well absorbed from the gastrointestinal tract. Its half-life is short and its protein-binding power is low.

Pharmacodynamics Cardioselective beta-adrenergic blockers block beta$_1$ receptors, thereby decreasing heart rate and blood pressure. The nonselective beta blockers block beta$_1$ and beta$_2$ receptors, which can result in bronchial constriction. Beta blockers cross the placental barrier and are excreted in breast milk.

The onset of action of oral beta blockers is usually 30 minutes or less, and the duration of action is 6 to 12 hours. When beta blockers are administered intravenously, the onset of action is immediate, peak time is 20 minutes (compared with 1.5 hours orally), and duration of action is 4 to 10 hours.

PROTOTYPE DRUG CHART 44-1

Metoprolol

Drug Class Antihypertensive: $beta_1$ blocker Trade Names: Lopressor, Toprol SR Pregnancy Category: C; D (second and third trimester)	**Dosage** Hypertension: A: PO: 50-100 mg/d in 1-2 divided doses; maint: 100-450 mg in divided doses; *max:* 450 mg/d in divided doses C: >6 y: PO: 1 mg/kg/d; *max:* 2 mg/kg/d SR: 50-100 mg/d; *max:* 400 mg/d Myocardial infarction: A: IV: 5 mg q2min × 3 doses; then 25-50 mg q6h for 48 h; maint: PO: 50-100 mg b.i.d.
Contraindications Hypersensitivity, second- and third-degree heart block, cardiogenic shock, hypotension, acute HF, sinus bradycardia. Caution: Hepatic, renal, or thyroid dysfunction; asthma; peripheral vascular disease; diabetes mellitus type 1	**Drug-Lab-Food Interactions** Drug: Increase bradycardia with digitalis; increase hypotensive effect with other antihypertensives, alcohol, anesthetics; NSAIDs decrease effect of beta blockers Lab: Increase in hepatic enzymes
Pharmacokinetics Absorption: PO: 95% Distribution: PB: 12% Metabolism: t½: 3-7 h Excretion: In urine	**Pharmacodynamics** PO: Onset: 15 min Peak: 1.5 h Duration: 10-19 h IV: Onset: Immediate Peak: 20 min Duration: 4-10 h
Therapeutic Effects/Uses To control hypertension Mode of Action: Promotes blood pressure reduction via $beta_1$-blocking effect	
Side Effects Fatigue, weakness, dizziness, nausea, vomiting, diarrhea, mental changes, drowsiness, headache, blurred vision, photosensitivity, nasal stuffiness, impotence, decreased libido, depression	**Adverse Reactions** Bradycardia, thrombocytopenia, hypoglycemia, diabetes mellitus Life-threatening: Complete heart block, bronchospasm, agranulocytosis

A, Adult; *b.i.d.,* twice a day; *d,* day; *h,* hour; *HF,* heart failure; *IV,* intravenous; *maint,* maintenance; *max,* maximum; *min,* minute; *PB,* protein-binding; *PO,* by mouth; *SR,* sustained release; *t ½,* half-life.

Side Effects and Adverse Reactions. Side effects and adverse reactions include decreased pulse rate, markedly decreased blood pressure, and (with noncardioselective $beta_1$ and $beta_2$ blockers) bronchospasm. Beta blockers should not be abruptly discontinued, because rebound hypertension, angina, dysrhythmias, and myocardial infarction can result. Beta blockers can cause dizziness, insomnia, depression, fatigue, nightmares, and sexual dysfunction. Other side effects are discussed in Chapter 42. Table 44-1 lists the beta blockers used to treat hypertension and their dosages, uses and considerations.

Noncardioselective beta blockers inhibit the liver's ability to convert glycogen to glucose in response to hypoglycemia. Because of this side effect, beta blockers should be used with caution in patients with diabetes mellitus. In addition, the depression of heart rate masks the symptom (tachycardia) of hypotension.

Nursing Process
Patient-Centered Collaborative Care

Antihypertensives: Beta Blockers

Assessment

- Obtain a medication and herbal history from patient. Report if a drug-drug or drug-herbal interaction is probable.
- Obtain vital signs. Report abnormal blood pressure and bradycardia. Compare vital signs with baseline finding.
- Check laboratory values related to renal and liver function periodically. Elevated blood urea nitrogen (BUN) and serum creatinine may be caused by beta blockers or cardiac disorder. Elevated cardiac enzymes, such as aspartate transaminase (AST) and lactate

TABLE 44-1 ANTIHYPERTENSIVES: BETA BLOCKERS AND CENTRAL $ALPHA_2$ AGONISTS

GENERIC (BRAND)	ROUTE AND DOSAGE	USES AND CONSIDERATIONS
Beta-Adrenergic Blockers		
acebutolol HCl (Sectral) Cardioselective $beta_1$	A: PO: 400-800 mg/d in 1-2 divided doses; *max:* 1200 mg/d	For hypertension and cardiac dysrhythmia. Used alone or with a thiazide diuretic. Side effects include dizziness, fatigue, hypotension, bradycardia, and constipation/diarrhea. Closely monitor vital signs. Pregnancy category: B (D in second and third trimesters); PB: 10%-26%; t½: 3-13 h
atenolol (Tenormin) Cardioselective $beta_1$	A: PO: 25-100 mg/d; *max:* 100 mg/d Older adults: PO: 25-50 mg/d; *max:* 100 mg/d C: PO: 0.8-1.5 mg/kg/d; *max:* 2 mg/kg/d	For hypertension and angina. Similar side effects as acebutolol. Pregnancy category: D; PB: 5%-15%; t½: 6-7 h
betaxolol HCl (Kerlone, Betoptic-S) Cardioselective $beta_1$	Hypertension: A: PO: 5-20 mg/d; *max:* 20 mg/d Also used for glaucoma	For hypertension and glaucoma. Ophthalmic preparation used to decrease IOP. Pregnancy category: C; PB: 50%; t½: 15 h
bisoprolol fumarate (Zebeta) $Beta_1$ blocker	A: PO: Initially: 2.5-5 mg/d; *max:* 20 mg/d	For hypertension and angina pectoris. Long-acting $beta_1$ blocker. May decrease heart rate and blood pressure. Pregnancy category: C; PB: 30%-36%; t½: 9-12 h
carvedilol (Coreg) Alpha blocker Nonselective $beta_1$ and $beta_2$	A: PO: Initially: 6.25 mg, b.i.d. for 2 wk; *max:* 50 mg/d ER: A: PO: Initially: 20 mg/d; *max:* 80 mg/d	For treating hypertension and congestive heart failure. Food delays absorption. Pregnancy category: C (D in second and third trimesters); PB: 98%; t½: 7-10 h
metoprolol (Lopressor) Cardioselective $beta_1$	See Prototype Drug Chart 44-1.	
nadolol (Corgard) Nonselective $beta_1$ and $beta_2$	A: PO: 40-80 mg/d; *max:* 320 mg/d	For hypertension and angina pectoris. Similar to carteolol HCl. Pregnancy category: C; PB: 30%; t½: 10-24 h
penbutolol sulfate (Levatol) Nonselective $beta_1$ and $beta_2$	A: PO: 10-20 mg/d; *max:* 80 mg/d	Contraindicated in patients with asthma. Pregnancy category: C; PB: 80%-98%; t½: 5 h
pindolol (Visken) Nonselective $beta_1$ and $beta_2$	A: PO: 5 mg b.i.d.; *max:* 60 mg/d in divided doses	For hypertension and angina pectoris. Used alone or with a thiazide diuretic. Pregnancy category: B; PB: 40%-60%; t½: 3-4 h
propranolol (Inderal) Nonselective $beta_1$ and $beta_2$	A: PO: 40 mg b.i.d.; *max:* 640 mg/d SR: 80 mg/d; *max:* 640 mg/d	For hypertension, angina, and cardiac dysrhythmias. First beta blocker. May cause bronchospasm because of $beta_2$-blocker effect. Pregnancy category: C; PB: 90%; t½: 3-6 h
Central $Alpha_2$ Agonists		
clonidine HCl (Catapres)	A: PO: Initially: 0.1 mg b.i.d. or t.i.d.; *max:* 2.4 mg/d A: Transdermal patch: 0.1 mg/24 h q7d	For hypertension. Long duration of action. Well absorbed from GI tract. Used alone or with a thiazide diuretic. Decreases sympathetic effect. Drowsiness, dizziness, and dry mouth may occur. Pregnancy category: C; PB: 20%-40%; t½: 12-16 h
guanfacine HCl (Tenex)	A: PO: 1 mg/d h.s.; may increase to 2-3 mg/d; *max:* 4 mg/d	For hypertension. Long duration of action. Used alone or with a thiazide diuretic. Pregnancy category: B; PB: 70%; t½: 17 h
methyldopa	A: PO: 250 mg b.i.d.; *max:* 4 g/d IV: 250-1000 mg q6-8h; *max:* 4 g/d C: PO: 10 mg/kg/d in 2-4 divided doses	Used alone or with a thiazide diuretic. Can be given IV. Take with food if GI upset occurs. Pregnancy category: B; PB: 15%; t½: 1.7 h

A, Adult; *b.i.d.,* twice a day; *C,* child; *d,* day; *GI,* gastrointestinal; *h,* hour; *h.s.,* at bedtime; *IOP,* intraocular pressure; *IV,* intravenous; *maint,* maintenance; *max,* maximum; *PB,* protein-binding; *PO,* by mouth; *SR,* sustained- release; *t½,* half-life; *t.i.d.,* three times a day; *UK,* unknown; *wk,* week; >, greater than; <, less than.

dehydrogenase (LDH), may be caused by beta blockers or cardiac disorder.

Nursing Diagnoses

- Decreased cardiac output related to variations in blood pressure readings
- Noncompliance with drug regimen related to cost of multiple drugs ordered
- Sexual dysfunction related to side effect of beta blockers
- Deficient knowledge related to inexperience with beta blockers

Planning

- Patient's blood pressure will be decreased or will return to normal value.
- Patient states he or she will take medication as prescribed.
- Patient will verbalize importance of following beta blocker regimen.

Nursing Interventions

- Monitor vital signs, especially blood pressure and pulse.
- Monitor laboratory results, especially BUN, serum creatinine, AST, and LDH.

Patient Teaching

General

- Encourage patient to comply with drug regimen. Abrupt discontinuation of antihypertensive drug may cause rebound hypertension.
- Inform patient that herbs can interfere with beta blockers (Herbal Alert 44-1).
- Advise that patient avoid OTC drugs without first checking with health care provider. Many OTC drugs carry warnings against use in presence of hypertension or concurrent use with antihypertensives.
- Suggest that patient wear a MedicAlert bracelet or carry card indicating health problem and prescribed drugs.
- Teach patient in trauma situation to inform health care provider of drugs taken daily (such as beta blocker). Beta blockers block compensatory effects of the body to the shock state. Glucagon may be needed to reverse effects so patient can be resuscitated.

Self-Administration

- Teach patient or family member how to take a radial pulse and blood pressure and to report abnormal findings to health care provider.

Side Effects

- Advise patient that antihypertensives may cause dizziness (orthostatic hypotension). Warn patient to rise slowly from lying or sitting to a standing position.
- Advise patient to report dizziness, slow pulse rate, changes in blood pressure, heart palpitation, confusion, or gastrointestinal upset to health care provider.
- Alert patient with diabetes mellitus to possible hypoglycemic symptoms.
- Inform patient that antihypertensives may cause sexual dysfunction (e.g., impotence).

Diet

- Teach patient and family members nonpharmacologic methods to decrease blood pressure, such as low-salt diet, relaxation techniques, exercise, smoking cessation, and decreased alcohol ingestion (1 to 2 oz daily).
- Advise patient to report constipation. Foods high in fiber, a stool softener, and increased water intake (except in patients with heart failure) are usually indicated.

Cultural Considerations

- Explain to African-American patients that monotherapy with beta blockers is generally less effective in controlling their hypertension. However, taking a diuretic together with a beta blocker can increase effectiveness of therapy.

Evaluation

- Evaluate effectiveness of drug therapy (decreased blood pressure, absence of side effects).
- Determine that patient adheres to drug regimen.

HERBAL ALERT 44-1

Antihypertensives

- Ma-huang and ephedra decrease or counteract the effect of antihypertensive drugs. When taken with beta blockers, hypertension may continue or increase.
- Ephedra increases hypertension when taken with beta blockers.
- Black cohosh increases the hypotensive effect of antihypertensive drugs.
- Hawthorn may increase the effects of beta blockers and angiotensin-converting enzyme inhibitors.
- Licorice antagonizes the effects of antihypertensive drugs.
- Goldenseal may increase the effects of antihypertensive drugs.
- Parsley may potentiate hypotension when taken with an antihypertensive drug.

Centrally Acting Alpha$_2$ Agonists

Centrally acting alpha$_2$ agonists decrease the sympathetic response from the brainstem to the peripheral vessels. They stimulate the alpha$_2$ receptors, which in turn decreases sympathetic activity; increases vagus activity; decreases cardiac output; and decreases serum epinephrine, norepinephrine, and renin release. All of these actions result in reduced peripheral vascular resistance and increased vasodilation. This group of drugs has minimal effects on cardiac output and blood flow to the kidneys. Beta blockers are not given with centrally acting sympatholytics, because accentuation of bradycardia during therapy and rebound hypertension on discontinuing therapy can occur.

Drugs in this group include methyldopa, clonidine, and guanfacine. Methyldopa was one of the first drugs widely used to control hypertension. In high doses, methyldopa and clonidine can cause sodium and water retention. Frequently methyldopa and clonidine are administered with diuretics. Clonidine is available in a transdermal preparation that provides a 7-day duration of action. Transdermal patches are replaced every 7 days and may be left on while bathing; skin irritations may occur. Guanfacine has effects similar to clonidine. Guanfacine has a long half-life and usually is taken once a day. Table 44-1 lists centrally acting $alpha_2$ agonists along with beta blockers.

Side Effects and Adverse Reactions. Side effects and adverse reactions of $alpha_2$ agonists include drowsiness, dry mouth, dizziness, and slow heart rate (bradycardia). Methyldopa should not be used in patients with impaired liver function, and serum liver enzymes should be monitored periodically in all patients. This group of drugs must not be abruptly discontinued, because a rebound hypertensive crisis can result. If the drug needs to be stopped immediately, another antihypertensive drug is usually prescribed to avoid rebound hypertensive symptoms (e.g., restlessness, tachycardia, tremors, headache, increased blood pressure). Rebound hypertension is less likely to occur with guanfacine. The nurse should emphasize the need to take the medication as prescribed. This group of drugs can cause sodium and water retention, resulting in peripheral edema. A diuretic may be ordered with methyldopa or clonidine to decrease water and sodium retention (edema). Patients who are pregnant or contemplating pregnancy should avoid clonidine. Methyldopa is frequently used to treat chronic or pregnancy-induced hypertension; however, it crosses the placental barrier, and small amounts may enter the breast milk of a lactating patient.

Alpha-Adrenergic Blockers

This group of drugs blocks the alpha-adrenergic receptors (alpha blockers), resulting in vasodilation and decreased blood pressure. They help maintain the renal blood flow rate. Alpha blockers are useful in treating hypertension in patients with lipid abnormalities. They decrease the very-low-density lipoproteins (VLDL) and the low-density lipoproteins (LDL) that are responsible for the buildup of fatty plaques in the arteries (atherosclerosis). In addition, they increase high-density lipoprotein (HDL) levels. Alpha blockers are safe for patients with diabetes, because they do not affect glucose metabolism. They also do not affect respiratory function.

The selective $alpha_1$-adrenergic blockers—prazosin, terazosin, and doxazosin—are used mainly to reduce blood pressure and can be used to treat benign prostatic hypertrophy. Prazosin is a commonly prescribed drug. Terazosin and doxazosin have longer half-lives than prazosin, and they are normally given once at bedtime. When prazosin is taken with alcohol or other antihypertensives, the hypotensive state can be intensified. These drugs, like the centrally acting $alpha_2$ agonists, cause sodium and water retention with edema; therefore, diuretics are frequently given concomitantly to decrease fluid accumulation in the extremities.

The more potent alpha blockers—phentolamine and phenoxybenzamine—are used primarily for hypertensive crisis and severe hypertension resulting from catecholamine-secreting tumors of the adrenal medulla (pheochromocytomas).

Pharmacokinetics Prazosin is absorbed through the GI tract, but a large portion of prazosin is lost during hepatic first-pass metabolism. The half-life is short, so the drug should be administered twice a day. Prazosin is highly protein-bound, and when it is given with other highly protein-bound drugs, the patient should be assessed for adverse reactions.

Pharmacodynamics Selective alpha-adrenergic blockers dilate the arterioles and venules, decreasing peripheral resistance and lowering blood pressure. With prazosin, the heart rate is only slightly increased, whereas with nonselective alpha blockers such as phentolamine, the blood pressure is greatly reduced, and reflex tachycardia can occur. Nonselective alpha blockers are more effective for acute hypertension; selective alpha blockers are more useful for long-term essential hypertension.

The onset of action of prazosin occurs between 30 minutes and 2 hours. The duration of action of prazosin is 10 hours. Table 44-2 presents drug data for selective and nonselective alpha blockers.

Side Effects and Adverse Reactions. Side effects of prazosin, doxazosin, and terazosin include orthostatic hypotension (dizziness, faintness, lightheadedness, and increased heart rate, which may occur with first dose), nausea, headache, drowsiness, nasal congestion caused by vasodilation, edema, and weight gain.

Side effects of phentolamine include hypotension, reflex tachycardia caused by the severe decrease in blood pressure, nasal congestion caused by vasodilation, and GI disturbances.

Drug Interactions. Drug interactions occur when alpha-adrenergic blockers are taken with antiinflammatory drugs and nitrates (e.g., nitroglycerin for angina). Peripheral edema is intensified when prazosin and an antiinflammatory drug are taken daily. Nitroglycerin taken for angina lowers blood pressure. If prazosin is taken with nitroglycerin, syncope (faintness) caused by a decrease in blood pressure can occur. The selective alpha-adrenergic blocker prazosin is shown in Prototype Drug Chart 44-2.

Adrenergic Neuron Blockers (Peripherally Acting Sympatholytics)

Adrenergic neuron blockers are potent antihypertensive drugs that block norepinephrine release from the sympathetic nerve endings, causing a decrease in norepinephrine release that results in a lowering of blood pressure. There is a decrease in both cardiac output and peripheral vascular resistance. Reserpine (the most potent drug) is used to control severe hypertension. Orthostatic hypotension is a common side effect, so the patient should be advised to rise slowly from a reclining or sitting position. The adrenergic neuron blockers are considered the last choices for treatment of chronic hypertension, because these drugs can cause orthostatic hypotension. Use of reserpine may cause vivid dreams, nightmares, and suicidal ideation. The drugs in this group can cause sodium and water retention. These drugs can be taken alone or with a diuretic to decrease peripheral edema.

$Alpha_1$- and $Beta_1$-Adrenergic Blockers

This group of drugs blocks both the $alpha_1$ and $beta_1$ receptors. Labetalol (Normodyne) is an example of an alpha/beta blocker. Blocking the $alpha_1$ receptor causes vasodilation, decreasing resistance to blood flow. The effect on the alpha receptor is stronger than the effect on the beta receptor;

TABLE 44-2 ANTIHYPERTENSIVES: SYMPATHOLYTICS: ALPHA ADRENERGIC AND PERIPHERALLY ACTING BLOCKERS AND DIRECT ACTING VASODILATORS

GENERIC (BRAND)	ROUTE AND DOSAGE	USES AND CONSIDERATIONS
Selective Alpha-Adrenergic Blockers		
doxazosin mesylate (Cardura)	A: PO: Initially: 1 mg/d; *max:* 16 mg/d Older adults: PO: 0.5 mg/d	Used alone or with another antihypertensive. Orthostatic hypotension, headache, dizziness, and GI upset may occur. Pregnancy category: C; PB: 98%; $t\frac{1}{2}$: 22 h
prazosin HCl (Minipress)	See Prototype Drug Chart 44-2.	
terazosin HCl (Hytrin)	A: PO: Initially: 1 mg h.s.; *max:* 20 mg/d	Used alone or with another antihypertensive. Dizziness and headache may occur. Pregnancy category: C; PB: 90%-94%; $t\frac{1}{2}$: 9-12 h
Nonselective Alpha-Adrenergic Blockers		
phenoxybenzamine HCl (Dibenzyline)	A: PO: Initially: 10 mg b.i.d.; maint: 20-40 mg/d;	For hypertension related to adrenergic excess, pheochromocytoma. Lowers peripheral resistance. Long duration of action. Pregnancy category: C; PB: UK; $t\frac{1}{2}$: 24 h
phentolamine (OraVerse)	Pheochromocytoma: A: IM/IV: 2.5-5 mg; repeat 5-mg dose PRN; test is positive if decreased SBP >35 mm Hg and decreased DBP >25 mm Hg C: IV: 0.05-0.1 mg/kg; repeat with 5 mg PRN Extravasation: 5-10 mg in 10 mL NS local injection within 12 h	For diagnosis of pheochromocytoma and prevention of tissue necrosis after norepinephrine or epinephrine extravasation. Pregnancy category: C; PB: UK; $t\frac{1}{2}$: 20 min
Adrenergic Neuron Blockers (Peripherally Acting Sympatholytics)		
reserpine	A: PO: Initially: 0.5 mg/d for 1-2 wk; maint: 0.1-0.25 mg/d	For hypertension. Rarely used. May cause nightmares and vivid dreams. Pregnancy category: C; PB: 96%; $t\frac{1}{2}$: 50-100 h
Alpha$_1$- and Beta$_1$-Adrenergic Blockers		
labetalol HCl (Trandate)	Hypertension: A: PO: Initially: 100 mg b.i.d.; maint: 200-400 mg/d; *max:* 2.4 g/d Hypertensive emergency: A: IV: 20 mg over 2 min; continuous infusion: 1-2 mg/min; *max:* 300 mg/dose	For hypertension. Used alone or with a thiazide diuretic. May cause orthostatic hypotension, palpitations, and syncope. Pregnancy category: C; PB: 50%; $t\frac{1}{2}$: 6-8 h
Direct-Acting Vasodilators		
hydralazine HCl	A: PO: Initially: 10 mg q.i.d.; maint: 25-50 mg q.i.d. Severe hypertension: IM/IV: 10-40 mg, repeat PRN C: PO: 0.75-1 mg/kg/d divided q12h; max: 7.5 mg/kg/d q12h	For hypertension. Short duration of action. May be used with a diuretic to decrease edema and a beta blocker to prevent tachycardia. Dizziness, tremors, headaches, tachycardia, and palpitations may occur. Closely monitor vital signs. Pregnancy category: C; PB: 87%; $t\frac{1}{2}$: 2-8 h
minoxidil	A: PO: Initially: 5 mg/d; *max:* 100 mg/d C: PO: Initially: 0.2 mg/kg/d; *max:* 50 mg/d Alopecia: Topical: 2% sol b.i.d.	For hypertension. May be used with a diuretic to reduce edema and with a beta blocker to prevent tachycardia. Long duration of action. Do not discontinue drug abruptly; withdraw drug slowly to avoid rebound hypertension. Closely monitor vital signs. Pregnancy category: C; PB: 0%; $t\frac{1}{2}$: 4 h
sodium nitroprusside (Nipride, Nitropress)	Hypertensive emergency: A: IV: 0.25-5 mcg/kg/min in D_5W; *max:* 10 mcg/kg/min	For hypertensive crisis. Potent antihypertensive. Drug decomposes in light; container must be wrapped in aluminum foil. Good for 24 h. Discard drug if red or blue. Cyanide toxicity may occur. Measure cyanide and thiocyanate levels. May cause profound hypotension. Pregnancy category: C; PB: UK; $t\frac{1}{2}$: 2 min

A, Adult; *b.i.d.,* twice a day; *C,* child; *d,* day; *GI,* gastrointestinal; *h,* hour; *h.s.,* at bedtime; *IM,* intramuscular; *IV,* intravenous; *maint,* maintenance; *MAOI,* monoamine oxidase inhibitor; *max,* maximum; *min,* minute; *NB,* newborn; *PB,* protein-binding; *PO,* by mouth; *PRN,* as needed; *q.i.d.,* four times a day; *sec,* second; $t\frac{1}{2}$, half-life; *t.i.d.,* three times a day; *UK,* unknown; *wk,* week.

PROTOTYPE DRUG CHART 44-2

Prazosin HCl

Drug Class Antihypertensive: alpha-adrenergic blocker Trade Name: Minipress Pregnancy Category: C	**Dosage** A: PO: 1 mg b.i.d./t.i.d.; maint: 3-15 mg/d; *max:* 20 mg/d in divided doses
Contraindications Renal disease Caution: Angina	**Drug-Lab-Food Interactions** Drug: Increased hypotensive effect with other antihypertensives, nitrates, alcohol Lab: Increased hepatic enzymes
Pharmacokinetics Absorption: GI: 60% (5% to circulation) Distribution: PB: 95% Metabolism: t½: 3 h Excretion: In bile and feces; 10% in urine	**Pharmacodynamics** PO: Onset: 0.5-2 h Peak: 2-4 h Duration: 10 h
Therapeutic Effects/Uses To control hypertension, refractory HF; to treat benign prostatic hypertrophy Mode of Action: Dilates peripheral blood vessels by blocking alpha-adrenergic receptors	
Side Effects Dizziness, drowsiness, vertigo, blurred vision, tinnitus, fatigue, headache, depression, nasal congestion, dry mouth, nausea, vomiting, diarrhea, abdominal pain, impotence, urinary incontinence	**Adverse Reactions** Orthostatic hypotension, palpitations, bradycardia, tachycardia, pancreatitis

A, Adult; *b.i.d.,* twice a day; *d,* day; *h,* hour; *HF,* heart failure; *GI,* gastrointestinal; *maint,* maintenance; *max,* maximum; *PB,* protein-binding; *PO,* by mouth; *t ½,* half-life; *t.i.d.,* three times a day.

therefore blood pressure is lowered and pulse rate is moderately decreased. By blocking the cardiac $beta_1$ receptor, both heart rate and atrioventricular (AV) contractility are decreased. Large doses of alpha/beta blockers could block $beta_2$-adrenergic receptors, thus increasing airway resistance. Patients who have severe asthma should not take large doses of labetalol. Table 44-2 lists two alpha/beta blockers.

Nursing Process
Patient-Centered Collaborative Care

Antihypertensives: Alpha-Adrenergic Blockers

Assessment
- Obtain a medication history from patient, including current drugs. Report if drug-drug or drug-herbal interaction is probable. Prazosin is highly protein-bound and can displace other highly protein-bound drugs.
- Obtain baseline vital signs and weight for future comparison.
- Check urinary output. Report if it is decreased (less than 600 mL/day), because drug is contraindicated if renal disease is present.

Nursing Diagnoses
- Risk for activity intolerance related to drug regimen and/or cardiac status
- Deficient knowledge related to drug regimen
- Ineffective sexuality pattern related to beta-blocker or other drug therapy

Planning
- Patient's blood pressure will decrease.
- Patient will follow proper drug regimen.

Nursing Interventions
- Monitor vital signs. Desired therapeutic effect of prazosin may not fully occur for 4 weeks. Sudden marked decrease in blood pressure and tachycardia should be reported.
- Check daily for fluid retention in extremities and weight gain. Prazosin may cause sodium and water retention.

Patient Teaching
General
- Advise patient to comply with drug regimen. Abrupt discontinuation of antihypertensive drug may cause rebound hypertension.
- Inform patient that orthostatic hypotension may occur. Explain that before rising, patient should sit and dangle

feet. Drug may be taken at bedtime to avoid orthostatic hypotension.
- Teach patient to self-monitor daily weights. Prazosin may lead to edema.

Self-Administration
- Teach patient or family member how to take and record blood pressure. A blood pressure chart should be established, and blood pressure changes should be reported.

Side Effects
- Caution patient that dizziness, lightheadedness, and drowsiness may occur, especially when drug is first prescribed. If these symptoms occur, health care provider should be notified.
- Inform male patient that impotence may occur if high doses of drug are prescribed. This problem should be reported to the health care provider.
- Tell patient to report if edema is present in the morning. Water retention is a problem with alpha blockers.
- Inform patient not to take cold, cough, or allergy OTC medications without first contacting the health care provider.

Diet
- Encourage patient to decrease salt intake unless otherwise indicated by the health care provider.

Cultural Considerations
- Explain to African-American patients with hypertension that they can take alpha-adrenergic blockers and calcium channel blockers but should avoid taking beta blockers, because these agents are not generally effective in controlling their hypertension. However, taking a diuretic together with a beta blocker increases effectiveness for these patients.
- Caution Asian patients that they are twice as sensitive to effects of propranolol on the blood pressure and heart rate, so dose should be decreased or another antihypertensive drug may be given.

Evaluation
- Evaluate effectiveness of drug in controlling blood pressure; side effects should be absent.
- Evaluate patient's adherence to medication schedule.
- Evaluate patient's knowledge of medication.

Common side effects of these drugs include orthostatic hypotension, GI disturbances, nervousness, dry mouth, and fatigue. Large doses of labetalol may cause AV heart block.

Direct-Acting Arteriolar Vasodilators

Vasodilators are potent antihypertensive drugs. Direct-acting vasodilators act by relaxing the smooth muscles of the blood vessels, mainly the arteries, causing vasodilation. Vasodilators promote an increase in blood flow to the brain and kidneys. With vasodilation, the blood pressure decreases and sodium and water are retained, resulting in peripheral edema. Diuretics can be given with a direct-acting vasodilator to decrease the edema.

Two direct-acting vasodilators, hydralazine and minoxidil, are used for moderate to severe (dose-related) hypertension. These two drugs cause little orthostatic hypotension, because of minimum dilation of the arterioles. However, reflex tachycardia and release of renin can occur secondary to vasodilation and decreased blood pressure. Beta blockers are frequently prescribed with arteriolar vasodilators to decrease the heart rate; this counteracts the effect of reflex tachycardia.

Nitroprusside is prescribed for acute hypertensive emergency. This is a very potent vasodilator that rapidly decreases blood pressure. Nitroprusside acts on both arterial and venous vessels. Table 44-2 lists direct-acting vasodilators.

Side Effects and Adverse Reactions

The effects of hydralazine are numerous and include reflex tachycardia, palpitations, edema, nasal congestion, headache, dizziness, GI bleeding, lupus-like symptoms, and neurologic symptoms (tingling, numbness). Minoxidil has similar side effects, as well as tachycardia, edema, and excess hair growth. It can precipitate an anginal attack.

Nitroprusside can cause reflex tachycardia, palpitations, restlessness, agitation, nausea, and confusion. Nitroprusside is discussed in greater detail in Chapter 59.

Angiotensin-Converting Enzyme Inhibitors

ACE inhibitors inhibit ACE, which in turn inhibits the formation of angiotensin II (vasoconstrictor) and blocks the release of aldosterone. Aldosterone promotes sodium retention and potassium excretion. When aldosterone is blocked, sodium is excreted along with water, and potassium is retained. ACE inhibitors cause little change in cardiac output or heart rate, and they lower peripheral resistance. (Figure 44-1 illustrates the RAAS.) These drugs can be used in patients who have elevated serum renin levels.

The ACE inhibitors are used primarily to treat hypertension; some of these agents are also effective in treating heart failure. The ACE inhibitors are benazepril (Lotensin), captopril (Capoten), enalapril maleate (Vasotec), fosinopril (Monopril), lisinopril (Prinivil, Zestril), moexipril (Univasc), perindopril (Aceon), quinapril (Accupril), ramipril (Altace), and trandolapril (Mavik), which are all presented in Table 44-3. These drugs can be used for first-line antihypertensive therapy, but thiazide diuretics are recommended by JNC 7.

African Americans and older adults do not respond to ACE inhibitors with the desired reduction in blood pressure, but when taken with a diuretic, blood pressure usually will be lowered. ACE inhibitors should not be given during pregnancy, because they reduce placental blood flow. For patients with renal insufficiency, reduction of the drug dose (except for fosinopril), is necessary.

TABLE 44-3 ANTIHYPERTENSIVES: ACE INHIBITORS AND ANGIOTENSIN II RECEPTOR BLOCKERS

GENERIC (BRAND)	ROUTE AND DOSAGE	USES AND CONSIDERATIONS
Angiotensin Antagonists (ACE Inhibitors)		
benazepril HCl (Lotensin)	A: PO: 10-40 mg/d in 1-2 divided doses; *max:* 80 mg/d	Headache, dizziness, hypotension, nausea, diarrhea, or constipation may occur. Pregnancy category: D; PB: 97%; t½: 10 h
captopril (Capoten)	A: PO: Initially: 12.5-25 mg, b.i.d./t.i.d.; maint: 25-150 mg, b.i.d./t.i.d.; *max:* 450 mg/d	For hypertension and HF. Inhibits conversion of angiotensin I to angiotensin II. Irritating cough may occur; retains potassium. Pregnancy category: C and D; PB: 25%-30%; t½: 2-3 h
enalapril maleate (Vasotec); enalaprilat (Vasotec I.V.)	A: PO: Initially: 2.5-5 mg/d; maint: 10-40 mg/d Hypertensive emergencies: IV: 1.25-5 mg over 5 min q6h PRN	For hypertension and HF. Similar to captopril and benazepril. Give IV slowly over at least 5 min. Pregnancy category: C and D; PB: 50%-60%; t½: 2-11 h
fosinopril (Monopril)	A: PO: 5-40 mg/d; *max:* 80 mg/d	For hypertension and HF. Reduces peripheral resistance (afterload) and improves cardiac output. Dose does not need to be reduced because of renal insufficiency. Pregnancy category: D; PB: 97%; t½: 12 h
lisinopril (Prinivil, Zestril)	A: PO: Initially: 10 mg/d; maint: 20-40 mg/d; *max:* 80 mg/d	For hypertension and HF. Usually given with a diuretic. Long duration of action (24 h). Monitor vital signs. Pregnancy category: D; PB: 25%; t½: 12 h
moexipril (Univasc)	A: PO: 7.5 mg/d; *max:* 30 mg/d in divided doses	For hypertension. May increase serum lithium levels and cause toxicity. Pregnancy category: C and D; PB: 50%; t½: 2-9 h
perindopril (Aceon)	A: PO: 4-8 mg/d; *max:* 16 mg/d	For mild to moderate hypertension. Reduces vasoconstriction. Cough may occur. Pregnancy category: D; PB: 10%-60%; t½: 1-10 h
quinapril HCl (Accupril)	A: PO: 10-20 mg/d; *max:* 80 mg/d in divided doses Older adults: A: PO: Initially 2.5-5 mg/d	For hypertension and HF. Potent ACE inhibitor. Reduces systemic vascular resistance and increases cardiac output. Pregnancy category: C and D; PB: 97%; t½: 24 h
ramipril (Altace)	A: PO: 2.5-5 mg/d; *max:* 20 mg/d	For hypertension and HF. Similar to captopril. Long duration of action (24 hours). Pregnancy category: C and D; PB: 73%; t½: 2-3 h
trandolapril (Mavik)	A: PO: 1-2 mg/d; may increase weekly to 2-4 mg/d; *max:* 8 mg/d	For hypertension. May be used alone or with another antihypertensive. African Americans respond to trandolapril, including those with low-renin hypertension. Pregnancy category: C and D; PB: 80%; t½: 6-10 h
Combinations of ACE Inhibitors with Calcium Blockers		
benazepril with amlodipine (Lotrel)	A: PO: amlodipine/benazepril 2.5/10 mg/d; 5/10 mg/d; 5/20 mg/d	For hypertension
trandolapril with verapamil (Tarka)	A: PO: trandolapril/verapamil SR: 2/180 mg/d; 1/240 mg/d; 2/240 mg/d; 4/240 mg/d	For hypertension
Angiotensin II Receptor Blockers (ARBs)		
candesartan (Atacand)	A: PO: 16 mg/d; maint: 8-32 mg/d	For hypertension and HF. May be used when patient does not respond to or tolerate ACE inhibitors. May be combined with calcium blocker amlodipine for more effective response in decreasing high blood pressure. Pregnancy category: C and D; PB: 99%; t½: 9 h
eprosartan (Teveten)	A: PO: Initially: 600 mg/d; maint: 400-800 mg/d; *max:* 900 mg/d	For mild to moderate hypertension. Does not cause irritating cough associated with ACE inhibitors. Food can cause slight delay in drug absorption. Pregnancy category: C and D; PB: 98%; t½: 5-9 h
irbesartan (Avapro)	A: PO: 150 mg/d; maint: 150-300 mg/d	For hypertension. May be used alone or with other antihypertensives. Pregnancy category: C and D; PB: 90%; t½: 11-15 h
losartan potassium (Cozaar)	A: PO: 25-50 mg/d, in 1-2 divided doses; *max:* 100 mg/d	For hypertension. May be used alone or with other antihypertensives. Pregnancy category: C and D; PB: 98%; t½: 2 h
olmesartan medoxomil (Benicar)	A: PO: 20 mg/d; may increase to 40 mg/d	Inhibits binding angiotensin II to AT_1 receptors. Promotes vasodilation, and decreases peripheral resistance. Not recommended if patient is volume-depleted. Pregnancy category: C and D; PB: 99%; t½: 13 h
telmisartan (Micardis)	A: PO: 40-80 mg/d	For mild to moderate hypertension. Does not cause cough associated with ACE inhibitors. Angioedema rarely occurs. Pregnancy category: C and D; PB: 99.5%; t½: 24 h
valsartan (Diovan)	See Prototype Drug Chart 44-3.	
azilsartan (Edarbi)	A: PO: 40-80 mg/d; *max:* 80 mg/d	For hypertension as monotherapy or with other antihypertensives. Minimal adverse effects of diarrhea, orthostatic hypotension. Pregnancy category: C and D; PB: 99%; t½: 11 h

TABLE 44-3 ANTIHYPERTENSIVES: ACE INHIBITORS AND ANGIOTENSIN II RECEPTOR BLOCKERS—cont'd

GENERIC (BRAND)	ROUTE AND DOSAGE	USES AND CONSIDERATIONS
Aldosterone Receptor Antagonists		
eplerenone (Inspra)	A: PO: 50 mg/d; may increase to 50 mg b.i.d.	Binds aldosterone at mineralocorticoid receptor. Contraindications: serum potassium >5.5 mEq/L, creatinine clearance <50 mL/min, type 2 diabetes, and taking potassium-sparing diuretics. For hypertension, HF, and postmyocardial infarction. Pregnancy category: B; PB: 50%; t½: 4-6 h
Direct Renin Inhibitors		
aliskiren (Tekturna)	A: PO: 150-300 mg/d	First direct renin inhibitor for mild to moderate hypertension. Used either as monotherapy or with antihypertensive such as an ARB valsartan (Diovan). Hyperkalemia uncommon for monotherapy. Pregnancy category: C and D; PB: 49%; t½: 24 h

A, Adult; *ACE,* angiotensin-converting enzyme; *ARB,* angiotensin II receptor blocker; AT_1, angiotensin I; *b.i.d.,* two times a day; *d,* day; *ER,* extended-release; *h,* hour; *HF,* heart failure; *IV,* intravenous; *maint,* maintenance; *max,* maximum; *min,* minute; *PB,* protein-binding; *PO,* by mouth; *t½,* half-life; *t.i.d.,* three times a day; *UK,* unknown; >, greater than; <, less than.

With the exception of moexipril, which should be taken on an empty stomach for maximum effectiveness, ACE inhibitors can be administered with food.

Side Effects and Adverse Reactions. The primary side effect of ACE inhibitors is a constant, irritated cough. Other side effects include nausea, vomiting, diarrhea, headache, dizziness, fatigue, insomnia, serum potassium excess (hyperkalemia), and tachycardia. The persistent, nonproductive "ACE cough" may be relieved upon discontinuance of the drug. Often an ARB may be substituted without cough as a side effect. The major adverse effects are first-dose hypotension and hyperkalemia. Hypotension results because of the vasodilating effect. First-dose hypotension is more common in patients also taking diuretics. Angioedema (swelling of face, tongue, lips, mucous membranes, larynx, and extremity edema) may occur due to hypersensitivity and has a higher incidence in African Americans. This may occur within hours or 1 week after the first dose. Angioedema may be reversed with drug discontinuance. When laryngeal edema occurs, the patient may require rescue epinephrine.

Contraindications. ACE inhibitors should not be given during pregnancy; harm to the fetus due to reduction in placental blood flow could occur. This group of drugs should not be taken with potassium-sparing diuretics such as spironolactone (Aldactone) or salt substitutes that contain potassium, because of the risk of hyperkalemia (serum potassium excess).

Nursing Process
Patient-Centered Collaborative Care

Antihypertensives: Angiotensin-Converting Enzyme Inhibitors

Assessment
- Obtain a drug and herbal history from patient of current drugs taken. Report if drug-drug or drug-herbal interaction is probable.
- Obtain baseline vital signs for future comparisons.
- Check laboratory values for serum protein, albumin, blood urea nitrogen (BUN), creatinine, potassium, and white blood cell count, and compare with future serum levels.

Nursing Diagnoses
- Deficient knowledge related to drug regimen
- Anxiety related to hypertensive state
- Risk for falls related to orthostatic hypotension

Planning
- Patient's blood pressure will be within desired range.
- Patient will be free from moderate to severe side effects. Angioedema, cough, dysgeusia, weakness, hyperkalemia, orthostatic hypotension, and renal impairment may occur as side effects.

Nursing Interventions
- Monitor blood pressure. A sudden drop in blood pressure should be reported.
- Monitor laboratory tests related to renal function (BUN, creatinine, protein) and blood glucose levels. Caution: Watch for hypoglycemic reaction in patients with diabetes mellitus. Urine protein may be checked in the morning using a dipstick.
- Report to health care provider occurrences of bruising, petechiae, and/or bleeding. These may indicate a severe adverse reaction to an angiotensin antagonist such as captopril.

Patient Teaching
General
- Warn patient not to abruptly discontinue use of captopril without notifying health care provider. Rebound hypertension could result.

- Inform patient not to take OTC drugs (e.g., cold medication) without first contacting health care provider.
- Advise patient not to use salt substitute with potassium.
- Warn patient who is pregnant or contemplating becoming pregnant not to take ACE inhibitors or ARBs; they can cause harm to the fetus.
- Teach patient to rise slowly to avoid orthostatic hypotension.

Self-Administration

- Teach patient or family member how to take and record blood pressure. A blood pressure chart should be established, and blood pressure changes should be reported.

Side Effects

- Explain to patient that dizziness and/or lightheadedness may occur during the first week of captopril therapy. If dizziness persists, health care provider should be notified.
- Advise patient to report any occurrence of bleeding.

Diet

- Teach patient to take captopril 20 minutes to 1 hour before a meal. Food decreases 35% of captopril absorption.
- Warn patient that taste of food may be diminished during first month of drug therapy.
- Advise patient to avoid foods high in potassium because hyperkalemia is an adverse effect of ACE inhibitors.

Cultural Considerations

- Explain to African-American patients that they may not respond well to ACE inhibitors unless the drug is taken with a diuretic.

Evaluation

- Evaluate effectiveness of drug therapy (absence of severe side effects, blood pressure return to desired range).
- Evaluate patient's renal function.

Angiotensin II Receptor Blockers

Angiotensin II receptor blockers (ARBs) are similar to ACE inhibitors in that they prevent the release of aldosterone (sodium-retaining hormone). They act on the renin-angiotensin-aldosterone system (RAAS). The difference between ARBs and ACE inhibitors is that ARBs block angiotensin II from the angiotensin I (AT_1) receptors found in many tissues, whereas ACE inhibitors inhibit the angiotensin-converting enzyme in the formation of angiotensin II. ARBs cause vasodilation and decrease peripheral resistance. They do not cause the constant, irritated cough ACE inhibitors can. Like ACE inhibitors, ARBs should not be taken during pregnancy.

Losartan (Cozaar), valsartan (Diovan), irbesartan (Avapro), candesartan cilexetil (Atacand), eprosartan (Teveten), olmesartan medoxomil (Benicar), and telmisartan (Micardis) are examples of ARBs. These agents block the vasoconstrictor effects of angiotensin II at the receptor site. The combination of losartan potassium and hydrochlorothiazide tablets and valsartan and hydrochlorothiazide tablets and others should not cause serum potassium excess or loss. ARBs may be used as a first-line treatment for hypertension.

Prototype Drug Chart 44-3 gives the pharmacologic data related to valsartan.

SAFETY: Preventing Medication Errors

Do not confuse…

- **Diovan** and **Dioval.** Diovan (valsartan) is an angiotensin II receptor blocker. Dioval is an estradiol, an estrogen hormone. If both drugs are in the home, caution must be taken to select the correct drug, especially by the male patient taking Diovan and the female patient taking Dioval.

Pharmacokinetics Valsartan is prescribed primarily to manage hypertension. The combination drug Diovan HCT contains valsartan plus a low dose of hydrochlorothiazide. It is rapidly absorbed in the GI tract and undergoes first-pass metabolism in the liver to form active metabolites. It is highly protein-bound and should not be given during pregnancy, especially during the second and third trimester. The half-life is 6 to 9 hours. The drug is excreted in urine and feces.

Pharmacodynamics Valsartan is a potent vasodilator. It blocks the binding of angiotensin II to the AT_1 receptors found in many tissues. Its peak time is 4 to 6 hours, and it has a long duration of action: 24 hours.

Like ACE inhibitors, ARBs are less effective for treating hypertension in African-American patients. In addition, like ACE inhibitors, ARBs may cause angioedema. These agents can be taken with or without food and are suitable for patients with mild hepatic insufficiency.

Direct Renin Inhibitor

The first FDA-approved direct renin inhibitor for treating hypertension is aliskiren (Tekturna). Aliskiren binds with renin, causing a reduction of angiotensin I, angiotensin II, and aldosterone levels (see Figure 44-1). It is effective for mild and moderate hypertension. Aliskiren can be used alone or with another antihypertensive agent. It has an additive effect in reducing blood pressure when combined with a thiazide diuretic or an ARB.

This drug, when used as monotherapy, has not proven to be as effective in reducing blood pressure in the African-American population.

Calcium Channel Blockers

Slow calcium channels are found in the myocardium (heart muscle) and vascular smooth muscle (VSM) cells. Free calcium increases muscle contractility, peripheral resistance, and blood pressure. Calcium channel blockers, also called *calcium antagonists* and *calcium blockers,* block the calcium channel in the VSM, promoting vasodilation. The large central arteries are not as sensitive to calcium blockers as coronary and cerebral arteries and the peripheral vessels. Calcium blockers are highly protein-bound but have a short

PROTOTYPE DRUG CHART 44-3

Valsartan

Drug Class	Dosage
Antihypertensive: angiotensin II receptor blocker Trade Names: Diovan Pregnancy Category: C (first trimester); D (second and third trimesters)	Hypertension: A: PO: Initially 80-160 mg/d; maint: 80-320 mg/d; *max:* 320 mg/d C: >6 y: PO: Initially 1.3 m/kg/d; *max:* 2.7 mg/kg/d
Contraindications	**Drug-Lab-Food Interactions**
Hypersensitivity, pregnancy, breastfeeding Caution: Renal and hepatic impairments, hypotension, hypovolemia, hyperkalemia	Drug: Antihypertensives, diuretics, MAOIs, alcohol may increase hypotensive effects; ACE inhibitors and aspirin may increase hyperkalemia and renal dysfunction; digoxin, NSAIDs may increase renal dysfunction; lithium may increase lithium toxicity Lab: May increase AST, ALT, ALP, bilirubin, BUN, creatinine, Hct, Hgb
Pharmacokinetics	**Pharmacodynamics**
Absorption: Rapidly absorbed, 25-30 in blood circulation Distribution: PB: 94%-95% Metabolism: $t\frac{1}{2}$: 6-9 h Excretion: 13% in urine and 83% in bile/feces	PO: Onset: 2 h Peak: 4-6 h Duration: 24 h
Therapeutic Effects/Uses	
To treat hypertension Mode of Action: Potent vasodilator; inhibits binding of angiotensin II	
Side Effects	**Adverse Reactions**
Dizziness, drowsiness, cough (rare), blurred vision, headache, diarrhea, insomnia, arthralgia, fatigue	Orthostatic hypotension, hypoglycemia, hyperkalemia Life threatening: renal dysfunction

A, Adult; *ALP,* alkaline phosphatase; *ALT,* alanine aminotransferase; *AST,* aspartate aminotransferase; *BUN,* blood urea nitrogen; *C,* child; *d,* day; *h,* hour; *Hct,* hematocrit; *Hgb,* hemoglobin; *max,* maximum; *PO,* by mouth; *PB,* protein-binding; $t\frac{1}{2}$, half-life.

half-life. Slow-release preparations decrease frequency of administration. Table 44-4 lists the calcium blockers in three groups: diphenylalkylamine (verapamil), benzothiazepines (diltiazem), and dihydropyridine (amlodipine and others).

Verapamil (Calan) is used to treat chronic hypertension, angina pectoris, and cardiac dysrhythmias. Verapamil and diltiazem act on the arterioles and the heart. The dihydropyridines are the largest group of calcium channel blockers and consist of seven drugs; six of these are used to control hypertension. The calcium blocker nimodipine is used to prevent ischemic brain injury due to vasospasm that often accompanies subarachnoid hemorrhage.

Nifedipine (Procardia) decreases blood pressure in older adults and in those with low serum renin values. Nifedipine and verapamil are potent calcium blockers. Nifedipine, in its immediate-release form (10- and 20-mg capsules), has been associated with an increased incidence of sudden cardiac death, especially when prescribed for outpatients at high doses. This is not true of the sustained-release preparations (Procardia XL, Adalat CC). For this reason, immediate-release nifedipine is usually prescribed for acute rises in blood pressure only on an as-needed basis in the hospital setting. Like the vasodilators, calcium channel blockers can cause reflex tachycardia; it is more prevalent with nifedipine.

Pharmacokinetics Amlodipine (Norvasc), like other calcium blockers, is highly protein-bound. It is gradually absorbed via the GI tract. Because the half-life of amlodipine is longer than that of other calcium blockers, it is taken once a day.

Pharmacodynamics Amlodipine may be used alone or with other antihypertensive drugs. Peripheral edema may occur because of its vasodilator effect, so persons with edema may need to take another type of antihypertensive drug. This drug has a long duration of action, so it is prescribed only once a day. Amlodipine may be combined with the ACE inhibitor benazepril, forming Lotrel.

Normally beta blockers are not prescribed with calcium blockers, because both drugs decrease myocardium contractility. Calcium blockers lower blood pressure better in African Americans than drugs in other categories.

Side Effects and Adverse Reactions. The side effects and adverse reactions of calcium channel blockers include flushing, headache, dizziness, ankle edema, bradycardia, and AV block.

KEY WEBSITES

Antihypertensive agents: *www.nhlbi.nih.gov/hbp/treat/bpd_type.htm*

Captopril: *www.nlm.nih.gov/medlineplus/druginfo/meds/a682823.html*

Management of hypertension: *www.aafp.org/afp/2008/0715/p270.html*

TABLE 44-4 ANTIHYPERTENSIVES: CALCIUM CHANNEL BLOCKERS

GENERIC (BRAND)	ROUTE AND DOSAGE	USES AND CONSIDERATIONS
Phenylalkylamines		
verapamil (Calan SR, Isoptin SR)	A: PO: 40-80 mg t.i.d. A: PO: SR: 90-240 mg/d in 2 divided doses; *max:* 480 mg/d	For hypertension (SR form). One of first calcium blockers. Also used for variant angina and cardiac dysrhythmias. Dizziness, headache, hypotension, bradycardia, and constipation may occur. Pregnancy category: C; PB: 94%; t½: 3-8 h
Benzothiazepines		
diltiazem HCl (Cardizem CD, Tiazac)	A: PO SR: Initially: 120-240 mg/d; *max:* 540 mg/d	For hypertension (SR form) and angina pectoris; IV form for cardiac dysrhythmias (atrial fibrillation). Headache, bradycardia, and hypotension may occur. Pregnancy category: C; PB: 75%; t½: 3-8 h
Dihydropyridines		
amlodipine (Norvasc)	A: PO: 5-10 mg/d. Older adults: 2.5-5.0 mg/d; maint: 5-10 mg/d	For mild to moderate hypertension and angina pectoris. Decreases peripheral vascular resistance (vasodilation). Used alone or with other antihypertensives. Pregnancy category: C; PB: 95%; t½: 30-50 h
felodipine (Felendil XL)	A: PO: Initially: 2.5-5 mg/d; *max:* 10 mg/d	For hypertension, HF, and angina pectoris. Potent calcium blocker. Flushing, peripheral edema, palpitations, dizziness, and headache may occur. Long duration of action. Pregnancy category: C; PB: 99%; t½: 10-16 h
isradipine (DynaCirc CR)	Hypertension: A: PO: 2.5 mg b.i.d.; *max:* 20 mg/d Older adults: 2.5 mg b.i.d.; *max:* 10 mg/d	For management of hypertension, HF, and angina pectoris. Used alone or with a diuretic. Pregnancy category: C; PB: 95%-97%; t½: 5-11 h
nicardipine HCl (Cardene SR)	A: PO: 20-40 mg t.i.d. SR: 30-60 mg b.i.d. ER: A: PO: 30-60 mg b.i.d. A: IV: initially: 5 mg/h; *max:* 15 mg/h	For essential hypertension and vasospastic angina. IV therapy for short-term hypertension therapy. Decreases systemic resistance; heart rate and cardiac output increased. Pregnancy category: C; PB: 95%; t½: 2-4 h
nifedipine (Procardia XL, Adalat CC)	A: PO: XL: 30-60 mg once daily; *max:* Adalat CC: 90 mg/d; Procardia XL: 120 mg/d	For hypertension and angina pectoris. Potent calcium channel blocker. Dizziness, lightheadedness, headache, flushing, peripheral edema, and nausea may occur. May be taken alone or with a diuretic. Pregnancy category: C; PB: 92%-98%; t½: 2-5 h
nisoldipine (Sular)	A: PO: 17-20 mg/d in 2 divided doses; *max:* old Sular formulation: 60 mg/d; newer Sular formulation: 34 mg/d	For hypertension and angina pectoris. May be used alone or with another antihypertensive. Like nifedipine, causes vasodilation, but 10 times more potent than nifedipine. Considered a potent coronary vasodilator. Pregnancy category: C; PB: 99%; t½: 7-12 h

A, Adult; *b.i.d.,* twice a day; *C,* child; *ER,* extended-release; *HF,* heart failure; *d,* day; *h,* hour; *IV,* intravenous; *maint,* maintenance; *max,* maximum; *min,* minute; *PB,* protein-binding; *PO,* by mouth; *PRN,* as needed; *SR,* sustained-release; *t½,* half-life; *t.i.d.,* three times a day; >, greater than.

CRITICAL THINKING CASE STUDY

GG, a 72-year-old African-American patient, has heart failure and diabetes. Her vital signs are blood pressure 176/94, pulse 92, and respirations 30. Her medications include hydrochlorothiazide 50 mg/day, atenolol 50 mg/day, and digoxin 0.25 mg/day.

1. Why was hydrochlorothiazide prescribed for GG? Explain the effects of hydrochlorothiazide on blood pressure.
2. Abnormal electrolytes and other laboratory test results may occur when taking hydrochlorothiazide. Would the following serum electrolyte and laboratory values be expected to *increase* or *decrease?*
   a. Sodium
   b. Potassium
   c. Calcium
   d. Magnesium
   e. Glucose
   f. Uric acid
3. Why should GG's blood glucose level be monitored while she is taking hydrochlorothiazide?
4. What effect may result when GG takes digoxin and hydrochlorothiazide together? Explain your answer.
5. Atenolol is what type of antihypertensive? Would atenolol be effective in lowering GG's blood pressure if given as the only antihypertensive drug? Explain your answer.
6. How effective is the combination of hydrochlorothiazide and atenolol for controlling GG's blood pressure? Explain your answer.

7. When using a combination drug therapy to correct hypertension, would the dosage for each drug be the same? Explain your answer.
8. When abruptly discontinuing beta blockers for hypertension without the patient taking another antihypertensive, what might occur? Explain how adverse effects can be avoided.

GG's blood glucose is 229. Her drugs for controlling hypertension are changed to prazosin 10 mg t.i.d. Her cholesterol and LDL are elevated. Her serum potassium level is 3.2 mEq/L.

9. Why were GG's hydrochlorothiazide and atenolol discontinued? Explain your answer.
10. What type of antihypertensive is prazosin? Explain the physiologic action of prazosin for lowering the blood pressure.
11. Does prazosin have an effect on the blood glucose level? What effect could prazosin have on GG's abnormal lipid levels? Explain your answer.

GG's ankles have become edematous. Hydrochlorothiazide is prescribed.

12. Why was hydrochlorothiazide added again to the drug regimen?
13. Is the daily prazosin dose within the safe therapeutic prescribed range for GG? Explain your answer. (You may refer to Prototype Drug Chart 44-2.)
14. List the groups of antihypertensive drugs that can cause sodium and water retention.

NCLEX STUDY QUESTIONS

1. A patient's blood pressure (BP) is 130/84. The health care provider plans to suggest nonpharmacologic methods for the patient. Which should the nurse include in teaching? (Select all that apply.)
   a. Stress-reduction techniques
   b. Starting an exercise program
   c. Salt restriction
   d. Smoking cessation
   e. Diet with increased protein
2. A patient has developed mild hypertension. The nurse acknowledges that the first-line drug for treating this patient's blood pressure might be which drug?
   a. Diuretic
   b. Alpha blocker
   c. ACE inhibitor
   d. Alpha/beta blocker
3. An African-American patient has developed hypertension. The nurse is aware that which group(s) of antihypertensive drugs are *less effective* in African-American patients?
   a. Diuretics
   b. Calcium channel blockers and vasodilators
   c. Beta blockers and ACE inhibitors
   d. Alpha blockers
4. The nurse knows that which diuretic is most frequently combined with an antihypertensive drug?
   a. chlorthalidone
   b. hydrochlorothiazide
   c. bendroflumethiazide
   d. potassium-sparing diuretic
5. The nurse is administering a beta blocker to a patient. Which is an important assessment to perform before administration?
   a. Urine output
   b. Apical pulse
   c. Potassium level
   d. Serum level of medication
6. Captopril (Capoten) has been ordered for a patient. The nurse teaches the patient that angiotensin-converting enzyme (ACE) inhibitors have which common side effects?
   a. Nausea and vomiting
   b. Dizziness and headaches
   c. Upset stomach
   d. Constant, irritating cough
7. A patient is prescribed losartan (Cozaar). The nurse teaches the patient that an angiotensin II receptor blocker (ARB) acts by doing what?
   a. Inhibiting angiotensin-converting enzyme
   b. Blocking angiotensin II from AT_1 receptors
   c. Preventing the release of angiotensin I
   d. Promoting the release of aldosterone
8. During an admission assessment, a patient states that she takes amlodipine (Norvasc). The nurse wishes to determine whether the patient has any common side effects of a calcium channel blocker. The nurse asks the patient if she has which signs and symptoms? (Select all that apply.)
   a. Insomnia
   b. Dizziness
   c. Headache
   d. Angioedema
   e. Ankle edema
   f. Hacking cough

Answers: 1, a, b, c, d; 2, a; 3, c; 4, b; 5, b; 6, d; 7, b; 8, b, c, e.

CHAPTER

45

Anticoagulants, Antiplatelets, and Thrombolytics

evolve WEBSITE

http://evolve.elsevier.com/KeeHayes/pharmacology/

- Animations
- Content Updates
- Key Points
- Review Questions for the NCLEX® Examination
- References from the Textbook
- Unfolding Case Studies

OBJECTIVES

- Compare the action for anticoagulants, antiplatelets, and thrombolytics.
- Differentiate the side effects and adverse reactions of anticoagulants, antiplatelets, and thrombolytics.
- Apply the nursing process, including patient teaching, for anticoagulants and thrombolytics.

OUTLINE

KEY TERMS

activated partial thromboplastin time, p. 651
acute myocardial infarction, p. 657
aggregation, p. 650
anticoagulants, p. 651
antiplatelets, p. 657
fibrinolysis, p. 659
international normalized ratio, p. 653
ischemia, p. 657
myocardial infarction, p. 651
necrosis, p. 657
partial thromboplastin time, p. 651
prothrombin time, p. 653
thromboembolism, p. 657
thrombolytics, p. 657
thrombosis, p. 650

Various drugs are used to maintain or restore circulation. The three major groups of these drugs are (1) anticoagulants, (2) antiplatelets (antithrombotics), and (3) thrombolytics. The *anticoagulants* prevent the formation of clots that inhibit circulation. The *antiplatelets* prevent platelet **aggregation** (clumping together of platelets to form a clot). The *thrombolytics,* popularly called *clot busters,* attack and dissolve blood clots that have already formed. Each of these three drug groups are discussed separately.

PATHOPHYSIOLOGY: THROMBUS FORMATION

Thrombosis is the formation of a clot in an arterial or venous vessel. The formation of an arterial thrombus could be caused by blood stasis (decreased circulation), platelet aggregation on the blood vessel wall, or blood coagulation. Arterial clots are usually made up of both white and red clots with the white clots *(platelets)* initiating the process, followed by fibrin formation and the trapping of red blood cells in the fibrin mesh. Blood clots found in the veins are from platelet aggregation with fibrin that attaches to red blood cells. Both types of thrombus can be dislodged from the vessel and become an embolus (blood clot moving through the bloodstream).

Platelets do not usually stick together unless there is a break in the endothelial lining of a blood vessel. When platelets adhere to the broken surface of an endothelial lining, they synthesize thromboxane A_2, which is a product of prostaglandins and a potent stimulus for platelet aggregation (clumping of platelet cells). The platelet receptor protein that binds fibrinogen, known as *glycoprotein IIb/IIIa,* or GP IIb/IIIa, also promotes platelet aggregation. Thromboxane A_2 and adenosine diphosphate (ADP) increase the activation of this receptor.

As the thrombus inhibits blood flow, fibrin, platelets, and red blood cells (erythrocytes) surround the clot, building the clot's size and structure. As the clot occludes the blood vessel, tissue ischemia occurs.

The venous thrombus usually develops because of slow blood flow. The venous clot can occur rapidly. Small pieces of the venous clot can detach and travel to the pulmonary artery and then to the lung. Inadequate oxygenation and gas exchange in the lungs result.

Oral and parenteral anticoagulants (warfarin and heparin) act primarily to prevent venous thrombosis, whereas antiplatelet drugs act to prevent arterial thrombosis. However, both groups of drugs suppress thrombosis in general.

ANTICOAGULANTS

Anticoagulants are used to inhibit clot formation. Unlike thrombolytics, they do *not* dissolve clots that have already formed, but rather act prophylactically to prevent new clots from forming. Anticoagulants are used in patients with venous and arterial disorders that put them at high risk for clot formation. Venous problems include deep vein thrombosis (DVT) and pulmonary embolism, and arterial problems include coronary thrombosis, or **myocardial infarction;** presence of artificial heart valves; and cerebrovascular accidents (CVAs, or stroke).

Heparin

Anticoagulants are administered orally or parenterally (subcutaneously [subQ] and intravenously [IV]). Heparin, introduced in 1938, is a natural substance in the liver that prevents clot formation. It was first used in blood transfusions to prevent clotting. Heparin is indicated for rapid anticoagulant effect when a thrombosis occurs because of a deep vein thrombosis (DVT), pulmonary embolism (PE), or an evolving stroke. Heparin is also used in open-heart surgery to prevent blood from clotting and in the critically ill patient with disseminated intravascular coagulation (DIC). DIC occurs when fibrin clots form within the vascular system. These clots consume proteins and platelets, depleting clotting factors and causing excess bleeding. However, the primary use of heparin is to prevent venous thrombosis, which can lead to pulmonary embolism or stroke.

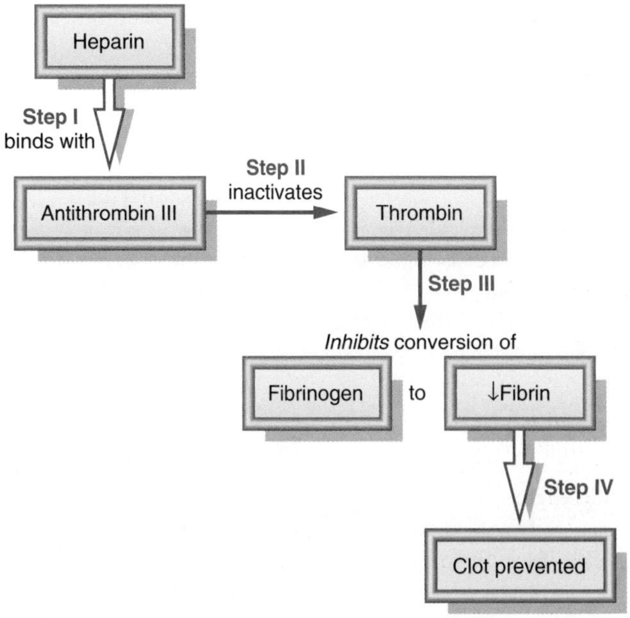

FIGURE 45–1 Action of the parenteral anticoagulant heparin.

Heparin combines with antithrombin III, which accelerates the anticoagulant cascade of reactions that prevents thrombosis formation. By inhibiting the action of thrombin, conversion of fibrinogen to fibrin does not occur and the formation of a fibrin clot is prevented (Figure 45-1).

Heparin is poorly absorbed through the gastrointestinal (GI) mucosa, and much is destroyed by heparinase, a liver enzyme. Because heparin is poorly absorbed orally, it is given subQ for prophylaxis or IV to treat acute thrombosis. It can be administered as an IV bolus or in IV fluid for continuous infusion. Heparin prolongs clotting time. **Partial thromboplastin time** (PTT) and **activated partial thromboplastin time** (aPTT) are laboratory tests used to detect deficiencies of certain clotting factors, and these tests are used to monitor heparin therapy. Heparin can decrease the platelet count, causing thrombocytopenia. If hemorrhage occurs during heparin therapy, the anticoagulant antagonist protamine sulfate is given IV. Protamine sulfate can be an anticoagulant, but in the presence of heparin, it is an antagonist to reverse the action of heparin. Before discontinuing heparin, oral therapy with warfarin therapy is begun.

Low–Molecular-Weight Heparins

These derivatives of standard heparin were introduced to prevent venous thromboembolism. Studies have shown that by extracting only the low–molecular-weight fractions of standard heparin through depolymerization, the equivalent of anticoagulation can be achieved with a lower risk of bleeding. Low–molecular-weight heparins (LMWHs) produce more stable responses at recommended doses. As a result, frequent laboratory monitoring of aPTT is not required, because LMWH does not have the standard effect of heparin. Heparin prevents coagulation by combining with

Antithrombin III to inactivate factor Xa and thrombin. Low–molecular-weight heparin inactivates the Xa factor, but it is less able to inactivate thrombin.

There are examples of LMWHs include enoxaparin sodium (Lovenox) and dalteparin sodium (Fragmin).

SAFETY: Preventing Medication Errors

Do not confuse...

- **Enoxaparin** (LMWH) and **enoxacin** (fluoroquinolone antibiotic)
- **Lovenox** (LMWH) and **Lotronex** (gastrointestinal drug)

The anticoagulant fondaparinux (Arixtra) is a synthetically engineered antithrombotic designed to be effective as a once-daily subcutaneous injection. Categorized as a *selective Factor Xa inhibitor,* fondaparinux is closely related in structure to heparin and LMW heparins and is used for the same purposes.

These agents are most commonly prescribed to prevent DVT and acute pulmonary embolism after orthopedic or abdominal surgery. Hip- and knee-replacement anticoagulant therapy often includes enoxaparin, and abdominal surgery includes dalteparin. The drugs can be administered at home, because aPTT monitoring is not necessary, whereas heparin must be given in the hospital. LMWHs are administered subQ once or twice a day, depending on the drug or drug regimen, and are available in prefilled syringes with attached needles. The patient or family member is taught how to administer the subQ injection, which is usually given in the abdomen. The average treatment period lasts 7 to 10 days. The LMWH is usually started in the hospital within 24 hours after surgery (Table 45-1).

The half-life of LMWHs is two to four times longer than that of heparin. Patients should be instructed not to take antiplatelet drugs such as aspirin while taking LMWHs or heparin. Bleeding because of LMWH use is less likely to occur than when heparin is given. LMWH overdose is rare; if bleeding occurs, protamine sulfate is the anticoagulant antagonist used. The dosage is 1 mg of protamine sulfate for every 100 units of unfractionated heparin or LMWH given.

Contraindications

The LMWHs are contraindicated for patients with strokes, peptic ulcers, and blood anomalies. These drugs should not be given to patients having eye, brain, or spinal surgery.

Direct Thrombin Inhibitors: Parenteral Anticoagulants II

Parenteral anticoagulants directly inhibit thrombin from converting fibrinogen to fibrin. These drugs differ from heparin-like anticoagulants. Three of these drugs are given intravenously: argatroban (Acova), bivalirudin (Angiomax), and lepirudin (Refludan). Bivalirudin binds with and inhibits free-flowing thrombin. The fourth drug, desirudin (Iprivask),

TABLE 45-1 ANTICOAGULANTS AND ANTICOAGULANT ANTAGONISTS

GENERIC (BRAND)	ROUTE AND DOSAGE	USES AND CONSIDERATIONS
Anticoagulants		
Heparins		
heparin sodium	See Prototype Drug Chart 45-1.	
Low–Molecular-Weight Heparins (LMWHs)		
dalteparin sodium (Fragmin)	Surgery: A: subQ: 2500 international units/d for 5-10 d starting 1-2 h before surgery DVT: A: subQ: 5000 units/d or q12h for 2-6 mo	For prevention of DVT before surgery and for those at risk of thromboembolism. Similar to enoxaparin. Pregnancy category: B; PB: <10%; t½: 3-5 h
enoxaparin sodium (Lovenox)	A: subQ: 40 mg daily for 5 to 10 d	For thromboembolism. Prevents and treats DVT and pulmonary embolism. Bleeding is an adverse reaction. Monitor CBC. Pregnancy category: B; PB: UK; t½: 4.5 h
Oral Anticoagulants		
Coumarin		
warfarin (Coumadin)	See Prototype Drug Chart 45-1.	
Selective Factor Xa Inhibitors		
fondaparinux (Arixtra)	A: subQ: 2.5-10 mg/d for 5-9 d	Indirectly inhibits factor Xa, preventing blood clots. Closely related to heparin and LMWHs. Used to prevent DVT after hip fracture, hip replacement surgery, and knee replacement surgery and treat pulmonary emboli. May cause more bleeding than LMWHs. Long duration of action. Pregnancy category: B; PB: 94%; t½: 17-21 h

TABLE 45-1 ANTICOAGULANTS AND ANTICOAGULANT ANTAGONISTS—cont'd

GENERIC (BRAND)	ROUTE AND DOSAGE	USES AND CONSIDERATIONS
rivaroxaban (Xarelto)	A: PO: 10-20 mg once daily with evening meal; *max:* 30 mg/d	For prophylaxis of DVT and PE in patients undergoing knee or hip replacement surgery, stroke, and atrial fibrillation. Not easily reversed. Does not require routine coagulation monitoring. Pregnancy category: C; PB: 92%-95%; t½: 5-9 h
apixaban (Eliquis)	A: PO: 5 mg b.i.d.	To prevent stroke and thromboembolism associated with nonvalvular atrial fibrillation. Routine coagulation monitoring not required. Pregnancy category: B; PB: 87%; t½: 5-12 h
Direct-Acting Thrombin Inhibitors: Anticoagulants II (Intravenous)		
argatroban (Argatroban)	A: IV: 2 mcg/kg/min; adjust dose to maintain aPTT 1.5-3 times baseline; *max:* 10 mcg/kg/min	Directly inhibits thrombin (thrombin inhibitor). Same effect as lepirudin. Decreases development of new thrombosis and treats heparin-induced thrombocytopenia (HIT). Pregnancy category: C; PB: 54%; t½: 40-52 min
bivalirudin (Angiomax)	A: IV bolus: 0.75 mg/kg; then IV infusion of 1.75 mg/kg/h during and within 4 h postprocedure; may require 0.2 mg/kg/h up to 20 h	Inhibits thrombin by binding to its receptor sites. Has been effective for use in preventing clot formation in patients with unstable angina who are undergoing cardiac angioplasty. Adverse effect is bleeding. Pregnancy category: B; PB: 0%; t½: 25 min
desirudin (Iprivask)	A: subQ: 15 mg/12 h for 9-12 d	Interferes with fibrin production, platelet aggregation, and factor XII activation, and inactivates thrombin. Given for DVT prophylaxis. Pregnancy category: C; PB: UK, t½: 2-3 h
lepirudin (Refludan)	A: IV bolus: 0.2-0.4 mg/kg over 15-20 sec; follow with 0.15 mg/kg/h for 2-10 d	Directly inhibits thrombin. Used for prophylaxis and treatment of thrombosis due to HIT. Titrated to aPTT ratio. Liver function should be normal. Adverse effect is bleeding. Pregnancy category: B; PB: UK; t½: 1.3 h
dabigatran (Pradaxa)	A: PO: 150 mg b.i.d.; *max:* 300 mg/d	For prevention of stroke and atrial fibrillation. Assess renal function before initiating drug and periodically throughout therapy. Pregnancy category: C; PB: 35%; t½: 12-17 h
Anticoagulant Antagonists		
protamine sulfate	A: IV: Initially: 1 mg/100 units heparin; administer 10-50 mg in 10-15 min IV push; *max:* 100 mg in 2-h period	Binds and neutralizes heparin. Antidote to heparin overdose. Pregnancy category: C; PB: UK; t½: 7.4 min
phytonadione, Vitamin K_1 (Mephyton)	A: PO/IM/IV: 1-10 mg, q12-24h PRN C: subQ/IM: 0.5-5 mg	Promotes liver synthesis of clotting factors. Antidote for warfarin overdose. Pregnancy category: C; PB: UK; t½: UK

A, Adult; *aPTT,* activated partial thromboplastin time; *b.i.d.,* twice a day; *C,* child; *CBC,* complete blood count; *d,* day; *DVT,* deep vein thrombosis; *h,* hour; *HIT,* heparin-induced thrombocytopenia; *IM,* intramuscular; *IV,* intravenous; *inf,* infusion; *INR,* international normalized ratio; *LD,* loading dose; *LMWH,* low–molecular-weight heparin; *maint,* maintenance; *min,* minute; *PB,* protein-binding; *PO,* by mouth; *PRN,* as needed; *PT,* prothrombin time; *sec,* second; *subQ,* subcutaneous; *t½,* half-life; *UK,* unknown.

is administered subcutaneously. Dabigatran (Pradaxa) is an oral anticoagulant that does not require routine coagulation monitoring (see Table 45-1). These drugs are more expensive than the other anticoagulants.

Oral Anticoagulants

Warfarin (Coumadin) is an oral anticoagulant from the coumarin drug family. Dicumarol, a coumarin drug, and anisindione from the indanedione group, have been discontinued because of their many side effects. Warfarin is synthesized from dicumarol. Before warfarin was available for human use, it was used in rodenticides to kill rats by causing hemorrhage.

Oral anticoagulants inhibit hepatic synthesis of vitamin K, thus affecting the clotting factors II, VII, IX, and X. Warfarin is used mainly to prevent thromboembolic conditions such as thrombophlebitis, pulmonary embolism, and embolism formation caused by atrial fibrillation, which can lead to stroke (CVA). Oral anticoagulants prolong clotting time and are monitored by the **prothrombin time** (PT), a laboratory test that measures the time it takes blood to clot in the presence of certain clotting factors, which warfarin affects. This laboratory test is usually performed immediately before administering the next drug dose until the therapeutic level has been reached. Today, **international normalized ratio** (INR) is the laboratory test most frequently used to report PT results. It was introduced to account for variability in reported PTs from different laboratories. Reagents used in the PT test are compared with an international reference standard and reported as the INR; normal INR is 1.3 to 2. Patients on warfarin therapy are maintained at an INR of 2 to 3. The desired INR for patients who have a mechanical heart valve or recurrent systemic embolism is 2.5 to 3.5, but the desired level could be as high as 4.5.

Monitoring INR at regular intervals is required for the duration of drug therapy. Warfarin (Coumadin) has a long half-life and very long duration. Drug accumulation can occur and lead to external or internal bleeding, so the nurse must observe for petechiae, ecchymosis, tarry stools, and hematemesis and teach the patient to do the same at home.

The antidote for warfarin overdose is Vitamin K, but it takes 24 to 48 hours to be effective. Usually a low dose of oral Vitamin K may be recommended for patients with an INR of 5.5. If excessive Vitamin K is given, it may take warfarin 1 to 2 weeks before it can be effective again. For acute bleeding, fresh frozen plasma is indicated.

Parenteral and oral anticoagulants (heparin and warfarin) are presented in Prototype Drug Chart 45-1.

Pharmacokinetics Heparin is poorly absorbed through the GI mucosa, and much is destroyed by heparinase, a liver enzyme. Heparin is given parenterally, either subcutaneously for prophylactic anticoagulant therapy or IV (bolus or continuous infusion) for an immediate response. Warfarin, an oral anticoagulant, is well absorbed through the GI mucosa; food will delay but not inhibit absorption.

PROTOTYPE DRUG CHART 45-1

Heparin and Warfarin Sodium

Drug Class Anticoagulant Trade Name (warfarin): Coumadin Pregnancy Category: C (heparin) Pregnancy Category: X (warfarin)	**Dosage** Heparin: A: subQ: 5000-10,000 units q4-12h IV: Bolus: 5000 units; inf: 20,000-40,000 units over 24 h based on APTT C: IV: 50 units/kg bolus; then 5-100 units/kg q4h based on APTT Warfarin: A: PO: LD: 5-10 mg/d for 2-5 d; *maint:* 2-10 mg/d C: PO: 0.05-0.2 mg/kg/d; titrate to INR
Contraindications Heparin/warfarin: Bleeding disorder, peptic ulcer, severe hepatic or renal disease, hemophilia Warfarin: Blood dyscrasias, eclampsia, alcoholism, bleeding, head trauma Caution: diabetes mellitus, leukemia	**Drug-Lab-Food Interactions** Drug: heparin: Increase effect with aspirin, NSAIDs, thrombolytics, probenecid; decrease effect with nitroglycerin, protamine sulfate Warfarin: Increase effect with amiodarone, aspirin, NSAIDs, sulfonamides, thyroid drugs, allopurinol, histamine$_2$ blockers, oral hypoglycemics, metronidazole, miconazole, methyldopa, diuretics, oral antibiotics, vitamin E; decrease effect with barbiturates, laxatives, phenytoin, estrogens, vitamins C and K, oral contraceptives, rifampin Lab: May increase AST, ALT Food: Decrease diet rich in vitamin K
Pharmacokinetics Absorption: heparin: subQ or IV; warfarin: PO: Well absorbed Distribution: PB: heparin: >80%; warfarin: 99% Metabolism: t½: heparin: 0.5-2.5 h; warfarin: 1-7 d Excretion: heparin: Slowly in urine and reticuloendothelial system; warfarin: in urine and bile	**Pharmacodynamics** Heparin: subQ: Onset: 20-60 min Peak: 2 h Duration: 8-12 h IV: Onset: immediate Peak: 5-10 min Duration: 2-6 h Warfarin: PO: Onset: >2 d Peak: 1-3 d Duration: 2.5-5 d
Therapeutic Effects/Uses Heparin/warfarin: To prevent blood clotting Mode of Action: heparin: Inhibits thrombin, which prevents conversion of fibrinogen to fibrin Warfarin: Depresses hepatic synthesis of vitamin K clotting factors (II [prothrombin], VII, IX, and X)	
Side Effects Heparin: Itching, burning, chills, injection site reaction Warfarin: Anorexia, nausea, vomiting, diarrhea, abdominal cramps, rash, alopecia, fever, stomatitis	**Adverse Reactions** Heparin: Bleeding, ecchymoses, hematuria, angioedema, osteoporosis, stroke, heparin-induced thrombocytopenia Life-threatening: Hemorrhage Warfarin: Purple-toe syndrome Life-threatening: Hemorrhage

A, Adult; *ALT,* alanine aminotransferase; *aPTT,* activated partial thromboplastin time; *AST,* aspartate aminotransferase; *C,* child; *CVA,* cerebrovascular accident; *d,* day; *h,* hour; *inf,* infusion; *INR,* international normalized ratio; *IV,* intravenous; *LD,* loading dose; *maint,* maintenance; *min,* minute; *NSAIDs,* nonsteroidal antiinflammatory drugs; *PB,* protein-binding; *PO,* by mouth; *subQ,* subcutaneous; *t½,* half-life, *>,* greater than.

The half-life of heparin is dose-related; high doses prolong the half-life. The half-life of warfarin is 1 to 7 days, in contrast to 0.5 to 2.5 hours for heparin. Because warfarin has a long half-life and is highly protein-bound, the drug can have cumulative effects. Bleeding can occur, especially if another highly protein-bound drug is administered together with warfarin. Kidney and liver disease prolong the half-life of both heparin and warfarin. Warfarin is metabolized to inactive metabolites that are excreted in urine and bile.

Pharmacodynamics Heparin, administered for acute thromboembolic disorders, prevents thrombus formation and embolism. It has been effectively used to treat DIC, which causes multiple thrombi in small blood vessels. Warfarin is effective for long-term anticoagulant therapy. The PT level should be 1.5 to 2 times the reference value to be therapeutic, or INR should be 2.0 to 3.0. INR has effectively replaced the use of PT, because PT can vary from laboratory to laboratory and reagent to reagent. Higher INR levels (up to 3.5) are usually required for patients with prosthetic heart valves, cardiac valvular disease, and recurrent emboli. Heparin does not cross the placental barrier, unlike warfarin; warfarin use is not recommended during pregnancy.

Intravenous heparin has a rapid onset; its peak time of action is reached in minutes, and its duration of action is short. After an IV heparin dose, the patient's clotting time will return to normal in 2 to 6 hours. SubQ heparin is more slowly absorbed through the blood vessels in fatty tissue. Warfarin (Coumadin) has a long onset of action, peak concentration, and duration of action, so drug accumulation may occur.

Table 45-2 gives the summary comparison between heparin and warfarin, including methods of administration, drug action, uses, contraindications, laboratory tests, side effects, adverse reactions, and antidotes.

Side Effects and Adverse Reactions. Bleeding (hemorrhage) is the major adverse effect of warfarin. Patients should be monitored closely for signs of bleeding (e.g., petechiae, ecchymosis, hematemesis). Laboratory testing of PT or INR should be scheduled at recommended intervals.

Drug Interactions. Because warfarin is highly protein-bound, it is affected by drug interactions. Aspirin, nonsteroidal antiinflammatory drugs (NSAIDs), other types of antiinflammatory drugs, sulfonamides, phenytoin (Dilantin), cimetidine (Tagamet), allopurinol (Zyloprim), and oral hypoglycemic drugs for diabetes can displace warfarin from the protein-bound site, causing more free-circulating anticoagulant. Numerous other drugs also increase the action of warfarin, and bleeding is likely to occur. Acetaminophen (Tylenol) should be used instead of aspirin by patients taking warfarin. For frank bleeding resulting from excess free drug, parenteral vitamin K is given as a coagulant to decrease bleeding and promote clotting. However, caution must be used with this approach, because the prothrombin can remain depressed for prolonged periods.

Table 45-1 lists the pharmacologic data for the anticoagulants.

Xa Inhibitor: Oral Anticoagulants. Two new oral anticoagulants form a new anticoagulant category called Xa inhibitors. Rivaroxaban (Xarelto) was FDA approved in July 2011, and apixaban (Eliquis) was FDA approved in December 2012. These drugs do not require routine coagulation monitoring and are given once or twice daily (see Table 45-1).

Anticoagulant Antagonists

Bleeding occurs in about 10% of patients taking oral anticoagulants. Vitamin K_1 (phytonadione), an antagonist of warfarin, is used for warfarin overdose or uncontrollable bleeding. Usually 1 to 10 mg of vitamin K_1 is given at once, and if it fails to control bleeding, then fresh whole blood or fresh-frozen plasma or platelets are generally given.

TABLE 45-2 COMPARISON OF PARENTERAL AND ORAL ANTICOAGULANTS

FACTORS TO CONSIDER	HEPARIN	WARFARIN (COUMADIN)
Methods of administration	Subcutaneously Intravenously	Primarily orally
Drug actions	Binds with antithrombin III, which inactivates thrombin and clotting factors, inhibiting fibrin formation	Inhibits hepatic synthesis of vitamin K, which decreases prothrombin and the clotting factors VII, IX, and X
Uses	Treatment of venous thrombosis, pulmonary embolism, thromboembolic complications (e.g., heart surgery, disseminated intravascular coagulation)	Treatment of deep vein thrombosis, pulmonary embolism, transient ischemic attack; prophylactic for cardiac valves
Contraindications/cautions	Hemophilia, peptic ulcer, severe (stage 3 or 4) hypertension, severe liver or renal disease, dissecting aneurysm	Hemophilia, peptic bleeding ulcer, blood dyscrasias, severe liver or kidney disease, acute myocardial infarction, alcoholism
Laboratory tests	PTT: 60-70 sec Anticoagulant therapeutic level: 1.5 to 2 × control in seconds aPTT: 20-35 sec Anticoagulant: aPTT: 30-85 sec	PT: 11-15 sec Anticoagulant therapeutic level: 1.25 to 2.5 × control in seconds INR: 1.3-2 Anticoagulant: INR 2-3 Prosthetic heart valves: INR up to 3.5
Side/adverse effects	Bleeding, hemorrhage, hematoma, severe hypotension	Bleeding, hemorrhage, GI bleeding, ecchymoses, hematuria
Antidote	Protamine sulfate: 1 mg per 100 units of heparin (see Table 45-1)	Vitamin K_1 PO/subQ/IM/IV: 2.5-10 mg, C: subQ/IM: 5-10 mg Infant: 1 mg

A, Adult; *aPTT,* activated partial thromboplastin time; *C,* child; *d,* day; *GI,* gastrointestinal; *IM,* intramuscular; *INR,* international normalized ratio; *IV,* intravenous; *PO,* by mouth; *PT,* prothrombin time; *PTT,* partial thromboplastin time; *sec,* second; *subQ,* subcutaneous.

Nursing Process
Patient-Centered Collaborative Care

Anticoagulants: Warfarin and Heparin

Assessment
- Obtain a history of abnormal clotting or health problems that affect clotting, such as severe alcoholism or severe liver or renal disease. Warfarin is contraindicated for patients with blood dyscrasias, peptic ulcer, cerebrovascular accident (CVA), hemophilia, or severe hypertension. Use with caution in patients with acute traumatic injury.
- Gather a drug and herbal history of current drugs and herbs patient takes. Report if drug-drug or drug-herbal interaction is probable. Warfarin is highly protein-bound and can displace other highly protein-bound drugs, or warfarin could be displaced, which may result in bleeding.
- Develop a flowchart that lists prothrombin time (PT) or international normalized ratio (INR) and warfarin dosages. A baseline PT or INR should be obtained before warfarin is administered.

Nursing Diagnoses
- Risk for injury related to bleeding due to adverse effect of heparin or warfarin
- Deficient knowledge related to lack of previous exposure to side effects of anticoagulants and their action

Planning
- Patient's PT will be 1.25 to 2.5 times control level, or INR will be 2 to 3.
- Patient will not have excessive bleeding.
- Patient's aPTT level will be within a therapeutic range.

Nursing Interventions
- Monitor vital signs. An increased pulse rate followed by a decreased systolic pressure can indicate a fluid volume deficit resulting from external or internal bleeding.
- Monitor PT or INR for warfarin (Coumadin) and aPTT for heparin before administering anticoagulant. PT should be 1.25 to 2.5 times control level or INR 2 to 3, except for prosthetic heart valves (up to INR 3.5). Monitor platelet count (anticoagulants can decrease platelet count).
- Examine patient's mouth, nose (epistaxis), urine (hematuria), and skin (petechiae, purpura) for bleeding. Watch older adults closely for bleeding; their skin is thin, and capillary beds are fragile.
- Check stools periodically for occult blood.
- Keep anticoagulant antagonists (protamine sulfate for heparin and vitamin K for warfarin) available when drug dose is increased or there are indications of frank bleeding. Fresh-frozen plasma may be needed for transfusion.

Patient Teaching
General
- Teach patient to inform dentist when taking an anticoagulant. Contacting health care provider may be necessary.
- Advise patient to use a soft toothbrush to prevent gums from bleeding.
- Warn patient to shave with an electric razor. Bleeding from shaving cuts may be difficult to control.
- Advise patient to have laboratory tests such as PT or INR performed as ordered by health care provider. Warfarin dose is regulated according to INR derived from PT.
- Suggest that patient carry medical identification card or wear MedicAlert bracelet that lists name, telephone number, and drug taken.
- Encourage patient *not* to smoke. Smoking increases drug metabolism, so warfarin dose may need to be increased. If patient insists on smoking, notify health care provider.
- Tell patient to check with health care provider before taking OTC drugs. Aspirin should *not* be taken with warfarin, because aspirin intensifies its action and bleeding is apt to occur. Suggest that patient use acetaminophen.
- Inform patient that many herbal products interact with anticoagulants and may increase bleeding (Herbal Alert 45-1). Closely monitor international normalized ratio (INR) or prothrombin time (PT).
- Teach patient to control external hemorrhage (bleeding) from accidents or injuries by applying firm, direct pressure for at least 5 to 10 minutes with a clean, dry, absorbent material.

Side Effects
- Warn patient to report frank or occult bleeding (petechiae, ecchymosis, purpura, tarry stools, bleeding gums, epistaxis, expectoration of blood).

Diet
- Advise patient to avoid large amounts of green, leafy vegetables; broccoli; legumes; soybean oil (rich in vitamin K); coffee, tea, cola (caffeine); excessive alcohol; and certain herbs and nutritional supplements (coenzyme Q10) or to be very consistent with their intake. Coenzyme Q10, fish oils, items high in vitamin K, St. John's wort, ginseng, and vitamin C may decrease effectiveness of warfarin. Garlic, ginger, kava kava, green tea, chamomile tea, ginkgo biloba, and acute alcohol intoxication decrease warfarin effectiveness.

Cultural Considerations

- Provide instructions in language patient speaks and reads most easily. Certain cultural groups may lack understanding of Western approaches to health problems, drug therapy, adverse effects, and follow-up care concerning thrombophlebitis or other conditions that cause thrombus formation.
- Identify conflicts in cultural values and beliefs of patient regarding method for treating a vascular problem. Respect traditional practices, and incorporate them into care plan if harmless. If method may be harmful, initiate explanations along with nursing plan.

Evaluation

- Evaluate effectiveness of drug therapy. Patient's PT or INR values are within desired range, and patient is free from significant side effects.

HERBAL ALERT 45-1

Anticoagulants: Warfarin and Heparin

- Dong quai, feverfew, garlic, ginger, green tea, chamomile tea, ginkgo, and bilberry may increase bleeding when taken with anticoagulants such as warfarin. Warfarin has an additive effect and increases the international normalized ratio and prothrombin time.
- Excessive doses of anise may interfere with anticoagulants.
- Ginseng may decrease the effects of warfarin, thereby decreasing INR.
- Alfalfa may decrease anticoagulant activity.
- Goldenseal may decrease the effects of heparin and oral anticoagulants.
- Black haw increases the action of anticoagulants.
- Valerian may decrease the effects of warfarin.

ANTIPLATELET DRUGS

Antiplatelets are used to prevent thrombosis in the arteries by suppressing platelet aggregation. Heparin and warfarin prevent thrombosis in the veins.

Antiplatelet drug therapy is mainly for prophylactic use in (1) prevention of myocardial infarction or stroke for patients with familial history, (2) prevention of repeat myocardial infarction or stroke, and (3) prevention of stroke for patients having transient ischemic attacks (TIAs).

Long-term, low-dose aspirin therapy has been found to be both an effective and inexpensive treatment for suppressing platelet aggregation. Aspirin inhibits cyclooxygenase, an enzyme needed by platelets to synthesize thromboxane A_2 (TxA_2). For patients with familial history of stroke or myocardial infarction, the recommended aspirin dose is 81, 162, or 325 mg/d. Because aspirin has prolonged antiplatelet activity, it should be discontinued at least 7 days before surgery.

Other antiplatelet drugs include dipyridamole (Persantine), ticlopidine (Ticlid), clopidogrel (Plavix), anagrelide HCl (Agrylin), abciximab (ReoPro), eptifibatide (Integrilin), tirofiban (Aggrastat), and ticagrelor (Brilinta). Clopidogrel, dipyridamole, and ticlopidine have similar effects as aspirin, but they are known as *adenosine diphosphate (ADP) antagonists* affecting platelet aggregation. Cilostazol (Pletal) inhibits platelet aggregation and is a vasodilator that may be used for intermittent claudication. Ticagrelor is taken in conjunction with aspirin 75 to 100 mg in a maintenance regime. Doses greater than 100 mg should be avoided. Table 45-3 lists the antiplatelets and their dosages, uses, and considerations.

Clopidogrel (Plavix) is an antiplatelet drug frequently used after myocardial infarction or stroke to prevent a second event. It may be prescribed singly or with aspirin. It has been stated that Plavix and aspirin are more effective in inhibiting platelet aggregation if used together than if used as separate antiplatelet therapies. Prototype Drug Chart 45-2 lists the pharmacologic data for clopidogrel (Plavix).

Pharmacokinetics Clopidogrel (Plavix) is rapidly absorbed and has a high protein-binding power. Studies have not established a relationship between the concentration of the main metabolite and platelet aggregation. The half-life is 8 hours; it is usually prescribed once a day. Excretion of the drug metabolite occurs equally in the urine and feces.

Pharmacodynamics Clopidogrel (Plavix) prevents platelet aggregation by blocking the binding of adenosine diphosphate (ADP) to the platelet ADP receptor. ADP-mediated activation of the glycoprotein (GP) IIb/IIIa complex inhibits platelet aggregation. Plavix prolongs bleeding time; therefore it should be discontinued for 7 days preceding surgery. The onset of action of Plavix is 1 to 2 hours, and its peak time is 2 to 3 hours. The drug should not be taken if the patient has a bleeding peptic ulcer, any active bleeding, or intracranial hemorrhage.

Abciximab, eptifibatide, and tirofiban are used primarily for acute coronary syndromes (unstable angina or non–Q-wave myocardial infarction) and for preventing reocclusion of coronary arteries following percutaneous transluminal coronary angioplasty (PTCA). These drugs are usually given before and after PTCA. The drug of choice for angioplasty is abciximab. Abciximab, eptifibatide, and tirofiban block the binding of fibrinogen to the glycoprotein IIb/IIIa receptor on the platelet surface. They are called *platelet glycoprotein (GP) IIb/IIIa receptor antagonists.* Following IV infusion, the antiplatelet effects for abciximab persist for 24 to 48 hours; for eptifibatide and tirofiban, the antiplatelet effects last for 4 hours.

Herbal products can interact with antiplatelet drugs (Herbal Alert 45-2).

THROMBOLYTICS

Thromboembolism (occlusion of an artery or vein caused by a thrombus or embolus) results in **ischemia** (deficient blood flow) that causes **necrosis** (death) of the tissue distal to the obstructed area. It takes approximately 1 to 2 weeks for the blood clot to disintegrate by natural fibrinolytic mechanisms. If a new thrombus or embolus can be dissolved more quickly, tissue necrosis is minimized, and blood flow to the area is reestablished faster. This is the basis for thrombolytic therapy.

Thrombolytics have been used since the early 1980s to promote the fibrinolytic mechanism (converting plasminogen to plasmin, which destroys the fibrin in the blood clot). The thrombus, or blood clot, disintegrates when a thrombolytic drug is administered within 4 hours after an **acute**

TABLE 45-3 **ANTIPLATELETS**

GENERIC (BRAND)	ROUTE AND DOSAGE	USES AND CONSIDERATIONS
anagrelide HCl (Agrylin)	A: PO: 1 mg, b.i.d. May increase by 0.5 mg/d every wk if necessary until platelet count: <600,000 mcL; *max:* 10 mg/d	Selectively inhibits platelet production. Inhibits platelet aggregation; affects aggregating agents ADP, cAMP PDE III, and collagen. Adverse reactions include HF, heart block, pulmonary hypertension, and cardiomyopathy. Pregnancy category: C; PB: UK; $t_{1/2}$: 3-4 d
aspirin, ASA (Bayer, Stanback, Aspergum)	A: PO: 75-100 mg/d	For prevention of thrombosis before or after CVA or MI. Patient should check with health care provider before taking aspirin for antiplatelet therapy. Aspirin not recommended for patients with peptic ulcer or liver dysfunction. Enteric-coated preparation decreases GI upset. Pregnancy category: D; PB: 76%-90%; $t_{1/2}$: 15-20 min
cilostazol (Pletal)	A: PO: 100 mg, b.i.d. 30 min before or 2 h after meals	Inhibits platelet aggregation and is a vasodilator. Indicated for intermittent claudication, peripheral vascular disease. Smoking may decrease serum levels. Adverse reactions include HF, tachycardia, cerebral ischemia, and atrial flutter or fibrillation. Pregnancy category: C; PB: 95%-98%, $t_{1/2}$: 11-13 h
clopidogrel (Plavix)	See Prototype Drug Chart 45-2.	
dipyridamole (Persantine)	A: PO: 75-100 mg q.i.d.	For prevention of thromboembolism post-MI and associated with prosthetic devices (heart valves and hip replacement); prevention of TIA. Monitor blood pressure. Pregnancy category: B; PB: 91%-99%; $t_{1/2}$: 10-12 h
prasugrel (Effient)	A: PO: Loading dose: 60 mg; maint: 10 mg/d	For prevention of thrombotic cardiovascular event. Patient should also take aspirin 75-325 mg/d with prasugrel. Monitor patient for bleeding. Pregnancy category: B; PB: 98%, $t_{1/2}$: 2-15 h
ticlopidine (Ticlid)	A: PO: 250 mg b.i.d.	To reduce risk of strokes and thrombin formation. To treat intermittent claudication and sickle cell disease. Not recommended for patients with hematopoietic disorders such as thrombocytopenia or bleeding peptic ulcer. Pregnancy category: B; PB: 98%: $t_{1/2}$: 8-12 h
ticagrelor (Brilinta)	A: PO: Loading dose: 180 mg with aspirin 325 mg; then 90 mg b.i.d. with aspirin 75-100 mg/d; *max:* 180 mg/d ticagrelor and 100 mg/d aspirin	For prevention of thrombotic cardiovascular event in acute coronary syndrome. Does not have irreversible effects on platelets. Given in combination with aspirin. Pregnancy category: C; PB: 99%: $t_{1/2}$: 7 h
Combination of Antiplatelet Drugs		
dipyridamole and aspirin (Aggrenox)	Stroke prevention: 1 cap b.i.d. (aspirin 25 mg and ER-dipyridamole 200 mg)	Combination of aspirin and ER-dipyridamole for stroke prevention in patients who have had TIA
Antiplatelets: Glycoprotein (GP) IIb/IIIa Receptor Antagonists		
abciximab (ReoPro)	A: IV bolus: 0.25 mg/kg given 10-60 min before PTCA. Inject 4.5 mL abciximab into 250 mL NSS or D_5W. Follow with continuous infusion of 0.125 mcg/kg/min for next 12 h; *max:* 10 mcg/min	To prevent acute cardiac ischemia before and following PTCA and for unstable angina. May cause intracranial hemorrhage. Pregnancy category: C; PB: UK; $t_{1/2}$: 10-30 min
eptifibatide (Integrilin)	A: IV bolus: 180 mcg/kg, then 2 mcg/kg/min for up to 72 h	For acute cardiac syndromes (unstable angina and non–Q-wave MI). Can be used with angioplasty. Pregnancy category: B; PB: 25%; $t_{1/2}$: 1.5-2 h
tirofiban (Aggrastat)	A: IV: 0.4 mcg/kg/min for 30 min, then 0.1 mcg/kg/min for 12-24 h after angioplasty	For acute cardiac syndromes (unstable angina and non–Q-wave MI). May be used with angioplasty. Pregnancy category: B; PB: 65%; $t_{1/2}$: 2 h

ADP, Adenosine diphosphate; *AV,* arteriovenous; *cAMP,* cyclic adenosine monophosphate; *cap,* capsule; *HF,* heart failure; *CVA,* cerebrovascular accident; *d,* day; *ER,* extended-release; *GI,* gastrointestinal; *h,* hour; *maint,* maintenance; *max,* maximum; *MI,* myocardial infarction; *NSS,* normal saline solution; *PTCA,* percutaneous transluminal coronary angioplasty; *q.i.d.,* four times a day; $t_{1/2}$, half-life; *TIA,* transient ischemic attack; *t.i.d.,* three times a day; *UK,* unknown; *wk,* week; >, greater than.

PROTOTYPE DRUG CHART 45-2

Clopidogrel Bisulfate

Drug Class	Dosage
Antiplatelet Trade Name: Plavix Pregnancy Category: B	A: PO: loading dose: 300 mg and then 75 mg/d
Contraindications	**Drug-Lab-Food Interactions**
Intracranial hemorrhage, peptic ulcer, GI bleeding, Caution: Liver disease, surgery, bleeding from trauma, renal disease	Drug: May increase bleeding when taken with NSAIDs, anticoagulants, antineoplastics, azole antifungals, barbiturates; interferes with metabolism of phenytoin, warfarin, fluvastatin, tamoxifen, tolbutamide, NSAIDs, torsemide Lab: Prolongs bleeding time Herb: May increase bleeding when taken with ginger, garlic, ginkgo, feverfew, green tea
Pharmacokinetics	**Pharmacodynamics**
Absorption: Rapid Distribution: PB: 94%-98% Metabolism: t½: 8 h Excretion: 50% in urine and 50% in feces	PO: Onset: 1-2 h Peak: 2-3 h Duration: 3 d or longer
Therapeutic Effects/Uses	
To prevent recurrence of MI, stroke; to prevent vascular death. Mode of Action: Inhibits platelet aggregation. Prevents ADP from binding with the ADP platelet receptor.	
Side Effects	**Adverse Reactions**
Abdominal pain, flulike symptoms, dizziness, epistaxis, headaches, fatigue, chest pain, diarrhea	Hypotension, bronchospasm Life-threatening: Agranulocytosis, aplastic anemia, thrombocytopenia

A, Adult; *ADP*, adenosine diphosphate; *GI*, gastrointestinal; *h*, hour; *PB*, protein-binding; *PO*, by mouth; *MI*, myocardial infarction; *NSAIDs*, nonsteroidal antiinflammatory drugs; *RTI*, respiratory tract infection; *t ½*, half-life.

HERBAL ALERT 45-2

Antiplatelets

Dong quai, feverfew, garlic, and *ginkgo biloba* interfere with platelet aggregation. When these herbs are taken with an antiplatelet drug such as aspirin, increased bleeding may occur.

myocardial infarction (AMI) (acute heart attack). Necrosis resulting from the blocked artery is prevented or minimized, and hospitalization time may be decreased. The need for cardiac bypass or coronary angioplasty can be evaluated soon after thrombolytic treatment. A thrombolytic drug should be administered within 3 hours of a thrombolic stroke. These drugs are also used for pulmonary embolism, DVT, noncoronary arterial occlusion from an acute thromboembolism, and thrombolic stroke.

Commonly used thrombolytics include urokinase (Abbokinase), alteplase tPA (Activase), reteplase rPA (Retavase), and tenecteplase TNK-tPA (TNKase). Streptokinase and urokinase are enzymes that act systemically to promote the conversion of plasminogen to plasmin. Alteplase, also known as *tissue plasminogen activator (tPA)*, is clot-specific and binds to the fibrin surface of a clot, promoting the conversion of plasminogen to plasmin. Plasmin, an enzyme, digests the fibrin in the clot. Plasmin also degrades fibrinogen, prothrombin, and other clotting factors. These five drugs all induce **fibrinolysis** (fibrin breakdown). Prototype Drug Chart 45-3 lists the pharmacologic data for alteplase.

Reteplase (Retavase) is a derivative of tPA. Anticoagulants and antiplatelet drugs increase the risk of hemorrhage; therefore they should be avoided until the thrombolytic effect has passed. The health care provider needs to determine whether the patient has taken any of these drugs before seeking treatment.

SAFETY: Preventing Medication Errors

Do not confuse...

Tenecteplase (TNKase) and **tissue plasminogen activator (tPA).** These two drugs look alike and are from the same class—thrombolytics—but they are different, and their dosages and administration time are different. TNKase is administered as a single dose; tPA is administered in three different doses and times. The first dose is a bolus, and the second and third doses are administered over 30 minutes and 60 minutes, respectively.

PROTOTYPE DRUG CHART 45-3

Alteplase (Tissue Plasminogen Activator [tPA])

Drug Class Thrombolytic agent Trade Names: Activase Pregnancy Category: C	**Dosage** A: IV bolus: 15 mg, then 50 mg infused over 30 min, then 35 mg infused over 60 min; *max:* 100 mg
Contraindications Internal bleeding, bleeding disorders, recent CVA, surgery or trauma, bacterial endocarditis, severe liver dysfunction, severe uncontrolled hypertension, brain tumor, head trauma Caution: Cardiac dysrhythmias, hepatic or renal disease	**Drug-Lab-Food Interactions** Drug: Increase bleeding when taken with oral anticoagulants, NSAIDs, cefotetan, plicamycin; decrease effect when taken with nitroglycerin Lab: Decrease in plasminogen, fibrinogen, hematocrit, and hemoglobin Herbs: Increased bleeding with ginkgo biloba, garlic, feverfew, ginger, green tea
Pharmacokinetics Absorption: Direct IV Distribution: PB: UK Metabolism: $t\frac{1}{2}$: 30-45 min Excretion: Urine	**Pharmacodynamics** PO: Onset: Immediate Peak: 5-10 min Duration: 3 h
Therapeutic Effects/Uses To dissolve clot following acute MI, pulmonary embolism, acute ischemic stroke. Mode of Action: Alteplase promotes conversion of plasminogen to plasmin. Plasmin, an enzyme, digests fibrin matrix of clots. Alteplase initiates fibrinolysis.	
Side Effects Bleeding, nausea, vomiting, fever	**Adverse Reactions** Anaphylactoid reactions, laryngeal edema, angioedema; cholesterol microembolization (purple-toe syndrome, gangrenous digitus, hypertension, spinal cord infarction, MI, cerebral infarction, bowel infarction, rhabdomyolysis) Life-threatening: Intracerebral hemorrhage, stroke, atrial or ventricular dysrhythmias, pulmonary edema

A, Adult; *CVA,* cerebrovascular accident; *IV,* intravenous; *PB,* protein-binding; *max,* maximum; *min,* minute; *NSAIDs,* nonsteroidal antiinflammatory drugs; *PO,* by mouth; $t\frac{1}{2}$, half-life; *tPA,* tissue plasminogen activator; *UK,* unknown.

Pharmacokinetics The commercial preparation of alteplase (tissue plasminogen activator [tPA]) is identical to natural human tPA, the enzyme that converts plasminogen to plasmin. Alteplase is initially administered as an IV bolus, then infused over 30 minutes, and then 60 minutes. A total dose of 100 mg is the recommended maximum; a larger dose could result in risk for intracranial bleeding. The half-life of alteplase (tPA) is 5 minutes, shorter than the half-life of streptokinase. Alteplase is very expensive but about the same as TNKase and reteplase. Allergic reactions to alteplase occur less frequently than to anistreplase and urokinase.

Pharmacodynamics Alteplase is similar to natural human tissue plasminogen activator (tPA). It promotes thrombolysis by converting plasminogen to plasmin. Plasmin degrades fibrin, fibrinogen, and factors V, VIII, and XII. Alteplase does not induce hypotension as streptokinase does. Peak action of Alteplase is 5 to 10 minutes. The duration of action is 3 hours.

Side Effects and Adverse Reactions. Allergic reactions can complicate thrombolytic therapy. Anaphylaxis (vascular collapse) occurs more frequently with streptokinase than with the other thrombolytics. If the drugs are administered through an intracoronary catheter after myocardial infarction, reperfusion dysrhythmia or hemorrhagic infarction at the myocardial necrotic area can result. The major complication of thrombolytic drugs is hemorrhage. The antithrombolytic drug aminocaproic acid (Amicar) is used to stop bleeding by inhibiting plasminogen activation, which inhibits thrombolysis.

Table 45-4 lists the thrombolytic drugs and their dosages, uses, and considerations.

Nursing Process
Patient-Centered Collaborative Care

Thrombolytics

Assessment
- Assess baseline vital signs for comparison with future values.
- Check baseline complete blood count (CBC), prothrombin time (PT), or international normalized ratio (INR) values before administration of thrombolytics.
- Obtain a medical and drug history. Contraindications for use of thrombolytics include recent cerebrovascular accident (CVA), active bleeding, severe hypertension, and anticoagulant therapy. Report if patient takes

TABLE 45-4 THROMBOLYTICS

GENERIC (BRAND)	ROUTE AND DOSAGE	USES AND CONSIDERATIONS
Thrombolytics		
reteplase, r-PA (Retavase)	A: IV bolus: 10 units over 2 min, then repeat 10 units in 30 min (total of 20 units)	For lysis of thrombi after AMI. Inhibits fibrin aspect of thrombus. Derivative of tPA (Alteplase). Considered more effective than tPA with less risk of hemorrhage. Pregnancy category: C; PB: UK; t½: 13-16 min
tenecteplase, TNK-tPA (TNKase)	A: IV: *max:* 30-50 mg Note: Dose is based on body weight.	To reduce mortality associated with AMI. A "clot buster" that can be administered in 5 seconds in one dose. Pregnancy category: C; PB: UK; t½: 11-138 min
alteplase (tPA, Activase)	See Prototype Drug Chart 45-3.	
urokinase (Abbokinase)	A: IV: LD: 4400 international units/kg diluted and infused over 10 min, then continuous infusion: 4400 international units/kg over 12 h	Same uses as streptokinase. Causes less allergic reaction but is more expensive than streptokinase. Not susceptible to antistreptokinase antibodies. May also be used for peripheral artery occlusion. Pregnancy category: B; PB: UK; t½: 10-20 min
Plasminogen Inactivators		
aminocaproic acid (Amicar)	A: PO/IV: LD: 4-5 g first h Inf: 1-1.25 g/h for 8 h; *max:* 30 g/d	To control excessive bleeding from hyperfibrinolysis. Side effects include orthostatic hypotension, headache, and thrombophlebitis. Pregnancy category: C; PB: 0%; t½: 1-2 h

A, Adult; *AMI,* acute myocardial infarction; *d,* day; *DVT,* deep vein thrombosis; *h,* hour; *inf,* infusion; *IV,* intravenous; *LD,* loading dose; *max,* maximum; *MI,* myocardial infarction; *min,* minute; *PB,* protein-binding; *PE,* pulmonary embolism; *t½,* half-life; *tPA,* tissue plasminogen activator; *UK,* unknown.

aspirin or nonsteroidal antiinflammatory drugs (NSAIDs). Thrombolytics are contraindicated for patients with a recent history of traumatic injury, especially head injury.

Nursing Diagnoses

- Decreased cardiac output related to excessive bleeding
- Anxiety related to fear of the unknown secondary to coronary artery disease
- Impaired tissue integrity related to a thrombus or embolus secondary to heart attack, or stroke
- Risk for injury related to thrombus or embolus

Planning

- Patient's blood clot will be dissolved.
- Patient's vital signs will be monitored for stability during and after thrombolytic therapy.
- Patient will not have excessive bleeding from thrombolytic therapy.

Nursing Interventions

- Monitor vital signs. Increased pulse rate followed by decreased blood pressure usually indicates blood loss and impending shock. Record vital signs, and report changes.
- Observe for signs and symptoms of active bleeding from the mouth or rectum. Hemorrhage is a serious complication of thrombolytic treatment. Aminocaproic acid can be given as an intervention to stop bleeding.
- Examine patient for active bleeding for 24 hours after thrombolytic therapy has been discontinued: q15min for first hour, q30min until eighth hour, and then hourly.
- Observe for signs of allergic reaction to thrombolytics, such as itching, hives, flush, fever, dyspnea, bronchospasm, hypotension, and/or cardiovascular collapse.
- Avoid administering aspirin or NSAIDs for pain or discomfort when patient is receiving a thrombolytic. Acetaminophen can be substituted.
- Monitor electrocardiogram for presence of reperfusion dysrhythmias as blood clot is dissolving; antidysrhythmic therapy may be indicated.
- Avoid venipuncture/arterial sticks.

Patient Teaching

General

- Explain thrombolytic treatment to patient and family. Be supportive.

Side Effects

- Advise patient to report any side effects, such as lightheadedness, dizziness, palpitations, nausea, pruritus, or urticaria.

Evaluation

- Determine effectiveness of drug therapy: clot has dissolved, vital signs are stable, no signs or symptoms of active bleeding, and patient is pain free.

KEY WEBSITES

Copidogrel: *www.medicinenet.com/clopidogrel-oral/article.htm*

Anticoagulation: *www.acforum.org*

CRITICAL THINKING CASE STUDY

TM, a 57-year-old man, has thrombophlebitis in the right lower leg. IV heparin, 5000 units by bolus, was given. Following the IV bolus, heparin 5000 units given subQ q6h was prescribed. Other therapeutic means to decrease pain and alleviate swelling and redness were also prescribed. An aPTT test was ordered.

1. Was TM's heparin order within the safe daily dosage range?
2. What are the various methods for administering heparin?
3. Why was an aPTT test ordered? How would you determine whether TM is within the desired range? Explain your answer.

After 5 days of heparin therapy, TM was prescribed warfarin (Coumadin) 5 mg PO daily. An INR test was ordered.

4. What is the pharmacologic action of warfarin? Is the warfarin dose within the safe daily dosage range? Explain your answer.
5. What are the half-life and protein-binding for warfarin? If a patient takes a drug that is highly protein-bound, would there be a drug interaction? Explain your answer.
6. Why was an INR ordered for TM? What is the desired range?
7. What serious adverse reactions could result with prolonged use or large doses of warfarin?
8. What patient teaching interventions should the nurse include? List three interventions.
9. Months later, TM has hematemesis. What nursing action should be taken?

NCLEX STUDY QUESTIONS

1. A patient is placed on heparin, and the nurse acknowledges that heparin is effective for preventing clot formation in patients who have which disorder(s)? (Select all that apply.)
   a. Coronary thrombosis
   b. Acute myocardial infarction
   c. Deep vein thrombosis
   d. Hemorrhagic cerebrovascular accident (stroke)
   e. Disseminated intravascular coagulation
2. A patient who received heparin begins to bleed. The nurse anticipates that the health care provider will order which antidote?
   a. protamine sulfate
   b. vitamin K_1 (Mephyton)
   c. aminocaproic acid (Amicar)
   d. potassium chloride (KCl)
3. A patient is prescribed enoxaparin (Lovenox). The nurse knows that low–molecular-weight heparin has what kind of half-life?
   a. A longer half-life than heparin
   b. A shorter half-life than heparin
   c. The same half-life as heparin
   d. A four times shorter half-life than heparin
4. The nurse is teaching a patient about clopidogrel (Plavix). Which information will the nurse include in the patient's teaching plan?
   a. Constipation may occur.
   b. Hypotension may occur.
   c. Bleeding may increase when taken with aspirin.
   d. Normal dose is 25 mg tablet per day.
5. A patient had an orthopedic surgery and is prescribed dalteparin (Fragmin). What would the nurse teach the patient and/or family about this low–molecular-weight heparin (LMWH) before discharge?
   a. How to administer the medication intramuscularly
   b. PT and INR monitoring will be done weekly.
   c. Avoidance of green leafy vegetables is recommended.
   d. Watch for bleeding or excessive bruising.
6. A patient is being changed from an injectable anticoagulant to an oral anticoagulant. Which anticoagulant does the nurse realize is administered orally?
   a. enoxaparin sodium (Lovenox)
   b. warfarin (Coumadin)
   c. bivalirudin (Angiomax)
   d. lepirudin (Refludan)
7. A patient is taking warfarin 5 mg/day for atrial fibrillation. The patient's international normalized ratio (INR) is 3.8. The nurse would consider the INR to be what?
   a. Within normal range
   b. Elevated range
   c. Low range
   d. Low-average range
8. Cilostazol (Pletal) is being prescribed for a patient with coronary artery disease. The nurse understands that which is the major purpose for antiplatelet drug therapy?
   a. Dissolve the blood clot
   b. Decrease tissue necrosis
   c. Inhibit hepatic synthesis of vitamin K
   d. Suppress platelet aggregation

9. A patient is to undergo a coronary angioplasty. The nurse acknowledges that which drug is used primarily for preventing reocclusion of coronary arteries following coronary angioplasty?
   a. clopidogrel (Plavix)
   b. abciximab (ReoPro)
   c. warfarin (Coumadin)
   d. cilostazol (Pletal)
10. A patient is admitted to the emergency department with an acute myocardial infarction. Which drug does the nurse anticipate the health care provider to order for prevention of tissue necrosis following blood clot blockage in a coronary artery?
   a. heparin sodium
   b. clopidogrel (Plavix)
   c. alteplase (rPA, Activase)
   d. aminocaproic acid (Amicar)

Answers: 1, a, b, c, d, e; 2, a; 3, a; 4, c; 5, d; 6, b; 7, b; 8, d; 9, b; 10, c.

CHAPTER

46

Antihyperlipidemics and Peripheral Vasodilators

evolve WEBSITE

http://evolve.elsevier.com/KeeHayes/pharmacology/

- Animations
- Content Updates
- Key Points
- Review Questions for the NCLEX® Examination
- References from the Textbook
- Unfolding Case Studies

OBJECTIVES

- Describe the action of the two main drug groups: antihyperlipidemics and peripheral vasodilators.
- Compare the side effects and adverse reactions of antihyperlipidemics.
- Differentiate the side effects and adverse reactions of peripheral vasodilators.
- Apply the nursing process, including patient teaching, for antihyperlipidemics and peripheral vasodilators.

OUTLINE

KEY TERMS

Various drugs are used to maintain or decrease blood lipid concentrations and promote dilation of vessels. Drugs that lower blood lipids are called *antihyperlipidemics, antilipidemics, antilipemics,* and *hypolipidemics.* In this chapter, drugs used to lower lipoproteins are called **antihyperlipidemics. Peripheral vasodilators** are drugs that dilate vessels that have been narrowed by vasospasm.

LIPOPROTEINS

Lipids (cholesterol, triglycerides, and phospholipids) are bound in the inner shell of protein, which is a carrier that transports lipids in the bloodstream. When there is an excess of one or more lipids in the blood, the condition is known as **hyperlipidemia** or *hyperlipoproteinemia.* The four major categories of **lipoprotein** are **high-density lipoprotein** (HDL), **low-density lipoprotein** (LDL), **very low-density lipoprotein** (VLDL), and chylomicrons. HDL, also known as "friendly" or "good" lipoprotein, is the smallest, most dense lipoprotein, meaning that it contains more protein and less fat than the others. The function of HDL is to remove cholesterol from the bloodstream and deliver it to the liver for excretion in bile. LDL, the "bad" lipoprotein, contains 50% to 60% of cholesterol in the bloodstream. With an elevated LDL,

TABLE 46-1 **LIPOPROTEIN GROUPS**

LIPOPROTEIN SUBGROUPS	COMPOSITION OF LIPOPROTEINS			
	PROTEIN (%)	CHOLESTEROL (%)	TRIGLYCERIDES (%)	PHOSPHOLIPIDS (%)
Chylomicrons	1-2	1-3	80-95	3-6
Very low density	6-10	8-20	45-65	15-20
Low density	15-20	50-60	4-8	16-20
High density	45-55	15-20	2-7	26-32

TABLE 46-2 **SERUM LIPID VALUES**

LIPIDS	DESIRABLE (mg/dL)	LEVEL OF RISK FOR CAD		
		LOW RISK (mg/dL)	MODERATE RISK (mg/dL)	HIGH RISK (mg/dL)
Cholesterol	150-200	200	200-240	>240
Triglycerides	40-150	Values vary with age	Values vary with age	>190
Lipoproteins				
LDL	<100	100-130	130-159	>160
HDL	>60	50-60	35-50	<35

CAD, Coronary artery disease; *HDL,* high-density lipoproteins; *LDL,* low-density lipoproteins.

there is greater risk for developing atherosclerotic plaques and heart disease. VLDL carries mostly triglycerides and less cholesterol. The **chylomicrons** are large particles that transport fatty acids and cholesterol to the liver. They are composed mostly of triglycerides. Table 46-1 presents the composition of the lipoproteins.

Serum cholesterol and triglyceride measurements are frequently part of a regular physical examination or readmission evaluation and are used as baseline test results. If the levels are high, a 12- to 14-hour fasting lipid profile may be ordered. When cholesterol, triglycerides, and LDL are elevated, the patient is at increased risk for coronary artery disease (CAD). Table 46-2 lists the various serum lipids and their reference values (normal serum levels) according to risk classification.

APOLIPOPROTEINS

Apolipoproteins are within the lipoprotein shell and contain apolipoprotein (apo) A-1, apoB, and apoE. The major component of apoA1 is HDL. The major component of apoB is LDL, which exists in two forms, apoB-100 and apoB-48. ApoB-100 has VLDL as well as LDL and is a better indicator of risk for coronary artery disease (CAD) than LDL alone.

NONPHARMACOLOGIC METHODS FOR CHOLESTEROL REDUCTION

Before drugs to lower LDL and raise HDL are prescribed, nondrug therapy should be initiated for decreasing cholesterol. Saturated fats and cholesterol in the diet should be reduced. Total fat intake should be 30% or less of caloric intake, and cholesterol intake should be 300 mg/d or less. The patient should be advised to read labels on containers and buy appropriate foods. Patients should choose lean meats, especially chicken and fish.

In many cases, diet alone will not lower blood lipid levels. Because 75% to 85% of serum cholesterol is endogenously (internally) derived, dietary modification alone will typically lower total cholesterol levels by only 10% to 30%. This and the fact that adherence to dietary restrictions is often short-lived explains why many patients do not respond to diet modification alone.

Exercise is an important aspect of the nonpharmacologic method to reduce cholesterol and increase HDL. For the older adult, exercise can be walking and bicycling. Smoking is another risk factor that should be eliminated. Smoking increases LDL cholesterol and decreases HDL.

If nonpharmacologic methods are ineffective for reducing cholesterol, LDL, and VLDL and hyperlipidemia remains, antihyperlipidemic drugs are prescribed to lower blood lipid levels. It must be emphasized to the patient that dietary changes need to be made and an exercise program followed even after drug therapy is initiated. The type of antihyperlipidemics ordered depends on the lipoprotein phenotype (Table 46-3).

ANTIHYPERLIPIDEMICS

Drugs that lower lipid levels include bile-acid sequestrants, fibrates (fibric acid), nicotinic acid, cholesterol absorption inhibitor, and hepatic 3-hydroxy-3-methylglutaryl-coenzyme A (HMG-CoA) reductase inhibitors (statins). The statins have fewer adverse effects and are well tolerated.

TABLE 46-3 HYPERLIPIDEMIA: LIPOPROTEIN PHENOTYPE

TYPE*	MAJOR LIPIDS
I	Increased chylomicrons and increased triglycerides. Uncommon.
IIA	Increased low-density lipoprotein (LDL) and increased cholesterol. Common.
IIB	Increased very low-density lipoprotein (VLDL), increased LDL, increased cholesterol and triglycerides. Very common.
III	Moderately increased cholesterol and triglycerides. Uncommon.
IV	Increased VLDL and markedly increased triglycerides. Very common.
V	Increased chylomicrons, VLDL, and triglycerides. Uncommon.

*Types II and IV are commonly associated with coronary artery disease.

One of the first antihyperlipidemics, cholestyramine (Questran), is a bile-acid sequestrant that reduces LDL cholesterol (LDL-C) levels by binding with bile acids in the intestine. It is effective against hyperlipidemia type II. This group may be used as an adjunct to the statins. The drug comes in a gritty powder, which is mixed thoroughly in water or juice. Colestipol (Colestid) is another resin antihyperlipidemic similar to cholestyramine. Both are effective in lowering cholesterol. Colesevelam HCl, another bile acid sequestrant similar to cholestyramine and colestipol, is an agent that has fewer side effects (less constipation, flatulence, and cramping). Colesevelam also has less effect on the absorption of fat-soluble vitamins than the older agents and is usually the first-choice bile-acid sequestrant drug.

Gemfibrozil (Lopid) is a fibric acid derivative that is more effective at reducing triglyceride and VLDL levels than reducing LDL. It is used primarily to reduce hyperlipidemia type IV, but it can also be used for type II hyperlipidemia. This drug is highly protein-bound and should not be taken with anticoagulants, because they compete for protein sites. The anticoagulant dose should be reduced during antihyperlipidemic therapy, and the international normalized ratio (INR) should be closely monitored. Fenofibrate has similar actions and some of the same side effects as gemfibrozil. If taken with warfarin, bleeding might occur. It is highly protein-bound.

Nicotinic acid, or niacin (vitamin B_3), reduces VLDL and LDL. Nicotinic acid is actually very effective at lowering cholesterol levels, and its effect on the lipid profile is highly desirable. Because it has numerous side effects and large doses are required, as few as 20% of patients can initially tolerate niacin. However, with proper counseling, careful drug titration, and concomitant use of aspirin, this number can be increased to as high as 60% to 70%.

Ezetimibe (Zetia) is a cholesterol absorption inhibitor that acts on the cells in the small intestine to inhibit cholesterol absorption. It decreases cholesterol from dietary absorption, reducing serum cholesterol, LDL, triglycerides, and apoB levels. Ezetimibe causes only a small increase in HDL. It must be combined with a statin for optimum effect (ezetimibe and simvastatin [Zocor], marketed as Vytorin).

Statins

The statin drugs inhibit the enzyme HMG CoA reductase in cholesterol biosynthesis; thus the statins are called *HMG CoA reductase inhibitors.* By inhibiting cholesterol synthesis in the liver, this group of antihyperlipidemics decreases the concentration of cholesterol, decreases LDL, and slightly increases HDL cholesterol. Reduction of LDL cholesterol may be seen as early as 2 weeks after initiating therapy. The statin group has been useful in decreasing CAD and reducing mortality rates.

Numerous statins have been approved since they were first introduced. The present group of statins includes atorvastatin calcium (Lipitor), fluvastatin (Lescol), lovastatin (Mevacor), pravastatin sodium (Pravachol), simvastatin (Zocor), and rosuvastatin calcium (Crestor). Lovastatin was the first statin used to decrease cholesterol. It is effective in lowering LDL (hyperlipidemia type II) within several weeks. Gastrointestinal (GI) disturbances, headaches, muscle cramps, and fatigue are early complaints. With all statins, serum liver enzymes should be monitored, and an annual eye examination is needed, because cataract formation may result. The patient should report immediately any muscle aches or weakness, which can lead to rhabdomyolysis, a muscle disintegration that can become fatal.

The statins have actions in decreasing serum cholesterol, LDL, VLDL, and triglycerides, and they slightly elevate HDL. Atorvastatin, lovastatin, and simvastatin are more effective at lowering LDL than the other statins. Atorvastatin and simvastatin are at the top of the list of most prescribed drugs in the United States.

The statin drugs can be combined with other drugs to decrease blood pressure and blood clotting and to enhance the antihyperlipidemic effect. Examples are Advicor (lovastatin and niacin), Caduet (atorvastatin and amlodipine), Vytorin (simvastatin and ezetimibe), and Liptruzet (ezetimibe and atorvastatin). Table 46-4 lists these combination drugs and their dosages, uses, and considerations.

If antihyperlipidemic therapy is withdrawn, cholesterol and LDL levels return to pretreatment levels. The patient taking an antihyperlipidemic drug should understand that antihyperlipidemic therapy is a lifetime commitment for maintaining a decrease in serum lipid levels. Abruptly stopping the statin drug could cause a threefold rebound effect that may cause death from acute myocardial infarction (AMI).

Laboratory Tests

Homocysteine reference values are 4 to 17 mmol/L (fasting). Homocysteine, an amino acid, is a by-product of protein and is found in eggs, chicken, beef, and cheddar cheese. A high level of homocysteine has been linked to cardiovascular disease, stroke, and the possibility of Alzheimer's disease. It may also promote blood clotting. It has been stated that an increase in serum homocysteine can damage the inner

TABLE 46-4 ANTIHYPERLIPIDEMICS

GENERIC (BRAND)	ROUTE AND DOSAGE	USES AND CONSIDERATIONS
Bile-Acid Sequestrants		
cholestyramine (Questran, Prevalite)	A: PO: 4 g 1-2 times/d; mix powder in 120-240 mL of fluid; *max:* 24 g/d C >6 y: PO: 80 mg/kg/d t.i.d.	For type II hyperlipoproteinemia (LDL). Decrease in LDL apparent in 1 week. Mix powder well in 4-6 oz fluid. Has no effect on VLDL and HDL, but could increase triglyceride levels. GI upset and constipation can occur. Vitamin A, D, or K deficiency may occur because of decreased GI absorption. Pregnancy category: C; PB: UK; t½: UK
colesevelam (Welchol)	A: PO: 3 tabs (625 mg/tab) b.i.d. or 6 tabs/d with meals	Cholesterol-lowering effect achieved by binding with bile salts in intestines to form insoluble complex with fecal excretions, reducing circulating cholesterol, including LDL. Triglycerides may be slightly increased. Contraindicated with bowel obstruction. May be used in combination with a statin drug. Pregnancy category: B; PB: UK; t½: UK
colestipol HCl (Colestid)	A: PO: 5-20 g/d in divided doses; *max:* 30 g/d	To reduce cholesterol and LDL levels. Same as cholestyramine. Pregnancy category: C; PB: UK; t½: UK
Fibrates (Fibric Acid)		
fenofibrate (TriCor)	A: PO: 48-145 mg/d; *max:* 148 mg/d	Treatment of type IV and V hyperlipidemia, and for hypertriglyceridemia. Specified diet should be part of drug therapy. Monitor serum creatinine levels. Pregnancy category: C; PB: 99%; t½: 20 h
gemfibrozil (Lopid)	A: PO: 600 mg b.i.d. 30 min before meals; *max:* 1,200 mg/d	For VLDL and elevated triglycerides; LDL may decrease, and HDL may increase. For types II (VLDL, LDL), III, IV, and V hyperlipidemia. Use in combination with lovastatin contraindicated because of increase in CPK. Pregnancy category: C; PB: 95%; t½: 1.5 h
Nicotinic Acid		
niacin (nicotinic acid) (Niaspan)	A: PO: Initially: 250 mg/d; maint: 1.5-2 g/d with meals in 3 divided doses; *max:* 6 g/d	For VLDL and LDL: types II, III, IV, and V hyperlipidemia. Doses are 100 times higher than RDA to lower VLDL. Pregnancy category: C; PB: <20%; t½: 45 min
Cholesterol Absorption Inhibitors		
ezetimibe (Zetia)	A/C >10 y: PO: 10 mg/d	Inhibits cholesterol absorption in small intestine. Reduces total cholesterol, LDL, and triglycerides. Increases HDL. Caution with liver dysfunction and elevated serum transaminase. Pregnancy category: C; PB: 90%; t½: 22 h
Statins (HMG-CoA Reductase Inhibitors)		
atorvastatin calcium (Lipitor)	A: PO: 10-40 mg/d; *max:* 80 mg/d	Treatment of dyslipidemia and hypercholesterolemia. Monitor liver enzymes for elevation. Pregnancy category: X; PB 98%; t½: 20-30 h
fluvastatin sodium (Lescol)	A: PO: Initially: 20-40 mg h.s.; maint: 20-80 mg/d; *max:* 80 mg/d	Treatment of types IIA and IIB hyperlipidemia, total cholesterol, and elevated triglycerides. HDL slightly increased. Monitor liver function (liver enzymes). Pregnancy category: X; PB: 98%; t½: 2.5 h
lovastatin (Mevacor)	A: PO: 10-20 mg/d with evening meal; *max:* 80 mg/d	Controls cholesterol by inhibiting cholesterol synthesis. Decreases LDL, increases some HDL. Monitor liver enzymes. Pregnancy category: X; PB: 95%; t½: 1-2 h
pravastatin sodium (Pravachol)	A: PO: 10-80 mg/d; *max:* 80 mg/d	Decreases serum cholesterol, LDL, VLDL, and triglycerides. HDL slightly increased. Monitor liver enzymes. Pregnancy category: X; PB: 50%; t½: 1.5-2.5 h
rosuvastatin calcium (Crestor)	See Prototype Drug Chart 46-1.	
simvastatin (Zocor)	A: PO: 5-40 mg/d in evening; *max:* 40 mg/d	Similar to lovastatin. Monitor liver enzymes. Pregnancy category: X; PB: 95%; t½: 2 h
pitavastatin (Livalo)	A: PO: Initially 2 mg/d; maint: 1-4 mg/d; *max:* 4 mg/d	Moderate reduction of LDLs and only modest increase in HDLs. May cause rhabdomyolysis. Monitor liver enzymes and muscle pain. Pregnancy category: X; PB: 99%; t½: 12 h
Miscellaneous Antilipemics		
icosapent ethyl (Vascepa)	A: PO: 2 g q12h; *max:* 4 g/d	For severe hypertriglyceridemia (triglyceride levels >500 mg/dL as an adjunct to diet. Monitor bleeding time for prolonged levels. Pregnancy category: C; PB: 99%; t½: 89 h
lomitapide (Juxtapid)	A: PO: 5 mg/d, may increase to 10 mg in 2 wks; *max:* 60 mg/d	For hypercholesterolemia. Most common adverse effects are GI disorders such as nausea, vomiting, abdominal pain, and diarrhea. Pregnancy category: X; PB: 99.8%; t½: 39.7 h
Omega 3 fatty acids (Lovaza)	A: PO: 4 g/d	For hypertriglyceridemia. Pregnancy category: C; PB: UK; t½: UK

TABLE 46-4 ANTIHYPERLIPIDEMICS—cont'd

GENERIC (BRAND)	ROUTE AND DOSAGE	USES AND CONSIDERATIONS
Combination Anticholesterol Drugs		
niacin and lovastatin (Advicor)	A: PO: 500 mg niacin/20 mg lovastatin Also available: 750 mg/20 mg; 1000 mg/20 mg; 1,000 mg/40 mg	Niacin raises HDL, triglycerides; lovastatin lowers LDL. Indicated for hypercholesterolemia and mixed dyslipidemia.
amlodipine and atorvastatin (Caduet)	A: PO: 2.5 mg amlodipine/20 mg atorvastatin/d; Also available: 2.5 mg/40 mg; 5 mg/10 mg to 5 mg/80 mg; 10 mg/10 mg to 10 mg/80 mg	Combination of calcium channel blocker and statin. Useful in treating hypertension and dyslipidemia. Helpful to patients who take these drugs separately.
ezetimibe/simvastatin (Vytorin)	A: PO: 10/10 mg to 10/80 mg	Combination of ezetimibe (Zetia) and simvastatin (Zocor). Ezetimibe decreases absorption of cholesterol in small intestine; simvastatin interferes with production of cholesterol in liver.
Ezetimibe and atorvastatin (Liptruzet)	A: PO: 10 mg daily	For hyperlipidemia. May cause increased ALT and AST. Pregnancy category: X; PB: 90%-98%; t½: 14 h

A, Adult; *a.c.,* before meals; *b.i.d.,* twice a day; *CPK,* creatine phosphokinase; *d,* day; *GI,* gastrointestinal; *h,* hour; *HDL,* high-density lipoprotein; *h.s.,* at bedtime; *LDL,* low-density lipoprotein; *maint,* maintenance; *max,* maximum; *min,* minute; *PB,* protein-binding; *p.c.,* after meals; *PO,* by mouth; *q.i.d.,* four times a day; *RDA,* recommended daily allowance; *t½,* half-life; *tab,* tablet; *t.i.d.,* three times a day; *UK,* unknown; *VLDL,* very low-density lipoprotein; >, greater than.

lining of blood vessels and promote a thickening and loss of flexibility in the vessel. Three vitamins that can lower serum homocysteine levels are vitamin B_6 (pyridoxine), vitamin B_{12} (cyanocobalamin), and folic acid.

High-sensitivity C-reactive protein (hsCRP) reference values are <0.175 mg/L; low risk are <1 mg/L; moderate risk are 1 to 3 mg/L; and high risk are >3 mg/L. The standard C-Reactive Protein (CP) is produced in the liver in response to tissue injury and inflammation. The hsCRP is a highly sensitive test for detecting the inflammatory protein that can be associated with cardiovascular and peripheral vascular disease. This test is frequently ordered along with cholesterol screen testing. Approximately one third of persons who have had a heart attack have normal cholesterol levels and normal blood pressure. A positive hsCRP test can indicate that the patient is at high risk for coronary artery disease (CAD), making it a valuable test for predicting CAD. This test can detect an inflammatory process caused by the buildup of atherosclerotic plaque in the arterial system, particularly the coronary arteries.

Prototype Drug Chart 46-1 lists the pharmacologic data for a frequently prescribed antihyperlipidemic, rosuvastatin.

Pharmacokinetics Rosuvastatin (Crestor) decreases LDL by 46% at a dose of 10 mg. It is highly protein-bound, so it usually is prescribed as a once-daily dose. Rosuvastatin has a half-life of 20 hours.

Pharmacodynamics The positive effect of lowering lipids with rosuvastatin is seen in about 2 weeks. The peak time after a dose of rosuvastatin is 3 to 5 hours; however, it takes 2 to 4 weeks to achieve therapeutic effect. When the patient is taking high doses of rosuvastatin or any statins, myopathy and rhabdomyolysis (disintegration of striated muscle fibers) may occur. If the patient complains of muscle pain or tenderness, it should be reported immediately.

Side Effects and Adverse Reactions. Side effects and adverse reactions of cholestyramine include constipation and peptic ulcer. Constipation can be decreased or alleviated by increasing intake of fluids and foods high in fiber. Early signs of peptic ulcer are nausea and abdominal discomfort, followed later by abdominal pain and distention. To avoid GI discomfort, the drug must be taken with and followed by sufficient fluids.

The many side effects of nicotinic acid (e.g., GI disturbances, flushing of the skin, abnormal liver function [elevated serum liver enzymes], hyperglycemia, hyperuricemia) decrease its usefulness. However, as mentioned, aspirin and careful drug titration can reduce side effects to a manageable level in most patients.

The statin drugs can cause a dose-related increase in liver enzyme levels. Serum liver enzyme levels (alkaline phosphatase, alanine aminotransferase, gamma-glutamyl transferase) should be monitored. Baseline liver enzyme studies should be obtained before initiating statin drug therapy. A slight transient increase in serum liver enzyme level may be within normal value for the patient, but it should be rechecked in 1 week or so. Patients with acute hepatic disorder should not take a statin drug.

The serious skeletal muscle adverse effect known as *rhabdomyolysis* has been reported with use of the statin drug class. Patients should be advised to promptly report to the health care provider any unexplained muscle tenderness or weakness, especially if accompanied by fever or malaise.

Table 46-4 lists the pharmacologic data for antihyperlipidemics.

PERIPHERAL VASODILATORS

A common problem in older adults is peripheral arterial (vascular) disease (PAD, PVD). It is characterized by numbness and coolness of the extremities, intermittent claudication (pain and weakness of limb when walking but no symptoms

PROTOTYPE DRUG CHART 46-1

Rosuvastatin

Drug Class	Dosage
Antihyperlipidemic: HMG-CoA reductase inhibitor Trade Name: Crestor Pregnancy Category: X	A: PO: 5-40 mg/d; *max:* 40 mg/d
Contraindications	**Drug-Lab-Food Interactions**
Active liver disease, pregnancy Caution: History of liver disease, increased alcohol ingestion, trauma, severe metabolic diabetes mellitus, uncontrolled seizures	Drug: Decrease effect with antacids, phenytoin, and propranolol. May increase digoxin level, oral contraceptives. Increase effects with macrolide antibiotics, antifungals
Pharmacokinetics	**Pharmacodynamics**
Absorption: Rapid Distribution: PB: 88% Metabolism: t½: 20 h Excretion: Primarily in bile; some in urine	PO: Onset: UK Peak: 3-5 h Duration: UK
Therapeutic Effects/Uses	
To decrease cholesterol levels and to decrease serum lipids, especially LDL and triglycerides Mode of Action: Inhibits HMG-CoA reductase, the enzyme necessary for hepatic production of cholesterol.	
Side Effects	**Adverse Reactions**
Rare. Headache, rash/pruritus, constipation, diarrhea	Rhabdomyolysis, myalgia, photosensitivity, hyperglycemia, elevated liver enzymes

A, Adult; *C,* child; *h,* hour; *HMG-CoA,* 3-hydroxy-3-methyl-glutaryl coenzyme A; *PO,* by mouth; *PB,* protein-binding; *t½,* half-life; *LDL,* low-density lipoproteins.

at rest), and possible leg ulcers. The primary cause is arteriosclerosis and hyperlipidemia, resulting in atherosclerosis. The arteries become occluded.

Peripheral vasodilators increase blood flow to the extremities. They are used in peripheral vascular disorders of venous and arterial vessels. They are more effective for disorders resulting from vasospasm (Raynaud's disease) than from vessel occlusion or arteriosclerosis (arteriosclerosis obliterans, thromboangiitis obliterans [Buerger's disease]). In Raynaud's disease, cold exposure or emotional upset can trigger vasospasm of the toes and fingers; these patients have benefited from vasodilators. Patients with diabetes mellitus are more likely to have PAD by two to four times the usual rate and are at risk of intermittent claudication.

Papaverine (Para-Time SR) is a direct-acting peripheral vasodilator. The alpha-blocker prazosin (Minipress) and the calcium channel blocker nifedipine (Procardia) have also been used as peripheral vasodilators.

Individuals with PAD who are treated with HMG-CoA reductase inhibitors (statins) for dyslipidemia may get improvement for intermittent claudication symptoms as well as a decrease in serum lipids. Also, patients with PAD who are hypertensive receive improvement for both conditions when taking the antihypertensive drug ramipril (Altace), an ACE inhibitor. The antiplatelet drugs clopidogrel (Plavix) and aspirin have been used to decrease PAD symptoms. Another antiplatelet drug, cilostazol (Pletal), has been approved by the U.S. Food and Drug Administration (FDA) for treating intermittent claudication. It decreases arterial thrombi. The herb ginkgo biloba, taken with an antiplatelet drug, has been used to treat intermittent claudication, because of its vasodilating and antioxidant effects, although this herb has not been approved by the FDA. Most of the drugs used for treating PAD do not cure the health problem, but they can aid in relieving PAD symptoms.

Cilostazol is an antiplatelet that has a dual purpose of inhibiting platelet aggregation as well as causing vasodilation to treat intermittent claudication. Prototype Drug Chart 46-2 lists the pharmacologic data for cilostazol.

Nursing Process
Patient-Centered Collaborative Care

Antihyperlipidemics (Statins)

Assessment

- Assess vital signs and baseline serum chemistry values (cholesterol, triglycerides, aspartate aminotransferase [AST], alanine aminotransferase [ALT], and creatine phosphokinase [CPK]).
- Obtain a medical history. Statin drugs are contraindicated for patients with a liver disorder. Pregnancy category is X.

PROTOTYPE DRUG CHART 46-2

Cilostazol

Drug Class Direct-acting vasodilator Trade Name: Pletal Pregnancy Category: C	**Dosage** A: PO: 100 mg q12h 30 min before or 2 h after meals; max: 200 mg/d
Contraindications Class III-IV congestive heart failure, hypersensitivity, bleeding disorders, thrombocytopenia Caution: Bleeding disorders, liver and renal disease, leucopenia	**Drug-Lab-Food Interactions** Drug: Increased effects with aspirin, cimetidine, clarithromycin, erythromycin, enoxaparin, ticlopidine, warfarin Food: Grapefruit and green tea will increase levels; ginger and ginkgo biloba may prolong bleeding time.
Pharmacokinetics Absorption: PO: Readily absorbed Distribution: PB: 95%-98% Metabolism: t½: 11-13 h Excretion: In urine (74%), feces (20%)	**Pharmacodynamics** PO: Onset: 2-12 weeks Peak: UK Duration: UK
Therapeutic Effects/Uses To treat peripheral vascular disease Mode of Action: Acts directly to inhibit platelet aggregation and cause vasodilation, especially in femoral vasculature	
Side Effects Nausea, vomiting, dizziness, syncope, blood in eye, headache, abdominal pain, abnormal stools, peripheral edema	**Adverse Reactions** Tachycardia, palpitations

A, Adult; *h,* hour; *PB,* protein-binding; *PO,* by mouth; *q.i.d.,* four times a day; *t ½,* half-life; *t.i.d.,* three times a day; *UK,* unknown.

Nursing Diagnoses

- Impaired tissue integrity related to atherosclerosis because of hyperlipidemia
- Anxiety related to elevated cholesterol level because of possible coronary artery disease
- Knowledge deficit related to inexperience with statin medications

Planning

- Patient's cholesterol level will be <200 mg/dL in 6 to 8 weeks.
- Patient will be able to choose foods low in fat, cholesterol, and complex sugars.

Nursing Interventions

- Monitor patient's blood lipid levels (cholesterol, triglycerides, LDL, and high-density HDL) every 6 to 8 weeks for first 6 months after statin therapy, then every 3 to 6 months. For lipid level profile, patient should fast for 12 to 14 hours. Desired cholesterol value is <200 mg/dL; triglyceride value is <150 mg/dL (can vary); LDL is <100 mg/dL; and HDL is >60 mg/dL. Cholesterol levels >240 mg/dL, LDL levels >160 mg/dL, and HDL levels <35 mg/dL can lead to severe cardiovascular event or cerebrovascular accident (CVA).
- Monitor laboratory tests for liver function (ALT, ALP, and gamma-glutamyl transferase [GGT]). Antihyperlipidemic drugs may cause liver disorder.
- Observe for signs and symptoms of GI upset. Taking the drug with sufficient water or with meals may alleviate some of the GI discomfort.

Patient Teaching

General

- Emphasize need to comply with drug regimen to lower blood lipids.
- Inform patient that it may take several weeks before blood lipid levels decline.
- Explain that laboratory tests for blood lipids (cholesterol, triglycerides, LDL, and HDL) are usually ordered every 3 to 6 months.
- Advise patient to have serum liver enzymes monitored as indicated by health care provider. Lovastatin, pravastatin, and simvastatin are contraindicated in acute hepatic disease and pregnancy.
- Instruct patient to have annual eye examination and to report changes in visual acuity.
- Advise patient taking gemfibrozil that it may increase risk for bleeding when concurrently taking oral anticoagulant, so bleeding should be reported. Drug dosage

can be changed or another antihyperlipidemic may be ordered.

- Instruct patients with diabetes or those at risk for developing diabetes to monitor blood glucose levels if they take gemfibrozil. Dietary changes or insulin adjustment may be necessary.
- Instruct patient to take nicotinic acid with meals to decrease GI discomfort.

Self-Administration

- Teach patient to mix cholestyramine/colestipol powder well in water or juice.

Side Effects of Cholestyramine, Colestipol, and Nicotinic Acid (Niacin)

- Advise patient that constipation may occur with cholestyramine and colestipol. Increasing fluid intake and food bulk should help alleviate the problem.
- Explain to patient that flush is common with niacin and should decrease with continued use of drug. Usually drug is started at a low dose.
- Advise patient that large doses of nicotinic acid can cause vasodilation, producing dizziness and faintness (syncope).

Side Effects of Ezetimibe

- Explain to patient that ezetimibe may cause headaches and GI upset. If it continues, notify the health care provider.

Side Effects of Statins

- Explain to patient that serum liver enzyme levels are periodically monitored.
- Encourage patient to report promptly any unexplained muscle tenderness or weakness that may be caused by rhabdomyolysis.
- Caution patient not to abruptly stop taking statin drug, because serious rebound effect might occur that could lead to AMI and possible death. Before stopping a statin, patient should talk to his or her health care provider.

Diet

- Explain to patient that GI discomfort is a common problem with most antihyperlipidemics. Suggest increasing fluid intake when taking medication.
- Encourage patient to maintain low-fat diet by eating foods that are low in animal fat, cholesterol, and complex sugars. Lovastatin and other antihyperlipidemics are adjuncts to, not substitutes for, a low-fat diet.

Cultural Considerations

- Respect patient's belief of how to control his or her cholesterol level.
- Avoid criticizing traditional practices. Explanations and modifications to plan of care may be necessary if method patient uses is not effective or is unsafe.

Evaluation

- Evaluate effectiveness of antihyperlipidemic drug. Patient's cholesterol level is within desired range.
- Determine that patient is on a low-fat, low-cholesterol diet.

Cilostazol

Pharmacokinetics Cilostazol is a direct-acting vasodilator that is absorbed from GI tract. It has a half-life of 11 to 13 hours. Cilostazol is usually taken two times a day.

Pharmacodynamics Cilostazol causes vasodilation of arteries, especially within the femoral vasculature. Common adverse effects include headache, diarrhea, and abnormal stools. This drug has an onset of action with 2 to 12 weeks.

Side Effects and Adverse Reactions. Lightheadedness, dizziness, tachycardia, palpitation, and GI distress may occur.

The effectiveness of peripheral vasodilators in increasing blood flow by vasodilation is questionable in the presence of arteriosclerosis. These drugs may decrease some of the symptoms of cerebrovascular insufficiency. Table 46-5 lists the peripheral vasodilators and their dosages, uses, and considerations.

Pentoxifylline

Pentoxifylline (Trental), classified as a *hemorrheologic agent,* improves microcirculation and tissue perfusion by decreasing blood viscosity and improving the flexibility of erythrocytes, thus increasing tissue oxygenation. It inhibits aggregation of platelets and red blood cells and helps increase flow through peripheral vessels, because it decreases blood viscosity. It is a derivative of the xanthine group. Pentoxifylline has been approved by the FDA for patients with intermittent claudication and has been prescribed for those with Buerger's disease resulting from arterial occlusions. However, in one research study, pentoxifylline was not determined to be more effective than a placebo.

Reactions to an overdose of pentoxifylline include flushing of the skin, faintness, sedation, and GI disturbances. The drug should be taken with food. The patient should avoid smoking, because nicotine increases vasoconstriction. Patients taking an antihypertensive drug along with pentoxifylline may need to have the antihypertensive dosage decreased to avoid side effects.

Nursing Process
Patient-Centered Collaborative Care

Vasodilators: Cilostazol

Assessment

- Obtain baseline vital signs for future comparison.
- Assess for signs of inadequate blood flow to the extremities: pallor, coldness of extremity, and pain.

TABLE 46-5 PERIPHERAL VASODILATORS

GENERIC (BRAND)	ROUTE AND DOSAGE	USES AND CONSIDERATIONS
Direct-Acting Peripheral Vasodilators		
ergoloid mesylates	A: PO/SL: 1 mg t.i.d.; *max:* 3 mg/d	For cerebrovascular insufficiency. To improve cognitive skills, self-care, and mood, especially in the older adult. SL tablets should be placed under the tongue. May cause GI distress, orthostatic hypotension. Pregnancy category: X; PB: UK; t½: 2.6-5 h
Hemorrheologic		
cilostazol (Pletal)	See Prototype Drug Chart 46-2.	
pentoxifylline (Trental)	A: PO: 400 mg t.i.d. with meals	For peripheral vascular disorders. Alleviates intermittent claudication. Improves cerebral function for those with cerebrovascular insufficiency. May decrease stroke incidence for those having recurrent TIAs. Pregnancy category: C; PB: UK; t½: 0.5-1.8 h

A, Adult; *b.i.d.,* twice a day; *d,* day; *GI,* gastrointestinal; *h,* hour; *max,* maximum; *min,* minute; *PB,* protein-binding; *PO,* by mouth; *SL,* sublingual; *t½,* half-life; *TIA,* transient ischemic attack; *t.i.d.,* three times a day; *UK,* unknown.

Nursing Diagnoses

- Impaired tissue integrity related to insufficient blood supply
- Acute pain related to inadequate blood flow to extremity

Planning

- Patient's blood flow to the extremities will improve, and patient's pain will be controlled.

Nursing Interventions

- Monitor vital signs, especially blood pressure and heart rate. Tachycardia and orthostatic hypotension can be problematic with peripheral vasodilators.

Patient Teaching

General

- Inform patient that a desired therapeutic response may take 1.5 to 3 months.
- Advise patient not to smoke; smoking increases vasospasm.
- Instruct patient to use aspirin or aspirin-like compounds only with the health care provider's approval. Salicylates help prevent platelet aggregation.

Side Effects

- Encourage patient to change position slowly but frequently to avoid orthostatic hypotension. Orthostatic hypotension is common when taking high doses of a vasodilator.
- Instruct patient to report side effects of cilostazol , such as flushing, headaches, and dizziness.

Diet

- Suggest that patient with GI disturbances take cilostazol with meals.
- Advise patient not to ingest alcohol with a vasodilator, because it may cause a hypotensive reaction.

Evaluation

- Evaluate effectiveness of cilostazol therapy; blood flow is increased in extremities, and pain has subsided.
- Patient experiences no side effects from the prescribed drug.

KEY WEBSITES

Cholesterol: *www.nhlbi.nih.gov/health/prof/heart/index.htm#chol*

Lipid-lowering treatment: *www.nhlbi.nih.gov/health/allhat*

CRITICAL THINKING CASE STUDY

JH had a myocardial infarction (MI) 3 years ago. He was prescribed gemfibrozil (Lopid) 600 mg, twice daily, before meals. His cholesterol remained between 220 and 240 mg/dL, and his LDL was 140 mg/dL. His anticholesterol drug was changed to simvastatin (Zocor) 20 mg/day in the evening.

1. How does simvastatin differ from gemfibrozil?
2. Why do you think JH's cholesterol drug, gemfibrozil, was changed to simvastatin?
3. While JH is taking simvastatin, which group of serum levels should be monitored?
4. How long after JH took simvastatin should his cholesterol and lipoproteins be checked?
5. What is the maximum dose for simvastatin?
6. JH complains of muscle pain and muscle weakness. What might this indicate?
7. Could JH receive both gemfibrozil and simvastatin? Explain your answer.
8. JH is on vacation and does not have enough simvastatin tablets. What should he do?

NCLEX STUDY QUESTIONS

1. A patient has a serum cholesterol level of 265 mg/dL, triglyceride level of 235 mg/dL, and LDL of 180 mg/dL. What do these serum levels indicate?
   a. Hypolipidemia
   b. Normolipidemia
   c. Hyperlipidemia
   d. Alipidemia
2. The nurse knows that a patient's total cholesterol level should be within which range?
   a. 150 to 200 mg/dL
   b. 200 to 225 mg/dL
   c. 225 to 250 mg/dL
   d. >250 mg/dL
3. A patient has a low-density lipoprotein (LDL) of 175 mg/dL and a high-density lipoprotein (HDL) of 30 mg/dL. What teaching should the nurse implement for this patient?
   a. Discuss medications ordered, dietary changes, and exercise.
   b. No changes in lifestyle are needed and continue with current plan.
   c. Discuss how to have fat intake be 40% of caloric intake.
   d. Begin keeping a food diary and schedule lab work to be repeated in 6 months.
4. Which laboratory test value does the nurse realize can contribute to the development of cardiovascular disease and stroke?
   a. Decreased antidiuretic hormone
   b. Increased homocysteine level
   c. Decreased triglycerides
   d. Increased HDL level
5. A patient is taking lovastatin (Mevacor). Which serum level is most important for the nurse to monitor?
   a. Blood urea nitrogen
   b. Complete blood count
   c. Cardiac enzymes
   d. Liver enzymes
6. For what severe skeletal muscle adverse reaction should the nurse observe in a patient taking rosuvastatin (Crestor)?
   a. Myasthenia gravis
   b. Rhabdomyolysis
   c. Dyskinesia
   d. Agranulocytosis
7. A patient is taking ezetimibe (Zetia) and asks the nurse how it works. The nurse should explain that ezetimibe does what?
   a. Inhibits absorption of dietary cholesterol in the intestines.
   b. Binds with bile acids in the intestines to reduce LDL levels.
   c. Inhibits HMG-CoA reductase, which is necessary for cholesterol production in the liver.
   d. Forms insoluble complexes and reduces circulating cholesterol in the blood.
8. A patient is diagnosed with peripheral arterial disease. He is prescribed pentoxifylline (Trental). What does the nurse realize are the effects of pentoxifylline? (Select all that apply.)
   a. May lead to hypertension and bradycardia
   b. Improves microcirculation and tissue perfusion
   c. Decreases blood viscosity and improves flexibility of erythrocytes
   d. Alleviates intermittent claudication
   e. Commonly causes an adverse effect of rhabdomyolysis
   f. Allows vasodilation of arteries in skeletal muscles

Answers: 1, c; 2, a; 3, a; 4, b; 5, d; 6, b; 7, a; 8, b, c.

UNIT XV

Gastrointestinal Agents

The gastrointestinal (GI) system (tract), comprising the alimentary canal and the digestive tract, begins at the oral cavity and ends at the anus. Major structures of the GI system are (1) the oral cavity (mouth, tongue, and pharynx), (2) the esophagus, (3) the stomach, (4) the small intestine (duodenum, jejunum, and ileum), (5) the large intestine (cecum, colon, and rectum), and (6) the anus. The accessory organs and glands that contribute to the digestive process are (1) the salivary glands, (2) the pancreas, (3) the gallbladder, and (4) the liver (Figure XV-1). The main functions of the GI system are digestion of food particles and absorption of the digestive contents (nutrients, electrolytes, minerals, and fluids) into the circulatory system for cellular use. Digestion and absorption take place in the small intestine and to a lesser extent in the stomach. Undigested material passes through the lower intestinal tract with the aid of peristalsis to the rectum and anus, where it is excreted as feces, or stool.

ORAL CAVITY

The oral cavity, or mouth, starts the digestive process by (1) breaking up food into smaller particles; (2) adding saliva, which contains the enzyme amylase for digesting starch (the beginning of the digestive process); and (3) swallowing, a voluntary movement of food that becomes involuntary (peristalsis) in the esophagus, stomach, and intestines. Swallowing occurs in the pharynx (throat), which connects the mouth and esophagus.

ESOPHAGUS

The esophagus, a tube that extends from the pharynx to the stomach, is composed of striated muscle in its upper portion and smooth muscle in its lower portion. The inner lining of the esophagus is a mucous membrane that secretes mucus. The peristaltic process of contraction begins in the esophagus and ends in the lower large intestine. There are two sphincters, the superior esophageal (hyperpharyngeal) sphincter and the lower esophageal sphincter. The lower esophageal sphincter prevents gastric reflux into the esophagus, a condition called *reflux esophagitis.*

STOMACH

The stomach is a hollow organ that lies between the esophagus and the intestine. The body of the stomach has lesser and greater curvatures. It can hold 1000 to 2000 mL of gastric contents and empties in 2 to 6 hours (average is 3 to 4 hours), depending on gastric content and motility. Two sphincters, the *cardiac sphincter,* which lies at the upper opening of the stomach, and the *pyloric sphincter,* located at the lower portion of the stomach or the head of the duodenum, regulate the entrance of food into the stomach.

The interior lining of the stomach has mucosal folds that contain glands that secrete gastric juices. The four types of cells in the stomach mucosa that secrete these juices are (1) *chief cells,* which secrete the proenzyme pepsinogen (pepsin); (2) *parietal cells,* which secrete hydrochloric acid (HCl); (3) *gastrin-producing cells,* which secrete gastrin, a hormone that regulates enzyme release during digestion; and (4) *mucus-producing cells,* which release mucus to protect the stomach lining (which extends into the duodenum).

SMALL INTESTINE

The small intestine begins at the pyloric sphincter of the stomach and extends to the ileocecal valve at the cecum. Most drug absorption occurs in the duodenum, but lipid-soluble drugs and alcohol are absorbed from the stomach. The lower digestive process begins in the stomach, but most of the digestive contents are absorbed from the small intestine. The duodenum releases the hormone secretin, which suppresses gastric acid secretion, causing the intestinal juices to have a higher pH than the gastric juices. The intestinal cells also release the hormone cholecystokinin, which in turn stimulates the release of pancreatic enzymes and the contraction of the gallbladder to release bile into the duodenum. Hormones, bile, and pancreatic enzymes (trypsin, chymotrypsin, lipase, and amylase) complete the digestion of carbohydrates, protein, and fat in preparation for absorption.

LARGE INTESTINE

The large intestine accepts undigested material from the small intestine, absorbs water, secretes mucus, and with peristaltic contractions moves the remaining intestinal contents to the rectum for elimination. Defecation completes the process.

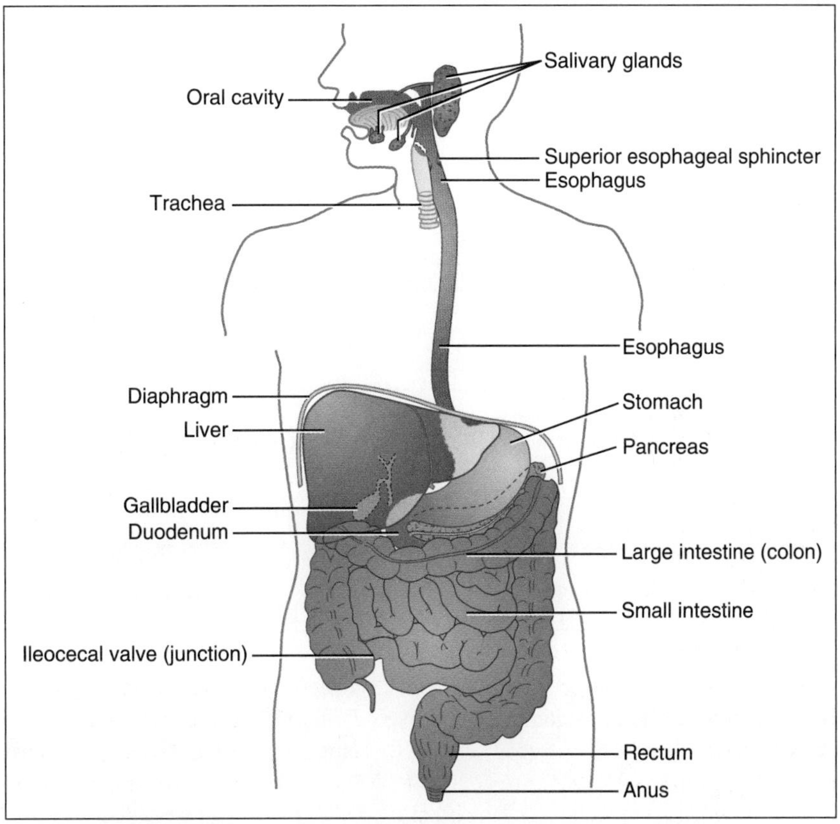

FIGURE XV–1 The gastrointestinal system and alimentary canal.

DRUGS FOR GASTROINTESTINAL DISORDERS

Vomiting, diarrhea, and constipation are GI problems that frequently require drug intervention. Chapter 47, Drugs for Gastrointestinal Tract Disorders, describes the antiemetics used to control vomiting. This chapter also discusses emetics used to eliminate ingested toxins and drugs, antidiarrheal drugs, and laxatives. The nursing process is considered in relation to each of these drug groups.

Chapter 48, Antiulcer Drugs, discusses drugs used to prevent and treat peptic ulcers (gastric and duodenal). These drugs include tranquilizers, anticholinergics, antacids, histamine$_2$ blockers, proton pump inhibitors, a pepsin inhibitor, and a prostaglandin analogue antiulcer drug.

CHAPTER

47

Drugs for Gastrointestinal Tract Disorders

evolve WEBSITE

http://evolve.elsevier.com/KeeHayes/pharmacology/

- Animations
- Content Updates
- Key Points
- Review Questions for the NCLEX® Examination
- References from the Textbook
- Unfolding Case Studies

OBJECTIVES

- Compare the pharmacologic treatment of vomiting, diarrhea, and constipation.
- Differentiate the actions and side effects of antiemetics, emetics, antidiarrheals, and laxatives.
- Apply the nursing process for the patient taking antiemetics, antidiarrheals, and laxatives.
- Differentiate contraindications to the use of antiemetics, emetics, antidiarrheals, and laxatives.

OUTLINE

KEY TERMS

Drug groups used to correct or control vomiting, diarrhea, and constipation are antiemetics, emetics, antidiarrheals, and laxatives. Each of these drug groups is discussed separately. Drugs used to treat peptic ulcers are discussed in Chapter 48.

VOMITING

Vomiting (emesis), the expulsion of gastric contents, has a multitude of causes, including motion sickness, viral and bacterial infection, food intolerance, surgery, pregnancy, pain,

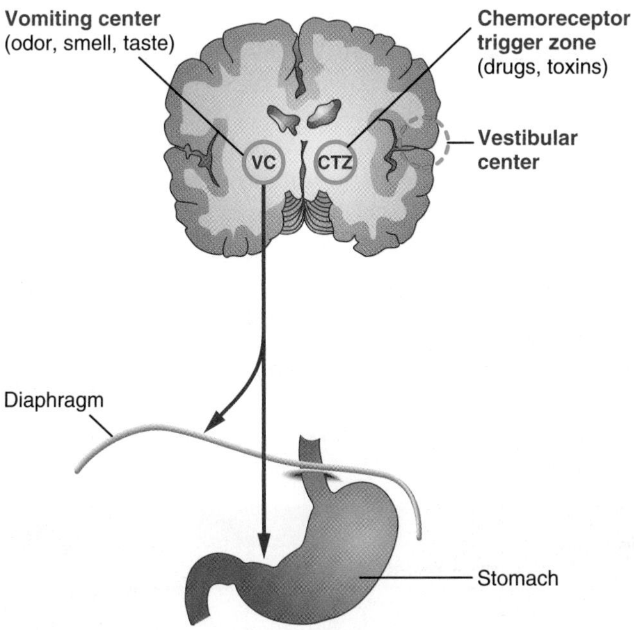

FIGURE 47–1 The chemoreceptor trigger zone and vomiting center.

shock, effects of selected drugs (e.g., antineoplastics), radiation, and disturbances of the middle ear that affect equilibrium. Nausea, a queasy sensation, may or may not precede the expulsion. The cause of the vomiting must be identified. Antiemetics can mask the underlying cause of vomiting and should not be used until the cause has been determined, unless the vomiting is so severe as to cause dehydration and electrolyte imbalance.

Two major cerebral centers—the **chemoreceptor trigger zone (CTZ),** which lies near the medulla, and the **vomiting center** in the medulla—cause vomiting when stimulated (Figure 47-1). The CTZ receives most of the impulses from drugs, toxins, and the vestibular center in the ear and transmits them to the vomiting center. The neurotransmitter dopamine stimulates the CTZ, which in turn stimulates the vomiting center. Levodopa, a drug with dopamine-like properties, can cause vomiting by stimulating the CTZ. Some sensory impulses, such as odor, smell, taste, and gastric mucosal irritation, are transmitted directly to the vomiting center. The neurotransmitter acetylcholine is also a vomiting stimulant. When the vomiting center is stimulated, the motor neuron responds by causing contraction of the diaphragm, the anterior abdominal muscles, and the stomach. The glottis closes, the abdominal wall moves upward, and vomiting occurs.

Nonpharmacologic measures should be used first when nausea and vomiting occur. If the nonpharmacologic measures are not effective, antiemetics are combined with nonpharmacologic measures. The two major groups of antiemetics are *nonprescription* (antihistamines, bismuth subsalicylate, and phosphorated carbohydrate solution) and *prescription* (antihistamines, dopamine antagonists, benzodiazepines, serotonin antagonists, glucocorticoids, cannabinoids, and miscellaneous antiemetics).

Nonpharmacologic Measures

The nonpharmacologic methods of decreasing nausea and vomiting include administration of weak tea, flat soda, gelatin, Gatorade, and Pedialyte (for use in children). Crackers and dry toast may be helpful. When dehydration becomes severe, intravenous (IV) fluids are needed to restore body fluid balance.

Nonprescription Antiemetics

Nonprescription **antiemetics** (antivomiting agents) can be purchased as over-the-counter (OTC) drugs. These drugs are frequently used to prevent motion sickness but have minimal effect on controlling severe vomiting resulting from anticancer agents (antineoplastics), radiation, and toxins. To prevent motion sickness, the antiemetic should be taken 30 minutes before travel. These drugs are not effective in relieving motion sickness if taken after vomiting has occurred.

Selected antihistamine antiemetics, such as dimenhydrinate (Dramamine), cyclizine hydrochloride (Marezine), meclizine hydrochloride (Antivert), and diphenhydramine hydrochloride (Benadryl) can be purchased OTC to prevent nausea, vomiting, and dizziness (vertigo) caused by motion. These drugs inhibit vestibular stimulation in the middle ear. Benadryl is also used to prevent or alleviate allergic reactions to drugs, insects, and food by acting as an antagonist to histamine$_1$ (H_1) receptors.

The side effects of antihistamine antiemetics are similar to those of anticholinergics: drowsiness, dryness of the mouth, and constipation. Table 47-1 lists the nonprescription antiemetics used for vomiting caused by motion sickness.

Several nonprescription drugs such as bismuth subsalicylate (Pepto-Bismol) act directly on the gastric mucosa to suppress vomiting. They are marketed in liquid and chewable tablet forms and can be taken for gastric discomfort or diarrhea. Phosphorated carbohydrate solution (Emetrol), a hyperosmolar carbohydrate, decreases nausea and vomiting by changing the gastric pH; it may also decrease smooth-muscle contraction of the stomach. Its effectiveness as an antiemetic has not been verified. Patients with diabetes mellitus should avoid this drug because of its high sugar content.

Antiemetics were once frequently used for the treatment of nausea and vomiting during the first trimester of pregnancy, but they are no longer recommended because they may cause harm to the fetus. Instead, nonpharmacologic methods should be used to alleviate nausea and vomiting during pregnancy, and OTC antiemetics should be avoided. If vomiting becomes severe and threatens the well-being of the mother and fetus, an antiemetic such as trimethobenzamide (Tigan) can be administered, although this drug is classified as *pregnancy category C.* Other antiemetics may be prescribed cautiously.

Prescription Antiemetics

Common prescription antiemetics are classified into the following groups: (1) antihistamines, (2) anticholinergics, (3) dopamine antagonists, (4) benzodiazepines, (5) serotonin antagonists, (6) glucocorticoids, (7) cannabinoids (for patients with cancer), and (8) miscellaneous. Many of these drugs act as antagonists to dopamine, histamine, serotonin, and acetylcholine, which are associated with vomiting. Antihistamines and anticholinergics act primarily on the vomiting center; they also act by decreasing stimulation of the CTZ and vestibular pathways. The cannabinoids act on the cerebral cortex. Phenothiazines, the miscellaneous antiemetics (e.g., metoclopramide), and trimethobenzamide act on the CTZ center. Drug combination therapy is commonly used to manage chemotherapy-induced nausea and vomiting. Lorazepam (Ativan), glucocorticoids, and serotonin (5-HT_3) receptor antagonists are quite effective in combination therapy. Lorazepam, haloperidol, and glucocorticoids are not approved by the U.S. Food and Drug Administration (FDA) as antiemetics but are extremely effective when combined for this unlabeled use.

Antihistamines and Anticholinergics

Only a few prescription antihistamines and anticholinergics are used in the treatment of nausea and vomiting. Table 47-2 lists these drugs and their dosages, uses, and considerations.

TABLE 47-1 NONPRESCRIPTION ANTIEMETICS: ANTIHISTAMINE

GENERIC (BRAND)	ROUTE AND DOSAGE	USES AND CONSIDERATIONS
Motion Sickness		
cyclizine HCl (Marezine)	A: PO: 50 mg q4-6 h; *max:* 200 mg/d C: 6-12 y: PO: 25 mg q6-8h; *max:* 75 mg/d	Used for prevention and treatment of nausea, vomiting, and motion sickness. Pregnancy category: B; PB: UK; t½: 13 h
dimenhydrinate (Dramamine)	A: PO: 50-100 mg q4-6h; *max:* 400 mg/d; IM/IV: 50 mg PRN; *max:* 300 mg/d C: 6-12 y: PO: 25-50 mg q6-8h PRN; *max:* 150 mg/d C: 2-5 y: 12.5-25 mg q6-8h PRN; *max:* 75 mg/d	Primarily used to prevent motion sickness. Drowsiness, dizziness, dry mouth, and hypotension may occur. Pregnancy category: B; PB: 78%; t½: 3.5 h
meclizine HCl (Antivert)	A/C: >12 y: PO: 25-50 mg 1 h before travel, after meal; may repeat q24h Vertigo: A: PO: 25-100 mg/d in divided doses	Prevention of nausea, vomiting, and dizziness. Drowsiness and dry mouth may occur. Pregnancy category: B; PB: UK; t½: 5-6 h

A, Adult; *C,* child; *d,* day; *h,* hour; *IM,* intramuscular; *max,* maximum; *PB,* protein-binding; *PO,* by mouth; *PRN,* as needed; *t½,* half-life; *t.i.d.,* three times a day; *UK,* unknown; *y,* year; *>,* greater than; *<,* less than.

TABLE 47-2 PRESCRIPTION ANTIEMETICS

GENERIC (BRAND)	ROUTE AND DOSAGE	USES AND CONSIDERATIONS
Prescription Antihistamines		
hydroxyzine (Vistaril)	A: PO/IM: 25-100 mg t.i.d./q.i.d. PRN; *max:* 400 mg/d C: IM: 1.1 mg/kg q4-6h	For postoperative nausea and vomiting and vertigo (dizziness). Given preoperatively with narcotics to decrease nausea. Give hydroxyzine deep IM. Drowsiness and dry mouth usually occur. Pregnancy category: X; PB: UK; t½: 14-25 h
promethazine (Phenergan)	See Prototype Drug Chart 47-1.	
Anticholinergics		
scopolamine (Transderm-Scōp)	A: transdermal patch: 1.5 mg (1 mg dose over 3 d); apply patch behind ear at least 4 h before antiemetic effect is required.	For motion sickness. Anticholinergic side effects (dizziness, drowsiness, dry mouth, constipation). Patch effective for 3 days. Alternate ears if using for longer than 3 days. Wash hands after applying disc/patch. Wear no more than one disc/patch at a time. Pregnancy category: C; PB: <25%; t½: 8 h
Dopamine Antagonists		
Phenothiazines		
prochlorperazine maleate (Compazine)	A: PO/IM: 5-10 mg t.i.d./q.i.d., PRN (give deep IM) SR: 10-15 mg q12h PR: 25 mg/b.i.d.; *max:* 40 mg/d C: PO/PR: 2.5 mg 1-3 times/d; *max:* 15 mg/d	Primary use is for severe nausea and vomiting. Secondary use is to reduce anxiety and tension and for psychosis. Drowsiness, dizziness, EPS, and dry mouth may occur. Pregnancy category: C; PB: 91%-99%; t½: 3-7 h
promethazine (Phenergan)	See Prototype Drug Chart 47-1.	

TABLE 47-2 PRESCRIPTION ANTIEMETICS—cont'd

GENERIC (BRAND)	ROUTE AND DOSAGE	USES AND CONSIDERATIONS
Butyrophenones		
droperidol (Inapsine)	A: IM/IV: 0.625-1.25 mg; C: 2-12 y: IM/IV: 0.1 mg/kg; *max:* 0.1 mg/kg	Prevention of nausea and vomiting during surgical and diagnostic procedures. May cause hypotension, tachycardia, and EPS. Black Box Warning: Not approved for patients with dementia-related psychosis. Pregnancy category: C; PB: UK: $t\frac{1}{2}$: 2.5 h
Benzodiazepines		
lorazepam (Ativan)	A: PO: 0.5-2 mg q4-6h PRN; *max:* 10 mg/d A: IV: 0.025 mg/kg C: IV: 0.05 mg/kg q6h PRN	For prevention of nausea and vomiting resulting from cancer chemotherapy. Usually administered with an antiemetic such as metoclopramide. Pregnancy category: D; PB: 91%; $t\frac{1}{2}$: 12 h
Serotonin (5-HT_3) Receptor Antagonists		
dolasetron mesylate (Anzemet)	Cancer chemotherapy: A/C: >2 y: PO: 100 mg, 1 h before chemotherapy A/C: >2 y: IV: 1.8 mg/kg 1 h before chemotherapy; Pre- and postoperatively: A: PO: 100 mg 2 h before surgery; IV: 12.5 mg 15 min before end of anesthesia; *max:* 100 mg	To prevent nausea and vomiting before chemotherapy or pre- and postoperatively. Acts on serotonin 5-HT_3 receptor in stomach and CTZ. Pregnancy category: B; PB: 69%-77%; $t\frac{1}{2}$: 10 min
granisetron (Kytril)	Cancer chemotherapy: A: PO: 1 mg b.i.d. (1 h before and 12 h after chemotherapy) A/C: >2 y: IV: 10 mcg/kg 30 min before chemotherapy	Prevention of nausea and vomiting caused by cancer chemotherapy. Acts on CTZ and vomiting center. Headache may occur. Pregnancy category: B; PB: 65%; $t\frac{1}{2}$: 5-12 h
ondansetron HCl (Zofran)	A: PO: 8-24 mg 30 min before chemotherapy, then q8h × 2 A/C: IV: 0.15 mg/kg 30 min before, then q4h × 2	For nausea and vomiting related to cancer chemotherapy, especially treatment with cisplatin. Pregnancy category: B; PB: 70%-76%; $t\frac{1}{2}$: 3-6 h
palonosetron (Aloxi)	A: IV: 0.25 mg over 30 sec, 30 min before chemotherapy	To prevent nausea and vomiting associated with cancer chemotherapy. Pregnancy category: B; PB: 52%; $t\frac{1}{2}$: 40 h
Cannabinoids		
dronabinol (Marinol) CSS III	Chemotherapy-induced nausea: A: PO: 5 mg/m^2 1-3 h before chemotherapy, then q2-4h after; *max:* 15 mg/m^2/dose	For nausea and vomiting caused by cancer chemotherapy. Taken before and for 24 hours after chemotherapy. Can be an appetite stimulant for patients with AIDS. Common side effects include drowsiness, dizziness, dry mouth, impaired thinking, and euphoria. Pregnancy category: C; PB: 98%; $t\frac{1}{2}$: 25-36 h
Miscellaneous		
metoclopramide HCl (Reglan)	Chemotherapy: IV: 1-2 mg/kg 30 min before chemotherapy; then q2h × 2; then q3h × 3 Postoperative: A: IM/IV: 10-20 mg at end of surgery	For nausea and vomiting related to cancer chemotherapy and postoperatively. Increases gastric and intestinal emptying. Avoid alcohol and CNS depressants. EPS may occur. Pregnancy category: B; PB: 30%; $t\frac{1}{2}$: 4-6 h
trimethobenzamide HCl (Tigan)	A: PO: 250-300 mg t.i.d./q.i.d. PRN; *max:* 1200 mg/d A: IM: 200 mg t.i.d./q.i.d. PRN; *max:* 800 mg/d	For postoperative nausea and vomiting, motion sickness, and vertigo. Avoid with CNS depressants and if sensitive to benzocaine or similar local anesthetics. Pregnancy category: C; PB: UK; $t\frac{1}{2}$: 7-9 h
aprepitant (Emend)	A: PO: 125 mg 1 h before chemotherapy on day 1, 80 mg on days 2 and 3 in the morning	For nausea and vomiting related to cancer chemotherapy. Pregnancy category: B; PB: 95%; $t\frac{1}{2}$: 9-13 h

A, Adult; *a.c.,* before meals; *AIDS,* acquired immunodeficiency syndrome; *b.i.d.,* two times a day; *C,* child; *CNS,* central nervous system; *CSS,* Controlled Substances Schedule; *CTZ,* chemoreceptor trigger zone; *d,* day; *EPS,* extrapyramidal symptoms; *h,* hour; *IM,* intramuscular; *IV,* intravenous; *max,* maximum; *min,* minute; *PB,* protein-binding; *PO,* by mouth; *PR,* per rectum; *PRN,* as needed; *q.i.d.,* four times a day; *sec,* second; *SR,* sustained release; $t\frac{1}{2}$, half-life; *t.i.d.,* three times a day; *UK,* unknown; *y,* year; >, greater than; <, less than.

Side Effects and Adverse Reactions. Side effects include drowsiness, which can be a major problem, dry mouth, blurred vision caused by pupillary dilation, tachycardia (with anticholinergic use), and constipation. These drugs should *not* be used by patients with glaucoma.

Dopamine Antagonists

These agents suppress emesis by blocking dopamine$_2$ receptors in the CTZ. The categories of dopamine antagonists include phenothiazines, butyrophenones, and benzodiazepines. Common side effects of dopamine antagonists are extrapyramidal symptoms (EPS), which are caused by blocking dopamine receptors, and hypotension. See Chapter 27 for a more detailed description of EPS and phenothiazines.

Phenothiazine Antiemetics

Selected piperazine phenothiazines are used to treat nausea and vomiting resulting from surgery, anesthetics, chemotherapy, and radiation sickness. They act by inhibiting the CTZ. When used in patients with cancer, these drugs are commonly given the night before treatment, the day of treatment, and for 24 hours after treatment. Not all phenothiazines are effective antiemetic agents. When prescribed for vomiting, the drug dosage is usually smaller than when used for psychiatric disorders.

Chlorpromazine (Thorazine) and prochlorperazine edisylate (Compazine) were the first phenothiazines used for both psychosis and vomiting. Promethazine (Phenergan), a phenothiazine introduced as an antihistamine in the 1940s, has a sedative effect and can also be used for motion sickness and management of nausea and vomiting. Promethazine is the most frequently prescribed antiemetic drug. Prototype Drug Chart 47-1 lists the pharmacologic data for promethazine.

Pharmacokinetics Promethazine is readily absorbed in the gastrointestinal (GI) tract. It has 93% protein-binding capacity. Promethazine is metabolized by the liver and excreted in urine and feces.

Pharmacodynamics Promethazine blocks H$_1$-receptor sites on effector cells and impedes histamine-mediated responses. The onset of

PROTOTYPE DRUG CHART 47-1

Promethazine HCl

Drug Class Antiemetic: phenothiazine Trade Name: Phenergan Pregnancy Category: C	**Dosage** A: PO/PR/IM/IV: 12.5-25 mg q4-6h PRN C: >2 y: PO/PR/IM/IV: 0.25-1 mg/kg q4-6h PRN; *max:* 25 mg/dose
Contraindications Hypersensitivity, narrow-angle glaucoma, severe liver disease, intestinal obstruction, blood dyscrasias, bone marrow depression Caution: Cardiovascular disease, liver dysfunction, asthma, respiratory dysfunction, hypertension, older adults and debilitated patients	**Drug-Lab-Food Interactions** Drug: Increases CNS depression and anticholinergic effects when taken with alcohol and other CNS depressants; lowers seizure threshold with phenytoin (Dilantin) Lab: False pregnancy test
Pharmacokinetics Absorption: PO: easily absorbed from GI tract Distribution: PB: 93% Metabolism: t½: 10-14 h Excretion: In urine and feces	**Pharmacodynamics** PO: Onset: 20 min Peak: UK Duration: 4-6 h IM: Onset: 20 min Peak: UK Duration: 2-8 h IV: Onset: 3-5 min Peak: UK Duration: 4-6 h PR: Onset: 20 min Peak: UK Duration: 4-6 h
Therapeutic Effects/Uses To treat and prevent motion sickness, nausea, and vomiting Mode of Action: Blocks H$_1$ receptor sites; inhibits CTZ	
Side Effects Drowsiness, confusion, anorexia, dry mouth and eyes, constipation, blurred vision, photosensitivity, hypertension, hypotension, transient leukopenia, urinary retention	**Adverse Reactions** Extrapyramidal syndrome (tardive dyskinesia, akathisia) Life-threatening: Agranulocytosis, respiratory depression

A, Adult; *C,* child; *CNS,* central nervous system; *CTZ,* chemoreceptor trigger zone; *GI,* gastrointestinal; *h,* hour; *IM,* intramuscular; *IV,* intravenous; *min,* minute; *PB,* protein-binding; *PO,* by mouth; *PR,* per rectum; *PRN,* as needed; *t ½,* half-life; *UK,* unknown; *y,* year.

action of oral and intramuscular (IM) administration is 20 minutes, and the duration of action is from 4 to 6 hours. The onset of action of intravenous (IV) promethazine is 3 to 5 minutes; the duration of action is the same as for the oral preparation.

Drug and Laboratory Interactions. Central nervous system (CNS) depression increases when promethazine is taken with alcohol, narcotics, sedative-hypnotics, and general anesthetics. Anticholinergic effects increase when promethazine is combined with antihistamines, anticholinergics such as atropine, and other phenothiazines. Promethazine may interfere with urinary pregnancy tests, producing false results.

Side Effects and Adverse Reactions. Phenothiazines have antihistamine and anticholinergic properties. The side effects of phenothiazine antiemetics are moderate sedation, hypotension, EPS, CNS effects (restlessness, weakness, dystonic reactions, agitation), and mild anticholinergic symptoms (dry mouth, urinary retention, and constipation). Because the dose is lower for vomiting than for psychosis, the side effects are not so severe. Promethazine is relatively free of EPS at antiemetic doses. Table 47-2 lists the pharmacologic data for phenothiazines and other prescription antiemetics.

Butyrophenones

Haloperidol (Haldol) and droperidol (Inapsine), like phenothiazines, block the dopamine$_2$ receptors in the CTZ. They are used to treat postoperative nausea and the vomiting and emesis associated with toxins, cancer chemotherapy, and radiation therapy. Antiemetic doses of haloperidol are smaller than those required for antipsychotic effects. Like phenothiazines, haloperidol and droperidol are likely to cause EPS if used for an extended time. Hypotension may result; therefore blood pressure should be monitored.

Benzodiazepines

Selected benzodiazepines indirectly control nausea and vomiting that may occur with cancer chemotherapy. Lorazepam (Ativan) is the drug of choice. Previously diazepam (Valium) was the preferred benzodiazepine. Lorazepam effectively provides emesis control, sedation, anxiety reduction, and amnesia when used in combination with a glucocorticoid and serotonin 5-HT$_3$ receptor antagonist.

Serotonin (5-HT$_3$) Receptor Antagonists

Serotonin antagonists suppress nausea and vomiting by blocking the serotonin receptors (5-HT$_3$) in the CTZ and the afferent vagal nerve terminals in the upper GI tract.

Serotonin antagonists—ondansetron (Zofran), granisetron (Kytril), dolasetron (Anzemet), and palonosetron (Aloxi)—are the most effective of all antiemetics in suppressing nausea and vomiting caused by cancer chemotherapy–induced emesis or emetogenic anticancer drugs. Ondansetron (the first serotonin antagonist), granisetron, and dolasetron do not block the dopamine receptors; therefore, they do not cause EPS as do the phenothiazine antiemetics. These drugs can be administered orally and IV. They are also effective in preventing nausea and vomiting before and after surgery. Common side effects include headache, diarrhea, dizziness, and fatigue.

Glucocorticoids (Corticosteroids)

Dexamethasone (Decadron) and methylprednisolone (Solu-Medrol) are two agents that are effective in suppressing emesis associated with cancer chemotherapy. Because these glucocorticoids are administered IV and for only a short while, side effects normally associated with glucocorticoids are minimized. Glucocorticoids are discussed in Chapter 51.

Cannabinoids

Cannabinoids, the active ingredients in marijuana, were approved for clinical use in 1985 to alleviate nausea and vomiting resulting from cancer treatment. These agents may be prescribed for patients receiving chemotherapy who do not respond to or are unable to take other antiemetics. They are contraindicated for patients with psychiatric disorders. Cannabinoids can be used as an appetite stimulant for patients with acquired immunodeficiency syndrome (AIDS). The cannabinoid dronabinol (Marinol) is described in Table 47-2.

Side Effects and Adverse Reactions. Side effects occurring as a result of cannabinoid use include mood changes, euphoria, drowsiness, dizziness, headaches, depersonalization, nightmares, confusion, incoordination, memory lapse, dry mouth, orthostatic hypotension or hypertension, and tachycardia. Less common symptoms are depression, anxiety, and manic psychosis.

Miscellaneous Antiemetics

Diphenidol (Vontrol) and trimethobenzamide (Tigan) are in the class of miscellaneous antiemetics, because they do not act strictly as antihistamines, anticholinergics, or phenothiazines. These drugs suppress impulses to the CTZ. Diphenidol also prevents vertigo by inhibiting impulses to the vestibular area.

Side Effects and Adverse Reactions. The side effects and adverse reactions of the miscellaneous antiemetics are drowsiness and anticholinergic symptoms (dry mouth, increased heart rate, urine retention, constipation, and blurred vision). Trimethobenzamide can cause hypotension, diarrhea, and EPS (abnormal involuntary movements, postural disturbances, and alteration in muscle tone).

Nursing Process
Patient-Centered Collaborative Care

Antiemetics

Assessment

- Determine a history of the onset, frequency, and amount of vomiting and contents of the vomitus. If appropriate, elicit from patient possible causative factors such as food (e.g., seafood, mayonnaise).

- Obtain a history of present health problems. Patients with glaucoma should avoid many of the antiemetics.
- Record vital signs for abnormalities and for future comparison.
- Assess urinalysis before and during therapy.

Nursing Diagnoses

- Imbalanced nutrition: less than body requirements related to inability to ingest food
- Risk for deficient fluid volume related to vomiting

Planning

- Patient will adhere to nonpharmacologic methods and/or drug regimen to alleviate vomiting.
- Patient's underlying cause of vomiting will be corrected.
- Patient will retain small amounts of food.

Nursing Interventions

- Check vital signs. If vomiting is severe, dehydration may occur, and shocklike symptoms may be present.
- Monitor bowel sounds for hypoactivity or hyperactivity.
- Provide mouth care after vomiting. Encourage patient to maintain oral hygiene.

Patient Teaching

General

- Instruct patient to store drug in airtight, light-resistant container if required.
- Tell patient to avoid OTC preparations.
- Warn patient not to consume alcohol while taking antiemetics. Alcohol can intensify sedative effect.
- Advise pregnant patients to avoid antiemetics during first trimester because of possible teratogenic effects on the fetus. Encourage these patients to seek medical advice about OTC or prescription antiemetics.

Side Effects

- Tell patient to report sore throat, fever, and mouth sores; notify health care provider and have blood drawn for complete blood count (CBC).
- Alert patient to avoid driving a motor vehicle or engaging in dangerous activities, because drowsiness is common with antiemetics. If drowsiness becomes a problem, a decrease in dosage may be indicated.
- Caution patient with hepatic disorder to seek medical advice before taking phenothiazines. Instruct patient to report dizziness.
- Suggest to patient nonpharmacologic methods of alleviating nausea and vomiting such as flat soda, weak tea, crackers, and dry toast.

Cultural Considerations

- Respect patients' cultural beliefs and alternative methods for treating nausea and vomiting. Discuss with patients the safety of their methods, other nondrug methods, and purpose of antiemetic if prescribed.
- Procure an interpreter to assist non–English-speaking patients to understand the drug schedule for prescribed antiemetics and their side effects when needed.

Evaluation

- Evaluate effectiveness of nonpharmacologic methods or antiemetic by noting absence of vomiting. Identify any side effects that may result from drug.

Metoclopramide

Metoclopramide (Reglan) suppresses emesis by blocking the dopamine receptors in the CTZ. It is used in the treatment of postoperative emesis, cancer chemotherapy, and radiation therapy. High doses can cause sedation and diarrhea. With this agent, the occurrence of EPS is more prevalent in children than in adults. Metoclopramide should not be given if the patient has GI obstruction, hemorrhage, or perforation.

Table 47-2 lists pharmacologic data for the miscellaneous antiemetics along with other prescription antiemetics.

SAFETY: Preventing Medication Errors

Do not confuse ...

- **Antivert** (antiemetic) with **Axert** (antimigraine)
- **Lorazepam** (controls nausea and vomiting) with **alprazolam** (anxiolytic)
- **Hydroxyzine** (antiemetic) with **hydralazine** (antihypertensive)

EMETICS

Emetics are drugs used to induce vomiting. When an individual has consumed certain toxic substances, induced vomiting (emesis) may be indicated to expel the substance before absorption occurs. There are many ways to induce vomiting without using drugs, such as putting the finger in the back part of the throat.

Vomiting should not be induced if caustic substances, such as ammonia, chlorine bleach, lye, toilet cleaners, or battery acid, have been ingested. Regurgitating these substances can cause additional injury to the esophagus. To prevent aspiration, vomiting should also be avoided if petroleum distillates are ingested; these include gasoline, kerosene, paint thinners, and lighter fluid. Activated charcoal is given when emesis is contraindicated.

Ipecac

Administration of ipecac has diminished greatly but it is still used when indicated. The American Academy of Clinical Toxicology and the European Association of Poisons Centres and Clinical Toxicologists issued guidelines in 2004 that ipecac syrup should not be administered routinely in the management of poisoned individuals; no new guidelines have

TABLE 47-3 EMETICS AND ADSORBENTS

GENERIC (BRAND)	ROUTE AND DOSAGE	USES AND CONSIDERATIONS
Emetics		
ipecac syrup (OTC preparation)	A: PO: 15-30 mL, followed by 8-16 oz of water C: 1-12 y: PO: 15 mL, followed by 8-16 oz of water C: 6-11 mo: PO: 5-10 mL, followed by 4-8 oz of water	Induces vomiting after poisoning. Administer within 60 minutes of poisoning to an alert and conscious individual. Pregnancy category: C; PB: NA; t½: 2 h
Adsorbents		
charcoal (CharcoAid, CharcoCaps)	For poisoning, use CharcoAid: A: PO: 30-100 g in 6-8 oz of water C: PO: 1-2 g/kg in 6-8 oz of water C: <1 y: PO: 1 g/kg	Promotes absorption of poison/toxic substances. Neither drug is systemically absorbed. Pregnancy category: C; PB: NA; t½: NA

A, Adult; *C,* child; *CNS,* central nervous system; *d,* day; *max,* maximum; *mo,* month; *NA,* not applicable; *OTC,* over-the-counter; *PB,* protein-binding; *PO,* by mouth; *PRN,* as necessary; *t½,* half-life; *y,* year.

been issued since 2004. Ipecac is considered appropriate in isolated cases for the patient who is alert and if administered within 60 minutes of poisoning.

When the patient purchases ipecac, instruct the patient to buy ipecac *syrup* and *not* ipecac fluid extract, which is more potent and may cause fatalities. When ipecac is kept in the household, it should be kept out of the reach of children. Ipecac syrup induces vomiting by stimulating the CTZ in the medulla and acting directly on the gastric mucosa. Ipecac should be taken with a glass of water (do not give with milk or carbonated beverages). The onset of emesis production following administration of ipecac syrup is usually 15 to 30 minutes. When vomiting is not induced, patients should be treated with an adsorbent, such as activated charcoal, or gastric lavage (Table 47-3). Individuals with bulimia and anorexia nervosa often abuse ipecac, which may lead to cardiomyopathy, ventricular fibrillation, and death.

DIARRHEA

Diarrhea (frequent liquid stool) is a symptom of an intestinal disorder. Causes include (1) foods (spicy, spoiled), (2) fecal impaction, (3) bacteria *(Escherichia coli, Salmonella)* or viruses (parvovirus, rotavirus), (4) toxins, (5) drug reaction, (6) laxative abuse, (7) malabsorption syndrome caused by lack of digestive enzymes, (8) stress and anxiety, (9) bowel tumor, and (10) inflammatory bowel disease such as ulcerative colitis or Crohn's disease. Diarrhea can be mild to severe. Antidiarrheals should not be used for more than 2 days and should not be used if fever is present.

Because intestinal fluids are rich in water, sodium, potassium, and bicarbonate, diarrhea can cause minor or severe dehydration and electrolyte imbalances. The loss of bicarbonate places the patient at risk for developing metabolic acidosis. Patients with diarrhea should avoid milk products and foods rich in fat. Diarrhea can develop very quickly and can be life threatening to young patients and older adults, who may not be able to compensate for the fluid and electrolyte losses.

Nonpharmacologic Measures

The cause of diarrhea should be identified. Nonpharmacologic treatment for diarrhea is recommended until the underlying cause can be determined. This includes use of clear liquids and oral solutions (Gatorade; Pedialyte or Rehydralyte [both for use in children]) and IV electrolyte solutions. Antidiarrheal drugs are frequently used in combination with nonpharmacologic treatment.

Traveler's Diarrhea

Traveler's diarrhea, also called *acute diarrhea,* is usually caused by *E. coli.* It ordinarily lasts less than 2 days; however, if it becomes severe, fluoroquinolone antibiotics are usually prescribed. Loperamide (Imodium) may be used to slow peristalsis and decrease the frequency of defecation, but it can also slow the exit of the organism from the GI tract. Traveler's diarrhea can be reduced by drinking bottled water, washing fruit, and eating cooked vegetables. Meats should be cooked until well done.

Antidiarrheals

There are various **antidiarrheals** for treating diarrhea and decreasing hypermotility (increased peristalsis). Usually there is an underlying cause of the diarrhea that needs to be corrected as well. The antidiarrheals are classified as (1) opiates and opiate-related agents, (2) somatostatin analogue, (3) adsorbents, and (4) miscellaneous antidiarrheals.

Opiates and Opiate-Related Agents

Opiates decrease intestinal motility, thereby decreasing peristalsis. Constipation is a common side effect of opium preparations. Codeine is an example. Opiates are frequently combined with other antidiarrheal agents. Opium antidiarrheals can cause CNS depression when taken with alcohol, sedatives, or tranquilizers. The duration of action of opiates is approximately 2 hours.

Diphenoxylate with atropine (Lomotil) is an opiate that has less potential for causing drug dependence than other opiates such as codeine. Difenoxin (Motofen) is an active metabolite of diphenoxylate, but it is more potent than

PROTOTYPE DRUG CHART 47-2

Diphenoxylate with Atropine

Drug Class Antidiarrheal Trade Name: Lomotil Pregnancy Category: C CSS V	**Dosage** A: PO: 2.5-5 mg t.i.d./q.i.d. PRN C: 2-12 y: PO: 0.3-0.4 mg/kg/d in 4 divided doses
Contraindications Severe diarrhea due to poisoning or pseudomembranous colitis Severe hepatic or renal disease, glaucoma, severe electrolyte imbalance; children <2 y	**Drug-Lab-Food Interactions** Drug: Increase CNS depression with alcohol, antihistamines, opioids, sedative-hypnotics; MAOIs may enhance hypertensive crisis Lab: Increase serum liver enzymes, amylase
Pharmacokinetics Absorption: PO: Well absorbed Distribution: PB: UK Metabolism: t½: 3-14 h Excretion: In feces and urine	**Pharmacodynamics** PO: Onset: 45-60 min Peak: 2 h Duration: 3-4 h
Therapeutic Effects/Uses To treat diarrhea by slowing intestinal motility Mode of Action: Inhibits gastric motility	
Side Effects Drowsiness, dizziness, constipation, dry mouth, weakness, flush, rash, blurred vision, mydriasis, urine retention	**Adverse Reactions** Angioedema Life-threatening: Paralytic ileus, toxic megacolon, severe allergic reaction

A, Adult; *b.i.d.,* twice a day; *C,* child; *CNS,* central nervous system; *CSS,* Controlled Substances Schedule; *d,* day; *h,* hour; *MAOIs,* monoamine oxidase inhibitors; *min,* minute; *PB,* protein-binding; *PO,* by mouth; *PRN,* as necessary; *q.i.d.,* four times a day; *t ½,* half-life; *UK,* unknown; *y,* year; >, greater than; <, less than.

diphenoxylate. Both drugs are combined with atropine to decrease abdominal cramping, intestinal motility, and hypersecretion. Diphenoxylate with atropine (Lomotil) is frequently prescribed for traveler's diarrhea, and difenoxin with atropine (Motofen) is prescribed to treat nonspecific and chronic diarrhea. With prolonged use of these drugs, physical dependence may occur. Diphenoxylate antidiarrheal products are approximately 50% atropine, which will discourage drug abuse. Prototype Drug Chart 47-2 lists the parmacologic data for diphenoxylate with atropine (Lomotil).

Loperamide (Imodium) is structurally related to diphenoxylate but causes less CNS depression than diphenoxylate and difenoxin. It can be purchased as an OTC drug, and it protects against diarrhea, reduces fecal volume, and decreases intestinal fluid and electrolyte losses.

Patients with severe hepatic impairment should not take products containing diphenoxylate, difenoxin, or loperamide. Children and older adults who take diphenoxylate are more susceptible to respiratory depression than other age groups.

Pharmacokinetics Diphenoxylate with atropine is well absorbed from the GI tract. The diphenoxylate is metabolized by the liver mainly as metabolites. There are two half-lives: 3 hours for diphenoxylate and 3 to 14 hours for the diphenoxylate metabolites. The drug is excreted in the feces and urine.

Pharmacodynamics Diphenoxylate with atropine is an opium agonist with anticholinergic properties (atropine); it decreases GI motility (peristalsis). It has a moderate onset of action of 45 to 60 minutes, and the duration of action is 3 to 4 hours. Many side effects are caused by the anticholinergic atropine. Patients with severe glaucoma should take another antidiarrheal that does not have an anticholinergic effect. If this drug is taken with alcohol, narcotics, or sedative-hypnotics, CNS depression can occur.

Adsorbents

Adsorbents act by coating the wall of the GI tract and adsorbing bacteria or toxins that cause diarrhea. Adsorbent antidiarrheals include kaolin and pectin. These agents are combined as a mild or moderate antidiarrheal that can be purchased OTC and used in combination with other antidiarrheals. Bismuth subsalicylate (Pepto-Bismol) is considered an adsorbent because it adsorbs bacterial toxins. Pepto-Bismol can also be used as an antacid for gastric discomfort. Pepto-Bismol is an OTC drug commonly used to treat traveler's diarrhea. Colestipol and cholestyramine (Questran) are prescription drugs that have been used to treat diarrhea due to excess bile acids in the colon. They are effective, although they have not been approved by the FDA for this purpose. Table 47-4 lists the pharmacologic data for antidiarrheal adsorbents.

Miscellaneous Antidiarrheals

Various miscellaneous antidiarrheals are prescribed to control diarrhea. This group includes rifaximin. Table 47-4 includes these other antidiarrheals.

TABLE 47-4 ANTIDIARRHEALS: OPIATES AND OPIATE-RELATED, ADSORBENTS, AND MISCELLANEOUS

GENERIC (BRAND)	ROUTE AND DOSAGE	USES AND CONSIDERATIONS
Opiates and Opiate-Related		
deodorized opium tincture CSS II	A: PO: 0.6-1 mL q.i.d. mixed with water; *max:* 6 mL/d C: PO: 0.005-0.01 mL/kg q3-4 h; *max:* 6 doses/d	For acute, nonspecific diarrhea. To treat withdrawal symptoms in neonates of mothers who are addicted to opiates. Not recommended for diarrhea caused by poison. Avoid taking alcohol and CNS depressants. Pregnancy category: C; PB: UK; $t\frac{1}{2}$: 2-3 h
difenoxin and atropine (Motofen) CSS IV	A: PO: Initially: 2 mg; then 1 mg after each loose stool; *max:* 8 mg/d for 2 d	For acute nonspecific and chronic diarrhea. Combination of a synthetic narcotic and atropine. Avoid use in patients with narrow-angle glaucoma. Dry mouth, flush, and tachycardia may occur. Pregnancy category: C; PB: UK; $t\frac{1}{2}$: 12-24 h
loperamide HCl (Imodium)	A: PO: Initially: 4 mg; then 2 mg after each loose stool; *max:* 16 mg/d C: 9-11 y: PO: 2 mg t.i.d. on day 1, then 0.1 mg/kg after unformed stool; *max:* 6 mg/d C: 6-8 y: PO: 2 mg b.i.d. on day 1, then 0.1 mg/kg after unformed stool; *max:* 4 mg/d	For diarrhea. Newest OTC drug. Does not affect CNS. Less than 1% reaches systemic circulation. Pregnancy category: C; PB: 97%; $t\frac{1}{2}$: 11-24 h
Adsorbents		
bismuth subsalicylate (Pepto-Bismol, Kapectolin, Kaopectate)	A: PO: 2 tab or 30 mL q30-60 min PRN; *max:* 8 doses/d	For diarrhea, gastric distress. OTC liquid and tab form. Pregnancy category: C; PB: UK; $t\frac{1}{2}$: UK
kaolin-pectin (Kaolin with Pectin)	A: 60-120 mL after each loose stool C: 6-12 y: 30-60 mL after each loose stool	For diarrhea. Administer after each loose stool. OTC drug. Pregnancy category: C; PB: UK; $t\frac{1}{2}$: UK
Miscellaneous		
rifaximin (Xifaxan)	A: PO: 200 mg t.i.d. for 3 days	For treatment of travelers' diarrhea caused by noninvasive strains of *E. coli.* Pregnancy category: C; PB: 67.5%; $t\frac{1}{2}$: 5-6 h

A, Adult; *a.c.,* before meals; *b.i.d.,* twice a day; *C,* child; *CNS,* central nervous system; *CSS,* Controlled Substances Schedule; *d,* day; *GI,* gastrointestinal; *h,* hour; *h.s.,* at bedtime; *max,* maximum; *min,* minute; *mo,* month; *OTC,* over-the-counter; *PB,* protein-binding; *PO,* by mouth; *PRN,* as needed; *q.i.d.,* four times a day; *subQ,* subcutaneous; $t\frac{1}{2}$, half-life; *tab,* tablet; *t.i.d.,* three times a day; *UK,* unknown; *wk,* week; *y,* year; >, greater than; <, less than.

CONSTIPATION

Constipation (accumulation of hard fecal material in the large intestine) is a relatively common complaint and a major problem for older adults. Insufficient water intake and poor dietary habits are contributing factors. Other causes include (1) fecal impaction, (2) bowel obstruction, (3) chronic laxative use, (4) neurologic disorders (paraplegia), (5) ignoring the urge to defecate, (6) lack of exercise, and (7) selected drugs, such as anticholinergics, narcotics, and certain antacids.

Nursing Process
Patient-Centered Collaborative Care

Antidiarrheals

Assessment

- Obtain a history of any viral or bacterial infection, drugs taken, and foods ingested that could be contributing factors to diarrhea. Many antidiarrheals are contraindicated if patient has liver disease, narcotic dependence, ulcerative colitis, or glaucoma.
- Check vital signs to provide baseline for future comparison and to determine body fluid and electrolyte losses.
- Determine frequency and consistency of bowel movements.
- Assess bowel sounds. Hyperactive sounds can indicate increased intestinal motility.
- Report if patient has a narcotic drug history. If opiate or opiate-related antidiarrheals are given, drug misuse or abuse may occur.

Nursing Diagnoses

- Diarrhea related to laxative abuse
- Imbalanced nutrition: less than body requirements related to misconceptions regarding OTC drugs
- Risk for imbalanced fluid volume related to diarrhea

Planning

- Patient will have bowel movements that are formed.
- Patient's body fluids will be restored.

Nursing Interventions

- Record vital signs. Report tachycardia or systolic blood pressure decrease of 10 to 15 mm Hg. Monitor respirations. Opiates and opiate-related drugs can cause central nervous system (CNS) depression.
- Monitor frequency of bowel movements and bowel sounds. Notify health care provider if intestinal hypoactivity occurs when taking drug.
- Check for signs and symptoms of dehydration resulting from persistent diarrhea. Fluid replacement may be necessary. With prolonged diarrhea, check serum electrolytes.
- Administer antidiarrheals cautiously to patients with glaucoma, liver disorders, or ulcerative colitis and to pregnant patients.
- Recognize that drug may need to be withheld if diarrhea continues for more than 48 hours or acute abdominal pain develops.

Patient Teaching

- Instruct patient not to take sedatives, tranquilizers, or other narcotics with drug. CNS depression may occur.
- Tell patient to avoid OTC preparations (they may contain alcohol promoting liver damage and concurrent use with loratadine and loperamide may lead to significant interaction).
- Advise patient to take the drug only as prescribed. Drug may be habit-forming; do not exceed recommended dose.
- Encourage patient to drink clear liquids.
- Advise patient not to ingest fried foods or milk products until diarrhea has stopped.
- Teach patient that constipation can result from overuse of antidiarrheal drugs.

Cultural Considerations

- Do not assume that lack of eye contact means that patient is not listening or does not care. It might indicate respect. The more traditional and older individuals in some cultures may not maintain eye contact.

Evaluation

- Evaluate the effectiveness of the drug; diarrhea has stopped.
- Monitor long-term use of opiates and opiate-related drugs for possible abuse and physical dependence.
- Continue to monitor vital signs. Report abnormal changes.

Nonpharmacologic Measures

Nonpharmacologic management includes diet (high fiber), water, exercise, and routine bowel habits. A "normal" number of bowel movements ranges between one and three per day to three per week. What is normal varies from person to person; the nurse should determine what normal bowel habits are for each patient. At times a laxative may be needed, but the patient should also use nonpharmacologic measures to prevent constipation.

Laxatives

Laxatives and **cathartics** are used to eliminate fecal matter. Laxatives promote a soft stool, cathartics result in a soft to watery stool with some cramping, and frequently dosage determines whether a drug acts as a laxative or cathartic. Because these terms are often used interchangeably, *laxative* will cover both classes in this chapter. **Purgatives** are "harsh" cathartics that cause a watery stool with abdominal cramping. There are four types of laxatives: (1) osmotics (saline), (2) stimulants (contact or irritants), (3) bulk-forming, and (4) emollients (stool softeners).

Laxatives should be avoided if there is any question that the patient may have intestinal obstruction; if abdominal pain is severe; or if symptoms of appendicitis, ulcerative colitis, or diverticulitis are present. Most laxatives stimulate peristalsis. Laxative abuse from chronic use is a common problem, especially in older adults. Laxative dependence can become a problem, so patient teaching is an important nursing responsibility.

Osmotic (Saline) Laxatives

Osmotics (hyperosmolar laxatives) include salts or saline products, lactulose, and glycerin. Saline products consist of sodium or magnesium, and a small amount is systemically absorbed. Serum electrolytes should be monitored to avoid electrolyte imbalance. Hyperosmolar salts pull water into the colon and increase water in the feces to increase bulk, which stimulates peristalsis. Saline cathartics cause a semiformed to watery stool according to low or high doses. Good renal function is needed to excrete any excess salts. Saline cathartics are contraindicated for patients with heart failure.

Osmotic laxatives contain electrolyte salts, including (1) sodium salts (sodium phosphate or Phospho-Soda, sodium biphosphate) and (2) magnesium salts (magnesium hydroxide [milk of magnesia], magnesium citrate). High doses of salt laxatives are used for bowel preparation for diagnostic and surgical procedures. Another laxative used for bowel preparation is polyethylene glycol (PEG) with electrolytes, marketed as GoLYTELY. With PEG, however, a large volume of solution, approximately 3 to 4 liters over 3 hours, must be ingested. Patients may be advised to keep GoLYTELY refrigerated to make it more palatable. The positive aspect is that the solution is an isotonic, nonabsorbable osmotic substance that contains sodium salts and potassium chloride; thus it can be used by patients with renal impairment or cardiac disorder.

Lactulose, another saline laxative that is not absorbed, draws water into the intestines to form a soft stool. It decreases the serum ammonia level and is useful in liver diseases, such as cirrhosis. Glycerin acts like lactulose, increasing water in the feces in the large intestine. The bulk that results from the increased water in the feces stimulates peristalsis and defecation.

Side Effects and Adverse Reactions. Adequate renal function is needed to excrete excess magnesium. Patients who have renal insufficiency should avoid magnesium salts. Hypermagnesemia can result from continuous use of magnesium salts, causing symptoms such as drowsiness, weakness, paralysis, complete heart block, hypotension, flush, and respiratory depression.

The side effects of excess lactulose use include flatulence, diarrhea, abdominal cramps, nausea, and vomiting. Patients who have diabetes mellitus should avoid lactulose, because it contains glucose and fructose.

Stimulant (Contact) Laxatives

Stimulant (contact or irritant) laxatives increase peristalsis by irritating sensory nerve endings in the intestinal mucosa. Types include those containing bisacodyl (Dulcolax), senna (Senokot), and castor oil (purgative). Bisacodyl is the most frequently used and abused laxative and can be purchased OTC. Bisacodyl and several others of these drugs are used to empty the bowel before diagnostic tests (barium enema). Prototype Drug Chart 47-3 lists the pharmacologic data for the stimulant laxative bisacodyl.

Castor oil is a harsh laxative (purgative) that acts on the small bowel and produces a watery stool. The action is quick, within 2 to 6 hours, so the laxative should not be taken at bedtime. Castor oil is seldom used to correct constipation. It is used mainly for bowel preparation.

Pharmacokinetics The contact laxative bisacodyl is minimally absorbed from the GI tract. It is excreted in feces, but because of the small amount of bisacodyl absorption, a portion is excreted in urine.

Pharmacodynamics Bisacodyl promotes defecation. Bisacodyl irritates the colon, causing defecation, and psyllium compounds increase fecal bulk and peristalsis. The onset of action of oral bisacodyl occurs within 6 to 8 hours, and with the suppository (rectal administration) it occurs within 15 to 60 minutes.

Side Effects and Adverse Reactions. Side effects include nausea, abdominal cramps, weakness, and reddish brown urine caused by excretion of phenolphthalein, senna, or cascara.

With excessive and chronic use of bisacodyl, fluid and electrolyte (especially potassium and calcium) imbalances are likely to occur. Systemic effects occur infrequently, because absorption of bisacodyl is minimal. Mild cramping and diarrhea are side effects of bisacodyl.

Castor oil should not be used in early pregnancy, because it stimulates uterine contraction. Spontaneous abortion may result. Prolonged use of senna can damage nerves, which may result in loss of intestinal muscular tone. Table 47-5 lists the osmotic and stimulant laxatives with their dosages, uses, and considerations.

PROTOTYPE DRUG CHART 47-3

Bisacodyl

Drug Class Laxative: stimulant Trade Name: Dulcolax Pregnancy Category: C	**Dosage** A: PO: 5-15 mg PRN; *max:* 30 mg C: >6 y: PO: 5-10 mg A/C: 6 y: rectal supp: 10 mg/d C: >2 y: 5 mg
Contraindications Hypersensitivity, fecal impaction, intestinal/biliary obstruction, GI bleeding, appendicitis, abdominal pain, nausea, vomiting, rectal fissures	**Drug-Lab-Food Interactions** Drug: Decrease effect with antacids, histamine$_2$ blockers, proton pump inhibitors Food: milk
Pharmacokinetics Absorption: Minimal (5%-15%) Distribution: PB: UK Metabolism: t½: UK Excretion: In bile and urine	**Pharmacodynamics** PO: Onset: 6-8 h Peak: N/A Duration: N/A PR: Onset: 15-60 min Peak: N/A Duration: N/A
Therapeutic Effects/Uses Short-term treatment for constipation; bowel preparation for diagnostic tests Mode of Action: Increases peristalsis by direct effect on smooth muscle of intestine	
Side Effects Anorexia, nausea, vomiting, cramps, diarrhea	**Adverse Reactions** Dependence, hypokalemia Life-threatening: Tetany

A, Adult; *C,* child; *d,* day; *h,* hour; *max,* maximum; *min,* minute; *PB,* protein-binding; *PO,* by mouth; *PR,* per rectum; *PRN,* as needed; *supp,* suppository; *t ½,* half-life; *UK,* unknown; *y,* year; >, greater than; <, less than.

TABLE 47-5 LAXATIVES: OSMOTICS (SALINE), STIMULANTS, AND SELECTIVE CHLORIDE CHANNEL ACTIVATOR

GENERIC (BRAND)	ROUTE AND DOSAGE	USES AND CONSIDERATIONS
Osmotics: Saline		
glycerin	A: Supp: 1 supp into rectum; retain 15 min C: <6 y: supp: 1 infant supp	For constipation. Use with caution in patients with cardiac, renal, or liver disease and for older adults or dehydrated patients. Pregnancy category: C; PB: UK; t½: 30-45 min
lactulose (Cephulac, Chronulac)	Chronic constipation: A: PO: 15-30 mL/d, may increase to 60 mL/d PRN	For constipation. Also used in liver disease for ammonia elimination. May be used for constipation after barium studies. Poorly absorbed. Pregnancy category: B; PB: UK; t½: UK
magnesium citrate (Citroma)	A: PO: 150-300 mL in single or divided dose C: 6-12 y: PO: 100-150 mL in single or divided dose C: 2-5 y: PO: 60-120 mL in single or divided dose	For constipation or to complete bowel elimination before diagnostic procedures and surgery. Pregnancy category: B; PB: UK; t½: UK
magnesium hydroxide (milk of magnesia)	A: PO: 15-60 mL/d C: 6-11 y: PO: 15-30 mL/d C: 2-5 y: PO: 5-15 mL/d	For constipation. Take with a glass of water in morning or evening. With frequent use, good renal function is necessary. Pregnancy category: B; PB: UK; t½: UK
magnesium oxide (Mag-Ox)	A: PO: 2-4 g h.s. with 8 oz water	Similar to magnesium hydroxide. Contraindicated in patients with renal failure. Pregnancy category: A; PB: UK; t½: UK
sodium biphosphate (Fleet Phospho-Soda)	A: PO: 15-30 mL mixed in water Enema: A: 60-120 mL C: 30-60 mL	For constipation or bowel preparation. Contraindicated in patients with HF. Pregnancy category: C; PB: UK; t½: UK
Stimulants		
bisacodyl (Dulcolax)	See Prototype Drug Chart 47-3.	
castor oil (Neoloid, Purge)	A: PO: 15-60 mL/d C: 2-12 y: 5-15 mL/d	For bowel preparation for diagnostic tests. Harsh cathartic or purgative. Not commonly used for constipation. Pregnancy category: X; PB: UK; t½: UK
senna (Senokot)	A: PO: 1-2 tab or 1-2 tsp (granules) diluted in water; *max:* 4 tab/d	For constipation. Available in granules, syrup, and suppository. Prolonged use may cause fluid and electrolyte imbalances. Flatus and abdominal cramps may occur. Pregnancy category: C; PB: UK; t½: UK
Selective Chloride Channel Activator		
lubiprostone (Amitiza)	A: PO: 24 mcg b.i.d.	For treatment of chronic idiopathic constipation in adults. Pregnancy category: C; PB: 94%; t½: 0.9-1.4 h

A, Adult; *b.i.d.,* twice a day; *C,* child; *HF,* heart failure; *h.s.,* at bedtime; *d,* day; *h,* hour; *IV,* intravenous; *max,* maximum; *min,* minute; *PB,* protein-binding; *PO,* by mouth; *PRN,* as needed; *supp,* suppository; *t½,* half-life; *tab,* tablet; *tsp,* teaspoon; *UK,* unknown; *y,* year; >, greater than; <, less than.

Bulk-Forming Laxatives

Bulk-forming laxatives are natural fibrous substances that promote large, soft stools by absorbing water into the intestine, increasing fecal bulk and peristalsis. These agents are nonabsorbable. Defecation usually occurs within 8 to 24 hours; however, it may take up to 3 days after drug therapy is started for the stool to be soft and well formed. Powdered bulk-forming laxatives, which sometimes come in flavored and sugar-free forms, should be mixed in a glass of water or juice, stirred, drunk immediately, and followed by a half to a full glass of water. Insufficient fluid intake can cause the drug to solidify in the GI tract, which can result in intestinal obstruction. This group of laxatives does not cause laxative dependence and may be used by patients with diverticulosis, irritable bowel syndrome, and ileostomy and colostomy.

Polycarbophil (FiberCon), polyethylene glycol (MiraLax), methylcellulose (Citrucel), and psyllium (Metamucil) are examples of bulk-forming laxatives. Patients with hypercalcemia should avoid calcium polycarbophil because of the significant amount of calcium in the drug. Prototype Drug Chart 47-4 lists the pharmacologic data for the bulk-forming laxative psyllium (Metamucil).

Pharmacokinetics The bulk-forming laxative Metamucil is a nondigestible and nonabsorbent substance that, when mixed with water, becomes a viscous solution. Because it is not absorbed, there is no protein-binding or half-life for the drug. Metamucil is excreted in the feces.

Pharmacodynamics The onset of action for Metamucil is 12 to 72 hours. Peak action is 1 to 3 days. The duration of action is unknown.

Side Effects and Adverse Reactions. Bulk-forming laxatives are not systemically absorbed; therefore there is no systemic effect. If bulk-forming laxatives are excessively used, nausea, vomiting, flatus, or diarrhea may occur. Abdominal cramps may occur if the drug is used in dry form.

PROTOTYPE DRUG CHART 47-4

Psyllium

Drug Class Laxative: bulk forming Trade Name: Metamucil Pregnancy Category: B	**Dosage** A: PO: 1-2 tsp in 8 oz water followed by 8 oz water 1-3 times/d C: >6 y: PO: 0.5-1 tsp in 8 oz water, followed by at least 4 oz water 1-3 times/d
Contraindications Hypersensitivity, fecal impaction, intestinal obstruction, abdominal pain, GI bleeding, dysphagia, appendicitis	**Drug-Lab-Food Interactions** Drug: Decrease absorption of oral anticoagulants, aspirin, and digoxin
Pharmacokinetics Absorption: Not absorbed Distribution: PB: NA Metabolism: t½: NA Excretion: In feces	**Pharmacodynamics** PO: Onset: 12-72 h Peak: 1-3 d Duration: UK
Therapeutic Effects/Uses To control chronic constipation Mode of Action: Acts as bulk-forming laxative by drawing water into intestine	
Side Effects Anorexia, nausea, vomiting, cramps, flatulence, diarrhea	**Adverse Reactions** Esophageal or intestinal obstruction if not taken with adequate water Life-threatening: Bronchospasm, anaphylaxis

A, Adult; *C*, child; *d*, day; *h*, hour; *NA*, not applicable; *PB*, protein-binding; *PO*, by mouth; *t ½*, half-life; *tsp*, teaspoon; *UK*, unknown; *y*, year; >, greater than; ≥, greater than or equal to.

Chloride Channel Activators

Selective chloride channel activators are a new category of laxatives used to treat idiopathic constipation in adults. The first drug in this category is lubiprostone, manufactured by Sucampo Pharmaceuticals. Lubiprostone was approved by the FDA in January 2006. This drug activates chloride channels in the lining of the small intestine, leading to an increase in intestinal fluid secretion and motility. By enhancing the passage of stool, lubiprostone relieves constipation, as well as accompanying symptoms of abdominal discomfort, pain, and bloating. Lubiprostone is contraindicated for patients with a history of mechanical GI obstruction, Crohn's disease, diverticulitis, and severe diarrhea. Adverse effects of lubiprostone include nausea, which seems to be dose-dependent, diarrhea, headache, abdominal distention, and flatulence.

Emollients (Stool Softeners)

Emollients are lubricants and stool softeners (surface-acting or wetting drugs) used to prevent constipation. These drugs decrease straining during defecation. Lubricants such as mineral oil increase water retention in the stool. Mineral oil absorbs essential fat-soluble vitamins A, D, E, and K. Some of the minerals can be absorbed into the lymphatic system.

Stool softeners work by lowering surface tension and promoting water accumulation in the intestine and stool. They are frequently prescribed for patients after myocardial infarction or surgery. They are also given before administration of other laxatives in treating fecal impaction. Docusate calcium (Surfak), docusate sodium (Colace), and docusate sodium with senna (Peri-Colace) are examples of stool softeners.

Side Effects and Adverse Reactions. Side effects of mineral oil include nausea, vomiting, diarrhea, and abdominal cramping. This laxative is not indicated for children, older adults, or patients with debilitating diseases, because they might aspirate the mineral oil, resulting in lipid pneumonia. The docusate group of drugs may cause mild cramping.

Contraindications. Contraindications to the use of laxatives include inflammatory disorders of the GI tract (appendicitis, ulcerative colitis, undiagnosed severe pain that could be caused by inflammation within the intestine [diverticulitis, appendicitis]), pregnancy, spastic colon, or bowel obstruction. Laxatives are contraindicated when any of these conditions is suspected. Table 47-6 lists the laxatives and their dosages, uses, and considerations.

Nursing Process
Patient-Centered Collaborative Care

Laxative: Stimulant

Assessment

- Obtain a history of constipation and possible causes (insufficient water or fluid intake, diet deficient in bulk

TABLE 47-6 LAXATIVES: BULK FORMING, EMOLLIENTS, AND EVACUANTS

GENERIC (BRAND)	ROUTE AND DOSAGE	USES AND CONSIDERATIONS
Bulk Forming		
polycarbophil (FiberCon)	A: PO: 1 g 1-4 times/d; *max:* 6 g/d C: 6-12 y: PO: 500 mg/d 1-4 times/d; *max:* 2 g C: 2-5 y: PO: 500 mg 1-2 times/d; *max:* 1 g/d	For prevention of constipation. Also used to treat acute nonspecific diarrhea or diarrhea associated with irritable bowel syndrome. For diarrhea, absorbs water and produces formed stool. For constipation, chew tablet and follow with a full glass of water. Pregnancy category: C; PB: NA; $t\frac{1}{2}$: NA
polyethylene glycol (MiraLax, GoLytely)	A: PO: 17 g (1 Tbsp) in 4-8 oz water qd; *max:* 1 week C: >6 months: PO: 0.5-1.5 g/kg qd; *max:* 17 g/d, 2 weeks	For constipation. May be used for bowel preparation. Pregnancy category: C; PB: NA; $t\frac{1}{2}$: NA
methylcellulose (Citrucel)	A: PO: 5-20 mL t.i.d. in 8-10 oz of water C: 5-10 mL b.i.d. with 8 oz of water	For constipation. Effects similar to Metamucil. Mix in at least 8 oz of water, and take immediately. Pregnancy category: C; PB: NA; $t\frac{1}{2}$: NA
psyllium hydrophilic mucilloid (Metamucil)	See Prototype Drug Chart 47-4.	
Emollient: Stool Softeners		
docusate calcium; docusate sodium (Surfak, Dialose, Colace)	Docusate calcium: A: PO: 240 mg/d Docusate sodium: A: PO: 50-300 mg/d C: 2-12 y: 50-150 mg/d	For prevention of constipation. Stool softener. Acts on small and large intestines; little absorption. When first used, may take 1-5 days for effect. Available with calcium, potassium, or sodium. Pregnancy category: C; PB: NA; $t\frac{1}{2}$: NA
docusate sodium with senna (Peri-Colace)	A: PO: 2-4 tabs/d C: PO: 1-2 tabs/d C: PO: 1 tab/d	For prevention of constipation. Combination drug: docusate sodium 100 mg with casanthranol 30 mg. Pregnancy category: C; PB: NA; $t\frac{1}{2}$: NA
Emollient: Lubricant		
mineral oil (Kondremul Plain)	A: PO: 15-45 mL h.s.	For constipation and fecal impaction. May be useful for those with cardiac disorders and following anorectal surgery. Avoid prolonged use because vitamins A, D, E, and K may be lost. Pregnancy category: UK; PB: NA; $t\frac{1}{2}$: NA
Evacuant/Bowel Preparation		
polyethylene glycol-electrolyte solution (GoLYTELY)	Preparation for GI examination requires 3-4 h; fasting A: PO: 240 mL q10-15min for total of 4 L	For bowel preparation before GI examination. Pregnancy category: C; PB: NA; $t\frac{1}{2}$: NA

A, Adult; *b.i.d.,* twice a day; *C,* child; *HF,* heart failure; *h.s.,* at bedtime; *d,* day; *h,* hour; *GI,* gastrointestinal; *max,* maximum; *min,* minute; *NA,* not applicable; *PB,* protein-binding; *PO,* by mouth; $t\frac{1}{2}$, half-life; *tab,* tablet; *t.i.d.,* three times a day; *UK,* unknown; *y,* year; >, greater than.

or fiber, inactivity), frequency and consistency of stools, and general health status.
- Record baseline vital signs for identification of abnormalities and for future comparison.
- Evaluate renal function.
- Assess electrolyte balance of patients who frequently use laxatives.

Nursing Diagnoses
- Constipation related to ignoring urge to defecate
- Risk for deficient fluid volume related to diuretic therapy
- Deficient knowledge related to overuse of laxatives
- Ineffective health maintenance related to lack of ability to make thoughtful judgments

Planning
- Patient will have a normal bowel elimination pattern.
- Patient will exercise, eat foods high in fiber, and have adequate fluid intake to avoid constipation.

Nursing Interventions
- Monitor fluid intake and output.
- Note signs and symptoms of fluid and electrolyte imbalances that may result from watery stools. Habitual use of laxatives can cause fluid volume deficit, electrolyte losses, and loss of urge to defecate.

Patient Teaching

General
- Encourage patient to increase water intake (if not contraindicated), which will decrease hard, dry stools.

- Advise patient to avoid overuse of laxatives, which can lead to fluid and electrolyte imbalances and drug dependence. Suggest exercise to help increase peristalsis.
- Teach patient not to chew tablets but to swallow them whole.
- Direct patient to store suppositories at less than 86° F (30° C).
- Council patient to take drug only with water to increase absorption.
- Educate patient not to take drug within 1 hour of any other drug.
- Warn patient that drug is not for long-term use; bowel tone may be lost.
- Encourage patient to time administration of drug so as not to interfere with activities or sleep.

Side Effects

- Advise patient to discontinue use if rectal bleeding, nausea, vomiting, or cramping occurs.

Diet

- Inform patient to increase foods high in fiber, such as bran, whole grains, and fruits.

Cultural Considerations

- Provide explanation and written information as needed related to the use and abuse of stimulant laxatives. Respect values and beliefs of patients from various cultural groups, and incorporate their traditional practices into treatment plan when possible.

Evaluation

- Determine effectiveness of nonpharmacologic methods for alleviating constipation.
- Evaluate patient's use of laxatives in managing constipation. Identify laxative abuse.

Nursing Process
Patient-Centered Collaborative Care

Laxative: Bulk Forming

Assessment

- Obtain a history of constipation and possible causes (insufficient water or fluid intake, diet deficient in bulk or fiber, inactivity), frequency and consistency of stools, and general health status.
- Record baseline vital signs for identification of abnormalities and for future comparisons.
- Assess renal function, urine output, blood urea nitrogen (BUN), and serum creatinine.

Nursing Diagnoses

- Constipation related to inadequate fiber in diet
- Risk for deficient fluid volume related to overuse of laxatives

Planning

- Patient will have a normal bowel elimination pattern.
- Patient will exercise, eat foods high in fiber, and have adequate fluid intake to avoid constipation.

Nursing Interventions

- Check fluid intake and output. Note signs and symptoms of fluid and electrolyte imbalances that may result from watery stools. Habitual use of laxatives can cause fluid volume deficit and electrolyte losses.
- Monitor bowel sounds.
- Identify cause of constipation.
- Avoid inhalation of psyllium dust.

Patient Teaching

General

- Teach patient to mix drug with water immediately before use to avoid GI obstruction.
- Advise patient *not* to swallow drug in dry form.
- Counsel patient to avoid overuse of laxatives, which can lead to fluid and electrolyte imbalances and drug dependence. Suggest exercise to help increase peristalsis.
- Advise patient to avoid inhaling psyllium dust; it may cause watery eyes, runny nose, and wheezing.

Side Effects

- Encourage patient to discontinue use if nausea, vomiting, cramping, or rectal bleeding occurs.

Diet

- Instruct patient to mix drug in 8 to 10 oz of water, stir, and drink immediately. At least one glass of extra water should follow. Insufficient water can cause drug to solidify and lead to dry, hard stools, and fecal impaction.
- Encourage patient to increase foods rich in fiber (bran, grains, vegetables, fruits).
- Inform patient to increase water intake (at least 8 oz of fluids per day), which will decrease hard, dry stools.

Cultural Considerations

- Respect patient's cultural beliefs and alternative methods for treating constipation. Suggest nonpharmacologic methods that might be of benefit.
- Provide additional explanation about use and abuse of laxatives, and provide written materials in a language that patient speaks and reads most easily.

Evaluation

- Determine effectiveness of nonpharmacologic methods for alleviating constipation.
- Evaluate patient's use of laxatives in managing constipation.
- Identify laxative abuse.

KEY WEBSITES

Activated charcoal: *www.mayoclinic.com/health/drug-information/DR602267*

Promethazine: *www.nlm.nih.gov/medlineplus/druginfo/meds/a682284.html*

CRITICAL THINKING CASE STUDY

CS, a 34-year-old woman, has been vomiting for 48 hours. In the last 12 hours, CS has had vomiting and diarrhea. Prochlorperazine (Compazine) 10 mg was administered intramuscularly.

1. What nonpharmacologic measures should the nurse suggest when vomiting occurs?
2. Why was CS given prochlorperazine intramuscularly and not orally or rectally? Prochlorperazine should be given deep intramuscularly. Why?
3. What electrolyte imbalances may occur as a result of vomiting and diarrhea? Explain how they can be replaced.
4. What are the side effects of prochlorperazine? Could these occur to CS? Explain your answer.
5. Could a serotonin antagonist be given to CS instead of prochlorperazine? Explain your answer.
   CS was prescribed diphenoxylate with atropine (Lomotil) 2.5 mg t.i.d.
6. Is the diphenoxylate with atropine (Lomotil) dosage for CS within the normal prescribed range? Explain your answer.
7. What clinical conditions are contraindicated for the use of Lomotil?
8. What are some combination drugs that may be prescribed to control diarrhea? Give their advantages and disadvantages.
9. Explain the similarities of two over-the-counter antidiarrheals. Explain how frequently they should be administered.
10. Do you think CS should receive an adsorbent? Explain your answer.
11. Explain the similarities and differences between ipecac and charcoal.

NCLEX STUDY QUESTIONS

1. A patient complains of constipation and requires a laxative. In providing teaching for this patient, the nurse reviews the common causes of constipation, including which cause?
   a. Motion sickness
   b. Poor dietary habits
   c. Food intolerance
   d. Bacteria *(Escherichia coli)*
2. A patient with nausea is taking ondansetron (Zofran). She asks the nurse how this drug works. The nurse is aware that this medication has which action?
   a. Enhances histamine$_1$ receptor sites
   b. Blocks serotonin receptors in the CTZ
   c. Blocks dopamine receptors in the CTZ
   d. Stimulates anticholinergic receptor sites
3. A patient who has constipation is prescribed a bisacodyl (Dulcolax) suppository. Which explanation will the nurse use to explain the action of bisacodyl?
   a. Acts on smooth intestinal muscle to gently increase peristalsis
   b. Absorbs water into the intestines to increase bulk and peristalsis
   c. Lowers surface tension and increases water accumulation in the intestines
   d. Pulls salts into the colon and increases water in the feces to increase bulk
4. A patient is using scopolamine (Transderm-Scōp) to prevent motion sickness. About which common side effect should the nurse teach the patient?
   a. Diarrhea
   b. Vomiting
   c. Insomnia
   d. Dry mouth
5. When metoclopramide (Reglan) is given for nausea, the nurse plans to caution the patient to avoid which substance?
   a. Milk
   b. Coffee
   c. Alcohol
   d. Carbonated beverages
6. The nurse is administering diphenoxylate with atropine (Lomotil) to a patient. Which should be included in the patient teaching regarding this medication? (Select all that apply.)
   a. Caution the patient to avoid laxative abuse.
   b. Record the frequency of bowel movements.
   c. Caution the patient against taking sedatives concurrently.
   d. Encourage the patient to increase fluids.
   e. Instruct the patient to avoid this drug if he or she has narrow-angle glaucoma.
   f. Teach the patient that the drug acts by drawing water into the intestine.

Answers: 1, b; 2, b; 3, a; 4, d; 5, c; 6, a, b, c, d, e.

CHAPTER

48

Antiulcer Drugs

evolve WEBSITE

http://evolve.elsevier.com/KeeHayes/pharmacology/

- Animations
- Content Updates
- Key Points
- Review Questions for the NCLEX® Examination
- References from the Textbook
- Unfolding Case Studies

OBJECTIVES

- Explain the predisposing factors for peptic ulcers.
- Differentiate between peptic ulcer, gastric ulcer, duodenal ulcer, and gastroesophageal reflux disease.
- Compare the actions of seven groups of antiulcer drugs used in the treatment of peptic ulcer: tranquilizers, anticholinergics, antacids, histamine$_2$ blockers, proton pump inhibitors, pepsin inhibitor, and prostaglandin analogue.
- Plan patient teaching for the following drug groups: anticholinergics, antacids, and histamine$_2$ blockers.
- Differentiate between the side effects of anticholinergics and systemic and nonsystemic antacids.
- Apply the nursing process, including teaching, to antiulcer drugs.

OUTLINE

KEY TERMS

Peptic ulcer is a broad term for an ulcer occurring in the esophagus, stomach, or duodenum within the upper gastrointestinal (GI) tract. Ulcers are more specifically named according to the site of involvement: esophageal, gastric, and duodenal ulcers. Duodenal ulcers occur 10 times more frequently than gastric and esophageal ulcers. The release of **hydrochloric acid** (HCl) from the parietal cells of the stomach is influenced by histamine, gastrin, and acetylcholine. Peptic ulcers occur when there is a hypersecretion of hydrochloric acid and pepsin, which erode the GI mucosal lining.

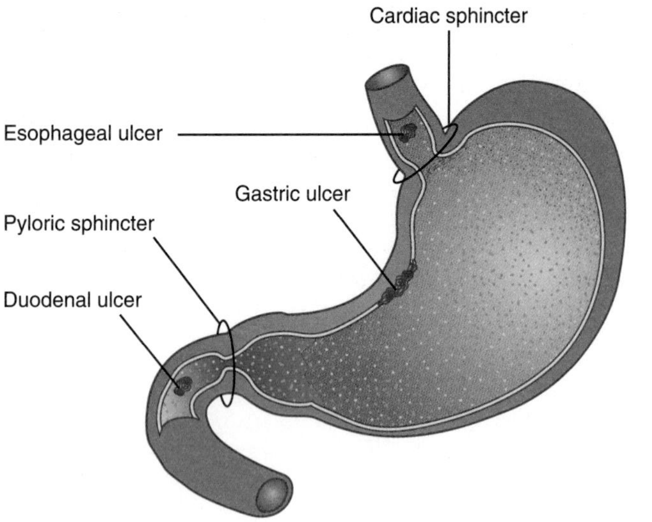

FIGURE 48–1 Common sites of peptic ulcers.

The gastric secretions in the stomach strive to maintain a pH of 2 to 5. **Pepsin,** a digestive enzyme, is activated at a pH of 2, and the acid-pepsin complex of gastric secretions can cause mucosal damage. If the pH of gastric secretions increases to pH 5, the activity of pepsin declines. The **gastric mucosal barrier (GMB)** is a thick, viscous, mucous material that provides a barrier between the mucosal lining and acidic gastric secretions. The GMB maintains the integrity of the gastric mucosal lining and is a defense against corrosive substances. The two sphincter muscles—the *cardiac,* located at the upper portion of the stomach, and the *pyloric,* located at the lower portion of the stomach—act as barriers to prevent reflux of acid into the esophagus and duodenum. Figure 48-1 shows common sites of peptic ulcers.

An **esophageal ulcer** results from reflux of acidic gastric secretions into the esophagus as a result of a defective or incompetent cardiac sphincter. A **gastric ulcer** frequently occurs because of a breakdown of the GMB. A **duodenal ulcer** is caused by hypersecretion of acid from the stomach passing into the duodenum because of (1) insufficient buffers to neutralize gastric acid in the stomach, (2) a defective or incompetent pyloric sphincter, or (3) hypermotility of the stomach. **Gastroesophageal reflux disease (GERD)** is inflammation or erosion of the esophageal mucosa caused by a reflux of gastric acid content from the stomach into the esophagus.

PREDISPOSING FACTORS IN PEPTIC ULCER DISEASE

The nurse needs to assist the patient in identifying possible causes of the ulcer and to teach ways to alleviate them. Predisposing factors include mechanical disturbances, genetic influences, bacterial organisms, environmental factors, and certain drugs. Healing of an ulcer takes 4 to 8 weeks. Complications can occur as the result of scar tissue. Table 48-1 lists the predisposing factors for peptic ulcers and their effects.

TABLE 48-1 PREDISPOSING FACTORS FOR PEPTIC ULCER DISEASE

PREDISPOSING FACTORS	EFFECTS
Mechanical disturbances	Hypersecretion of acid and pepsin. Inadequate GMB mucous secretion. Impaired GMB resistance. Hypermotility of the stomach. Incompetent (defective) cardiac or pyloric sphincter.
Genetic influences	Increased number of parietal cells in the stomach. Susceptibility of mucosal lining to acid penetration. Susceptibility to excess acetylcholine and histamine. Excess hydrochloric acid caused by external stimuli.
Environmental influences	Foods and liquids containing caffeine; fatty, fried, and highly spiced foods; alcohol. Nicotine, especially from cigarette smoking. Stressful situations. Pregnancy, massive trauma, major surgery.
Helicobacter pylori	A gram-negative bacterium, *H. pylori,* infects gastric mucosa and can cause gastritis, gastric ulcer, and duodenal ulcer. If not eradicated, peptic ulcer may return as frequently as every year. *H. pylori* can lead to atrophic gastritis in some patients. Serology and special breath tests can detect the presence of *H. pylori.*
Drugs	NSAIDs, including aspirin and aspirin compounds, ibuprofen (Motrin, Advil, Nuprin), and indomethacin (Indocin); corticosteroids (cortisone, prednisone); potassium salts; antineoplastic drugs.

GMB, Gastric mucosal barrier; *NSAIDs,* nonsteroidal antiinflammatory drugs.

The classic symptom of peptic ulcers is gnawing, aching pain. With a gastric ulcer, pain occurs 30 minutes to 1.5 hours after eating, and with a duodenal ulcer, 2 to 3 hours after eating. Small, frequent meals of nonirritating foods decrease the pain. With treatment, pain usually subsides in 10 days; however, the healing process may take 1 to 2 months.

A **stress ulcer** usually follows a critical situation such as extensive trauma or major surgery (e.g., burns, cardiac surgery). Prophylactic use of antiulcer drugs decreases the incidence of stress ulcers.

Helicobacter pylori

Helicobacter pylori, a gram-negative bacillus, is linked with the development of peptic ulcer and is known to cause gastritis, gastric ulcer, and duodenal ulcer. When a peptic ulcer recurs after antiulcer therapy, and the ulcer is not caused by nonsteroidal antiinflammatory drugs (NSAIDs) such as aspirin or ibuprofen, the patient should be tested for the presence of the bacterium *H. pylori,* which may have infected the gastric mucosa. In the past, endoscopy and a biopsy of the gastric antrum were needed to check for *H. pylori*. Currently a noninvasive breath test, the Meretek UBT, can detect *H. pylori*. This test consists of drinking a liquid containing 13C urea and breathing into a container. If *H. pylori* is present, the bacterial urease hydrolyzes the urea, releasing 13CO_2, which is detected by a spectrometer. This test is 90% to 95% effective for detecting *H. pylori*. In addition, a serology test may be performed to check for antibodies to *H. pylori*.

There are various protocols for treating *H. pylori* infection, but antibacterial agents are the treatment of choice. The use of only one antibacterial agent is not effective for eradicating *H. pylori*, because the bacterium can readily become resistant to that drug. Treatment to eradicate this bacterial infection includes using a dual-, triple-, or quadruple drug therapy program in a variety of drug combinations, such as amoxicillin (Amoxil), tetracycline (Achromycin V), clarithromycin (Biaxin), omeprazole (Prilosec), lansoprazole (Prevacid), metronidazole (Flagyl), bismuth subsalicylate (Pepto-Bismol), and ranitidine bismuth citrate (Tritec), on a 7- to 14-day treatment plan. The combination of drugs differs for each patient according to the patient's drug tolerance. A common treatment protocol is the triple therapy of metronidazole (or amoxicillin), omeprazole (or lansoprazole), and clarithromycin (MOC). The drug regimen eradicates more than 90% of peptic ulcer caused by *H. pylori* (Herbal Alert 48-1).

HERBAL ALERT 48-1

Herbs and Tetracycline

St. John's wort may increase the risk for photosensitivity when taken with tetracycline.

One of the proton pump inhibitors (PPIs) (e.g., omeprazole, lansoprazole) is frequently used as a component of combination drug therapy, because each suppresses acid secretion by inhibiting the enzyme hydrogen or potassium ATPase, which makes gastric acid. These agents block the final steps of acid production. If triple therapy fails to eradicate *H. pylori*, then quadruple therapy using two antibiotics, a PPI, and a bismuth or histamine$_2$ (H_2) blocker is recommended. After completion of the treatment regimen, 6 weeks of standard acid suppression, such as H_2 blocker therapy, is recommended. Table 48-2 lists agents used to treat *H. pylori* with their dosages, uses, and considerations.

Gastroesophageal Reflux Disease

Gastroesophageal reflux disease (GERD), also called *reflux esophagitis*, is an inflammation of the esophageal mucosa caused by reflux of gastric acid content into the esophagus. Its main cause is an incompetent lower esophageal sphincter. Smoking tends to accelerate the disease process.

Medical treatment for GERD is similar to the treatment for peptic ulcers. This includes use of the common antiulcer drugs to neutralize gastric contents and reduce gastric acid secretion. Drugs used in treatment include H_2 blockers such as ranitidine (Zantac), and PPIs such as omeprazole (Prilosec), lansoprazole (Prevacid), rabeprazole (Aciphex), pantoprazole (Protonix), or esomeprazole (Nexium). A PPI relieves symptoms faster and maintains healing better than an H_2 blocker. Once the strictures are relieved by dilation, they are less likely to recur if the patient was taking PPIs rather than an H_2 blocker.

Effective management of GERD keeps the esophageal mucosa healed and the patient free from symptoms, but GERD is a chronic disorder that requires continuous care.

TABLE 48-2 PHARMACOLOGIC AGENTS USED TO TREAT *HELICOBACTER PYLORI*

GENERIC (BRAND)	ROUTE AND DOSAGE	USES AND CONSIDERATIONS
Antiinfective Agents		
metronidazole HCl (Flagyl)	A: PO: 250 q.i.d.	To treat numerous organisms, including *H. pylori*. Used in combination with other drugs to treat *H. pylori*.
amoxicillin (Amoxil)	A: PO: 1000 mg b.i.d	Used in triple or quadruple therapy for *H. pylori*
clarithromycin (Biaxin)	A: PO: 500 mg b.i.d.	Used in dual and triple therapy for *H. pylori*
tetracycline (Sumycin)	A: PO: 500 mg q.i.d.	Used in triple and quadruple therapy for *H. pylori*
Proton Pump Inhibitors (PPIs)		
omeprazole (Prilosec)	A: PO: 20 mg/b.i.d. or 40 mg/d	Used in dual, triple, and quadruple therapy for *H. pylori*
lansoprazole (Prevacid)	A: PO: 30 mg b.i.d.	Used in dual and triple therapy for *H. pylori*
esomeprazole (Nexium)	A: PO: 40 mg/d	Used in therapy for *H. pylori*
pantoprazole (Protonix)	A: PO: 40 mg/d	Used in therapy for *H. pylori*
rabeprazole (Aciphex)	A: PO: 20 mg b.i.d.	Used in therapy for *H. pylori*
Antacids		
bismuth subsalicylate	A: PO: 525 mg q.i.d. (or 2 tabs q.i.d.)	Used in combination with other drugs to treat *H. pylori*
bismuth subcitrate potassium	A: PO: 420 mg (or 3 caps) q.i.d.	Used in combination with other drugs to treat *H. pylori*

A, Adult; *b.i.d.*, twice a day; *d*, day; *PO*, by mouth; *q.i.d.*, four times a day; *t.i.d.*, three times a day; *tab*, tablet.

NONPHARMACOLOGIC MEASURES FOR MANAGING PEPTIC ULCER AND GASTROESOPHAGEAL REFLUX DISEASE

Nonpharmacologic measures, along with drug therapy, are an important part of treatment for a GI disorder. Once the GI problem is resolved, the patient should continue to follow nonpharmacologic measures to avoid recurrence of the condition.

Avoiding tobacco and alcohol can decrease gastric secretions. With GERD, nicotine relaxes the lower esophageal sphincter, permitting gastric acid reflux. Obesity enhances GERD; weight loss is helpful in decreasing symptoms. The patient should avoid hot, spicy, and greasy foods, which could aggravate the gastric problem. Certain drugs like NSAIDs, which include aspirin, should be taken with food or in a decreased dosage. Glucocorticoids can cause gastric ulceration and should be taken with food.

To relieve symptoms of GERD, the patient should raise the head of the bed, not eat before bedtime, and wear loose-fitting clothing.

SAFETY: Preventing Medication Errors

Do not confuse ...

- **ranitidine** (H_2 blocker) with **rimantadine** (an antiviral) or **amantadine** (an antiviral and antiparkinsonism agent)
- **Zantac** (H_2 blocker) with **Xanax** (anxiolytic)

ANTIULCER DRUGS

There are seven groups of antiulcer agents: (1) tranquilizers, which decrease vagal activity; (2) anticholinergics, which decrease acetylcholine by blocking the cholinergic receptors; (3) antacids, which neutralize gastric acid; (4) H_2 blockers, which block the H_2 receptor; (5) PPIs, which inhibit gastric acid secretion, regardless of acetylcholine or histamine release; (6) the pepsin inhibitor sucralfate; and (7) the prostaglandin E_1 analogue misoprostol, which inhibits gastric acid secretion and protects the mucosa. Currently, tranquilizers and anticholinergics are used infrequently due to potential adverse effects and much more effective drugs on the market. Figure 48-2 shows the action of the antiulcer drug groups, each of which is discussed separately.

Tranquilizers

Tranquilizers have minimal effect in preventing and treating ulcers; however, they reduce vagal stimulation and decrease anxiety. Generic versions of Librax, a reformulated product of the anxiolytic chlordiazepoxide (Librium) and the anticholinergic clidinium bromide (Quarzan), may be used in the treatment of ulcers. Adverse effects may include edema, ataxia, confusion, extrapyramidal syndrome (EPS), and agranulocytosis.

Anticholinergics

Anticholinergics (antimuscarinics, parasympatholytics) and antacids were the drugs of choice for peptic ulcers for many

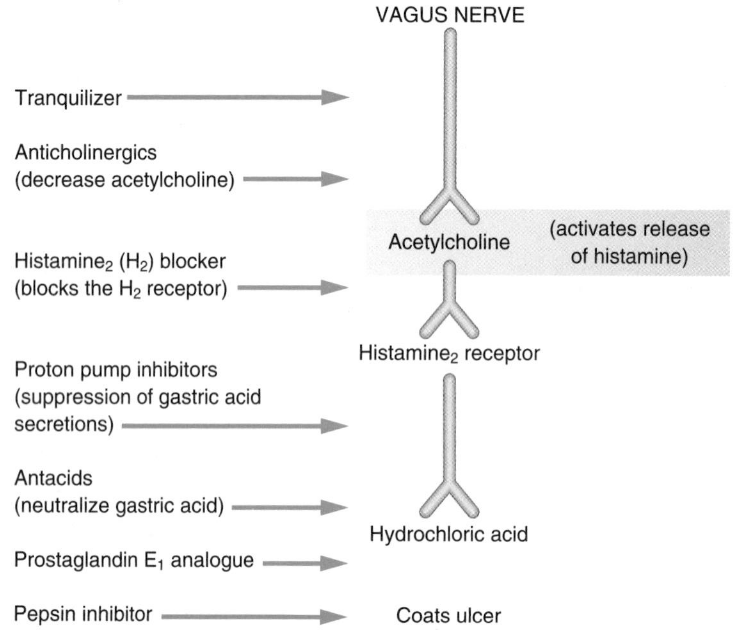

FIGURE 48–2 Actions of the antiulcer drug groups.

TABLE 48-3 ANTIULCER DRUGS: ANTICHOLINERGICS

GENERIC (BRAND)	ROUTE AND DOSAGE	USES AND CONSIDERATIONS
clidinium bromide and chlordiazepoxide HCl	A: PO: 1-2 cap t.i.d./q.i.d. a.c./h.s.	Decreases anxiety and GI distress. Contains a benzodiazepine. Pregnancy category: D; PB: UK; $t\frac{1}{2}$: 5-100 h
glycopyrrolate (Robinul)	A/C: >12 y: PO: 1-2 mg b.i.d./t.i.d.; *max:* 6 mg/d IM/IV: 0.1-0.2 mg t.i.d./q.i.d.	For peptic ulcers and gastric disorders caused by hyperacidity. Used as a preanesthetic drug. Same contraindications as belladonna. Pregnancy category: B; PB: UK; $t\frac{1}{2}$: UK
propantheline bromine (Pro-Banthine)	A: PO: 15 mg t.i.d. 30 min a.c. and 30 mg h.s.; *max:* 120 mg/d Older adults: PO: 7.5 mg b.i.d./t.i.d. a.c.; *max:* 90 mg/d	For peptic ulcers; decreases gastric secretions, irritable bowel syndrome, pancreatitis, and urinary bladder spasm. Standard anticholinergic side effects. Pregnancy category: C; PB: UK; $t\frac{1}{2}$: 1.6 h

A, Adult; *a.c.,* before meals; *b.i.d.,* twice a day; *C,* child; *cap,* capsule; *d,* day; *GI,* gastrointestinal; *h,* hour; *h.s.,* at bedtime; *IM,* intramuscular; *IV,* intravenous; *max,* maximum; *PB,* protein-binding; *PO,* by mouth; *q.i.d.,* four times a day; $t\frac{1}{2}$, half-life; *t.i.d.,* three times a day; *UK,* unknown.

years. However, anticholinergic use has declined with the introduction of H_2 blockers in 1975. These drugs relieve pain by decreasing GI motility and secretion. They act by inhibiting acetylcholine and blocking histamine and hydrochloric acid. Anticholinergics delay gastric emptying time, so they are used more frequently for duodenal ulcers than for gastric ulcers. The anticholinergic propantheline bromine (Pro-Banthine) inhibits gastric secretions in the treatment of peptic ulcers.

Anticholinergics should be taken before meals to decrease the acid secretion that occurs with eating. Antacids can slow the absorption of anticholinergics and therefore should be taken 2 hours after anticholinergic administration.

Table 48-3 lists selected the anticholinergic drugs used to treat peptic ulcer. Anticholinergics should be used as adjunctive therapy and not as the only antiulcer drug. Anticholinergics are discussed in more detail in Chapter 19.

Side Effects and Adverse Reactions

Anticholinergics have many side effects, including dry mouth, decreased secretions, headache, blurred vision, drowsiness, dizziness, lethargy, palpitations, bradycardia, tachycardia, urinary retention, and constipation. Because anticholinergics decrease GI motility, gastric emptying time is delayed, which can stimulate gastric secretions and aggravate the ulceration.

Antacids

Antacids promote ulcer healing by neutralizing hydrochloric acid and reducing pepsin activity; they do not coat the ulcer. There are two types of antacids: those that have a *systemic* effect and those that have a *nonsystemic* effect.

Sodium bicarbonate, a systemically absorbed antacid, was one of the first antiulcer drugs. Because it has many side effects (sodium excess, causing hypernatremia and water retention; metabolic alkalosis caused by excess bicarbonate; and acid rebound [excess acid secretion]), sodium bicarbonate is seldom used to treat peptic ulcers. An example of a sodium bicarbonate compound is Alka-Seltzer.

Calcium carbonate is most effective in neutralizing acid; however, one third to one half of the drug can be systemically absorbed and can cause acid rebound. Hypercalcemia and Burnett's syndrome, formerly called *milk-alkali syndrome,* can result from excessive use of calcium carbonate. Burnett's syndrome is intensified if milk products are ingested with calcium carbonate. It is identified by the presence of alkalosis, hypercalcemia, and in severe cases crystalluria and renal failure.

The nonsystemic antacids are composed of alkaline salts such as aluminum (aluminum hydroxide) and magnesium (magnesium hydroxide, magnesium trisilicate). There is a small degree of systemic absorption with these drugs, mainly of aluminum. Magnesium hydroxide has greater neutralizing power than aluminum hydroxide. Magnesium compounds can cause diarrhea, and aluminum and calcium compounds can cause constipation with long-term use. A combination of magnesium and aluminum salts neutralizes gastric acid without causing severe diarrhea or constipation. Simethicone (an antigas agent) is found in many antacids, including Mylanta Gas, Maalox Antigas, and Mylicon. Prototype Drug Chart 48-1 lists the pharmacologic data for aluminum hydroxide antacids.

Pharmacokinetics Aluminum hydroxide (Amphojel) was one of the first antacids used to neutralize hydrochloric acid. Aluminum products are frequently used to lower high serum phosphate (hyperphosphatemia). Because aluminum hydroxide alone can cause constipation, and magnesium products alone can cause diarrhea, combination drugs such as aluminum hydroxide and magnesium hydroxide (Maalox Caplet) have become popular, because they decrease these side effects.

Only a small amount of aluminum hydroxide is absorbed from the GI tract. It is primarily bound to phosphate and excreted in the feces. The small portion that is absorbed is excreted in the urine.

Pharmacodynamics Aluminum hydroxide neutralizes gastric acid, including hydrochloric acid, and increases the pH of gastric secretions (an elevated pH inactivates pepsin). The onset of action is fairly rapid, but the duration of action varies, depending on whether the antacid is taken with or without food. If the antacid is taken after a meal, the duration of action may be up to 3 hours, because food delays gastric emptying time. Frequent dosing may be necessary if the antacid is given during a fasting state or early in the course of treatment.

PROTOTYPE DRUG CHART 48-1

Aluminum Hydroxide

Drug Class Antiulcer: antacid Trade Name: Amphojel Pregnancy Category: C	**Dosage** Antacid: A: PO: susp: 5-15 mL 1 h p.c. and h.s. Hyperphosphatemia: A: PO: 10-30 mL (suspension) t.i.d./q.i.d. with meals
Contraindications Hypersensitivity to aluminum products, hypophosphatemia Caution: In older adults	**Drug-Lab-Food Interactions** Drug: Decrease effects with tetracycline, phenothiazine, isoniazid, phenytoin, digitalis, quinidine, amphetamines. May increase effect of benzodiazepines Lab: Increase urine pH
Pharmacokinetics Absorption: PO: Small amount absorbed Distribution: PB: UK Metabolism: t½: UK Excretion: In feces; small amount in urine	**Pharmacodynamics** PO: Onset: 15-30 min Peak: 0.5 h Duration: 1-3 h
Therapeutic Effects/Uses To treat hyperacidity, peptic ulcer, and reflux esophagitis; to reduce hyperphosphatemia Mode of Action: Neutralizes gastric acidity	
Side Effects Anorexia, constipation	**Adverse Reactions** Hypophosphatemia, osteoporosis, nephrolithiasis; long-term use can result in GI obstruction

A, Adult; *cap*, capsule; *GI*, gastrointestinal; *h*, hour; *h.s.*, at bedtime; *min*, minute; *PB*, protein-binding; *p.c.*, after meals; *PO*, by mouth; *q.i.d.*, four times a day; *susp*, suspension; *t½*, half-life; *t.i.d.*, three times a day; *UK*, unknown.

The ideal dosing interval for antacids is 1 and 3 hours after meals (maximum acid secretion occurs after eating) and at bedtime. Antacids taken on an empty stomach are effective for 30 to 60 minutes before passing into the duodenum. Chewable tablets should be followed by water. Liquid antacids should also be taken with water (2 to 4 ounces) to ensure that the drug reaches the stomach; however, no more than 4 ounces of water should be taken, because water quickens gastric emptying time.

Antacids containing magnesium salts are contraindicated in patients with impaired renal function because of the risk for hypermagnesemia. Magnesium is primarily excreted by the kidneys; however, hypermagnesemia is usually not a problem unless a patient with renal insufficiency is ingesting magnesium. Prolonged use of aluminum hydroxides can cause hypophosphatemia (low serum phosphate), osteoporosis, nephrolithiasis, and osteomalacia. If hyperphosphatemia occurs because of poor renal function, aluminum hydroxide can be given to decrease the phosphate level. In patients with renal insufficiency, aluminum salt ingestion can cause encephalopathy from accumulation of aluminum in the brain. Table 48-4 lists the antacids and their dosages, uses, and considerations.

Histamine$_2$ Blockers

The histamine$_2$ (H_2) blockers (**histamine$_2$ receptor antagonists**) are popular drugs used in the treatment of gastric and duodenal ulcers. Histamine$_2$ blockers prevent acid reflux in the esophagus (reflux esophagitis). These drugs block the H_2 receptors of the parietal cells in the stomach, thus reducing gastric acid secretion and concentration. Antihistamines, used to treat allergic conditions, act against histamine$_1$ (H_1); they are not the same as H_2 blockers.

The first H_2 blocker was cimetidine (Tagamet), introduced in 1975. Cimetidine, which has a short half-life and a short duration of action, blocks about 70% of acid secretion for 4 hours. Good kidney function is necessary, because approximately 50% to 80% of the drug is excreted unchanged in the urine. In patients with renal insufficiency, the dose and frequency may need to be reduced. Antacids can be given 1 hour before or after cimetidine as part of an antiulcer drug regimen; however, if they are given at the same time, the effectiveness of the H_2 blocker is decreased.

Nursing Process
Patient-Centered Collaborative Care
Antiulcer: Antacids

Assessment
- Evaluate patient's pain, including type, duration, severity, and frequency.
- Check patient's renal function.
- Assess for fluid and electrolyte imbalances, especially serum phosphate and calcium levels.

TABLE 48-4 ANTIULCER DRUGS: ANTACIDS

GENERIC (BRAND)	ROUTE AND DOSAGE	USES AND CONSIDERATIONS
aluminum hydroxide (Amphojel, AlternaGEL)	See Prototype Drug Chart 48-1.	
calcium carbonate (Tums)	A: PO: 0.5-2 g b.i.d./t.i.d.	To alleviate heartburn, acid indigestion, esophagitis, and hiatal hernia caused by hyperacidity. Also used to treat hyperphosphatemia in patients with renal disorders. OTC drug. One third of drug dose absorbed from GI tract. Constipation can be a problem. Pregnancy category: C; PB: 40%; t½: UK
magaldrate (Riopan)	A: PO: 5-10 mL PRN or 1-2 tab PRN; *max:* 100 mL/d or 20 tab/d	To alleviate heartburn, gastritis, esophagitis, and peptic ulcers caused by hyperacidity. Contains aluminum and magnesium hydroxide. Low sodium content. Simethicone decreases flatus. Drug is minimally absorbed. Pregnancy category: B; PB: UK; t½: UK
calcium carbonate and magnesium hydroxide (Rolaids, Mylanta, Tums)	A: PO: Chew 2-4 tabs between meals and h.s.	For heartburn, dyspepsia, and flatulence. Pregnancy category: C; PB: UK; t½: UK
magnesium hydroxide and aluminum hydroxide (Maalox Caplet, Mylanta Ultimate Strength)	A: PO: 2-4 tab PRN; *max:* 16 tab/d or 10-30 mL, 1-3 h p.c. and h.s.	Same as magaldrate. Caution for patients with renal disorder caused by magnesium content. OTC drug. Pregnancy category: B; PB: UK; t½: UK
magnesium hydroxide and aluminum hydroxide with simethicone (Mylanta, Maalox, Gelusil)	A: PO: 10-20 mL PRN; *max:* 120 mL/d; or 2-4 tab PRN; *max:* 24 tab/d	Same as magaldrate. Also contains simethicone, which decreases flatus. OTC drug. Pregnancy category: B; PB: UK; t½: UK
magnesium trisilicate with aluminum hydroxide (Gaviscon Regular Strength)	A: PO: 2-4 tab q.i.d.; *max:* 16 tab/d	To relieve gastric disorders caused by hyperacidity. OTC drug. Contains magnesium trisilicate and aluminum hydroxide. Pregnancy category: UK; PB: UK; t½: UK
sodium bicarbonate (Alka-Seltzer Heartburn Relief)	A: PO: 300 mg-2 g 1-4 times/d	Previously used for gastric hyperacidity. Short-acting, potent antacid that is systemically absorbed. Acid-base imbalance could occur. Pregnancy category: C; PB: UK; t½: UK

A, Adult; *cap*, capsule; *d*, day; *GI*, gastrointestinal; *h*, hour; *h.s.*, at bedtime; *max*, maximum; *OTC*, over-the-counter; *PB*, protein-binding; *p.c.*, after meals; *PO*, by mouth; *PRN*, as needed; *t½*, half-life; *tab*, tablet; *tsp*, teaspoon; *UK*, unknown.

- Obtain drug history; report probable drug-drug interactions.

Nursing Diagnoses

- Acute pain related to repeated spicy food and alcohol ingestion
- Ineffective health maintenance related to misuse of antacids
- Deficient knowledge related to misinterpretation of information

Planning

- Patient's abdominal pain will decrease after 1 to 2 weeks of antiulcer drug management.

Nursing Interventions

- Avoid administering antacids with other oral drugs, because antacids can delay their absorption. Do not give an antacid with tetracycline, digoxin, or quinidine, because it binds with and inactivates most of the drug. Antacids are given 1 to 2 hours after other medications.
- Shake suspension well before administering; follow with water.
- Monitor electrolytes and urinary pH, calcium, and phosphate levels.

Patient Teaching

General

- Teach patient to report pain, coughing, or vomiting of blood.
- Encourage patient to drink 2 oz of water after antacid to ensure that drug reaches stomach.
- Direct patient to take antacid 1 to 3 hours after meals and at bedtime. Instruct patient not to take antacids at mealtime; they slow gastric emptying time, causing increased GI activity and gastric secretions.
- Advise patient to notify health care provider if constipation or diarrhea occurs; the antacid may have to be changed. Self-treatment should be avoided.
- Warn that taking an unlimited amount of the antacid is contraindicated.
- Warn patient to avoid taking antacids with milk or foods high in vitamin D.
- Advise patient to avoid taking antacids within 1 to 2 hours of other oral medications, because they may interfere with absorption.

- Guide patient on a sodium-restricted diet to check antacid labels for sodium content.
- Alert patient to consult with health care provider before taking self-prescribed antacids for longer than 2 weeks.
- Inform patient on use of relaxation techniques.

Self-Administration

- Teach patient how to take antacids correctly. Chewable tablets must be thoroughly chewed and followed with water. With liquid antacid, patient should follow antacid with 2 to 4 ounces of water. Increased amount of water with antacids increases gastric emptying time.

Side Effects

- Direct patient to avoid food and beverages that can cause gastric irritation (high-fat or spicy meals; caffeine-containing coffee and soda; alcohol).
- Explain to patient that stools may become speckled or white.

Cultural Considerations

- Respect patient's cultural beliefs and alternative methods for treating GI discomfort.
- Discuss with patient the safety of those methods and the use of drugs prescribed to heal and lessen the symptoms.
- Recognize that patients of various cultural backgrounds may need guidance in understanding the disease process of their GI disturbance. Use of a written plan of care with modifications should be considered.

Evaluation

- Determine the effectiveness of the antiulcer treatment and the presence of side effects. Patient should be free of pain, and healing should progress.

Three H_2 blockers, ranitidine (Zantac), famotidine (Pepcid), and nizatidine (Axid), are more potent than cimetidine. In addition to blocking gastric acid secretions, they promote healing of the ulcer by eliminating its cause. Their duration of action is longer, decreasing the frequency of dosing, and they have fewer side effects and fewer drug interactions than cimetidine. Prototype Drug Chart 48-2 lists the pharmacologic data for ranitidine (Zantac), the most frequently prescribed H_2 blocker.

Pharmacokinetics Ranitidine is 5 to 12 times more potent than cimetidine but less potent than famotidine. It is rapidly absorbed and reaches its peak concentration after a single dose in 1 to 3 hours. Ranitidine has a low protein-binding power and a short half-life. With liver disease, the half-life of ranitidine is prolonged. About 50% of the absorbed drug is excreted unchanged in the urine.

Ulcer healing occurs in 4 weeks for 70% of patients and in 8 weeks for 90% of patients taking ranitidine. Large doses of ranitidine are effective for controlling Zollinger-Ellison syndrome, whereas cimetidine is not effective in controlling the symptoms of this disorder.

Pharmacodynamics Ranitidine inhibits histamine at the H_2 receptor site. The drug is effective in treating gastric and duodenal ulcers and can be used prophylactically. It is also useful in relieving symptoms of reflux esophagitis, preventing stress ulcers that can occur following major surgery, and preventing aspiration pneumonitis that can result from aspiration of gastric acid secretions.

Ranitidine has a longer onset of action and duration of action (up to 12 hours) than cimetidine. Because the duration of action of cimetidine is only 4 to 5 hours, it is frequently given three to four times a day.

Famotidine (Pepcid) is 50% to 80% more potent than cimetidine and is five to eight times more potent than ranitidine. It is indicated for short-term use (4 to 8 weeks) for duodenal ulcer and for Zollinger-Ellison syndrome.

Nizatidine (Axid) is an H_2 blocker that can relieve nocturnal gastric acid secretion for 12 hours. This drug is similar to famotidine and ranitidine, and none of these agents suppresses the metabolism of other drugs. To prevent recurrence of duodenal ulcers, administer nizatidine 150 mg/day at bedtime or famotidine 20 mg/day at bedtime. Both nizatidine and famotidine have similar protein-binding times and half-lives.

Table 48-5 lists the H_2 blockers and their dosages, uses, and considerations.

Side Effects and Adverse Reactions. Side effects and adverse reactions of H_2 blockers include headache, dizziness, constipation, pruritus, skin rash, gynecomastia, decreased libido, and impotence. Ranitidine and famotidine have fewer side effects than cimetidine.

Drug and Laboratory Interactions. Cimetidine interacts with many drugs. By inhibiting hepatic drug metabolism, it enhances the effects of oral anticoagulants, theophylline, caffeine, phenytoin (Dilantin), diazepam (Valium), propranolol (Inderal), phenobarbital, and calcium channel blockers. Cimetidine can cause an increase in blood urea nitrogen (BUN), serum creatinine, and serum alkaline phosphatase. Neither cimetidine nor ranitidine should be taken with antacids, because their H_2 blocking action could be decreased. Ranitidine can increase the effect of oral anticoagulants. Table 48-5 lists the H_2 blockers and their dosages, uses, and considerations.

Nursing Process
Patient-Centered Collaborative Care

Antiulcer: Histamine$_2$ Blocker

Assessment

- Determine patient's pain, including type, duration, severity, frequency, and location.
- Evaluate GI complaints.
- Check mental status.
- Assess fluid and electrolyte imbalances, including intake and output.

PROTOTYPE DRUG CHART 48-2

Ranitidine

Drug Class	Dosage
Antiulcer: histamine$_2$ blocker Trade Name: Zantac Pregnancy Category: B	A: PO: 150 mg q12h or 300 mg h.s.; maint: 150 mg h.s. A: IM: 50 mg q6-8h A: IV: 50 mg q6-8h diluted C: PO: 2-4 mg/kg/d divided q12h C: IV: 1-2 mg/kg/d divided q6-8h
Contraindications	**Drug-Lab-Food Interactions**
Hypersensitivity, severe renal or liver disease Caution: Pregnancy, lactation	Drug: Decrease absorption with antacids; decrease absorption of ketoconazole; toxicity with metoprolol Lab: Increase serum alkaline phosphatase
Pharmacokinetics	**Pharmacodynamics**
Absorption: PO: well absorbed, 50% Distribution: PB: 15% Metabolism: t½: 2-3 h Excretion: In urine and feces	PO: Onset: 15 min Peak: 1-3 h Duration: 8-12 h IM/IV: Onset: 10-15 min Peak: 15 min Duration: 8-12 h
Therapeutic Effects/Uses	
To prevent and treat peptic ulcers, gastroesophageal reflux, and stress ulcers Mode of Action: Inhibits gastric acid secretion by inhibiting histamine at histamine$_2$ receptors in parietal cells	
Side Effects	**Adverse Reactions**
Headache, confusion, nausea, vertigo, diarrhea or constipation, depression, rash, blurred vision, malaise, decreased libido	Life-threatening: Hepatotoxicity, cardiac dysrhythmias, blood dyscrasias

A, Adult; *C,* child; *d,* day; *h,* hour; *h.s.,* at bedtime; *IM,* intramuscular; *IV,* intravenous; *maint,* maintenance; *min,* minute; *PB,* protein-binding; *PO,* by mouth; *t½,* half-life.

TABLE 48-5 ANTIULCER DRUGS: HISTAMINE$_2$ BLOCKERS

GENERIC (BRAND)	ROUTE AND DOSAGE	USES AND CONSIDERATIONS
cimetidine (Tagamet)	A: PO: 200 mg q.i.d. OR 800 mg h.s.; maint: 300 mg h.s. IV: 300 mg q6-8h diluted in 50 mL (administered over 15-30 min) IV: continuous infusion: 37.5 mg/h over 24 h; *max:* 900 mg/d C: PO: 10-40 mg/kg/d divided q6h	For peptic ulcers (gastric and duodenal). First H_2 blocker marketed. Many drug interactions and side effects. Duration of action 4-6 h. Pregnancy category: B; PB: 20%; t½: 2 h
famotidine (Pepcid)	A: PO: 20 mg b.i.d. or 40 mg h.s.; maint: 20 mg h.s. IV: 20 mg b.i.d. diluted	For active duodenal ulcer. Inhibits gastric secretion. More potent than cimetidine. Pregnancy category: B; PB: 15%-20%; t½: 2.5-4 h
nizatidine (Axid)	A: PO: 150 mg b.i.d. or 300 mg h.s.; maint: 150 mg h.s.	Same as famotidine. Also used to treat gastroesophageal reflux. Give drug after meals or at bedtime. Do not give within 1 h of antacids. Pregnancy category: B; PB: 35%; t½: 1-2 h
ranitidine (Zantac)	See Prototype Drug Chart 48-2.	

A, Adult; *C,* child; *d,* day; *h,* hour; *h.s.,* at bedtime; *IV,* intravenous; *maint,* maintenance; *max,* maximum; *PB,* protein-binding; *PO,* by mouth; *q.i.d.,* four times a day; *t½,* half-life.

- Monitor gastric pH (>5 is desired), blood urea nitrogen (BUN), and creatinine.
- Determine drug history; report probable drug-drug interactions.

Nursing Diagnoses

- Acute pain related to excess gastric secretion

Planning

- Patient's abdominal pain will decrease after 1 to 2 weeks of drug therapy.

Nursing Interventions

- Administer drug just before meals or at bedtime to decrease food-induced acid secretion.

- Be alert that older adults have less gastric acid and need reduced doses of drug. Metabolic acidosis must be prevented.
- Administer IV drug in 20 to 100 mL of solution.

Patient Teaching

General

- Teach patient to report pain, coughing, or vomiting of blood.
- Advise patient to avoid smoking, because it can hamper effectiveness of drug.
- Remind patient that drug must be taken exactly as prescribed to be effective.
- Direct patient to separate ranitidine and antacid dosage by at least 1 hour.
- Warn patient not to drive a motor vehicle or engage in dangerous activities until stabilized on the drug.
- Tell patient that drug-induced impotence and gynecomastia are reversible.
- Educate patient in use of relaxation techniques to decrease anxiety.

Diet

- Teach patient to eat foods rich in vitamin B_{12} to avoid deficiency as a result of drug therapy.
- Alert patient to avoid foods and liquids that cause gastric irritation, such as caffeine-containing beverages, alcohol, and spices.

Cultural Considerations

- Respect patient's cultural beliefs and alternative methods for treating GI discomfort. Discuss safety of these methods and use of drugs prescribed to heal and lessen symptoms.
- Recognize that patients of various cultural backgrounds may need guidance in understanding the disease process of their GI disturbance. Use of a written plan of care with modifications should be considered.

Evaluation

- Determine effectiveness of drug therapy and presence of any side effects or adverse reactions. Patient should be free of pain, and healing should progress.

Proton Pump Inhibitors (Gastric Acid Secretion Inhibitors, Gastric Acid Pump Inhibitors)

PPIs suppress gastric acid secretion by inhibiting the hydrogen/potassium adenosine triphosphatase (ATPase) enzyme system located in the gastric parietal cells. They tend to inhibit gastric acid secretion up to 90% greater than the H_2 blockers (histamine antagonists). These agents block the final step of acid production.

Omeprazole (Prilosec) was the first PPI marketed, followed by lansoprazole (Prevacid), rabeprazole (Aciphex), pantoprazole (Protonix), esomeprazole (Nexium), and dexlansoprazole (Dexilant), a delayed-release oral capsule. These agents are effective in suppressing gastric acid secretions and are used to treat peptic ulcers and GERD. With lansoprazole, ulcer relief usually occurs in 1 week. Rabeprazole is more effective in treating duodenal ulcers than gastric ulcers, but it is most effective for treating GERD and hypersecretory disease (Zollinger-Ellison syndrome). Pantoprazole is prescribed to treat short-term erosive GERD. Intravenous pantoprazole is also reported as effective in treating Zollinger-Ellison syndrome. Esomeprazole has the highest success rate for healing erosive GERD, more so than omeprazole. Omeprazole promotes irreversible hydrogen or potassium ATPase inhibition until new enzyme is synthesized, which could take days, whereas rabeprazole causes reversible ATPase inhibition. Dexlansoprazole is prescribed to treat erosive esophagitis and symptomatic nonerosive GERD. All PPIs in large doses can be combined with antibiotics to treat *H. pylori.* Prototype Drug Chart 48-3 lists the pharmacologic data for esomeprazole.

SAFETY: Preventing Medication Errors

Do not confuse ...

- **Protonix** (proton pump inhibitor) with **Lotronex** (serotonin 5-HT3 receptor antagonist used for irritable bowel syndrome)
- **Aciphex** (proton pump inhibitor) with **Aricept** (Alzheimer's agent)
- **Nexium** (proton pump inhibitor) with **Nexavar** (biologic response modifier) **Rabeprazole** (proton pump inhibitor) with **Aripiprazole** (atypical antipsychotic)
- **Misoprostol** (antiulcer agent) with **mifepristone** (postcoital contraceptive agent)

Two combination medications involving PPIs are omeprazole with sodium bicarbonate (Zegerid) and esomemprazole with Naproxen (Vimovo). Zegerid is the only drug given to prevent stress ulcers in critically ill patients. It also is used to treat GERD, erosive esophagitis, and gastric or duodenal ulcers. Zegerid can now be found over the counter as well. Vimovo is an immediate-release PPI layered over an enteric-coated NSAID in one tablet used to prevent NSAID-associated gastric ulcers.

Pharmacokinetics and Pharmacodynamics The duration of action for esomemprazole is 24 hours. These drugs have a short half-life and are highly protein-bound (97%). PPIs should usually be taken before meals. Caution should be used in patients with hepatic impairment; liver enzymes should be monitored. Possible side effects include headache, dizziness, diarrhea, abdominal pain, and rash. Prolonged use of PPIs may increase the risk for cancer, although this has only been proven in mice, not humans.

Table 48-6 lists the PPIs and their dosages, uses, and considerations.

Drug Interactions. PPIs can enhance the action of digoxin, oral anticoagulants, certain benzodiazepines, and phenytoin, because they interfere with liver metabolism of these drugs.

PROTOTYPE DRUG CHART 48-3

Esomeprazole

Drug Class Antiulcer: proton pump inhibitor Trade Name: Nexium Pregnancy Category: B	**Dosage** Erosive esophagitis: A: PO: 20-40 mg/d for 4-8 wk, then 20 mg daily GERD: A: PO: 15 mg/d for 4 wk C: PO: 1-11 y: 1.5 mg/kg/d *max:* 30 mg/d *H. pylori:* A: PO: 40 mg b.i.d. for 2 wk in combination therapy for 10-14 d Duodenal ulcer: A: PO: 15 mg/d for 4 wk
Contraindications Hypersensitivity, pregnancy, lactation Caution: Hepatic disease	**Drug-Lab-Food Interactions** Drug: May decrease theophylline levels; sucralfate decreases lansoprazole bioavailability; may interfere with absorption of ampicillin, ketoconazole, digoxin Food: Food decreases peak levels
Pharmacokinetics Absorption: Rapidly absorbed in GI tract Distribution: PB: 97% Metabolism: $t\frac{1}{2}$: 1.5 h Excretion: Primarily in urine; also in bile and feces	**Pharmacodynamics** PO: Onset: 2 h Peak: 1.5-3 h Duration: 24 h
Therapeutic Effects/Uses To treat peptic and duodenal ulcers, GERD, erosive esophagitis, *H. pylori,* and Zollinger-Ellison syndrome Mode of Action: Suppresses gastric acid secretion by inhibiting hydrogen/potassium ATPase enzyme in gastric parietal cells	
Side Effects Headache, dizziness, blurred vision, fatigue, thirst, dry mouth, increased appetite, anorexia, nausea, hiccups, diarrhea, constipation, rash	**Adverse Reactions** Elevated AST, ALT

A, Adult; *ALT,* alanine aminotransferase; *AST,* aspartate aminotransferase; *ATP,* adenosine triphosphate; *b.i.d.,* two times a day; *C,* child; *d,* day; *GERD,* gastroesophageal reflux disease; *GI,* gastrointestinal; *h,* hour; *max,* maximum; *PB,* protein-binding; *PO,* by mouth; $t\frac{1}{2}$, half-life; *wk,* weeks; *y,* years.

Pepsin Inhibitor (Mucosal Protective Drug)

Sucralfate (Carafate), a complex of sulfated sucrose and aluminum hydroxide, is classified as a pepsin inhibitor, or *mucosal protective drug.* It is nonabsorbable and combines with protein to form a viscous substance that covers the ulcer and protects it from acid and pepsin. This drug does not neutralize acid or decrease acid secretions.

The dosage of sucralfate is 1 gram, usually four times a day before meals and at bedtime. If antacids are added to decrease pain, they should be given either 30 minutes before or 30 minutes after the administration of sucralfate. Because sucralfate is not systemically absorbed, side effects are few; however, it can cause constipation. If the drug is stored at room temperature in an airtight container, it will remain stable for up to 2 years. Prototype Drug Chart 48-4 lists the pharmacologic data for sucralfate.

Pharmacokinetics Less than 5% of sucralfate is absorbed by the GI tract. It has a half-life of 6 to 20 hours. Ninety percent of the drug is excreted in feces.

Pharmacodynamics Sucralfate promotes healing by adhering to the ulcer surface. Onset of action occurs within 30 minutes, and duration of action is short. Sucralfate decreases the absorption of tetracycline, phenytoin fat-soluble vitamins, and the antibacterial agents, ciprofloxacin and norfloxacin. Antacids decrease the effects of sucralfate.

Nursing Process
Patient-Centered Collaborative Care

Antiulcer: Pepsin Inhibitor

Assessment

- Evaluate patient's pain, including type, duration, severity, and frequency. Ulcer pain usually occurs after meals and during the night.
- Determine patient's renal function. Report urine output of <600 mL/d or <30 mL/h.
- Assess for fluid and electrolyte imbalances.
- Measure gastric pH (>5 is desired).

Nursing Diagnosis

- Acute pain related to excess gastric secretion

TABLE 48-6 ANTIULCER DRUGS: PROTON PUMP INHIBITORS, PEPSIN INHIBITOR, AND PROSTAGLANDIN ANALOGUE

GENERIC (BRAND)	ROUTE AND DOSAGE	USES AND CONSIDERATIONS
Proton Pump Inhibitors (Gastric Acid Secretion Inhibitors)		
esomeprazole magnesium (Nexium)	See Prototype Drug Chart 48-3.	
lansoprazole (Prevacid)	A: PO: 15 mg/d	For treatment of duodenal and gastric ulcers, GERD, and esophagitis. Pregnancy category: B; PB: 97%-99%; t1/2: 1-1.5 h
omeprazole (Prilosec)	GERD and peptic ulcer: A: PO: 20 mg/d for 4-8 wk Hypersecretory: A: PO: Initially: 60 mg/d; may increase to 120 mg t.i.d.	For GERD, esophagitis, Zollinger-Ellison syndrome, and *H. pylori.* Poorly absorbed, only 35%-40% in circulation. Antacids can be taken with drug. Pregnancy category: C; PB: 95%; t½: 0.5-1.5 h
pantoprazole (Protonix)	A: PO/IV: 20-40 mg/d for up to 14 days	For gastric and duodenal ulcers and GERD. Action same as rabeprazole: suppresses gastric acid secretion. Pregnancy category: B; PB: 99%; t½: 3.5-10h.
rabeprazole (AcipHex)	Duodenal ulcer/GERD: A: PO: 20 mg/d Hypersecretory disease: A: PO: 60 mg/d or 60 mg b.i.d.	For duodenal ulcer, GERD, and hypersecretory syndrome (Zollinger-Ellison syndrome). Decreases gastric acid production by inhibiting hydrogen/potassium ATPase enzyme at gastric parietal cells. Pregnancy category: B; PB: 96.3%; t½: 1-2 h
dexlansoprazole (Dexilant)	A: PO: 30-60 mg/d for up to 8 weeks	For erosive esophagitis and symptomatic nonerosive GERD. May be given without regard to food. Pregnancy category: B; PB: 96%-98%; t½: 1-2 h
Pepsin Inhibitor		
sucralfate (Carafate)	See Prototype Drug Chart 48-4.	
Prostaglandin Analogue		
misoprostol (Cytotec)	A: PO: 100-200 mcg q.i.d. p.c.	Prevention of NSAID-induced gastric ulcer. May be taken during NSAID therapy, including with aspirin. Side effects include diarrhea, abdominal pain, flatulence, nausea, vomiting, constipation, and menstrual spotting. Short duration of action. Pregnancy category: X; PB: 85%; t½: 20-40 min

A, Adult; *a.c.,* before meals; *ATP,* adenosine triphosphate; *b.i.d.,* two times a day; *C,* child; *d,* day; *GERD,* gastroesophageal reflux disease; *h,* hour; *IV,* intravenous; *NSAIDs,* nonsteroidal antiinflammatory drugs; *p.c.,* after meals; *PB,* protein-binding; *PO,* by mouth; *q.i.d.,* four times a day; *t½,* half-life; *t.i.d.,* three times a day; *UK,* unknown; *wk,* week; *y,* year; *<,* less than.

Planning

- Patient will have relief of abdominal pain after 1 to 2 weeks of antiulcer drug management.

Nursing Interventions

- Administer drug on empty stomach.
- Administer antacid 30 minutes before or 30 minutes after sucralfate. Allow 1 to 2 hours to elapse between sucralfate and other prescribed drugs; sucralfate binds with certain drugs (e.g., tetracycline, phenytoin), reducing their effect.

Patient Teaching

General

- Advise patient to take drug exactly as ordered. Therapy usually requires 4 to 8 weeks for optimal ulcer healing. Advise patient to continue to take drug even if feeling better.
- Increase fluids, dietary bulk, and exercise to relieve constipation.
- Educate patient in use of relaxation techniques.
- Monitor for severe, persistent constipation.
- Encourage need for follow-up medical care.
- Emphasize cessation of smoking as indicated.

Side Effects

- Direct patient to report pain, coughing, or vomiting of blood.

Diet

- Teach patient to avoid liquids and foods that can cause gastric irritation, such as caffeine-containing beverages, alcohol, certain fats, and spices.

PROTOTYPE DRUG CHART 48-4

Sucralfate

Drug Class	Dosage
Antiulcer: pepsin inhibitor Trade Names: Carafate, ♣ Apo-Sucralfate Pregnancy Category: B	Active disease: A: PO: 1 g q.i.d. 1 h a.c. and h.s. Maint: A: PO: 1 g b.i.d.
Contraindications	**Drug-Lab-Food Interactions**
Hypersensitivity Caution: Renal failure	Drug: Decrease effects with tetracycline, phenytoin, fat-soluble vitamins, digoxin; altered absorption with ciprofloxacin, norfloxacin, antacids
Pharmacokinetics	**Pharmacodynamics**
Absorption: PO: Minimal absorption (<5%) Distribution: PB: UK Metabolism: t½: 6-20 h Excretion: In urine	PO: Onset: 30 min Peak: UK Duration: 5 h
Therapeutic Effects/Uses	
To prevent gastric mucosal injury from drug-induced ulcers (aspirin, NSAIDs); to manage ulcers Mode of Action: In combination with gastric acid, forms a protective covering on the ulcer surface	
Side Effects	**Adverse Reactions**
Dizziness, headache, nausea, flatulence, constipation, dry mouth, rash, pruritus, sleepiness	Hyperglycemia, hypomagnesemia

A, Adult; *a.c.*, before meals; *b.i.d.*, twice a day; *h*, hour; *h.s.*, at bedtime; *maint*, maintenance; *min*, minute; *NSAIDs*, nonsteroidal antiinflammatory drugs; *PB*, protein-binding; *PO*, by mouth; *q.i.d.*, four times a day; *t ½*, half-life; *UK*, unknown; ♣, Canadian drug name; <, less than.

Cultural Considerations

- Greet the patient by name with appropriate title (e.g., Mr., Ms., Dr.). Wait until patient gives permission to use his or her first name.
- Orthodox Jewish men do not touch women other than their wives, so their failure to take a hand offered in greeting should not be interpreted as impoliteness.

Evaluation

- Determine the effectiveness of the antiulcer treatment and the presence of any side effects. Patient should be free of pain, and healing should progress.

Prostaglandin Analogue Antiulcer Drug

Misoprostol, a synthetic prostaglandin analogue, is a drug used to prevent and treat peptic ulcer. It appears to suppress gastric acid secretion and increase cytoprotective mucus in the GI tract. It causes a moderate decrease in pepsin secretion. Misoprostol is considered as effective as cimetidine. Patients who complain of gastric distress from NSAIDs such as aspirin or indomethacin prescribed for long-term therapy can benefit from misoprostol. When a patient takes high doses of NSAIDs, misoprostol is frequently recommended for the duration of the NSAID therapy. Misoprostol is contraindicated during pregnancy and for women of childbearing age.

Table 48-6 lists the pharmacologic data for the PPIs, pepsin inhibitors, and a prostaglandin analogue.

KEY WEBSITES

Gastritis and peptic ulcer disease: *www.emedicine.com/emerg/topic820.htm*

Proton pump inhibitors: *www.aafp.org/afp/20020715/273.html*

CRITICAL THINKING CASE STUDY

JH, a 48-year-old patient, complains of a gnawing, aching pain in the abdominal area that usually occurs several hours after eating. He says that over-the-counter antacids help somewhat but that the pain has recently intensified. Diagnostic tests indicate that the patient has a duodenal ulcer.

1. Differentiate between peptic ulcer, gastric ulcer, and duodenal ulcer. Explain your answer.
2. What are the predisposing factors related to peptic ulcers? What additional information do you need from JH?
3. What nonpharmacologic measures can you suggest to alleviate symptoms related to peptic ulcer?

The health care provider prescribed Mylanta 2 tsp to be taken 2 hours after meals, and ranitidine (Zantac) 150 mg twice a day. The dose of magnesium hydroxide and aluminum hydroxide with simethicone (Mylanta) is to be taken either 1 hour before or 1 hour after the ranitidine.

4. JH asks the nurse the purposes for Mylanta and ranitidine. What is the nurse's best response?
5. Why does the health care provider suggest that the patient take ranitidine with meals? Why should Mylanta and ranitidine not be taken at the same time?
6. In what ways are ranitidine and cimetidine (Tagamet) the same, and how do they differ? Explain your answer.
7. As part of patient teaching, the nurse discusses side effects of ranitidine with JH. What is the most effective way to present this information? Develop a plan.

JH states that he drinks beer at lunch and has two gin and tonics in the afternoon. He states that the drinks help him relax.

8. What nursing intervention should be taken in regard to his alcohol intake?
9. What foods should he avoid?

A week later JH states that he discontinued the prescribed medications because he "felt better." However, the pain recurred and he asked whether he should resume taking the medications.

10. What is the nurse's best response? What should be included in the patient teaching?

NCLEX STUDY QUESTIONS

1. A patient is diagnosed with peptic ulcer disease. The nurse realizes that which factor is a predisposing factor for this condition?
   a. *Helicobacter pylori*
   b. Hyposecretion of pepsin
   c. Decreased hydrochloric acid
   d. *Escherichia coli*
2. A student nurse is preparing to administer sucralfate (Carafate) to a patient. Which statement by the student nurse demonstrates understanding of sucralfate's mode of action?
   a. "Sucralfate neutralizes gastric acidity."
   b. "Gastric acid secretion is decreased by inhibiting histamine at H_2 receptors in parietal cells."
   c. "Gastric acid secretion is suppressed by inhibiting the hydrogen/potassium ATPase enzyme."
   d. "Sucralfate combines with protein to form a viscous substance that forms a protective covering of ulcer."
3. A patient is taking ranitidine (Zantac). What information should the nurse teach the patient about this drug? (Select all that apply.)
   a. Drug-induced impotence is irreversible.
   b. The drug must be administered 30 minutes before meals.
   c. The drug must be administered separately from an antacid by at least 1 hour.
   d. The drug must always be administered with magnesium hydroxide.
   e. Smoking should be avoided while taking this drug.
   f. Foods high in vitamin B_{12} should be increased in diet.
4. When a patient complains of pain accompanying a peptic ulcer, why should the nurse give an antacid?
   a. Antacids decrease GI motility.
   b. Antacids decrease gastric acid secretion.
   c. Antacids strengthen the lower esophageal sphincter's action.
   d. Antacids neutralize HCl and reduce pepsin activity.
5. A patient is taking famotidine (Pepcid) to inhibit gastric secretions. Which side effects of famotidine will the nurse teach the patient? (Select all that apply.)
   a. Diarrhea
   b. Dizziness
   c. Dry mouth
   d. Headaches
   e. Blurred vision
   f. Decreased libido
6. The patient is taking esomeprazole magnesium (Nexium) for an erosive GERD. Which should the nurse include in patient teaching?
   a. Take with breakfast daily.
   b. Healing should occur in one week.
   c. This medication decreases stomach acid secretion.
   d. Blood test to check kidney function should be done.

Answers: 1, a; 2, d; 3, c, e, f; 4, d; 5, b, d, f; 6, c.

UNIT XVI

Eye, Ear, and Skin Agents

Drugs used to treat eye and ear disorders are also discussed in other chapters. Antibiotics are covered in Chapter 29, Penicillins and Cephalosporins; Chapter 30, Macrolides, Tetracyclines, Aminoglycosides, and Fluoroquinolones; and Chapter 31, Sulfonamides. Unit XVI discusses in detail the agents used to treat disorders of the eye, ear, and skin. Chapter 49, Drugs for Eye and Ear Disorders, presents medications used to treat eye disorders, particularly glaucoma and ocular infections. Drugs used to treat ear disorders are also covered. Chapter 50, Drugs for Dermatologic Disorders, presents the agents used to treat skin conditions such as acne and psoriasis.

OVERVIEW OF THE EYE

The eyeballs, protected within the orbits of the skull, are controlled by the third, fourth, and sixth cranial nerves and are connected to six extraocular muscles. The eye has three layers: (1) the cornea and sclera; (2) the choroid, iris, and ciliary body; and (3) the retina. Figure XVI-1 illustrates the basic structures of the eye.

The cornea, the anterior covering of the eye, is transparent, enabling light to enter the eye. It has no blood vessels and receives nutrition from the aqueous humor. An abraded cornea is susceptible to infection. Loss of corneal transparency is usually caused by increased intraocular pressure (IOP).

The sclera is the opaque, white fibrous envelope of the eye. Within the sclera are the posterior chamber and the anterior chamber. The posterior chamber has a blind spot, which is not sensitive to light, around the optic nerve. The lens, held in place by ligaments, separates these two chambers. The normally transparent lens focuses light on the retina by changing its shape through a process called *accommodation.*

The anterior chamber, filled with aqueous humor secreted by the ciliary body, lies in front of the lens. The fluid flows into the anterior chamber through a space between the lens and iris. The excess fluid drains into the canal of Schlemm. An increase in IOP, resulting in glaucoma, occurs with increased production or decreased drainage of aqueous humor.

The choroid, iris, and ciliary body (thickened part of the vascular covering of the eye that provides attachment to ligaments and support to the lens) constitute the second layer. The choroid absorbs light. The iris surrounds the pupil and gives the eye its color. By dilating and constricting, the iris controls the quantity of light reaching the lens.

The retina, the third layer, consists of nerves, rods, and cones that serve as visual sensory receptors. The retina is connected to the brain via the optic nerve.

The eyebrows, eyelashes, eyelids, tears, and corneal and conjunctival reflexes all serve to protect the eye. Bilateral blinking occurs every few seconds during waking hours to keep the eye moist and free of foreign material.

OVERVIEW OF THE EAR

The ear is divided into the external, middle, and inner ear. Figure XVI-2 illustrates the basic structures of the ear.

The *external ear* consists of the pinna and the external auditory canal. The external auditory canal transmits sound to the tympanic membrane (eardrum), a transparent partition between the external and middle ear. The eardrum in turn transmits sound to the bones of the middle ear; it also serves a protective function.

The *middle ear,* an air-filled cavity, contains three auditory ossicles (malleus, incus, and stapes) that transmit sound waves to the inner ear. The tip of the malleus is attached to the eardrum; its head is attached to the incus, which is attached to the stapes. The Eustachian tube provides a direct connection to the nasopharynx and equalizes air pressure on both sides of the eardrum to prevent it from rupturing. Swallowing, yawning, and chewing gum help the Eustachian tube relieve pressure changes during airplane flights.

The *inner ear,* a series of labyrinths (canals), consists of a bony section and a membranous section. The vestibule, cochlea, and semicircular canals make up the bony labyrinth. The vestibular area is responsible for maintaining equilibrium and balance. The cochlea is the principal hearing organ.

Professional evaluation of ear problems is essential, because hearing loss can result from untreated disorders. Middle ear problems require prescription medications and are not treated with over-the-counter preparations.

OVERVIEW OF THE SKIN

Skin, the largest organ of the body, consists of two major layers: the *epidermis* (the outer layer of skin) and the *dermis* (the layer of skin beneath the epidermis). The functions of the skin include (1) protecting the body from the environment, (2) aiding in body temperature control, and (3) preventing body fluid loss.

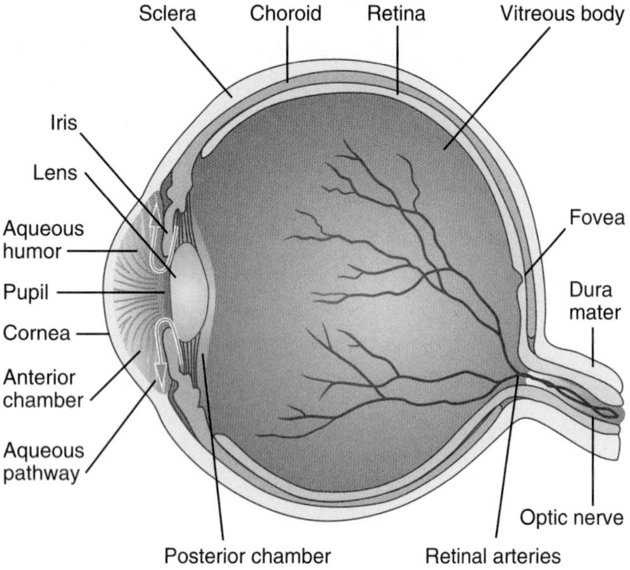

FIGURE XVI–1 Basic structures of the eye.

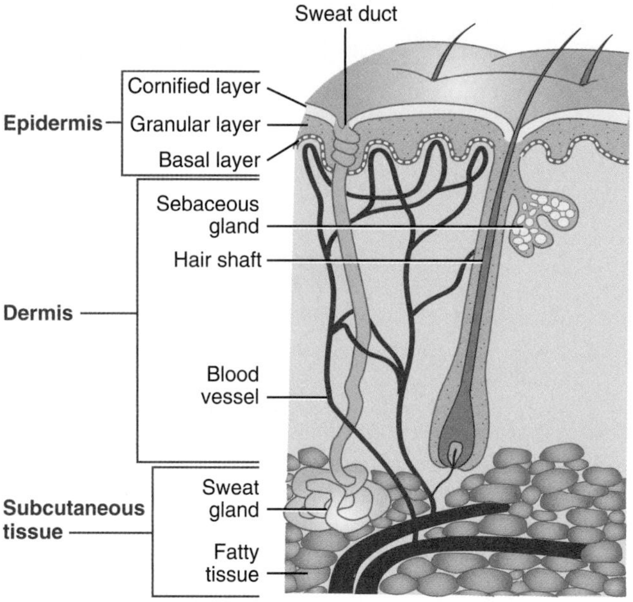

FIGURE XVI–3 Basic structures of the skin.

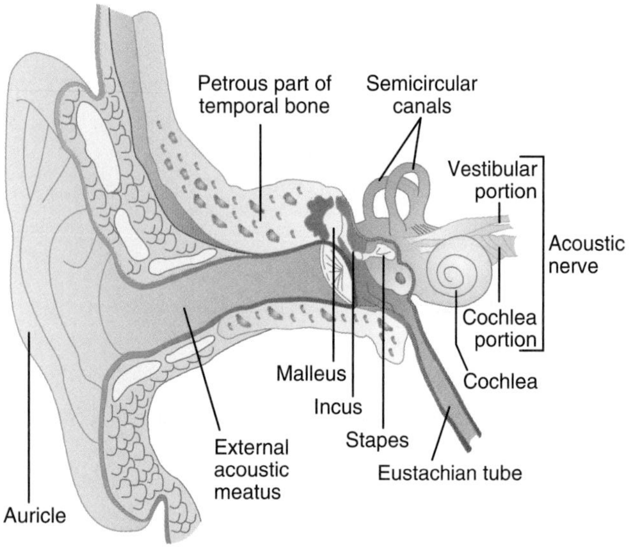

FIGURE XVI–2 Basic structures of the ear.

The epidermis has four layers: (1) the basal layer (stratum germinativum), the deepest layer lying over the dermis; (2) the spinous layer (stratum spinosum); (3) the granular layer (stratum granulosum); and (4) the cornified layer (stratum corneum), the outer layer of the epidermis. As the epidermal cells migrate to the surface, they die, and their cytoplasm converts to keratin (hard and rough texture), forming keratinocytes. Eventually the keratinocytes slough off as new layers of epidermal cells migrate upward.

The dermis has two layers: (1) the papillary layer, next to the epidermis, and (2) the reticular layer, which is the deeper layer of the dermis. The dermal layers consist of fibroblasts, collagen fibers, and elastic fibers. The collagen and elastic fibers give the skin its strength and elasticity. Within the dermal layer, there are sweat glands, hair follicles, sebaceous glands, blood vessels, and sensory nerve terminals. Figure XVI-3 shows the layers of the skin.

The subcutaneous tissue, primarily fatty tissue, lies under the dermis. Besides fatty cells, subcutaneous tissue contains blood and lymphatic vessels, nerve fibers, and elastic fibers. It supports and protects the dermis.

CHAPTER

49

Drugs for Eye and Ear Disorders

evolve WEBSITE

http://evolve.elsevier.com/KeeHayes/pharmacology/

- Animations
- Content Updates
- Key Points
- Review Questions for the NCLEX® Examination
- References from the Textbook
- Unfolding Case Studies

OBJECTIVES

- Describe the medication groups commonly used for disorders of the eye and ear.
- Discuss the mechanisms of action, route, side effects and adverse reactions, and contraindications for selected drugs in each group.
- Develop teaching plans for the drug groups presented.
- Describe the nursing process related to drugs used in treating and managing disorders of the eye and ear.

OUTLINE

KEY TERMS

carbonic anhydrase inhibitors, p. 718
cerumen, p. 725
ceruminolytics, p. 725
conjunctivitis, p. 710
cycloplegics, p. 720
glaucoma, p. 714
intraocular pressure, p. 714
lacrimal duct, p. 710
miosis, p. 715
mydriatics, p. 720
narrow-angle glaucoma, p. 714
ocular, p. 710
open-angle glaucoma, p. 714
ophthalmic, p. 710
osmotics, p. 718
otitis externa, p. 722
prostaglandin analogues, p. 715

The authors gratefully acknowledge the work of Jacqueline Rosenjack Burchum, who updated this chapter for the eighth edition.

DRUGS FOR DISORDERS OF THE EYE

Problems associated with the eyes may occur as the result of injuries, infections, and specific eye disorders like glaucoma and macular degeneration. Most drugs used to treat these conditions are topical medications in formulations developed specifically for sensitive eyes. Drugs designed to be applied to the eyes are known as **ocular** or **ophthalmic** drugs.

Diagnostic Stains

Diagnostic stains (Table 49-1) are frequently used to locate lesions or foreign objects, evaluate dry eye, or evaluate eye changes from poorly fitting contact lenses. Stains may be combined with local anesthetics to allow more thorough examination when pain is present. Patients should be informed that these drugs may stain nasal secretions if the **lacrimal ducts** (tear ducts) are patent; they can also discolor soft contact lenses. Contact lenses should be removed before administration. After the procedure, the stain should be flushed out with normal saline; contact lenses can be replaced after 1 hour.

Topical Anesthetics

Topical anesthetics are used in selected aspects of a comprehensive eye examination and in a variety of ophthalmic procedures. The two most common topical ophthalmic anesthetics are proparacaine HCl and tetracaine HCl (Pontocaine). Both medications are administered as drops.

Corneal anesthesia is achieved within 1 minute and generally lasts about 15 minutes. The blink reflex is temporarily lost; therefore, the corneal epithelium may become dry. To protect the eye, a patch is usually worn until the effects of the drug are gone. However, because patching of the eye may impede healing, the patch should be removed once sensation and the blink reflex return.

TABLE 49-1 DIAGNOSTIC STAINS FOR EYE DISORDERS

DIAGNOSTIC AID	PURPOSE
Fluorescein sodium (Fluorescite)	Demonstration of defects in corneal epithelium. When viewed through the cobalt blue filter of the ophthalmoscope or under a Wood's lamp, corneal scratches and lesions fluoresce a bright yellow-green.
Rose Bengal	Demonstration of defects and dryness of the conjunctival tissues. Defects are stained a pink-violet color. Stinging and mild tissue toxicity limits use.
Lissamine green	Demonstration of defects and dryness of the conjunctival tissues. Defects are stained green. Because it is not toxic to tissues and does not usually cause stinging, it has largely replaced Rose Bengal.

Ophthalmic anesthetics are *not* to be self-administered by the patient. Repeated doses are given only under strict medical supervision.

Antiinfectives

Antiinfectives (Table 49-2) are frequently used for eye infections. **Conjunctivitis,** an inflammation of the delicate membrane covering the eye and inner eyelids, is the most common eye condition requiring antibiotic therapy. Examples of other ocular conditions treated with ophthalmic antiinfective drugs include the following:

- Blepharitis (infection of margins of eyelid)
- Chalazion (infection of meibomian glands of the eyelids that may produce cysts, causing blockage of the ducts)
- Bacterial and fungal endophthalmitis (infection and inflammation of structures of the inner eye)
- Hordeolum (local infection of eyelash follicles and glands on lid margins, also known as a *stye*)
- Infectious keratitis (corneal infection and inflammation)
- Infectious uveitis (infection of vascular layer of eye [ciliary body, choroid, and iris])

Before administering ophthalmic antiinfectives, the nurse should screen the patient for previous allergic reactions. Noninfectious conjunctivitis and local skin and eye irritation are possible side effects of topical antiinfective drugs.

Antiinflammatories

Inflammatory conditions of the eye often require treatment with antiinflammatory drugs (Table 49-3) such as NSAIDs and corticosteroids. If the inflammation is secondary to a bacterial or fungal infection, an antibiotic or antifungal agent is included in the medication regimen. Antiinflammatories should not be given if the patient has a viral infection.

When allergies are the cause of eye inflammation, ophthalmic antihistamines and mast cell stabilizers are commonly prescribed to treat the underlying cause. Antihistamines block histamine from activating histamine receptors in the tissues. Examples of ophthalmic antihistamines include emedastine (Emadine) and epinastine (Elestat). Mast cell stabilizers prevent mast cells from breaking open and releasing histamine and other inflammatory mediators. Ophthalmic mast cell stabilizers include cromolyn (Crolom) and nedrocromil ophthalmic (Alocril). Some drugs, such as azelastine (Optivar), epinastine, ketotifen (Zaditor) and olopatadine (Patanol), have both antihistamine and mast cell stabilizer effects. Burning, headache, and stinging may occur in some patients and are the most frequent adverse effects of these drugs.

Decongestants

Eye inflammation typically presents with redness due to vascular congestion of the conjunctiva. Ophthalmic decongestants are vasoconstrictors that manage these effects by narrowing these blood vessels. Examples of ophthalmic decongestants are phenylephrine (Neo-Synephrine Ophthalmic), naphazoline (Clear Eyes), tetrahydrozoline (Opti-Clear), and oxymetazoline (Ocuclear). If these are absorbed

TABLE 49-2 OPHTHALMIC ANTIINFECTIVES

GENERIC (BRAND)	ROUTE AND DOSAGE*	USES AND CONSIDERATIONS
Antibacterials		
chloramphenicol	A/C: Ophthalmic: Instill 1-2 gtt or ½-inch ribbon of oint q3-4h for 48 h; increase interval to b.i.d./t.i.d.	For severe ophthalmic infections that are unresponsive to other antibiotics. Effective against gram-negative and gram-positive bacteria. Boxed warning: Bone marrow suppression and deaths have resulted from topical administration. Continue treatment for at least 48 h after eye appears normal. Contact lenses should not be worn for duration of treatment. Pregnancy category: C
ciprofloxacin (Ciloxan) 5 mg/mL sol	Bacterial conjunctivitis: Solution: A/C: >1 y: 1-2 gtt q2h while awake for 2 d, then q4h while awake for 5 d Bacterial conjunctivitis: Ointment: A/C: >2 y: ½-inch ribbon t.i.d for 2 d, then ½-inch ribbon b.i.d for 5 d Corneal ulcer: A/C: >1 y: Day 1: 2 gtt q15min for 6 h, then 2 gtt q30min for rest of day Day 2: 2 gtt q1h Days 3-14: 2 gtt q4h	For bacterial conjunctivitis and corneal ulceration. Contact lenses should not be worn for duration of treatment. Pregnancy category: C
erythromycin	Chlamydial conjunctivitis or ophthalmia neonatorum caused by *Chlamydia trachomatis:* Oral dosage: Neonates/infants: CDC recommends 50 mg/kg/d PO divided q.i.d. for 14 d. Second course may be required. CDC states that topical therapy alone is inadequate and unnecessary when systemic therapy is administered. Ophthalmia neonatorum caused by *Neisseria gonorrhoeae* or *Chlamydia trachomatis:* Ophthalmic dosage: A: Instill 1-2 gtt of 0.25% sol into each affected eye b.i.d., or instill 1-2 gtt of 0.5% sol into each affected eye once/d. Greater than 1 gtt of 0.5% preparation b.i.d. generally does not further reduce IOP and is not recommended. Neonates: Apply a ribbon of 0.5% ophthalmic ointment into each lower conjunctival sac no later than 1 hour after birth	For chlamydial conjunctivitis caused by *C. trachomatis* and ophthalmia neonatorum caused by *C. trachomatis* or *N. gonorrhoeae*. Prolonged use can lead to acquired sensitivity. Contact lenses should not be worn for duration of treatment. Pregnancy category: B
gentamicin sulfate (Garamycin Ophthalmic, Gentak)	A/C: Sol 0.3%: 1-2 gtt q4h; may increase to 2 gtt q1h for severe infections Oint 0.3%: ½-inch ribbon b.i.d./t.i.d.	For blepharitis, blepharo-conjunctivitis, bacterial conjunctivitis, corneal ulcer, dacryocystitis, keratitis, kerato-conjunctivitis, and acute meibomianitis. Ophthalmia neonatorum secondary to *N. gonorrhoeae* May cause ototoxicity (toxic effect on eighth cranial nerve), which may be permanent. Contact lenses should not be worn for duration of treatment. Pregnancy category: C
levofloxacin	A: 1-2 gtts q2h; *max:* 8 doses/d for 1-2 d; then q4h; *max:* 4 doses/d for 5 d	For bacterial conjunctivitis and corneal ulcers (Systemic therapy is required for treatment of hordeolum, dacryocystitis, and meibomianitis). Contact lenses should not be worn for duration of treatment. Pregnancy category: C
silver nitrate 1% (Dey-Drop)	Neonate: Instill 2 gtt in each eye within 1 h of birth	For prophylaxis of ophthalmia neonatorum caused by *N. gonorrhoeae* Pregnancy category: C
sulfacetamide (Bleph-10)	A/C: >12 y: Sol: 1 gtt q1-3h while awake; then q3-4h while sleeping	For conjunctivitis, corneal ulcer, and adjunctive therapy for chlamydial conjunctivitis. Effectiveness of sulfonamides decreased in presence of PABA and purulent drainage; hence, remove exudates before instilling drops. Contact lenses should not be worn for duration of treatment. Pregnancy category: C

Continued

TABLE 49-2 OPHTHALMIC ANTIINFECTIVES—cont'd

GENERIC (BRAND)	ROUTE AND DOSAGE*	USES AND CONSIDERATIONS
tobramycin (Tobrex)	A/C: >12 y: Oint 0.3%: ½-inch ribbon b.i.d./t.i.d Sol 0.3%: 1-2 gtt q4h For severe infections: Oint: ½-inch ribbon q3-4h Sol: 2 gtt q30-60min until improvement, then decrease frequency	For external ocular infections. Contact lenses should not be worn for duration of treatment. Pregnancy category: D
tetracycline HCl	A: Instill 1-2 gtt b.i.d./q.i.d. A: Instill ½-inch ribbon q2-12h	Bacteriostatic action; alternative to silver nitrate for prevention of ophthalmia neonatorum. Contact lenses should not be worn for duration of treatment. Pregnancy category: D
triple antibiotic ophthalmic ointment (neomycin, polymyxin B Sulfate, bacitracin ophthalmic)	A/C: >12 y: 1 cm applied in conjunctival sac q3-4h	Combination antibiotic effective against many gram-positive and gram-negative organisms. Do not use longer than 10 d. Contact lenses should not be worn for duration of treatment. Pregnancy category: C
Antifungals		
natamycin (Natacyn Ophthalmic)	A/C: Sol 5%: 1 gt q2h for 3-4 d; then 1 gt q3h for 14-21 d	May cause transient stinging or temporary blurring of vision. Pregnancy category: C
Antivirals		
idoxuridine (IDU, Herplex Liquifilm)	A/C: Sol 1%: Initially: 1 gt q1h during day and q2h at night; when definite improvement occurs, use 1 gt q2h during day and q4h at night; continue 3-7 d after healing occurs Oint 0.5%: Place ½-inch ribbon q4h while awake	For cytomegalovirus and herpes simplex keratitis. Store in refrigerator; do not mix with boric acid. Discontinue if no response in 1 wk. Pregnancy category: C
trifluridine (Viroptic)	A: Sol 1%: Instill 1 gt into infected eye q2h while awake; *max:* 9 gtt/d until corneal ulcer reepithelialized; then 1 gt q4h for 7 d; *max:* 21 d of treatment	For herpetic ophthalmic infections and keratoconjunctivitis caused by HSV-1 and HSV-2. Pregnancy category: C

*To minimize systemic absorption, gently apply pressure on inner canthus.
A, Adult; *b.i.d.,* twice a day; *C,* child; *d,* day; *IOP,* intraocular pressure; *HSV,* herpes simplex virus; *gt,* drop; *gtt,* drops; *h,* hour; *max,* maximum; *NA,* not applicable; *oint,* ointment; *PABA,* paraaminobenzoic acid; *PB,* protein-binding; *q.i.d.,* four times a day; *sol,* solution; *t½,* half-life; *t.i.d.,* three times a day; *wk,* week; *y,* year; >, greater than.

TABLE 49-3 OPHTHALMIC ANTIINFLAMMATORIES

GENERIC (BRAND)	ROUTE AND DOSAGE*	USES AND CONSIDERATIONS
Nonsteroidal Antiinflammatory Drugs (NSAIDs)		
diclofenac sodium (Voltaren Ophthalmic)	A: 1 gt to affected eye q.i.d. for 2 wk; start 24 h after cataract surgery	For postoperative inflammation and photophobia after cataract surgery. May increase bleeding and delay healing. Increased risk for keratitis and elevated IOP. Pregnancy category: C
flurbiprofen sodium (Ocufen)	A: Instill 1 gt q30min starting 2 h before surgery; total dose is 4 gtt	For prevention of intraoperative miosis. May increase bleeding and delay healing. Pregnancy category: C
ketorolac tromethamine (Acular)	Allergic conjunctivitis: A/C >2 y: Sol 0.5%: Instill 1 gt q.i.d. Following cataract surgery: A: Begin q.i.d 24 h postop, and continue for 2 weeks	For relief of itching due to allergic conjunctivitis and management of inflammation post–cataract surgery. May increase bleeding and delay healing. Pregnancy category: C
suprofen (Profenal) (Maple Leaf)	Preoperative: A: Instill 2 gtt in sac q4h while awake on day preceding surgery; instill 2 gtt in conjunctival sac at 3, 2, and 1 h before surgery	For prevention of intraoperative miosis. May increase bleeding and delay healing. Pregnancy category: C
Corticosteroids		
dexamethasone (Maxidex)	A/C: Oint: Apply into conjunctival sac t.i.d./q.i.d.; gradually decrease to discontinue Susp: Instill 2 gtt q1h while awake and q2h during night; taper to q3-4h; then t.i.d./q.i.d.	For uveitis; allergic conditions; and inflammation of conjunctiva, cornea, and lids. Not recommended for minor abrasions and wounds. May delay healing. Avoid use with viral infections. Pregnancy category: C

TABLE 49-3 OPHTHALMIC ANTIINFLAMMATORIES—cont'd

GENERIC (BRAND)	ROUTE AND DOSAGE*	USES AND CONSIDERATIONS
medrysone (HMS Liquifilm)	A/C: Susp: Initially: Instill 1 gt in conjunctival sac q1-2h (1-2 d); then 1 gt b.i.d./q.i.d.	For allergic conditions, burns, and inflammation of conjunctiva, cornea, and lids. May delay healing. Avoid use with viral infections. Pregnancy category: C
prednisolone acetate (Econopred Plus)	A: Initially instill 1-2 gtt in conjunctival sac q1h while awake, q2h during night until desired effect; maint: 1 gt q4-6h Susp: 0.125% and 1%	For uveitis; allergic conditions; burns; and inflammation of conjunctiva, cornea, and lids. May delay healing. Avoid use with viral infections. Pregnancy category: C
prednisolone sodium phosphate	A/older adults: Sol 0.125% and 1%: 1-2 gtt q1h during day; q2h at night; with response, give 1 gt q4-6h Oint: thin coat t.i.d./q.i.d.; with response, decrease to b.i.d., then daily	To prevent or decrease tissue response to inflammatory process. May delay healing. Avoid use with viral infections. Pregnancy category: C
Ophthalmic Antihistamines		
emedastine (Emadine)	A/C ≥3 y: 1 gtt up to 4 times/d	For allergic conjunctivitis. Wait 10 minutes after administration before inserting contact lenses. Pregnancy category: B
epinastine (Elestat)	A/C ≥3 y: 1 gtt b.i.d.	For allergic conjunctivitis Wait 10 minutes after administration before inserting contact lenses. Pregnancy category: C
Ophthalmic Mast Cell Stabilizers		
cromolyn (Crolom)	A/C >4 y: 1-2 gtt in each eye 4-6 times/d	For allergic conjunctivitis Contact lenses should not be worn for duration of therapy Pregnancy category: B
nedrocromil ophthalmic (Alocril)	A/C ≥3 y: 1-2 gtt b.i.d.	For allergic conjunctivitis About 40% experience headache; 10%-30% experience burning sensation Contact lenses should not be worn for duration of therapy Pregnancy category: B
Ophthalmic Drugs with Both Antihistamines and Mast Cell Stabilizer Properties		
azelastine (Optivar)	A/C ≥3 y: 1 gtt in each eye b.i.d.	For allergic conjunctivitis. Has both antihistamine and mast-cell stabilizing actions. 11.5% experience drowsiness; enhances CNS depressants Wait 10 minutes after administration before inserting contact lenses. Pregnancy category: C
epinastine (Elestat)	A/C ≥3 y: 1 gtt each eye b.i.d.	For allergic conjunctivitis. Has both antihistamine and mast-cell stabilizer actions 1%-10% develop coldlike symptoms. Wait 10 minutes after administration before inserting contact lenses. Pregnancy category: C
ketotifen (Zaditor)	A/C ≥3 y: 1 gtt in each eye q8-12h	For allergic conjunctivitis. 10%-25% experience mild hyperemia and headache. Wait 10 minutes after administration before inserting contact lenses. Pregnancy category: C
olopatadine (Patanol)	A/C ≥3 y: 0.1% sol: 1 drop in each affected eye b.i.d. at an interval of 6-8 h	For allergic conjunctivitis. May potentiate CNS depressants if systemically absorbed. Wait 10 minutes after administration before inserting contact lenses. If eyes turn red, do not wear contact lenses. Pregnancy category: C

*To minimize systemic absorption, gently apply pressure on inner canthus.

A, Adult; *b.i.d.,* twice a day; *C,* child; *d,* day; *gt,* drop; *gtt,* drops; *h,* hour; *maint,* maintenance; *max,* maximum; *min,* minute; *NA,* not applicable; *oint,* ointment; *PB,* protein-binding; *q.i.d.,* four times a day; *sol,* solution; *susp,* suspension; $t\frac{1}{2}$, half-life; *t.i.d.,* three times a day; *q.i.d.,* four times a day; *wk,* week.

in significant amounts, their sympathetic nervous system effects may pose problems for patients with hypertension. Patients who have narrow-angle glaucoma should not use these drugs because they may contribute to acute angle-closure, which is a medical emergency.

Lubricants

Eye lubricants replace tears to alleviate discomfort associated with eye dryness. They are also used to moisten contact lenses and artificial eyes. During anesthesia and in acute or chronic central nervous system (CNS) disorders that result in unconsciousness or decreased blinking, lubricants keep eyes moist and maintain the integrity of the epithelial surface of the eye.

Most lubricants are available over the counter (OTC) in both liquid and ointment form. Popular lubricants include Isopto Tears, Tearisol, Ultra Tears, Tears Naturale, Tears Plus, Lens Mate, and Lacri-Lube. While these agents typically are safe, the nurse must be alert to potential allergic reactions to preservatives in lubricants.

Immunosuppressants

Cyclosporine ophthalmic emulsion (Restasis) relieves dry eyes by a mechanism that is different from lubricants. It is prescribed for patients who have decreased tear production due to inflammation. Cyclosporine suppresses the immune response that leads to inflammation, allowing tear production to resume.

Ophthalmic corticosteroids are another type of immunosuppressant. Corticosteroids are used to treat a number of conditions that manifest as significant eye inflammation. Examples include prednisolone (Pred Forte), dexamethasone (Maxidex), loteprednol (Lotemax), rimexolone (Vexol), and fluorometholone (FML). Refer to Chapter 25 for more information on corticosteroids.

Because they suppress the immune response, ophthalmic immunosuppressants should not be given to patients with bacterial infections of the eye unless accompanied by an antibiotic that treats the underlying infection. Ophthalmic immunosuppressants are contraindicated for viral eye infections such as herpes.

Antiglaucoma Agents

Glaucoma is an eye condition in which optic nerve damage occurs as a result of increased **intraocular pressure (IOP),** which is a buildup of pressure within the eye that occurs when there is too much aqueous humor. Without treatment, permanent loss of vision can occur.

Typically, as aqueous humor is formed, excess fluid drains though the trabecular meshwork structure of the eye and out the canal of Schlemm, with a much smaller fraction of the fluid exiting through the uveoscleral structure at the root of the iris (Figure 49-1, *A*). In glaucoma, excess fluid is prevented from draining through the trabecular structure.

There are two types of glaucoma. In **open-angle glaucoma,** the trabecular network becomes clogged (Figure 49-1, *B*). Over time, as blockage of the trabecular network worsens, the IOP gradually increases.

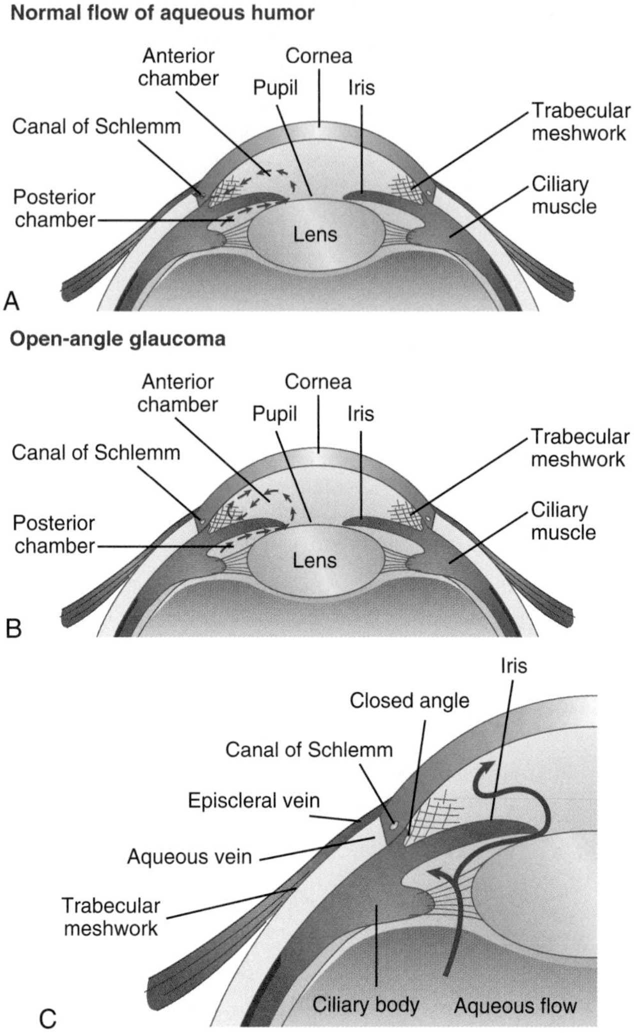

FIGURE 49–1 *A,* Normal flow of aqueous humor. *B,* Open-angle glaucoma. *C,* Closed-angle glaucoma.

In **narrow-angle glaucoma,** also known as closed-angle or angle-closure glaucoma, the iris bows and blocks the trabecular network by narrowing or closing the angle where fluid typically exits the eye (Figure 49-1, *C*). Because the excess aqueous humor cannot drain, it builds up within the eye, increasing IOP. Management of narrow-angle glaucoma is often surgical; however, pharmacologic management is sometimes indicated.

Glaucoma is further classified as either primary or secondary. Primary glaucoma occurs due to a pathologic change within the eye that happens without a known cause. Primary open-angle glaucoma (POAG), the most common type of glaucoma, is a chronic condition that develops slowly over time as the trabecular meshwork becomes clogged for unknown reasons. Secondary glaucoma occurs in response to a known cause such as injury, disease, or medication. While a number of drugs can increase the risk of secondary glaucoma, those that cause pupillary dilation are particularly problematic because they give the iris more flexibility to move in a way that blocks the trabecular meshwork. Certain herbal preparations can also create problems when given to patients who have glaucoma (Herbal Alert 49-1).

HERBAL ALERT 49-1

Herbs and Antiglaucoma Agents

The following herbs should be avoided in patients with glaucoma: bitter orange, blood root, celandine, coffee, corkwood, ephedra, goldenseal, and jimsonweed. Because all herbs have inherent risks, it is important to receive approval from the patient's health care provider before recommending herbal preparations.

Antiglaucoma drugs belong to one of the following categories: **prostaglandin analogues,** beta-adrenergic blockers, alpha-adrenergic agonists, cholinergic agents, carbonic anhydrase inhibitors, or systemic hyperosmotic drugs. Prostaglandin analogues and beta-adrenergic blockers are typically first-line therapy, followed by alpha-adrenergic agonists. Each category acts in different ways to decrease IOP.

Prostaglandin Analogues

Prostaglandin analogues (Table 49-4) are first-line drugs used primarily in the treatment of open-angle glaucoma; however, studies suggest a role in management of narrow-angle glaucoma, as well. These drugs decrease IOP by improving trabecular outflow and by increasing the uveoscleral pathway, which is an alternate pathway of aqueous humor outflow. Examples of prostaglandin analogues include bimatoprost (Lumigan), latanoprost (Xalatan) (Prototype Drug Chart 49-1), tafluprost (Zioptan), and travoprost (Travatan).

Side Effects and Adverse Reactions. Prostaglandin analogues used for glaucoma have unique side effects. These drugs gradually change the color of the iris by increasing brown pigmentation. This effect, most noticeable in individuals with green-brown and yellow-brown irises, may be permanent. Darkening of the eyelids may also occur. Another unusual side effect is the development of eyelash hypertrichosis, which is a growth in the number, length, thickness, and pigmentation of eyelashes. Up to 15% of patients may also develop blurred vision, redness of the conjunctiva, and itching or stinging of the eye. Systemic effects are rare, however, and these drugs are generally better tolerated than alternative antiglaucoma drugs.

Cholinergic Agents

Ophthalmic cholinergic agents cause **miosis**, which is a constriction of the pupil, and contraction of the ciliary muscle. These actions result in a widening of the trabecular meshwork to improve outflow of excess aqueous humor. Additionally, as the pupil constricts, it straightens the iris, thus opening or widening the angle to relieve narrow-angle glaucoma. There are two types of cholinergics: cholinergic agonists and cholinesterase inhibitors. Although their outcomes are the same, cholinergic agonists and cholinesterase inhibitors differ in their mechanism of action.

Cholinergic agonists are direct-acting cholinergics. Direct-acting cholinergics directly stimulate cholinergic receptors.

TABLE 49-4 PROSTAGLANDIN ANALOGUES USED TO TREAT GLAUCOMA

GENERIC (BRAND)	ROUTE AND DOSAGE	USES AND CONSIDERATIONS
latanoprost (Xalatan)	A: 1 gt 0.005% sol h.s.	Decreases IOP in open-angle glaucoma; may have a role in narrow-angle glaucoma, but more studies needed. Few adverse effects. Not recommended for patients with torn or absent lens or with eye trauma. Do not insert contact lenses for 15 minutes after administration. Pregnancy category: C
bimatoprost (Lumigan)	A: 1 gt 0.03% sol h.s.	Decreases IOP in open-angle glaucoma; may have a role in narrow-angle glaucoma, but more studies are needed. Few adverse effects. Not recommended for patients with torn or absent lens or with eye trauma. May worsen intraocular inflammation. Onset is 4 h, and peak action occurs in 4-12 h. Pregnancy category: C
travoprost (Travatan Z)	A: 1 gt 0.004% sol h.s.	Decreases IOP in open-angle glaucoma; may have a role in narrow-angle glaucoma, but more studies needed. Few adverse effects. Avoid use in patients with torn or absent lens or with eye trauma. More effective in African Americans than in non–African Americans. Onset is 2 h, with peak action occurring in 12 h.
tafluprost (Zioptan)	A: 1 gt every evening	Decreases IOP in open-angle glaucoma; may have a role in narrow-angle glaucoma, but more studies needed. Few adverse effects. Avoid use in patients with torn or absent lens or with eye trauma. Information on contact lenses not available in prescribing information/package insert.

A, Adult; *b.i.d.,* twice a day; *gt,* drop; *h,* hour; *h.s.,* at bedtime; *IOP,* intraocular pressure; *sol,* solution.

PROTOTYPE DRUG CHART 49-1

Latanoprost

Drug Class Prostaglandin analogue Generic Name: Latanoprost Trade Name: Xalatan Pregnancy Category: C	**Dosage** 1 gtt (1.5 mcg)/d in affected eye(s)
Contraindications No absolute contraindication. Use caution in patients with a torn or absent lens, intraocular inflammation, or risk of macular edema. Drug is absorbed by soft contact lenses, so advise patient to use alternate means of vision correction. Indicated only for open-angle glaucoma because only limited testing has taken place with narrow-angle glaucoma, neovascular glaucoma, and inflammatory glaucoma. Patients with history of diabetic retinopathy who took latanoprost experienced retinal detachment, retinal embolus, and vitreous hemorrhage. This may or may not be related to the latanoprost, but caution is urged.	**Drug-Lab-Food Interactions** Drugs: Concomitant administration with eyedrops containing thimerosal causes latanoprost to precipitate out of solution. Bromfenac ophthalmic solution, an NSAID, may reduce latanoprost's ability to lower IOP. Bimatoprost ophthalmic solution (Latisse), which is prescribed to promote growth of eyelashes, may decrease the ability of latanoprost to lower IOP.
Pharmacokinetics Absorption: Latanoprost is a prodrug. After absorption through the cornea, it is hydrolyzed to its active form. Distribution: 0.16 ± 0.02 L/kg. Primary measurable concentration is in the eye. Levels are often undetectable in serum. Metabolism: Hepatic Excretion: Primarily in urine (88%) with remainder in feces	**Pharmacodynamics** Onset: 3-4 h Peak: 8-12 h Duration: 24 h
Therapeutic Effects/Uses Reduction of IOP in glaucoma	
Mechanism of Action Prostaglandin FP receptor stimulation promotes aqueous humor outflow via uveoscleral pathway.	
Side Effects Brown pigmentation of iris; darkening of eyelid; increased number, length, thickness, and darkening of eyelashes; 5%-15% experience blurred vision; itching, burning, or stinging; conjunctival hyperemia; 1%-4% experience dry eye or excessive tearing, eye pain, eyelid discomfort and/or crusting, sensitivity to light. Macular edema has occurred when administered to patients with lens injuries.	**Adverse Reactions** Rare reports of retinal problems (embolus, detachment, and vitreous hemorrhage) in patients with diabetic retinopathy. Up to 4% of patients taking latanoprost reported respiratory problems. Up to 2% of patients taking latanoprost reported chest pain, musculoskeletal discomfort, and skin rashes.

h, Hour; *IOP,* intraocular pressure; *NSAID,* nonsteroidal antiinflammatory drug.

As a result, these drugs have the same action as the parasympathetic neurotransmitter acetylcholine. Pilocarpine (Isopto Carpine) is an example of a cholinergic agonist.

Cholinesterase inhibitors are indirect-acting cholinergics, which inactivate the enzyme cholinesterase that typically breaks down acetylcholine. By inhibiting enzymatic destruction of acetylcholine, more acetylcholine is available to stimulate cholinergic receptors in the eye. Echothiophate (Phospholine Iodide) is an example of a cholinesterase inhibitor. Figure 49-1, *B* and 49-1, *C* illustrate increased IOP resulting in open-angle and narrow-angle glaucoma. Table 49-5 lists the commonly prescribed ophthalmic cholinergic drugs and their dosages, uses, and considerations. Refer to Chapter 19 for more information on cholinergic drugs.

Beta-Adrenergic Blockers

Beta-adrenergic blockers, also known as beta blockers, are one of the first-line drugs used in the treatment of glaucoma. Beta-adrenergic blockers decrease IOP by decreasing the production of aqueous humor. Examples of ophthalmic beta-adrenergic blockers include betaxolol (Betoptic), carteolol, levobunolol (Betagan), metipranolol (OptiPranolol), and timolol (Timoptic).

Side Effects and Adverse Effects

In the eye, beta-adrenergic blockers (see Table 49-5) may cause some eye discomfort, which is possible with most eye medications. Some types cause miosis. Because the pupil does

TABLE 49-5 CHOLINERGICS AND BETA-ADRENERGIC BLOCKERS

GENERIC (BRAND)	ROUTE AND DOSAGE (TO AFFECTED EYE[S])	USES AND CONSIDERATIONS
Direct-Acting Cholinergics		
pilocarpine HCl (Isopto Carpine, Pilopine HS)	A/C: Sol: 1%-2%, 1 gtt, up to q.i.d. Gel: Apply ½-in ribbon in lower eyelid h.s.	Decreases IOP in both open-angle and acute angle-closure glaucoma; prevents postoperative IOP elevation. Miosis decreases vision in darkened environments. Retinal detachment may occur in patients with preexisting retinal disease. May worsen preexisting iritis. Pregnancy category: C
Indirect-Acting Cholinesterase Inhibitors		
echothiophate iodide (Phospholine Iodide)	A: Sol 0.03%-0.25%: 1 gt 1-2 times/d	Decreases IOP in chronic open-angle glaucoma and chronic angle-closure glaucoma after cataract and glaucoma surgery. Miosis decreases vision in darkened environments. May have additive effects in patients with myasthenia gravis who take systemic cholinesterase inhibitors. May cause retinal detachment, iris cysts, and lens opacities. Pregnancy category: C
Beta-Adrenergic Blockers		
betaxolol HCl (Betoptic S)	A: Susp 0.25% or sol 0.5%: Usual dose 1-2 gtts b.i.d.	Decreases IOP in chronic open-angle glaucoma and ocular hypertension. Does not produce miosis like some beta blockers. Relatively contraindicated in patients with asthma, bradycardia, and HF due to systemic effects of beta blockers if absorbed. May have additive effect in patients receiving oral beta blockers. Wait 15 minutes after administration before inserting contact lenses. Pregnancy category: C
carteolol HCl	A: Sol 1%: 1 gtt b.i.d.	Decreases IOP in chronic open-angle glaucoma and ocular hypertension. Less effective in narrow angle glaucoma. Relatively contraindicated in patients with asthma, bradycardia, and HF. May have additive effect in patients receiving oral beta blockers. Miosis decreases night vision. Wait 15 minutes after administration before inserting contact lenses. Pregnancy category: C
levobunolol HCl (Betagan Liquifilm)	A: Instill 1-2 drops of the 0.25% solution into each affected eye b.i.d., or instill 1-2 drops of the 0.5% solution into each affected eye once daily. A dosage greater than 1 drop of the 0.5% preparation b.i.d. generally does not further reduce intraocular pressure (IOP) and is not recommended	Decreases IOP regardless of glaucoma. Decreased miotic effect. Relatively contraindicated in patients with asthma, bradycardia, and HF. May have an additive effect in patients receiving oral beta blockers. Wait 15 minutes after administration before inserting contact lenses. Pregnancy category: C
timolol maleate (Timoptic)	A: Sol 0.25%-0.5%: Initially: 1 gt b.i.d.; maint: 1 gt/d once response occurs with initial dosage	Decreases IOP in chronic open-angle glaucoma and ocular hypertension. Relatively contraindicated in patients with asthma, bradycardia, and HF. May have additive effect in patients receiving oral beta blockers. Wait 15 minutes after administration before inserting contact lenses. Pregnancy category: C

A, Adult; *b.i.d.*, twice a day; *C*, child; *d*, day; *gt*, drop; *gtt*, drops; *HF*, heart failure; *IOP*, intraocular pressure; *maint*, maintenance; *NA*, not applicable; *oint*, ointment; *PB*, protein-binding; *q.i.d.*, four times a day; *sol*, solution; *susp*, suspension; *t½*, half-life; *t.i.d.*, three times a day; *wk*, week.

not dilate adequately in dark environments, patients taking these drugs may experience vision problems at night.

While ophthalmic drugs do not typically enter the general circulation in large amounts, it can occur to the extent that systemic effects occur. Beta-adrenergic blockers can slow the heart rate, which can worsen bradycardia, AV heart block, and heart failure. Also, these drugs can prevent adequate bronchodilation in patients who have asthma and other obstructive pulmonary diseases. Refer to Chapter 18 for more information on adrenergic blockers.

Alpha-Adrenergic Agonists

Alpha-adrenergic agonists decrease IOP by decreasing production and improving outflow of aqueous humor. Examples include apraclonidine (Iopidine), brimonidine (Alphagan), epinephrine, and dipivefrin, a prodrug of epinephrine.

Side Effects and Adverse Effects

The most common effects of topical administration are burning, stinging, blurred vision, and headache. Epinephrine and dipivefrin cause adverse cardiovascular effects such as tachycardia and hypertension; these are less common with dipivefrin. Patients with narrow-angle glaucoma should not take epinephrine and dipivefrin because dilation of the pupil may allow the iris to block the outflow of aqueous humor, triggering acute closed-angle glaucoma. Apraclonidine and brimonidine, on the other hand, are selective $alpha_2$ agonists that decrease IOP without causing mydriasis or adverse cardiovascular effects. Because of the relative safety of $alpha_2$ adrenergic agonists, they are often used when ophthalmic beta-adrenergic antagonists are contraindicated.

Carbonic Anhydrase Inhibitors

Carbonic anhydrase inhibitors (CAIs) decrease IOP by decreasing the production of aqueous humor. These drugs, initially developed as diuretics, are sometimes used for adjunctive treatment of glaucoma. They are indicated for both open-angle and acute closed-angle glaucoma. Carbonic anhydrase inhibitors are not as effective as other antiglaucoma drugs, though, and they carry a greater risk of adverse effects. For these reasons, they are generally added to a therapeutic regimen only after other treatment options have been exhausted. Both topical and systemic formulations are available. Examples of topical carbonic anhydrase inhibitors are brinzolamide (Azopt) and dorzolamide (Trusopt). Acetazolamide (Diamox) and methazolamide are systemic forms. Table 49-6 presents additional information on these drugs.

Side Effects and Adverse Reactions. Adverse effects of carbonic anhydrase inhibitors, particularly for the systemic forms, include CNS effects such as lethargy, drowsiness, headache, seizures, paresthesias, and mental status changes. GI effects such as nausea, vomiting, diarrhea, altered taste, and anorexia may occur. Because they have diuretic effects, polyuria and increased thirst are common, and fluid and electrolyte disturbances may occur as a result. They may promote hyperuricemia, which may precipitate gout attacks. They may also worsen liver disease, resulting in hepatic encephalopathy and even hepatic necrosis. Because they are sulfonamides, they should not be given to patients who have experienced allergic reactions to other sulfonamide drugs.

Osmotics

Osmotics are generally used preoperatively and postoperatively to decrease vitreous humor volume, reducing IOP. These drugs are primarily used in the emergency treatment of acute closed-angle glaucoma because of their ability to rapidly reduce IOP. Commonly prescribed osmotic drugs are presented in Table 49-7.

Side Effects and Adverse Reactions. Osmotic medications can cause headache, nausea, vomiting, and diarrhea. Disorientation resulting from electrolyte imbalances can result from use of mannitol and urea, especially in older adults.

Nursing Process
Patient-Centered Collaborative Care

Antiglaucoma Drugs

Assessment

- Obtain a thorough medical history.
- Obtain a thorough drug history, including allergies and use of herbal preparations and recreational drugs.
- Check baseline vital signs for future comparison.
- Check baseline visual acuity.
- Obtain, or assist with obtaining, baseline IOP measurements.

TABLE 49-6 CARBONIC ANHYDRASE INHIBITORS

GENERIC (BRAND)	ROUTE AND DOSAGE	USES AND CONSIDERATIONS
acetazolamide (Diamox)	A: PO: 250-1000 mg/d in divided doses for amounts >250 mg; doses >1000 mg show no increased benefit	Reduces IOP in both open- and narrow-angle glaucoma. Volume loss may cause dehydration and postural hypotension. Electrolyte imbalance may occur. Pregnancy category: C
brinzolamide ophthalmic susp 1% (Azopt)	A: 1 gt t.i.d.	Topical: For elevated IOP in patients with ocular hypertension or open-angle glaucoma by suppressing production of aqueous humor. Pregnancy category: C
Cosopt (timolol/dorzolamide 0.5%/2%)	A: 1 gt 0.25% in affected eye(s) b.i.d.	Decreases aqueous production. Contraindicated with sulfa allergy. Adverse effects include asthma, bronchospasm, bradycardia, and dyspnea.
dorzolamide (Trusopt)	A: sol 2%: 1 gt t.i.d.	Do not use with oral carbonic anhydrase inhibitors. Side effects include burning, stinging, and bitter taste.

A, Adult; *b.i.d.,* two times a day; *C,* child; *d,* day; *gt,* drop; *h,* hour; *IOP,* intraocular pressure; *PB,* protein-binding; *PO,* by mouth; *t½,* half-life; *t.i.d.,* three times a day; *UK,* unknown; >, greater than.

TABLE 49-7 OSMOTICS

GENERIC (BRAND)	ROUTE AND DOSAGE	USES AND CONSIDERATIONS
Glycerin (Osmoglyn, Ophthalgan)	Osmoglyn: A/C: PO: 1-1.8 g/kg given 1-1.5 h before surgery Ophthalgan: A: 1-2 gtt before examination of edematous cornea	Decreases volume of intraocular fluid to lower ocular tension. Carbohydrate; use with caution in patients with diabetes. Pregnancy category: C; PB: UK; $t\frac{1}{2}$: 30-45 min
mannitol (Osmitrol)	A: IV: sol 15%-20%, 1.5-2 g/kg over 0.5-1 h	Monitor I&O; weigh daily. Contraindicated in severe pulmonary congestion, anuria, and dehydration. Use with caution in patients with HF. Pregnancy category: C; PB: UK; $t\frac{1}{2}$: 15-100 min

A, Adult; *b.i.d.,* twice a day; *C,* child; *HF,* heart failure; *h,* hour; *I&O,* intake and output; *IV,* intravenous; *min,* minute; *PB,* protein-binding; *PO,* by mouth; *q.i.d.,* four times a day; *sol,* solution; $t\frac{1}{2}$, half-life; *UK,* unknown.

- Assess for conditions in which antiglaucoma drugs are contraindicated or relatively contraindicated.
  - Prostaglandin analogues may worsen respiratory conditions.
  - Beta-adrenergic blockers may worsen conditions such as bradycardia, heart block, and obstructive respiratory conditions such as asthma and chronic bronchitis.
  - Alpha adrenergic agonists may worsen conditions such as narrow-angle glaucoma, tachyarrhythmias, and hypertension.
  - Cholinergic agonists and cholinesterase inhibitors may worsen conditions such as acute iritis, bradycardia or heart block, cardiac disease, and obstructive respiratory conditions such as asthma and chronic bronchitis.
  - Carbonic anhydrase inhibitors may worsen conditions such as dehydration, electrolyte imbalances, diabetes, obstructive respiratory conditions such as asthma and chronic bronchitis, bone marrow suppression, hepatic disease, and narrow-angle glaucoma.
  - Systemic hyperosmotic drugs such as mannitol may worsen conditions such as dehydration, electrolyte imbalance, pulmonary edema, heart failure, and obstructive respiratory conditions such as asthma and chronic bronchitis.

Nursing Diagnoses

- Deficient knowledge related to purpose of and administration of antiglaucoma drugs
- Disturbed sensory perception (visual) related to drug-induced visual changes
  - Prostaglandin analogues, beta-adrenergic blockers, alpha-adrenergic agonists, and cholinergic agents may cause blurred vision.
  - Beta-adrenergic blockers typically cause miosis, which impairs vision in dark environments.
  - Alpha adrenergic agonists typically cause mydriasis, which increases sensitivity to light.
  - Cholinergic agonists and cholinesterase inhibitors may cause myopia and will impair vision in dark environments.
  - Carbonic anhydrase inhibitors may cause swelling of the lens.
- Risk for injury related to impaired vision
- Risk for electrolyte imbalance secondary to carbonic anhydrase inhibitors and systemic osmotic
- Anxiety related to drug-induced visual changes

Planning

- Patient will take antiglaucoma medications in dose and times prescribed.
- Patient will demonstrate proper method of ophthalmic drug administration.
- Patient will avoid contamination of tip of tube or dropper.
- Patient's IOP will decrease to within target range.

Nursing Interventions

- Monitor for significant alterations in patient status.
  - Monitor patients taking prostaglandin analogues for blurred vision, dyspnea, and pulmonary crackles and wheeze.
  - Monitor patients taking beta-adrenergic antagonists for blurred vision, bradycardia, and pulmonary wheeze.
  - Monitor patients taking alpha-adrenergic agonist analogues for blurred vision, tachycardia, and elevated blood pressure.
  - Monitor patients taking cholinergics for blurred vision, dry mouth, bradycardia, and pulmonary wheeze.
  - Monitor patients taking carbonic anhydrase inhibitors for blurred vision, dehydration, and electrolyte imbalances, hyperglycemia, blood dyscrasias, and pulmonary wheeze.
  - Monitor patients taking systemic hyperosmotic drugs for dehydration, electrolyte imbalances, pulmonary crackles or wheeze, and peripheral edema.

Patient Teaching

General

- Advise patient to never stop medication suddenly without prior approval of health care provider.

- Advise patient to avoid driving or operating machinery while vision is impaired.
- Explain importance of follow-up appointments for subsequent ophthalmologic examination and reevaluation of intraocular pressure.
- Counsel patients with glaucoma to avoid drugs with potential to increase IOP (Table 49-8).
- If both eyedrops and eye ointment are prescribed, instruct patient to put in eyedrops first.
- If more than one kind of eyedrop is ordered, instruct patient to wait at least 5 minutes before instilling second medication.
- Refer to Chapter 13 for more information on medication administration; Box 13-1 and Figure 13-3 provide information on eyedrops, and Box 13-2 and Figure 13-4 provide information on eye ointments.

Cultural Considerations

- Depending on patient's culture, include appropriate support person in health teaching and decisions. This need is heightened in conditions with possible loss of vision or diminished vision.
- Use an interpreter as needed.
- Provide printed materials in language patient reads and speaks most easily.

Evaluation

- Evaluate patient and family knowledge of purpose and administration of medications.
- Evaluate effectiveness of drug therapy. IOP should be reduced from baseline measurements.
- Evaluate for alleviation or decrease in adverse effects after interventions targeted to unwanted effects of antiglaucoma therapy.

Anticholinergic Mydriatics and Cycloplegics

Mydriatics dilate the pupils; **cycloplegics** paralyze the muscles of accommodation. Both are used in diagnostic procedures and ophthalmic surgery. (See the Unit 5 opener for a review of the autonomic nervous system and a comprehensive discussion of anticholinergics.) Anticholinergics actively block acetylcholine from attaching to cholinergic receptors, resulting in both dilation of the pupils and paralysis of the muscles of accommodation by blocking the response of sphincter muscles that normally constrict the pupil when cholinergic receptors are stimulated. Commonly prescribed anticholinergic mydriatics and cycloplegics are presented in Table 49-9.

Side Effects and Adverse Reactions

Side effects of topical anticholinergics include xerophthalmia (dry eyes), photophobia (sensitivity to light), and blurred vision. Systemic effects, while uncommon with topical use, are typical of all anticholinergic drugs and include dry mouth, increased heart rate, and constipation. These drugs are contraindicated in patients with narrow-angle glaucoma because the paralyzed iris may block the outlet for outflow of aqueous humor (see Figure 49-1, *C*).

TABLE 49-8 DRUGS WITH THE POTENTIAL TO WORSEN GLAUCOMA

DRUG	EFFECT
acetazolamide (Diamox)	While appropriate for *acute* narrow-angle glaucoma, long-term use can worsen *chronic* narrow-angle glaucoma.
Anticholinergics	Anticholinergics cause mydriasis, which can exacerbate narrow-angle glaucoma.
Corticosteroids	Corticosteroids can reduce the outflow of aqueous humor. Steroid-induced IOP does not occur in all patients, but primarily affects those with open-angle glaucoma.
Drugs for Mental Health Disorders • Monoamine oxidase inhibitors • Phenothiazines • Serotonin-norepinephrine reuptake inhibitors • Selective serotonin reuptake inhibitors • Tricyclic antidepressants • trihexyphenidyl (Artane)	These drugs have anticholinergic properties. Anticholinergics typically cause mydriasis, which can exacerbate narrow-angle glaucoma.
Miscellaneous Drugs with Anticholinergic Properties • cyclobenzaprine (Flexeril) • First-generation antihistamines • Opthalmic, nasal, and systemic decongestants • scopolamine (Transderm Scōp) • Urinary antispasmodics	These drugs have anticholinergic properties. Anticholinergics typically cause mydriasis, which can exacerbate narrow-angle glaucoma.
Sulfonamides	These drugs can cause swelling of the lens and anterior rotation of the ciliary body, which can precipitate acute narrow-angle glaucoma.

Drugs for Macular Degeneration

Age-related macular degeneration (ARMD) is a leading cause of vision loss in those age 65 years and older. The macula is that part of the eye responsible for sharp central vision; damage to the macula blurs central vision in the affected eye. There are two forms of ARMD: (1) wet (neovascular or exudative), which progresses quite rapidly, and (2) dry (atrophic), which slowly destroys vision over a period of years.

Dry ARMD is more common. It occurs in response to the deposit of extracellular material, called *drusen,* in the macula

SAFETY: Preventing Medication Errors

Do not confuse...

- betaxolol ophthalmic (Betoptic) with timolol ophthalmic (Timoptic)
- bevacizumab (Avastin) with Avostatin
- cyclopentolate (Cyclogyl) with cyclopentolate/phenylephrine (Cyclomydril)
- loteprednol ophthalmic (Lotemax) with alosetron (Lotronex)
- ofloxacin ophthalmic (Ocuflox) with flurbiprofen ophthalmic (Ocufen)
- prednisolone ophthalmic (Pred Forte) with chlorzoxazone (Parafon Forte)
- prednisone (Deltasone) with prednisolone ophthalmic (Pred Forte)
- timolol ophthalmic (Timoptic) with atenolol (Tenormin)
- timolol/dorzolamide (Cosopt) with dorzolamide (Trusopt)
- tobramycin ophthalmic (Tobrex) with dexamethasone/tobramycin (TobraDex)
- different strengths of a solution (e.g., Isopto Carpine 1% with Isopto Carpine 2%)
- ophthalmic solutions with otic or other topical solutions of the same name (e.g., cortisporin ophthalmic solution with cortisporin otic solution)

of the eye. This is coupled with areas of atrophy in the macula. Occasionally, dry ARMD will progress to wet ARMD.

Wet ARMD is associated with the growth of abnormal blood vessels behind the retina. Leakage of fluid from these vessels collects behind the retina and shifts the macula from its normal position. Wet ARMD accounts for 10% to 15% of ARMD cases; however, it causes greater destruction and is responsible for 80% of cases in which patients suffer severe vision loss or become legally blind.

An effective drug has not been identified to treat dry ARMD, but several drugs are currently in the trial stages. Some studies suggest that antioxidants and zinc supplements may have a role in preventing or slowing progression of dry ARMD.

Pharmacologic management of wet ARMD targets vascular endothelial growth factor (VEGF), a substance that plays a role in the formation of abnormal vessels in the eye. These VEGF inhibitors are intravitreal drugs that are injected into

TABLE 49-9 MYDRIATICS AND CYCLOPLEGICS

GENERIC (BRAND)	ROUTE AND DOSAGE*	USES AND CONSIDERATIONS
atropine sulfate (Atropisol, Isopto Atropine)	A: sol 1%: 1-2 gtt up to q.i.d. C: sol 0.5%: 1-2 gtt up to t.i.d. Oint 1%: Apply in lower eyelid sac up to t.i.d.	Most potent cycloplegic. For refraction, especially in children; for iritis and uveitis. Not for use with glaucoma or tachycardia. Wait 5 minutes before using other drugs. Pregnancy category: C
cyclopentolate HCl (Cyclogyl)	A: sol 0.5%-2%: 1-2 gtt; then 1 gt in 5 min C: 1-2 gtt × 1; may repeat × 1 in 5-10 min with 0.5% or 1% sol	Mydriasis and cycloplegia for eye examination. Pregnancy category: C
epinephrine HCl (Epifrin, Glaucon)	A/C: sol 0.1%-2%: 1-2 gtt 1-2 times/d	For open-angle glaucoma and during eye surgery. Discard brown or precipitate solution. Pregnancy category: C
epinephrine borate (Epinal)	Surgery: A: sol 0.5-1%: Instill 1-2 gtt three times Open-angle glaucoma: A: sol 0.5% or 1.0%: Instill 1 gt in eye b.i.d.	For treatment of open-angle glaucoma and during ocular surgery. Contraindicated in narrow-angle glaucoma. Monitor tonometer readings with long-term use. Increased pressor effects. Pregnancy category: C
homatropine hydrobromide (Isopto Homatropine)	A/C: sol 2% and 5%: 1-2 gtt q3-4h Cy: Use only 2%	Similar to atropine but faster onset and shorter duration. Mydriasis and cycloplegia for eye examination. Pregnancy category: C
phenylephrine HCl (AK-Dilate)	Mydriasis: A/C: sol 2.5% or 10%: Instill 1 gt in eye before examination Mydriasis with vasoconstriction: A/C >12 y: Instill 1 gt in eye; repeat once in 1 h PRN Cy: 2.5% sol: Instill 1 gt in eye; repeat once in 1 h PRN	For eye examination or surgery and treatment of wide-angle glaucoma and uveitis. Pregnancy category: C
scopolamine hydrobromide (Isopto Hyoscine)	A: sol 0.25%: 1-2 gtt 1 h before examination; 1-2 gtt for treatment up to q.i.d.	Used for patients sensitive to atropine sulfate. More rapid onset and shorter duration than atropine. Pregnancy category: C
tropicamide (Mydriacyl Ophthalmic)	Refraction: A: 1%: 1-2 gtt; repeat in 5 min Fundus examination: 0.5%: 1-2 gtt 15-20 min before examination	Mydriasis and cycloplegia for eye examination. Pregnancy category: C

*To minimize systemic absorption, apply gentle pressure to the lacrimal duct.

A, Adult; *b.i.d.*, twice a day; *C*, child; *Cy*, cycloplegic; *gt*, drop; *gtt*, drops; *h*, hour; *IOP*, intraocular pressure; *min*, minute; *oint*, ointment; *PB*, protein-binding; *PRN*, as needed; *q.i.d.*, four times a day; *sol*, solution; $t\frac{1}{2}$, half-life; *t.i.d.*, three times a day; *NA*, not applicable; *UK*, unknown; *y*, year; >, greater than.

the eye by ophthalmologists; trials to evaluate topical agents are in progress. Examples of VEGF inhibitors are ranibizumab (Lucentis), bevacizumab (Avastin), pegaptanib (Macugen), and aflibercept (Eylea).

Administration of Eyedrops and Ointments

Techniques for administering eyedrops and ophthalmic ointments are described in Chapter 13. Patients who wear contact lenses should be knowledgeable about the products associated with the lenses.

Patients with Eye Disorders: General Suggestions for Teaching

- Listen to patient concerns. Eye disorders carrying the possibility of blindness promote high anxiety in patients.
- Provide patient education regarding expected drug effect, dosage, side effects, and when to notify the health care provider.
- Use lay terms rather than medical terminology when providing education.
- Provide written instructions for confused or forgetful patients.
- When developing patient education materials, write them at a fifth- to eighth-grade reading level. Use a large, easily-read font. Give instructions in patient's native language.
- Supplement written instructions with images or pictograms to clarify instructions.
- Instruct patient or family member that one drop of eye medication is the preferred amount with prescriptions written for one to two drops; the conjunctival sac of the lower lid typically holds the volume of one drop without overflowing. The second drop may cause overflow, greater chance of systemic toxicity, and increased cost of treatment.
- If a second topical medication is ordered to be given at the same time, instruct patient to wait at least 5 minutes before instilling the second medication.
- Instruct patient or family member on proper administration of eyedrops or ointment. Teach them how to maintain sterile technique and prevent dropper contamination.
- Ask patient for a return demonstration of any procedure to ensure patient's ability to carry it out properly and to determine if additional teaching is needed.
- Advise patient to apply ointments at bedtime, if possible, to avoid safety problems from diminished vision that occurs from looking through the film it places over the eye.
- Instruct patient to store the drug away from heat.
- Counsel patient not to stop medication suddenly without prior approval from the prescribing health care provider.
- Advise patient to check labels on OTC drugs with a pharmacist.
- Instruct patient to carry an identification card or wear a MedicAlert bracelet at all times if allergic to any medications.
- Encourage patient to keep health care appointments. Recommend that patient bring a list of questions about their condition or medications.
- Tailor instructions for patients who wear contact lenses. Notify them regarding any special procedures that need to be done regarding use of contact lenses and the various ophthalmic medications. Advise patients to avoid wearing contact lenses in the presence of eye infections.

DRUGS FOR DISORDERS OF THE EAR

Antiinfectives

Common ear conditions requiring antibacterial drugs are acute otitis media (AOM) and acute otitis externa, commonly known as *swimmer's ear.* AOM occurs more often in children. *Streptococcus pneumoniae* is the most common pathogen, followed by *haemophilus influenzae* and *moraxella catarralis.* AOM may also be caused by other microorganisms, such as viruses.

Risk factors for the development of AOM include age younger than 2 years, attending day care centers, and exposure to tobacco smoke and air pollution. A significant decline in AOM has occurred since the pneumococcal conjugate vaccine (PCV) was introduced in 2000. Because it provides immunization against *S. pneumoniae*, families should be urged to have children receive the scheduled PCV13 as a prophylactic measure against AOM, as well as against the other more serious conditions that this vaccine prevents.

Amoxicillin is usually the drug of choice when antibiotics are indicated for AOM. The recommended dose is 40 to 45 mg/kg twice daily for 5 to 10 days depending on severity of condition and age of patient. Azithromycin and clarithromycin are often ordered if the patient has a severe allergy to penicillin. For more mild penicillin allergies, a cephalosporin may be ordered; however, the nurse should be alert to any signs or symptoms of penicillin-cephalosporin cross-sensitivity.

Otitis externa (OE) is an infection of the external auditory canal (EAC) that occurs when excess moisture and breaks in skin allow bacteria or fungi to invade the tissues. *Pseudomonas aeruginosa* and *Staphylococcus aureus* are the pathogens most often responsible. Treatment is usually with topical antibacterial or antifungal drugs, depending on the source of the infection. These are often prescribed as a combination product containing an antiinflammatory drug. An analgesic may also be needed.

If the EAC becomes so swollen that eardrops cannot reach the inner recesses of the EAC, a wick must be inserted (Figure 49-2). A wick is a thin cylinder composed of highly compressed absorbable material. It is inserted into the edematous canal, and eardrops are applied to the tip of the wick that is exposed. Sufficient drops should be administered to keep the wick moist. The wick pulls the medication down the length of the wick as it is absorbed, exposing the medication to tissues along the EAC. Wicks should be replaced every 24 to 48 hours. Once the swelling resolves, the wick will fall out, or it may be manually removed.

Topical antibacterial preparations are preferred. Oral antibiotics are required if the OE extends to the pinna.

Patency of the tympanic membrane (TM) presents a special concern when antibiotic eardrops are used. This is especially true when an edematous EAC prevents adequate visualization of the TM. Topical antibiotics such as neomycin-polymyxin B-hydrocortisone are very effective in treating OE because polymyxin B is effective against *P. aeruginosa* and neomycin is effective against *S. aureus*. However, if this drug combination is given to a patient with a perforated TM, there is a significant risk of ototoxicity. Chloramphenicol is another drug sometimes ordered for OE but contraindicated with a perforated TM. Fluoroquinolones, on the other hand, are effective against both organisms and are safe to use when the TM is incompetent; therefore, they are usually the first drug of choice when prescribing treatment for OE. When OE is caused by the growth of fungi, restoring an acidic environment with an acidifying solution such as acetic acid is usually sufficient. A topical antifungal otic solution such as clotrimazole is typically used if the fungal infection is severe.

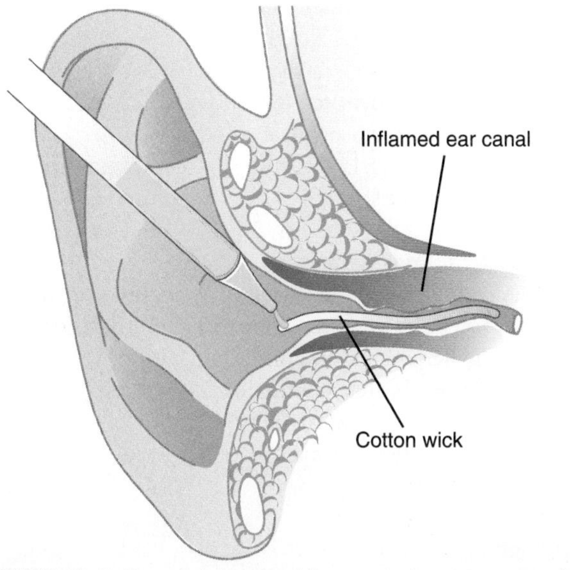

FIGURE 49–2 Ear wick inserted into an edematous canal.

Side Effects and Adverse Reactions

The most common side effect of otic antimicrobials is burning and stinging. Ototoxicity can occur with aminoglycoside antibiotics. Chloroamphenical may cause bone marrow suppression resulting in decreased erythrocytes, leukocytes, and platelets. Opportunistic overgrowth of nonsusceptible organisms may occur with any of these drugs. Hypersensitivity is a contraindication.

Table 49-10 lists selected antibacterial medications used to treat ear disorders and their dosages, uses, and considerations.

TABLE 49-10 OTIC: ANTIINFECTIVES

GENERIC (BRAND)	ROUTE AND DOSAGE	USES AND CONSIDERATIONS
Topical (Otic)		
acetic acid (Acetasol, Borofair, VoSol)	A/C >3 y: sol 2%: Insert saturated wick, keep moist × 24 h; instill 4-6 gtt q2-3h	For OE. Acidity of solution provides antibacterial and antifungal activity. May cause stinging and irritation, especially if tissues are inflamed or sloughing. Contraindicated with tympanic membrane perforation. Pregnancy category: C
chloramphenicol (Chloromycetin Otic)	A/C: Otic sol 0.5%: Instill 2-3 gtt into ear every 6-8 h	For OE. Boxed warning of bone marrow suppression after topical administration. Use restricted to serious infections that are resistant to other antimicrobials. Pregnancy category: C
Fluoroquinolones ciprofloxacin (Cetraxal, Floxin Otic) ofoxacin (Ocuflox)	A/C: Otic sol 0.2% in single-use 0.25-mL container: Instill contents into ear every 12 h for 7 d	Drug of choice for treatment of OE. Discontinue if superinfection from overgrowth of unsusceptible organisms such as fungi occurs. Pregnancy category: C
polymyxin B and neomycin	A/C: 3-4 gtt t.i.d./q.i.d. for 7-10 d	For OE. Combination product; each drug provides coverage for a different primary causative organism of OE. A corticosteroid is usually included in otic combinations. Discontinue after 10 days to prevent superinfection from fungal overgrowth. Contraindicated with tympanic membrane perforation due to an increased risk of irreversible ototoxicity. Pregnancy category: C

A, Adult; *b.i.d.*, twice a day; *C*, child; *d*, day; *GI*, gastrointestinal; *gtt*, drops; *h*, hour; *IM*, intramuscular; *IV*, intravenous; *max*, maximum; *min*, minute; *NA*, not applicable; *OE*, otitis externa; *OTC*, over-the-counter; *PB*, protein-binding; *PO*, by mouth; *q.i.d.*, four times a day; *sol*, solution; $t\frac{1}{2}$, half-life; *t.i.d.*, three times a day; *UK*, unknown; *y*, year; >, greater than.

Nursing Process
Patient-Centered Collaborative Care
Topical Antiinfectives: Ear Conditions

Assessment
- Obtain a medical history.
- Obtain a thorough drug history, including any allergies and use of herbal preparations and recreational drugs.
- Check vital signs. Obtain baseline data that can be compared with future findings.
- Conduct an otoscopic exam and record findings for future comparison.
- Check audiometry and tympanometry, and perform other testing as indicated.
- Assess for conditions in which selected antiinfectives are contraindicated or relatively contraindicated.

Nursing Diagnoses
- Deficient knowledge related to drug regimen (purpose, taking medications as ordered, administration of meds)
- Disturbed sensory perception (auditory) due to diagnosis
- Pain related to infection
- Risk for injury related to adverse drug effects.

Planning
- Patient will be free from ear infection after completion of drug regimen.
- Adverse effects will be minimized.

Nursing Interventions
- Complete culture and sensitivity testing, if ordered, before starting drug.
- Ensure TM patency before administering eardrops other than fluoroquinolones.
- Provide relief of associated pain, if present.
- Monitor for significant alterations in patient status
  - Monitor patients taking acetic acid solutions for burning and ear discomfort.
  - Monitor patients taking chloramphenicol for infections, increased bruising or bleeding, and pallor that could indicate bone marrow suppression. Assess for the development of superinfections.
  - Monitor patients taking fluoroquinolones for superinfections in the ear.
  - Monitor patients taking neomycin-polymyxin B-hydrocortisone for evidence of ototoxicity manifested by worsening of hearing or of alterations in balance.

Patient Teaching
- Instruct patient to complete entire course of medication (usually 10 to 14 days) and *not* to stop medication when the ear(s) feels better.
- If patient is prone to OE after swimming or showers, give instruction on prevention of OE. The Centers for Disease Control and Prevention recommends the following:
  - Keep water out of ears by using custom-fitted ear plugs.
  - If water enters the ear, tilt the ear downward to allow water to drain out. Pull the ear in different directions to enhance water drainage.
  - Use a portable hair dryer to facilitate drying.
- Instruct the patient to wear a MedicAlert bracelet at all times if allergic to medications.
- Refer to Chapter 13 for information on the administration of eardrops.

Cultural Considerations
- Depending on patient's culture, include appropriate support person in health teaching and decisions. This need is heightened in conditions with possible loss of hearing or diminished hearing.
- Use interpreter as needed.
- Provide printed materials in language patient reads and speaks most easily.

Evaluation
- Evaluate patient and family's knowledge of drug regimen.
- Determine effectiveness of drug therapy.
- Inquire regarding alleviation of side effects.

Antihistamines and Decongestants

For years, antihistamine and decongestants were thought to reduce middle-ear congestion and Eustachian tube dysfunction associated with otitis media with effusion (OME), a noninfectious collection of fluid in the middle ear. The rationale was that these drugs would reduce edema of the Eustachian tube which would promote drainage from the middle ear.

In 2006, a landmark Cochrane review of the medical literature concluded that antihistamines and decongestants were not as effective as once assumed and that the risks of adverse effects outweighed the benefits. Shortly thereafter, the American Academy of Pediatrics recommended against their use for ear conditions in young children. A 2012 report by the Agency for Healthcare Research and Quality makes the following statement regarding the use of these drugs in the management of OME: "The effects on multiple short- and long-term outcomes repeatedly demonstrated no benefit for use of these medications over placebo for treating OME. … The reviewed studies found evidence of increased side effects and harms with use of these medications." Unfortunately, many patients are not aware of these findings and may continue to take these drugs.

The importance of the nurse's role in educating patients regarding this concern cannot be overstated. Numerous

OTC antihistamine-decongestant medications are readily available to unknowing patients. Examples of antihistamines include chlorphenamine (Chlor-Trimeton), clemastine (Tavist), diphenhydramine (Benadryl), and many others. Examples of decongestants are phenylephrine (Neo-Synephrine) and pseudoephedrine (Sudafed). (Pseudoephedrine requires a prescription in some states.) Of even greater concern is that most of these are available as combination products that contain both an antihistamine and decongestant. (Refer to Chapter 40 for a discussion of upper respiratory agents.)

Ceruminolytics

Cerumen (earwax) is produced by glands in the outer half of the EAC. Usually it moves to the external os by itself and is washed away; however, sometimes cerumen accumulates due to overproduction or narrowing of the EAC. In these instances, cerumen can harden in the EAC, creating a cerumen impaction.

Ceruminolytics are topical otic agents that soften or break up the cerumen so that it can be removed. They are usually composed of mineral oil with hydrogen peroxide. An example is carbamide peroxide (Auro Ear Drops, Debrox), which is available OTC. Patients may also elect to use regular mineral oil to soften the wax or prevent cerumen impaction. Generally two to five drops applied twice a day for 4 days is sufficient.

Administration of Ear Medications

Ear medications are usually contained in a liquid vehicle for ease of administration. Guidelines for the administration of eardrops are given in Chapter 13.

Irrigation

Sometimes ceruminolytics alone are insufficient. In these instances, ear irrigation can be used to flush the cerumen deposits out of the ear canal. Irrigation is best accomplished when there is direct visualization of the tympanic membrane (TM). It must be done *gently* to avoid damage to the TM. It is also important to warm the water to prevent nausea and vomiting.

Frequently used irrigating solutions include hydrogen peroxide 3% in a 1:1 solution with warm water, normal saline solution, or acetic acid (vinegar) solution mixed with warm water. Contraindications to irrigation include perforation of the IM and prior hypersensitivity.

Patients with Ear Disorders: General Suggestions for Teaching

- Instruct patient not to insert any foreign objects into the ear canal.
- Instruct patient to keep drug away from heat.
- Provide education regarding the expected drug effect, dosage, side effects, and when to notify health care provider.
- Teach patient about OTC drug concerns, particularly antihistamines and decongestants. OTC drugs may interact with prescribed drug and may have risks that outweigh any drug benefit.
- Advise patient to contact health care provider before using OTC drugs or herbal preparations to treat ear disorders.
- Encourage patient to keep follow-up appointments.

KEY WEBSITES

American Society of Ophthalmic Registered Nurses: *www.asorn.org*

Society of Otorhinolaryngology and Head-Neck Nurses: *www.sohnnurse.com*

U.S. Pharmacopeia: *www.usp.org/usp-healthcare-professionals/related-topics-resources/usp-pictograms*

CRITICAL THINKING CASE STUDY

MH, a 70-year-old woman with POAG, is prescribed one drop of latanoprost (Xalatan) 0.005% ophthalmic solution each evening and one drop of timolol (Timoptic) 0.25% ophthalmic solution each morning and evening.

1. What is the purpose of giving two different medications to manage MH's glaucoma?
2. What special concerns related to medication timing are important for MH to consider when administering the evening dose of these medications?
3. Although systemic absorption of ophthalmic beta-adrenergic antagonists is usually small, it may potentially create problems for patients with certain conditions. Which conditions create a risk, and how will the nurse monitor for complications?
4. After a few months on these medications, MH notices changes in the appearance of her eyes. Describe the changes that MH is likely experiencing, and explain which drug is responsible.

NCLEX STUDY QUESTIONS

1. The ophthalmologist prescribes mannitol 20% to be administered IV at a dose of 1.5 g/kg to a patient with acute narrow-angle glaucoma who is awaiting surgery. Before administration, the nurse will assess the patient for which condition?
   a. Dehydration
   b. Constipation
   c. Gastrointestinal bleeding
   d. Allergies to sulfonamides
2. A patient is taking oral acetazolamide, a carbonic anhydrase inhibitor to decrease intraocular pressure. When providing drug education, what will the nurse advise the patient to anticipate?
   a. Increased weight
   b. Light sensitivity
   c. Burning or stinging of the eyes
   d. Increased urine output
3. The camp nurse is reviewing the shopping list of supplies needed for the upcoming camping season. Which product will the nurse purchase to prevent and treat cerumen impaction?
   a. Hydrogen peroxide
   b. Rubbing alcohol
   c. Charcoal
   d. Clove oil
4. A patient is about to undergo a diagnostic eye exam. The ophthalmologist asks the nurse to prepare to assist in the administration of tetracaine (Pontocaine), fluorescein stain (Fluorescite), and atropine (Isopto Atropine). Before assisting in the procedure, it is most important for the nurse to inform the ophthalmologist if the patient has a history of which condition?
   a. Cataracts
   b. Narrow-angle glaucoma
   c. Open-angle glaucoma
   d. Macular degeneration
5. The nurse has a patient demonstrate self-administration of eyedrops. Place the steps in the order in which the patient will perform them.
   a. Pull the lower lid away from the eye so that a pouch is formed.
   b. Gently shake the bottle to evenly distribute the drug.
   c. Press a finger against the inner corner of the eye for 2 to 3 minutes.
   d. Remove the cap.
   e. Tilt the head backward, and look upward.
   f. Place the dropper just above the pouch without touching the tip to the eye or finger.
   g. Wash hands.
   h. Gently squeeze one drop of medicine into the pouch.
6. When collecting a medication history from a patient with primary open angle glaucoma, the nurse identifies several drugs that could exacerbate glaucoma. Which drug poses a priority concern for this particular patient?
   a. cyclobenzaprine (Flexeril), an antispasmodic
   b. oxymetazoline (Afrin nasal spray), a decongestant
   c. prednisone (Deltasone), a corticosteroid
   d. sulfamethoxasole with trimethoprim (Bactrim), a sulfonamide antibiotic combination
7. The nurse asks a parent to demonstrate administration of eardrops on a toddler. Which steps by the parent indicate the need for additional education? (Select all that apply.)
   a. Position with the affected ear upward.
   b. Pull the ear backward and upward.
   c. Instill one drop of medication at a time allowing 3 to 5 minutes between each drop.
   d. Apply gentle pressure to the flap (tragus) over the ear canal.
   e. Keep the ear positioned upward for 5 minutes.

Answers: 1, a; 2, d; 3, a; 4, b; 5, g, b, d, e, a, f, h, c; 6, c; 7, b, c.

CHAPTER

50

Drugs for Dermatologic Disorders

evolve WEBSITE

http://evolve.elsevier.com/KeeHayes/pharmacology/

- Animations
- Content Updates
- Key Points
- Review Questions for the NCLEX® Examination
- References from the Textbook
- Unfolding Case Studies

OBJECTIVES

- Differentiate acne vulgaris, psoriasis, drug-induced dermatitis, and contact dermatitis.
- Describe nonpharmacologic measures used to treat mild acne vulgaris.
- Describe at least three drugs that can cause drug-induced dermatitis and their characteristic symptoms.
- Compare the topical antibacterial agents used to prevent and treat burn tissue infection.
- Discuss the nursing process, including teaching, related to commonly used drugs for acne vulgaris, psoriasis, and burns.

OUTLINE

KEY TERMS

Numerous skin lesions and eruptions require mild to aggressive drug therapy. Some skin disorders include acne vulgaris, psoriasis, eczema dermatitis, contact dermatitis, drug-induced dermatitis, and burn infection. Skin eruptions may result from viral infections (e.g., herpes simplex, herpes zoster), fungal infections (e.g., **tinea pedis** [athlete's foot], **tinea capitis** [ringworm]), and bacterial infections.

Most treatments for skin eruptions include topical creams, ointments, pastes, gels, lotions, and solutions. Skin lesions may appear as **macules** (flat with varying colors), **papules** (raised, palpable, and less than 1 cm in diameter), **vesicles** (raised, filled with fluid, and less than 1 cm in diameter), or **plaques** (hard, rough, raised, and flat on top). Selected skin disorders and their drug therapy regimens are discussed separately.

ACNE VULGARIS

Acne is the most common skin disorder in the United States. **Acne vulgaris** is the formation of papules, nodules, and cysts on the face, neck, shoulders, and back resulting from keratin plugs at the base of the pilosebaceous oil glands near the hair follicles. Of persons with acne, 90% are adolescents. The increase in androgen production that occurs during adolescence increases the production of sebum, an oily skin lubricant. The sebum combines with keratin to form a plug, which results in acne. Table 50-1 lists the drugs commonly used to control acne vulgaris and their dosages, uses, and considerations.

Nonpharmacologic Approach

Nonpharmacologic measures should be tried before drug therapy is initiated. A prescribed or suggested cleansing agent is necessary for all types of acne. The skin should be gently cleansed several times a day; vigorous scrubbing should be avoided. A well-balanced diet is indicated. Decreasing emotional stress and increasing emotional support are suggested. If drug therapy is necessary, nonpharmacologic measures should be maintained as well.

Topical Antiacne Drugs

Mild acne may require gentle cleansing and the use of keratolytics (keratin dissolvers such as benzoyl peroxide, resorcinol, and salicylic acid). Benzoyl peroxide is applied as a cream, lotion, or gel once or twice a day. This agent loosens the outer horny layer of the epidermis.

Tretinoin (Retin-A, Renova), a derivative of vitamin A, is a topical drug for mild to moderate acne that alters keratinization. Other antiacne agents, such as adapalene (Differin), azelaic acid (Azelex), and tazarotene (Tazorac), are used to treat mild to moderate acne. Adapalene is similar in action to tretinoin. It has antiinflammatory and comedolytic (eliminates blackheads) properties and tends to be more effective than tretinoin in reducing the number of acne lesions. Adapalene should not be used before or after extended sun exposure or sunburn. It can increase the risk of sunburn and intensify existing sunburn. Azelaic acid is as effective as benzoyl peroxide and tretinoin. Adapalene and azelaic acid can cause burning, pruritus, and erythema after several applications; however, this is less common with azelaic acid. Adapalene and tazarotene bind to select retinoid receptors; thus fewer adverse effects are anticipated.

Moderate acne requires a stronger concentration of benzoyl peroxide (10%), and topical antibiotics (e.g., tetracycline, erythromycin, clindamycin) may be added to the treatment regimen. Erythromycin and clindamycin are the most frequently prescribed topical antibiotics and have the fewest side effects.

Systemic Antiacne Drugs

For severe acne, oral antibiotics (doxycycline and minocycline [drugs of choice], tetracycline, erythromycin) and topical glucocorticoids may be prescribed. Pregnant patients should not take tetracycline because of possible teratogenic effects on the fetus. Once the condition is stabilized, the patient commonly progresses to the use of a topical preparation.

TABLE 50-1 DRUGS FOR ACNE VULGARIS AND PSORIASIS

GENERIC (BRAND)	ROUTE AND DOSAGE	USES AND CONSIDERATIONS
Acne Vulgaris		
Systemic Preparations		
tetracycline HCl	A/C: >12 y: PO: Initially, 125-250 mg every 6 h for 1-2 wk (or 250-500 mg b.i.d)., then decrease slowly to 125-500 mg/d or q.o.d.	For moderate to severe acne. Inexpensive. Contraindicated during pregnancy. Take 1 h before or 2 h after meals. Do not take with milk products or antacids. Pregnancy category: D; PB: 65%; $t\frac{1}{2}$: 6-12 h
erythromycin (Ery-Tab)	A: PO: 250 mg q.i.d. Topical dosage: Apply 1.5% or 2% solution, 2% gel, or 2% ointment to affected area b.i.d.	For moderate to severe acne. Substitute for tetracycline. Pregnancy category: B; PB: 73%-81%; $t\frac{1}{2}$: 1.5-2 h
minocycline HCl (Solodyn)	A: PO: ER: 1 mg/kg once daily	Once-daily treatment for nonnodular moderate to severe acne. Take with food to decrease esophageal irritation. Do not cut/crush/chew/tabs Pregnancy category: D; PB: >90%; $t\frac{1}{2}$: UK.
doxycycline (Adoxa)	A: PO: 100 mg/d; start 100 mg every 12 h for 1 d	For treatment of mild to moderate acne. Adjunct treatment for severe acne. Pregnancy category: D; PB: 90%; $t\frac{1}{2}$: 15-24 h
isotretinoin (Amnesteem, Claravis, Sotret, Absorica)	A: PO: 0.5-1 mg/kg/d in 2 divided doses. Treat for 15-20 wk or less if nodule count reduced by >70%; *max:* 2 mg/kg/d. Take with meals. May repeat course PRN after at least 2 mo of being drug free.	For severe acne. Decreases sebum secretion. Used when oral antibiotics have failed. Avoid sunlight, contact lenses, and use with tetracycline and vitamin A to reduce toxic effects. Monitor CBC, glucose, and lipid levels. Swallow whole tab. Pregnancy category: X; PB: 99%; $t\frac{1}{2}$: 10-20 h

TABLE 50-1 DRUGS FOR ACNE VULGARIS AND PSORIASIS—cont'd

GENERIC (BRAND)	ROUTE AND DOSAGE	USES AND CONSIDERATIONS
Topical Preparations		
Keratolytic Agents		
azelaic acid (Azelex)	A/C: >12 y: Topical: cream 20%; apply b.i.d.	For mild to moderate acne. Inhibits hyperactivity of normal melanocytes. Mild pruritus, erythema, dryness, and peeling of skin might result. Pregnancy category: B; PB: UK; t½: 12 h
benzoyl-peroxide (Benzac, Persa-Gel)	A/C: 2.5%-10% 1-4 times/d (cream, gel, or lotion)	For mild to moderate acne. Promotes **keratolysis** (removal of horny layer of epidermis). May cause skin irritation (burning, blistering, swelling).
salicylic acid (Sebulex)	Antiacne/antiseborrheic: A/C: 2%-6% cream, gel, and shampoo. Use as directed.	For mild to moderate acne; promotes desquamation.
resorcinol (Bicozene)	A/C: 1%-10% cream, ointment, lotion, and shampoo	For mild to moderate acne.
resorcinol and sulfur	A/C: 2% resorcinol + 5% sulfur A/C: 2% resorcinol + 8% sulfur Use as directed.	For mild to moderate acne.
Antibiotics: Topical		
tetracycline	Ointment: 3% Sol: 2.2 mg/mL Use as directed	For moderate acne. Pregnancy category: B; PB: N/A; t½: N/A
erythromycin	Ointment: 2% Gel: 1.5%-2% Use as directed	For moderate acne. Pregnancy category: B; PB: N/A; t½: N/A
clindamycin (Cleocin)	Gel: 1/5 Lotion: 1% Sol: 1% Use as directed	For moderate acne. Pregnancy category: B; PB: N/A; t½: N/A
Topical Vitamin A Derivatives		
tretinoin (Retin-A)	Cream: 0.0.25%-0.1% Gel: 0.025%-0.1% Apply h.s.	For mild to moderate acne. Vitamin A derivative. May be used with benzoyl peroxide or topical antibiotic. Do not apply to open wounds. Cleanse area first. Pregnancy category: B; PB: UK; t½: UK
adapalene (Differin)	A/C: >12 y: topical: 0.1% creme, gel, or lotion; 0.3% gel apply after washing h.s.	For mild to moderate acne. Do not use before or after extended sun exposure (it intensifies sunburn). Pruritus may occur. Pregnancy category: C; PB: UK; t½: UK
adapalene 0.1% + benzoyl peroxide 2.5% gel (Epiduo)	A: After washing, apply thin film to affected areas of face and/or trunk daily. Decrease frequency or discontinue if severe irritation occurs C: Not recommended	For acne vulgaris in patients >12 years. Pregnancy category: C; PB: N/A; t½: N/A
Oral Contraceptives		
Estrostep	A: PO: 1 tab/d for 21 d; no tab for 7 d; Take as OC schedule	FDA approved for treatment of acne. Pregnancy category: X; PB: N/A; t½: 5-14 h with norethindione; 26 h with ethinyl estradiol
Ortho Tri-Cyclen	A: PO: 1 tab/d for 21 d; then no tab for 7 d; take as OC schedule	FDA approved for treatment of acne. Pregnancy category: X; PB: N/A; t½: 12-30 h with deacetyl norgestimate; 26 h with ethinyl estradiol
Drospirenone/ ethinylestradiol (Yaz, and others)	A: PO: 3 mg/0.02 mg, 1 active tab daily for 24 d, then 1 inert tab daily for 4 d	To treat moderate acne in female patients ≥14 y. Take at same time each day.
Psoriasis		
methoxsalen (Oxsoralen, 8MOP, Oxsoralen Ultra, Uvadex)	A: PO: 10-70 mg (according to body weight) 2 h before exposure to therapeutic ultraviolet rays. Topical application before exposure to ultraviolet rays.	For severe psoriasis. Systemic antimetabolite. Avoid during pregnancy. Avoid sunlight during drug therapy; sunlight could cause burning and blistering. Pregnancy category: C/D; PB: 80%-90%; t½: >2 h

Continued

TABLE 50-1 DRUGS FOR ACNE VULGARIS AND PSORIASIS—cont'd

GENERIC (BRAND)	ROUTE AND DOSAGE	USES AND CONSIDERATIONS
acitretin (Soriatane)	A: PO: Initial: 25-50 mg once daily with main meal. Maintenance doses of 25-50 mg/d may be given, dependent upon person's response to initial treatment. Trials found that 25 mg/d for Rx of psoriasis vulgaris are similar in efficacy to 50 mg/d with fewer and less severe adverse clinical and laboratory events.	For recalcitrant psoriasis, including plaque, guttate, erythrodermic, palmar-plantar and pustular types. May take up to 6 mo for response to treatment. Pregnancy category: X; PB: 99%; $t\frac{1}{2}$: 4-8 d
Topical Preparations		
anthralin (Psoriatec)	A: Topical: 1.0%-1.2% cream	For moderate psoriasis. Inhibits DNA synthesis thus suppressing proliferation of epidermal cells. May stain clothing, skin, and hair.
calcipotriene (Dovonex)	A: Topical: cream, ointment, and scalp sol: 0.005%; apply daily or b.i.d.	For mild to moderate plaque psoriasis. Burning, stinging, and erythema may occur. Excess use may increase serum calcium level. Pregnancy category: C; PB: UK; $t\frac{1}{2}$: UK
calcipotriol/betamethasone dipropionate (Taclonex)	Psoriatic plaque: A: Topical: ointment; apply once daily to affected areas for up to 4 wk; *max:* 100g/wk	First once-daily topical ointment
clobetasol propionate (Clobex)	A: Lotion: Apply thin layer b.i.d.; *max:* 50 g/wk Spray: Spray on b.i.d., rub in gently and completely; *max:* 50g/wk for 4 consecutive wk; avoid occlusion in both forms. Neither product recommended for children <18 y	Super-high-potency corticosteroid for moderate to severe plaque psoriasis of <20% BSA. Adverse effects include reversible hypothalamic-pituitary-adrenal axis suppression and local site burning. Reassess lesions after 2 weeks of treatment. Contraindicated for application to axilla, face, or groin. Pregnancy category: C
coal tar (Scytera)	A: Topical: shampoo, paste, soap, ointment, lotion, solution, foam	For mild to moderate psoriasis. Suppresses DNA synthesis, decreasing mitotic activity. May stain clothing, skin, and hair.
tazarotene (Tazorac)	A: Topical: 0.05% and 0.1% gel. Apply in evening to lesions. Indicated for up to 20% BSA.	For mild to moderate psoriasis; can also be used for acne. Reduces epidermal inflammation. Photosensitivity can occur.
Biologic Agents		
alefacept (Amevive)	A: IM: 15 mg q1wk for 12 weeks	For severe chronic plaque psoriasis. Inhibits T-cell activation. Pregnancy category: B; PB: UK; $t\frac{1}{2}$: 270 h
adalimumab (Humira)	Moderate to severe psoriasis: A: subQ: 40 mg q other wk Start 80 mg subQ for 1 wk on wk 0; then 40 mg subQ q2wk on wk 1. Psoriasis arthritis: A: 40 mg subQ q2wk	Human IgG1 monoclonal TNF-alpha antibody. Pregnancy category: B; PB: UK; $t\frac{1}{2}$: 10-20 d
etanercept (Enbrel)	A: subQ: Psoriatic arthritis: 50 mg b.i.w. Psoriasis: Start with 50 mg b.i.w. for 3 mo; then 50 mg/wk	For moderate to severe psoriasis. Pregnancy category: B; PB: UK; $t\frac{1}{2}$: 115 h
infliximab (Remicade)	A: IV: Psoriasis: 5 mg/kg IV infusion (>120 min) weeks 0, 2, 6, then q8wk	FDA approved in 1999 for treatment of psoriasis Pregnancy category: C; PB: UK; $t\frac{1}{2}$: 9.5 d
ustekinumab (Stelara)	A: >18 y: <100 kg: 45 mg subQ once, then 4 wk later, and then once q12wk. >100 kg: 90 mg subQ once, then 4 wk later, and then once q12wk. C: Not recommended for children <18 y	For moderate to severe plaque psoriasis. May affect CYP450 substrates. Pregnancy category: B.
Keratolytic Agents		
salicylic acid, sulfur, resorcinol		See acne vulgaris.

A, Adult; *BSA*, body surface area; *b.i.d.*, twice a day; *b.i.w.*, twice weekly; *C*, child; *d*, day; *DNA*, deoxyribonucleic acid; *ER*, extended-release; *FDA*, U.S. Food and Drug Administration; *h*, hour; *h.s.*, at bedtime; *IR*, immediate release; *IV*, intravenous; *max*, maximum; *mo*, month; *N/A*, not available; *OC*, oral contraceptive; *PB*, protein-binding; *PO*, by mouth; *q.o.d.*, every other day; *sol*, solution; *subQ*, subcutaneous; $t\frac{1}{2}$, half-life; *tab*, tablet; *TNF*, tumor necrosis factor; *UK*, unknown; *wk*, week; *y*, year; >, greater than; <, less than.

Isotretinoin (Amnesteem) is used for treatment of severe cystic acne. It can be administered orally or topically. It decreases sebum formation and secretion and has antiinflammatory and antikeratinizing (keratolytic) effects. The typical patient takes this drug for 4 to 6 months. It can cause adverse reactions such as chelitis (90%), dizziness, conjunctivitis, skin irritation, pruritus, epistaxis, hirsutism, and photosensitivity. Isotretinoin must not be used during pregnancy because of teratogenic effects. Using vitamin A or tetracycline with isotretinoin may increase its adverse effects. Baseline blood tests are required before initiating isotretinoin therapy and at intervals throughout therapy. Additional cautions associated with isotretinoin include the following: Do not breastfeed, give blood during or for 1 month after therapy, take other medications or herbal products without first consulting the health care provider, drive at night without knowing the effect of isotretinoin on night vision, or have cosmetic procedures to smooth skin. Instruct the patient to avoid excessively vigorous activity and to contact the health care provider and stop taking isotretinoin if experiencing muscle weakness, which may be an indication of serious muscle damage. Monitoring of complete blood count (CBC), glucose and lipid levels, and urinalysis on a regular basis is important. Isotretinoin must not be used during pregnancy; its pregnancy category is X. Because of this drug's powerful teratogenicity, a risk-management system to prevent isotretinoin-related teratogenicity was designed by the FDA Dermatologic and Ophthalmic Advisory Committee in 2002. Named the System to Manage Accutane-Related Teratogenicity (SMART), its purpose was to ensure that no patient is pregnant when treatment is initiated and no patient becomes pregnant while taking the drug or for at least 1 month after completing a course of isotretinoin. The iPLEDGE program replaced SMART in December 2005. An Internet-based registry system, iPLEDGE uses a central database to track isotretinoin users and account for all information and access to the drug. This comprehensive program has rules for the health care provider, patient, pharmacist, and wholesaler, as follows:

- Female patient responsibilities: Female patients must receive warnings of teratogenicity both orally and in writing before use. Two negative pregnancy tests are required before starting the drug, and one negative test is required before each monthly refill. Two effective methods of contraception are required 1 month before, throughout, and 1 month after isotretinoin treatment. (Exceptions are total abstinence from intercourse or following hysterectomy.) Patients must review iPLEDGE educational materials on a variety of topics, including reasons for contraception when using a drug known to be teratogenic. A signed patient information/informed consent document is also required.
- Health care provider responsibilities: Registration by the health care provider for the iPLEDGE program is required, and the patient must follow up by telephone or Internet before treatment, monthly during treatment, and 1 month after treatment. During these contacts, the patient must indicate both birth control methods and respond to questions related to program requirements. After registering and agreeing to follow iPLEDGE, the health care provider must enter the two methods of birth control the patient is using and the results of monthly pregnancy tests. Initial and refill prescriptions must also be entered.
- Pharmacist responsibilities: Pharmacists must be registered with the iPLEDGE program. Isotretinoin must be obtained from a wholesaler also registered with the iPLEDGE program. The pharmacist for each prescription must get authorization from iPLEDGE, confirm with iPLEDGE that the prescription date is within 7 days, dispense a 30-day supply (maximum), and indicate the risk-management authorization number on the prescription.
- Wholesaler responsibilities: Wholesalers must be registered with the iPLEDGE program.

iPLEDGE has recently become less stringent for female patients not of childbearing age and for male patients.

PSORIASIS

Psoriasis is a chronic skin disorder that affects 2% to 4% of the U.S. population. Onset usually occurs before age 30 years, but it may occur as early as age 10 years. Psoriasis is characterized by erythematous papules and plaques covered with silvery scales. It appears on the scalp, elbows, palms of the hands, knees, and soles of the feet. With psoriasis, epidermal cell growth and epidermal turnover are accelerated to approximately five times the normal expected epidermal growth. Antipsoriatic drug therapy uses preparations such as coal tar products and anthralin to keep the psoriasis in check; however, there are usually periods of remission and exacerbation.

Topical and Systemic Preparations

Psoriatic scales may be loosened with keratolytics (salicylic acid, sulfur). Topical glucocorticoids are sometimes used for mild psoriasis. Other topical preparations for psoriasis include anthralin (Dithro-Crème Psoriatec, Zithranol-RR) and coal tar (Estar), Oxipor VHC, Balnetar, and Scytera. Applications of 1% anthralin may cause erythema to occur. This agent can stain clothing, skin, and hair. Coal tar products are available in shampoos, lotions, and creams. They have an unpleasant odor and can cause burning and stinging, so they are rarely used. A topical product for mild to moderate psoriasis is calcipotriene (Dovonex), a synthetic vitamin D_3 derivative useful for suppressing cell proliferation. This drug may cause local irritation and the serious adverse effects of hypercalciuria and hypercalcemia (increased urine and serum calcium levels). A topical antipsoriatic, tazarotene (Tazorac), is used to treat mild to moderate psoriasis. Photosensitivity is a side effect of tazarotene; therefore, the patient should use sunscreen to avoid severe sunburn.

The anticancer drug methotrexate is a systemic drug that slows high growth fraction. It is prescribed to decrease the acceleration of epidermal cell growth in severe psoriasis.

Ultraviolet A (UVA) may be used to suppress mitotic (cell division) activity. Photochemotherapy, a combination of ultraviolet radiation and the psoralen derivative methoxsalen (photosensitive drug), is used to decrease proliferation of epidermal cells. This type of therapy is called *psoralen and ultraviolet A* (PUVA). PUVA permits lower doses of methoxsalen and ultraviolet A to be given.

High-cost biologic agents are helpful in the management of psoriasis in patients who are refractory to ultraviolet B (UVB) phototherapy and need improved control. FDA-approved agents include the T-cell antagonist alefacept (Amevive) and the tumor necrosis factor (TNF) inhibitors etanercept (Enbrel), infliximab (Remicade), adalimumab (Humira), and interleukin antagonist ustekinumab (Stelara). All TNF inhibitors have a risk of severe opportunistic infection. These biologic agents are expensive but tend to have fewer side effects with comparable efficacy to other systemic treatments.

Alefacept (Amevive) is a recombinant protein that modifies the inflammatory process and inhibits the activation of memory effector T lymphocytes. No increased rate of opportunistic infections or malignancy has been observed. The drug is administered IM weekly for 12 weeks. Chills are the most common side effect. A second 12-week cycle may be initiated, but with decreased benefits from the first cycle. Weekly monitoring of CBC and T-cell counts is required, and alefacept must be discontinued if the CD4+ T-cell count falls lower than 250 cells per microliter.

Etanercept (Enbrel) is a soluble recombinant human TNF-alpha inhibitor. This agent worsens infections, especially tuberculosis (TB). A tuberculin test (PPD) is required before initiation of therapy. Etanercept may also worsen heart failure (HF). The drug is administered twice weekly for 12 weeks, and then weekly.

Infliximab (Remicade) is a monoclonal antibody that neutralizes TNF-alpha purified protein derivative (PPD). The drug is administered IV at 0, 2, and 6 weeks, and then every 8 weeks as tolerated. Opportunistic infection rate is higher than with other agents. A tuberculin test before the start and during treatment is recommended. This drug is associated with demyelinating disease. The major side effect is increased risk for infection.

Adalimumab (Humira) is a TNF-alpha inhibitor. The drug is administered subcutaneously every other week.

Table 50-1 lists the drugs used to control psoriasis.

Side Effects and Adverse Reactions

- Anthralin: Erythema (redness) to normal skin, inflamed eyes, and staining effect.
- Coal tar: Skin irritation, such as burning; photosensitivity; and staining effect.
- Methoxsalen: Nausea, headache, vertigo, rash, pruritus, and burning and peeling of skin. Adverse reactions: Anemia, leukopenia, thrombocytopenia, ulcerative stomatitis, bleeding, alopecia, and cystitis.
- Alefacept: Injection site reaction (erythema, itching, pain, swelling), dizziness, throat inflammation, nausea, muscle pain, and chills.
- Etanercept: Injection site reaction (erythema, itching, pain, swelling) and infections, including reactivation of TB.
- Infliximab: Infusion reactions and infections, including reactivation of TB.
- Adalimumab: Injection site reaction (erythema, itching, pain, swelling) and infections, including reactivation of TB.
- Ustekinumab: Nasopharyngitis, URI, headache, fatigue

VERRUCA VULGARIS (WARTS)

The common wart is a hard, horny nodule that may appear anywhere on the body, particularly on the hands and feet. Warts may be benign lesions, or they may be precursors to cancerous lesions, especially those in the genital region. They may be removed by freezing, electrodesiccation, or surgical excision. Drugs commonly used in the treatment of warts include salicylic acid and podophyllum resin. Salicylic acid promotes desquamation. It can be absorbed through the skin, and salicylism (toxicity) might occur. Podophyllum resin is indicated mainly for venereal warts and is not as effective against the common wart. This drug also can be absorbed through the skin; toxic symptoms such as peripheral neuropathy, blood dyscrasias, and kidney impairment may result if a large area is treated. Podophyllum can cause teratogenic effects and should not be used during pregnancy. Imiquimod (Aldara, Zyclara) and podofilox (Condylox) may be prescribed as alternative agents for podophyllin. Both drugs may be used for topical treatment of external genital and perianal warts.

Nursing Process
Patient-Centered Collaborative Care

Acne Vulgaris and Psoriasis

Assessment

- Obtain history from patient of the onset of skin lesions. Note whether or not there is a familial history of the disorder.
- Assess patient's skin eruptions. Describe lesions, location, and drainage, if present.
- Obtain culture of a purulent draining skin lesion.
- Determine baseline vital signs. Report any elevation in temperature.
- Assess the psychological effects of skin lesions and changes in body image.
- Assess type of psoriatic lesions (pustules, plaques, or guttate)

Nursing Diagnoses

- Deficient knowledge related to management of skin lesions and adverse effects of medications used to treat skin lesions
- Risk for impaired skin integrity related to side effects of some medications
- Risk for infection due to selected medications
- Risk for disturbed body image related to skin lesions

- Risk for situational low self-esteem related to skin lesions

Planning

- Patient will have increased knowledge of management of skin condition.
- Patient's lesions will be decreased in size or will be absent after drug therapy and skin care.
- Patient will report improved body image.

Nursing Interventions

- Establish rapport, because patient may be embarrassed.
- Apply topical medications to skin lesions using aseptic technique.
- Monitor vital signs, and report abnormal findings.
- Check lesion sites during drug therapy for improvement or adverse reactions to drug therapy.

Patient Teaching

General

- Advise patient not to use harsh cleansers. Tell patient to gently cleanse the skin several times a day.
- Teach patient to apply topical ointments and creams using clean technique.
- Inform patient about side effects and adverse reactions associated with drugs taken.
- Advise patient to report abnormal findings immediately.
- Instruct patient to notify health care provider if pregnant or if there is possibility of pregnancy. Many agents used to treat acne can cause teratogenic effects on the fetus.
- Advise patient to keep health care appointments and have laboratory tests performed as prescribed.

Self-Administration

- Teach patient and family about how to administer biologic agents given via the parenteral route (e.g., preparation and administration of Amevive: store diluted solution in refrigerator, and use within 4 hours; do not shake medication; rotate injection sites, leaving at least 1 inch between sites).

Cultural Considerations

- Respect patient's cultural beliefs and alternative methods for treating acne vulgaris or psoriasis. Plan may need modification to include pharmacologic treatment for acne or psoriasis.
- Obtain an interpreter when necessary; do not rely on family members, who may not fully disclose because of cultural norms.

Evaluation

- Evaluate patient's knowledge of management of condition.
- Evaluate effectiveness of drug therapy. If improvement is not apparent, drug therapy and skin care regimen may need to be changed.
- Be aware of the different time periods for improvement with various drug therapies.

Cantharidin (Cantharone, Verr-Canth) is used to remove the common wart; however, it can be harmful to normal skin. For treating the common wart, cantharidin is applied to the wart, allowed to dry, and then the wart is covered with nonporous tape for 24 hours. The procedure may be repeated in 1 to 2 weeks.

Many OTC agents are used to remove warts. The efficacy of some of these is questionable; however, some that contain chemical compounds such as salicylic acid may be effective.

DRUG-INDUCED DERMATITIS

An adverse reaction to drug therapy may result in skin lesions that vary from a rash, urticaria, papules, and vesicles to life-threatening skin eruptions such as erythema multiforme (red blisters over a large portion of the body), Stevens-Johnson syndrome (large blisters in the oral and anogenital mucosa, pharynx, eyes, and viscera), and toxic epidermal necrolysis (widespread detachment of the epidermis from underlying skin layers). A hypersensitive reaction to a drug is caused by the formation of sensitizing lymphocytes. If multiple drug therapy is used, the last drug given may be the cause of the hypersensitivity and skin eruptions. The usual skin reactions are a rash, which may take several hours or a day to appear, and urticaria (hives), which usually takes a few minutes to appear. Certain drugs, such as penicillin, are known to cause hypersensitivity.

Other drug-induced dermatitides include discoid lupus erythematosus and exfoliative dermatitis. Hydralazine hydrochloride (isoniazid, phenothiazines, anticonvulsants, and antidysrhythmics), such as procainamide, may cause lupus-like symptoms. If lupus symptoms occur, the drug should be discontinued. Certain antibacterials and anticonvulsants may cause exfoliative dermatitis, resulting in erythema of the skin, itching, scaling, and loss of body hair (e.g., sulfa antibiotics are one cause of toxic epidermal necrolysis).

CONTACT DERMATITIS

Contact dermatitis, also called *exogenous dermatitis,* is caused by chemical or plant irritation. Skin rash with itching, swelling, blistering, oozing, or scaling at the affected skin sites characterizes this disorder. Chemical contacts include cosmetics, cleaning products, perfume, clothing, dyes, and topical drugs. Plant contacts include poison ivy, oak, or sumac.

Nonpharmacologic measures include avoiding direct contact with the causative irritant. Protective gloves or clothing may be necessary if the chemical is associated with work;

skin that has been in contact with the irritant should be immediately cleansed. Patch testing may be needed to determine the causal factor.

Treatment may consist of wet dressings containing Burow's solution (aluminum acetate); lotions, such as calamine, that contain zinc oxide; calcium hydroxide solution; and glycerin. Calamine lotion may contain the antihistamine diphenhydramine and is used primarily for plant irritations. If itching persists, antipruritics (systemic diphenhydramine [Benadryl]) may be used. Topical Benadryl is not recommended, as it increases the risk of allergic reaction to systemic Benadryl. Topical antipruritics should not be applied to open wounds or near the eyes or genital area. Other antipruritic treatments include baths of oatmeal and application of glucocorticoid ointments, creams, or gels.

Dexamethasone (Decadron) cream, hydrocortisone ointment or cream, methylprednisolone acetate (Medrol) ointment, triamcinolone acetonide (Aristocort), and flurandrenolide (Cordran) are examples of topical glucocorticoids that aid in alleviating dermatitis. Box 50-1 lists selected topical glucocorticoids according to their potency for relieving the itching and inflammation associated with dermatitis.

A portion of topical glucocorticoids can be systemically absorbed into the circulation. The amount and rate of absorption depend on the vehicle (cream, lotion), drug concentration, drug composition, and skin area to which the glucocorticoid is applied. Absorption is greater where the skin is more permeable—the face, scalp, eyelids, neck, axilla, and genital area. Side effects and adverse reactions may occur with prolonged use of the topical drug or if the drug is continuously covered with a dressing. Prolonged use of topical glucocorticoids can cause thinning of the skin with atrophy of the epidermis and dermis and purpura from small-vessel eruptions; therefore, prolonged use is discouraged.

IMPETIGO

Impetigo, a common *Staphylococcus aureus* infection of the skin, is most commonly seen in children 2 to 5 years old. Topical agents are used in the treatment of mild and moderate infection, and oral agents are used for severe infection. The two drugs of choice are mupirocin (Bactroban) and retapamulin (Altabax). With multiple lesions and ineffective topical therapy, oral antibiotics are needed.

HAIR LOSS AND BALDNESS

When the hair shaft is lost and the hair follicle cannot regenerate, male-pattern baldness, or *alopecia*, occurs. Permanent hair loss is associated with a familial history and occurs during the aging process, earlier in some individuals than others. Drugs also known to cause alopecia include anticancer (antineoplastic) agents, sulfonamides, anticonvulsants, aminoglycosides, and some nonsteroidal antiinflammatory drugs (NSAIDs), such as indomethacin. Severe febrile illnesses, pregnancy, myxedema (condition resulting from hypothyroidism), and cancer therapies are some of the health conditions contributing to temporary hair loss.

A 2% minoxidil (Rogaine) solution has been approved by the FDA for treating baldness for men and women. A 5% solution is approved for men only. Minoxidil causes

BOX 50-1 TOPICAL GLUCOCORTICOIDS

Super High Potency

betamethasone dipropionate, augmented 0.05%
- Diprolene (o, g)

clobetasol propionate 0.05%
- Clobex (l, sh, s)
- Olux (f)
- Olux-E (f)
- Temovate (c, g, o, s app)
- Temovate E (e crm)

fluocinonide 0.1%
- Vanos (c)

flurandrenolide 4 mcg/sq cm
- Cordran (t)

halobetasol propionate 0.05%
- Ultravate 0.05% (c, o)

High Potency

amcinonide 0.1%

betamethasone dipropionate, augmented 0.05%
- Diprolene (l)
- Diprolene AF (e crm)

desoximetasone 0.05%
- Topicort (g)

desoximetasone 0.25%
- Topicort (e crm, o)

diflorasone diacetate 0.05%
- Psorcon E (e crm, e oint)

fluoc

halcinonide 0.1%
- Halog (c, o, sol)

triamcinolone acetonide 0.5%
- Kenalog (c)

Intermediate Potency

betamethasone valerate 0.12%
- Luxiq (f)

clocortolone pivalate 0.1%
- Cloderm (c)

desonide 0.5%
- DesOwen (c, l, o)
- Desonate (g)
- Verdeso (f)

desoximetasone 0.05%
- Topicort LP (e crm)

fluocinolone acetonide 0.01%
- Derma-Smoothe/FS (oil)
- Capex (sh)

fluocinolone acetonide 0.025%
- Synalar (c, o)

flurandrenolide 0.025%
- Cordran SP (c)
- Cordran (o)

flurandrenolide 0.05%
- Cordran (l, o)
- Cordran-SP (c)

fluticasone propionate 0.005%
- Cutivate (o)

fluticasone propionate 0.05%
- Cutivate (c, l)

hydrocortisone probutate 0.1%
- Pandel (c)

hydrocortisone butyrate 0.1%
- Locoid (c, o, sol)
- Locoid Lipocream

hydrocortisone valerate 0.2%
- Westcort (c, o)

mometasone furoate 0.1%
- Elocon (c, l, o)

prednicarbate 0.1%
- Dermatop (e crm, o)

triamcinolone acetonide 0.1%
- Kenalog (c, l)

triamcinolone acetonide 0.2%
- Kenalog (a)

Low Potency

alclometasone dipropionate 0.05%
- Aclovate (c, o)

fluocinolone acetonide 0.01%
- Synalar (sol)

hydrocortisone base or acetate 0.5%
- Cortisporin (c)

hydrocortisone base or acetate 1%
- Cortisporin (o)*
- Hytone (c, o)
- U-cort (c)
- Vytone (c)*

hydrocortisone base or acetate 2.5%
- Anusol-HC (crm)
- Hytone (c, o)

triamcinolone acetonide 0.025%
- Kenalog (c, l, o)

*More than 1 active ingredient.
C, Cream; *e crm,* emollient cream; *e oint,* emollient ointment; *f,* foam; *g,* gel; *l,* lotion; *o,* ointment; *s,* spray; *s app,* scalp application; *sh,* shampoo; *sol,* solution; *t,* tape.

vasodilation, increasing cutaneous blood flow. The increased blood flow tends to stimulate hair follicle growth. When the drug is discontinued, however, hair loss occurs within 3 to 4 months. Systemic absorption of minoxidil is minimal, so adverse reactions seldom occur. Occasionally, headaches and a slight decrease in systolic blood pressure occur.

Finasteride (Propecia, Proscar) is an oral drug used for male baldness. It is available in 1-mg tablets. (A 5-mg tablet is prescribed for benign prostatic hyperplasia.) For growing hair, finasteride is effective in 50% of men. It has been reported that it is relatively ineffective in growing hair in older men, even with an increased dose.

SUNSCREENS

Chemical screens are those that absorb ultraviolet (UV) radiation, and physical screens are those that scatter UV radiation. Chemical screens account for most FDA-approved sunscreens. Most absorb UV-UVB, less than half absorb UVA, and one (avobenzone) protects against UVA and UVB. Physical screens prevent skin penetration of UV. Examples of these products are titanium dioxide and zinc oxide, generally applied to limited areas of the body such as the nose and ears.

UV radiation causes many problems, including premature aging of the skin, burns, and skin cancer. Sunscreens protect against sunburn photosensitivity to selected drugs but do not guard against melanoma and basal cell carcinoma. Sun protection factor (SPF) is a rating on sunscreen products of protection against UVB radiation. The highest rating approved by the FDA is SPF 30+. A higher protection rating is not proportional to the amount of UVB radiation blocked. For example, SPF 15 blocks 93% of UVB, and SPF 30 blocks 96.7%. Sunscreens with SPF greater than 15 are recommended for children older than 6 months and all adults.

The FDA requires UVA ratings and separate labeling for UVB and UVA SPF protection. Use of the term *sunblock* is not permitted. Lack of UVA protection is to be clearly indicated on the product label. The FDA requirements for sunscreens are summarized in Table 50-2.

Using common sense is the best way to protect the skin. UV radiation is most intense between 10:00 AM and 3:00 PM. Apply a sunscreen appropriate for the circumstances at least 30 minutes before going out into the sun. (For sunscreens with PABA or padimate, allow 2 hours). Sunscreen will protect for about 2 hours when applied properly and not exposed to moisture through swimming or sweating. Wearing protective clothing (e.g., a wide-brimmed hat, sunglasses, long-sleeved shirt) is a good idea. When using DEET insect repellent with sunscreen, apply DEET first to avoid decreased effectiveness of sunscreen. Contact dermatitis and photosensitivity reaction are adverse effects and occur most commonly with PABA derivatives.

BURNS AND BURN PREPARATIONS

Burns from heat (thermal burns, most common kind of burn injury), electricity (electrical burns), and chemical agents (chemical burns) can cause skin lesions. Burns are classified according to degree and tissue depth (Table 50-3).

Moderately severe sunburn is an example of a first-degree burn. Severe sunburn can result in a second-degree burn. Burns needs immediate attention, regardless of the degree and tissue depth of the burn.

For first-degree (superficial epidermal and superficial partial thickness) and minor burns, a cold, wet compress is applied to the burned area to constrict blood vessels and decrease swelling. This treatment also decreases the amount of pain. The quicker the burn area is cooled, the less tissue damage occurs. No greasy ointment or dressing should be applied, because they can inhibit heat loss from the burn and increase damage to the tissues. A nonprescription antibiotic, such as bacitracin with polymyxin B (Polysporin), may be used for minor burns. Used separately, polymyxin B and neomycin are not drugs of choice, because they do not have a broad-spectrum effect. With chemical burns, clothing should be removed immediately and the skin thoroughly flushed with water.

Persons with second (deep thickness)—and third-degree (full thickness) burns that involve the dermis and subcutaneous tissue should undergo treatment at a burn center or other hospital setting. Intravenous therapy is started immediately, and a nonnarcotic or narcotic analgesic is given for pain.

TABLE 50-2 FDA REQUIREMENTS FOR SUNSCREENS

PROTECTION	UVB RATING AND LABELING	UVA RATING AND LABELING
Low	UVB SPF 2-14	*
Medium	UVB SPF 15-29	**
High	UVB SPF 30-50	***
Highest	UVB SPF 50+	****

FDA, U. S. Food and Drug Administration; *UV,* ultraviolet.

TABLE 50-3 DEGREE AND TISSUE DEPTH OF BURNS

TYPE	DEGREE	DEPTH	CHARACTERISTICS
Superficial epidermal	First	Epidermis	Erythema, painful
Partial-thickness superficial	First-second	Epidermis, upper dermis	Blistering, very painful
Deep-thickness	Second	Epidermis, lower dermis	Mottled, blistering, intense pain
Full-thickness	Third	Epidermis, dermis, nerve ending involvement, subcutaneous tissue	Pearly white skin, charred, no pain

Burn areas are cleansed with sterile saline solution and an antiseptic such as povidone-iodine (Betadine). If a povidone-iodine solution is used, it should be determined that the patient is not allergic to iodine or seafood. Broad-spectrum topical antibacterials, usually effective against many gram-positive and gram-negative organisms and yeast infections, are applied to burn areas to prevent infection. Examples of these antibacterials include mafenide acetate (Sulfamylon), silver sulfadiazine (Silvadene), and silver nitrate 0.5% solution. Prototype Drug Chart 50-1 lists the pharmacologic data for the antibacterial agent mafenide acetate (Sulfamylon).

Analgesics are required for pain control, usually controlled substances and NSAIDs.

Mafenide Acetate

Pharmacokinetics Mafenide acetate is absorbed through the skin and metabolized by the liver to a metabolite. The drug is excreted in the urine. The drug and its metabolite are strong carbonic anhydrase inhibitors, which may lead to acid-base imbalances (e.g., metabolic acidosis, respiratory alkalosis) and fluid loss from the mild diuretic effect. If respiration becomes rapid, labored, or shallow, the cream should be discontinued for a few days until the acid-base balance is restored.

Pharmacodynamics Mafenide, a sulfonamide derivative, interferes with bacterial cell-wall synthesis and metabolism and is bacteriostatic. It is used as a topical water-soluble antibacterial agent to prevent or combat burn infection. After the burn is cleansed and debrided, $\frac{1}{16}$-inch of mafenide cream is applied to the affected area one to two times daily and covered lightly with a dressing. The patient may complain of a burning sensation when the drug is applied.

Table 50-4 lists selected topical medications for burns and their dosages, uses, and considerations.

Silver Sulfadiazine

Silver sulfadiazine (Silvadene, SSD) is commonly used to prevent and treat sepsis in second- and third-degree burns. It acts on the cell membrane and cell wall to produce

PROTOTYPE DRUG CHART 50-1

Mafenide Acetate

Drug Class Topical antiinfective Trade Names: Sulfamylon Cream Pregnancy Category: C	**Dosage** A/C: Topical: Apply $\frac{1}{16}$-inch layer evenly to affected area b.i.d.; reapply PRN
Contraindications Hypersensitivity, inhalation injury Caution: Renal failure	**Drug-Lab-Food Interactions** None known
Pharmacokinetics Absorption: Some absorbed Distribution: PB: UK Metabolism: t½: UK Excretion: In urine	**Pharmacodynamics** Topical: Onset: On contact Peak: 2-4 h Duration: As long as applied
Therapeutic Effects/Uses To treat second- and third-degree burns; to prevent organism invasion of burned tissue areas; to treat burn infections Mode of Action: Inhibits bacterial cell wall synthesis	
Side Effects Rash, burning sensation, urticaria, pruritus, swelling	**Adverse Reactions** Metabolic acidosis, respiratory alkalosis, blistering, superinfection Life-threatening: Bone marrow suppression, fatal hemolytic anemia

A, Adult; *b.i.d.*, twice a day; *C*, child; *h*, hour; *PB*, protein-binding; *PRN*, as needed; *t½*, half-life; *UK*, unknown.

TABLE 50-4 TOPICAL ANTIINFECTIVES: BURNS

GENERIC (BRAND)	ROUTE AND DOSAGE	USES AND CONSIDERATIONS
mafenide acetate (Sulfamylon)	See Prototype Drug Chart 50-1.	
silver nitrate	0.5 sol; 10%, 25% sticks; apply only to affected area 2-3 times/wk for 2-3 wk	For second- and third-degree burns. Dressings are soaked in 0.5% silver nitrate solution and then removed before they dry. Effective against some gram-negative organisms. May cause electrolyte imbalance (hypokalemia) if used extensively. Pregnancy category: C; PB: NA; t½: NA
silver sulfadiazine (Silvadene, SSD)	1% Cream, apply b.i.d. in $\frac{1}{16}$-inch layer	To prevent and treat infection of second- and third-degree burns. Ten percent of drug is absorbed. Excessive use or extensive application area may cause sulfa crystals (crystalluria). Pregnancy category: C; PB: NA; t½: NA

b.i.d., Twice a day; *d*, day; *NA*, not applicable; *PB*, protein-binding; *t½*, half-life; *sol*, solution; *wk*, week.

bactericidal effects. Unlike mafenide, it is not a carbonic anhydrase inhibitor. It is contraindicated at or near term pregnancy.

One percent or less of the silver is absorbed, and up to 10% of sulfadiazine is absorbed. Side effects and adverse reactions may include skin discoloration, burning sensation, rashes, erythema multiforme, skin necrosis, and possible leukopenia.

Nursing Process
Patient-Centered Collaborative Care

Topical Antiinfectives: Burns

Assessment

- Assess burned tissue for infection (foul odor, purulent drainage, erythema, heat).
- Culture an oozing wound.
- Check patient's vital signs. Report abnormal findings, such as elevated temperature.
- Determine fluid status. Report signs and symptoms of hypovolemia or hypervolemia.

Nursing Diagnoses

- Impairment of skin integrity related to disruption of skin surface secondary to burns
- Risk for imbalanced fluid volume related to fluid shifts secondary to burns
- Deficient knowledge related to management of burns
- Risk for infection related to loss of skin integrity
- Acute pain related to thermal injury
- Risk for disturbed body image related to loss of skin integrity

Planning

- The patient will remain free from infection.
- The patient's pain will be decreased or tolerable.

Nursing Interventions

- Administer prescribed analgesia before application, if needed.
- Cleanse burned tissue sites using aseptic technique.
- Apply topical antibacterial drug and dressing with sterile technique.
- Monitor patient's fluid balance and renal function.
- Monitor patient for side effects and adverse reactions to topical drug.
- Monitor patient's vital signs, and be alert for signs of infection. Use with caution in patients with acute renal failure.
- Closely monitor patient's acid-base balance, especially in the presence of pulmonary or renal dysfunction.
- Store drug in dry place at room temperature.

Patient Teaching

General

- Instruct patient and family about pain management, medications used to treat burns, and signs of complications from burns, such as fluid excess or deficit.

Self-Administration

- Explain to patient and family the care given to the burned tissue areas using aseptic technique.
- Teach patient and family how to apply topical agent and dressings to burned areas.
- Teach patient and family about signs and symptoms of infection and to report them promptly to the health care provider.

Evaluation

- Evaluate patient and family knowledge of burn management.
- Patient will remain in normovolemic state and be free of complications from burns (e.g., hypervolemia, hypovolemia).
- Evaluate effectiveness of treatment interventions to burned tissue areas by determining whether healing is proceeding and sites are free from infection.

KEY WEBSITES

iPLEDGE: *www.ipledgeprogram.com*
National Psoriasis Foundation: *www.psoriasis.org*
Skin and skin disorders: *www.noah-health.org/en/skin*

CRITICAL THINKING CASE STUDY

MG, a 15-year-old patient, complains about blackheads and large, raised pimples on her face. She seeks help from a health care provider.

1. To assist in identifying her skin problem, what should the health history and assessment include?
2. Which nonpharmacologic measures might the nurse discuss with MG in caring for her skin condition?
   MG's skin disorder does not improve. Her health care provider says she has acne vulgaris and has prescribed benzoyl peroxide and oral tetracycline.

3. M.G. asks the nurse how to use benzoyl peroxide. What should the explanation of the method and frequency for use of benzoyl peroxide include?
4. What should be included in the patient teaching related to the use of oral tetracycline?
5. What other agents for acne might MG use? Explain their uses and side effects.
6. MG asks if she will have to remain on benzoyl peroxide and oral tetracycline for the rest of her life. What is the nurse's best response or course of action? Explain your answer.

NCLEX STUDY QUESTIONS

1. The nurse is reviewing a patient's list of medications. The patient asks, "What do kerolytic agents remove?" What is the nurse's best response?
   a. A horny layer of dermis
   b. A horny layer of epidermis
   c. Erythematous lesions
   d. Hair follicles
2. A male patient is to begin therapy with isotretinoin and asks, "What do I have to remember to do while taking this medicine?" What is the nurse's best response? (Select all that apply.)
   a. Avoid sunlight.
   b. Monitor your weight.
   c. Keep appointments for laboratory tests.
   d. Avoid pregnancy.
   e. Always take the drug with food.
3. The nurse is doing health teaching with a patient with psoriasis. Which is a nursing implication of a biologic agent such as infliximab (Remicade) for the management of psoriasis?
   a. Monitor daily weight.
   b. Monitor electrolytes.
   c. Monitor urine output.
   d. Monitor CBC.
4. A 55-year-old man is concerned about hair loss. The nurse expects that the patient's baldness may be treated with which oral drug?
   a. dexamethasone
   b. PABA
   c. mupirocin
   d. finasteride
5. The nurse reviews the patient's medication history. Based on the patient's prolonged use of topical glucocorticoids, what could the nursing assessment include? (Select all that apply.)
   a. Weight gain
   b. Thinning of the skin
   c. Erythematous lesions
   d. Purpura
   e. Urinary retention
6. A 20-year-old woman comes to the clinic for follow-up related to isotretinoin use. The nurse reviews the iPLEDGE program, which includes which important information? (Select all that apply.)
   a. One method of contraception must be used throughout treatment.
   b. A review of iPLEDGE educational materials
   c. A negative pregnancy test is required before each monthly refill.
   d. Informed consent is not required.
   e. A prescription for 60 days' worth of drug is to be given.
7. The school nurse prepares a program for junior high school students on sun safety. What is important information to include? (Select all that apply.)
   a. Sunscreen products should contain information about UVA and UVB SPF protection.
   b. UVB radiation is greatest between 10 AM and 3 PM.
   c. Clouds block radiation, so sunscreen is not needed on cloudy days.
   d. SPF should be at least 15 in sunscreen products.
   e. Sunscreen is to be applied once daily.
8. A patient is receiving etanercept (Enbrel). Which nursing interventions are appropriate for this patient? (Select all that apply.)
   a. Drug is administered by subQ route.
   b. PPD is required before start of therapy.
   c. Monitor for injection site reaction.
   d. Monitor for seizures.
   e. Monitor for heart failure.
9. The nurse is teaching the patient about the medication clobetasol (Clobex) to be started today. What information needs to be included in the teaching session? (Select all that apply.)
   a. Appropriate treatment for 6 months' duration
   b. Can apply lotion to all body parts
   c. Super–high-potency corticosteroid
   d. Maximum dose is 50 g/wk
   e. Occlusive dressing speeds healing

Answers: 1, b; 2, a, c, d; 3, d; 4, d; 5, b, d; 6, b, c; 7, a, b, d; 8, a, b, c, e; 9, c, d.

UNIT XVII

Endocrine Agents

The endocrine system consists of ductless glands that secrete hormones into the bloodstream. *Hormones* are chemical substances synthesized from amino acids and cholesterol that act on body tissues and organs and affect cellular activity. Hormones can be divided into two categories: (1) proteins or small peptides and (2) steroids. Hormones from the adrenal glands and the gonads are steroid hormones; the others are protein hormones. The *endocrine glands* include the pituitary (hypophysis), thyroid, parathyroid, adrenals, gonads, and pancreas. Figure XVII-1 illustrates the location and functions of these glands. This unit discusses the hormonal activity of the endocrine glands.

PITUITARY GLAND

The *pituitary gland,* or hypophysis, is located at the base of the brain and has two lobes, the anterior pituitary gland (adenohypophysis) and the posterior pituitary gland (neurohypophysis). The anterior pituitary gland is called the *master gland* because it secretes hormones that stimulate the release of other hormones from target glands, including the thyroid, adrenals, and gonads. The posterior pituitary gland secretes two neurohormones—antidiuretic hormone (ADH), or vasopressin, and oxytocin. Figure XVII-2 shows the anterior and posterior pituitary glands and the types of hormones secreted.

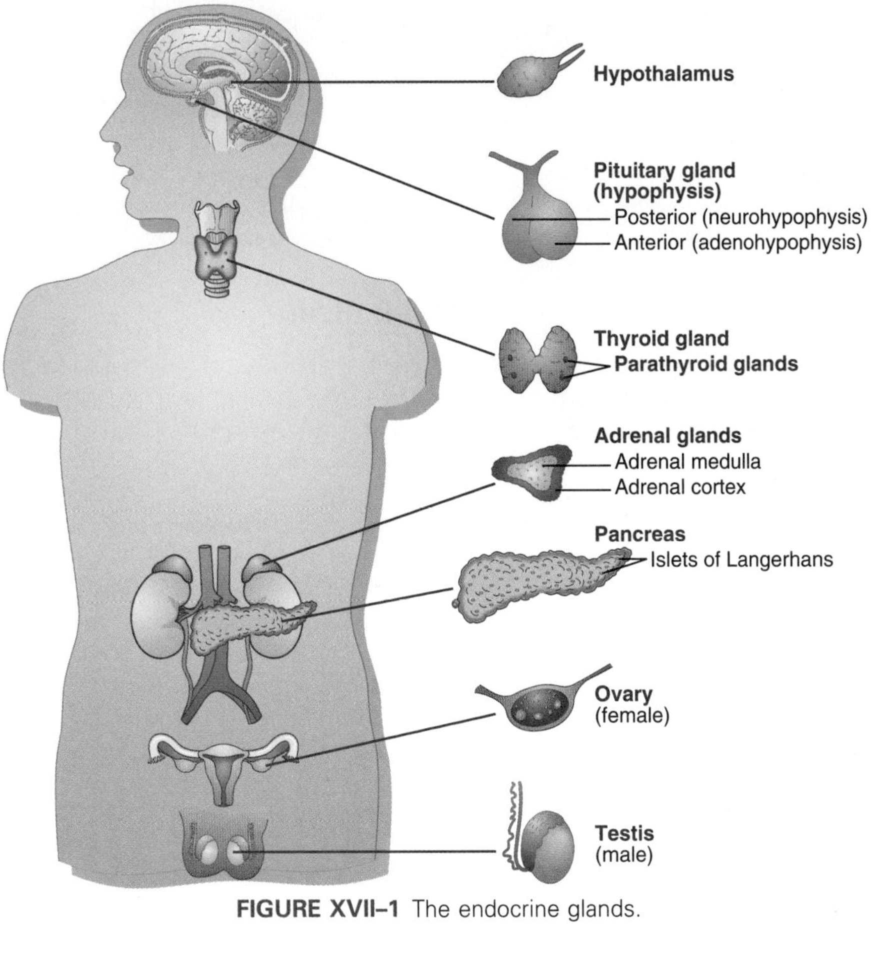

FIGURE XVII–1 The endocrine glands.

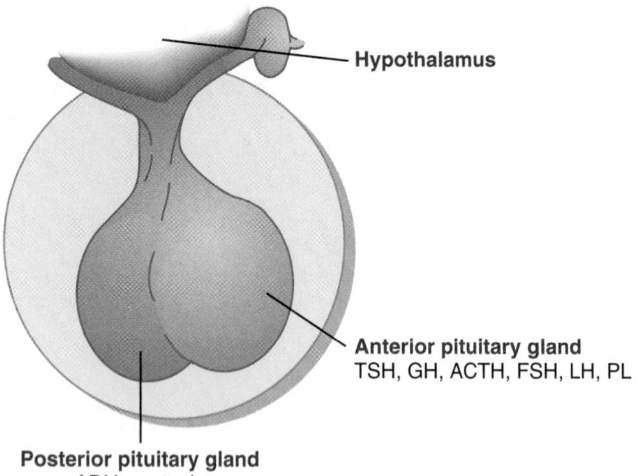

FIGURE XVII–2 The anterior and posterior pituitary glands. *ACTH,* Adrenocorticotropic hormone; *ADH,* antidiuretic hormone; *FSH,* follicle-stimulating hormone; *GH,* growth hormone; *LH,* luteinizing hormone; *PL,* prolactin; *TSH,* thyroid-stimulating hormone.

Anterior Pituitary Gland

The anterior pituitary hormones are (1) thyroid-stimulating hormone (TSH), (2) adrenocorticotropic hormone (ACTH), and (3) the gonadotropins (follicle-stimulating hormone [FSH] and luteinizing hormone [LH]). They control the synthesis and release of hormones from the thyroid, adrenals, and ovaries. Other hormones secreted from the anterior pituitary gland include growth hormone (GH), prolactin (PL), and melanocyte-stimulating hormone (MSH). The amount of each hormone secreted from the anterior pituitary gland is regulated by a negative feedback system. If excess hormone is secreted from the target gland, hormonal release from the anterior pituitary gland is suppressed. If there is a lack of hormone secretion from the target gland, there will be an increase in that particular anterior pituitary hormone.

Thyroid-Stimulating Hormone

The anterior pituitary gland secretes TSH in response to thyroid-releasing hormone (TRH) from the hypothalamus. TSH, or thyrotropic hormone, stimulates the release of thyroxine (T_4) and triiodothyronine (T_3) from the thyroid gland. Hypersecretion of TSH can cause hyperthyroidism and thyroid enlargement, and hyposecretion can cause hypothyroidism. Serum TSH levels should be checked to determine whether there is a TSH deficit or excess. TSH and T_4 levels are frequently measured to differentiate pituitary from thyroid dysfunction. A decreased T_4 level and a normal or elevated TSH level can indicate a thyroid disorder.

Adrenocorticotropic Hormone

Secretion of ACTH occurs in response to corticotropin-releasing factor (CRF) from the hypothalamus. ACTH from the anterior pituitary gland stimulates the release of glucocorticoids (cortisol), mineralocorticoids (aldosterone), and androgen from the adrenal cortex (adrenal glands). Elevated serum cortisol from the adrenal cortex inhibits ACTH and CRF release. When the cortisol level is low, ACTH secretion is stimulated, which in turn stimulates the adrenal cortex to release more cortisol. More ACTH is secreted in the morning than in the evening.

Gonadotropic Hormones

The gonadotropic hormones regulate hormone secretion from the ovaries and testes (the gonads). The anterior pituitary gland secretes the gonadotropic hormones FSH, LH, and prolactin. FSH promotes the maturation of follicles in the ovaries and initiates sperm production in the testes. LH combines with FSH in follicle maturation and estrogen production and promotes secretion of androgens from the testes. Prolactin stimulates milk formation in the glandular breast tissue after childbirth. Estrogen, progesterone, and testosterone are discussed in Chapter 56, Drugs for Women's Reproductive Health and Menopause, and Chapter 57, Drugs for Men's Health and Reproductive Disorders, respectively.

Growth Hormone

GH, or somatotropic hormone (STH), acts on all body tissues, particularly the bones and skeletal muscles. The amount of GH secreted is regulated by growth hormone–releasing hormone (GH-RH) and growth hormone–inhibiting hormone (GH-IH, or somatostatin) from the hypothalamus. Sympathomimetics, serotonin, and glucocorticoids can inhibit the secretion of GH.

Posterior Pituitary Gland

The posterior pituitary gland (neurohypophysis) secretes ADH (vasopressin) and oxytocin. Interconnecting nerve fibers between the hypothalamus and the posterior pituitary gland allow ADH and oxytocin to be synthesized in the hypothalamus and stored in the posterior pituitary gland. ADH increases the reabsorption of water from the renal tubules, returning it to the systemic circulation. Secretion of ADH is regulated by the serum osmolality (concentration of the vascular fluid). An increase in serum osmolality increases the release of ADH from the posterior pituitary gland; more water is then absorbed from the renal tubules to dilute the vascular fluid. Excess ADH can overload the vascular system. A decrease in serum osmolality decreases the release of ADH, promoting more water excretion from the renal tubules. Oxytocin stimulates contraction of the smooth muscle of the uterus; it is discussed in Chapter 54, Female Reproductive Cycle II: Labor, Delivery, and Preterm Neonatal Drugs.

THYROID GLAND

Located anterior to the trachea, the thyroid gland has two lobes that are connected by a bridge of thyroid tissue. The thyroid gland secretes two hormones, thyroxine (T_4) and triiodothyronine (T_3 liothyronine). These hormones affect nearly every tissue and organ by controlling their metabolic rate and activity. Stimulation by the thyroid hormones results in an increase in cardiac output, oxygen consumption, carbohydrate use, protein synthesis, and breakdown of fat (lipolysis). Thyroid hormones also affect body heat regulation and the menstrual cycle. Thyroid hormone levels in the blood are regulated by negative feedback. The anterior pituitary gland secretes TSH, which stimulates the thyroid gland to produce T_4 and T_3. An increased amount of circulating thyroid hormones suppresses the release of TSH, and a decreased amount increases the release of TSH by the adenohypophysis.

PARATHYROID GLANDS

There are four parathyroid glands (two pairs) that lie on the dorsal surface of the thyroid gland. The parathyroid gland secretes parathormone, or parathyroid hormone (PTH), which regulates calcium levels in the blood. A decrease in serum calcium stimulates the release of PTH. PTH increases calcium levels by (1) mobilizing calcium from the bone, (2) promoting calcium absorption from the intestine, and (3) promoting calcium reabsorption from the renal tubules. Calcitonin, a hormone produced primarily by the thyroid gland and to a lesser extent by the parathyroid and thymus glands, inhibits calcium reabsorption by bone and increases renal excretion of calcium. Calcitonin counteracts the action of PTH.

ADRENAL GLANDS

The adrenal glands, located at the top of each kidney, consist of two separate sections—the adrenal medulla (the inner section) and the adrenal cortex (the section surrounding the adrenal medulla). The adrenal medulla releases the catecholamines epinephrine and norepinephrine and is linked with the sympathetic nervous system. The adrenal cortex produces two major types of hormones (corticosteroids)—glucocorticoids and mineralocorticoids. The principal glucocorticoid is cortisol, and the principal mineralocorticoid is aldosterone. The adrenal cortex also produces small amounts of androgen, estrogen, and progestin. Glucocorticoids have a profound influence on electrolytes and the metabolism of carbohydrates, protein, and fat, and glucocorticoid deficiencies can result in serious illness and even death.

PANCREAS

The pancreas, located to the left of and behind the stomach, is both an exocrine and an endocrine gland. The exocrine section of the pancreas secretes digestive enzymes into the duodenum; these enzymes are discussed in Unit XV, Gastrointestinal Agents. The endocrine section has cell clusters called *islets of Langerhans.* The alpha islet cells produce glucagon, which breaks glycogen down to glucose in the liver, and the beta cells secrete insulin, which regulates glucose metabolism. Insulin, an antidiabetic agent, is used to control diabetes mellitus. Antidiabetic agents are discussed in Chapter 52.

DRUGS FOR ENDOCRINE DISORDERS

Chapter 51 (Endocrine Drugs: Pituitary, Thyroid, Parathyroid, and Adrenal Disorders) and Chapter 52 (Antidiabetics) discuss the drugs used to diagnose and treat endocrine disorders. Chapter 51 discusses the agents for disorders involving the pituitary gland, thyroid gland, parathyroid gland, adrenal gland, and ADH. The parenteral and oral antidiabetic drugs (hypoglycemic drugs) are described in Chapter 52.

CHAPTER

51

Endocrine Drugs: Pituitary, Thyroid, Parathyroid, and Adrenal Disorders

evolve WEBSITE

http://evolve.elsevier.com/KeeHayes/pharmacology/

- Animations
- Content Updates
- Key Points
- Review Questions for the NCLEX® Examination
- References from the Textbook
- Unfolding Case Studies

OBJECTIVES

- Compare the hormones secreted from the adenohypophysis and the neurohypophysis.
- Differentiate the actions and uses of the pituitary hormones: thyroxine (T_4), triiodothyronine (T_3), parathyroid hormone (PTH), and glucocorticoids.
- Differentiate the side effects of thyroxine (T_4) and triiodothyronine (T_3).
- Apply the nursing process, including patient teaching, of drug therapy related to hormonal replacement or hormonal inhibition for the pituitary, thyroid, parathyroid, and adrenal glands.

OUTLINE

KEY TERMS

acromegaly, p. 743
Addison's disease, p. 751
adenohypophysis, p. 743
adrenal glands, p. 751
adrenocorticotropic hormone, p. 743
antidiuretic hormone, p. 745
corticosteroids, p. 751
cretinism, p. 747
Cushing's syndrome, p. 751
diabetes insipidus, p. 745
endocrine, p. 743
gigantism, p. 743
glucocorticoids, p. 752
Graves' disease, p. 748
hyperthyroidism, p. 748
hypophysis, p. 743
hypothyroidism, p. 747
mineralocorticoids, p. 755
myxedema, p. 747
neurohypophysis, p. 745
parathyroid hormone, p. 749
thyroid-stimulating hormone, p. 743
thyrotoxicosis, p. 748
thyroxine, p. 746
triiodothyronine, p. 746

This chapter describes drugs used for hormonal replacement and for inhibition of hormonal secretion from the pituitary, thyroid, parathyroid, and adrenal glands. Before reading Chapters 51 and 52, review the introduction to Unit XVII, which describes the locations of the endocrine glands and the hormones they secrete. Knowledge of the various **endocrine** (ductless glands that produce internal secretions that flow to all parts of the body) hormones and their functions facilitates an understanding of the drugs that act on the endocrine glands.

PITUITARY GLAND

Anterior Lobe

The pituitary gland, or **hypophysis,** has an anterior and a posterior lobe. The anterior pituitary gland, called the **adenohypophysis,** secretes the following hormones that target glands and tissues:

- Growth hormone (GH), which stimulates growth in tissue and bone
- Thyroid-stimulating hormone (TSH), which acts on the thyroid gland
- Adrenocorticotropic hormone (ACTH), which stimulates the adrenal gland
- Gonadotropins (follicle-stimulating hormone [FSH] and luteinizing hormone [LH]), which affect the ovaries.

Drugs with adenohypophyseal properties used to stimulate or inhibit glandular activity are discussed according to their therapeutic use. The negative feedback system that controls the amount of hormonal secretion from the pituitary gland and the target gland is discussed in the introduction to Unit XVII.

Growth Hormone

Two hypothalamic hormones regulate GH: (1) growth hormone–releasing hormone (GH-RH) and (2) growth hormone–inhibiting hormone (GH-IH; somatostatin). Growth hormone does not have a specific target gland. It affects body tissues and bone; GH replacement stimulates linear growth when there is a GH deficiency. Growth hormone drugs cannot be given orally, because they are inactivated by gastrointestinal enzymes. Subcutaneous (subQ) or intramuscular (IM) administration of GH is necessary.

If a child's height is well below the standard for a specified age, GH deficiency may be diagnosed, and dwarfism can result. Growth hormone replacement is very expensive; therefore, various tests are performed to determine if this therapy is essential. Because GH acts on newly forming bone, it must be administered before the epiphyses are fused. Administration of GH over several years can increase height by a foot. Prolonged GH therapy can antagonize insulin secretion and eventually cause diabetes mellitus. Athletes should be advised not to take GH to build muscle and physique because of its effects on blood sugar and other side effects.

Drug Therapy: Growth Hormone Deficiency

Somatropin (Genotropin) is a growth hormone used to treat growth failure in children because of pituitary GH deficiency. Somatropin is a product that has the identical amino acid sequence as human growth hormone. Somatropin is contraindicated in pediatric patients who have growth deficiency due to Prader-Willi syndrome and are severely obese or who have severe respiratory impairment, because fatalities associated with these risk factors have been reported.

Drug Therapy: Growth Hormone Excess

Gigantism (excessive growth during childhood) and **acromegaly** (excessive growth after puberty) can occur with GH hypersecretion and are frequently caused by a pituitary tumor. If the tumor cannot be destroyed by radiation, the prolactin-release inhibitor bromocriptine can inhibit the release of GH from the pituitary gland.

Octreotide (Sandostatin) is a potent synthetic somatostatin used to suppress GH release. It can be used alone or with surgery or radiation. This drug is expensive. GI side effects are common. This drug can also be used for severe diarrhea resulting from carcinoid tumors.

Table 51-1 lists the drugs used to replace or inhibit GH and their dosages, uses, and considerations.

Thyroid-Stimulating Hormone

The adenohypophysis secretes **thyroid-stimulating hormone** (TSH) in response to thyroid-releasing hormone (TRH) from the hypothalamus, and TSH stimulates the thyroid gland to release thyroxine (T_4) and triiodothyronine (T_3, or liothyronine). Excess TSH secretion can cause hyperthyroidism, and a TSH deficit can cause hypothyroidism. Hypothyroidism may be caused by a thyroid gland disorder (primary cause) or a decrease in TSH secretion (secondary cause). Thyrotropin (Thytropar), a purified extract of TSH, is used as a diagnostic agent to differentiate between primary and secondary hypothyroidism (see Table 51-1).

Adrenocorticotropic Hormone

The hypothalamus releases corticotropin-releasing factor (CRF), which stimulates the pituitary corticotrophs to secrete **adrenocorticotropic hormone** (ACTH). ACTH secretion stimulates the release of glucocorticoids (cortisol), mineralocorticoids (aldosterone), and androgen from the adrenal cortex. Usually ACTH and cortisol secretions follow a diurnal rhythm in which the ACTH and cortisol secretion is higher in the early morning and then decreases throughout the day. Stresses such as surgery, sepsis, and trauma override the diurnal rhythm, causing an increase in secretions of ACTH and cortisol.

The ACTH drug corticotropin (Acthar) is used to diagnose adrenal gland disorders, to treat adrenal gland insufficiency, and as an antiinflammatory drug in the treatment of allergic response. Administration of ACTH intravenously (IV) should increase the serum cortisol level in 30 to 60 minutes if the adrenal gland is functioning. If steroid

TABLE 51-1 ANTERIOR AND POSTERIOR PITUITARY HORMONES

GENERIC (BRAND)	ROUTE AND DOSAGE	USES AND CONSIDERATIONS
Anterior Lobe		
Growth Hormone (GH)		
somatropin (Nutropin, Genotropin)	C: subQ/IM: Nutropin: 0.006 mg/kg/d; Genotropin: 0.04 mg/kg in 6-7 equal daily doses; *max:* 0.08 mg/kg/wk	For growth hormone deficiency. Promotes bone growth at epiphyseal plates of long bones. Pregnancy category: Nutropin: C; Genotropin: B; PB: 20%; $t\frac{1}{2}$: 15-60 min
Growth Hormone Suppressant Drugs		
bromocriptine mesylate (Parlodel)	A: PO: 1.25-2.5 mg/d for 3 d; range: 10-30 mg/d; *max:* 100 mg/d	For acromegaly. Also used with pituitary radiation or surgery to decrease GH levels. Decreases lactation and prolactinoma. Pregnancy category: B; PB: 93%; $t\frac{1}{2}$: 3-6 h
octreotide acetate (Sandostatin)	A: subQ: 50-100 mcg t.i.d.	For acromegaly. To treat severe diarrhea associated with metastatic carcinoid and other tumors. Pregnancy category: B; PB: 65%; $t\frac{1}{2}$: 1.5 h
lanreotide acetate (Somatuline Depot)	A: subQ: Initially 90 mg q4wk for 3 mo; then 60-120 mg q4wk for 4 mo	To suppress GH. Monitor glucose levels. Pregnancy category: C; PB: 69%-78%; $t\frac{1}{2}$: 23-30 d
Thyroid-Stimulating Hormone (TSH)		
thyrotropin (Thyrogen)	Thyroid cancer: A: IM: 0.9 mg into gluteus maximus, repeat in 24 h for 2 doses; *max:* 0.9 mg/d	For thyroid cancer. . Radioiodine study follows last injection. Pregnancy category: C; PB: UK; $t\frac{1}{2}$: 15-35 h
Adrenocorticotropic Hormone (ACTH)		
corticotropin (H.P. Acthar gel)	See Prototype Drug Chart 51-1.	
cosyntropin (Cortrosyn)	A/C: >2 y: IM/IV: 0.25 mg over 2 min or slow infusion over 6 h C: <2 y: IM/IV: 0.125 mg slow infusion over 6 h	For diagnostic testing to differentiate between pituitary and adrenal cause of adrenal insufficiency. Obtain plasma cortisol level before and 30 min after administration. Pregnancy category: C; PB: UK; $t\frac{1}{2}$: 15 min
Posterior Lobe		
Antidiuretic Hormone (ADH)		
desmopressin acetate (DDAVP, Stimate)	DDAVP: A: Intranasal: 0.1-0.4 mL/d in divided doses Stimate: A: subQ/IV: 0.2-0.4 mcg A/C: >11 mo: intranasal: 150 mcg/kg	For DI, hemophilia A, and von Willebrand disease. Can have a long duration of action (5-21 h). Pregnancy category: B; PB: UK; $t\frac{1}{2}$: 1.5-2.5 h
vasopressin (aqueous) (Pitressin)	Diabetes insipidus: A: subQ/IM: 5-10 units, b.i.d./q.i.d. C: subQ/IM: 2.5-10 units, b.i.d./q.i.d.	For DI. For relief of intestinal distention. Decreases GI bleeding from esophageal varices. Can also be given intranasally. Promotes reabsorption of water from renal tubules. Duration of action is 2-8 h. Pregnancy category: C; PB: UK; $t\frac{1}{2}$: 15 min
demeclocycline (Declomycin)	A: PO: 600 mg/d in 3-4 divided doses	For treatment of SIADH. Inhibits ADH-induced water reabsorption in renal distal tubules. Closely monitor sodium levels. Pregnancy category: C; PB: 99%; $t\frac{1}{2}$: 12 h
conivaptan (Vaprisol)	A: IV: LD 20 mg over 30 min; maint: 20 mg continuous IV over 24 h; then 20 mg/d for 1-3 d; *max:* 4 days therapy	For hypervolemic hyponatremia associated with SIADH. Closely monitor sodium levels. Pregnancy category: C; PB: 99%; $t\frac{1}{2}$: 5 h
tolvaptan (Samsca)	A: PO: Initially 15 mg/d; then 15-30 mg/d; *max:* 60 mg/d	For hyponatremia associated with SIADH. Closely monitor sodium levels. Pregnancy category: C; PB: 99%; $t\frac{1}{2}$: 12 h

A, Adult; *ADH,* antidiuretic hormone; *b.i.d.,* twice a day; *C,* child; *d,* day; *DI,* diabetes insipidus; *GI,* gastrointestinal; *h,* hour; *IM,* intramuscular; *IV,* intravenous; *LD,* loading dose; *min,* minute; *NSS,* normal saline solution; *PB,* protein-binding; *PO,* by mouth; *q.i.d.,* four times a day; *subQ,* subcutaneous; $t\frac{1}{2}$, half-life; *t.i.d.,* three times a day; *UK,* unknown; *wk,* week; *y,* year; >, greater than; <, less than.

deficiency is caused by pituitary insufficiency, ACTH should eventually stimulate cortisol production. ACTH decreases the symptoms of multiple sclerosis during its exacerbation phase. Prototype Drug Chart 51-1 lists the pharmacologic data for repository corticotropin.

Pharmacokinetics Corticotropin stimulates the adrenal gland to secrete corticosteroids. The aqueous and gel preparations are well absorbed into the circulation. Zinc is added to some formulations to slow the absorption rate. A portion of the drug is bound to protein; however, the percentage is unknown. The half-life of the drug is 15 to 20 minutes. It is excreted in the urine.

PROTOTYPE DRUG CHART 51-1

Repository Corticotropin

Drug Class Pituitary adrenocorticotropic hormone Trade Name: H.P. Acthar Gel Pregnancy Category: C	**Dosage** Inflammation: A/C: subQ/IM: 40-80 units, q24-72h; *max:* 80 units/d Acute multiple sclerosis (MS): A: subQ/IM: 80-120 units/d for 2-3 wk; *max:* 120 units/d
Contraindications Severe fungal infection, adrenal insufficiency, Cushing's syndrome, HF, peptic ulcer, osterporosis, scleroderma, ocular herpes simplex, recent surgery Caution: Hepatic disease, psychiatric disorders, cardiac disease, diabetes mellitus, renal impairment, hypertension, hypothyroidism, myasthenia gravis	**Drug-Lab-Food Interactions** Drug: Increase potential for ulcer formation and hypoprothrombinemia with aspirin and NSAIDs; may increase potassium loss with thiazide and loop diuretics; barbiturates, phenytoin decrease corticotropin effects; estrogens increase corticotropin effects
Pharmacokinetics Absorption: IM: Well absorbed Distribution: PB: UK Metabolism: t½: 15-20 min Excretion: In urine	**Pharmacodynamics** IM: Onset: <6 h Peak: 6-18 h Duration: 12-24 h IV: Onset: UK Peak: 1 h Duration: UK
Therapeutic Effects/Uses To diagnose adrenocortical disorders; acts as antiinflammatory agent; to treat acute MS Mode of Action: Stimulates adrenal cortex to secrete cortisol	
Side Effects Nausea, vomiting, diarrhea, constipation, mood swing (euphoria to depression), petechiae, water and sodium retention, hypokalemia, hypocalcemia, acne	**Adverse Reactions** Edema, ecchymosis, osteoporosis, muscle atrophy, growth retardation, decreased wound healing, cataracts, glaucoma, seizures, menstrual irregularities, hypertension, Life-threatening: Ulcer perforation, pancreatitis

A, Adult; *HF,* heart failure; *d,* day; *h,* hour; *IM,* intramuscular; *IV,* intravenous; *MS,* multiple sclerosis; *q.i.d.,* four times a day; *subQ,* subcutaneous; *PB,* protein-binding; *t ½,* half-life; *UK,* unknown; *wk,* week; <, less than.

Pharmacodynamics Corticotropin suppresses the inflammatory and immune responses. It is also prescribed to treat adrenal insufficiency secondary to inadequate corticotropin secretion. The drug is administered IM and IV. Its onset of action, peak concentration time, and duration of action are prolonged when it is injected IM. The IV preparation is in aqueous form; therefore its actions are faster than those of the gel and zinc-additive preparations.

Drug Interactions. Corticotropin has numerous drug interactions. Diuretics and anti-*Pseudomonas* penicillins such as piperacillin can decrease the serum potassium level (hypokalemia). If the patient is taking a digitalis preparation and hypokalemia is present, digitalis toxicity can result. Phenytoin, rifampin, and barbiturates increase the metabolic rate, which can decrease the effect of the ACTH drug. Persons with diabetes may need increased insulin and oral antidiabetic (hypoglycemic) drugs because ACTH stimulates cortisol secretion, which increases the blood sugar level.

Posterior Lobe

The posterior pituitary gland, known as the **neurohypophysis,** secretes **antidiuretic hormone (ADH)** (vasopressin) and oxytocin. (Oxytocin is discussed in Chapter 54.)

ADH promotes water reabsorption from the renal tubules to maintain water balance in the body fluids. When there is a deficiency of ADH, large amounts of water are excreted by the kidneys. This condition, called **diabetes insipidus (DI),** can lead to severe fluid volume deficit and electrolyte imbalances. Head injury and brain tumors resulting in trauma to the hypothalamus and pituitary gland can also cause DI. Fluid and electrolyte balance must be closely monitored in these patients, and ADH replacement may be needed. The ADH preparations vasopressin (Pitressin) and desmopressin acetate (DDAVP) can be administered intranasally or by injection.

Nursing Process
Patient-Centered Collaborative Care

Pituitary Hormones

Assessment
- Obtain baseline vital signs for future comparison. Report abnormal results.
- Determine patient's urinary output and weight.

- Assess patient for an infectious process. Corticotropin can suppress signs and symptoms of infection.
- Note patient's physical growth. Compare child's growth with reported standards. Report findings.

Nursing Diagnoses
- Ineffective health maintenance related to lack of ability to maintain drug regimen
- Delayed growth and development related to deficient stimulation of growth hormone
- Deficient knowledge related to inexperience with medication regimen

Planning
- Patient will be free from pituitary disorder with appropriate drug regimen.

Nursing Interventions
Antidiuretic Hormone (ADH)
- Monitor vital signs. Increased heart rate and decreased systolic pressure can indicate fluid volume loss resulting from decreased ADH production. With less ADH secretion, more water is excreted, decreasing vascular fluid (hypovolemia).
- Record urinary output. Increased output can indicate fluid loss caused by a decrease in ADH.

Repository Corticotropin
- Avoid administering corticotropin to patients with adrenocortical hyperfunction. Corticotropin stimulates the release of cortisol from the adrenal glands.
- Monitor the growth and development of a child receiving corticotropin.
- Observe patient's weight. Check for edema if weight gain occurs. A side effect of repository corticotropin is sodium and water retention.
- Watch carefully for adverse effects when corticotropin is discontinued. Dose should be tapered and not stopped abruptly, because adrenal hypofunction may result.
- Check laboratory findings, especially electrolyte levels. Electrolyte replacement may be necessary.

Growth Hormone (GH)
- Monitor blood sugar and electrolyte levels in patients receiving GH. Hyperglycemia can occur with high doses.

Patient Teaching
Adrenocorticotropic Hormone (ACTH)
- Advise patient to adhere to drug regimen. Discontinuation of certain drugs, such as corticotropin, can cause hypofunction of gland being stimulated.
- Direct patient to decrease salt intake to decrease or avoid edema. Potassium supplement may be needed.
- Teach patient to report side effects such as muscle weakness, edema, petechiae, ecchymosis, decrease in growth, decreased wound healing, and menstrual irregularities.

Growth Hormone (GH)
- Advise athletes not to take GH because of side effects. GH can be effective for children whose height is markedly below expected norm for their age. Because GH acts on newly forming bone, administer before epiphyses are fused.
- Inform patient with diabetes to closely monitor blood sugar levels. Insulin regulation may be necessary.
- Suggest that patient or family monitor patient's growth rate.

Cultural Considerations
- Individuals in some cultural groups may misunderstand purpose and use of GH. Health care provider needs to emphasize that these are not drugs for building muscles and that they can cause many serious side effects, such as diabetes mellitus, when abused.

Evaluation
- Evaluate effectiveness of drug therapy.

When there is excess secretion of ADH from the posterior pituitary gland, the most common cause is small cell carcinoma of the lung. Medications, other malignancies, and stressors (e.g., pain, infection, anxiety, trauma) may also be causative factors. These conditions lead to an excessive amount of water retention expanding the intracellular volume. This increased fluid volume causes enhanced glomerular filtration and decreased tubular sodium reabsorption. Natriuresis (excretion of urinary sodium) results, leading to hyponatremia.

SIADH can be treated by fluid restriction, demeclocycline, conivaptan, and tolvaptan. Serum sodium levels must be monitored closely. Table 51-1 lists the drugs used for pituitary disorders and their dosages, uses, and considerations.

THYROID GLAND

Thyroxine (T_4) and **triiodothyronine** (T_3) are secreted by the thyroid gland. The functions of T_4 and T_3 are to regulate protein synthesis and enzyme activity and to stimulate mitochondrial oxidation. Approximately 20% of circulating T_3 is secreted from the thyroid gland, and 80% of T_3 comes from the degradation of about 40% of T_4, which occurs in the periphery. T_4 and T_3 are carried in the blood by thyroxine-binding globulin (TBG) and albumin, which protect the hormones from being degraded. T_3 is more potent than T_4, and only unbound free T_3 and T_4 are active and produce a hormonal response.

Feedback mechanisms regulate T_4 and T_3 secretion from the thyroid gland. The hypothalamus releases thyrotropin-releasing hormone (TRH), which stimulates the release of TSH from the pituitary gland. TSH stimulates the synthesis and release of T_4 and T_3 from the thyroid gland. Excess free T_4 and T_3 inhibit the hypothalamus-pituitary-thyroid (HPT) axis, which results in decreased TRH and TSH secretion. Likewise, too low an amount of T_4 and T_3 increases the function of the HPT axis.

For thyroid deficiency (hypothyroidism), synthetic T_4 and T_3 may be prescribed, either alone or in combination. When the thyroid gland secretes an overabundance of thyroid hormones (hyperthyroidism), antithyroid drugs are usually indicated.

Hypothyroidism

Hypothyroidism, a decrease in thyroid hormone secretion, can have either a primary cause (thyroid gland disorder) or a secondary cause (lack of TSH secretion). Primary hypothyroidism occurs more frequently. Decreased T_4 and elevated TSH levels indicate primary hypothyroidism, the causes of which are acute or chronic inflammation of the thyroid gland, radioiodine therapy, excess intake of antithyroid drugs, and surgery. **Myxedema** is severe hypothyroidism in the adult; symptoms include lethargy, apathy, memory impairment, emotional changes, slow speech, deep coarse voice, edema of the eyelids and face, dry skin, cold intolerance, slow pulse, constipation, weight gain, and abnormal menses. In children, hypothyroidism can have a congenital (**cretinism**) or prepubertal (juvenile hypothyroidism) onset. Drugs containing T_4 and T_3, alone or in combination, are used to treat hypothyroidism.

Drug Therapy: Hypothyroidism

Levothyroxine sodium (Synthroid) is the drug of choice for replacement therapy for the treatment of hypothyroidism. It increases the levels of T_3 and T_4. Levothyroxine is also used to treat simple goiter and chronic lymphocytic (Hashimoto) thyroiditis.

Liothyronine (Cytomel) is a synthetic T_3 that has a short half-life and duration of action; it is not recommended for maintenance therapy. Liothyronine is better absorbed from the GI tract than levothyroxine, and because of its rapid onset of action and short half-life, it is frequently used as initial therapy for treating myxedema.

Liotrix (Thyrolar) is a mixture of levothyroxine sodium and liothyronine sodium in a 4 : 1 ratio. For treating hypothyroidism, there is no significant advantage to using liotrix over levothyroxine sodium alone, because levothyroxine converts T_4 to T_3 in the peripheral tissues.

Prototype Drug Chart 51-2 lists the pharmacologic data for levothyroxine.

PROTOTYPE DRUG CHART 51-2

Levothyroxine Sodium

Drug Class Thyroid hormone Trade Names: T_4, Synthroid Pregnancy Category: A	**Dosage** A: PO: Initially: 25-50 mcg/d; maint: 50-200 mcg/d; A: IV: 50-100 mcg/d C: >12 y: PO: 2-3 mcg/kg/d
Contraindications Thyrotoxicosis, myocardial infarction, severe renal disease, adrenal insufficiency Caution: Cardiovascular disease, hypertension, angina pectoris, diabetes mellitus, osteoporosis	**Drug-Lab-Food Interactions** Drug: Increase cardiac insufficiency with epinephrine; increase effects of anticoagulants, tricyclic antidepressants, vasopressors, decongestants; decrease effects of antidiabetics (oral and insulin), digitalis products; decrease absorption with estrogens, antacids, cholestyramine, colestipol; increase risk of digitalis toxicity Food: Should be taken on an empty stomach, t½-1 h before eating
Pharmacokinetics Absorption: PO: 50%-75% Distribution: PB: 99% Metabolism: t½: 6-7 days Excretion: In bile and feces	**Pharmacodynamics** PO: Onset: UK Peak: 24 h-1 wk Duration: 1-3 wk IV: Onset: 6-8 h Peak: 24-48 h Duration: UK
Therapeutic Effects/Uses To treat hypothyroidism, myxedema, and cretinism Mode of Action: Increases metabolic rate, oxygen consumption, and body growth	
Side Effects Nausea, vomiting, anorexia, diarrhea, cramps, tremors, nervousness, irritability, insomnia, headache, weight loss, diaphoresis, amenorrhea	**Adverse Reactions** Tachycardia, hypertension, palpitations, osteoporosis, seizures Life-threatening: Thyroid crisis, angina pectoris, cardiac dysrhythmias (atrial fibrillation), cardiovascular collapse

A, Adult; *C,* child; *d,* day; *h,* hour; *IV,* intravenous; *maint,* maintenance; *PB,* protein-binding; *PO,* by mouth; *t½,* half-life; *UK,* unknown; *wk,* week; *y,* year; >, greater than.

Pharmacokinetics Levothyroxine (T_4) is a synthetic thyroid hormone preparation. The GI mucosa absorbs 50% to 75% of levothyroxine. It is highly protein-bound, and when administered with other highly protein-bound drugs like oral anticoagulants, side effects can result. The half-life of levothyroxine is longer than that of liothyronine. Levothyroxine is excreted in the bile and feces.

Pharmacodynamics Levothyroxine increases metabolic rate, cardiac output, protein synthesis, and glycogen use. The peak concentration time and duration of action are much longer with levothyroxine than with liothyronine. Liotrix is a combination of T_4 and T_3 with a greater concentration of T_4.

Drug Interactions. Many drug interactions are associated with T_4 and T_3 drugs. Thyroid preparations increase the effect of oral anticoagulants because of drug displacement from the protein-binding sites. When these thyroid replacement drugs are taken with an adrenergic agent (e.g., decongestant or vasopressor), the cardiac and central nervous system (CNS) actions are increased. Levothyroxine and liothyronine can decrease the effectiveness of digitalis preparations. Estrogen can increase the effect of liothyronine. Insulin and oral antidiabetic drug dosages may need to be increased.

Table 51-2 lists the natural and synthetic thyroid preparations and their dosages, uses, and considerations.

Hyperthyroidism

Hyperthyroidism is an increase in circulating T_4 and T_3 levels, which usually results from an overactive thyroid gland or excessive output of thyroid hormones from one or more thyroid nodules. Hyperthyroidism may be mild with few symptoms or severe, as in thyroid storm in which death may occur from vascular collapse. **Graves' disease,** or **thyrotoxicosis,** is the most common type of hyperthyroidism caused by hyperfunction of the thyroid gland. It is characterized by a rapid pulse *(tachycardia),* palpitations, excessive perspiration, heat intolerance, nervousness, irritability, exophthalmos (bulging eyes), and weight loss.

Hyperthyroidism can be treated by surgical removal of a portion of the thyroid gland (subtotal thyroidectomy), radioactive iodine therapy, or antithyroid drugs, which inhibit either synthesis or release of thyroid hormone. Any of these treatments can cause hypothyroidism. Propranolol (Inderal) can control cardiac symptoms like palpitations and tachycardia that result from hyperthyroidism. It does not lower T_4 and T_3.

TABLE 51-2 THYROID HORMONE: REPLACEMENTS AND ANTITHYROID DRUGS

GENERIC (BRAND)	ROUTE AND DOSAGE	USES AND CONSIDERATIONS
Thyroid Replacements: Hypothyroidism		
levothyroxine sodium (Synthroid)	See Prototype Drug Chart 51-2.	
liothyronine sodium (Cytomel)	A: PO: Initially: 5-25 mcg/d; maint: 25-75 mcg/d C: PO: Initially: 5 mcg/d; >3 y: 25-75 mcg/d	For hypothyroidism. Synthetic T_3 drug. Faster acting than other thyroid drugs. Effects seen in 24-72 h. Cardiac side effects. Pregnancy category: A; PB: 99%; t½: 2.5 d
liotrix (Thyrolar)	A/C: PO: Initially: 50-100 mcg/d	For hypothyroidism. Synthetic T_4 and T_3 drug; 4:1 ratio. Common side effects include irritability, nervousness, insomnia, tachycardia, and weight loss. Pregnancy category: A; PB: 99%; t½: <7 d
thyroid (Armour, Thyrotab)	A: PO: Initially: 15-30 mg/d; maint: 60-120 mg/d C: >6 mo: PO: maint: 30-90 mg/d	For hypothyroidism to reduce goiter size. Natural form obtained from animals. T_4 and T_3: 4:1 ratio. Common side effects include irritability, nervousness, insomnia, tachycardia, and weight loss. Pregnancy category: A; PB: 99%; t½: <7 d (T_3: 1-2 h; T_4: 6-7 d)
Antithyroid Drugs: Hyperthyroidism		
Thioamides		
methimazole (Tapazole)	A: PO: 15-60 mg/d in 1-3 divided doses C: PO: 0.2-0.4 mg/kg/d in 1-3 divided doses	For hyperthyroidism. Inhibits thyroid hormone synthesis. Onset of action: 1 wk for effect. Rash, urticaria, headache, and GI upset may occur. Pregnancy category: D; PB: 0%; t½: 5-9 h
propylthiouracil (PTU)	A: PO: Initially 300 mg/d divided q8h; then 100-150 mg/d divided q8h C: >6 y: PO: 50-150 mg/d in divided doses	For hyperthyroidism, Graves' disease. Inhibits conversion of T_4 and T_3. May be used before surgery or radioactive iodine treatment and for palliative control of toxic goiter. May cause severe liver damage, liver failure, and death. Pregnancy category: D; PB: 80%; t½: 1-5 h
Iodine		
potassium iodide (SSKI)	A/C: PO: 250 mg t.i.d. for 10-14 d before surgery	For hyperthyroidism. To reduce size and vascularity of thyroid gland. Dilute drug and administer after meals; sip through straw to avoid discoloration of teeth. Maximum effect after 10-15 days. Pregnancy category: D; PB: UK; t½: UK

A, Adult; *C,* child; *d,* day; *GI,* gastrointestinal; *h,* hour; *maint,* maintenance; *PB,* protein-binding; *p.c.,* after meals; *PO,* by mouth; *t½,* half-life; *T_4,* thyroxine; *T_3,* triiodothyronine; *t.i.d.,* three times a day; *UK,* unknown; *wk,* week; *y,* year; >, greater than; <, less than.

Drug Therapy: Hyperthyroidism

The purpose of antithyroid drugs is to reduce the excessive secretion of thyroid hormones (T_4 and T_3) by inhibiting thyroid secretion. The use of surgery (subtotal thyroidectomy) and radioiodine therapy frequently leads to hypothyroidism. Thiourea derivatives (thioamides) are the drugs of choice used to decrease thyroid hormone production. This drug group interferes with synthesis of thyroid hormone. Thiourea derivatives do not destroy thyroid tissue, but rather block thyroid hormone action.

Propylthiouracil (PTU) and methimazole (Tapazole) are effective thioamide antithyroid drugs. They are useful for treating thyrotoxic crisis and in preparation for subtotal thyroidectomy. Methimazole does not inhibit peripheral conversion of T_4 to T_3 as does PTU; however, it is 10 times more potent and it has a longer half-life than PTU. Prolonged use of thioamides may cause goiter because of increased TSH secretion and inhibited T_4 and T_3 synthesis. Minimal doses of thioamides should be given when indicated to avoid goiter formation.

Strong iodide preparations such as potassium iodide have been used to suppress thyroid function for patients who have undergone subtotal thyroidectomy as a result of Graves' disease. Table 51-2 lists the antithyroid drugs used to treat hyperthyroidism and their dosages, uses, and considerations.

Drug Interactions. Antithyroid drugs interact with many other drugs. When used with oral anticoagulants (e.g., warfarin [Coumadin]), they can cause an increase in the anticoagulation effect. In addition, thyroid drugs decrease the effect of insulin and oral antidiabetics; digoxin and lithium increase the action of thyroid drugs; and phenytoin (Dilantin) increases serum T_3 level.

PARATHYROID GLANDS

The parathyroid glands secrete **parathyroid hormone** (PTH), which regulates calcium levels in the blood. A decrease in serum calcium stimulates the release of PTH. Calcitonin decreases serum calcium levels by promoting renal excretion of calcium. The functions of PTH and calcitonin are discussed in the introduction to Unit XVII.

Hypoparathyroidism

Parathyroid hormone agents treat hypoparathyroidism. Hypocalcemia (serum calcium deficit) can be caused by PTH deficiency, vitamin D deficiency, renal impairment, or diuretic therapy, and PTH replacement helps correct the calcium deficit. The action of PTH is to promote calcium absorption from the GI tract, promote reabsorption of calcium from the renal tubules, and activate vitamin D.

Calcitriol

Calcitriol is a vitamin D analogue that promotes calcium absorption from the GI tract and secretion of calcium from bone to the bloodstream. Prototype Drug Chart 51-3 lists the pharmacologic data for calcitriol.

PROTOTYPE DRUG CHART 51-3

Calcitriol

Drug Class Vitamin D analogue Trade Name: Rocaltrol Pregnancy Category: C	**Dosage** A/C: >6 y: PO: 0.25 mcg/d
Contraindications Hypersensitivity, hypercalcemia, hypervitaminosis D, malabsorption syndrome Caution: Cardiovascular disease, renal calculi, renal failure, hyperphosphatemia, dehydration, excess sunlight exposure	**Drug-Lab-Food Interactions** Drug: Increase cardiac dysrhythmias with digoxin, verapamil; decrease calcitriol absorption with cholestyramine Lab: Increase serum calcium with thiazide diuretics, calcium supplements
Pharmacokinetics Absorption: PO: Well absorbed Distribution: PB: UK; crosses placenta Metabolism: t½: 3-8 h Excretion: Mostly in feces	**Pharmacodynamics** PO: Onset: 2-6 h Peak: 10-12 h Duration: 3-5 d
Therapeutic Effects/Uses To treat hypoparathyroidism and manage hypocalcemia in chronic renal failure Mode of Action: Enhances calcium deposits in bones	
Side Effects Anorexia, nausea, vomiting, diarrhea, cramps, drowsiness, headache, dizziness, vertigo, metallic taste, lethargy, photophobia	**Adverse Reactions** Hypercalciuria, hypercalcemia, hyperphosphatemia, hematuria

A, Adult; *d,* day; *h,* hour; *PB,* protein binding; *PO,* by mouth; *t½,* half-life; *UK,* unknown.

Pharmacokinetics Calcitriol is readily absorbed from the GI tract. Its half-life is moderate (3 to 8 hours). Most of the drug is excreted in feces.

Pharmacodynamics Calcitriol is given for the management of hypocalcemia. It increases serum calcium levels by promoting calcium absorption from the intestines and renal tubules. Calcitriol has a long onset of action, peak action, and duration of action.

Nursing Process
Patient-Centered Collaborative Care

Thyroid Hormone: Replacement and Antithyroid Drugs

Assessment

- Determine baseline vital signs for future comparison. Report abnormal results.
- Check serum T_3, T_4, and TSH levels. Report abnormal results.

Thyroid Replacement

- Obtain history of drugs patient currently takes. Be aware that thyroid drugs enhance action of oral anticoagulants, sympathomimetics, and antidepressants and decrease action of insulin, oral hypoglycemics, and digitalis preparations. Phenytoin and aspirin can enhance action of thyroid hormone.

Antithyroid Drugs

- Assess for signs and symptoms of thyroid crisis (thyroid storm), including tachycardia, cardiac dysrhythmias, fever, heart failure, flushed skin, apathy, confusion, behavioral changes, and later hypotension and vascular collapse. Thyroid crisis can result from a thyroidectomy (excess thyroid hormones released), abrupt withdrawal of antithyroid drug, excess ingestion of thyroid hormone, or failure to give antithyroid medication before thyroid surgery.

Nursing Diagnoses

- Ineffective health maintenance related to inability to maintain drug regimen
- Ineffective peripheral tissue perfusion related to hyposecretion of thyroid hormone
- Activity intolerance related to generalized weakness
- Deficient knowledge related to inexperience with thyroid medication regimen

Planning

- Patient's signs and symptoms of hypothyroidism will be alleviated within 2 to 4 weeks with prescribed thyroid drug replacement, and patient will not experience side effects.
- Patient's signs and symptoms of hyperthyroidism will be alleviated in 1 to 3 weeks with prescribed antithyroid drug.

Nursing Interventions

- Record vital signs. With hypothyroidism, temperature, heart rate, and blood pressure usually decrease. With hyperthyroidism, tachycardia and palpitations usually occur.
- Monitor patient's weight. Weight gain commonly occurs in patients with hypothyroidism.

Patient Teaching

Thyroid Drug Replacement

- Encourage patient to take drug at same time each day, preferably before breakfast. Food will hamper absorption rate.
- Teach patient to check warnings on OTC drug labels. Avoid OTC drugs that caution against use by persons with heart or thyroid disease.
- Direct patient to report symptoms of hyperthyroidism (tachycardia, chest pain, palpitations, excess sweating) caused by drug accumulation or overdosing.
- Suggest that patient carry MedicAlert identification card, tag, or bracelet with condition and drug used.

Diet: Hypothyroidism

- Caution patient to avoid foods that can inhibit thyroid secretion (strawberries, peaches, pears, cabbage, turnips, spinach, kale, brussels sprouts, cauliflower, radishes, peas).

Antithyroid Drugs for Hyperthyroidism

- Teach patient to take drug with meals to decrease gastrointestinal symptoms.
- Advise patient about effects of iodine and its presence in iodized salt, shellfish, and OTC cough medicines.
- Emphasize importance of drug compliance; abruptly stopping antithyroid drug could bring on thyroid crisis.
- Teach patient signs and symptoms of hypothyroidism: lethargy, puffy eyelids and face, thick tongue, slow speech with hoarseness, lack of perspiration, and slow pulse. Hypothyroidism can result from treatment of hyperthyroidism.
- Advise patient to avoid antithyroid drugs if pregnant or breastfeeding. Antithyroid drugs taken during pregnancy can cause hypothyroidism in fetus or infant.

Self-Administration

- Demonstrate to patient how to take pulse rate. Instruct patient to monitor pulse rate and report increases or marked decreases in rate.

Side Effects

- Teach patient side effects of antithyroid drugs: skin rash, hives, nausea, alopecia, loss of hair pigment, petechiae or ecchymoses, and weakness.

- Advise patient to contact health care provider if sore throat and fever occur while taking antithyroid drugs. A serious adverse reaction of antithyroid drugs is agranulocytosis (loss of white blood cells). Complete blood count should be monitored for leukopenia.

Cultural Considerations

- Recognize that members of various cultural groups may need guidance in understanding disease process of hypothyroidism or hyperthyroidism. Support patients and family members, who may lack knowledge of prescribed drug therapy for management of thyroid condition. Additional time in explanations and written plan of care may be necessary for non–English-speaking persons.

Evaluation

Thyroid Replacement

- Evaluate effectiveness of thyroid drug and drug compliance.
- Continue monitoring for side effects from drug accumulation or overdosing.
- Evaluate patient's knowledge of medication regimen.

Antithyroid Drugs

- Evaluate effectiveness of antithyroid drug in decreasing signs and symptoms of hyperthyroidism. If signs and symptoms persist after 2 to 3 weeks of therapy, other methods for correcting hyperthyroidism may be necessary.

Hyperparathyroidism

Hyperparathyroidism can be caused by malignancies of the parathyroid glands or ectopic PTH hormone secretion from lung cancer, hyperthyroidism, or prolonged immobility, during which calcium is lost from bone. Synthetic calcitonin treats hyperparathyroidism. Table 51-3 lists the drugs used to treat hypoparathyroidism and hyperparathyroidism and their dosages, uses, and considerations.

ADRENAL GLANDS

The paired **adrenal glands** consist of the adrenal medulla and adrenal cortex. The adrenal cortex produces two types of hormones, or corticosteroids: glucocorticoids (cortisol) and mineralocorticoids (aldosterone). Cortisol is secreted by the adrenal glands in response to the hypothalamus-pituitary-adrenal (HPA) axis as a result of the feedback mechanism. A decrease in serum cortisol levels increases CRF and ACTH secretions, which stimulate the adrenal glands to secrete and release cortisol. An increased serum cortisol level exerts the negative feedback mechanism, which inhibits the HPA axis, resulting in less cortisol being released. Additional physiologic functions related to the hormones secreted from the adrenal medulla and adrenal cortex are described in the introduction to Unit XVII.

Corticosteroids promote sodium retention and potassium excretion. A sodium ion is reabsorbed from the renal tubule in exchange for a potassium ion; the potassium ion is then excreted. Because of their influence on electrolytes and carbohydrate, protein, and fat metabolism, a deficiency of corticosteroids can result in serious illness or death. A decrease in corticosteroid secretion is called *adrenal hyposecretion* (adrenal insufficiency, or **Addison's disease**), and an increase in corticosteroid secretion is called *adrenal hypersecretion* (**Cushing's syndrome**).

TABLE 51-3 DRUG THERAPIES FOR PARATHYROID DISORDERS

GENERIC (BRAND)	ROUTE AND DOSAGE	USES AND CONSIDERATIONS
Treatment for Hypoparathyroidism and Hypocalcemia: Vitamin D Analogues		
calcitriol (Rocaltrol)	See Prototype Drug Chart 51-3.	
ergocalciferol (Drisdol)	Hypoparathyroidism: A/C: PO: 1250-5000 mcg/d	For hypoparathyroidism and rickets. Enhances calcium and phosphorus absorption. Long duration of action. Pregnancy category: C; PB: UK; t½: 12-24 h
Treatment for Hyperparathyroidism and Hypercalcemia		
calcitonin-salmon (Miacalcin, Fortical)	Hyercalcemia: A: 200 units in 1 nostril/d, alternate nostrils	For Paget's disease (osteitis deformans), hyperparathyroidism, and hypercalcemia. Calcitonin decreases serum calcium by binding at receptor sites on osteoclast. Pregnancy category: C; PB: UK; t½: 1-1.5 h
etidronate	A: PO: 5-10 mg/kg/d; *max:* 20 mg/kg/d	For Paget's disease; for hypercalcemia caused by antineoplastic therapy. Pregnancy category: C; PB: UK; t½: 6 h
cinacalcet (Sensipar)	A: PO: Initially 30 mg/d; titrate individualized dose q2-4wk	For hyperparathyroidism and hypercalcemia. Pregnancy category: C; PB: 93%-97%; t½: 30-40 h

A, Adult; *b.i.d.,* two times a day; *C,* child; *d,* day; *h,* hour; *IM,* intramuscular; *maint,* maintenance; *max,* maximum; *PB,* protein-binding; *PO,* by mouth; *subQ,* subcutaneous; *t½,* half-life; *UK,* unknown; *wk,* week.

Nursing Process
Patient-Centered Collaborative Care

Parathyroid Hormone Insufficiencies

Assessment
- Note serum calcium level. Report abnormal results.
- Assess for symptoms of tetany in hypocalcemia: twitching of mouth, tingling and numbness of fingers, carpopedal spasm, spasmodic contractions, and laryngeal spasm.

Nursing Diagnoses
- Diarrhea related to adverse effects of calcitriol
- Deficient fluid volume related to fluid loss from vomiting and polyuria
- Deficient knowledge related to inexperience with parathyroid medication

Planning
- Patient's serum calcium level will be within normal range.

Nursing Interventions
- Monitor serum calcium level. Normal reference value is 4.5 to 5.5 mg/dL (ionized or free-flowing calcium in the blood) or 8 to 10 mg/dL (total calcium, including free-flowing calcium or calcium bound to albumin). Serum calcium <4.5 mg/dL or <8 mg/dL indicates hypocalcemia. Total serum calcium >10.5 mg/dL or ionized calcium >5.5 mg/dL indicates hypercalcemia. Serum ionized calcium levels are usually used because much of the calcium is protein-bound, non-ionized, and nonactive.

Patient Teaching

Hypoparathyroidism
- Direct patient to report symptoms of tetany (see Assessment).

Hyperparathyroidism
- Teach patient to report signs and symptoms of hypercalcemia: bone pain, anorexia, nausea, vomiting, thirst, constipation, lethargy, bradycardia, and polyuria.
- Advise women to inform health care provider about pregnancy status before taking calcitonin preparation.
- Encourage patient to check OTC drugs for possible calcium content, especially if patient has elevated serum calcium level. Some vitamins and antacids contain calcium. Tell patient to contact health care provider before taking drugs with calcium.

Cultural Considerations
- Obtain interpreter when necessary; do not rely on family members, who may not fully disclose because of cultural norms.
- Identify conflicts in values and beliefs, and engage in culturally sensitive patient dialogue and education.

Evaluation
- Monitor effectiveness of drug therapy.
- Continue monitoring for signs and symptoms of hypocalcemia (tetany) when commercially prepared calcitonin has been given.
- Evaluate patient's knowledge of medication regimen.

Glucocorticoids

Glucocorticoids are influenced by ACTH, which is released from the anterior pituitary gland. They affect carbohydrate, protein, and fat metabolism and muscle and blood cell activity. Because of their many mineralocorticoid effects, glucocorticoids can cause sodium absorption from the kidney, resulting in water retention, potassium loss, and increased blood pressure. Cortisol, the main glucocorticoid, has antiinflammatory, antiallergic, and antistress effects. Indications for glucocorticoid therapy include trauma, surgery, inflammation, emotional upsets, and anxiety. Table 51-4 lists the physiologic aspects of adrenal hyposecretion (Addison's disease) and hypersecretion (Cushing's syndrome).

Most of the wide variety of glucocorticoid drugs, frequently called *cortisone drugs,* is synthetically produced. These drugs have several routes of administration: oral, parenteral (IM or IV), topical (creams, ointments, lotions), and

TABLE 51-4 PHYSIOLOGIC DATA: ADRENAL HYPOSECRETION AND HYPERSECRETION

BODY SYSTEM	ADRENAL HYPOSECRETION	ADRENAL HYPERSECRETION
Metabolism		
Glucose	Hypoglycemia	Hyperglycemia
Protein	Muscle weakness	Muscle wasting; thinning of skin; poor wound healing; osteoporosis;
Fat		fat accumulation in face (moon face), back of neck (buffalo hump), and trunk (protruding abdomen); hyperlipidemia; high cholesterol
Central nervous system	Apathy, depression, fatigue	Increased neural activity; mood elevation; irritability; seizures
Gastrointestinal	Nausea, vomiting, abdominal pain	Peptic ulcers
Cardiovascular	Tachycardia, hypotension, cardiovascular collapse	Hypertension; edema; heart failure
Eyes	None	Cataract formation
Fluids and electrolytes	Hypovolemia; hyponatremia; hyperkalemia	Hypervolemia; hypernatremia; hypokalemia
Blood cells	Anemia	Increased red blood cell count and neutrophils; impaired clotting

aerosol (inhaler). The IM route, although seldom used, should be administered deep into the muscle. The subQ route is not recommended.

Glucocorticoids are used to treat many diseases and health problems, including inflammatory, allergic, and debilitating conditions. Among the inflammatory conditions that may require glucocorticoids are autoimmune disorders (e.g., multiple sclerosis, rheumatoid arthritis, myasthenia gravis); ulcerative colitis; glomerulonephritis; shock; ocular and vascular inflammations; polyarteritis nodosa; and hepatitis. Allergic conditions include asthma, drug reactions, contact dermatitis, and anaphylaxis. Debilitating conditions are mainly caused by malignancies. Organ transplant recipients may require glucocorticoids to prevent organ rejection.

There are many glucocorticoids, some more potent than others. Dexamethasone (Decadron) has been used to treat severe inflammatory response resulting from head trauma or allergic reactions. An inexpensive glucocorticoid frequently prescribed is prednisone. Prototype Drug Chart 51-4 lists the pharmacologic data for prednisone.

Pharmacokinetics Prednisone is readily absorbed from the GI tract. It has a short half-life of 3 to 4 hours, and it has a moderately high protein-binding power. Prednisone is excreted primarily in the urine.

Pharmacodynamics The major actions of prednisone are to suppress an sacute inflammatory process and for immunosuppression. It prevents cell-mediated immune reactions. Peak action occurs in 1 to 2 hours, and its duration of action is long (1 to 1.5 days).

Commonly used glucocorticoid drugs are listed in Table 51-5. Most of the glucocorticoids are pregnancy category C drugs. Agents used for adrenocortical insufficiency contain both glucocorticoids and mineralocorticoids, whereas drugs for antiinflammatory or immunosuppressive use contain mostly glucocorticoids.

Side Effects and Adverse Reactions. The side effects and adverse reactions of glucocorticoids that result from high doses or prolonged use include increased blood sugar, abnormal fat deposits in the face and trunk (so-called *moon face* and *buffalo hump*), decreased extremity size, muscle wasting, edema, sodium and water retention, hypertension, euphoria or psychosis, thinned skin with purpura, increased intraocular pressure (glaucoma), peptic ulcers, and growth retardation. Long-term use of glucocorticoid drugs can cause adrenal atrophy (loss of adrenal gland function). When drug therapy is discontinued, the dose should be tapered to allow the adrenal cortex to produce cortisol and other corticosteroids. Abrupt withdrawal of the drug can result in severe adrenocortical insufficiency.

Drug Interactions. Glucocorticoids increase the potency of drugs taken concurrently, including aspirin and nonsteroidal antiinflammatory drugs (NSAIDs), thus increasing the risk of GI bleeding and ulceration. Use of potassium-wasting diuretics (e.g., Lasix) with glucocorticoids increases potassium loss, resulting in hypokalemia.

PROTOTYPE DRUG CHART 51-4

Prednisone

Drug Class Adrenal hormone: glucocorticoid Trade Name: Deltasone Pregnancy Category: C	**Dosage** A: PO: 5-60 mg/d in single or divided doses C: PO: 0.1-0.15 mg/kg/d in single or divided doses
Contraindications Hypersensitivity, psychosis, fungal infection, peptic ulcer disease Caution: Diabetes mellitus, renal disease, HF, MI, hypertension, osteoporosis, seizures, cataracts, glaucoma	**Drug-Lab-Food Interactions** Drug: Increase effect with estrogens, diltiazem, ketoconazole; decrease effects with barbiturates, phenytoin, rifampin. Concurrent use of aspirin and NSAIDs increase GI toxicity; concurrent use of diuretics and amphotericin B increase K depletion; concurrent use with cardiac glycosides increases risk of dysrhythmias and digitalis toxicity
Pharmacokinetics Absorption: PO: Well absorbed Distribution: PB: 70%-90%; crosses placenta Metabolism: t½: 3.5 h Excretion: In urine	**Pharmacodynamics** PO: Onset: UK Peak: 1-2 h Duration: 24-36 d
Therapeutic Effects/Uses To decrease inflammatory occurrence; as an immunosuppressant; to treat dermatologic disorders Mode of Action: Suppresses inflammation and adrenal function	
Side Effects Nausea, diarrhea, abdominal distention, increased appetite, sweating, headache, depression, flushing, mood changes, cataracts, amenorrhea	**Adverse Reactions** Petechiae, ecchymosis, hypertension, tachycardia, osteoporosis, muscle wasting, sodium and fluid retention Life-threatening: GI hemorrhage, pancreatitis, circulatory collapse, thrombophlebitis, embolism

A, Adult; *C*, child; *d*, day; *GI*, gastrointestinal; *h*, hour; *PB*, protein-binding; *PO*, by mouth; *t ½*, half-life; *UK*, unknown.

TABLE 51-5 ADRENAL HORMONES: GLUCOCORTICOIDS, MINERALOCORTICOID, AND GLUCOCORTICOID INHIBITORS

GENERIC (BRAND)	ROUTE AND DOSAGE	USES AND CONSIDERATIONS
Glucocorticoids		
Short Acting		
cortisone acetate	A: PO: 10-37.5 mg/d	For adrenocortical insufficiency. Contains glucocorticoid and mineralocorticoid. Decreases inflammatory process. Oral dose rapidly absorbed from GI tract. Administer deep IM. Give oral dose with food. Pregnancy category: D; PB: UK; t½: 8-12 h
hydrocortisone (Cortef, Hydrocortone)	A: PO: 20-240 mg/d in 3-4 divided doses IV: 15-500 mg/d Rectal supp: 10-25 mg	For adrenocortical insufficiency and inflammation. Parenteral form: hydrocortisone sodium phosphate. Acetate form of drug may be injected into joints. Available in cream, ointment, lotion, and spray. Pregnancy category: C; PB: 79%; t½: 1.5-2 h
Intermediate Acting		
methylprednisolone (Solu-Medrol, Depo-Medrol)	A: PO: 2-60 mg/d in 1 or more divided doses A: IV: Succinate: 10-80 mg/d IM: Acetate: 10-80 mg/wk	For inflammatory conditions such as arthritis, bronchial asthma, allergic reactions, and cerebral edema. Pregnancy category: C; PB: UK; t½: 18-36 h
prednisolone (AK-Pred)	A: PO: 5-60 mg/d C: PO: 0.1-2 mg/kg/d in divided doses	For antiinflammatory or immunosuppressive effect. For parenteral use. Can be injected into joints and soft tissue. Potent steroid. Pregnancy category: C; PB: 65%-90%; t½: 3.5 h
prednisone (Deltasone)	See Prototype Drug Chart 51-4.	
Long Acting		
beclomethasone dipropionate (Qvar, Beclovent, Vanceril)	A: Inhal: 1-2 puffs b.i.d.	Inhalation for bronchial asthma, bronchial inflammation, and seasonal rhinitis. Like all glucocorticoid inhalants, for prophylactic use. Not for acute asthmatic attack. Pregnancy category: C; PB: 87%; t½: 15 h
betamethasone (Celestone)	A: PO: 0.6-7.2 mg/d in single or divided doses IM/IV: 1-9 mg/d; *max:* IM: 12 mg/d	Potent antiinflammatory steroid drug. May be injected into joints. Also effective for treating bronchial asthma, arthritis, severe allergic reactions, and cerebral edema. Should be taken with food. Pregnancy category: C; PB: 64%; t½: 35-54 h
dexamethasone (Decadron)	Inflammation: A: PO: 0.75-9 mg/d in 2-4 divided doses C: PO: 0.024-0.34 mg/kg/d in divided doses A: IV/IM: 0.5-9 mg/d in 2-4 divided doses	Potent antiinflammatory drug. For acute allergic disorders, asthma attack, cerebral edema, and unresponsive shock. For diagnosis of Cushing's syndrome and depression. Can be administered IV push or in IV fluids. Give oral dose with food. Pregnancy category: C; PB: 80%-90%; t½: 3-4.5 h
Mineralocorticoids		
fludrocortisone (Florinef)	A: PO: 0.1-0.2 mg/d	For adrenocortical insufficiency, Addison's disease. Also for salt-losing adrenogenital syndrome. Used only for its mineralocorticoid effects. Pregnancy category: C; PB: 92%; t½:18-36 h
Diagnosis for Adrenal Gland Dysfunction		
corticotropin (Acthar)	Diagnostic test for adrenal and pituitary function	See Prototype Drug Chart 51-1.
cosyntropin (Cortrosyn)	Diagnostic test for adrenal and pituitary function	See Table 51-1.

A, Adult; *ACTH,* adrenocorticotropic hormone; *b.i.d.,* twice a day; *C,* child; *d,* day; *GI,* gastrointestinal; *h,* hour; *IM,* intramuscular; *inhal,* inhalation; *IV,* intravenous; *PB,* protein-binding; *PO,* by mouth; *q.i.d.,* four times a day; *t½,* half-life; *t.i.d.,* three times a day; *UK,* unknown; *wk,* week.

Barbiturates, phenytoin, and rifampin decrease the effect of prednisone because they increase glucocorticoid metabolism. Larger doses of glucocorticoids may be required to achieve the desired effect. Prolonged use of prednisone can cause severe muscle weakness.

Dexamethasone, a potent glucocorticoid, interacts with many drugs. Phenytoin, theophylline, rifampin, barbiturates, and antacids decrease the action of dexamethasone, whereas NSAIDs, including aspirin, and estrogen increase its action. Dexamethasone decreases the effects of oral antidiabetics.

Glucocorticoids can increase blood sugar levels, so insulin or oral antidiabetic drug dosage may need to be increased. When the drug is given with diuretics or anti-*Pseudomonas* penicillin preparations, the serum potassium level may decrease markedly.

Mineralocorticoids

Mineralocorticoids, the second type of corticosteroid, secrete aldosterone. Aldosterone is controlled by the renin-angiotensin system, not by ACTH. These hormones maintain fluid balance by promoting the reabsorption of sodium from the renal tubules. Sodium attracts water, resulting in water retention. When *hypovolemia* (decrease in circulating fluid) occurs, more aldosterone is secreted to increase sodium and water retention and restore fluid balance. With sodium reabsorption, potassium is lost and hypokalemia (potassium deficit) can occur. Some glucocorticoid drugs also contain mineralocorticoids; these include cortisone and hydrocortisone. A severe decrease in the mineralocorticoid aldosterone leads to hypotension and vascular collapse, as seen in Addison's disease. Mineralocorticoid deficiency usually occurs with glucocorticoid deficiency, frequently called *corticosteroid deficiency.*

Fludrocortisone (Florinef) is an oral mineralocorticoid that can be given with a glucocorticoid. It can cause a negative nitrogen balance; therefore a high-protein diet is usually indicated. Because potassium excretion occurs with the use of mineralocorticoids and glucocorticoids, the serum potassium level should be monitored.

Nursing Process
Patient-Centered Collaborative Care

Adrenal Hormone: Glucocorticoids

Assessment
- Note baseline vital signs for future comparison.
- Assess laboratory test results, especially serum electrolytes and blood sugar. Serum potassium level usually decreases and blood sugar level increases when a glucocorticoid such as prednisone is taken over an extensive period.
- Obtain patient's weight and urine output for future comparison.
- Assess patient's medical and herbal history. Report if patient has glaucoma, cataracts, peptic ulcer, psychiatric problems, or diabetes mellitus. Glucocorticoids can intensify these health problems.

Nursing Diagnoses
- Deficient knowledge of drug discontinuation related to lack of recall
- Excess fluid volume related to fluid retention
- Risk for impaired skin integrity related to side effect of rash

Planning
- Patient's side effects of glucocorticoid therapy will be minimal.
- Patient's inflammatory process will decrease.
- Patient will have increased knowledge of medication regimen.

Nursing Interventions
- Determine vital signs. Glucocorticoids such as prednisone can increase blood pressure and sodium and water retention.
- Administer glucocorticoids only as ordered. Routes of administration include oral, IM (not in deltoid muscle), IV, aerosol, and topical. Apply topical glucocorticoids in thin layers. Rashes, infection, and purpura should be noted and reported.
- Record weight. Report weight gain of 5 lb in several days; this would most likely be caused by water retention.
- Monitor laboratory values, especially serum electrolytes and blood sugar. Serum potassium level could decrease to <3.5 mEq/L, and blood sugar level would probably increase.
- Watch carefully for signs and symptoms of hypokalemia: nausea, vomiting, muscular weakness, abdominal distention, paralytic ileus, and irregular heart rate.
- Assess for side effects from glucocorticoid drugs when therapy has lasted more than 10 days and drug is taken in high dosages. Cortisone preparation should not be abruptly stopped, because adrenal crisis can result.
- Monitor older adults for signs and symptoms of increased osteoporosis. Glucocorticoids promote calcium loss from bone.
- Report changes in muscle strength. High doses of glucocorticoids promote loss of muscle tone.

Patient Teaching

General
- Advise patient to take drug as prescribed. Caution patient not to abruptly stop drug. When drug is discontinued, dose is tapered over 1 to 2 weeks.
- Prepare schedule for patient to decrease dose over 4 to 5 days. For short-term use (<10 days) of glucocorticoids such as prednisone or other cortisone preparations, drug dose still needs to be tapered. For example, day 1: 1 tab four times a day; day 2: 1 tab three times a day; day 3: 1 tab twice a day; day 4: 1 tab once a day.
- Direct patient not to take cortisone preparations (oral or topical) during pregnancy unless necessary and prescribed by health care provider. Drugs may be harmful to fetus.
- Inform patient that certain herbal laxatives and diuretics may interact with glucocorticoid drug and may increase severity of hypokalemia (Herbal Alert 51-1).

- Teach patient to avoid persons with respiratory infections, because these drugs suppress immune system. This is especially important if patient is receiving high dose of glucocorticoids.
- Teach patient receiving glucocorticoids to inform other health care providers of all drugs taken, especially before surgery.
- Encourage patient to carry MedicAlert identification card, tag, or bracelet stating glucocorticoid taken.

Self-Administration

- Teach patient to use aerosol nebulizer. Warn patient against overuse of aerosol to avoid possible rebound effect.

Side Effects

- Teach patient to report signs and symptoms of drug overdose or Cushing's syndrome: moon face, puffy eyelids, edema in feet, increased bruising, dizziness, bleeding, and menstrual irregularity.

Diet

- Counsel patient to take cortisone preparations at mealtime or with food. Glucocorticoid drugs can irritate gastric mucosa and cause peptic ulcer.
- Advise patient to eat foods rich in potassium, such as fresh and dried fruits, vegetables, meats, and nuts. Prednisone promotes potassium loss and hypokalemia.

Cultural Considerations

- Recognize that members of various cultural groups may need guidance in understanding disease process of Cushing's syndrome. Explain to family that patient is not "dumb" or "uninterested" but has an adrenal problem. Explain that symptoms do not "go away" and may be progressive if prescribed therapy is not followed.

Evaluation

- Evaluate effectiveness of glucocorticoid therapy. If inflammation has not improved, change in drug therapy may be necessary.
- Continue monitoring for side effects, especially when patient is receiving high doses of glucocorticoids.
- Evaluate patient's knowledge of glucocorticoid therapy.

HERBAL ALERT 51-1

Herbs and Corticosteroids

- Herbal laxatives (cascara, senna) and herbal diuretics (celery seed, juniper) can decrease serum potassium levels. When these herbs are taken with corticosteroids, hypokalemia can become more severe.
- Ginseng taken with corticosteroids may cause central nervous system stimulation and insomnia.
- Echinacea may counteract the effects of corticosteroids.
- Licorice potentiates the effect of corticosteroids and may cause a substantial decrease in serum potassium level.

KEY WEBSITES

Levothyroxine: *www.nlm.nih.gov/medlineplus/druginfo/medmaster/a682461.html*

Myxedema coma: diagnosis and treatment: *www.aafp.org/afp/20001201/2485.html*

CRITICAL THINKING CASE STUDY

MP, a 68-year-old woman, had a severe allergic reaction to shellfish and was taken to the emergency department. A single dose of dexamethasone 100 mg IV (direct IV over 30 seconds) was ordered. MP weighs 65 kg.

1. Why is MP receiving dexamethasone IV? Is the dosage of dexamethasone within safe therapeutic range? Explain your answer.
2. Describe the various ways for administering dexamethasone IV. By what other routes can dexamethasone be administered?
3. What additional health information and assessment may aid the health care provider in treating MP's serious health problem?

   Twenty-one tablets of prednisone, 5 mg each, were prescribed to be taken over 5 days, with tapering daily doses. The dosage is as follows: Day 1: take 10 mg four times a day; day 2: take 10 mg three times a day; day 3: take 10 mg twice a day; day 4: take 10 mg once a day; and day 5: take 5 mg once a day.
4. Why was prednisone ordered and not oral dexamethasone? Explain your answer.
5. What is the purpose for tapering prednisone doses? Explain your answer.
6. Is the drug dose within safe therapeutic range? Explain your answer.
7. Should MP have side effects such as peripheral edema caused by water and sodium retention as a result of tapered prednisone doses? Explain your answer.
8. What is the difference between prednisone and prednisolone?
9. What are the adverse reactions from prolonged use of prednisone?
10. What are the nursing interventions and patient teaching for MP and for patients who take prednisone?

NCLEX STUDY QUESTIONS

1. A patient is receiving the drug somatropin (Genotropin). The nurse understands that the action of this drug is to do what?
   a. Act as an antiinflammatory agent
   b. Increase metabolic rate and oxygen consumption
   c. Stimulate growth in long bones at epiphyseal plates
   d. Promote water reabsorption from the renal tubules
2. A patient is given desmopressin acetate. The nurse knows that this drug is used to treat which condition?
   a. Gigantism
   b. Diabetes mellitus
   c. Diabetes insipidus
   d. Adrenal insufficiency
3. A patient is taking levothyroxine (Synthroid). For which adverse effect would the nurse monitor this patient?
   a. Tachycardia
   b. Drowsiness
   c. Constipation
   d. Weight gain
4. A patient has just begun taking calcitriol (Rocaltrol). Which is a nursing implication of this drug?
   a. Monitor the patient's weight.
   b. Monitor serum calcium levels.
   c. Teach side effects of alopecia and petechiae.
   d. Instruct the patient to avoid persons with respiratory infections.
5. A patient is given corticotropin (Acthar). The nurse knows to monitor the patient for which condition?
   a. Weight gain
   b. Hyperkalemia
   c. Hypoglycemia
   d. Dehydration
6. A nurse is administering prednisone (Deltasone) to a newly admitted patient who is taking multiple other drugs. The nurse should consider which drug interactions with prednisone? (Select all that apply.)
   a. Cardiac and CNS actions are increased when taken with an adrenergic agent.
   b. Potassium-wasting diuretics increase potassium loss, resulting in hypokalemia.
   c. Risk for GI bleeding and ulceration increases when taken with aspirin or other NSAIDs.
   d. Action of prednisone is decreased when taken with phenytoin (Dilantin) because phenytoin increases glucocorticoid metabolism.
   e. Risk for dysrhythmias and digitalis toxicity increases when taken with cardiac glycosides.
   f. Dosage of antidiabetic agents may need to be increased when taken concurrently with glucocorticoids.
7. The nurse is administering vasopressin (Pitressin) to a patient. The nurse realizes that nursing implications for this drug would include which implications? (Select all that apply.)
   a. Record urinary output.
   b. Observe the patient's weight, and note edema.
   c. Monitor the patient for decreased blood pressure.
   d. Closely monitor the patient's blood glucose levels.
   e. Monitor the patient's pulse for increased heart rate.
   f. Record the patient's daily calcium levels.

Answers: 1, c; 2, c; 3, a; 4, b; 5, a; 6, b, c, d, e, f; 7, a, b, c, e.

CHAPTER

52

Antidiabetics

evolve WEBSITE

http://evolve.elsevier.com/KeeHayes/pharmacology/

- Animations
- Content Updates
- Key Points
- Review Questions for the NCLEX® Examination
- References from the Textbook
- Unfolding Case Studies

OBJECTIVES

- Compare type 1 and type 2 diabetes mellitus.
- Describe the symptoms of diabetes mellitus.
- Differentiate symptoms of hypoglycemic reaction and hyperglycemia.
- Compare onset, peak and duration of rapid-acting, short-acting, intermediate-acting, and long-acting insulins.
- Compare the action of oral antidiabetic drugs and their side effects.
- Differentiate between the action of insulin, oral antidiabetic agents, and glucagon.
- Apply the nursing process to the patient taking insulin and oral antidiabetic agents.

OUTLINE

KEY TERMS

Antidiabetic drugs are used primarily to control diabetes mellitus, a chronic disease that affects carbohydrate metabolism. There are two groups of antidiabetic agents: (1) insulin and (2) oral hypoglycemic (antidiabetic) drugs. **Insulin,** a protein secreted from the beta cells of the pancreas, is necessary for carbohydrate metabolism and plays an important role in protein and fat metabolism. The beta cells make up 75% of the pancreas, and the alpha cells that secrete glucagon, a hyperglycemic substance, occupy approximately 20% of the pancreas. **Oral hypoglycemic drugs,** also known as **oral antidiabetic drugs** (to avoid confusion with the term *hypoglycemic reaction*), are synthetic preparations that stimulate insulin release or otherwise alter the metabolic response to hyperglycemia.

TABLE 52-1 TYPES AND OCCURRENCES OF DIABETES MELLITUS

TYPES OF DIABETES MELLITUS	PERCENTAGE OF OCCURRENCES
Type 1	10%-12%
Type 2	85%-90%
Secondary diabetes (medications, hormonal changes)	2%-3%
GDM	1% (2%-5% of all pregnancies)

GDM, Gestational diabetes mellitus;

DIABETES MELLITUS

Diabetes mellitus, a chronic disease resulting from deficient glucose metabolism, is caused by insufficient insulin secretion from the beta cells. This results in high blood glucose *(hyperglycemia).* Diabetes mellitus is characterized by the three *p*'s: **polyuria** (increased urine output), **polydipsia** (increased thirst), and **polyphagia** (increased hunger). Diabetes *mellitus* is a disorder of the pancreas, whereas diabetes *insipidus* is a disorder of the posterior pituitary gland, discussed in detail in Chapter 51.

The four types of diabetes are presented in Table 52-1. Viral infections, environmental conditions, and genetic factors contribute to the onset of **type 1 diabetes mellitus. Type 2 diabetes mellitus** is the most common type of diabetes. Some sources suggest that heredity and obesity are the major factors that cause type 2 diabetes. With type 2 diabetes, there is some beta-cell function with varying amounts of insulin secretion. Hyperglycemia may be controlled for some type 2 diabetes patients with oral antidiabetic *(hypoglycemic)* drugs and a diet prescribed by the American Diabetic Association; however, about one third of patients with type 2 diabetes need insulin. Patients with type 2 diabetes who use one or two oral antidiabetic drugs may become insulin-dependent years later.

Certain drugs increase blood glucose and can cause hyperglycemia in prediabetic persons. These include glucocorticoids (cortisone, prednisone), thiazide diuretics (hydrochlorothiazide [HydroDIURIL]), and epinephrine. Usually the blood glucose level returns to normal after the drug is discontinued.

During the second and third trimesters of pregnancy, the levels of the hormones progesterone, cortisol, and human placental lactogen (hPL) increase. These increased hormone levels can inhibit insulin usage. This is a contributing factor for the occurrence of gestational diabetes mellitus (GDM) during pregnancy. Glucose is then mobilized from the tissue and lipid storage sites. After pregnancy, the blood glucose level may decrease; however, some patients may develop diabetes mellitus, whereas others may develop type 2 diabetes in later years.

Insulin

Insulin is released from the beta cells of the islets of Langerhans in response to an increase in blood glucose. Oral glucose load is more effective in raising the serum insulin level than an intravenous (IV) glucose load. Insulin promotes the uptake of glucose, amino acids, and fatty acids and converts them to substances that are stored in body cells. Glucose is converted to glycogen for future glucose needs in the liver and muscle, thereby lowering the blood glucose level. The normal range for blood glucose is 60 to 100 mg/dL and 70 to 110 mg/dL for serum (or plasma) glucose. When the blood glucose level is greater than 180 mg/dL, *glycosuria* (glucose in the urine) can occur. Increased blood glucose acts as an osmotic diuretic, causing polyuria. When blood glucose remains elevated (>200 mg/dL), diabetes mellitus occurs.

In 2009, the American Diabetes Association (ADA) revised its recommendations to include hemoglobin A_{1c} (HbA_{1c}) for the diagnosis of diabetes. Previously, this test had been used to monitor treatment. HbA_{1c} is a derivative of the interaction of glucose with hemoglobin in red blood cells (RBCs). Because RBCs have a life span of approximately 120 days, the HbA_{1c} level reflects the average glucose level for up to 3 months. In monitoring treatment, the goal is to keep the diabetic patient's HbA_{1c} below 7%. For diagnostic purposes, an HbA_{1c} level of ≤5% indicates that the patient does not have diabetes, 5.7% to 6.4% indicates prediabetes, and ≥6.5% indicates a diagnosis of diabetes mellitus.

Beta Cell Secretion of Insulin

The beta cells in the pancreas secrete approximately 0.2 to 0.5 units/kg/day. A patient weighing 70 kg (154 pounds) secretes 14 to 35 units of insulin per day. More insulin secretion may occur if the person consumes a greater caloric intake. A patient with diabetes mellitus may require 0.2 to 1 units/kg/day. The higher range may be because of obesity, stress, or tissue insulin resistance.

Commercially Prepared Insulin

Insulins are all currently manufactured by using deoxyribonucleic acid (DNA) technology. Human insulin (Humulin) was introduced in 1983 and duplicates insulin produced by the pancreas of the human body. Examples of human insulin include Humulin R and Novolin N. The use of Humulin insulin has a low incidence of allergic effects and insulin resistance. Human insulin analogues are modifications of human insulin with alterations in onset and duration of action. Insulin lispro (Humalog) and insulin aspart (Novolog) are examples of human insulin analogues.

Insulins are usually administered subcutaneously (subQ). Abdominal injections of insulin are absorbed faster than other body sites and found to be more consistent. Newly diagnosed patients with insulin-dependent diabetes are usually prescribed human insulin. In addition, patients in whom hyperglycemia develops during pregnancy or who already have diabetes and become pregnant are usually prescribed human insulin.

The concentration of insulin is 100 units/mL or 500 units/mL (U100/mL or U500/mL, respectively), and the insulin is packaged in a 10-mL vial. Insulin 500 units is only available in short-acting regular insulin (Humulin R and Novolin R). Insulin 500 units is seldom used except in emergencies and for patients with serious insulin resistance (>200 units/day). Insulin 40 units is no longer used in the United States, although it is still used in other countries. Insulin syringes are typically marked in units of 100 units per 1 mL or 50 units per 0.5 mL for insulin U100. Insulin syringes must be used for accurate dosing. To prevent dosage errors, the nurse must be certain that there is a match of the insulin concentration with the calibration of units on the insulin syringe. Before use, the patient or nurse must roll, not shake, cloudy insulin bottles to ensure that the insulin and its ingredients are well mixed. Shaking a bottle of insulin can cause bubbles and an inaccurate dose. Insulin requirements vary; usually less insulin is needed with increased exercise, and more insulin is needed with infections and high fever.

Administration of Insulin

Insulin is a protein and cannot be administered orally because gastrointestinal (GI) secretions destroy the insulin structure. It is administered subQ, at a 45- to 90-degree angle. The 90-degree angle is made by raising the skin and fatty tissue; the insulin is injected into the pocket between the fat and the muscle. In a thin person with little fatty tissue, the 45- to 60-degree angle is used. Regular insulin is the *only* type that can be administered IV.

The site and depth of insulin injection affect absorption. Insulin absorption is greater when given in the abdominal areas than when given in the thigh and buttock areas. Heat and massage could increase subQ absorption. Cooling the subQ area can decrease absorption.

Insulin is usually given in the morning before breakfast. It can be given several times a day. Insulin injection sites should be rotated to prevent **lipodystrophy** (tissue atrophy or hypertrophy), which can interfere with insulin absorption. Lipoatrophy (tissue atrophy) is a depression under the skin surface that primarily occurs in women and children. Lipohypertrophy (tissue hypertrophy) is a raised lump or knot on the skin surface that is more common in men. It is frequently caused by repeated injections into the same subQ site. The patient needs to develop a "site rotation pattern" to avoid lipodystrophy and to promote insulin absorption. There are various insulin rotation programs, such as an 8-day rotation schedule (insulin is given at a different site each day). The ADA suggests that insulin be injected daily at a chosen site for 1 week. Injections should be 1.5 inches apart (a knuckle length) at a site area each day. When a patient requires two insulin injections a day (morning and evening), one site should be chosen on the right side (morning) and one site chosen on the left side (evening). Figure 52-1 illustrates the sites for insulin injections. A record of injection area sites and dates administered should be kept.

Illness and stress increase the need for insulin. Insulin doses should *not* be withheld during illness, including infections and stress. Hyperglycemia and ketoacidosis may result from insufficient insulin.

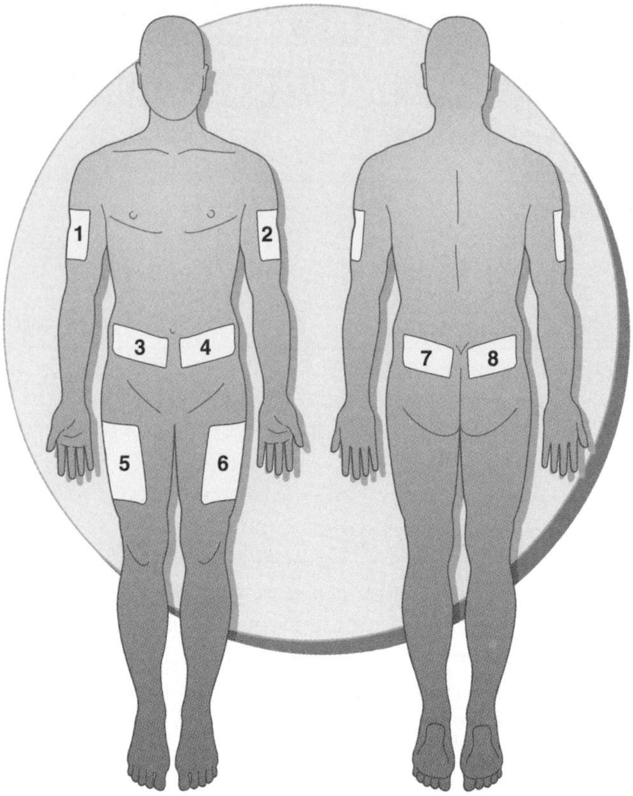

FIGURE 52–1 Sites for insulin injection.

Types of Insulin

There are several standard types of insulin: rapid acting, short acting, intermediate acting, long acting, and combinations. Rapid- and short-acting insulins are in a clear solution without any added substance to prolong insulin action. Intermediate-acting insulins are cloudy and may contain protamine, a protein that prolongs the action of insulin, or zinc, which also slows the onset of action and prolongs the duration of activity.

Rapid-acting insulins include insulin lispro (human analog) (Humalog) and human insulin aspart (rDNA origin) (NovoLog). Insulin lispro is formed by reversing two amino acids in human regular insulin (Humulin). Insulin aspart (rDNA origin) is another human insulin analogue in which a single amino acid (proline) has been substituted with aspartic acid to help prevent the molecules from clumping together to allow quicker entry into blood circulation. Insulin lispro and insulin aspart act faster than regular insulin, so they must not be administered more than 5 minutes before mealtime (food should be present before administering these insulins). Patients who are insulin-dependent and take rapid-acting insulin usually require intermediate-acting insulin as well.

Short-acting insulin has an onset of action in 30 minutes to 1 hour. The peak action occurs in 2.5 to 5 hours, and the duration of action is 6 to 8 hours. Regular (unmodified, crystalline) insulin is short-acting insulin that can be administered IV and subQ. Regular insulin is generally given 30 minutes before meals.

Intermediate-acting insulins include neutral-protamine-Hagedorn (NPH), Lente, and Humulin N. Isophane insulins like NPH and Humulin N contain protamine, a protein that prolongs the action of insulin. Humulin L insulin contains zinc, which also prolongs the insulin action time. The onset of intermediate-acting insulin is 1 to 2 hours, peak action occurs in 6 to 12 hours, and the duration of action is 18 to 24 hours.

Insulin glargine (Lantus) is long-acting insulin with an onset of 1 hour. It is evenly distributed over a 24-hour duration of action; thus it is administered once a day, usually at bedtime. Incidence of nocturnal hypoglycemia is not as common as with other insulins because of its continuous sustained release. Insulin detmir (Levemir) is another long-acting insulin that peaks in 6 to 8 hours and lasts for 12 to 24 hours. These two insulins are analogues of human insulin. Approved by the FDA in 2000, Glargine was the first long-acting recombinant DNA (rDNA origin) human insulin for patients with types 1 and 2 diabetes. Glargine and detmir are available in a prefilled 3-mL cartridge for the "OptiPen One" insulin pen device. Some patients complain of more pain at the injection site with the administration of glargine than with NPH insulin.

Combination insulins are commercially premixed. These include Humulin 70/30, Novolin 70/30, Humulin 50/50, and Humalog Mix 75/25. These combinations are widely used. The Humulin 70/30 vials or prefilled disposable pens contain 70% of human insulin isophane (intermediate-acting insulin, NPH) and 30% regular (fast-acting) insulin. The exterior of an insulin pen resembles a fountain pen. The Humulin 50/50 vial or pen contains 50% isophane (NPH) insulin and 50% regular insulin. The Humalog 75/25 mix is available in vials or prefilled disposable pens and contains 75% lispro protamine insulin and 25% lispro "rapid" insulin. Humalog 75/25 helps prevent hypoglycemia, which could occur with the 70/30 or 50/50 combination insulins, and helps control hyperglycemia more effectively. The 75/25 pen contains 300 units of insulin and does not require refrigeration after first use. It can be stored at room temperature for up to 10 days. With these combinations of insulin, the patient does not have to mix regular and NPH insulins as long as one of these combinations is effective. However, some patients need less than 25% or 30% regular insulin and more intermediate-acting insulin. These patients needs to mix the two insulins in the prescribed proportions.

Regular insulin can be mixed with protamine or zinc insulin in the same syringe. However, mixing insulin can alter the absorption rate.

Insulin Resistance

Antibodies develop over time in persons taking animal insulin. This can slow the onset of insulin action and extend its duration of action. Antibody development can cause insulin resistance and insulin allergy. Obesity can also be a causative factor for insulin resistance. Skin tests with different insulin preparations may be performed to determine whether there is an allergic effect. Human and regular insulins produce fewer allergens.

Storage of Insulin

Unopened insulin vials are refrigerated until needed. Once an insulin vial has been opened, it may be kept (1) at room temperature for 1 month or (2) in the refrigerator for 3 months. Insulin is less irritating to the tissues when injected at room temperature. Insulin vials should not be put in the freezer. In addition, insulin vials should not be placed in direct sunlight or in a high-temperature area. Prefilled syringes should be stored in the refrigerator and should be used within 1 to 2 weeks. Opened insulin vials lose their strength after approximately 3 months.

Prototype Drug Chart 52-1 lists the pharmacologic data for the different types of insulin.

Pharmacokinetics All insulins can be administered subQ, but only regular insulin can be given IV. The half-life varies. Insulin is metabolized by the liver and muscle and is excreted in the urine.

Pharmacodynamics Insulin lowers blood sugar by promoting the use of glucose by the body's cells. Insulin is also active in the storage of glucose as glycogen in muscles. The onset of action of rapid-acting insulin given subQ is 5 to 15 minutes. The onset of action of regular insulin is 30 minutes to 1 hour given subQ and 10 to 30 minutes given IV. The onset of action of intermediate-acting insulin is 1 to 2 hours. The peak action of insulins is important because of the possibility of hypoglycemic reaction (insulin shock) occurring during that time. The peak action for rapid-acting insulin is 30 minutes to 3 hours. The peak time for regular insulin is 2.5 to 5 hours; for intermediate-acting insulin, it is 6 to 12 hours. The nurse needs to assess for signs and symptoms of hypoglycemic reaction, such as nervousness, tremors, confusion, sweating, and increased pulse rate. Orange juice, sugar-sweetened beverages, or hard candy should be kept available and given if a reaction occurs. If patient is unable to ingest fast acting carbohydrates, glucagon may be given. Glucagon promotes the breakdown of glycogen in the liver, raising blood glucose within 10 minutes.

Regular insulin can be given several times a day, especially during the regulation of insulin dosage. Intermediate- and long-acting insulins are usually administered once a day. Regular insulin can be mixed with intermediate-acting insulin (Humulin N), especially if rapid onset of action is needed. When switching from one type of insulin to another, the patient may require a dose adjustment because human insulin has a shorter duration of action.

Sliding-Scale Insulin Coverage

Insulin may be administered in adjusted doses that depend on individual blood glucose test results. When the diabetic patient has extreme variances in insulin requirements (e.g., stress from hospitalization, surgery, illness, or infection), adjusted dosing or sliding-scale insulin coverage provides a more constant blood glucose level. Blood glucose testing is performed several times a day at specified intervals (usually before meals). A preset scale usually involves directions for the administration of rapid- or short-acting insulin.

Drug Interactions. Drugs such as thiazide diuretics, glucocorticoids (cortisone preparations), thyroid agents, and estrogen increase the blood sugar; therefore the insulin dosage may need adjustment. Drugs that decrease insulin needs are tricyclic antidepressants, monoamine oxidase inhibitors (MAOIs), aspirin products, and oral anticoagulants.

PROTOTYPE DRUG CHART 52-1

Insulins

Drug Class Antidiabetic: insulin Humalog (Lispro)—rapid-acting Regular Humulin R—short-acting Humulin N—intermediate-acting Glargine (Lantus)—long-acting Pregnancy Category: B	**Dosage** Must be individualized. Varies according to patient's blood sugar and health status
Contraindications Hypersensitivity, hypoglycemia Caution: Hypokalemia, fever, surgery or trauma, nausea or vomiting	**Drug-Lab-Food Interactions** Drug: Increased hypoglycemic effect with aspirin, oral anticoagulant, alcohol, oral hypoglycemics, beta blockers, tricyclic antidepressants, MAOIs, tetracycline; decreased hypoglycemic effect with thiazides, glucocorticoids, oral contraceptives, thyroid drugs, smoking
Pharmacokinetics Absorption: Lispro and Humulin R rapidly absorbed from subQ injection site. Humulin N absorbed at a slower rate. Glargine absorbed at a slow, evenly distributed rate. Distribution: PB: UK Metabolism: t½: varies with type of insulin Excretion: Mostly in urine	**Pharmacodynamics** Lispro (Humalog): subQ: Onset: 5-15 min Peak: 30-60 min Duration: 3-4 h Regular Humulin R: subQ: Onset: 30-60 min Peak: 2.5-5 h Duration: 4-8 h Humulin N: subQ: Onset: 1-2 h Peak: 4-12 h Duration: 18-24 h Glargine (Lantus): subQ: Onset: 1 h Peak: None Duration: 24 h
Therapeutic Effects/Uses To control diabetes mellitus; to lower blood sugar Mode of Action: Promotes use of glucose by body cells.	
Side Effects Confusion, agitation, tremors, headache, flushing, hunger, weakness, lethargy, fatigue, urticaria, redness, irritation or swelling at injection site	**Adverse Reactions** Tachycardia, palpitations, hypoglycemic reaction, rebound hyperglycemia (Somogyi effect), lipodystrophy Life-threatening: Shock, anaphylaxis, ketoacidosis

h, Hour; *MAOI,* monoamine oxidase inhibitor; *min,* minute; *PB,* protein-binding; *subQ,* subcutaneous; *t ½,* half-life; *UK,* unknown.

Table 52-2 lists the rapid-acting, short-acting, intermediate-acting, long-acting, and combination insulins with their dosages, uses, and considerations.

Side Effects and Adverse Reactions: Hypoglycemic Reactions and Ketoacidosis. When more insulin is administered than needed for glucose metabolism, a **hypoglycemic reaction,** or **insulin shock,** occurs. The person may exhibit nervousness, trembling, and lack of coordination; have cold and clammy skin; and complain of a headache. Some patients become combative and incoherent. Giving sugar orally or IV increases the use of insulin, and the symptoms disappear immediately.

In response to an excessive dose of insulin, diabetic patients may develop the Somogyi effect. This hypoglycemic condition usually occurs in the predawn hours of 2:00 AM to 4:00 AM. A rapid decrease in blood glucose during the nighttime hours stimulates a release of hormones (e.g., cortisol, glucagon, epinephrine) to increase blood glucose by lipolysis, gluconeogenesis, and glycogenolysis, thus creating the Somogyi effect. Management of the Somogyi effect involves monitoring blood glucose between 2:00 AM and 4:00 AM and reducing the bedtime insulin dosage.

Hyperglycemia on awakening is known as the *dawn phenomenon.* The patient usually awakens with a headache and

TABLE 52-2 ANTIDIABETICS: INSULINS

GENERIC (BRAND)	ROUTE AND DOSAGE	PREGNANCY CATEGORY	HALF-LIFE	ACTION: ONSET	ACTION: PEAK	ACTION: DURATION
Rapid-Acting Insulins						
insulin lispro (Humalog) insulin aspart [rDNA origin] (NovoLog) insulin glulisine (Apidra)	A: 0.5-1 unit/kg/d; dose individualized	Humalog: B NovoLog, Apidra: C	26-81 min	5-15 min	Humalog, Apidra: 30-90 min NovoLog: 1-3 h	Humalog: 2-5 h NovoLog: 3-5 h Apidra: 1-2.5 h
Short-Acting Insulins						
insulin regular (Humulin R, Novolin R, regular insulin)	A/C: subQ/IV: 100 units/mL; dose individualized	B	10 min-1 h	30 min	2.5-5 h	6-8 h
Intermediate-Acting Insulins						
insulin isophane NPH (Humulin N, Novolin N)	See Prototype Drug Chart 52-1.	B	13 h	1-2 h	6-12 h	18-24 h
Long-Acting Insulins						
insulin glargine (Lantus)	Dose individualized	C	UK	1 h	None	24 h
insulin detemir (Levemir)	Dose individualized	B	5-7 h	3-4 h	6-8 h	24 h
Combination Insulins*						
Humulin 70/30 (isophane NPH 70%, regular 30%)	Dose individualized	B	13 h	30 min	4-8 h	22-24 h
insulin isophane NPH 50/50 (Humulin NPH 50%, regular 50%)	Dose individualized	B	13 h	0.5 h	4-8 h	24 h
Humalog 75/25 (lispro protamine 75%, lispro 25%)	Dose individualized	B	<13 h	5-15 min	0.5-6 h	20-24 h

*Protamine suspensions are added to regular insulin.
A, Adult; *C,* child; *h,* hour; *IV,* intravenous; *min,* minute; *NPH,* neutral-protamine-Hagedorn; *subQ,* subcutaneous; *UK,* unknown; <, less than.

reports night sweats and nightmares. Management of the dawn phenomenon involves increasing the bedtime dose of insulin.

With an inadequate amount of insulin, sugar cannot be metabolized, and fat catabolism occurs. The use of fatty acids (ketones) for energy causes **ketoacidosis** (diabetic acidosis or diabetic coma). Table 52-3 lists the signs and symptoms of hypoglycemic reaction and ketoacidosis.

TABLE 52-3 HYPOGLYCEMIC REACTION AND DIABETIC KETOACIDOSIS

REACTION	SIGNS AND SYMPTOMS
Hypoglycemic reaction (insulin shock)	Headache, lightheadedness Nervousness, apprehension Tremor Excess perspiration; cold, clammy skin Tachycardia Slurred speech Memory lapse, confusion, seizures Blood sugar level <60 mg/dL
Diabetic ketoacidosis (hyperglycemic reaction)	Extreme thirst Polyuria Fruity breath odor Kussmaul breathing (deep, rapid, labored, distressed, dyspneac) Rapid, thready pulse Dry mucous membranes, poor skin turgor Blood sugar level 250 mg/dL

>, Greater than; <, less than.

Insulin Pen Injectors

An insulin pen resembles a fountain pen. The pen contains a disposable needle and a disposable insulin-filled cartridge. Insulin pens come in two types: prefilled and reusable. These insulin pens are considered to deliver a more accurate dose than the traditional 100-unit syringe and vial.

To operate the insulin pen, the insulin dose is obtained by turning the dial to the number of insulin units needed. The capacity of these prefilled and reusable-insulin pens is 150 to 300 units, or 1.5 to 3 mL. The 1.5-mL replaceable cartridges for insulin pens are being phased out. Insulin pens available on the market include Novolog FlexPen (Novo Nordisk), Humalog KwikPen (Lilly), Apidra SoloSTAR (Sanofi-Aventis), Lantus SoloSTAR (Sanofi), and Levemir FlexPen (Novo Nordisk). Insulin pens tend to be more expensive than other delivery systems, but their advantages may outweigh the extra cost.

The use of insulin pens increases the patient's compliance with the insulin regimen. The convenience of the pen is most appealing. The patient may choose to use the insulin pen for its portability (e.g., at work, while traveling). The traditional method for administering insulin may be used at other times. The cost of insulin in vials is somewhat less than the prefilled pens, but most patients state that less injection pain is associated with insulin pens than with the traditional insulin syringe.

Insulin Pumps

Insulin pumps are an alternative to daily insulin injections used in association with blood glucose monitoring and carbohydrate counting. These computerized devices have an insulin reservoir and programming capacity to deliver continuous rapid-acting insulin in varying amounts at different times throughout a 24-hour period. These pumps are smaller than most mobile phones. Types of insulin pumps include implantable and portable. The implantable insulin pump is surgically implanted in the abdomen. It delivers both basal infusion (continuous release of a small amount of insulin) and bolus (additional) doses with meals. It is administered intraperitoneally. With the use of implantable insulin pumps, fewer hypoglycemic reactions occur and blood glucose levels are controlled. Long-term effectiveness of the pump is currently under study.

Portable or external insulin pumps, also called *continuous subQ insulin infusion* (CSII), may have a tube (or infusion set) placed under the skin. The needle is inserted into the abdomen, upper thigh, or upper arm. This type of pump is worn outside the body and placed in a pocket or bra. The external tubeless pump lies directly on the skin and injects insulin through the skin without tubes. The external insulin pump keeps blood glucose levels as close to normal as possible. This insulin pump is a battery-operated device that uses rapid-acting insulin, which is stored in a reservoir syringe placed inside the device. It delivers both basal insulin infusion and bolus doses with meals. Infusions are programmed by the patient. About three basal rates are programmed per day; however, the patient can adjust the rate according to changes in activity. The insulin can be delivered by bolus (the patient pushes a button to deliver a bolus dose at meals). Only rapid-acting insulin is used. Modified insulins (NPH) are not used because of unpredictable control of blood sugars. The pump delivers exactly as much insulin as the patient programs.

The ongoing insulin delivery therapy helps decrease the risk of severe hypoglycemic reaction and maintains tight glucose (glycemic) control. Glucose levels should be monitored at least four times daily with an insulin pump. The patient must count carbohydrates and bolus prior to meals.

Most insulin pumps have a memory of the last 24 boluses (time and day). An alarm sounds so the patient can take appropriate action when insulin is not delivered or when there is an oncoming low or high. Newer pumps have an automatic shutoff for 1 to 2 hours during periods of low blood glucose. This feature is designed for the patient that may not hear the alarm and for whom blood glucose is allowed to elevate. The pump can be disconnected from the insertion site for bathing, swimming, and other activities; however, it is recommended that it not be discontinued for longer than 1 to 2 hours.

Success of insulin pump therapy depends on the individual's knowledge and compliance related to insulin use and the diabetic state. The person with type 1 diabetes mellitus may benefit most from the use of insulin pump therapy. This insulin delivery method is considered more effective than the use of multiple injections of regular and modified types of insulins and lessens the long-term diabetic complications. Studies have shown that myocardial infarction, renal disease, nerve damage, eye damage, and death have all been greatly reduced by tight blood glucose control. Also, HbA_{1c} levels, neuropathy pain, and sexual performance have improved with the use of insulin pump control.

Insulin Jet Injectors

Insulin jet injectors shoot insulin, without a needle, directly through the skin into the fatty tissue. Because the insulin is delivered under high pressure, stinging, pain, burning, and bruising may occur. This method of insulin insertion is not indicated for children or older adults. This type of device is also expensive, costing approximately 2 to 10 times as much as the subQ dose.

Nursing Process
Patient-Centered Collaborative Care

Antidiabetics: Insulin

Assessment

- Identify the drugs patient currently takes. Certain drugs such as alcohol, aspirin, oral anticoagulants, oral antidiabetics, beta-blockers, tricyclic antidepressants, monoamine oxidase inhibitors (MAOIs), and tetracycline increase the hypoglycemic effect when taken with insulin. Note that thiazides, glucocorticoids, oral contraceptives, thyroid drugs, and smoking can increase blood sugar.
- Assess the type of insulin and dosage. Note whether it is given once or multiple times a day.
- Note BP, heart rate, and blood glucose levels. Tachycardia and heart palpitations may occur with hypoglycemia. Hypotension may occur with hyperglycemia. Report abnormal findings.
- Determine patient's knowledge of diabetes mellitus and use of insulins.
- Check for signs and symptoms of hypoglycemic reaction (insulin shock), hyperglycemia, or ketoacidosis.

Nursing Diagnoses

- Risk for impaired skin integrity related to failure to rotate insulin injection sites

- Imbalanced nutrition, more than body requirements, related to excessive intake associated with metabolic need
- Risk for injury related to confusion from hypoglycemic reaction
- Deficient knowledge related to inexperience with insulin therapy

Planning
- Patient's blood glucose will be within normal values (70 to 110 mg/dL).
- Patient will self-administer insulin correctly.

Nursing Interventions
- Monitor vital signs. Tachycardia can occur during insulin reaction.
- Determine blood glucose levels, and report changes. The reference value is 60 to 100 mg/dL for blood glucose and 70 to 110 mg/dL for serum glucose.
- Monitor the patient's HbA_{1c} to provide feedback of diabetic control.
- Prepare a teaching plan based on patient's knowledge of health problem, diet, and drug therapy.

Patient Teaching

General
- Teach patient to recognize and immediately report symptoms of hypoglycemic (insulin) reaction, such as headache, nervousness, sweating, tremors, rapid pulse, and hyperglycemic reaction (diabetic acidosis), such as thirst, increased urine output, and sweet, fruity breath odor.
- Advise patient that hypoglycemic reactions are more likely to occur during peak action time. Most diabetic patients know whether they are having a hypoglycemic reaction, but some have higher tolerance to low blood glucose and can have a severe reaction without realizing it.
- Explain that orange juice, sugar-containing drinks, and hard candy may be used when a hypoglycemic reaction begins.
- Teach family members to administer glucagon by injection if patient has a hypoglycemic reaction and cannot drink sugar-containing fluid.
- Inform patient that certain herbs may interact with insulin and oral antidiabetic drugs. A hypoglycemic or hyperglycemic effect might occur (Herbal Alert 52-1).
- Teach patient about necessity for compliance with prescribed insulin therapy and diet. HbA_{1c} provides most accurate picture of optimal diabetic control.
- Advise patient to carry a MedicAlert card, tag, or bracelet indicating the health problem and insulin dosage.

Self-Administration
- Instruct patient on how to check blood glucose with a glucometer (Sure Touch, One Step, Accu-Chek).
- Teach patient about care of insulin container and syringes. Inform patient taking NPH insulin with regular insulin that regular insulin is drawn up before NPH insulin.

Diet
- Advise patient taking insulin to eat prescribed diet on a consistent schedule. Diet information may be obtained from ADA or a nutritionist.

Cultural Considerations
- Provide additional instructions about insulin action, administration, reactions, and possible complications in language patient speaks and reads most easily.
- Determine if follow-up by community health nurse is needed to assist with patient's compliance with insulin use, diet, and exercise regimen.

Evaluation
- Evaluate effectiveness of insulin therapy by noting if blood sugar level is within accepted range.
- Establish patient's self-care ability.
- Determine patient's knowledge of signs and symptoms of hypoglycemic or hyperglycemic reaction.

HERBAL ALERT 52-1

Antidiabetic Agents

- Chromium may decrease insulin requirements.
- Black cohosh may potentiate hypoglycemic effects of insulin and oral antidiabetic drugs.
- Garlic, bitter melon, aloe, and gymnema can increase insulin levels and therefore may cause hypoglycemia when used with insulin or oral antidiabetic drugs. They can have a direct hypoglycemic effect.
- Ginseng can lower blood glucose levels. When taken with insulin or an oral antidiabetic (hypoglycemic) drug, hypoglycemic effects or reaction may occur.
- Bilberry may increase hypoglycemia when taken with insulin or oral antidiabetics.
- Rosemary and stinging nettle decrease the therapeutic effect of insulin and oral antidiabetic drugs (have a hyperglycemic effect).

Oral Antidiabetic Drugs (Oral Hypoglycemic Drugs)

First- and Second-Generation Sulfonylureas

Oral antidiabetic drugs, also called *oral hypoglycemics,* should be used by those with type 2 diabetes; persons with type 1 diabetes should not use them. Patients with type 2 diabetes have some degree of insulin secretion by the pancreas. The sulfonylureas, a group of antidiabetics chemically related to sulfonamides but lacking antibacterial activity, stimulate pancreatic beta cells to secrete more insulin. This increases the insulin cell receptors, increasing the ability of the cells to bind insulin for glucose metabolism.

The sulfonylureas are classified as first- and second-generation. First-generation sulfonylureas are divided into short-acting, intermediate-acting, and long-acting antidiabetics. Tolbutamide (Orinase) is a first-generation short-acting sulfonylurea. Tolazamide (Tolinase) is a first-generation intermediate-acting sulfonylurea. Chlorpropamide (Diabinese) is a first-generation long-acting sulfonylurea.

Second-generation sulfonylureas increase the tissue response to insulin and decrease glucose production by the liver. They have greater hypoglycemic potency than the first-generation sulfonylureas. Effective doses for the second-generation drugs are lower than for the first-generation drugs. They have a longer duration of action and cause fewer side effects. The second-generation drugs have less displacement potential from protein-binding sites by other highly protein-bound drugs, such as salicylates and warfarin (Coumadin), than first-generation drugs. Second-generation sulfonylureas should not be used when liver or kidney dysfunction is present. A hypoglycemic reaction is more likely to occur in older adults.

Second-generation sulfonylureas include glimepiride (Amaryl) and glipizide (Glucotrol, Glucotrol XL), which directly stimulate the beta cells to secrete insulin, thus decreasing the blood glucose level. Glimepiride improves postprandial glucose levels. It may be used in combination with insulin in persons with type 2 diabetes. Side effects include GI disturbances such as nausea, vomiting, diarrhea, and abdominal pain.

Table 52-4 lists the sulfonylureas and their dosages, uses, and considerations. Prototype Drug Chart 52-2 lists the pharmacologic data for the second-generation sulfonylurea glipizide.

Pharmacokinetics Glipizide is well absorbed from the GI tract and highly protein-bound. Glipizide is metabolized by the liver. The primary metabolites are inactive and excreted mainly in urine.

Pharmacodynamics Glipizide is the most common sulfonylurea drug prescribed for type 2 diabetes mellitus. It lowers blood sugar by stimulating pancreatic beta cells to secrete insulin. The onset of action usually occurs within 15 to 30 minutes, and the peak action time is between 1 and 2 hours. Glipizide is normally given once a day in the morning because of its long duration of action of 24 hours.

TABLE 52-4 ANTIDIABETICS

GENERIC (BRAND)	ROUTE AND DOSAGE	USES AND CONSIDERATIONS
First-Generation Sulfonylureas: Short Acting		
tolbutamide (Orinase)	A: PO: 250-3,000 mg/d in 1-2 divided doses	For managing type 2 diabetes mellitus. Chemically related to sulfonamides, but no antiinfective effect. Hypoglycemic reaction may occur if overdosed. Pregnancy category: C; PB: 98%; $t_{1/2}$: 4-7 h
First-Generation Sulfonylureas: Intermediate Acting		
tolazamide (Tolinase)	A: PO: 100-250 mg 1-2 times/d *max:* 1 g/d	Diet and exercise should be part of diabetic therapy. Duration of action is 10-20 hours. Pregnancy category: C; PB: 90%; $t_{1/2}$: 7 h
First-Generation Sulfonylureas: Long Acting		
chlorpropamide (Diabinese)	A: PO: 100-250 mg/d; *max:* 750 mg/d	For managing type 2 diabetes. May be given to selected type 1 patients for reducing insulin doses. Diet and exercise should be a part of diabetic therapy. Duration of action is 24 h. May cause water and sodium retention. Pregnancy category: C; PB: 60%-90%; $t_{1/2}$: 25-60 h
Second-Generation Sulfonylureas		
glipizide (Glucotrol)	See Prototype Drug Chart 52-2.	
glyburide (DiaBeta, Glynase, Micronase)	A: PO: Initially: 1.25-5 mg/d; maint: 1.25-20 mg/d; *max:* 20 mg/d	Same as chlorpropamide. Potent drug. Duration of action 10-24 h. Pregnancy category: C; PB: 99%; $t_{1/2}$: 10 h
glimepiride (Amaryl)	A: PO: Initially: 1-2 mg a.c.; maint: 1-4 mg/d a.c.; *max:* 8 mg/d a.c.	For managing type 2 diabetes. May be used in combination with insulin. Can lower 2-hour postprandial glucose levels significantly. GI disturbances may occur. Pregnancy category: C; PB: 99%; $t_{1/2}$: 5-9 h
Nonsulfonylureas		
Biguanides		
metformin (Glucophage)	See Prototype Drug Chart 52-3.	
Alpha-Glucosidase Inhibitors		
acarbose (Precose)	A: PO: Initially 25 mg t.i.d. with first bite of each meal; *max:* 150 mg/d if <60 kg, 300 mg/d if >60 kg	For managing hyperglycemia in type 2 diabetes mellitus. Used as monotherapy or in combination with a sulfonylurea. Pregnancy category: B; PB: UK; $t_{1/2}$: 2 h
miglitol (Glyset)	A: PO: 25-100 mg t.i.d. a.c.	For managing type 2 diabetes. May be taken with a sulfonylurea or as monotherapy with diet and exercise. GI disturbances may occur. Pregnancy category: B; PB: <4%; $t_{1/2}$: 2 h

TABLE 52-4 ANTIDIABETICS—cont'd

GENERIC (BRAND)	ROUTE AND DOSAGE	USES AND CONSIDERATIONS
Thiazolidinediones (Insulin-Enhancing Agents)		
pioglitazone HCl (Actos)	A: PO: 15-45 mg/d	For managing type 2 diabetes. Improves glycemic control and decreases insulin resistance. Inhibits gluconeogenesis and increases sensitivity to insulin in muscle and fatty tissues. For monotherapy; can be combined with sulfonylurea or insulin. Monitor liver enzymes. Contraindicated for patients with symptomatic heart disease and Class III and IV CHF. Pregnancy category: C; PB: 99%; t½: 16-24 h
Meglitinides		
repaglinide (Prandin)	A: PO: 0.5-4 mg t.i.d./q.i.d. a.c.; *max:* 16 mg/d	For managing type 2 diabetes. May be taken alone or in combination with metformin. Similar in action to sulfonylureas but not in structure. Increases beta cell secretion of insulin. Pregnancy category: C; PB: 98%; t½: 1 h
nateglinide (Starlix)	A: PO: 60-120 mg t.i.d. a.c.; *max:* 360 mg/d	For managing type 2 diabetes. Increases release of insulin from beta cells. May be used alone or in combination with metformin. Pregnancy category: C; PB: 98%; t½: 1.5 h
DPP-4 Inhibitors		
sitagliptin phosphate (Januvia) Combination form: sitagliptin/metformin (Janumet)	A: PO: 100 mg/d	For managing type 2 diabetes. Used in combination with exercise and diet. Pregnancy category: B; PB: 38%; t½: 12 h
saxagliptin (Onglyza)	A: PO: 2.5-5 mg/d	For managing type 2 diabetes. Used in combination with exercise and diet. Pregnancy category: B; PB: UK; t½: 2.5 h
linagliptin (Tradjenta)	A: PO: 5 mg/d	For managing type 2 diabetes. Used in combination with exercise and diet. Pregnancy category: B; PB: 75%-99%; t½: 12 h
alogliptin (Nesina)	A: PO: 25 mg/d	For managing type 2 diabetes. Used in combination with exercise and diet. Pregnancy category: B; PB: 20%; t½: 21 h
Selective Sodium-Glucose Transporter 2		
canagliflozin (Invokana)	A: PO: 100 mg/d before first meal of day; *max:* 300 mg/d	For managing type 2 diabetes. Used in combination with exercise and diet. Pregnancy category: C; PB: 99%; t½: 10.6-13.1 h
Amylin Analogue		
pramlintide (Symlin)	Type 1: A: subQ: Initially 15 mcg a.c., then 30-60 mcg; *max:* 120 mcg/dose Type 2: A: subQ: Initially 60 mcg a.c., then 60-120 mcg; *max:* 120 mcg/dose	For managing types 1 and 2 diabetes as adjunct to insulin therapy. Decreases postmeal glucagon and glucose. Give subQ in abdomen and thigh immediately before each major meal. Never administer in arm as absorption is unpredictable. Pregnancy category: C; PB: 40%; t½: 48 min
Glucagon-Like Peptide-1 Agonists		
exenatide (Byetta, Bydureon)	Injectable suspension (Byetta): A: subQ: 5 mcg b.i.d within 60 min before morning and evening meal; *max:* 20 mcg/d Injectable suspension (Bydureon): A: subQ: 2 mg/week	For managing type 2 diabetes. Suppresses glucagon secretion. May be given in abdomen, arm, or thigh. Pregnancy category: C; PB: 40%; t½: 2.4 h
liraglutide (Victoza)	A: subQ: 0.6 mg/d for 1 wk, then 1.2-1.8 mg/d	For managing type 2 diabetes. Monitor patient closely; may cause thyroid C-cell tumors. Pregnancy category: C; PB: 98%; t½: 12-13 h
Fixed Combination Oral Antidiabetic Drugs		
glyburide/metformin (Glucovance)	A: PO: Initially: 1.25/250 mg (glyburide/metformin) once daily or b.i.d. a.c. Increase dose at 2-wk intervals; maint: 2.5/510 mg/d or 5/510 mg/d or b.i.d. a.c.; *max:* 20/2,000 mg/d	For managing type 2 diabetes. May be used when glucose is not controlled with either drug alone. Contraindicated for patients with renal insufficiency because of risk for lactic acidosis. Pregnancy category: B; PB: UK; t½: 6-10 h

A, Adult; *a.c.,* before meals; *b.i.d.,* twice a day; *CHF,* congestive heart failure; *d,* day; *GI,* gastrointestinal; *h,* hour; *maint,* maintenance; *max,* maximum; *PB,* protein-binding; *PO,* by mouth; *q.i.d.,* four times a day; *t½,* half-life; *t.i.d.,* three times a day; *UK,* unknown; *wk,* week; >, greater than; <, less than.

PROTOTYPE DRUG CHART 52-2

Glipizide

Drug Class	Dosage
Glipizide: sulfonylurea, second-generation Trade Names: Glucotrol, Glucotrol XL Pregnancy Category: C	A: PO: Initially 2.5-5 mg/d a.c.; maint: 10-15 mg/d a.c. (dose is divided if >15 mg); *max:* 40 mg/d A: PO: ER: 5-10 mg/d; *max:* 20 mg/d
Contraindications	**Drug-Lab-Food Interactions**
Diabetic ketoacidosis Caution: Hepatic or renal dysfunction, older adults, debilitated or malnourished patients, adrenal or pituitary insufficiency	Drug: Alcohol may produce disulfiram-like reaction (flushing, headache, sweating, nausea, violent vomiting, weakness); beta blockers, systemic azole antifungals, clarithromycin, oral anticoagulants, MAOIs, atypical antipsychotics, salicylates, probenecid, sulfonamides, antacids, cimetidine, clofibrate, and phenylbutazone may potentiate hypoglycemia; oral contraceptives, thiazide diuretics, and anticonvulsants may enhance hyperglycemia. Lab: Altered liver function tests Food: Green tea may potentiate hypoglycemia
Pharmacokinetics	**Pharmacodynamics**
Absorption: Rapidly absorbed from GI tract Distribution: PB: 92%-99% Metabolism: t½: 2-4 h Excretion: Primarily in urine	PO: Onset: 15-30 min Peak: 1-2 h Duration: 12-24 h
Therapeutic Effects/Uses	
To control hyperglycemia in type 2 diabetes mellitus Mode of Action: Directly stimulates beta cells in pancreas to secrete insulin; indirectly alters sensitivity of peripheral insulin receptors, allowing increased insulin binding	
Side Effects	**Adverse Reactions**
Drowsiness, headache, confusion, visual disturbances, anxiety, hunger, anorexia, nausea, constipation, diarrhea	Hypoglycemia, tachycardia Life-threatening: Seizures, coma, respiratory depression

A, Adult; *a.c.,* before meals; *d,* day; *GI,* gastrointestinal; *h,* hour; *MAOIs,* monoamine oxidase inhibitors; *max,* maximum; *min,* minute; *PB,* protein-binding; *PO,* by mouth; *ER,* extended-release; *t ½,* half-life; >, greater than.

Side Effects, Adverse Reactions, and Contraindications. The side effects of most oral antidiabetic drugs are similar to those of insulin. Taking antidiabetic drugs without adequate food can lead to an insulin reaction with signs and symptoms such as nervousness, tremors, and confusion. Adverse reactions include hematologic disorders, such as aplastic anemia, leukopenia, and thrombocytopenia. Weight gain, seizures, and coma may also occur. Sulfonylureas are contraindicated in type 1 diabetes (no functioning beta cells), diabetic ketoacidosis, pregnancy, and lactation and during stress, surgery, or severe infection.

The major side effect of sulfonylureas is hypoglycemia. Acarbose does not cause hypoglycemia unless it is taken with a sulfonylurea or insulin. It can cause increased flatulence (gas), diarrhea, and abdominal distention.

Drug Interactions. Aspirin, oral anticoagulants, MAOIs, sulfonamides, cimetidine, and some NSAIDs can increase the action of sulfonylureas, especially first-generation ones, by binding to plasma proteins and displacing sulfonylureas. Because this causes increased free sulfonylurea, insulin reaction can result. The action of sulfonylureas is decreased by concurrent administration of thiazide diuretics, isoniazid, phenytoin, and corticosteroids. Patients should be alerted not to drink alcohol while taking sulfonylureas, because alcohol increases the half-life, and a hypoglycemic reaction can result.

Nonsulfonylureas

Expanding knowledge of glucose metabolism has revealed new mechanisms for the management of type 2 diabetes. The drugs metformin and acarbose use different methods to control serum glucose levels following a meal. Unlike the sulfonylureas, which enhance insulin release and receptor interaction, these drugs affect the hepatic and GI production of glucose.

Biguanides: Metformin (Glucophage)

Metformin is a biguanide compound that acts by decreasing hepatic production of glucose from stored glycogen. This diminishes the increase in serum glucose following a meal and blunts the degree of postprandial hyperglycemia. Metformin also decreases the absorption of glucose from the small intestine, and there is evidence that it increases insulin receptor sensitivity as well as peripheral glucose uptake at the cellular level. Unlike sulfonylureas, metformin does not produce hypoglycemia or hyperglycemia. It can cause GI disturbances.

Metformin is 51% to 60% bioavailable and is absorbed primarily from the small intestine. It does not undergo hepatic metabolism and is eliminated unchanged in the urine. It is not recommended for patients with renal impairment. Monotherapy with metformin is effective; however, when combined with a sulfonylurea, the drug is useful in cases that are resistant to oral antidiabetics (hypoglycemics). Metformin therapy should be withheld for 48 hours before and after the patient undergoes IV contrast dye, because lactic acidosis or acute renal failure may develop.

Alpha-Glucosidase Inhibitors: Acarbose (Precose) and Miglitol (Glyset)

Acarbose acts by inhibiting the digestive enzyme in the small intestine that is responsible for the release of glucose from complex carbohydrates (CHO) in the diet. By inhibiting alpha glucosidase, absorption of complex CHO is delayed. Acarbose has no demonstrated systemic effects and is not absorbed into the body in significant amounts. It does not cause hypoglycemic reaction. Acarbose is intended for use in patients who do not achieve results with diet alone. Miglitol, like acarbose, inhibits alpha glucosides. Miglitol is absorbed from the GI tract. This drug will not cause hypoglycemia, but if taken with a sulfonylurea or insulin, hypoglycemia could occur.

Thiazolidinediones

Pioglitazone (Actos) and rosiglitazone (Avandia) were considered safe thiazolidinedione drugs. However, in 2007 a warning was added to the Avandia packaging after the FDA issued a statement that Avandia users may be at greater risk for heart attack and possibly death. Both drugs are contraindicated in symptomatic heart disease and Classes III and IV congestive heart failure. These two drugs can be prescribed for monotherapy or combined with other oral antidiabetic drugs. Pioglitazone can be taken in combination with sulfonylurea or insulin, and rosiglitazone may be combined with metformin (Prototype Drug Chart 52-3). These drugs do not induce hypoglycemic reactions if taken alone. They decrease insulin resistance and improve blood glucose control.

Meglitinides

Repaglinide (Prandin) and nateglinide (Starlix) are classified as meglitinide oral antidiabetic agents. They stimulate the beta cells to release insulin. The action of repaglinide and nateglinide is similar to that of sulfonylureas. These agents can be used alone or in combination with metformin for patients with type 2 diabetes mellitus. They are short-acting antidiabetic drugs. Repaglinide and nateglinide should not be

PROTOTYPE DRUG CHART 52-3

Metformin

Drug Class Metformin: biguanide Trade Names: Glucophage, Glucophage XR Pregnancy Category: B	**Dosage** A: PO: Initial: 500 mg 1-3 times/d with or shortly after meals; increase dose gradually; *max:* 2550 mg/d A: PO: ER: 500 mg/d with evening meal; *max:* 2,000 mg/d
Contraindications Hypersensitivity, diabetic ketoacidosis, radiographic contrast administration, concurrent infection, hepatic or renal dysfunction, cardiopulmonary insufficiency, alcoholism Caution: Pregnancy, lactation	**Drug-Lab-Food Interactions** Drug: ACE inhibitors, ARBs, calcium channel blockers, beta-blockers, procainamide, quinidine, digoxin, furosemide, alcohol, cimetidine, ranitidine, azole antifungals, trimethoprim, vancomycin, and quinine may potentiate hypoglycemia; iodinated contrast dyes, nicotine, morphine, triamterene, thiazide diuretics may cause lactic acidosis or acute kidney failure Lab: Altered liver function tests Food: Green tea may lead to hypoglycemia
Pharmacokinetics Absorption: 51%-60% absorbed Distribution: PB: 0% Metabolism: $t\frac{1}{2}$: 6-17 h Excretion: Primarily in urine	**Pharmacodynamics** PO: Onset: UK Peak: 1-3 h Duration: UK
Therapeutic Effects/Uses To control hyperglycemia in type 2 diabetes mellitus Mode of Action: Increases binding of insulin to receptors, improves tissue sensitivity to insulin, increases glucose transport to skeletal muscles and fatty tissues, decreases glucose production in liver by reducing gluconeogenesis, and reduces glucose absorption from intestines	
Side Effects Dizziness, fatigue, headache, agitation, bitter or metallic taste, anorexia, nausea, vomiting, diarrhea, weight loss	**Adverse Reactions** Lactic acidosis; malabsorption of amino acids, vitamin B_{12}, and folic acid Life-threatening: Lactic acidosis

A, Adult; *d,* day; *h,* hour; *max,* maximum; *PB,* protein-binding; *PO,* by mouth; *ER,* extended-release; $t\frac{1}{2}$, half-life; *t.i.d.,* three times a day; *UK,* unknown.

prescribed for patients with liver dysfunction because of possible decreased liver metabolism rate. More of the drug could remain in the body, which may cause a hypoglycemic reaction.

Incretin Modifier

The oral antidiabetics sitagliptin phosphate (Januvia) and saxagliptin (Onglyza) are classified as incretin modifiers (also called *dipeptidyl peptidase-4 [DPP-4] inhibitors* and *gliptins*) for treatment of type 2 diabetes mellitus. The action of DPP-4 inhibitors is to increase the level of incretin hormones, increase insulin secretion, and decrease glucagon secretion to reduce glucose production. This incretin modifier is used as adjunct treatment with exercise and diet to reduce both fasting and postprandial plasma glucose levels.

Guidelines for Oral Antidiabetic (Hypoglycemic) Therapy for Type 2 Diabetes

The following are criteria for the use of oral antidiabetic drugs:

- Onset of diabetes mellitus at age 40 years or older
- Diagnosis of diabetes for <5 years
- Normal weight or overweight
- Fasting blood glucose ≤200 mg/dL
- <40 units of insulin required per day
- Normal renal and hepatic function

Other Antidiabetic Agents

Exenatide (Byetta) and liraglutide (Victoza) are in a classification of antidiabetic drugs known as *incretin mimetics* (also called *glucagon-like peptide-1 agonists* or *GLP-1 agonists*). These drugs improve beta-cell responsiveness, which improves glucose control in people with type 2 diabetes mellitus. The actions of exenatide and liraglutide are to enhance insulin secretion, increase beta-cell responsiveness, suppress glucagon secretion, slow gastric emptying, and reduce food intake. Exenatide and liraglutide are not a substitute for insulin and should not be administered to patients with type 1 diabetes mellitus, diabetic ketoacidosis, severe renal dysfunction, or severe GI disease. Common adverse effects that occur with exenatide include headache, dizziness, jitteriness, nausea, vomiting, and diarrhea. Exenatide is administered by injectable prefilled pens in twice-a-day dosing and has significantly improved A_{1c} levels and weight loss in many patients. Liraglutide is given subcutaneously once a day.

Nursing Process
Patient-Centered Collaborative Care

Oral Antidiabetics

Assessment

- Identify drugs patient currently takes. Aspirin, alcohol, sulfonamides, oral contraceptives, and monoamine oxidase inhibitors (MAOIs) increase hypoglycemic effect; a decrease in oral antidiabetic drug may be needed. Glucocorticoids (cortisone), thiazide diuretics, and estrogen increase blood glucose.
- Note vital signs and blood glucose levels. Report abnormal findings.
- Determine patient's knowledge of diabetes mellitus and use of oral antidiabetics.

Nursing Diagnoses

- Risk for injury related to side effect of visual disturbances
- Imbalanced nutrition, more than body requirements, related to excessive food intake
- Deficient knowledge related to lack of exposure to teaching about taking adequate food with oral antidiabetics

Planning

- Patient's blood sugar will be within normal serum levels (70 to 110 mg/dL).
- Patient will adhere to prescribed diet, blood testing, and drug.
- Patient will demonstrate knowledge of oral hypoglycemics and their importance.

Nursing Interventions

- Determine vital signs. Oral antidiabetics increase cardiac function and oxygen consumption, which can lead to cardiac dysrhythmias.
- Administer oral antidiabetics with food to minimize gastric upset.
- Monitor blood glucose levels, and report changes. Reference value is 60 to 100 mg/dL for blood glucose and 70 to 110 mg/dL for serum glucose.
- Prepare a teaching plan based on patient's knowledge of health problems, diet, and drug therapy.

Patient Teaching

General

- Advise patient that hypoglycemic (insulin) reaction can occur when taking an oral hypoglycemic drug, especially sulfonylureas. This drug stimulates the release of insulin from beta cells of the pancreas. Oral antidiabetics are not insulin. Normally, patients with diabetes mellitus type 1 do not have functioning beta cells and should not take oral antidiabetics, only insulin. Sulfonylureas are prescribed for patients with diabetes mellitus type 2.
- Teach patient to recognize symptoms of hypoglycemic reaction (headache, nervousness, sweating, tremors, and rapid pulse) and hyperglycemic reaction (thirst, increased urine output, sweet, fruity breath odor).
- Explain that insulin might be needed instead of oral antidiabetic drug during stress, surgery, or serious infection. Blood glucose levels are usually elevated during stressful times.

- Tell patient about necessity for compliance to diet and drug.
- Advise patient to carry MedicAlert card, tag, or bracelet indicating health problem and antidiabetic dosage.

Self-Administration

- Teach patient how to check blood glucose level with a glucometer. Patient should record and report abnormal results.

Side Effects

- Advise patient to report side effects such as vomiting, diarrhea, and rash.

Diet

- Caution patient not to ingest alcohol with antidiabetic drugs to avoid hypoglycemic reaction.
- Advise patient taking oral antidiabetics to eat prescribed diet on schedule. Delaying or missing a meal can cause hypoglycemia.
- Explain use of orange juice, sugar-containing drinks, or hard candy when hypoglycemic reaction begins. Explain importance of reporting such problems to health care provider.
- Direct patient to take oral antidiabetics with food to decrease gastric irritation.

Cultural Considerations

- Respect patient's cultural beliefs and alternative methods for treating diabetes and elevated blood glucose levels. Discuss safety of methods and use of oral antidiabetic drugs to correct problem (an interpreter may be necessary). If patient takes an oral antidiabetic drug to decrease blood glucose level, emphasize importance of checking blood glucose levels daily or as indicated. Hypoglycemic reaction can result from increased doses of oral antidiabetic agents and insufficient dietary intake.

Evaluation

- Evaluate effectiveness of drug therapy by noting if blood glucose levels are within accepted range.
- Determine patient knowledge of diabetic regimen.

Pramlintide acetate (Symlin) is another antidiabetic agent in a classification called *amylin analogue*, approved by the FDA for adults with type 1 and type 2 diabetes mellitus. The primary purpose of pramlintide is to improve postprandial glucose control in diabetic patients who are using insulin but are unable to achieve and maintain glucose control. The actions of pramlintide are to suppress glucagon secretion, slow gastric emptying, and modulate appetite by inducing satiety. Suppression of glucagon secretion reduces postprandial hepatic glucose for approximately 3 hours. By slowing gastric emptying, the absorption rate of glucose is reduced. Satiety promotes reduced food intake. Common adverse effects include dizziness, anorexia, nausea, vomiting, and fatigue. Pramlintide is administered by subcutaneous injection before meals in the abdomen or thigh; it is never given in the arm.

Hyperglycemic Drugs

Glucagon

Glucagon is a hyperglycemic hormone secreted by alpha cells of the islets of Langerhans in the pancreas. Glucagon increases blood sugar by stimulating glycogenolysis (glycogen breakdown) in the liver. It protects the body cells, especially those in the brain and retina, by providing the nutrients and energy needed to maintain body function.

Glucagon is available for parenteral use (subQ, IM, and IV). It is used to treat insulin-induced hypoglycemia when other methods of providing glucose are not available. For example, the patient may be semiconscious or unconscious and unable to ingest sugar-containing products. Patients with diabetes who are prone to severe hypoglycemic reactions (insulin shock) should keep glucagon in the home, and family members should be taught how to administer subQ or IM injections during an emergency hypoglycemic reaction. The blood glucose level begins to increase within 10 minutes after administration.

Diazoxide

Oral diazoxide (Proglycem), which is chemically related to thiazide diuretics, increases blood sugar by inhibiting insulin release from the beta cells and stimulating release of epinephrine (Adrenalin) from the adrenal medulla. This drug is not indicated for hypoglycemic reaction; rather, it is used to treat chronic hypoglycemia caused by hyperinsulinism due to islet cell cancer or hyperplasia. The parenteral form of diazoxide (Hyperstat) is prescribed for malignant hypertension. Hypotension does not usually occur with oral diazoxide.

Diazoxide has a long half-life and is highly protein-bound. Its onset of action is 1 hour, and the duration of action is 8 hours. Most of the drug is excreted unchanged in urine.

KEY WEBSITES

Insulin Lispro Injection: *www.humalog.com*
Lantus: *www.lantus.com*
Diabetes: *www.diabetes.org*

CRITICAL THINKING CASE STUDY

TC, a 32-year-old patient, was diagnosed with diabetes mellitus after the birth of her first child; her blood sugar level was 180 mg/dL. Her serum glucose level has been maintained within the normal range with metformin (Glucophage) 500 mg/day.

1. Why was TC, at 32 years of age, taking an oral antidiabetic drug instead of insulin?
2. Metformin is indicated for what type of diabetes mellitus? When should metformin not be taken?
3. Why should TC monitor her blood sugar using a home glucometer?

Two years later, TC became pregnant again. Metformin was discontinued, and Humulin N insulin 25 units was prescribed. Since the birth of her second child, she has remained on Humulin N 25 units/day.

4. Give a possible reason why the health care provider changed the antidiabetic drug to insulin when TC became pregnant.
5. Humulin N is similar to what other type of insulin? How do these two types differ?
6. Give the onset, peak, and duration of action for Humulin N insulin. When is an insulin reaction most likely to occur with Humulin N?
7. What are the pros and cons for TC to receive Humulin 70/30 insulin?
8. What are the signs and symptoms of hypoglycemic reaction?
9. What should be included in patient teaching?

TC asks the nurse if she can take metformin again instead of insulin, because she is eating the "right foods."

10. What is the nurse's best response?

NCLEX STUDY QUESTIONS

1. A patient is diagnosed with type 2 diabetes mellitus. The nurse is aware that which statement is true about this patient?
   a. Patient is most likely a teenager.
   b. Patient is most likely a child younger than 10 years.
   c. Heredity and obesity are major causative factors.
   d. Viral infections contribute most to disease development.
2. Antidiabetic drugs are designed to control signs and symptoms of diabetes mellitus. The nurse primarily expects a decrease in which?
   a. Blood glucose
   b. Fat metabolism
   c. Glycogen storage
   d. Protein mobilization
3. A patient is to receive insulin before breakfast, and the time of breakfast tray delivery is variable. The nurse knows that which insulin should not be administered until the breakfast tray has arrived and the patient is ready to eat?
   a. Humulin N
   b. lispro (Humalog)
   c. glargine (Lantus)
   d. Humulin R
4. A patient is receiving a daily dose of Humulin N insulin at 7:30 AM. The nurse expects the peak effect of this drug to occur at which time?
   a. 8:15 AM
   b. 10:30 AM
   c. 5:00 PM
   d. 11:00 PM
5. A patient is prescribed glipizide (Glucotrol). The nurse knows that which side effects and adverse effects may be expected? (Select all that apply.)
   a. Tachypnea
   b. Tachycardia
   c. Increased alertness
   d. Increased weight gain
   e. Visual disturbances
   f. Hunger
6. A nurse is teaching a patient how to recognize symptoms of hypoglycemia. Which symptoms should be included in the teaching? (Select all that apply.)
   a. Headache
   b. Nervousness
   c. Bradycardia
   d. Sweating
   e. Thirst
   f. Sweet breath odor
7. A patient is newly diagnosed with type 1 diabetes mellitus and requires daily insulin injections. Which instruction should the nurse include in the teaching of insulin administration?
   a. Teach family members how to administer glucagon by injection when the patient has a hyperglycemic reaction.
   b. Instruct the patient about the necessity for compliance with prescribed insulin therapy.
   c. Teach the patient that hypoglycemic reactions are more likely to occur at the onset of action time.
   d. Instruct the patient in the care and handling of the insulin container and syringe.

Answers: 1, c; 2, a; 3, b; 4, c; 5, b, e, f; 6, a, b, d; 7, b.

UNIT XVIII

Reproductive and Gender-Related Agents

This unit comprises six chapters that focus on reproductive and gender-related drugs. Chapters 53, 54, 55, and 56 address agents specifically associated with female health and disorders. Drugs used throughout the female reproductive cycle, including pregnancy and preterm labor, are comprehensively discussed in Chapter 53, Female Reproductive Cycle I: Pregnancy and Preterm Labor Drugs. Chapter 54, Female Reproductive Cycle II: Labor, Delivery, and Preterm Neonatal Drugs, covers labor and delivery. Chapter 55, Postpartum and Newborn Drugs, focuses on the pharmacology of the postpartum and neonatal period. Chapter 56, Drugs for Women's Reproductive Health and Menopause, details the variety of oral contraceptive products and the drugs used to treat menopausal discomforts. Chapter 57, Drugs for Men's Health and Reproductive Disorders, describes androgens and anabolic steroids, antiandrogens, and other drugs related to male reproductive health and disorders. Chapter 58, Drugs for Disorders in Women's Health, Infertility, and Sexually Transmitted Infections, concludes this unit with a discussion of drugs used to treat specific reproductive health issues, including endometriosis, premenstrual syndrome, infertility, and sexually transmitted infections.

FEMALE REPRODUCTIVE PROCESSES

The uterus is a pear-shaped, hollow, very muscular organ located in the pelvic cavity between the rectum and the bladder; it is connected to the vagina by the cervix (Figure XVIII-1). Three distinct layers compose the uterine wall: the outer layer (perimetrium); the muscular middle layer (myometrium); and the inner mucosal layer (endometrium).

The myometrium is a network of involuntary (smooth) muscles divided into three layers, with the muscles of each layer configured in different patterns. For example, the outer muscles are arranged longitudinally to assist with cervical effacement (thinning and shortening) and to expel the fetus at the time of delivery. Muscles in the middle layer are arranged in a figure-8 design. These muscles are extremely important in the control of bleeding (hemostasis). Blood vessels are threaded throughout these muscles, and when a contraction occurs, the vessels are compressed, creating a hemostatic effect. Circular muscle fibers are found in the area of the internal os and help control its sphincter. These circular muscles keep the fetus contained in the uterus for the normal gestational period. It is these muscles that stretch (dilate) the cervix to a diameter of 10 cm during labor. When all three muscle layers work together during labor, contractions cause cervical dilation and descent and delivery of the infant.

The Menstrual Cycle

The reproductive cycle is hormonally controlled by interactions between the endocrine and reproductive systems. The hypothalamus secretes gonadotropin-releasing hormone (Gn-RH), which stimulates the anterior pituitary gland to synthesize and release follicle-stimulating hormone (FSH) and luteinizing hormone (LH). These gonadotropins stimulate the ovaries to produce estrogen and progesterone, respectively.

In most women, the menstrual cycle lasts 28 days (range of 22 to 34 days). The ovarian hormones estrogen and progesterone regulate the cycle, which has three ovarian phases: follicular, ovulatory, and luteal. Endometrial phases occur simultaneously with these ovarian phases.

The *follicular phase* occurs during days 1 to 14 of the cycle. Days 1 to 6 of this period constitute the menstrual phase, and days 7 to 14 constitute the proliferative phase. During the total 14-day period, FSH increases and follicles begin to mature within the ovary. One graafian follicle from the group matures and swells by days 10 to 13, ruptures on day 14, and releases the ovum to the fallopian tube. The *ovulatory phase* occurs on day 14 when the ovum is released. The *luteal phase* occurs from days 15 to 28 and includes the secretory phase of the endometrial cycle. During this period, estrogen and progesterone are produced by the ovarian corpus luteum (the ruptured graafian follicle), reaching peak levels 8 days into the phase. Changes occur in the endometrium for optimal implantation of a fertilized ovum. FSH and LH levels decrease, mediated by dopamine, norepinephrine, and serotonin. Estrogen and progesterone are withdrawn immediately before menstruation, and the endometrial prostaglandin level increases. The cycle begins anew with the follicular phase. In cycles that are nonovulatory, hormonal secretion of estrogen, FSH, and LH is erratic; there is also an alteration in the usual amount of progesterone. These physiologic alterations become the basis for planning and implementing pharmacologic interventions.

MALE REPRODUCTIVE PROCESSES

There are three male reproductive processes: spermatogenesis, or sperm production; regulation of male sexual functioning; and sexual intercourse.

Male Reproductive Anatomy and Physiology

The anatomy of the male sexual organs is depicted in Figure XVIII-2. The external reproductive organs include the penis, the scrotum, and the testes. The penis consists of three cylindrical bodies of erectile tissue: two corpora cavernosa and the corpus spongiosum. With sexual excitement, the vascular spaces fill with blood to produce an erection (Figure XVIII-3).

The scrotum has two compartments, each of which holds a testis, epididymis, and spermatic cord. The spermatic cord supports the testis and includes the vas deferens, blood vessels, nerves, and muscle fibers.

Each testis contains seminiferous tubules in which spermatogenesis occurs. The sperm then move into the epididymis. This leads into the vas deferens, the source of about 20% of ejaculate, or semen. On either side of the prostate gland, a seminal vesicle empties seminal fluid into the ampulla. Seminal fluid contains fructose to provide energy for the sperm, prostaglandins, fibrinogen, and a sperm-activating factor.

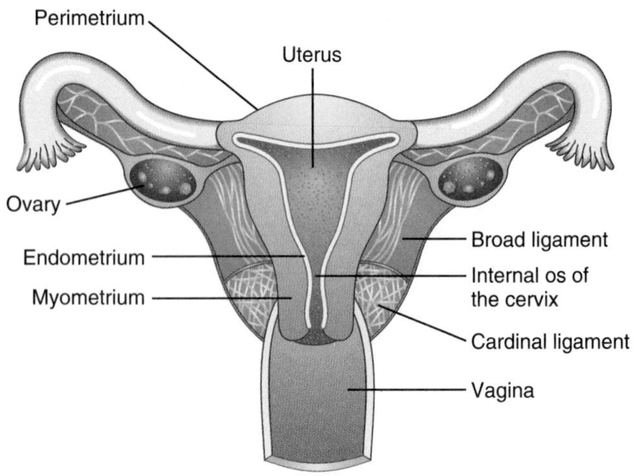

FIGURE XVIII-1 Anatomy of the female reproductive system.

The contents of the ampulla and the seminal vesicles empty into an ejaculatory duct that leads through the body of the prostate to empty into the urethra. Prostatic fluid, which constitutes about 20% of semen, empties from the prostate gland into the ejaculatory duct. The urethra carries semen to its distal end. The urethral glands along the length of the urethra and the bulbourethral glands near the prostatic end of the urethra supply the urethra with mucus. The bulbourethral glands secrete alkaline preejaculatory fluid to protect sperm from the acidity of the urethra.

Hormonal Regulation of Male Reproductive Functioning and Spermatogenesis

Gn-RH from the hypothalamus stimulates the anterior pituitary gland to secrete two major gonadotropins, LH and FSH, in both men and women. LH stimulates the interstitial Leydig cells of the testes to mature and produce testosterone. There is a direct relationship between the amount of circulating LH and the amount of testosterone produced. Testosterone is also produced to a lesser extent in the adrenal cortex and in the ovaries of women.

In men, FSH stimulates the Sertoli cells to begin conversion of spermatids into mature sperm. In addition, the Sertoli cells are stimulated to secrete estrogens, which may promote spermatogenesis. For spermatogenesis to be complete, testosterone must be secreted simultaneously by the Leydig cells and diffused into the seminiferous tubules.

Testosterone is the precursor of two classes of sex steroids: 5-alpha-reduced androgens and estrogens. The net effect of endogenous androgens is the sum of the effects of the 5-alpha-reduced metabolite dihydrotestosterone and its estrogen derivative, estradiol. Most testosterone is loosely bound by plasma protein and circulates for 15 to 30 minutes before it is fixed to target tissues or metabolized. Most testosterone fixed to target cells is then converted to its active form, dihydrotestosterone.

The rate of testosterone production is controlled by a negative feedback loop. With increased testosterone, the hypothalamus decreases production of Gn-RH (Figure XVIII-4). With sperm production, the Sertoli cells release a hormone called *inhibin,* which suppresses FSH production by the anterior

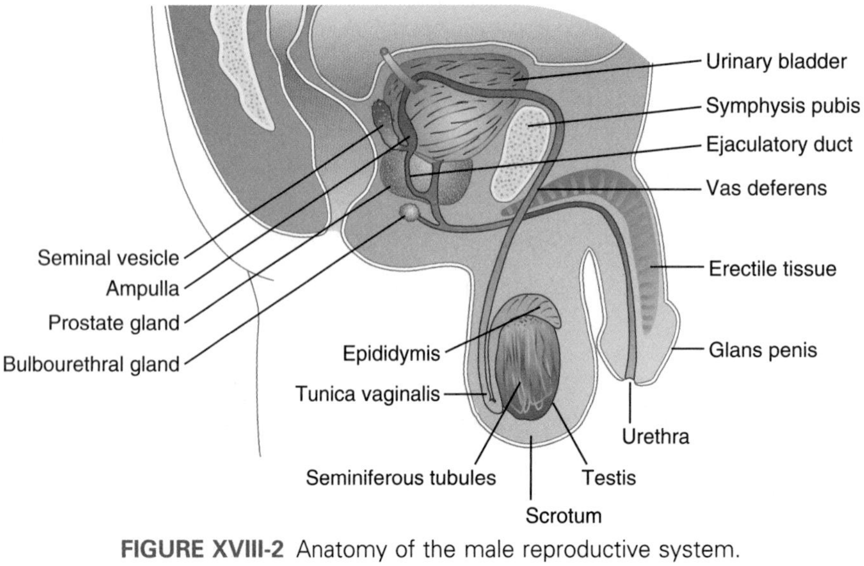

FIGURE XVIII-2 Anatomy of the male reproductive system.

pituitary gland, maintaining a constant rate of spermatogenesis. It is not known how, before puberty, the brain stimulates the hypothalamus to begin Gn-RH secretion, but if the brain is not intact, this may not occur.

Sexual Function

The human sexual response cycle consists of five phases: desire, excitement, plateau, orgasm, and resolution. Sexual desire is the stimulus that causes an individual to initiate or be receptive to sexual activity. During the excitement phase, the man experiences penile erection. Men are incapable of engaging in sexual intercourse without this arousal. The plateau phase is characterized by genital enlargement, mucous secretion, generalized muscle tension, hyperventilation, tachycardia, and increased blood pressure. During the orgasmic phase, the vas deferens, seminal vesicles, ejaculatory duct, and penile urethra contract three or four times over a few seconds, which causes the man to ejaculate. During resolution, there is a refractory period in which pelvic vasocongestion declines and generalized muscle relaxation takes place.

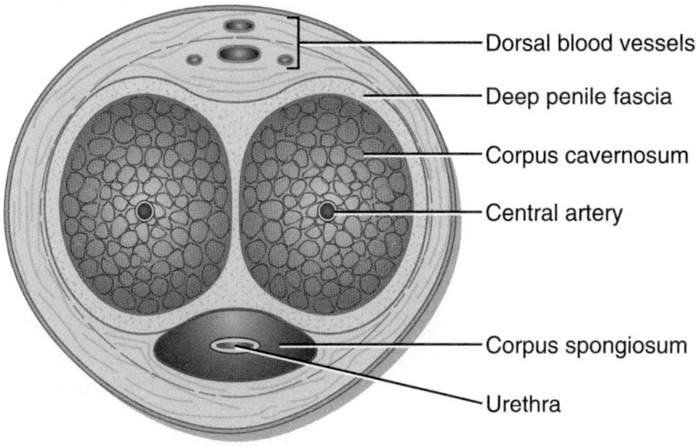

FIGURE XVIII-3 Erectile tissue of the penis.

PROCESS OF FERTILIZATION

Fertilization, or conception, occurs when a sperm penetrates an ovum, usually in the distal third of the fallopian tube.

In a single ejaculation, between 200 and 400 million spermatozoa are deposited in the vagina. Sperm move up the female reproductive tract using the flagellar motion of their tails. It takes an average of 4 to 6 hours for the sperm to reach the distal fallopian tube. Semen contains prostaglandins that may enhance uterine motility to facilitate sperm migration. The ciliary action of the fallopian tubes enhances migration of the ovum to the uterus and of sperm toward the ovary.

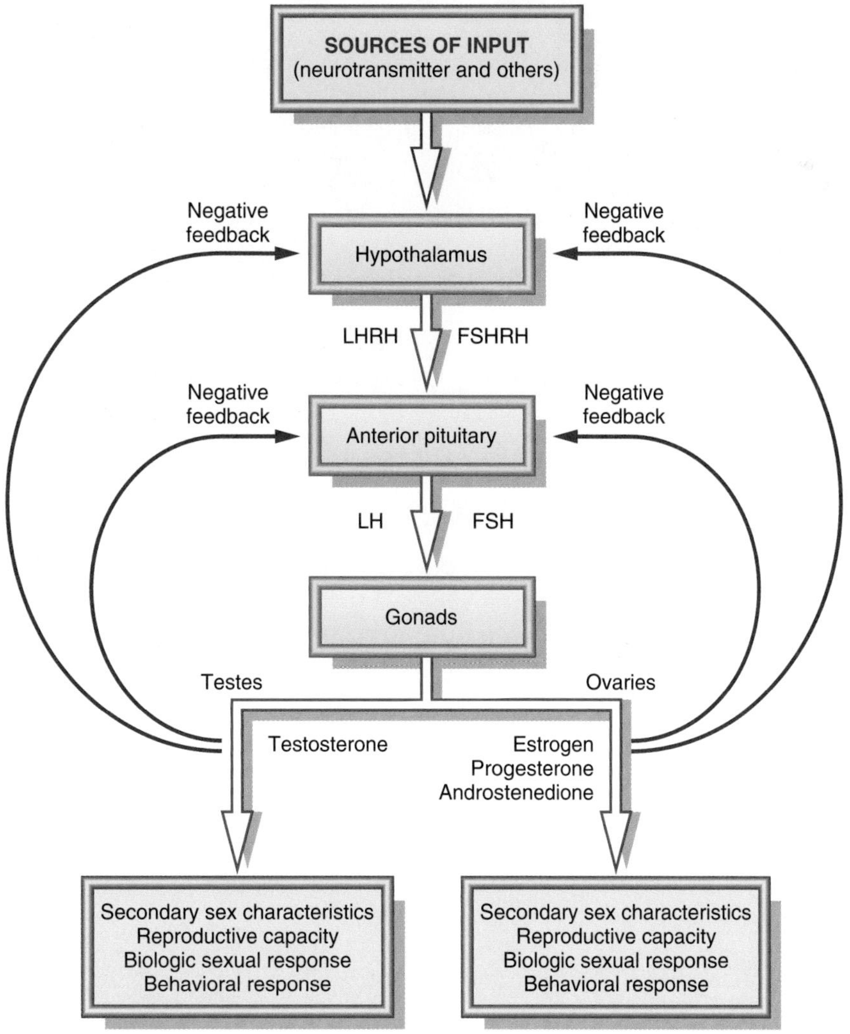

FIGURE XVIII-4 Hypothalamic-pituitary-gonadal feedback loops.

Uterine enzymes capacitate the sperm by altering their glycoprotein coat. In an acrosomal reaction, the sperm release the enzyme hyaluronidase, which breaks through the outer layer of the ovum. The moment one sperm penetrates the ovum, a chemical reaction occurs that blocks other sperm from entering. Cellular division begins immediately in what is now called the *zygote,* or fertilized egg.

After 3 days, the zygote enters the uterus. It has now differentiated into an inner solid mass of cells, the blastocyst, and an outer layer, the trophoblast. Progesterone secreted by the corpus luteum of the ovary maintains a favorable uterine environment to nourish the blastocyst until implantation in the uterine lining occurs. The blastocyst develops into the embryo and the amniotic membrane, whereas the trophoblast develops into the chorionic membrane and the fetal side of the placenta. The maternal portion of the placenta develops under the site of the blastocyst's implantation. The placenta is the structure through which oxygen, nutrients, and metabolic wastes pass between the maternal and fetal circulations for the duration of pregnancy. The placenta begins to function by the fourth week of pregnancy. Within the first 8 weeks of pregnancy, organ systems are differentiated, and it is during this period that the fetus is most vulnerable to teratogens. Growth of the fetus throughout pregnancy depends on adequate oxygenation and nutrition, the metabolic environment, freedom from infection, and integrity of the mother's reproductive tract.

CHAPTER

53

Female Reproductive Cycle I: Pregnancy and Preterm Labor Drugs

Robin Webb Corbett and Laura K. Williford Owens

evolve WEBSITE

http://evolve.elsevier.com/KeeHayes/pharmacology/

- Animations
- Content Updates
- Key Points
- Review Questions for the NCLEX® Examination
- References from the Textbook
- Unfolding Case Studies

OBJECTIVES

- Explain potential health-promoting and detrimental effects of substances ingested by the patient during the prenatal period.
- Describe the drugs that alter uterine muscle contractility.
- Discuss drug therapy used during preterm labor to decrease the incidence or severity of neonatal respiratory dysfunction.
- Compare systemic and regional medications for pain control during labor.
- Describe the drugs used in gestational hypertension.
- Describe the nursing process, including patient teaching, associated with the drugs used during pregnancy and preterm labor.

OUTLINE

KEY TERMS

PHYSIOLOGY OF PREGNANCY

Because pregnancy is a change in the normal physiology of the body, the normal and expected pharmacokinetics and pharmacodynamics of medications also change. Changes in drug action during pregnancy include (1) effect of circulating steroid hormones on the liver's metabolism of drugs; (2) reduced gastrointestinal motility and increased gastric pH; (3) increased glomerular filtration rate and increased renal perfusion, resulting in more rapid renal excretion of drugs; (4) expanded maternal circulating blood volume, resulting in dilution of drugs; and (5) alteration in the clearance of drugs in later pregnancy, resulting in a decrease in serum and tissue concentrations of drugs. Because of alterations in the normal physiology of the body, medications should not be ordered in lower doses with longer intervals between doses because of the possibility of subtherapeutic serum and tissue concentrations.

Other factors, such as late pregnancy and labor, can alter the half-lives of some medications. Antibiotics and barbiturates are examples of medications that have shorter half-lives during pregnancy. In contrast to later pregnancy, labor can actually increase the half-life of some medications (e.g., analgesics, hypnotics, antibiotics); it is believed that drug clearance decreases as a result of transient reduced blood flow associated with uterine contractions when the patient is in a supine position. There is also concern about the effects of certain disease states on medication during pregnancy. Disorders like diabetes mellitus and gestational hypertension may result in decreased renal perfusion and subsequent drug accumulation.

The placenta plays an important role in drug use and metabolism. It was once thought that the placenta played a barrier role, but it is now known that the placenta has an important function as the organ of exchange for numerous substances, including medications. It allows some substances to transfer quickly or slowly between mother and fetus, depending on variables such as (1) maternal and fetal blood flow; (2) molecular weight of the substance (low–molecular-weight substances cross more readily than do high–molecular-weight substances; most medications have a low molecular weight, so they readily cross the placenta); (3) degree of ionization of the drug molecule (the more ionized the molecule, the less readily it crosses the placenta); (4) degree of protein-binding (highly bound drugs do not cross readily); (5) metabolic activity of the placenta (the metabolic activity can biotransform molecules into active metabolites that can affect the fetus); and (6) maternal dose.

Guidelines for medication administration during pregnancy must include determination that the benefits of prescribing a drug outweigh potential short- or long-term risks to the maternal-fetal system. Careful selection and monitoring for the minimum effective dose for the shortest interval in the therapeutic range are required. Consideration must be given to alterations related to the physiologic changes of pregnancy.

Liver metabolism of medications is much slower in the fetus as a result of immaturity of the liver. Therefore, drug metabolism is slower in the fetus, which can cause more evident or longer drug effects than on the mother. The degree of fetal exposure to a drug and its breakdown products are more important to fetal outcome than the rate at which the drug is transported to the fetus.

The mechanisms by which drugs cross the placenta are analogous to the way in which drugs infiltrate breast tissue. Lactation results in increased blood flow to the breasts, and drugs accumulate in adipose breast tissue through simple diffusion. Long-term effects on infants from drugs in breast milk are unknown, but medications that accumulate in breast milk are known, and the breastfeeding patient should be alerted to the potential accumulation.

Despite prenatal education, public service announcements, and information conveyed through the media, use of legal and illicit drugs by pregnant patients continues. Additionally, health care providers may prescribe drugs for maternal disorders that indirectly affect the fetus. However, it is important to note that most drugs required by pregnant patients can be used safely. It is estimated that half the medications taken by pregnant patients are over-the-counter (OTC) drugs. The drugs most commonly ingested during pregnancy are iron supplements and vitamins, antiemetics, antacids, stool softeners, nasal decongestants, mild analgesics, and antibiotics. Pregnant patients should be discouraged from using OTC medications until they consult with their health care provider or pharmacist.

Drugs conclusively determined to be safe for the embryo are limited in number. Clinical trials can be resources for reliable drug information; however, it is unethical to test for the safety and efficacy of medications in pregnant patients. Animal studies are required during drug testing, but the information obtained from such studies is difficult to extrapolate to humans. Case reports used for such information can be of limited value because they usually present isolated occurrences. A commonly used source of information about drug safety in pregnancy is the U.S. Food and Drug Administration's (FDA) category system. The categories were created to assist with safe prescribing and informed counseling of the pregnant patient requiring medication.

There are many known **teratogens** (substances that cause developmental abnormalities). Timing, dose, and duration of exposure are of crucial importance in determining the teratogenicity of a given drug. In humans, the teratogenic period begins 2 weeks after conception. During the first 2 weeks, the embryo is not susceptible to teratogenesis. At this time of development, exposure to teratogens may result in either death of the embryo or minor cellular damage without congenital birth defects. From 2 gestational weeks through the next 10 weeks is the period of organogenesis (development of major structures and organs). Table 53-1 shows adverse effects of selected illicit substances commonly used during pregnancy.

TABLE 53-1 GENERAL ADVERSE EFFECTS OF SUBSTANCES COMMONLY ABUSED DURING PREGNANCY

SUBSTANCE	MATERNAL EFFECTS	FETAL EFFECTS*
Alcohol (high risk: 6 oz or more/d)	1 oz (2 drinks) absolute alcohol 2 times/wk: increased risk for spontaneous abortion (2-4 times)	Fetal alcohol syndrome (FAS): mild to moderate mental retardation, altered facial features, growth retardation, low birth weight, small head circumference, hypotonia, and poor motor coordination. Full FAS seen only in some children; others display only fetal alcohol effect (FAE).
Caffeine	2 cups increase epinephrine concentrations after 30 min and decrease intervillous blood flow with potential for spontaneous abortion (dosage and gestational period related)	Excess consumption (>6-8 cups/d) likely toxic to embryo. No evidence of teratogenicity
Cocaine	48-h clearance via urine. Increased incidence of spontaneous abortion in first trimester. Continued use or sporadic use related to premature delivery and abruptio placentae secondary to placental vasoconstriction and hyperextension	4-5 d clearance time via urine of newborn because of liver immaturity and lack of cholinesterase. Intrauterine growth retardation, decreased head circumference, intrauterine cerebral infarction. No true withdrawal syndrome, but increased irritability, hyperreflexia, and tremulousness. Deficient organization and interactive abilities. By month 4, still exhibits hypertonicity, tremulousness, and impaired motor development. By month 6, effects may appear self-limiting, but long-term research is needed.
Heroin	First-trimester spontaneous abortion, premature delivery, inadequate maternal calorie and protein intake	Neonatal meconium aspiration syndrome; decreased weight and length through postnatal month 9 (weight and length catch up by month 12); smaller head circumference (with no catch-up); impaired interactive abilities (hard to console and engage); inconsistent behavioral responses; increased tremulousness and irritability
Marijuana	Heavy use (5 or more marijuana cigarettes per week): shortened gestation (<37 wk); may hasten delivery through uterine stimulation	No higher incidence of serious birth defects caused solely by marijuana. Higher incidence of meconium passage during labor
Tobacco/nicotine	Degenerative placental lesions with areas of poor oxygen exchange; higher incidence of abruptio placentae; placenta previa, vaginal bleeding during pregnancy; possible PROM; possible amnionitis; less likely to choose to breastfeed	Short stature, smaller head and arm circumferences; no increase in mortality rate or congenital anomalies (some evidence of increased oral clefts); increased respiratory infections beyond perinatal period; possible shorter attention span beyond perinatal period
Methadone	If taken before pregnancy, will need to slow detoxification during pregnancy and decrease dose 5 mg every 2 wk. Do not detoxify before week 14 of gestation because of increased risk for spontaneous abortion	Smaller weight and length through postnatal month 9 (catch up on weight and length by month 12); smaller head circumference (no catch-up); withdrawal-induced fetal distress if mother detoxifies after 32 weeks' gestation
Barbiturates	CNS depression; lethargy; sleepiness; subtle mood alterations and impaired judgment/fine-motor skills for 24 h No known inhibitory effect on uterine tone or contractility. Selective anticonvulsant activity without anesthesia effects may warrant use in pregnancy for seizure disorders Active labor with imminent delivery is a contraindication, because no antagonist drug is available	Rapidly cross placenta; with excessive use/high doses cause CNS depression, leading to respiratory depression, hyperactivity, and decreased sucking reflex
Tranquilizers	Dose-dependent; toxic reactions include ataxia, syncope, vertigo, and drowsiness; control of acute eclamptic seizures during labor	Benzodiazepine (diazepam [Valium]) use in first trimester not associated with oral clefts or other anomalies. Chronic third trimester or labor exposure in high doses associated with hypotonia, hypothermia, hyperbilirubinemia, and poor sucking reflex. Effects may be enhanced if systemic analgesics also given to mother. Fetal effects are prolonged.

*Children with prenatal drug exposure scored significantly lower on measures of language, school readiness skills, impulse control, and visual attention span/sequencing at age 5 years when compared with nondrug-exposed children from a comparable environment.
CNS, Central nervous system; *d,* day; *h,* hour; *min,* minute; *PROM,* premature rupture of fetal membranes; *wk,* week; <, less than; >, greater than.

THERAPEUTIC DRUG AND HERBAL USE IN PREGNANCY

The most common indications for use of medications during pregnancy are nutritional supplementation with iron, vitamins, and minerals and treatment of nausea and vomiting, gastric acidity, and mild discomforts, but caution must be exercised (Herbal Alert 53-1).

HERBAL ALERT 53-1

Pregnancy

Herbal preparations are not generally recommended during pregnancy. In particular, the following herbs should be avoided:

- Feverfew and sage are emmenagogues that stimulate blood flow in the uterus.
- Kava kava decreases platelets.
- Dong quai, garlic, and gingko biloba increase bleeding when used with anticoagulants.
- Ginseng may decrease the action of anticoagulants.
- St. John's wort has mutagenic effects on cells of the developing embryo and fetus.

Iron

During pregnancy, approximately twice the normal amount of iron is needed to meet fetal and maternal daily requirements: 27 mg/day during pregnancy compared with 18 mg/day for nonpregnant patients 19 to 30 years of age. Supplementation with iron is not generally necessary until the second trimester, when the fetus begins to store iron; the goal is to prevent maternal iron-deficiency anemia, not to supply the fetus. The fetus is adequately supplied through the placenta, although the mother is deficient. Greatest iron demand occurs in the third trimester: 22.4 mg/day compared with 6.4 mg/day and 18.8 mg/day for the first and second trimesters, respectively.

Although a normal diet generally provides the 18-mg recommended daily allowance (RDA) of iron for nonpregnant patients, nonanemic pregnant patients are usually instructed to supplement using a dosage that provides 60 mg of elemental iron; anemic patients should receive 120 mg of elemental iron. The elemental iron content of the most common iron salts includes ferrous sulfate 20% (300 mg of ferrous sulfate is equivalent to 60 mg elemental iron), exsiccated ferrous sulfate 30%, ferrous gluconate 12%, and ferrous fumarate 33%. The estimated net iron cost of pregnancy is approximately 800 to 1000 mg. This iron cost is calculated as 250 mg basal losses + 320 mg deposition in fetal and placental tissue + 500 mg increased hemoglobin mass + 350 mg iron loss in blood associated with delivery. Patients are advised to continue supplements for 6 weeks postpartum.

Pregnant patients generally have decreased hematocrit early in the third trimester. Those with levels less than 30% will have their supplemental iron dosages increased and complete blood counts with platelet and ferritin measured. In those with true iron-deficiency anemia, response to iron supplementation is usually noted in 5 to 7 days, with a modest reticulocytosis and an increase in hemoglobin in 3 weeks. No teratogenic effects have been reported with physiologic doses. In contrast, increasing evidence has associated prenatal iron supplementation with glucose impairment and hypertension in midpregnancy. Many OTC and prescription iron products (Table 53-2) are available in varying dosages, which differ in the amount of elemental iron contained in the form of iron salts.

TABLE 53-2 IRON PRODUCTS

GENERIC (BRAND)	ROUTE AND DOSAGE	USES AND CONSIDERATIONS
ferrous sulfate (Fer-In-Sol, Feosol, Fero-Gradumet, Mol-Iron, Fer-Iron)	A: PO: 300-600 mg/d in divided doses 325 mg/d sufficient to meet needs of non–iron-deficient pregnant patient; with iron deficiency, administer 325 mg 2-3 times/d	Hematinic; for iron-deficiency anemia; prophylaxis for iron deficiency in pregnancy. Replaces iron stores needed for RBC development Absorption PO is 5%-30% in intestines; therefore GI side effects. Toxic reactions include pallor, hematemesis, shock, cardiovascular collapse, and metabolic acidosis. Contraindicated in patients with hypersensitivity and peptic ulcer. Decreased absorption of tetracycline, penicillamine, and antacids; increased absorption with ascorbic acid; decreased absorption with eggs, milk, coffee, tea. Can reduce availability of zinc from diet Take at bedtime to avoid GI upset. Absorption promoted when taken with orange juice or other vitamin C source. Use straw (elixir); swallow tab/cap whole; take with water on empty stomach. Sit upright 30 min after dose to decrease reflux. Increase fluids, activity, and dietary bulk. Keep out of reach of children Peak reticulocytosis: 5-10 d; hemoglobin values increase: 2-4 wk Pregnancy category: A; PB: UK; $t\frac{1}{2}$: UK; onset: 3-10 d; duration: 3-4 mo
ferrous gluconate (Fergon)	A: PO: 200-600 mg t.i.d.	Same as above
ferrous fumarate (Fumasorb, Femiron, Feostat, Fumerin)	A: PO: 200 mg t.i.d./q.i.d.	Same as above

A, Adult; *cap,* capsule; *d,* day; *GI,* gastrointestinal; *min,* minute; *mo,* month; *PB,* protein-binding; *PO,* by mouth; *q.i.d.,* four times a day; *RBC,* red blood cell; *t½,* half-life; *t.i.d.,* three times a day; *tab,* tablet; *UK,* unknown; *wk,* week.

Adverse Reactions

Common side effects of iron supplements include nausea, constipation, black tarry stools, gastrointestinal irritation, epigastric pain, vomiting, discoloration of urine, and diarrhea.

Nursing Implications

Liquid forms can cause temporary tooth discoloration and therefore should be diluted and administered through a plastic straw. Iron supplements are best absorbed on an empty stomach and when administered with water or juice (concurrent administration of 200 mg ascorbic acid/vitamin C per 30 mg of elemental iron increases the absorption of iron). However, if gastric irritation does occur, administer with food. Iron supplementation may inhibit the absorption of several medications, and appropriate separation of doses should be followed (e.g., iron supplementation should be administered 2 hours before or 4 hours after antacids). Additional examples of medications that may require separation in dose include levodopa, levothyroxine (Levothroid, Synthroid), methyldopa, penicillamine (Cuprimine, Depen), quinolones, and tetracyclines. For the same reasons, do not administer iron with milk, cereal, tea, coffee, or eggs.

Folic Acid

Folic acid supplementation as part of preconception planning improves the outcome of pregnancy. During pregnancy, folic acid (vitamin B_9, folate) is needed in increased amounts. Folic acid deficiency early in pregnancy can result in spontaneous abortion or birth defects, especially neural tube defects (failure of the embryonic neural tube to close properly, leading to spina bifida or skull and brain malformations). Deficiency of folic acid may also contribute to premature birth, low birth weight, and premature separation of the placenta *(abruptio placentae)*. In the United States, approximately 4,000 pregnancies a year are affected by neural tube defects. Controlled clinical trials have demonstrated that folic acid supplementation can reduce this incidence by as much as 50%.

Normally, the RDA for folic acid is 180 mcg, but the United States Preventive Services Task Force recommends that women who are planning pregnancy take a supplement containing 0.4 mg to 0.8 mg of folic acid 1 month before and for the first 2 to 3 months after conception. The American College of Obstetricians and Gynecologists (ACOG) recommends that all women of childbearing age ingest 400 mcg of folic acid daily for birth defect prevention (during pregnancy, the RDA rises to 600 mcg). The reasoning behind the ACOG's recommendation is the high incidence of unplanned and unrecognized pregnancies.

The neural tube closes within the first 4 weeks of pregnancy (18 to 26 days after conception); therefore, it is important that women consume the recommended amounts of folic acid per day. For patients who have had a pregnancy that was affected by a neural tube defect, higher doses of folic acid are recommended: 4 mg starting 1 to 3 months before conception.

The recommended amount should be ingested from folate-enriched foods and supplementation, because the amount of naturally occurring folic acid ingested in foods varies from day to day, and the folic acid from these sources is not well absorbed. Examples of folate-enriched foods are bread, cornmeal, rice, pasta, and cereal.

Adverse Reactions

Side effects of folic acid supplementation are not common but include allergic bronchospasm, rash, pruritus, erythema, and general malaise. Patients should be aware that folic acid supplementation may cause urine to turn more intensely yellow.

Multiple Vitamins

Prenatal vitamin preparations are routinely recommended for pregnant women. These preparations generally supply vitamins A, D, E, C, B complex, B_{12}, iron, calcium, and other minerals. The role of prenatal vitamins in preventing congenital defects (e.g., cleft lip or palate, limb defects) has not been determined.

Inadequate nutrition cannot be rectified through supplements alone; vitamins are used most effectively by the body when taken with meals, and calories and protein are not supplied by supplements.

Megadoses of vitamins and minerals during pregnancy will not improve health and may cause harm to the pregnant patient, the fetus, or both. Large doses of vitamin A can be teratogenic, and excessive ingestion of vitamins D, E, and K may also be toxic.

Drugs for Minor Discomforts of Pregnancy

The average prenatal patient uses three drugs during pregnancy, two of which are vitamin and mineral supplements. Drug ingestion is most likely during the first and third trimesters, when the discomforts of pregnancy tend to be most bothersome. Many complaints associated with pregnancy are related to the gastrointestinal (GI) tract (nausea and vomiting, heartburn, constipation). The etiology of nausea and vomiting is unclear. Physiologically, nausea is purported to be related to increased human chorionic gonadotropin (hCG) levels during pregnancy. Increased progesterone during pregnancy, which relaxes smooth muscle, contributes to heartburn and constipation. The physiologic reason is that elevated female sex hormones during pregnancy change the motility of the GI tract. Additionally, the enlarging uterus displaces the bowel.

Nausea and Vomiting

Nausea and vomiting (morning sickness) during early pregnancy are major complaints for most (about 88%) pregnant patients, but *hyperemesis gravidarum* (severe nausea and vomiting that may require hospitalization for hydration and nutrition) occurs with much lower incidence (1% to 3%). Nonpharmacologic measures to decrease nausea and vomiting include (1) eating crackers, dry toast, or other carbohydrates before rising; (2) avoiding high-fat or highly seasoned foods; (3) eating small, frequent meals; (4) drinking fluids between rather than with meals; (5) drinking apple juice or flat soda between meals; (6) eating a high-protein bedtime snack; (7) stopping smoking; and (8) taking an iron supplement at bedtime. These measures work well for most patients, but if vomiting is severe, fluid replacement and pharmacologic measures may be necessary.

The FDA has approved one drug for morning sickness, doxylamine succinate and pyridoxine hydrocholoride (Diclegis). Antiemetic drug studies often find that affected patients rate even placebo agents as helpful. Table 53-3 lists drugs used for management of nausea and vomiting during pregnancy with their dosages, uses, and considerations.

Many patients may use ginger to help treat nausea and vomiting associated with pregnancy, but there is insufficient evidence of its safety and efficacy during pregnancy. Ingestion of large amounts may act as an abortifacient. Studies suggest that ginger can be safely used in moderation, but as with all medications and herbal supplements, encourage the pregnant patient to discuss use of ginger with her health care provider. Ginger can increase the risk for bleeding, particularly if the patient has a history of bleeding disorder. Research has demonstrated safe dosage levels up to 1,000 mg/day in pregnancy; therefore, pregnant patients are advised not to take more than 1,000 mg/day.

Women who experience nausea and vomiting may experience gastric distress if they are also taking supplemental iron; taking the iron supplement with food or at bedtime, or temporarily suspending therapy, may help. Prenatal vitamins should be taken at the time of day the patient is least likely to experience emesis, because a high incidence of nausea and vomiting is associated with prenatal vitamins. For patients with continued iron-induced gastric distress, many health care providers recommend taking two children's chewable multivitamins with iron. Salting food to taste may help replace vomited chloride; foods rich in potassium and magnesium may also help replace lost nutrients.

Patients whose symptoms persist and who experience weight loss and dehydration may require intravenous (IV) rehydration, including replacement of electrolytes and vitamins. Antiemetic therapy (probably with phenothiazines) may be used, and ondansetron (Zofran) may be administered in severe cases of *hyperemesis gravidarum.*

Heartburn

Heartburn *(pyrosis)* is a burning sensation in the epigastric and sternal regions that occurs with reflux of acidic stomach contents. The incidence of heartburn during pregnancy is common, up to 80%. Pregnant patients experience decreased motility in the GI tract as a result of the normal increase in the hormone **progesterone.** Progesterone also relaxes the cardiac sphincter (the sphincter leading into the stomach from the esophagus, also called the *lower esophageal sphincter),* making reflux activity *(reverse peristalsis)* more likely. Digestion and gastric emptying are slower than in the nonpregnant state. Heartburn is common when a pregnant patient sits or lies down soon after eating a normal meal, only to have her gravid uterus exert upward pressure on her stomach, causing increased reflux activity and the perception of hyperacidity. Heartburn is a disorder of the second and third trimesters of pregnancy.

Nonpharmacologic measures are preferred in the management of heartburn. These include (1) limiting the size of meals; (2) avoiding highly seasoned or greasy foods; (3) avoiding gas-forming foods (e.g., cabbage, onions); (4) eating slowly and chewing thoroughly; (5) avoiding citrus juices; (6) drinking adequate fluids, but not with meals; and (7) avoiding reclining immediately after eating.

Antacids should be considered first-line therapy if the patient does not respond to nonpharmacologic therapy. The antacids of choice for the pregnant patient include nonsystemic low-sodium products (those considered dietetically sodium-free) containing aluminum and magnesium (in the form of hydroxide) in combination. Discourage long-term use or large doses of magnesium antacids, because fetal renal, respiratory, cardiovascular, and muscle problems may result. Sucralfate (Carafate) is likely safe during pregnancy, because the drug is not systemically absorbed. Calcium carbonate antacid preparations may be avoided in pregnancy because of the rebound effect following acid neutralization. TUMS are frequently taken by pregnant patients for heartburn, but because TUMS are calcium based, excessive use may contribute to constipation.

Most patients do not realize that remedies commonly used by nonpregnant patients (e.g., baking soda, antacids such as Alka-Seltzer) can be harmful during pregnancy. Selection of the wrong antacid can result in diarrhea, constipation, or electrolyte imbalance. A combination of nonpharmacologic measures and minimal use of safe antacids should effectively meet the pregnant patient's needs.

Liquid antacids are the preparations most commonly used in pregnancy because of their uniform dissolution, rapid action, and greater activity. Tablets are also acceptable, particularly for convenience, provided they are thoroughly chewed and the patient maintains adequate fluid intake.

Histamine$_2$ receptor antagonists can be used during pregnancy, but only if their use is recommended by a health care provider and initial treatment with antacids has failed. The teratogenicity of these medications is unknown; however, cimetidine (Tagamet), ranitidine (Zantac), famotidine (Pepcid), and nizatidine (Axid) have received the FDA's pregnancy category B rating. H_2 receptor antagonists work by competitively and reversibly binding to the histamine receptors of the parietal cells, causing a reduction in gastric acid secretion. The onset of action is generally in 1 hour and can persist for 6 to 12 hours.

There is even less experience with the use of proton pump inhibitors. These medications work to suppress gastric acid secretion by inhibiting the proton pump on the surface of the parietal cells. With the release of omeprazole (Prilosec OTC), pregnant patients may wonder about its use for heartburn during pregnancy. Encourage patients to discuss the options with their health care provider. Currently, the use of

TABLE 53-3 DRUGS FOR MANAGEMENT OF NAUSEA AND VOMITING DURING PREGNANCY*

GENERIC (BRAND)	ROUTE AND DOSAGE	USES AND CONSIDERATIONS
Vitamin		
pyridoxine (B_6)	PO: Up to 25 mg t.i.d.	Coenzyme for various metabolic functions, including metabolism of proteins, carbohydrates, and fats. Side effects are rare and include headache, nausea, somnolence, and sensory neuropathy Pregnancy category: A; absorbed in jejunum and metabolized primarily in the liver.excreted in urine; t½: 0.5 d; Peak plasma time: 5-6 h (pyridoxine)
Antihistamines		
meclizine (Antivert)	PO: 20-50 mg/d	Blocks CTZ, which acts on vomiting center; available OTC. Sites of action are labyrinth and CNS. Side effects include dizziness, drowsiness, dry mouth and nose, blurred vision, diplopia, urinary retention, urticaria, rash, and headache. Cardiovascular effects include hypotension, palpitations, and tachycardia Contraindicated in patients with hypersensitivity to drug or any component Contraindicated in patients with closed-angle glaucoma Increased effect of alcohol, tranquilizers, and narcotics Pregnancy category: B; metabolized in liver and excreted unchanged in feces and as metabolites in urine. t½: 6 h; Onset: 1-2 h; Duration: 8-24 h
doxylamine (Unisom) (unlabeled use)	PO: 25 mg (½ tab b.i.d.)	Considered mild, available OTC. Competes with free histamine for binding at H_1 receptor sites. If pyrixodine (B_6) 25 mg is not effective, health care provider may suggest docylamine 25 mg and pyridoxine 25 mg t.i.d. (1 tab h.s. and ½ tab in morning and afternoon). May cause sedative effects, thick bronchial secretions, drowsiness, dizziness, headache, constipation, abdominal pain with cramps, blurred vision, decreased coordination, and dry mouth Contraindicated in patients with acute asthma and possibly hypertension, cardiovascular disorders, and hyperthyroidism Caution: Take only under direction of health care provider. Pregnancy category: A; t½:1.25 h; Onset: 1-2 h
Antihistamine Plue Vitamin B_6 Analog		
doxylamine succineate (10 mg)/pyridoxine 10 mg (Diclegis)	PO: 2 tablets h.s. If dose controls symptoms the next day, continue taking 2 tablets at h.s. If symptoms persist into the afternoon of day 2, take 2 tablets at h.s., then 3 tablets starting on day 3 (1 tablet in the morning and 2 tablets at h.s.). If 3 tablets adequately control symptoms on day 4, continue taking 3 tablets daily. If symptoms persist, take 4 tablets starting on day 4 (1 tablet in morning, 1 tablet in mid-afternoon, and 2 tablets at h.s.	Mechanism of action: Unknown Side effects: Somnolence, falls or other accidents in combined use with CNS depressants, including alcohol Warnings/precautions: Contraindicated in women with known hypersensitivity to doxylamine succinate, other ethanolamine derivative antihistamines, and pyridoxine hydrochloride. Monoamine oxidase (MAO) inhibitors intensify and prolong the adverse central nervous system effects of Diclegis. Has anticholinergic properties and should be used with caution in women with asthma, increased intraocular pressure, narrow angle glaucoma, stenosing peptic ulcer, pyloroduodenal obstruction, and urinary bladder-neck obstruction. Nursing mothers should not use. Pregnancy category: A; absorbed in the jejunum and primarily metabolized in the liver; doxylamine is primarily excreted by the kidney; t½: 0.5 h; Peak plasma time: 7-8 h (doxylamine); 5-6 h (pyridoxine)

Continued

TABLE 53-3 DRUGS FOR MANAGEMENT OF NAUSEA AND VOMITING DURING PREGNANCY—cont'd

GENERIC (BRAND)	ROUTE AND DOSAGE	USES AND CONSIDERATIONS
Phenothiazines		
promethazine (Phenergan)	PO/IV/IM/PR: 12.5-25 mg q4-6h PRN	Blocks postsynaptic mesolimbic dopaminergic receptors in brain; exhibits strong alpha-adrenergic blocking effect and depresses release of hypothalamic and hypophyseal hormones; competes with histamine for H_1 receptor Side effects include dizziness, drowsiness, excitation, fatigue, insomnia, photosensitivity reactions, nausea, vomiting, and constipation Contraindicated in patients with hypersensitivity to drug or any component, CNS depression, or coma Use caution in patients with cardiovascular disease; not recommended for subQ or intraarterial administration; injection may contain sulfites, which may cause allergic reaction Pregnancy category: C; t½: 9-16 h; Onset: IM: 20 min; IV: 3-5 min; Duration: 2-6 h
Anticholinergics		
scopolamine	PO/IM/IV/subQ: 0.3-0.65 mg q4-6h	Antagonizes histamine and serotonin Side effects include confusion, drowsiness, headache, fatigue, dry skin, constipation, vomiting, and bloated feeling. Cardiovascular side effects include orthostatic hypotension, ventricular fibrillation, tachycardia, and palpitations Contraindicated in patients with hypersensitivity to drug or any component and those with narrow-angle glaucoma, acute hemorrhage, GI or GU obstruction, tachycardia secondary to cardiac insufficiency, and myasthenia gravis Use with caution in patients with hepatic or renal impairment Pregnancy category: C; Onset: IM: 0.5-1 h; Duration: 4-6 h
Prokinetic Agents		
metoclopramide (Reglan)	PO: 10-15 mg q.i.d. 30 min a.c.	Blocks dopamine receptors in CTZ of CNS; causes enhanced motility and accelerated gastric emptying without stimulating secretions Side effects include restlessness, drowsiness, diarrhea, weakness, and insomnia Contraindicated in patients with hypersensitivity to drug or any component; GI obstruction, perforation, or hemorrhage; pheochromocytoma; or history of seizure disorder Pregnancy category: B; t½: 4-7 h; Onset: 0.5-1 h; Duration: 1-2 h
Other		
trimethobenzamide (Tigan, T-Gen)	200 mg PR q6-8h	Obscure action; may be mediated through CTZ. Does not inhibit direct impulse to vomiting center. Chemically classified as ethanolamine derivative. Contraindicated in patients with cardiac dysrhythmias, narrow-angle glaucoma, asthma, and pyloroduodenal obstruction. Rectal doses of drug are more unpredictable Side effects include drowsiness, headache, blurred vision, diarrhea, depression, hypotension, muscle cramps, allergic reactions, extrapyramidal symptoms, and blood dyscrasias Contraindicated with benzocaine and in patients with hypersensitivity to drug. Use suppository form in neonates or preterm infants Caution: Do not use in patients with acute emesis to avoid masking symptoms Drug interactions with phenothiazines/barbiturates, belladonna Pregnancy category: C; t½: UK; Onset: PO/PR: 10-40 min; IM: 15-35 min; Duration: 3-4 h

TABLE 53-3 DRUGS FOR MANAGEMENT OF NAUSEA AND VOMITING DURING PREGNANCY—cont'd

GENERIC (BRAND)	ROUTE AND DOSAGE	USES AND CONSIDERATIONS
ondansetron (Zofran)	8 mg PO/IV every 8 h	Antiemetic; selective 5-HT_3 receptor antagonist. Blocks serotonin, both peripherally on vagal nerve terminals and centrally in CMZ of CNS Side effects include headache, constipation, diarrhea, malaise/fatigue Contraindicated in patients with hypersensitivity to drug or other selective 5-HT_3 antagonists Caution: Use as scheduled, not PRN. Use with caution in patients who have congenital/medical conditions that cause prolonged QT interval or take medications that prolong QT interval Drug interactions: drugs altering activity of liver enzymes Pregnancy category: B; t½: 3-6 h; Onset: 30 min; Duration: 4-8 h

*Recommendation not implied.
a.c., Before meals; *b.i.d.,* twice a day; *CNS,* central nervous system; *CTZ,* chemoreceptor trigger zone; *d,* day; *GI,* gastrointestinal; *GU,* genitourinary; H_1, histamine$_1$; *h,* hour; *h.s.,* at bedtime; *IM,* intramuscular; *IV,* intravenous; *min,* minute; *OTC,* over-the-counter; *PO,* by mouth; *PR,* by rectum; *PRN,* as needed; *subQ,* subcutaneously; *t½,* half-life; *t.i.d.,* three times a day; *tab,* tablet; *q.i.d.,* four times a day; *UK,* unknown.

omeprazole is limited to cases in which the benefits of therapy far outweigh the risks.

Table 53-4 presents medications for heartburn commonly used during pregnancy.

Constipation

Constipation is a frequent occurrence during pregnancy. Its cause may be related to hormonal changes—specifically progesterone, which decreases GI motility. As with heartburn, nonpharmacologic treatments for constipation should be tried first. These include (1) increased fluid intake, (2) increased dietary fiber intake, and (3) moderate physical exercise. If these methods do not work, treatment is indicated, and the safest agents are bulk-forming preparations containing fiber (e.g., Metamucil), because they are not systemically absorbed. Also, docusate sodium (Colace), a stool softener, would be appropriate as first-line treatment during pregnancy. Agents that should be reserved for occasional use include milk of magnesia, magnesium citrate, lactulose (Constulose, Enulose), sorbitol, bisacodyl (Correctol, Dulcolax), and senna (Senokot, Ex-Lax).

Castor oil should be avoided during pregnancy, because it can stimulate uterine contractions. Mineral oil should also be avoided, because it can reduce the absorption of fat-soluble vitamins like vitamin K. (Low levels of vitamin K in the neonate can result in hemorrhage.)

Pain

Through week 26 of pregnancy, headaches resulting from hormonally induced body changes, sinus congestion, or eye strain are quite common. It is not unusual for the pregnant patient to experience backaches, joint pains, round ligament pain (resulting in mild abdominal aches and twinges), and pain from minor injuries. Nonpharmacologic pain relief measures should be tried initially, including rest; calming environment; relaxation exercises; alteration in routine; mental imagery; ice packs; warm, moist heat; postural changes; correct body mechanics; and changes in footwear.

Acetaminophen

Acetaminophen (Tylenol), a para-aminophenol analgesic, is a pregnancy category B drug. It is the most commonly ingested nonprescription drug during pregnancy. Acetaminophen may be used during all trimesters of pregnancy in therapeutic doses on a short-term basis for its analgesic and antipyretic effects. The drug is a weak prostaglandin inhibitor and does not have significant antiinflammatory effects. Prototype Drug Chart 26-1 lists the pharmacologic data for acetaminophen.

Pharmacokinetics The rate of absorption of acetaminophen is dependent on the rate of gastric emptying. Acetaminophen is 20% to 50% protein-bound and crosses the placenta during pregnancy; it is also found in low concentrations in breast milk. Acetaminophen is partially hepatically metabolized into inactive metabolites; however, a highly active metabolite (N-acetyl-*p*-benzoquinone) produced when the drug is taken in large doses can have potential liver and kidney toxicity. The half-life is 2 to 3 hours. There is no concrete evidence of fetal anomalies associated with the use of acetaminophen, and no adverse effects have been noted in breastfed infants of patients who used the drug while pregnant or breastfeeding.

Pharmacodynamics The maximum daily dose of acetaminophen (Tylenol) is 4000 mg per day, and the use of acetaminophen during pregnancy should not exceed 12 tablets per 24 hours of a 325-mg formulation (regular strength) or 8 tablets per 24 hours of a 500-mg (extra strength) formulation (because of the potential for kidney and liver toxicity). The drug should be taken at 4- to 6-hour intervals. Onset of effects after oral ingestion is within 10 to 30 minutes; peak action occurs at 1 to 2 hours; duration is from 3 to 5 hours.

Manufacturers of OTC products containing acetaminophen have lowered the maximum daily dose recommendation to 3,000 mg due to the frequency of overdose with acetaminophen. One reason for the high frequency of overdose is that patients may take multiple OTC products that all contain acetaminophen.

TABLE 53-4 OVER-THE-COUNTER ANTACIDS COMMONLY USED IN PREGNANCY

GENERIC (BRAND)	ROUTE AND DOSAGE	USES AND CONSIDERATIONS
aluminum hydroxide (Amphojel)	A: PO: As directed*	Contains 320 mg of aluminum hydroxide gel per 300-mg tab or per 5 mL; ANC 8; contains saccharin and sorbitol. OTC preparation. For heartburn secondary to reflux Neutralizes gastric acidity Side effects include constipation; adverse reactions include dehydration, hypophosphatemia (long-term use), GI obstruction Decreased effects with tetracycline, phenothiazine, benzodiazepines, isoniazid, digoxin; follow dose with water Pregnancy category: C; PB: UK; $t\frac{1}{2}$: UK; Onset: 15-30 min; Peak: 0.5 h; Duration: 1-3 h
magnesium hydroxide and aluminum hydroxide with simethicone (Mylanta Extra Strength Liquid, Almacone)	40-125 mg PO q.i.d. after meals and h.s.; up to 500 mg/d	Mylanta Extra Strength Liquid: Each 5 mL contains 400 mg aluminum hydroxide, 400 mg magnesium hydroxide, 40 mg simethicone, parabens, saccharin, sorbitol, and 2 mg sodium OTC preparation Almacone tabs: Each tab contains 200 mg aluminum hydroxide, 200 mg magnesium hydroxide, and 20 mg simethicone OTC preparation. Tabs must be chewed thoroughly. Same as above with addition of antiflatulence action. Neutralizes gastric acidity and antiflatulent. Adverse effects include acid rebound. Aluminum-based antacids may cause constipation, while magnesium-based antacids have a laxative effect. Aluminum and magnesium–based combination antacids are given to balance the constipation and laxative effects. Do not administer magnesium-based antacids in patients with renal disease. Drug interactions: Concurrent administration with digoxin, indomethacin (Indocin), or iron salts may decrease absorption of these drugs. Concurrent administration with chlordiazepoxide hydrochloride decreases rate of chlordiazepoxide absorption. Decreased pharmacologic effect with antacids and benzodiazepines, captopril, corticosteroids, fluoroquinolones, histamine H_2 antagonists, hydantoins, ketoconazole, penicillamine (Cuprimine, Depen), phenothiazines, salicylates, and ticlopidine (Ticlid). Increased pharmacologic effect with levodopa, sulfonylureas, and valproic acid. Pregnancy category: C; PB: UK; $t\frac{1}{2}$: UK

*Dosage recommendations for antacid preparations should be clarified by the health care provider; however, as a general rule, no more than 12 tablets or 12 tsp should be taken in a 24-hour period, depending on the strength of the product. Major side effects are change in bowel habits (diarrhea or constipation), nausea, vomiting, alkalosis, and hypermagnesemia. Antacids figure in numerous drug interactions because of their increased action on gastric pH and their propensity to bind with other drugs to form poorly absorbed complexes. Antacids should not be taken within 2 hours of taking iron, digitalis products, tetracycline, or phenothiazine.

A, Adult; *ANC,* acid-neutralizing capacity (per tablet or 5 mL); *d,* day; *GI,* gastrointestinal; *h,* hour; *min,* minute; *OTC,* over-the-counter; *PB,* protein-binding; *PO,* by mouth; *q.i.d.,* four times a day; $t\frac{1}{2}$, half-life; *tab,* tablet; *tsp,* teaspoon; *UK,* unknown.

Most patients without preexisting renal or hepatic disease tolerate acetaminophen well. Patients with hypersensitivity to the compound should not use it. Acetaminophen should be used cautiously in patients who are at risk for infection because of the possibility of masking signs and symptoms. The most frequent adverse reactions are skin eruptions, urticaria, unusual bruising, erythema, hypoglycemia, jaundice, hemolytic anemia, neutropenia, leukopenia, pancytopenia, and thrombocytopenia.

Aspirin and Ibuprofen

Aspirin, a salicylate, is classified as a mild analgesic. Aspirin is a pregnancy category C drug (which changes to category D if full-dose aspirin is used in the third trimester). It is a prostaglandin synthetase inhibitor with antipyretic, analgesic, and antiinflammatory properties. Teratogenic effects have not been shown conclusively, but the risk for anomalies is perceived to be small.

Aspirin can inhibit the initiation of labor and actually prolong labor through its effects on uterine contractility; therefore, its use is not recommended during pregnancy. Aspirin use late in pregnancy is also associated with greater maternal blood loss at delivery, and there may be increased risk for anemia in pregnancy and of antepartum hemorrhage. Hemostasis is affected in the newborn whose mother ingested aspirin during the last 2 months of pregnancy (even without use during the week of delivery). Platelets are unable to aggregate to form clots, and it appears that this is not a reversible effect after delivery; the infant must wait for its own bone marrow to produce new platelets. (Refer to Chapter 26 for more information on aspirin.)

Ibuprofen is classified as a pregnancy category C drug (which changes to category D if used in the third trimester). If taken late in pregnancy, it may cause premature closure of the ductus arteriosus. Ibuprofen is a prostaglandin synthetase inhibitor with antipyretic, analgesic, and antiinflammatory properties. Bleeding risks are similar to those reported with aspirin, though ibuprofen causes less inhibition of platelet aggregation than aspirin formulations.

Antidepressant Drugs

Exposure to antidepressant drugs and depressive disorders have both been associated with adverse birth outcomes. Adverse outcomes have included low birth weight, small for gestational age, preterm delivery, and increased neonatal irritability and decreased attentiveness. Use of selective serotonin reuptake inhibitors (SSRIs) in pregnancy is associated with low birth weight and small for gestational age infants. Preterm delivery (before 37 gestational weeks) is significantly higher in patients taking SSRIs and tricyclics. Although tricyclic antidepressant use in pregnancy has not been associated with structural malformations, in utero exposure has been linked to neonatal jitteriness and irritability. *Poor neonatal adaptation,* a term for transient symptoms like tachypnea, irritability, hypoglycemia, and weak cry, has been reported in neonates exposed to SSRIs in late pregnancy. Options for treatment for pregnant patient include psychotherapy alone or in conjunction with pharmacologic therapy as determined by the health care provider.

Nursing Process
Patient-Centered Collaborative Care

Antepartum Drugs

Assessment

- Gather comprehensive medical and drug (illicit, herbal, nonpharmacologic, and pharmacologic) history.
- Obtain baseline vital signs.
- Identify patients at risk for substance abuse, and collaborate with other professionals to plan strategies to minimize risks.
- Assess drug history to determine if antacid use will interfere with absorption.
- Review history of aspirin use when admitting patient in labor. If aspirin has been used, alert staff and monitor for increased bleeding.
- Ascertain any medical history of alcoholism, liver disease, viral infection, or renal deficiencies. Acetaminophen should be used cautiously in these patients.
- Assess Group B colonization in pregnancy for treatment and neonatal prevention.

Nursing Diagnoses

- Deficient knowledge related to health maintenance needs during pregnancy
- Deficient knowledge related to potential adverse fetal outcomes from exposure to teratogens

Planning

- Patient will use or avoid various drugs during pregnancy as advised.
- Patient will discuss drug and herb use with health care provider or pharmacist before use.

Nursing Interventions

General

- Be cognizant that drug use may be part of multiple-substance abuse and may also involve maternal-neonatal infections.
- Stress the importance of prenatal care, and discuss patient's fears about health care professionals and concerns about legal action in the event of substance abuse.

Specific

- Advise on nonpharmacologic and pharmacologic measures to relieve common pregnancy discomforts.
- Refer patient to tobacco, alcohol, or drug treatment program if appropriate.
- Counsel patient on nutritional and therapeutic supplements needed during pregnancy.
- Monitor hemoglobin/hematocrit of prenatal patients per agency protocol.

Iron

- Question patient about nausea, constipation, and bowel habit changes if taking iron preparations.
- Give diluted liquid iron preparation through a plastic straw to prevent discoloration of teeth. Giving iron with orange juice, which is high in ascorbic acid, enhances absorption.
- Store iron in a light-resistant container.
- Recognize that patient may have false-positive result of occult blood in stool if taking iron.

Patient Teaching

General

- Advise patient that tobacco, alcohol, and heavy caffeine use may have adverse effects on the fetus.
- Encourage patient to speak with health care provider before taking drugs (illicit, OTC, prescribed) secondary to teratogenic potential.
- Counsel patient planning to breastfeed to discuss drugs (illicit, OTC, prescribed) with health care provider.

Aspirin/Acetaminophen/Ibuprofen

- Advise patient to take acetaminophen rather than aspirin during pregnancy; aspirin and ibuprofen are particularly contraindicated during the third trimester.

- Counsel patient against ingesting multiple OTC pain or cough/cold preparations, because many OTC products contain acetaminophen.

Antepartum Drugs

- Advise patient not to take nonsteroidal antiinflammatory drugs (NSAIDs) with acetaminophen.
- Advise patient not to take NSAIDS after second trimester.

Caffeine/Alcohol/Nicotine

- Advise patient to limit coffee ingestion to 1 to 2 cups per day and to limit other sources of caffeine (tea, cola, chocolate, certain drugs).
- If caffeine is allowed by health care provider, encourage patient to space limited caffeine intake evenly throughout day, because caffeine passes readily to fetus, who cannot metabolize it. Caffeine can decrease intervillous placental blood flow.
- Advise patient to use decaffeinated products or dilute caffeinated products.
- Suggest that patient use herbal products carefully because of occasionally harmful ingredients (see Herbal Alert 53-1).
- If patient plans to breastfeed, explain that 1% of caffeine consumed will appear in breast milk within 15 minutes. Therefore, although one cup of coffee is fine, it is not wise to drink several cups of coffee in succession; excess caffeine will accumulate in the infant's tissues. The infant lacks enzymes to adequately clear the caffeine for 7 to 9 months after birth.
- Advise pregnant patient not to drink alcohol, because no safe level has been determined, and that even minimal exposure may result in fetal alcohol effect, and moderate/excessive exposure may result in fetal alcohol syndrome.
- Advise patient that smoking can cause loss of nutrients such as vitamins A and C, folic acid, cobalamin, and calcium. Tobacco use may contribute to shortened gestation and low-birth-weight infants.

Antacids

- Advise patient that antacids should not be taken within 1 hour of taking an enteric-coated tablet, because the acid-resistant coating may dissolve in the increased alkaline condition of the stomach, and the medication will not be released in the intestine as intended. Stomach upset may result.
- Instruct patient to store antacid liquid suspension at room temperature (or place under refrigeration to improve palatability), not to freeze it, and to shake bottle well before ingesting.

Iron

- Advise patient about dietary sources of iron, including red meat, nuts and seeds, wheat germ, spinach, broccoli, prunes, and iron-fortified cereal.
- Explain to patient that if supplemental iron is taken between meals, increased absorption (and also increased side effects) may result. Taking iron 1 hour before meals is suggested. Give with orange juice or water, but not with milk or antacids.

Self-Administration for Iron and Antacids

- Advise patient to swallow iron tablets whole, not crush them. Liquid iron preparations are taken with a plastic straw to avoid staining teeth.
- Caution patient not to take antacids with iron, because antacids impair absorption and are generally discouraged during pregnancy. Iron and antacids should be taken 2 hours apart if both are prescribed.

Side Effects for Iron and Antacids

- Advise patient to keep iron tablets away from children. Iron tablets look like candy, and death has been reported in small children who have ingested 2 g or less of ferrous sulfate. Iron is a leading cause of fatal poisoning in children.
- Advise patient that there may be a change in bowel habits when taking antacids. Aluminum and calcium carbonate products can cause constipation, whereas magnesium products can cause diarrhea. Many antacids contain a combination of ingredients to reduce adverse effects.

Cultural Considerations

- Consider cultural food practices and beliefs in regard to the use of prenatal vitamins. For example, in Mexico, some may view vitamins as a "hot food" that should not be ingested during pregnancy.

Evaluation

- Evaluate effectiveness of prescribed drug therapy. Report side effects.
- Evaluate patient's understanding of possible effects on fetus from maternal use of drugs (prescribed, OTC, and illicit) and tobacco or alcohol.

DRUGS THAT DECREASE UTERINE MUSCLE CONTRACTILITY

Preterm Labor

Preterm labor (PTL) is labor that occurs between 20 and 37 weeks of pregnancy, involving a fetus with an estimated weight between 500 and 2499 g. Regular contractions occur at less than 10-minute intervals over 30 to 60 minutes and are strong enough to result in 2-cm cervical dilation and 80% effacement. PTL occurs in approximately 8% to 10% of all pregnancies. Preterm infants who survive very early delivery have significant physiologic challenges to overcome, so PTL that progresses to preterm delivery accounts for most perinatal morbidity and mortality (excluding fetuses with anomalies) in the United States.

Although PTL has no single known cause, certain risk factors have been identified: maternal age younger than 18 years or older than 40 years, low socioeconomic status, previous history of preterm delivery (17% to 37% chance of recurrence), intrauterine infections (e.g., bacterial vaginosis), polyhydramnios, multiple gestation, uterine anomalies, antepartum hemorrhage, smoking, drug use, urinary tract infections, and incompetent cervix. Attempts to arrest PTL are contraindicated in (1) pregnancy of less than 20 weeks' gestation (confirmed by ultrasound), (2) bulging or premature rupture of membranes (PROM), (3) confirmed fetal death or anomalies incompatible with life, (4) maternal hemorrhage and evidence of severe fetal compromise, and (5) chorioamnionitis.

Nonpharmacologic treatment measures for PTL include bed rest, hydration (ingestion of six to eight glasses of fluids daily or more, IV fluid bolus), pelvic rest (no sexual intercourse or douching), and screening for intrauterine and urinary tract infections. Patient assessment includes uterine activity (frequency, duration, and intensity), vaginal bleeding or discharge, and fetal monitoring.

Tocolytic Therapy

When patients in true PTL (with cervical change) have no contraindications, they become candidates for **tocolytic therapy** (drug therapy to decrease uterine muscle contractions) using beta$_2$-adrenergic receptor agonists (e.g., terbutaline) or, more commonly, the calcium antagonist magnesium sulfate. Other tocolytics less commonly used are calcium channel blockers (e.g., nifedine, [Procardia]) and prostaglandin inhibitors (e.g., indomethacin [Indocin]). Calcium channel blockers prevent the influx of calcium ions, resulting in relaxation of the myometrium. Prostaglandin or cyclooxygenase (COX, or prostaglandin synthase) is the enzyme responsible for converting acrachidonic acid and increasing available intracellular calcium. Therefore, prostaglandin inhibitors limit the available calcium for uterine contractions. With concerns regarding the safety profiles of beta-sympathomimetics and magnesium sulfate comes an increased interest in the latter two drug categories for tocolysis. The goals in tocolytic therapy are to (1) interrupt or inhibit uterine contractions to create additional time for fetal maturation in utero, (2) delay delivery so antenatal corticosteroids can be delivered to facilitate fetal lung maturation, and (3) allow safe transport of the patient to an appropriate facility if required. The use of progesterone, administered vaginally or intramuscularly to prevent preterm birth, is under investigation. Table 53-5 lists the drugs used to decrease preterm uterine contractions and their dosages, uses, and considerations.

Beta-Sympathomimetic Drugs

Beta-sympathomimetic drugs act by stimulating beta$_2$-receptors on uterine smooth muscle. The frequency and intensity of uterine contractions decrease as the muscle relaxes. Terbutaline is used in the late second and early third trimesters, more commonly limited to a single dose therapy as an acute tocolytic. It is approved for medicinal use but not specifically as a tocolytic. Terbutaline can effectively decrease uterine contractions; however, use of terbutaline in the United States has waned with increased awareness of its effects on maternal and fetal cardiovascular systems and free placental passage. The U.S. Food and Drug Administration (FDA) is recommending that *injectable* terbutaline should not be used in pregnant women for prevention or prolonged treatment (beyond 48 to 72 hours) of preterm labor secondary to the risk of maternal cardiac problems and death *(www.fda.gov/drugs/drugsafety/ucm243539.htm)*.

> **SAFETY: Preventing Medication Errors**
>
> **Do not confuse...**
>
> - **methylergonovine** (Methergine) (used to stimulate uterine contractions in the prevention and treatment of postpartum hemorrhage) with **terbutaline sulfate** (used to decrease uterine contractions in preterm labor). These drugs have the same packaging but opposite actions. Both are amber ampules with amber plastic packaging and colored neckbands wrapped in foil. Do not store together.

Pharmacokinetics Patients with contractions may be initially given subcutaneous terbutaline. Some health care providers may repeat every 1 to 6 hours if the maternal pulse is less than 130 beats/min. Less commonly, health care providers administer continuous intravenous infusions, starting with dosages from 2.5 to 5 mcg/min, which may be increased 2.5 to 5 mcg/min every 20 to 30 minutes with a maximum of 25 mcg/min. Patients are monitored to determine whether and when contractions diminish or cease. Terbutaline is minimally protein-bound (25%) and metabolized via the liver to inactive metabolites. Its half-life is 11 to 16 hours.

Pharmacodynamics Oral terbutaline has an onset of action of 30 to 45 minutes, a peak plasma/serum concentration of 1 to 2 hours, and a duration of action of 4 to 8 hours. IV and subcutaneous terbutaline have an onset of action within 15 minutes, a peak serum concentration level in 30 to 60 minutes, and a duration of action of 1.5 to 4 hours subcutaneously.

Adverse Reactions. Maternal side effects include tremors, malaise, weakness, dyspnea, tachycardia, increased systolic blood pressure, decreased diastolic blood pressure, chest pain, nausea, vomiting, diarrhea, constipation, erythema, sweating, hyperglycemia, and hypokalemia. Many of these effects are associated with terbutaline's cross-reactivity with beta$_1$-adrenergic receptors. More serious adverse reactions include pulmonary edema, dysrhythmias, ketoacidosis, and anaphylactic shock. Fetal side effects include tachycardia and potential hypoglycemia resulting from fetal hyperinsulinemia caused by maternal hyperglycemia. Terbutaline is contraindicated in patients with cardiac disease and those with poorly controlled hyperthyroidism or diabetes mellitus.

Drug Interactions. The increased effects of general anesthetics can produce additive hypotension. Pulmonary edema can occur with concurrent use of corticosteroids. Cardiovascular effects may be additive with other sympathomimetic drugs, such as epinephrine, albuterol,

TABLE 53-5 DRUGS USED TO DECREASE UTERINE CONTRACTILITY

GENERIC (BRAND)	ROUTE AND DOSAGE	USES AND CONSIDERATIONS
Beta-Adrenergic Agents		
terbutaline	Follow agency protocol for specific directives plus individual health care provider's order; may be given subQ; usually therapy is 0.25-0.5 mg subQ every 3-4 h	Sympathomimetic $beta_2$-adrenergic agonist. Partially metabolized in liver; excreted by kidneys. May require repeat therapy; 40%-50% rate of tocolytic breakthrough and recurrence of preterm labor 3 wk after start of PO therapy (possibly due to desensitization of beta receptors over time). Monitor MHR. Current research focuses on use of portable low-dose continuous subcutaneous pumps that deliver intermittent bolus doses based on data reflecting peak need periods. Increases in maternal pulse and FHR. Rapidly crosses placenta; breastfeeding not contraindicated because of short half-life Additive effect with CNS depressants (narcotics, sedative-hypnotics) and neuromuscular blocking agents Pregnancy category: B; t½: 11-16 h; Onset: 15 min IV/subQ and 30-45 min PO; Duration: 4-8 h PO and 1.5-4 h subQ; peak serum levels: 0.5-1 h IV/subQ and 1-2 h PO
Calcium Antagonists		
magnesium sulfate	Follow agency protocol for specific directives plus individual health care provider's order for concentration and mL/h IV. Usual LD: 4-6 g in 100 mL over 15-20 min; maint: 40 g in 1 L IVF at 2-4 g/h. Dose based on serum magnesium levels, DTR assessment, and uterine response	Calcium antagonist and CNS depressant. Relaxes uterine smooth muscle through calcium displacement. Must be given by infusion pump for accurate dosing. Freely crosses placenta. Few contraindications allow for use in patients with life-threatening complications. Monitor maternal magnesium levels through serum analyses, DTR, respiratory rate, and urinary output. Elevated levels may be evident in newborn for 7 d; observe newborn for 24-48 h for signs of toxicity if mother treated close to delivery; breastfeeding not contraindicated Antidote: IV: calcium gluconate 1 g over 3 min Pregnancy category: B; Onset: immediate by IV; Duration: 30 min

CNS, Central nervous system; *d,* day; *DTR,* deep tendon reflex; *FHR,* fetal heart rate; *h,* hour; *IV,* intravenous; *IVF,* intravenous fluid; *LD,* loading dose; *maint,* maintenance; *MHR,* maternal heart rate; *min,* minute; *PO,* by mouth; *subQ,* subcutaneously; *t½,* half-life; *wk,* week.

and isoproterenol. Beta-adrenergic blocking agents, such as propranolol HCl (Inderal), nadolol (Corgard), pindolol timolol maleate and metoprolol tartrate (Lopressor), antagonize beta-sympathomimetics.

Magnesium Sulfate

Magnesium sulfate, a calcium antagonist and central nervous system depressant, relaxes the smooth muscle of the uterus through calcium displacement and is more commonly given as a tocolytic. Administered IV, the drug has a direct depressant effect on uterine muscle contractility. It increases uterine perfusion, which has a therapeutic effect on the fetus. It is also less expensive and may be safer to use than the beta-sympathomimetics because it has fewer adverse effects. It can also be used when beta-sympathomimetics are contraindicated (e.g., in patients with diabetes and cardiovascular disease). The drug is excreted by the kidneys and crosses the placenta. Magnesium sulfate is administered as a 4 to 6 intravenous load over 20 minutes followed by a continuous infusion over 20 minutes of 2 to 4 g/h. The maintenance dose must be titrated to keep uterine contractions under control, and magnesium levels are drawn based on clinical response of the patient. Magnesium sulfate therapy is contraindicated in patients who have myasthenia gravis; impaired kidney function and recent myocardial infarction are relative contraindications. Patients with renal impairment may require adjusted dosages.

Adverse Reactions. Dosage-related side effects in the patient include flushing, feelings of increased warmth, perspiration, dizziness, nausea, headache, lethargy, slurred speech, sluggishness, nasal congestion, heavy eyelids, blurred vision, decreased GI action, increased pulse rate, and hypotension. Increased severity is evidenced by depressed reflexes, confusion, and magnesium toxicity (respiratory depression and arrest, circulatory collapse, cardiac arrest). Side effects in the fetus are decreased fetal heart rate (FHR) variability, and in the neonate are respiratory depression, slight hypotonia with diminished reflexes, and lethargy for 24 to 48 hours. If maternal neurologic, respiratory, or cardiac depression is evidenced, the antidote is calcium gluconate (1 g IV push over 3 minutes).

Nursing Interventions during Tocolytic Therapy

- Monitor vital signs, FHR, fetal activity, and uterine activity as ordered. Report respirations fewer than 12 per minute, which may indicate magnesium sulfate toxicity.

- Monitor intake and output (I&O). Report urinary output <30 mL/hr.
- Assess breath and bowel sounds as ordered, or at least every 4 hours.
- Assess deep tendon reflexes (DTRs) and clonus before initiation of therapy and as ordered. Notify health care provider of changes in DTRs (areflexia or hyporeflexia) and clonus.
- Assess pain and uterine contractions
- Weigh daily at the same time.
- Monitor serum magnesium levels as ordered (therapeutic level is 4 to 7 mg/dL).
- Have calcium gluconate (1 g given IV over 3 minutes) available as an antidote.
- Observe newborn for 24 to 48 hours for magnesium effects if drug was given to mother before delivery.

Nursing Process
Patient-Centered Collaborative Care

Beta$_2$-Adrenergic Agonists: Terbutaline

Assessment
- Identify risks for PTL early in pregnancy.
- When a patient has preterm uterine contractions, obtain a history, complete physical assessment, vital signs, FHR, and urine specimen for screening for intrauterine infection and urinary tract infection.

Nursing Diagnoses
- Anxiety related to potential for early labor and birth and pregnancy loss.
- Deficient knowledge related to etiology and nonpharmacologic and pharmacologic interventions for PTL
- Ineffective self-health management related to nonpharmacologic and pharmacologic interventions for PTL and long-term implications for patient and fetus or infant
- Risk for activity intolerance related to nonpharmacologic and pharmacologic interventions for PTL

Planning
- Patient's preterm uterine contractions will cease by resting in left side-lying position, increasing fluid intake, assuming pelvic rest, and following tocolytic therapy as directed.
- Patient has no progressive cervical change.

Nursing Interventions
- Monitor and assess uterine activity and FHR.
- Maintain patient in left lateral position as much as possible to facilitate uteroplacental perfusion.
- Monitor vital signs per unit protocol, specifically maternal pulse. Report maternal heart rate greater than 130 beats/min.
- Report auscultated cardiac dysrhythmias. An electrocardiogram (ECG) may be ordered.
- Auscultate breath sounds (anteriorly, posteriorly, and bilaterally) every 4 hours. Notify health care provider if respirations are more than 30 per minute or if quality changes (wheezes, rales, coughing).
- Monitor daily weight (at the same time of day) to assess fluid overload; implement strict I&O measurement.
- Report baseline FHR over 180 beats/min or any significant increase in uterine contractions from pretreatment baseline.
- Report persistence of uterine contractions despite tocolytic therapy.
- Report leaking of amniotic fluid, any vaginal bleeding or discharge, or complaints of rectal pressure.
- Be alert to presence of maternal hyperglycemia and hypokalemia and hypoglycemia in the newborn delivered within 5 hours of discontinued beta-sympathomimetic drugs.

Patient Teaching

General
- Advise patient of signs and symptoms of PTL (menstrual-type cramps, sensation of pelvic pressure, low backache, increased vaginal discharge, abdominal discomfort).
- Advise patient that if she experiences PTL contractions, initial action should be to void, recline on her left side to increase uterine blood flow, and drink extra fluids. Emphasize that she should notify her health care provider if uterine contractions do not cease or if they increase in frequency.
- Explain side effects of beta-sympathomimetic drugs. Report heart palpitations or dizziness to health care provider.
- Advise patient to contact health care provider before taking any other drugs while on tocolytic drug therapy.

Cultural Considerations
- Provide an interpreter with same ethnic background and gender as patient if possible, especially when dealing with sensitive topics or stressful situations.

Evaluation
- Evaluate effectiveness of tocolytic drug by noting six or fewer uterine contractions in 1 hour or per health care provider order.
- Evaluate patient's understanding of nonpharmacologic measures for decreasing preterm contractions: bed rest, increasing oral fluid intake, pelvic rest, and lying on her left side.
- Continue monitoring patient's vital signs, FHR, and uterine activity. Report any change immediately.

CORTICOSTEROID THERAPY IN PRETERM LABOR

The desired outcome of tocolytic therapy is prevention or cessation of PTL. Patients at risk for preterm delivery (24 to 34 weeks' gestation) should receive antenatal corticosteroid therapy with betamethasone (Celestone) or dexamethasone. An off-label use, administration of antenatal corticosteroids accelerates lung maturation and lung surfactant development in the fetus in utero, decreasing the incidence and severity of respiratory distress syndrome (RDS) and increasing survival of preterm infants. Antenatal therapy decreases infant mortality, RDS, and intraventricular bleeds in neonates born between 24 and 34 gestational weeks. The effects and benefits of corticosteroid administration are believed to begin 24 hours after administration and last for up to 1 week. The goal is to delay delivery by 48 hours to maximize the effect of the glucocorticoids. Research by the Agency for Healthcare Research and Quality has found that approximately one fifth of patients do not receive the recommended corticosteroids before delivery of premature births.

Surfactant is made up of two major phospholipids: sphingomyelin and lecithin. Sphingomyelin initially develops in greater quantity (from about the 24th week) than lecithin. However, by the 33rd to 35th weeks of gestation, lecithin production peaks, making the ratio of the two substances about 2:1 in favor of lecithin. This is called the **L/S (lecithin/sphingomyelin) ratio**, measured in the amniotic fluid. The L/S ratio is a predictor of fetal lung maturity and risk for neonatal RDS.

Patients with gestational hypertension, PROM, placental insufficiency, some types of diabetes, or narcotic abuse may have amniotic fluid with higher than expected L/S ratios for the gestational date because of a stress-induced increase in endogenous corticosteroid production.

Betamethasone

When PTL occurs before the 32nd week of gestation, corticosteroid therapy with betamethasone may be prescribed. The usual dose is 12 mg intramuscularly (IM) every 24 hours for 2 doses.

Adverse Reactions

Side effects of betamethasone are rare but include seizures, headache, vertigo, edema, hypertension, increased sweating, petechiae, ecchymoses, and facial erythema.

Dexamethasone

In clinical controlled trials, evidence is insufficient to recommend betamethasone over dexamethasone, because the two have not been directly compared. Investigations have noted a trend of decreased risk of neonatal cystic periventricular leukomalacia and intraventricular hemorrhage with exposure to betamethasone over dexamethasone. Dexamethasone has a rapid onset of action and a shorter duration of action; therefore, it must be prescribed in a shorter frequency compared with betamethasone. The recommended antepartum regimen for dexamethasone is 6 mg IM every 12 hours for 4 doses.

SAFETY: Preventing Medication Errors

Do not confuse…

- **Dexamethasone,** a corticosteroid used to accelerate fetal lung maturity during weeks 24 to 34 of gestation, with **desoximetasone** (Topicort), which is used to treat inflammation from corticosteroid responsive dermatoses.

Adverse Reactions

The potential adverse reactions associated with dexamethasone therapy include insomnia, nervousness, increased appetite, headache, hypersensitivity reactions, and arthralgias. Table 53-6 lists the prenatal drugs used for surfactant development and their dosages, uses, and considerations.

TABLE 53-6 PRENATAL THERAPY FOR SURFACTANT DEVELOPMENT

GENERIC (BRAND)	ROUTE AND DOSAGE	USES AND CONSIDERATIONS
betamethasone (Celestone)	IM: 12 mg IM	Corticosteroid. Given to prevent RDS in preterm infants by injecting mother before delivery to stimulate surfactant production in fetal lung. Not effective in treating preterm infant after delivery. Most effective if given at least 24 h (preferably 48-72 h) but less than 7 d before delivery in week 33 or before. Contraindicated in severe gestational hypertension and in systemic fungal infection. Simultaneous use with terbutaline may enhance risk for pulmonary edema. May mask signs of chorioamnionitis, so not usually given with ruptured membranes. Metabolized in liver and excreted by kidneys; crosses placenta; enters breast milk. Therapy less effective with multifetal birth and with male infants. Pregnancy category: C; PB: 64%; $t_{1/2}$: 6.5 h; Onset: 1-3 h; Peak: IV: 10-36 min; Duration: 7-14 d
dexamethasone	IM: 6 mg q12h × 4 doses	Same as betamethasone but shorter half-life and more significant variation in circulating serum levels

d, Day; *h,* hour; *IM,* intramuscular; *IV,* intravenous; *min,* minute; *PB,* protein-binding; *RDS,* respiratory distress syndrome; $t_{1/2}$, half-life.

Nursing Process
Patient-Centered Collaborative Care

Betamethasone (Celestone)

Assessment
- Assess for history of hypersensitivity.
- Assess vital signs; report abnormal findings.
- Assess FHR.

Nursing Diagnoses
- Anxiety related to potential for preterm labor and birth with uncertain fetal outcome secondary to fetal immaturity
- Deficient knowledge related to use of antenatal corticosteroids for promotion of fetal lung maturity in preterm delivery.

Planning
- Patient will not deliver within 24 hours of receiving betamethasone.

Nursing Interventions
- Shake the suspension well. Avoid exposing to excessive heat or light.
- Inject into large muscle (not deltoid) to avoid local atrophy.
- Monitor maternal vital signs.
- Maintain accurate I&O.
- Check blood glucose if used for patient with diabetes mellitus.

Cultural Considerations
- Provide an interpreter with same ethnic background and gender as patient if possible, especially when dealing with sensitive topics or stressful situations.

Evaluation
- Continue monitoring patient's vital signs. Report changes.
- Continue monitoring FHR. Report changes.
- Monitor neonate for hypoglycemia and presence of neonatal sepsis.

BOX 53-1 PREDISPOSING FACTORS IN PREECLAMPSIA
- African American
- Primigravida (first pregnancy)
- History of preeclampsia
- Younger than 20 years or older than 35 years (especially primigravida)
- Multifetal gestation
- Family history of preeclampsia
- Gestational trophoblastic disease
- Pregestational diabetes mellitus
- Preexisting hypertensive, vascular, or renal disease
- Antiphospholipid antibody syndrome

DRUGS FOR GESTATIONAL HYPERTENSION

Gestational hypertension (elevated blood pressure without proteinuria after 20 gestational weeks in patients normotensive before pregnancy), the most common serious complication of pregnancy, can have devastating maternal and fetal effects. Gestational hypertension has replaced the term *pregnancy-induced hypertension,* still commonly used in clinical discussions but no longer correct. With proper management of gestational hypertension, the prognosis for both patient and infant is good. Hypertensive disorders are reported in 10% to 20% of all pregnant patients, with 5% to 8% of all pregnancies reflecting incidence of **preeclampsia** (gestational hypertension with proteinuria). The condition is most often observed after 20 weeks gestation, intrapartum, and during the first 72 hours postpartum, though late postpartum preeclampsia-eclampsia may present more than 48 hours but less than 4 weeks postpartum.

The cause of preeclampsia remains unknown, although numerous hypotheses exist. The pathophysiology of preeclampsia and **eclampsia** (new-onset grand mal seizures in a patient with preeclampsia) is believed to be related to decreased levels of vasodilating prostaglandins with resulting vasospasm. The major predisposing risk factors for the development of preeclampsia are listed in Box 53-1.

The two categories of gestational hypertension—preeclampsia and eclampsia—are based on clinical manifestations. Preeclampsia is the presence of hypertension (systolic blood pressure >140 mm Hg or diastolic blood pressure >90 mm Hg) and proteinuria (≥300 mg in 24-hour urine collection) in a normotensive pregnant patient after 20 weeks' gestation. Preeclampsia is subdivided into *mild* preeclampsia and *severe* preeclampsia (Table 53-7).

About 5% of preeclamptic patients, notably those without adequate prenatal care, progress to eclampsia, in which seizure activity occurs and maternal mortality rate is about 10% to 15% in low- and middle-income countries. Early diagnosis of preeclampsia with appropriate treatment keeps most preeclamptic patients from progressing to this stage. Approximately 13% to 16% of eclampsia occurs postpartum.

A severe sequela of preeclampsia is known as **HELLP syndrome** (defined by *H*emolysis, *E*levated *L*iver enzymes, and *L*ow *P*latelet count), which occurs in about 2% to 12% of patients with gestational hypertension. Patients who manifest severe preeclampsia are most likely to also have HELLP syndrome.

Two primary treatment goals in preeclampsia, in addition to delivery of an uncompromised fetus and psychological support for the patient and family, are reduction of vasospasm and prevention of seizures.

Delivery of the infant and placenta (products of conception) is the only known cure for preeclampsia. Vaginal

TABLE 53-7 COMPARISON OF MILD AND SEVERE PREECLAMPSIA AND ECLAMPSIA

MILD PREECLAMPSIA	SEVERE PREECLAMPSIA	ECLAMPSIA
Blood pressure increase to >140 and/or >90 diastolic but <160 systolic	Blood pressure increase of >160/110 on two occasions at least 6 h apart (patient on bed rest)	Signs and symptoms of mild or severe preeclampsia and one grand mal seizure
Proteinuria >300 mg in 24 h or +1 ± 2 on dipstick; edema not generalized; noted in hands, feet	Proteinuria >5 g in 24 h or 3+ or greater in two random samples 4 hours apart; edema generalized; found in face (periorbital, coarse features), hands, lower extremities (ankles), abdomen, and dependent areas	
Weight gain >1 lb/wk before 32 wk or >2.5 lb/wk after 34 wk	Weight gain up to 10 lb in 1 wk	
Deep tendon reflexes in arms and legs only slightly increased (0: no response; 1+: sluggish/low; 2+: normal active; 3+: brisk)	Deep tendon reflexes in arms and legs hyperactive (4+: hyperactive/transient clonus; 5+: brisk; clonus sustained)	
Adequate urinary output (1 mL/kg/h)	Oliguria present (<400 mL per 24 h)	
No major cerebral or visual symptoms	Cerebral or visual symptoms, particularly blurred vision, spots, flashing lights, and/or persistent and severe headache in frontal area	
May have mild frontal headache	Severe headache	
No epigastric pain	Epigastric pain may be present; pulmonary edema, cyanosis	

h, Hour; *wk,* week; >, greater than; <, less than.

delivery is preferred so that anesthesia or surgical risks will not be added. Labor induction via cervical ripening may be initiated to facilitate labor. For a vaginal delivery, epidural anesthesia or combined epidural and spinal anesthesia is frequently performed for pain management while promoting uteroplacental circulation. Maternal hypotension is a significant concern for hypertensive patients who have epidurals. In contrast, parturients with worsening preeclampsia or fetal distress may be delivered via cesarean section. Patients with HELLP syndrome may have their labor induced for a vaginal delivery at 32 or more weeks' gestation. For patients with HELLP syndrome who are at less than 32 weeks' gestation, cesarean delivery may be considered.

If a patient's disease progresses to the point of eclampsia (maternal seizure), delivery is generally postponed for 1 to 3 hours if fetal status allows. The labor induction or cesarean delivery is an additional stressor for the patient who exhibits acidosis and hypoxia resulting from seizure. Ideally, once vital signs are stabilized with improved urinary output and decreased acidosis/hypoxia, delivery is pursued.

Nonpharmacologic treatments for preeclampsia include activity reduction, lying on the left side, increased dietary protein (supplemental 90 g/day), psychosocial therapy, and biofeedback, but the aforementioned recommendations have been studied and shown not to have clinically beneficial effects. Therefore, drug therapy is commonly used for treatment.

Methydopa, Hydralazine, and Magnesium Sulfate

Methyldopa , hydralazine , and Labetalol (Trandate) are considered first-line therapy for preeclampsia, because they have been most widely used in pregnant patients and their safety and efficacy have been established. Additional alternatives include the beta blocker prazosin (Minipress), the calcium channel blocker nifedipine (Procardia), and the centrally acting alpha agonist clonidine (Catapres). Beta blockers are generally considered safe, but there is potential for impaired fetal growth if used early in pregnancy. Nifedipine has been used with no major problems. Patients should avoid diuretics because of the potential alteration in plasma volume. Patients in the second and third trimesters should avoid taking angiotensin-converting enzyme inhibitors because of the potential for fetal renal toxicity. Table 53-8 lists the two most commonly used drugs for treating preeclampsia, magnesium sulfate and hydralazine, and their dosages, uses, and considerations.

Adverse Reactions of Methyldopa

Observe the patient for peripheral edema, anxiety, nightmares, drowsiness, headache, dry mouth, drug fever, and mental depression. These are the most common potential adverse reactions.

Adverse Reactions of Hydralazine

Observe the patient for headache, nausea, vomiting, nasal congestion, dizziness, tachycardia, palpitations, and angina pectoris. Avoid a sudden decrease in maternal blood pressure, which may cause fetal hypoxia. Hydralazine has no known direct adverse effects on the fetus.

Adverse Reactions of Magnesium Sulfate

Early signs of increased magnesium levels include lethargy, flushing, feelings of increased warmth, perspiration, thirst, sedation, heavy eyelids, slurred speech, hypotension, DTR,

TABLE 53-8 DRUGS USED IN SEVERE PREECLAMPSIA

GENERIC (BRAND)	ROUTE AND DOSAGE	USES AND CONSIDERATIONS
magnesium sulfate	LD: IV: 6 g in 20 min; piggyback via infusion pump; maint: 2-3 g/h IV via infusion pump	Prevention and treatment of seizures related to preeclampsia. Acts as CNS depressant. Decreases acetylcholine from motor nerves, which blocks neuromuscular transmission and decreases incidence of seizures. Secondary effect is reduction in blood pressure as magnesium sulfate relaxes smooth muscle. Secondarily affects peripheral vascular system with increased uterine blood flow caused by vasodilation and some transient BP decrease during first hour; also inhibits uterine contractions. Depresses DTRs and respiration; maintenance dose depends on reflexes, respiratory rate, urinary output, and magnesium level. Main risk is production of abnormally high serum magnesium levels. Therapeutic levels range from 4-7 mEq/L; effective in preventing seizures. Patient at risk if respiratory rate <12/min, urinary output <30 mL/h, DTR absent or hyporeflexic. Patellar reflexes disappear with serum magnesium levels of 8-10 mEq/L. Maternal respiratory depression may occur with levels >10-15 mEq/; cardiac arrest with levels >20-25 mEq/L. Notify health care provider of any of the above occurs Can be given IV or IM (infrequent). Do not give parenterally to patients with heart block or myocardial damage. Use with caution in patients with renal impairment. Absorbed magnesium is excreted by kidneys; excreted in breast milk, but breastfeeding not contraindicated. Contraindicated in patients with myasthenia gravis. Relative contraindications: myocardial damage or heart block Antidote: IV: calcium gluconate 1 g slow IV push over 3 min Pregnancy category: B; PB: UK; t½: UK; Onset: IV immediate, IM 1 h; Duration: IV 30 min, IM 3-4 h; infusion usually stopped 24 h postpartum
hydralazine hydrochloride	IV: IV push: 5-10 mg doses every 20 min; *max cumulative total:* 20 mg or until blood pressure controlled IM and PO routes not usually used	Antihypertensive agent. Causes arteriolar vasodilation. Usually lowers diastolic BP more than systolic BP. Objective is to maintain diastolic BP of 90-110 mm Hg. Usually not given to pregnant preeclamptic patients with diastolic BP >105 mm Hg because of risk for reduced intervillous blood flow. Patients with impaired renal function may require lower doses Parenteral: Onset: 5-20 min; Peak: 10-80 min; Duration: 2-6 h; well tolerated; maternal tachycardia and increased cardiac output and oxygen consumption may occur. Oral: Onset: 20-30 min; Peak: 1-2 h; Duration: 2-4 h
methyldopa (♣ Apo-Methyldopa)	IV: 250-500 mg every 6-8 h, *max:* 1 g every 6 h PO: 250 mg b.i.d., *max:* 3 g/d	Stimulates central alpha-adrenergic receptors, resulting in decreased sympathetic outflow to heart, kidneys, and peripheral vasculature. Contraindicated in patients with hypersensitivity to drug or any component. Active hepatic disease, liver disorders previously associated with use of methyldopa, concurrent use with MAOIs Caution: Sedation is usually transient during initial treatment and dosage increases
labetalol (Trandate)	IV: 20 mg, followed by 40 mg, then 80 mg, and then 80 mg every 10 min until blood pressure controlled or max cumulative dose of 220 mg given	Pregnancy category: C; t½: 75-80 min; Onset 3-6 h; Duration 12-24 h

b.i.d., Two times a day; *BP,* blood pressure; *CNS,* central nervous system; *d,* day; *DTR,* deep tendon reflex; *h,* hour; *IM,* intramuscular; *IV,* intravenous; *LD,* loading dose; *maint,* maintenance; *MAOIs,* monoamine oxidase inhibitors; *max,* maximum; *min,* minute; *PB,* protein-binding; *PO,* by mouth; *t½,* half-life; *UK,* unknown; *>,* greater than; *<,* less than, ♣, Canadian drug.

and decreased muscle tone. Adverse reactions generally occur with serum magnesium sulfate levels greater than 10 mEq/L. Therapeutic levels are 4 to 7 mEq/L. Loss of patellar reflexes is often the first sign of magnesium toxicity and may be seen at 8 to 10 mEq/L. Respiratory depression may manifest at levels greater than 10 to 15 mEq/L, and cardiac arrest may manifest at levels greater than 20 to 25 mEq/L.

Decreased variability is commonly seen on the FHR tracing. If the patient received magnesium sulfate close to the time of delivery, the neonate may exhibit low Apgar scores, hypotonia, lethargy, weakness, and potential respiratory distress. The fetal level of magnesium generally reaches more than 90% of maternal levels within 3 hours of administration. There is no evidence linking congenital defects and maternal hypocalcemia or hypermagnesemia. The greater risk to the fetus is from maternal preeclampsia with resulting decreased placental blood flow and intrauterine growth retardation.

Nursing Process
Patient-Centered Collaborative Care

Gestational Hypertension

Assessment
- Review baseline vital signs from early pregnancy and BP readings during prenatal visits.
- Identify patient history that may predispose patient to preeclampsia.

Nursing Diagnoses
- Deficient knowledge related to preeclampsia, diagnosis, treatment modalities, and common outcomes for patient and infant
- Ineffective renal perfusion and perfusion of cerebral and peripheral tissue; risk to fetal well-being secondary to vasospasm
- Anxiety related to possible preterm hospitalization and delivery with possible adverse fetal or maternal outcomes
- Risk for injury related to maternal seizure activity and magnesium toxicity
- Deficient fluid volume related to shift of intravascular fluid to extravascular space as outcome of vasospasm with subsequent elevated arterial hypertension

Planning
- Patient's BP will be maintained within acceptable ranges.
- Patient will verbalize understanding of preeclampsia, etiology, signs and symptoms, and nonpharmacologic and pharmacologic treatment measures.
- Patient will understand and comply with planned preeclampsia treatment regimen.
- Fetus will tolerate impaired uteroplacental perfusion and subsequent delivery without injury.
- Therapeutic magnesium levels will be maintained.
- Magnesium sulfate infusion will be planned for at least 24 hours postpartum.

Patient Teaching

General
- Explain to patient preeclampsia and its implications for patient, fetus, and newborn.
- Provide patient with information about nonpharmacologic and pharmacologic treatment measures for preeclampsia.
- Advise patient to avoid exposure to infection.
- Remind patient with diabetes to check her glucose level as ordered.

Side Effects
- Advise patient to report immediately any breathing difficulty, weakness, or dizziness.
- Advise patient to report changes in stool, easy bruising, bleeding, blurred vision, unusual weight gain, and emotional changes.

Safety
- Advise patient to lie in left lateral recumbent position, and explain rationale.
- Educate patient on signs and symptoms of progressive preeclampsia and when to seek medical assistance.
- Explain to patient that fetal well-being will be assessed through biophysical profile (BPP), nonstress test (NST), or contraction stress test at frequent intervals, depending on health care provider and preeclampsia severity (e.g., NST and/or BPP 1 to 2 times per week).
- Educate family regarding possibility of seizures and appropriate actions if seizure occurs.

Diet
- Provide nutritional counseling on need for additional protein intake (90 g) to make up for urinary protein losses; normal sodium diet; and importance of adequate fluid intake.
- Explain to patient the rationale for daily weights.

Magnesium Sulfate
- Explain to patient why she will have an indwelling catheter, infusion pump, continuous fetal monitoring, and assessment of DTRs and clonus. Explain that therapy will extend into postpartum period 24 to 48 hours, depending on agency and health care provider.
- Explain to patient about visitor restrictions and need for low-stimulation environment.
- Advise patient that she will likely experience flush, warm sensation, and possibly nausea and vomiting during initial loading dose.
- Advise patient that evidence of magnesium levels within therapeutic range includes decreased appetite, some speech slurring, double vision, and weakness.

Hydralazine

- Explain to patient that nurses will be monitoring pulse and BP almost constantly until they become stable after administration, then every 15 minutes thereafter. Explain that an electronic BP monitor may be used to obtain constant readings. Some health care providers will request manual BP measurements.
- Explain to patient the need for careful measuring of I&O.
- Inform patient she may experience headache as a side effect of the drug.

Nursing Interventions

Magnesium Sulfate

- Provide continuous electronic fetal monitoring.
- Monitor for maternal toxicity. Lethargy and weakness result from blocking of neuromuscular transmission. Diaphoresis, flushing, feelings of warmth, and nasal congestion are results of vasodilation from relaxation of smooth muscle.
- Have airway suction, resuscitation equipment, and emergency drugs available.
- Have antidote available. Calcium gluconate (1 g) IV is given over 3 minutes.
- Maintain patient in left lateral recumbent position in low-stimulation environment. Provide close observation.
- For IM administration, use Z-track technique and rotate sites (drug is painful and irritating). Rarely is magnesium sulfate administered IM.
- Monitor BP, pulse, and respiratory rate per agency protocol; monitor DTRs, clonus, and I&O (with urimeter) every hour. Some health care providers will request manual BP measurements.
- Monitor temperature, breath sounds, and bowel sounds every 4 hours.
- Check urine for protein every hour.
- Assess for epigastric pain, headache, visual symptoms (blurred vision and scotoma), sensory changes, edema, level of consciousness, and seizure activity on ongoing basis.
- Monitor serum magnesium levels according to agency protocol for range between 4 to 7 mEq/L.
- Notify health care provider if you observe: decreased or changed level of consciousness; respirations <12/min; absence of DTR; urinary output <30 mL/h; systolic BP ≥160 mm Hg, unless ordered otherwise; magnesium level >7 mEq/L; absent bowel sounds or altered breath sounds; epigastric pain or right upper quadrant pain (associated with hepatic edema causing stretching of the liver capsule); headache; visual symptoms (blurred vision and scotoma); sensory changes; change in affect or level of consciousness, seizure activity.
- Monitor laboratory reports for low platelet count, elevated liver enzymes (AST, LDH), and bilirubin levels. Observe for evidence of excessive bleeding.
- Monitor fetal status. FHR baseline should remain at 110 to 160 beats/min.
- Monitor 24-hour urinary protein laboratory results if ordered (≥300 mg/day is abnormal).
- Monitor patient for magnesium toxicity.
- Monitor newborn for effects of placental exposure to excess magnesium sulfate. Although infrequent, newborn side effects include lethargy, neurologic or respiratory depression, and muscle hypotonia.

Hydralazine

- Take pulse and BP every 5 minutes when drug is administered, or monitor with electronic BP device until stabilized, then every 15 minutes. Some health care providers will request manual BP measurements.
- Observe for maintenance of diastolic BP between 90 and 110 mm Hg or as ordered.
- Observe for change in level of consciousness and headache.
- Monitor I&O to avoid hypotensive episodes or overload.
- Monitor FHR.

Cultural Considerations

- Provide an interpreter with same ethnic background and gender as patient if possible, especially when dealing with sensitive topics or stressful situations.

Evaluation

- Evaluate effectiveness of therapy to reduce BP.
- Continue monitoring vital signs. Report changes.
- Document effect of teaching and learning opportunities on patient's knowledge deficit about preeclampsia treatment modalities and outcomes.
- Note fetal well-being secondary to treatment with drugs as evidenced by fetal monitoring and fetal movement assessment.
- Monitor maternal physiologic changes in relation to magnesium sulfate levels.
- Continue monitoring FHR. Report changes.

KEY WEBSITES

American College of Obstetricians and Gynecologists: *www.acog.org*

Fetal development: *www.pregnancy.org/fetaldevelopment*

Pregnancy and drugs: *www.fda.gov*

CRITICAL THINKING CASE STUDY

TA (gravida 3, para 0) has a history of spontaneous abortion at 10 weeks' gestation and a preterm delivery and demise of a neonate at 21 weeks' gestation. At her 28-week prenatal visit, she reports increased clear vaginal discharge and feelings of pelvic pressure. Examination of her cervix reveals 2-cm dilation and a presenting fetal part low in the pelvis. TA is admitted to the hospital, and uterine activity is documented. Magnesium sulfate therapy is ordered for treatment of preterm labor. The nurse prepares for magnesium sulfate administration by the intravenous route.

1. How will magnesium sulfate therapy be initiated? What intervals and dosages should be anticipated?
2. What maternal and fetal side effects will the nurse expect to observe?
3. What should TA be told about the drug effects she will experience?
4. How would the nurse respond to TA's questions about the risks of preterm delivery?

After 24 hours of magnesium sulfate therapy, uterine contractions have been reduced to two to three per hour. TA is to be discharged home. The nurse is preparing TA's discharge teaching.

5. What instructions should the nurse give TA about her activity and diet?
6. TA asks whether the side effects of magnesium sulfate will continue. What is an appropriate nursing response?
7. What signs and symptoms should TA be advised to report?

NCLEX STUDY QUESTIONS

1. A patient at 33 weeks' gestation is diagnosed with preterm labor. The nurse prepares to administer betamethasone 12 mg. The nurse knows that this patient understands the patient education when she states, "This medication will help my baby's lungs mature…" and what else?
   a. "and is effective within 24 hours and up to 1 week."
   b. "if I remain in bed for the next 6 weeks on my side."
   c. "if I take my medicine at the same time every day."
   d. "if I avoid sexual intercourse for the remainder of my pregnancy."
2. The nurse notes that a prenatal patient is Rh negative, has hemoglobin 9.7 g/dL, positive HIV test, positive rubella titer, and positive PPD. Based on these results, after the patient's aminocentesis, the nurse prepares to administer what?
   a. RhO(D) immune globulin
   b. Measles-mumps-rubella vaccine
   c. hepatitis B (Engerix-B, Recombivax HB) vaccine
   d. isoniazid (INH)
3. The nurse is teaching a prenatal patient how to decrease the gastrointestinal distress she experiences with prenatal vitamins. The nurse instructs the patient to do what?
   a. "Take the vitamins between meals."
   b. "Eat when you take your vitamins."
   c. "Drink orange juice when you take your vitamins."
   d. "Drink milk when you take your vitamins."
4. The nurse at an infertility clinic is working with a preconceptual couple. The nurse advises the woman to take which supplement for at least 3 months before becoming pregnant?
   a. Iron
   b. Ginger
   c. Folic acid
   d. Vitamin B_6
5. The nurse at a prenatal clinic is reviewing messages to be returned to patients that afternoon. Which patient will the nurse call first?
   a. Primigravida, 10 gestational weeks, with nausea and vomiting, who requests information about ginger
   b. Gravida 2, 35 gestational weeks, with Braxton Hicks contractions, who requests information about caffeine
   c. Gravida 2, 32 gestational weeks, who has gestational diabetes with a blood sugar of 132 and requests information about her insulin
   d. Primigravida, 28 gestational weeks, with preeclampsia, who requests information about taking Motrin for headache
6. A patient with severe preeclampsia is on magnesium sulfate. The laboratory report shows a magnesium sulfate level of 7 mEq/L. Which is the most appropriate initial nursing intervention?
   a. Continue to monitor the patient because this level is therapeutic.
   b. Contact the health care provider, and report the level.
   c. Prepare to administer 1 g of calcium gluconate.
   d. Turn the patient on her left side, and administer 10 L of oxygen by nasal cannula.
7. The nurse is assessing a patient in preterm labor who is receiving magnesium sulfate. What is the finding of most concern?
   a. Lethargy
   b. Feelings of warmth
   c. Loss of patellar reflexes
   d. Positive clonus +2 bilaterally
8. The patient has been receiving magnesium sulfate IV for 24 hours to treat severe preeclampsia. On assessment, the nurse finds the following: temperature 37.3° C (99° F), pulse 88, respirations 14, BP 138/76, 21 patellar reflexes, and negative ankle clonus. What is the priority nursing intervention?
   a. Obtain a stat magnesium sulfate level.
   b. Discontinue magnesium sulfate.
   c. Contact the health care provider.
   d. Continue to monitor.

9. A primigravida patient, 8 gestational weeks, is at the prenatal clinic for her first examination. She complains of nausea and vomiting "every morning." Which comment made by the patient would indicate the need for further instruction?
   a. "My friend gave me ginger cookies to eat."
   b. "I have been eating dry crackers before I get up."
   c. "I have tried to avoid foods with strong smells."
   d. "I have been drinking chamomile tea every day."
10. The nurse in labor and delivery is reviewing messages to be returned to patients. Which patient should the nurse call first?
   a. "I'm 32 weeks pregnant and taking TUMS for my heartburn. Is there anything else I can take?"
   b. "I'm 38 weeks pregnant and taking Motrin for my backache. Should I take aspirin too?"
   c. "I'm 8 weeks pregnant and taking folic acid. Will it hurt me or the baby if I stop?"
   d. "I checked my blood sugar with a friend's machine and it was 120 mg. I'm not diabetic. Is that normal?"
11. A young adolescent, gravida 1, para 0, is admitted to labor and delivery with preterm labor at 29 weeks' gestation. Which nursing interventions should the nurse include? (Select all that apply.)
   a. Administration of antenatal glucocorticoid
   b. Liver function tests
   c. Bed rest in the left lateral position
   d. Administration of bolus IV fluids
   e. Administration of tocolytics
   f. Administration of an antihypertensive
12. A patient is planning to become pregnant. Which actions should the nurse counsel the patient to initiate before she stops taking her oral contraceptive? (Select all that apply.)
   a. Stop smoking.
   b. Take omega-6 fatty acid every day.
   c. Take a multivitamin every day.
   d. Stop taking over-the-counter acetaminophen.
   e. See her health care provider.

Answers: 1, c; 2, a; 3, b; 4, c; 5, d; 6, a; 7, c; 8, d; 9, d; 10, b; 11, a, c, d, e; 12, a, c, e.

CHAPTER 54

Female Reproductive Cycle II: Labor, Delivery, and Preterm Neonatal Drugs

Robin Webb Corbett and Laura K. Williford Owens

evolve WEBSITE

http://evolve.elsevier.com/KeeHayes/pharmacology/

- Animations
- Content Updates
- Key Points
- Review Questions for the NCLEX® Examination
- References from the Textbook
- Unfolding Case Studies

OBJECTIVES

- Critique systemic and regional medications for pain control during labor, their action, side effects, and nursing implications.
- Describe the nursing process, including patient teaching, associated with the drugs used during labor and delivery.
- Compare drugs used to enhance uterine contractility during labor and after placental expulsion, their action, side effects, and nursing implications.
- Describe the nursing process associated with the administration of surfactant therapy for preterm neonates.

OUTLINE

KEY TERMS

DRUGS FOR PAIN CONTROL DURING LABOR

Labor and delivery are divided into four stages, the first three specific to labor and delivery. During the first stage, the dilating stage, cervical effacement and dilation occur; the cervix thins and becomes fully dilated at 10 cm. The first stage consists of three phases categorized by cervical dilation: the latent phase (0 to 4 cm), the active phase (4 to 7 cm), and the transition phase (8 to 10 cm). The second stage of labor, the pelvic stage, begins with complete cervical dilation and ends with delivery of the newborn (Figure 54-1). During the third stage of labor, the placenta separates from the uterine wall and is delivered. The fourth stage of labor, or the first 1 to 4 hours postpartum, is a period of physiologic stabilization for the mother and initiation of familial attachment.

During the first stage of labor, uterine contractions produce progressive cervical effacement and dilation. As the first stage of labor progresses, uterine contractions become stronger, longer, and more frequent, and discomfort increases. Pain and discomfort in labor are caused by uterine contraction, cervical dilation and effacement, hypoxia of the contracting myometrium, and perineal pressure from the presenting part. Pain perception is influenced by physiologic, psychological, social, and cultural factors, in particular, the woman's past experience with pain, anticipation of pain, fear and anxiety, knowledge deficit of the labor and delivery process, and involvement of support persons.

Before administering pharmacologic treatment, nonpharmacologic measures should be initiated. Nonpharmacologic measures for pain relief during labor include (1) ambulation, (2) supportive positioning of the gravid uterus and promotion of uterine perfusion, (3) touch and massage, (4) hygiene and comfort measures, (5) support persons, (6) breathing and relaxation techniques, (7) transcutaneous electrical nerve stimulation, (8) hypnosis, (9) acupuncture, and (10) hydrotherapy (warm-water baths or showers).

Other nonpharmacologic measures include alternative and complementary medicine. Of particular concern is the use of herbal supplements by the pregnant patient later in pregnancy to stimulate labor. For example, some women ingest pregnancy toner tea, which includes raspberry, nettles, dandelion, alfalfa, and peppermint leaf. Other herbal supplements used include blue cohosh, castor oil, and evening primrose oil. Pregnant patients may self-administer, or the practice may be part of their traditional beliefs and framework of health. Concerns with herbal supplements are related to the often numerous physiologic active components of the herbs, adulterants, inconsistent dosing, and lack of proven efficacy. Herbs taken in late pregnancy may contribute to preterm labor or increased bleeding during delivery. Nurses must be

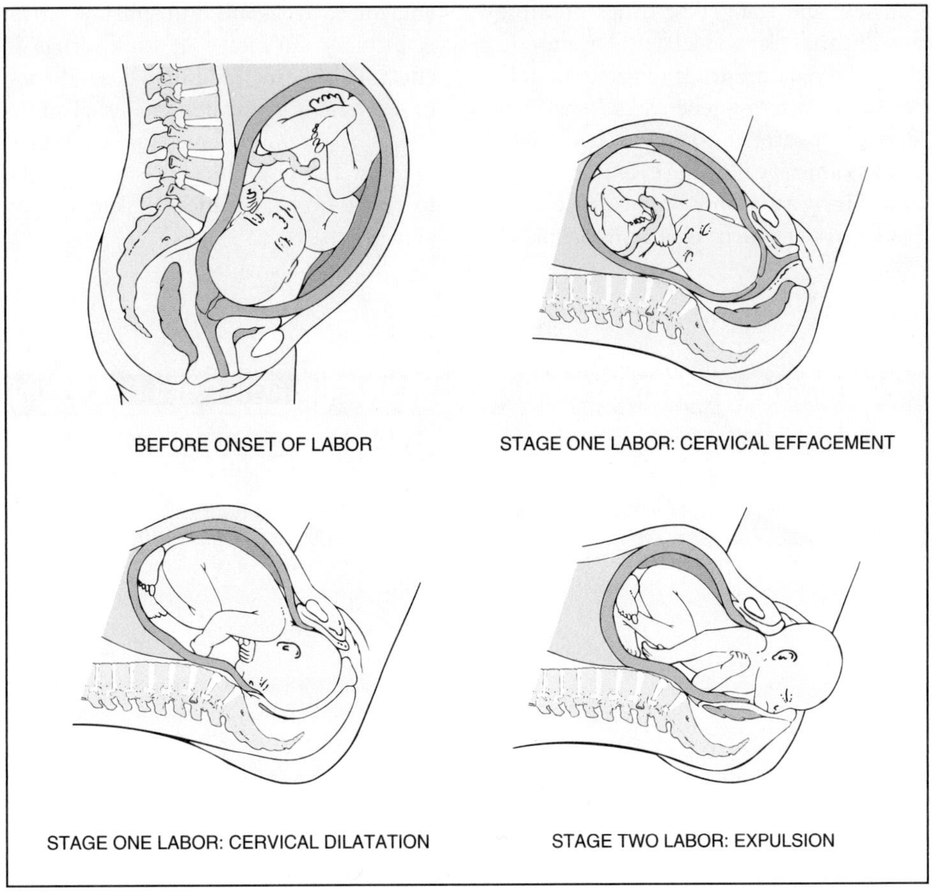

FIGURE 54–1 First and second stages of labor.

culturally sensitive to the use of herbal supplements and health practices during pregnancy, specifically in the latter gestational weeks.

When pharmacologic intervention is needed for pain relief, drugs are used as an adjunct to nonpharmacologic measures. Drugs should be selected not only to decrease the patient's pain but also to minimize side effects for the patient and the fetus or neonate. Pain relief in labor can be obtained with systemic analgesics and regional anesthesia. Analgesics alter the patient's perception and sensation of pain without producing unconsciousness.

Analgesia/Sedation

Systemic medications used during labor include sedative-tranquilizers, narcotics agonists, and mixed narcotic agonist-antagonists; these may be administered orally (sedative-hypnotic drugs), intravenously (IV), or intramuscularly (IM) (Table 54-1). Because of the variable response and blood levels with intramuscular administration, these drugs are more commonly administered intravenously. These medications should be administered at the onset of the uterine contraction, because parenteral administration at the onset of the contraction decreases neonatal drug exposure as blood flow is decreased to the uterus and fetus.

The sedative-tranquilizer drugs are most commonly given for false labor, latent labor, or with ruptured membranes without true labor. These drugs may also be administered to minimize maternal anxiety and fear. These drugs promote rest and relaxation and decrease fear and anxiety, but they do not provide pain relief. The sedative drugs most commonly used are barbiturates or hypnotics—generally secobarbital sodium (Seconal) and pentobarbital sodium (Nembutal). Other drugs, such as phenothiazine derivatives and hydroxyzine, can be given alone during early labor or in combination with narcotic agonists when the patient is in active labor. In addition to decreasing anxiety and apprehension, these drugs potentiate the analgesic action of the opioids and minimize emesis. These drugs include promethazine (Phenergan), a phenothiazine, and hydroxyzine hydrochloride (Vistaril), a sedative-hypnotic.

The second group of drugs given for active labor are the narcotic agonists. These drugs may be administered parenterally or via regional blocks. When administered with neuraxial anesthesia, a lower dose of anesthetic is required for effective pain relief, thereby minimizing side effects. These drugs interfere with pain impulses at the subcortical level of the brain. To effect pain relief, opioids interact with mu and kappa receptors. For example, morphine sulfate activates both mu and kappa receptors.

Meperidine (Demerol) is the most commonly prescribed synthetic opioid for pain control during labor. A second narcotic agonist used for pain relief during labor is fentanyl (Sublimaze). Fentanyl is a short-acting synthetic opioid that is best administered IV because of its short duration of action. Morphine sulfate may also be used for pain control in active labor, but it is less frequently used. High doses of opioids are required for effective labor analgesia when administered parenterally.

The third group of systemic medications used for pain relief in labor are opioids with mixed narcotic agonist-antagonist effects. These drugs exert their effects at more than one site—often an agonist at one site and an antagonist at another. The two most commonly used narcotic-agonist-antagonist drugs are butorphanol tartrate and nalbuphine. A primary advantage of these drugs is their dose-ceiling effect. This means additional doses do not increase the degree of respiratory depression, maternal and/or neonatal, so there is less respiratory depression with these drugs than with opioids. The respiratory depression ceiling effect is believed to result from activation of kappa agonists and weak mu antagonists.

TABLE 54-1 COMMON SYSTEMIC MEDICATIONS USED FOR PAIN RELIEF IN LABOR

GENERIC (BRAND)	ROUTE AND DOSAGE	USES AND CONSIDERATIONS
Sedative-Hypnotics		
secobarbital (Seconal)	IM: 50-100 mg; PO: 100-200 mg	To decrease anxiety during latent phase of labor. Onset: 15-30 min; peak: 15-30 min; duration: 1-4 h. No effects on uterine tone or contractility; rapidly crosses placenta; can cause decreased variability in FHR because of decreased CNS control over heart rate. No antagonist for barbiturates, so secobarbital administered only if delivery not expected for 24-48 h. May have prolonged depressant effects on neonate. Excreted in breast milk. Compatible with breastfeeding. May increase CNS depression with alcohol, narcotics, antihistamines, tranquilizers, and monoamine oxidase inhibitors (MAOIs). Avoid valerian, St. John's wort, kava kava, gotu kola. Pregnancy category: D; PB: 45%-60%; $t\frac{1}{2}$: 15-40 h
pentobarbital (Nembutal)	IV: Initial: 100-200 mg	Short-acting barbiturate. Sedative. Pregnancy category: D; PB: Varying degree based upon lipid solubility; $t\frac{1}{2}$: 15-50 h; Onset: IV: Immediate-5 minutes

TABLE 54-1 COMMON SYSTEMIC MEDICATIONS USED FOR PAIN RELIEF IN LABOR—cont'd

GENERIC (BRAND)	ROUTE AND DOSAGE	USES AND CONSIDERATIONS
promethazine (Phenergan)	IM/IV: 12.5-50 mg q3-4h or IM: 25-50 mg with 25-75 mg meperidine or IV: 15-25 mg with 25-75 mg meperidine; repeat if needed; *max:* 100 mg in 24 h	A phenothiazine antihistamine; used as an adjunct to narcotic analgesics during first stage of labor; antiemetic properties. Onset: IM: 20 min; IV: 3-5 min. Do not give subQ. To prevent or minimize tissue damage during IV administration, dilute, administer via running IV line at port furthest from vein, and administer through large bore vein if possible. Instruct patient to report signs of pain and burning with administration. Used alone to promote rest and sleep; potentiates action of narcotic agonists, reducing narcotic doses. May cause decreased variability in FHR; contraindicated during lactation. At term, rapidly crosses placenta; fetal and maternal blood concentrations in equilibrium in 15 min, with infant levels persisting for 4 h. Transient hypotonia, lethargy, and electroencephalographic changes for 3 days in newborn. May cause maternal tachycardia; may impair newborn platelet aggregation. If given with meperidine, administer slowly at beginning of contraction over several minutes to decrease amount of drug perfused immediately to fetus via placenta. Adverse reactions: dizziness, dry mouth, excessive sedation, weakness, blurred vision, and restlessness. Pregnancy category: C; PB: 35%-55%; $t\frac{1}{2}$: 22 h
promethazine HCl (Phenergan)	IV: 12.5-25 mg IM: 25-50 mg q4-6h; repeat if needed For sedation in obstetrics: IM or IV dosage Note: Deep IM injection is the preferred parenteral route of administration. IV administration is the most common route in clinical settings. IV administration has been associated with severe tissue damage. Do not give at a rate >25 mg/min IV; consider dilution prior to administration and giving over 10-15 minutes. Pregnant females: 25-50 mg IM or IV during the early stages of labor and 25-75 mg after labor is established; repeat dosage once or twice every 4 hours as needed; maximum total dose is 100 mg per 24-hour period for patients in labor.	Antianxiety agent; antihistamine; antiemetic; sedative-hypotonic. Used alone early in labor or later to potentiate action of narcotic agonists. Onset: IV: 3-5 min; IM: 20 min; peak: IV/IM: UK; duration: 2-6 h. IV is not preferred route for administration but is frequent route for obstetric patients. Solution for IV may be diluted in 25-100 mL NS or D_5W and infused slowly over 15-30 min at a rate <25 mg/min Use Z-track injection for IM to reduce pain. Intraarterial or subQ administration not recommended (thrombus and digital gangrene can occur). Extravasation can result in sterile abscesses and marked tissue induration. Use with caution in patients with chronic obstructive pulmonary disease and asthma. Crosses placenta. Possible respiratory depression if drug administered near delivery. Can cause decreased variability in FHR. Breastfeeding not recommended. No effect on labor or neonatal Apgar scores. Adverse reactions: hypotension, drowsiness, dizziness, ataxia; may cause CNS depression with alcohol, analgesics, barbiturates, narcotics; may decrease effects of epinephrine. Pregnancy category: C; PB: 93%; $t\frac{1}{2}$: 3 h
hydroxyzine pamoate (Vistaril)	Anxiety: PO: 25-100 mg Preoperative sedation: 50-100 mg IM: 25-100 mg	Anxiolytic; antiemetic; antihistamine. Used for anxiety and preoperative and postoperative adjunct for sedation. Onset: 15-30 min; Peak: 2 h; Duration: 4-6 hours. Administer deep in large muscle. Do not give IV or subQ. Additive effects may occur with use of ethanol, St. John's wort, kava kava, anticholinergics, and CNS depressants. Pregnancy category: C; PB: UK; $t\frac{1}{2}$: 3-7 h
Narcotic Agonists		
fentanyl citrate (Sublimaze)	IM/IV: 50-100 mcg	IV: Onset: 1-2 min; Peak: 3-5 min; Duration: 30-60 min; IM Onset: 7-15 min; Peak: 20-30 min; Duration: 1-2 h. Is 50-100 times as potent as morphine. Muscle rigidity may occur with too-rapid IV administration. Inject over 3-5 min. Crosses placenta and excreted in breast milk. Watch for respiratory depression in neonates of mothers who receive this drug in labor. May see withdrawal symptoms in neonate if mother was regular opioid user during pregnancy. Be alert to risk of overdose in patients using CNS depressants, phenothiazines, ethanol, and tricyclic antidepressants. Herbal interactions include increased CNS depression with use of St John's wort, kava kava, and gotu kola. Contraindicated in patients with severe asthma. Pregnancy category: C; PB: UK; $t\frac{1}{2}$: 2-4 h

Continued

TABLE 54-1 COMMON SYSTEMIC MEDICATIONS USED FOR PAIN RELIEF IN LABOR—cont'd

GENERIC (BRAND)	ROUTE AND DOSAGE	USES AND CONSIDERATIONS
morphine sulfate (Duramorph)	IM/IV: 5-10 mg or IV 2-5 mg q4h	Opioid; binds to CNS opiate receptors and inhibits ascending pain pathways. Used for relief of moderate to severe pain, for preoperative medication, and as supplement to anesthesia. Onset: IM: 20-30 min; IV: 3-10 min. Peak: IM: 0.5-1 h; IV: 20 min. Duration: IM: 3-4 h; IV: 3-5 h. Have naloxone available as antidote. If naloxone is necessary for maternal and fetal respiratory depression, give to mother and infant. CNS depressants and tricyclic antidepressants may potentiate effects of morphine. Cautious use with MAOIs and meperidine. Use of selective serotonin reuptake inhibitors (SSRIs) or meperidine may precipitate serotonin syndrome. Use with caution in patients with biliary tract disease and seizure disorders. Withdrawal symptoms may occur in narcotic-dependent patients and in neonates of narcotic-dependent patients. May cause drowsiness and respiratory depression, sedation, euphoria, hallucinations, headache, and palpitations. Do not give if respirations <12/min. Morphine crosses placenta. Use with caution in patients delivering a preterm infant, because fetus may exhibit decreased beat-to-beat variability on FHR monitor. Newborn may have moderate CNS depression, hypotonia at birth, and mild behavioral depression. When giving IV, dilute in 4-5 mL of sterile water and administer slowly (15 mg over 3-5 min). Herbal interactions include increased CNS depression with valerian, St. John's wort, kava kava, and gotu kola. Enters breast milk; compatible with breastfeeding for single doses of morphine. Chronic morphine use may have adverse neonatal effects and is not recommended. Pregnancy category: C (D, if prolonged use or high at-term dose); PB: 30%-35%; $t\frac{1}{2}$: 2-4 h
Mixed Narcotic Agonist-Antagonists		
butorphanol tartrate	IV: 0.5-1 mg q1.5-2h or 1-2 mg q4h	Mixed opioid agonist/antagonist. IV onset: 5-10 min; peak: 4-5 min; duration: 3-4 h. Herbal interactions include increased CNS depression with valerian, St John's wort, kava kava, and gotu kola. Contraindicated for opiate-dependent patients who have not been detoxified; may cause withdrawal syndrome. Cautious use in patients with renal or hepatic dysfunction. For use in pregnancies >37 gestational weeks with no fetal distress. Use alternative analgesic if delivery anticipated in 4 h or less. If breastfeeding, take dose immediately after breastfeeding or 3-4 hours prior to next feeding. Pregnancy category: C/D; PB: 80%; $t\frac{1}{2}$: 2.5-4 h
nalbuphine	IV: 10 mg q2-3h	Mixed opioid agonist/antagonist. Narcotic. Onset: 2-3 m; Peak: 2-3 min; Duration: 3-6 h. Limited respiratory depression. Less analgesic effect than morphine. About 10%-15% of laboring women experience hallucinations with nalbuphine. Cautious use in patients with renal or hepatic dysfunction. Avoid use in opiate-dependent patients; may cause withdrawal syndrome. Monitor for fetal bradycardia. Monitor newborn for respiratory depression or bradycardia. Inject slowly over at least 2-3 min. If breastfeeding, take immediately after breastfeeding or 3-4 h prior to next feeding. Herbal interactions include increased CNS depression with valerian, St. John's wort, kava kava, and gotu kola. Toxicity can be reversed with naloxone. Pregnancy category: B; PB: UK; $t\frac{1}{2}$: 5 h

CNS, Central nervous system; *d,* day; *FHR,* fetal heart rate; *h,* hour; *IM,* intramuscular; *IV,* intravenous; *MAOI,* monoamine oxidase inhibitor; *max,* maximum; *min,* minute; *PB,* protein-binding; *PO,* by mouth; *PRN,* as needed; *subQ,* subcutaneously; $t\frac{1}{2}$, half-life; *UK,* unknown; <, less than, >, greater than.

Adverse Reactions

Adverse effects of sedative-hypnotic drugs (secobarbital, pentobarbital) include paradoxically increased pain and excitability, lethargy, subdued mood, decreased sensory perception, and hypotension. Fetal and neonatal side effects include decreased fetal heart rate (FHR) variability and neonatal respiratory depression, sleepiness, hypotonia, and delayed breastfeeding with poor sucking response for up to 4 days.

Side effects of phenothiazine derivatives and antiemetics/antihistamines (promethazine, hydroxyzine) include confusion, disorientation, excess sedation, dizziness, hypotension, tachycardia, blurred vision, headache, restlessness, weakness, and urinary retention with promethazine, and drowsiness, dry mouth, dizziness, headache, blurred vision, dysuria, urinary retention, and constipation with hydroxyzine. Decreased FHR variability occurs, and the neonate can experience moderate central nervous system (CNS) depression, hypotonia, lethargy, poor feeding, and hypothermia.

The adverse effects of opioids depend on the responses activated by the mu and kappa receptors. Activation of mu receptors results in analgesia, decreased gastrointestinal (GI) motility, euphoria, respiratory depression, sedation, and physiologic dependence. In contrast, activation of kappa receptors results in analgesia, decreased gastrointestinal motility, miosis, and sedation. When parenterally administered, the side effects of opioids include nausea, vomiting, sedation, orthostatic hypotension, pruritus, and maternal and neonatal respiratory depression. The associated nausea and vomiting result from stimulation of the chemoreceptor trigger zone in the medulla. Motor block is another concern. Mothers may not walk after delivery until they are able to maintain a straight leg raise against downward pressure as applied by the practitioner. Fetal and neonatal effects include decreased FHR variability and depression of neonatal respirations and Apgar scores. Depression of neonatal neurobehavior is evidenced by lowered Apgar scores. For example, with meperidine, neonatal respiration occurs within 2 to 3 hours after administration. Neonatal respiratory depression may require reversal by administration of naloxone (Narcan). Through inhibition of both mu and kappa receptors, naloxone may reverse the effects of opioids. NOTE: With maternal administration of naloxone, there will be a subsequent increase in pain.

Narcotic agonist drugs (morphine, fentanyl) can cause orthostatic hypotension, nausea, vomiting, headache, sedation, hypotension, and confusion. Decreased FHR variability and neonatal CNS depression can occur with meperidine.

Mixed narcotic agonist-antagonist drugs (butorphanol tartrate, nalbuphine) can cause nausea, clamminess, sweating, sedation, respiratory depression, vertigo, lethargy, headache, and flush. Side effects in the fetus and neonate include decreased FHR variability, moderate CNS depression, hypotonia at birth, and mild behavioral depression.

Nursing Process
Patient-Centered Collaborative Care

Pain-Control Drugs

Assessment
- Assess patient's level of pain using agency pain scale.
- Assess patient's cultural framework to determine use of complementary and alternative medicine in later pregnancy and beliefs regarding labor.
- Assess laboring patient's behavior for relaxation and progress of labor in relation to expected norms.
- Assess patient's verbal and nonverbal behavior for data supportive or nonsupportive of coping with labor.
- To determine effectiveness of pain management, obtain baseline vital signs, blood pressure (BP), breath sounds, quality of uterine contractions, degree of effacement and dilation, and FHR before administering analgesic.
- Ask patient regarding use of complementary and alternative medicines (including herbal supplements) during pregnancy.
- Screen for drug history to ascertain potential for drug-drug interactions.
- Assess cultural expectations related to pain experiences.

Nursing Diagnoses
- Anxiety related to uncertainty about labor experience and personal coping ability
- Acute pain related to processes of labor and birth
- Fear related to deficient knowledge of processes and birth and expected sensations with analgesic interventions

Planning
- Patient will verbalize desired amount of pain relief during labor.
- Patient will demonstrate minimal to no side effects from pain-control drugs during labor.
- Patient will verbalize a decrease in pain on a scale of 1 to 10 or per agency pain scale.

Nursing Interventions
- Offer appropriate analgesia for stage and phase of labor and anticipated method of delivery. Encourage patient and support persons to participate in decision making about analgesia.
- Document administration of drug per agency protocol.
- Provide appropriate safety measures after administration of drugs.
- Check compatibility chart for any mixing of drugs.
- Verify that correct antidote drugs are available.
- Within agency protocol, safe obstetric practice, and patient preferences, administer drugs before maximum intensity of pain and anxiety.
- Assess patient's level of pain using agency-appropriate pain scale 30 to 60 minutes after analgesic administration.

Sedative-Hypnotics: Barbiturates
- Do not give if active labor is imminent.
- Monitor FHR; expect decreased variability.

Phenothiazine Derivatives
Promethazine (Phenergan)
- If administered by IV route, give at onset of uterine contraction. Administer at a rate not to exceed 25 mg/min.

- Monitor amount of promethazine patient receives in 24 hours; monitor maternal heart rate after administration.

Hydroxyzine (Vistaril)

- Administer IM (Z-track technique) only. Do not give subcutaneously or IV.

Narcotic Agonists and Mixed Narcotic Agonist-Antagonists

- Assess patient parity, obstetric delivery history, and anticipated time until delivery.
- Because of risk of neonatal respiratory depression, do not administer when delivery is likely within 2 hours.
- Monitor urine output.
- Monitor FHR, assessing for fetal well-being before and during drug administration.

Fentanyl

- Generally not given before active labor. Have naloxone available as antidote if needed.
- If drug is administered IV, administer slowly at beginning of contraction over several minutes to decrease amount of drug perfused to the fetus via the placenta.
- Assess respirations. Must be >12 before administration.
- Provide restful environment as adjunctive therapy.
- Keep bed rails up when patient is nonambulatory, and have patient solicit assistance with ambulation.
- Monitor FHR, assessing for fetal well-being before and during drug administration.
- Have neonatal naloxone available.

Butorphanol Tartrate

- Monitor for signs of narcotic withdrawal in narcotic-dependent patients.
- Monitor for maternal and/or neonatal respiratory depression.
- Assess respirations. Must be >12 before administration.
- IM: Inject deep into muscle. IV: Give slowly at onset contraction. Do not administer subcutaneously.
- Provide restful environment as adjunctive therapy.
- Monitor FHR tracing, assessing for fetal well-being before and during drug administration.
- Keep bed rails up when patient is nonambulatory, and have patient solicit assistance with ambulation.
- Have naloxone available.

Patient Teaching

General

- Advise patient concerning (1) drugs ordered, (2) route of administration and reason, (3) expected effects of drug on labor, and (4) potential drug effects on patient and fetus or neonate.
- Educate patient that most drugs used for pain relief in labor and delivery are not given by mouth, because the gastrointestinal tract functions more slowly during labor, and drug absorption is decreased, making the oral route ineffective.
- Advise patient about safety precautions to be used while receiving the drug, including (1) positioning in bed, (2) use of side rails, and (3) assistance with ambulation.

Cultural Considerations

- Acknowledge and incorporate patient's cultural belief framework into nursing care.
- Assess patient's use of complementary and alternative medicine (to include herbal supplements) during pregnancy and labor.
- Recognize cultural influences on patient's expression of discomfort and pain.
- Provide an interpreter as appropriate.

Evaluation

- Evaluate effectiveness of drug in alleviating pain.
- Evaluate fear and anxiety in regard to pain and ability to cope with labor.
- Monitor maternal respirations, heart rate, BP, uterine contractions, dilatation and effacement, and FHR for alterations from baseline. Report deviations beyond those expected with normally progressing labor.
- Document findings, using agency protocol and obstetric nursing standards of care.

Anesthesia

Anesthesia in labor and delivery represents the loss of painful sensations with or without loss of consciousness. Two types of pain are experienced in childbirth. Visceral pain from the cervix and uterus is carried by sympathetic fibers and enters the neuraxis at the thoracic 10, 11, 12, and lumbar 1 spinal levels. Early labor pain is transmitted to T11 and T12 with later progression to T10 and L1. Somatic pain is caused by pressure of the presenting part and stretching of the perineum and vagina. This pain is the pain of the transition phase and the second stage of labor and is transmitted to the sacral 2, 3, and 4 areas by the pudendal nerve.

Regional Anesthesia

Regional anesthesia achieves pain relief during labor and delivery without loss of consciousness. Injected local anesthetic agents temporarily block conduction of painful impulses along sensory nerve pathways to the brain (Table 54-2). Regional anesthesia allows the patient to experience labor and childbirth with relief from discomfort in the blocked area. There are primarily two types of anesthesia: (1) local anesthetic agents for local infiltration (e.g., episiotomy) and (2) regional blocks (e.g., epidural; Table 54-3). The most common peridural anesthesias are spinal, epidural, and combined spinal-epidural (Figure 54-2). Other less commonly administered regional blocks include caudal, paracervical, and pudendal blocks. The anesthesiologist or nurse anesthetist is responsible for administering regional anesthesia.

TABLE 54-2 ANESTHETIC AGENTS USED IN OBSTETRICS

ANESTHETIC AGENT	USUAL CONCENTRATION	USUAL DOSE (mg)	ONSET	AVERAGE DURATION (min)	CLINICAL USE
Chloroprocaine	1-2	400-600	Rapid	15-30	Local or pudendal block
(Nesacaine)	2-3	300-750		30-60	Epidural
Tetracaine	0.2	4	Slow	70-150	Low spinal block
(Pontocaine)	0.5	7-10	Fast	75-150	Spinal for cesarean
Lidocaine	1	200-300	Rapid	30-60	Local or pudendal block
(Xylocaine)	2	300-450		60-90	Epidural for cesarean
	5	50-75		45-60	Spinal for cesarean, PP tubal ligation, and vaginal delivery
Bupivacaine	0.5	50-100	Slow-moderate	90-150	Epidural for cesarean
(Marcaine)	0.25	20-25	Moderate	60-90	Epidural for labor
	0.75	7.5-11		60-120	Spinal for cesarean
Ropivacaine	0.5	75-100	Slow-moderate	90-150	Epidural for cesarean
(Naropin)	0.25	20-25	Slow-moderate	60-90	Epidural for labor

min, Minute; *PP,* postpartum.

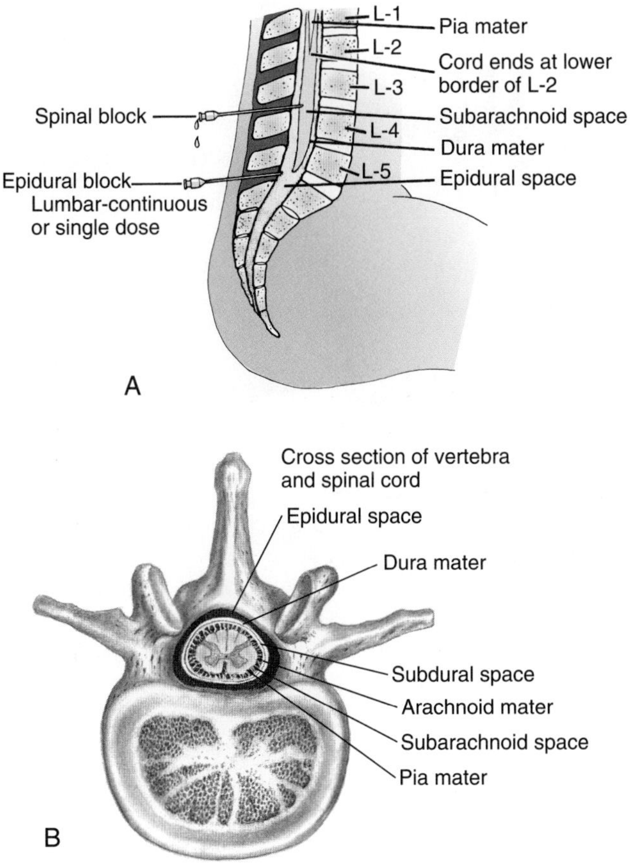

FIGURE 54–2 A, Membranes and spaces of spinal cord and levels of sacral, lumbar, and thoracic nerves. **B,** Cross-section of vertebra and spinal cord. (From Lowdermilk D, Perry S, Cashion C, Alden K: *Maternity and women's health care,* ed 10, St. Louis, 2012, Mosby.)

Nurses may assist with administration of anesthesia and monitor the patient for drug effectiveness and side effects during and after administration.

Women receiving parenteral analgesic for labor and delivery may require more focused anesthesia for episiotomies and repair of perineal lacerations. Local anesthetic agents may be administered alone, and the anesthetic agent primarily administered is lidocaine (Xylocaine). Burning at the site of injection is the most common side effect.

Spinal anesthesia, also known as a *saddle block,* is injected in the subarachnoid space at the T10 to S5 dermatome. This anesthesia may be a single dose or administered as a combined spinal-epidural. Spinal anesthesia is administered immediately before delivery or late in the second stage when the fetal head is on the perineal floor. Drugs frequently administered either alone or in combination with the local anesthetic for a vaginal delivery include bupivacaine (Marcaine) (2.5 to 3 mg) with fentanyl (25 mcg). Dosages vary depending on whether administration of the anesthetic agent is plain or with epinephrine. Spinal anesthesia has a rapid onset, requires less local anesthetic, and may be used with high-risk patients. Postdural puncture headache is a primary concern, occurring 6 to 48 hours after dural puncture; it may also occur after accidental dural puncture with epidural anesthesia. Treatment for postdural headache includes analgesics, increased fluids, and bed rest. With resistant headaches, some health care providers may give 500 mg of caffeine in 1000 to 2000 mL of normal saline over 2 hours, though caffeine preparations have not been proved to be effective. An epidural blood patch (10 to 20 mL) is the most effective means to treat postdural headache.

Lumbar epidurals may be administered as a single injection, intermittent injections, continuous patient-controlled epidural anesthesia (PCEA), and as a combined spinal-epidural. Epidurals may be administered as a single anesthetic agent or with opioids or epinephrine. Single-dose epidural anesthesia is infrequently used as analgesia and is limited to the single dosing action. Intermittent epidural bolus dosing was once commonly used for pain relief. Doses of the local anesthetic were injected intermittently via an epidural catheter. Limitations of this method included the need for frequent injections and decreased pain control because of the dosing schedule. Most frequently, patients now

TABLE 54-3 TYPES OF ANESTHESIA

TYPE OF ANESTHESIA	INDICATIONS	ADVERSE REACTIONS/ SIDE EFFECTS*	NORMAL DOSE	NURSING IMPLICATIONS†
Spinal block (subarachnoid block)	Need for high degree of pain relief for delivery.	High/spinal block (respiratory muscles impaired by block), neuritis, block failure, apnea with total spinal	Vaginal delivery: 2.5 or 3 mg bupivacaine (Marcaine) with 25 mcg fentanyl (Sublimaze). Epinephrine 0.2 mg and fentanyl 10-25 mcg or sufentanil (Sufenta) 5-10 mcg or morphine (Duramorph) 0.1-0.25 mg Cesarean delivery: 12 mg bupivacaine mixed with 8.25% dextrose with 10-25 mcg fentanyl. Postoperatively 0.1-0.25 mg morphine may be added	Cervix should be fully dilated before administration. Anesthetic should be given immediately after a contraction to avoid impairing neonate's respiratory efforts. Patient is generally placed sitting or in curled side-lying position for administration. Monitor BP every 1-2 minutes for first 10 minutes. After administration, monitor BP every 5-10 minutes. Assess level of analgesia. Treat maternal hypotension due to uterine displacement by placing a wedge under hip. Contraindications: Infection at site, increased intracranial pressure, allergy to local anesthetics, coagulopathies, severe hypovolemia, severe aortic or mitral stenosis, or lack of patient consent.
Lumbar epidural block (single dose)	Pain relief in first and second stages of labor.	Neuritis, epidural hematoma, high/ spinal block, catheter complications, intravascular injection, direct spinal cord injury, bloody tap.	Vaginal delivery: bupivacaine (Marcaine) 0.125% to 0.25%, lidocaine (Xylocaine) 1.5%, with 1 : 200,000 epinephrine followed by 0.1%-0.2% ropivacaine (Naropin) with fentanyl (Sublimaze) 2 mcg/mL. Cesarean delivery: 5 mL boluses of 2% lidocaine with 1 : 400,000 epinephrine, alternatively, 5 mL boluses of 0.5% bupivacaine or 0.5% ropivacaine or 3% 2-chloroprocaine (boluses of lidocaine or 2-chloroprocaine every 1-2 minutes, boluses of bupivacaine or ropivacaine every 2-5 minutes)	Of particular importance is the assessment of bilateral analgesia for pain relief during labor. If unilateral analgesia occurs, patient is turned to opposite side and more anesthetic is injected. Contraindications: Same as spinal block.

Continuous lumbar epidural block using indwelling catheter in epidural space	Pain relief during first and second stages. The most widely used anesthesia method for labor pain management. Useful for prolonged labor.	Pruritus, catheter complications, intravascular injection, direct spinal cord injury, bloody tap.	Continuous infusion options (rate is 12-15 mL/h): 0.1% or 0.15% ropivacaine or bupivacaine (Marcaine) with 1-2 mcg/mL fentanyl (Sublimaze)	Breakthrough pain is treated by increased infusion rate of rescue dose of anesthetic.
Patient-controlled epidural administration	Pain relief during first and second stages. Useful for prolonged labor.	Same as above.		Same as above.
Combined spinal-epidural	Pain relief during first and second stages. Spinal can help with early labor pain and epidural with pain management during active labor.	Same as above.	Spinal: 10-25 mcg fentanyl (Sublimaze) or 2.5-10 mcg sufentanil (Sufenta) alone or in combination with 1 mL bupivacaine (Marcaine) 0.25% epidural is initiated with bupivacaine 0.03%-0.0625% with fentanyl 1-2 mcg/mL or sufentanil 0.1-0.3 mcg/mL.	Same as above.
Local infiltration	For episiotomy and perineal laceration repair. When given: Just before delivery or repair. Area blocked: Local area adjacent to injection. Injection site: Perineal subcutaneous tissue.	Mild discomfort and/or burning during injection. Fetus or neonate: None.		May not obtain complete pain relief, and may need additional injections; requires large amount of local anesthetic agent.

*The following adverse reactions/side effects apply to each of the above: *Patient:* hypotension; paresthesia or nerve injury, postdural puncture headache, infection, nausea, vomiting, backache, urinary retention. Headache is less common because of the small size (25 gauge) of needle used. *Fetus or neonate:* Few, unless secondary to maternal hypotension, then FHR late decelerations.

†The following nursing considerations apply to all types of epidurals: Test dose (3 mL of lidocaine 1.5% with 1:200,000 epinephrine) is used to confirm correct placement of catheter; if local anesthetic is injected into vein, patient may experience dizziness, ringing in ears, numb mouth, metallic taste, or toxic response. Maternal lateral positioning is done to prevent aortocaval compression. Maternal diastolic BP should be less than 110 mm Hg before initiating the epidural. When maternal hypotension occurs, place patient on her left side, infuse IV fluids rapidly, and administer ephedrine 5 to 15 mg IV or 40 to 80 mcg phenylephrine IV. Repeat as necessary. Monitor BP every 1 to 2 minutes for first 10 minutes, then every 10 to 30 minutes until block wears off. Assess level of analgesia. After administration of the anesthetic, assess motor strength prior to ambulation.

TABLE 54-4 **PARENTERAL OPIOIDS FOR LABOR AND DELIVERY**

OPIOID	DOSAGE	ANALGESIC EFFECT BEGINS	PEAK ANALGESIC EFFECT	DURATION OF ACTION
meperidine (Demerol)	IM: 50-100 mg IV: 25-50 mg	IM: 10-45 min IV: <5 min	IM: 30-50 min IV: 5-10 min	IM: 2-4 h IV: 2-3 h
fentanyl (Sublimaze)	IM: 50-100 mcg IV: 50-100 mcg	IM: 7-15 min IV: Almost immediately	IM: 30 min IV: 3-5 min	IV: 30-60 min IM: 1-2 h
morphine sulfate (Duramorph)	IM: 10 mg IV: 2-5 mg	IM: 15-60 min IV: 5-10 min	IM: 1-2 h IV: 20 min	IM: 3-5 h IV: 3-5 h
nalbuphine	subQ: 5-10 mg IV: 5-10 mg	subQ: <15 min IV: <1-3 min	subQ: N/A IV: 30 min	subQ: 3-6 h IV: 3-4 h
butorphanol	IM: 1-2 mg IV: 1-2 mg	IM: 5-10 min IV: <10 min	IM: 30-60 min IV: 4-5 min	IM: 3-4 h IV: 2-4 h

h, Hour; *IM,* intramuscular; *IV,* intravenous; *min,* minute; *subQ,* subcutaneously; <, less than.

receive a continuous epidural infusion, which provides more consistent drug levels and more effective pain relief. Rescue doses are given as necessary to achieve pain relief.

Opioids are administered with the local anesthetic to more effectively control the somatic pain of transition and second-stage labor pain. The opioids most frequently used in combination with the local anesthetic (e.g., 0.125% bupivacaine, 0.2% ropivacaine) are fentanyl or sufentanil (Sufenta). Fentanyl or sufentanil are lipophilic opioids commonly used with continuous or PCEA epidural. These opioids offer rapid analgesia and fewer side effects than hydrophilic opioids. In contrast, morphine sulfate and hydromorphone are hydrophilic opioids. They have a slower onset of action, variable duration, and increased side effects, specifically respiratory depression (Table 54-4).

Another additive to the local anesthetic is epinephrine. Epinephrine increases the duration of the local anesthetic and decreases its uptake and clearance from the cerebrospinal fluid (CSF), while enhancing the intensity of the neural blockade. Single and intermittent injections have wide variations in drug levels and less effectively controlled pain. A continuous lumbar epidural allows a more evenly spaced drug level; less anesthetic is required to provide more effective pain control. Continuous-infusion PCEA gives the patient control of her anesthesia at a basal infusion rate of 10 mL/h, a 5-mL bolus dose, and a 10-minute lockout. Frequently single, intermittent, and PCEA will require rescue doses to improve analgesia.

Lastly, combined spinal-epidural analgesia couples the rapid analgesia and specificity of catheter placement of spinal anesthesia with the continuous infusion via catheter of epidural anesthesia, providing pain relief for later labor.

Controversy exists regarding the effect of regional analgesia, specifically epidurals, on the progress of labor. Some studies indicate no significant effect on labor, whereas other research has demonstrated a decreased maternal urge to push and increased length of labor.

Anesthesia for cesarean deliveries may be general, spinal, or epidural. General anesthesia may be necessary for emergency deliveries, when spinal or epidural anesthesias are contraindicated. It allows for rapid anesthesia induction and control of the airway. Before the administration of general anesthesia, citric acid/sodium citrate (Bicitra) 30 mL is orally administered to decrease gastric acidity. Antacids are administered to decrease complications from gastric acid aspiration. Other medications that may be used in place of citric acid/sodium citrate are cimetidine (Tagamet) 300 mg, ranitidine (Zantac) 50 mg, or metoclopramide 10 mg.

More commonly, spinal or epidural anesthesia is administered for cesarean births. Spinal anesthesia is the more common choice for cesareans because of rapid onset, increased reliability, and improvement in spinal needle design (smaller gauge and shape [Sprotte needle]) with subsequent reduction in postdural headaches. With spinal anesthesia, the local anesthetic most commonly administered is 2.5 or 3 mg bupivacaine (Marcaine) with fentanyl 25 mcg. Pain relief begins in 5 minutes and lasts for approximately 2 hours. The opioids fentanyl 10 to 25 mcg or sufentanil 5 to 10 mcg or morphine (Duramorph) 0.10 to 0.25 mg may also be administered. With the additives, spinal anesthesia provides 18 to 24 hours of pain relief. For epidural inductions, the test dose is given, 3 mL of lidocaine (Xylocaine) 1.5% with 1:200,000 epinephrine followed by administration of local anesthetics: 0.125% to 0.25% bupivacaine or 0.1% to 0.2% ropivacaine with fentanyl 2 mcg/mL. This is followed by a bolus of 15 to 20 mL in divided doses. For an epidural maintenance infusion, 0.1% or 0.15% ropivacaine or bupivacaine with 1 to 2 mcg of fentanyl is continuously infused at 12 to 15 mL/h. Pain relief should begin in 5 to 10 minutes and improve over the next 15 to 20 minutes. The epidural provides pain relief for 18 to 24 hours.

Contraindications to peridural anesthesia are patients with skin infection at the injection site, coagulopathies, active neurologic disease, severe aortic or mitral stenosis, prior sensitivity to an anesthetic agent, and hypovolemia. Of particular importance is patient understanding of the procedure and informed consent.

Adverse effects from local anesthetic agents depend on their chemical properties, but primarily the CNS and cardiovascular systems are affected. CNS effects generally precede cardiovascular effects, with the exception of bupivacaine, in which adverse effects occur at the same drug level. Maternal systemic hypotension is the most frequent complication of regional anesthesia. Adverse CNS effects include dizziness, confusion, headache, slurred speech, metallic taste, nausea, vomiting, seizures, and coma. Cardiovascular symptoms include hypertension and tachycardia initially, followed by hypotension, cardiac arrhythmias, and cardiac arrest. Fetal distress occurs secondary to maternal hypotension and subsequent reduced uteroplacental perfusion.

Adverse effects from regional anesthetics vary, depending on the agent and mode of delivery. With spinal and epidural anesthesia, a primary concern is maternal hypotension. Hypotension is defined as a decrease in systolic BP greater than 20% to 30% of baseline BP or below 100 mm Hg. To decrease maternal hypotension before epidural placement, an IV bolus of 500 to 1000 mL of crystalloids is given. Patients with hypotension are positioned on their left side to facilitate placental perfusion, and then are given a rapid bolus dose of crystalloid IV solution. If the hypotension does not improve with the fluid bolus, then 5 to 10 mg of ephedrine or 40 to 80 mcg of phenylephrine is administered IV and repeated as necessary. Maternal block is a primary consideration and is decreased with administration of lower concentrations of the regional local anesthetics. Women receiving morphine frequently complain of pruritus, which may be effectively relieved with diphenhydramine (Benadryl) administration.

Nursing Process
Patient-Centered Collaborative Care

Regional Anesthetics

Assessment

- Check history for drug sensitivity to local anesthetic agents.
- Assess patient's "labor plan" with expectations for coping with labor and beliefs about use of analgesia and anesthesia.
- Assess knowledge about regional anesthesia.
- Assess cervical dilation and effacement and labor progress.
- Monitor fetal status.
- Review history for contraindications to regional anesthesia; notify anesthesia provider.

Nursing Diagnoses

- Fear related to deficient knowledge of regional anesthesia/analgesia and expected sensations
- Acute pain related to processes of labor and delivery
- Risk for impaired fetal gas exchange, due to maternal hypotension secondary to epidural block
- Ineffective tissue perfusion, maternal/fetal, related to effects of analgesia/anesthesia and maternal position
- Impaired physical mobility secondary to regional anesthesia
- Risk for urinary retention secondary to regional anesthesia

Planning

- Patient will verbalize desired amount of pain relief during labor.
- Patient will remain normotensive and maintain a normal pulse rate; FHR will remain within normal parameters.
- Patient will not experience bladder distention.
- Patient will be able to discuss use of regional anesthesia for labor and delivery pain control.

Nursing Interventions

General

- Assess hydration status before regional anesthesia is given; monitor for anesthetic hypotensive effects. Provide bolus IV fluids as ordered, usually 500 to 1000 mL before regional anesthesia administration.
- Insert an indwelling urinary catheter before administration to monitor maternal fluid status.
- Position and support patient on her left side or as instructed by anesthesia provider.
- Monitor progress of labor for any decrease in frequency or intensity of uterine contractions.
- Monitor maternal vital signs and FHR.
- Have emergency drugs and ephedrine, antihistamines, oxygen, and resuscitation equipment available.
- Be aware of how to place patient in Trendelenburg position (supine on a surface inclined 45 degrees, head at the lower end and legs flexed over the upper end) if necessary.
- Monitor for postdural puncture headache; notify anesthesia provider.

Spinal

- Assess uterine contractions; anesthetic agent must be given immediately after a contraction.
- Monitor BP for hypotensive effects per agency protocol. Have oxygen with positive pressure ventilation equipment readily available.
- Assess level of analgesia following administration and sensory and motor status following delivery.
- Document procedure per agency protocol.

Epidural

- Ensure that patient has 500 to 1000 mL IV bolus of an isotonic solution before the procedure to increase circulatory volume and prevent maternal hypotension.
- Monitor FHR and progress of labor, and keep in mind that anesthetic can inhibit fetal descent.
- Monitor BP for hypotensive effects per agency protocol.
- Assess level of analgesia following administration.
- If maternal hypotension occurs, maintain patient on left side and increase rate of IV fluids. Notify health care provider.

- Assess for bladder distention. If voiding cues are unsuccessful (e.g., placement in semi-Fowler position, privacy, running water over the perineum, running water over the hand), then catheterize.
- Before allowing patient to ambulate after delivery, assess sensory and motor status.
- Conduct ongoing pain assessment. If nature of pain changes, contact anesthesia provider to evaluate anesthesia needs.
- Document procedure per agency protocol.

Caudal

- Place patient in position requested by anesthesia provider for administration.

Paracervical Block

- Maintain continuous FHR monitoring for fetal bradycardia after administration.
- Monitor maternal BP.

Patient Teaching

General

- Discuss technique, potential benefits, and side effects of patient's particular method of anesthesia.

Side Effects

- Instruct patient that regional anesthetics may slow labor and that patient may need a drug to enhance uterine contractions.
- Assess patient for postdural puncture headache after spinal anesthesia or after accidental dural puncture with epidural anesthesia. Instruct patient that bed rest, oral analgesics, caffeine, or an autologous blood patch may be used for headache pain relief.

Skill

- Teach patient how to curl into position for epidural administration.
- Advise patient that forceps or vacuum extraction may be needed for delivery (because of reduction of "urge to push" sensation).
- Teach patient how to assume the left lateral or other position as requested by anesthesia provider for caudal anesthesia.
- Advise patient receiving epidural anesthesia that she will have an IV and close monitoring of FHR and uterine contractions secondary to anesthesia.

Evaluation

- Evaluate BP compared with preprocedure baseline; evaluate FHR for alterations in variability and for decelerations.
- Evaluate effectiveness of anesthetic in relieving discomfort. Evaluate for uniformity of anesthesia; if there is lateralization or if it is "patchy," notify anesthesia provider.

- Assess for bladder distention. If voiding cues are unsuccessful, then catheterize.
- Before allowing patient to ambulate after delivery, assess sensory and motor status.
- Evaluate uterine fundus for firmness.

Spinal Block (Subarachnoid Block)

Adverse Reactions

Patient: Hypotension; paresthesia or nerve injury, high/spinal block (respiratory muscles are impaired by block), postdural puncture headache, neuritis, block failure. Headache is less common because of small size (25 gauge) of needle used. Patient may have nausea, vomiting, backache, urinary retention, apnea with total spinal, or infection. Fetus or neonate: None, unless secondary to maternal hypotension, then FHR late decelerations.

Normal Dose

Vaginal delivery: Fentanyl 25 mcg with or without bupivacaine 2.5 to 3 mg injected intrathecally into subarachnoid space. Cesarean delivery: 12 mg bupivacaine mixed with 8.25% dextrose for T2 to T4 sensory levels, with fentanyl 10 to 25 mcg added to minimize visceral discomfort. Postoperatively, 0.1 to 0.25 mg morphine may be added to local anesthetic.

Nursing Implications

Patient must be well hydrated; administer bolus of 500 to 1000 mL crystalloid solution as ordered. Cervix should be fully dilated before administration. Anesthetic should be given immediately after a contraction to avoid impairing neonate's respiratory efforts. Patient is generally placed sitting or in curled side-lying position for administration. Monitor BP every 1 to 2 minutes for the first 10 minutes. After administration, monitor BP every 5 to 10 minutes. Assess level of analgesia. Place a wedge under the patient's hip to treat maternal hypotension caused by uterine displacement. If patient receives morphine, monitor for respiratory depression and pruritus.

Contraindications

Infection at puncture site, increased intracranial pressure, allergy to local anesthetics, coagulopathies, severe hypovolemia, severe aortic or mitral stenosis, or lack of patient consent.

Indication

Need for high degree of pain relief for delivery. Used primarily for cesarean delivery, forceps delivery, or in the postpartum period for repair of traumatic lacerations of the perineum or removal of retained placenta; infrequently used for labor. When given: Immediately before delivery; late in second stage when fetal head is on the perineum (for vaginal delivery). Area blocked: Umbilicus to toes with vaginal delivery. Immediately below xyphoid process to toes with cesarean delivery.

Injection site: With patient in sitting or side-lying position, anesthetic injected into subarachnoid space at L4-L5.

Lumbar Epidural Block (Single Dose)

Adverse Reactions

Patient: Hypotension, paresthesia or nerve injury, neuritis, postdural headache with accidental puncture of dura, epidural hematoma, and high/total block (respiratory muscles are impaired by block). Headache is less common because of small size (25 gauge) of needle used. Patient may have nausea, vomiting, backache, urinary retention, infection, catheter complications, intravascular injection, direct spinal cord injury, and bloody tap. Fetus or neonate: Few, unless secondary to maternal hypotension, then FHR late decelerations.

Normal Dose

Vaginal delivery: A test dose is given, 3 mL of lidocaine 1.5% with 1:200,000 epinephrine, followed by administration of local anesthetics: 0.1% or 0.125% bupivacaine or ropivacaine with fentanyl 2 mcg/mL). This is followed by a bolus of 15 to 20 mL in divided doses and a continuous infusion at 12 to 15 mL/h; cesarean delivery: nonemergent cesarean: 2% lidocaine (with or without sodium bicarbonate) with 1:400,000 epinephrine. Fentanyl 50 to 100 mcg may be added to minimize pain with uterine manipulation. For patients who have an epidural catheter already placed and then require an emergent cesarean, a bolus dose of 15 to 20 mL of 3% 2-chloroprocaine (boluses of lidocaine or 2-chloroprocaine 3% every 1 to 2 minutes, boluses of bupivacaine or ropivacaine (Naropin) every 2 to 5 minutes) is used. As with the spinal, 3 mg morphine may be added and the need to monitor for respiratory depression and pruritus.

Nursing Implications

Before epidural, patient is well hydrated with 500 to 1000 mL of dextrose-free intravenous fluids. A test dose (3 mL of lidocaine with 1:200,000 epinephrine) is administered by the anesthesiologist or nurse anesthetist and used to confirm correct placement of catheter; if local anesthetic is injected into vein, patient may experience dizziness, ringing in ears, numb mouth, metallic taste, or toxic response. Loss or reduction of bearing-down reflex means low forceps or vacuum extraction may be needed for delivery. It may slow progress of labor. Maternal lateral positioning is done to prevent aortocaval compression. Maternal diastolic BP should be less than 110 mm Hg before initiating the epidural. When maternal hypotension occurs, place the patient on her left side, infuse IV fluids rapidly, and administer ephedrine 5 to 15 mg IV or 40 to 80 mcg phenylephrine IV and repeated as necessary. Monitor BP every 1 to 2 minutes for the first 10 minutes, and then every 10 to 30 minutes until the block wears off. Assess level of analgesia. After delivery, assess motor strength prior to ambulation. Of particular importance is the assessment of bilateral analgesia for pain relief during labor. If unilateral analgesia occurs, patient is turned to opposite side, and more anesthetic is injected.

Contraindications

Infection at site, increased intracranial pressure, allergy to local anesthetics, coagulopathies, severe hypovolemia, severe aortic or mitral stenosis, or lack of patient consent.

Indication

Pain relief in first and second stages of labor. When given: Active labor, 5 to 6 cm dilated in a primipara, 3 to 4 cm in a multipara. Area blocked: T12-S5 (entire pelvis) in area of dorsal root ganglion, with varying degrees of motor and sensory loss depending on dosage and agent injected. Injection site: Epidural space (potential space between the dura mater and vertebral canal from cranium to sacrum) at L2-L3, L3-L5, or L4-L5; not in the dura. Never injected above L1, where the spinal cord ends. Nerves run off and down the spinal canal, where they free-float and are easily moved aside by the epidural needle. The goal is to bathe the nerves with dispersed local anesthetic.

Continuous Lumbar Epidural Block Using Indwelling Catheter in Epidural Space

Adverse Reactions

Patient: Hypotension, paresthesia or nerve injury, postdural headache with accidental puncture of dura. Headache is less common because of small size (25 gauge) of needle used. Patient may have nausea, vomiting, backache, urinary retention, infection, catheter complications, intravascular injection, direct spinal cord injury, and bloody tap. Fetus or neonate: Few, unless secondary to maternal hypotension, then FHR late decelerations.

Normal Dose

Continuous infusion options (rate is 12 to 15 mL/h): bupivacaine or ropivacaine 0.1% or 0.15% 0.0625% to 0.2% with fentanyl 1 to 2 mcg.

Nursing Implications

Before epidural, patient is well hydrated with 500 to 1000 mL of dextrose-free IV fluids. Test dose (3 mL of lidocaine with 1:200,000 epinephrine) is administered by the anesthesiologist or nurse anesthetist and used to confirm correct placement of catheter; if local anesthetic is injected into vein, patient may experience dizziness, ringing in ears, numb mouth, metallic taste, or toxic response. Loss or reduction of bearing-down reflex means low forceps or vacuum extraction may be needed for delivery. May slow progress of labor. Maternal lateral positioning is done to prevent aortocaval compression. Maternal diastolic BP should be less than 110 mm Hg before initiating the epidural. When maternal hypotension occurs, place the patient on her left side, infuse IV fluids rapidly, and administer ephedrine 5 to 15 mg IV. Monitor BP every 1 to 2 minutes for the first 10 minutes and then every 10 to 30 minutes until the block wears off. Assess level of analgesia. After administering the anesthetic, assess motor strength before ambulation. Breakthrough pain is treated by increased infusion rate of rescue dose of anesthetic.

Indication
Pain relief during first and second stages. This is the most widely used anesthesia method for labor pain management. Useful for prolonged labor. When given: Progressive active labor, 5 to 6 cm dilated in a primipara, 3 to 4 cm in a multipara. Area blocked: Same as for lumbar epidural block. Injection site: Same as for lumbar epidural block.

Advantages
Provides continuous anesthesia from stage 1 through delivery and perineal repair. Patient can feel movement and pressure but no pain. Can be used for vaginal delivery or cesarean birth. Sensory level can be altered and density of the block can be manipulated. Can be used to deliver epidural morphine PF or fentanyl into epidural space for regional analgesia (highly effective). Patients may experience pruritus, which may be effectively relieved with diphenhydramine or naloxone intravenous infusions.

Considerations
Loss or reduction of bearing-down reflex means that forceps or vacuum extraction may be needed for delivery. Requires an increased amount of local anesthetic agent. Bupivacaine is used in low concentration (as low as 1/16%) and may be combined with fentanyl.

Complications
Same as for lumbar epidural block.

Side Effects
Pruritus (in 2 to 3 hours when drug reaches upper thoracic segments), urinary retention, and nausea and vomiting related to ineffective hydration to prevent hypotension during labor.

Patient-Controlled Epidural Administration (PCEA)
Adverse Reactions
Patient: Hypotension, paresthesia or nerve injury, postdural headache with accidental puncture of dura. Headache is less common because of small size (25 gauge) of needle used. Patient may have nausea, vomiting, backache, urinary retention, infection, catheter complications, intravascular injection, direct spinal cord injury, and bloody tap. Fetus or neonate: Few, unless secondary to maternal hypotension, then FHR late decelerations.

Nursing Implications
Before epidural, patient should be well hydrated with 500 to 1000 mL of dextrose-free IV fluids. Test dose (3 mL of lidocaine with 1 : 200,000 epinephrine) is used to confirm correct placement of catheter; if local anesthetic is injected into vein, patient may experience dizziness, ringing in ears, numb mouth, metallic taste, or toxic response. Loss or reduction of bearing-down reflex means low forceps or vacuum extraction may be needed for delivery. May slow progress of labor. Maternal lateral positioning is done to prevent aortocaval compression. Maternal diastolic BP should be less than 110 mm Hg before initiating the epidural. When maternal hypotension occurs, place the patient on her left side, infuse IV fluids rapidly, and administer ephedrine 5 to 15 mg IV or phenylephrine 40 to 80 mcg IV. Repeat as necessary. Monitor BP every 1 to 2 minutes for the first 10 minutes and then every 10 to 30 minutes until the block wears off. Assess level of analgesia. After delivery, assess motor strength before ambulation. Breakthrough pain is treated by increased infusion rate of rescue dose of anesthetic.

Indication
Pain relief during first and second stages. Useful for prolonged labor. When given: Progressive active labor, 5 to 6 cm dilated in a primipara, 3 to 4 cm in a multipara. Area blocked: Same as for lumbar epidural block. Injection site: Same as for lumbar epidural block.

Advantages
Provides continuous anesthesia from stage 1 through delivery and perineal repair. Patient can feel movement and pressure but no pain. Patient is in control, and dose may be self-titrated according to her perception of pain. Sensory level can be altered and density of the block can be manipulated. Can be used to deliver epidural morphine PF or fentanyl into epidural space for regional analgesia (highly effective). Patients may experience pruritus, which may be effectively relieved with diphenhydramine or naloxone infusions.

Considerations
Loss or reduction of bearing-down reflex means that forceps or vacuum extraction may be needed for delivery. Requires an increased amount of local anesthetic agent. Bupivacaine is used in low concentration (as low as 1/16%) and may be combined with fentanyl.

Complications
Same as for lumbar epidural block.

Side Effects
Pruritus (in 2 to 3 hours when drug reaches upper thoracic segments), urinary retention, and nausea and vomiting related to ineffective hydration to prevent hypotension during labor.

Combined Spinal-Epidural
Adverse Reactions
Patient: Hypotension, paresthesia or nerve injury, postdural headache. Headache is less common because of small size (25 gauge) of needle used. Patient may have nausea, vomiting, backache, urinary retention, infection, catheter complications, intravascular injection, direct spinal cord injury, and

bloody tap. Proper catheter placement is not assured; this becomes a problem if an epidural catheter is needed for emergency analgesic administration. Fetus or neonate: Few, unless secondary to maternal hypotension, then FHR late decelerations.

Normal Dose

Spinal: 10 to 25 mcg fentanyl or 2.5 to 10 mcg sufentanil alone or in combination with 1 mL bupivacaine 0.25% epidural is initiated with bupivacaine 0.03% to 0.0625% with fentanyl 1 to 2 mcg/mL or sufentanil 0.1 to 0.3 mcg/mL.

Nursing Implications

Before epidural, patient is well hydrated with 500 to 1000 mL of dextrose-free IV fluids. Test dose (3 mL of lidocaine with 1 : 200,000 epinephrine) is used to confirm correct placement of catheter; if local anesthetic is injected into vein, patient may experience dizziness, ringing in ears, numb mouth, metallic taste, or toxic response. Loss or reduction of bearing-down reflex means low forceps or vacuum extraction may be needed for delivery. May slow progress of labor. Maternal lateral positioning is done to prevent aortocaval compression. Maternal diastolic BP should be less than 110 mm Hg before initiating the epidural. When maternal hypotension occurs, place the patient on her left side, infuse IV fluids rapidly, and administer ephedrine 5 to 15 mg IV or phenylephrine 40 to 80 mcg IV. Repeat as necessary. Monitor BP every 1 to 2 minutes for the first 10 minutes and then every 10 to 30 minutes until the block wears off. Assess level of analgesia. After delivery, assess motor strength before ambulation. Breakthrough pain is treated by increased infusion rate of rescue dose of anesthetic.

Indication

Pain relief during first and second stages. Spinal can help with early labor pain and epidural with pain management during active labor. When given: Progressive active labor. Area blocked: Same as for spinal and lumbar epidural block. Injection site: Same as for spinal and lumbar epidural block.

Advantages

Provides continuous anesthesia from stage 1 through delivery and perineal repair. Patient can feel movement and pressure but no pain. Sensory level can be altered and density of the block can be manipulated. Can be used to deliver epidural morphine PF or fentanyl into epidural space for regional analgesia (highly effective). Patients may experience pruritus, which may be effectively relieved with diphenhydramine or naloxone. Administration of a combination of local anesthetic and opioid more effectively blocks the somatic pain of transition and second-stage labor.

Considerations

Loss or reduction of bearing-down reflex means that forceps or vacuum extraction may be needed for delivery. Requires an increased amount of local anesthetic agent. Bupivacaine is used in low concentration (as low as 1/16%) and may be combined with fentanyl.

Complications

Same as for lumbar epidural block.

Side Effects

Pruritus (in 2 to 3 hours when drug reaches upper thoracic segments), urinary retention, and nausea and vomiting related to ineffective hydration to prevent hypotension during labor.

Caudal (Type of Epidural Anesthesia)

Indication

Pain in first and second stages of labor. Infrequently used. When given: Active labor. Area blocked: Perineum; masks uterine contractions. Injection site: Epidural space through sacral hiatus (S4).

Advantages

Useful for women with metabolic, lung, and heart disease. Very rapid perineal anesthesia and muscle relaxation. Can be used continuously.

Considerations

Increased need to use forceps or vacuum extraction because there is a loss of urge to push. Risk of systemic toxic reactions. Level of anesthesia is more difficult to obtain.

Paracervical Block

Indication

Pain during first stage of labor. Due to high incidence of fetal bradycardia, paracervical block is infrequently administered. When given: Active phase of first stage; may be repeated periodically until 8-cm dilated. Area blocked: Uterus, cervix, and vagina; masks uterine contractions. Injection site: Submucosa of the fornix of the vagina lateral to the cervix.

Advantages

Rapid onset. Lasts 60 to 90 minutes. Relieves pain of cervical dilation and contractions. Does not block lower vagina or perineum.

Considerations

Rapid absorption (because injected into a very vascular area). Does not provide anesthesia for delivery or episiotomy repair. Has variable effects on labor progress.

Side Effects

Patient: Hematomas in tissue around injection site. Fetus: Mild to severe bradycardia or prolonged FHR deceleration with decreased variability are common.

Pudendal Block

Indication

For low forceps deliveries, episiotomy, and laceration repair. Infrequently used. When given: Immediately before birth.

Area blocked: Perineum; pudendal nerves. Injection site: Transvaginally, behind each sacrospinous ligament to block pudendal nerves.

Considerations

Not useful for pain management in first stage of labor.

Local Infiltration

Indication

For episiotomy and perineal laceration repair. When given: Just before delivery or repair. Area blocked: Local area adjacent to injection. Injection site: Perineal subcutaneous tissue.

Advantage

No effect on FHR or patient's vital signs.

Considerations

May not obtain complete pain relief, and may need additional injections; requires large amount of local anesthetic agent.

Adverse Effects and Side Effects

Patient: Mild discomfort and/or burning during injection. Fetus or neonate: None.

Relative Contraindications to Regional Anesthesia

The following are relative contraindications to regional anesthesia:

- Severe gestational hypertension (increased risk of profound hypotension associated with underlying disease state)
- Coagulation disorders and risk of bleeding secondary to decreased platelets (patient should have a normal partial thromboplastin time and platelet count)
- Generalized sepsis or local infection at needle insertion site

DRUGS THAT ENHANCE UTERINE MUSCLE CONTRACTILITY

Uterotropic drugs enhance uterine contractility by stimulating the smooth muscle of the uterus. Oxytocin, the ergot alkaloids, and some prostaglandins constitute the uterotropics.

Oxytocin is synthesized in the hypothalamus and is transported to nerve endings in the posterior pituitary gland. The hormone is released by the nerve endings under appropriate stimulation; capillaries absorb the substance and carry it into the general circulation, where it facilitates uterine smooth muscle contraction.

In the presence of adequate estrogen levels (those normally achieved by the third trimester), IV oxytocin stimulates uterine contraction. Oxytocin, prepared in synthetic form and marketed as Pitocin, is approved by the U.S. Food and Drug Administration (FDA) for labor induction and labor augmentation. Box 54-1 presents common medical indications for labor induction.

Before **labor induction** (process of causing or initiating labor) begins, risks and benefits and the status of mother and fetus must be assessed. Informed consent for induction must be obtained. The gestational age of the fetus must be considered, together with position of the fetus (head down and deep in the pelvis) and size of the fetus in relation to the patient's pelvis. The patient's **cervical ripening** (softening of the cervix) is also assessed; the cervix is ripe, and thus ready for induction, when it is soft and progressing in effacement and partial dilation. An objective scoring system called the **Bishop score** (scoring system to assist in predicting whether labor induction may be successful) is used to assess readiness for induction. Elements assessed in the modified Bishop Scoring System are dilation, effacement, station, cervical consistency, and cervical position. Modified Bishop scores of 8 or greater are associated with a successful labor induction.

Some patients are not suitable candidates for labor induction, because the risks of the procedure outweigh the potential benefits. Box 54-2 presents some major contraindications to labor induction.

BOX 54-1 INDICATIONS FOR LABOR INDUCTION

- Gestational hypertension
- Chronic hypertension
- Membrane rupture >24 hours
- Chorioamnionitis
- Postdates (>42 weeks' gestation)
- Intrauterine growth retardation
- Positive contraction stress test
- Maternal diabetes mellitus (classes B-F)
- Maternal renal disease
- Isoimmunization
- Intrauterine fetal death

BOX 54-2 CONTRAINDICATIONS TO LABOR INDUCTION

- Disproportion between fetal head and maternal pelvis (cephalopelvic disproportion)
- Unfavorable fetal presentation (transverse or breech)
- Documented fetal intolerance of uterine contractions
- Prematurity
- Placenta previa or suspected abruptio placentae
- Severe gestational hypertension
- Multiparity (six or more)
- Multifetal gestation
- History of uterine trauma
- Previous major surgery in the area of the cervix or uterus
- Prior classical uterine incision
- Active genital herpes infection
- Umbilical cord prolapse
- Excessive amniotic fluid causing overdistended uterus

Two approaches of labor induction are used to ripen, efface, and begin cervical dilation in pregnant women at term (or near term) with a medical or obstetric indication for labor induction: mechanical methods and *prostaglandins.*

One mechanical method involves insertion of a 36F indwelling catheter through an undilated cervix and internal os with subsequent inflation of the 30-mL balloon. The indwelling catheter bulb provides a mechanical stimulation similar to "stripping of the membranes." When the catheter "falls out," the patient is started on IV oxytocin. A second mechanical method is insertion of an extraamniotic saline infusion with a balloon catheter into the space between the internal cervical os and the placental membrane to induce labor. A third mechanical method is membrane "stripping." With membrane stripping, there is release of prostaglandin F2 from the decidua or prostaglandin E2 from the cervix. Spontaneous labor has been induced within 72 hours of membrane stripping with no increase in infection rates. Amniotomy, artificial rupture of the membranes, is commonly performed in patients with a partially dilated and effaced cervix. When done at 5 cm, dilated spontaneous labor is shortened by 1 to 4 hours without an increase in maternal or fetal complications. With rupture of the membranes, nursing assessment includes assessment of FHR and umbilical cord prolapse. Chorioamnionitis and cord compression have been reported.

The second approach to labor induction uses administration of dinoprostone, the naturally occurring form of prostaglandin E2 (PGE2). It is thought that intracervically or intravaginally administered PGE2 acts to create cervical effacement and softening through a combination of contraction-inducing and cervical-ripening properties, possibly secondary to an increased submucosal water content and collagen degradation resulting from collagenase secretion in response to PGE2. One approach uses prefilled syringes of commercially prepared dinoprostone cervical gel 0.5 mg (Prepidil gel), which is introduced just inside the cervical os. A second approach is the placement in the posterior vaginal fornix of a vaginal insert dinoprostone (Cervidil) containing 10 mg of controlled-release dinoprostone at 0.3 mg/h.

Prostaglandin E1 is also effective in stimulating cervical ripening, although administration is an off-label use. Cytotec or misoprostol (prostaglandin E1) may be administered intravaginally or orally. Dosing ranges from 25 to 100 mcg every 3 to 6 hours.

Side effects associated with the use of prostaglandins include uterine hyperstimulation, which may be treated with terbutaline sulfate. Uncommonly, some patients may experience chills, fever, vomiting, and diarrhea. Contraindications to the use of prostaglandins include active vaginal bleeding and known allergies to prostaglandins. With hepatic or renal disease, cautious use of prostaglandin E2 is recommended; its use is contraindicated in patients with glaucoma. Contraindications for prostaglandin E1 include a previous cesarean delivery or hysterotomy.

Table 54-5 lists the dosages, uses, and considerations for administration of dinoprostone for cervical ripening.

Oxytocin

In addition to labor induction, IV oxytocin can also be used for labor augmentation. It facilitates smooth-muscle contraction in the uterus of a patient already in labor but experiencing inadequate **uterine contractility** (tightening and shortening of uterine muscles). The patient with **uterine inertia** (uterine inactivity or hypotonic contractions) may be more responsive to oxytocin than the patient who has not begun labor; therefore a lower starting dose will be needed.

In both labor induction and **labor augmentation** (stimulation of effective uterine contractions once labor has begun), oxytocin is infused at a prescribed individualized dosage rate, and this rate is increased, decreased, or maintained at fixed intervals based on uterine and fetal response. The objective is to establish an adequate contraction pattern that promotes labor progress, generally represented by contractions every 2 to 3 minutes that last for 50 to 60 seconds with moderate intensity. It is important that the patient receiving oxytocin not experience uterine hyperstimulation, which causes markedly increased pain and compromised FHR patterns secondary to impaired placental perfusion. Continuous nursing observation during labor induction or augmentation is critical. The need for an accurate infusion rate requires the use of an infusion pump with oxytocin as an IV piggyback line. Once cervical dilation has reached 5 to 6 cm, and an adequate contraction pattern is evident, the rate of oxytocin infusion can often be slowed or stopped.

After delivery, oxytocin 20 mg is usually added to an existing IV solution to help the uterus stay contracted and close the uterine sinuses at the placental site. The drug can also be given IM after delivery of the placenta. Prototype Drug Chart 54-1 lists the pharmacologic data for oxytocin.

Oxytocin is well absorbed from the nasal mucosa when administered intranasally for milk letdown. The protein-binding percent is low, and the half-life is 1 to 9 minutes. It is rapidly metabolized and excreted by the liver.

The onset of action of oxytocin administered IM is in 3 to 5 minutes, the peak concentration time is unknown, and the duration of action is 2 to 3 hours. The onset of action of oxytocin administered IV is immediate, the peak concentration time is unknown, and the duration of action is 1 hour. The onset of action of intranasally administered oxytocin is a few minutes, the peak concentration time is unknown, and the duration of action is 20 minutes.

The medication is diluted and administered IV piggyback for induction or augmentation of labor. Oxytocin is diluted in a variety of ways and administered via infusion pump in mL/min dosing with the volume determined by the dilution. IV administration of undiluted oxytocin is not recommended because of the risk of a sudden, acute hypotensive response.

Concurrent use of vasopressors can result in severe hypertension. Hypotension can occur with concurrent use of cyclopropane anesthesia and with undiluted IV push administration. The Institute for Safe Medication Practices (ISMP) includes this medication on its list of high-alert medications that have a heightened risk of causing significant harm when used in error.

TABLE 54-5 DINOPROSTONE FOR CERVICAL RIPENING

GENERIC (BRAND)	ROUTE AND DOSAGE	USES AND CONSIDERATIONS
dinoprostone cervical gel, 0.5 mg (Prepidil gel)	Intracervical: Contains 0.5 mg of dinoprostone in 2.5 mL of gel for intracervical use. Repeat in 6-12 h if negative cervical or uterine response. Maximum 24- h dose is 1.5 mg, supplied in 3 doses. Before beginning oxytocin (Pitocin, Oxytocin) after the Prepidil administration, there should be a 6- to 12-h delay	Naturally occurring form of prostaglandin E2 (PGE2). Used to ripen unfavorable cervix at or near term in pregnant women needing labor induction. Metabolized in lung, liver, and kidney; eliminated by kidney. Patients may have reactive nonstress test before first dose. Monitor uterine activity and FHR; suggest 20-min FHR strip before doses. Must be at room temperature before administration and administered by sterile technique. Must not be placed above level of cervical os. Patient is to remain recumbent 15-30 min following administration of gel and 2 h after insert. May augment other oxytocic agents; therefore no concomitant use; sequential use 6-12 h after gel is recommended. Insert may be inserted with minimal amount of water-soluble lubricant. Wear sterile gloves when administering. See below.* Pregnancy category: C; PB: UK; $t\frac{1}{2}$: UK; Onset: 10-60 min; Peak: UK; Duration: 12 h
dinoprostone (Cervidil vaginal inserts)	Vaginal: Contains 10 mg of dinoprostone in a timed-release insert, releasing 0.3 mg/h. Insert is left in place for 12 h. Oxytocin (Pitocin) may be started 30-60 min after removal of insert. In contrast to gel, insert may be removed with FHR decelerations or uterine hyperstimulation. Ripening unfavorable cervix: Intravaginal: 10 mg over 12 h; remove 12 h after insertion or at onset of active labor	Remove insert, and have oxygen or beta-adrenergic drugs to treat uterine hyperstimulation. Use insert at room temperature. Wear sterile gloves to decrease risk of absorption as inserted high into vagina, posterior fornix. Assess cervical dilation and effacement at time of insertion. After administration, patient remains in lying position for 30 min to 2 h. Monitor FHR and uterine stimulation. Have medication available for frequent gastrointestinal side effects of abdominal cramping, diarrhea, nausea, and vomiting. See below.* Assess vaginal discharge. Onset: UK; Peak: UK; Duration: up to 2-3 h. Pregnancy category: C; PB: UK; $t\frac{1}{2}$: UK
*dinoprostone cervical gel, 0.5 mg (Prepidil gel) and dinoprostone (Cervidil vaginal inserts)		Wear sterile gloves when administering. Contraindicated in patients with prostaglandin hypersensitivity, cephalopelvic disproportion (CPD), ruptured membranes, and unexplained vaginal bleeding. Use with caution in patients with asthma; seizures; glaucoma; increased intraocular pressure; or cardiovascular, renal, or hepatic disease. Not recommended for patients in whom oxytocic drugs are contraindicated or with prolonged uterine contractions, placenta previa, or active genital herpes (vaginal delivery not indicated). Adverse reactions: uterine hyperstimulation, nausea, vomiting, diarrhea, back pain, warm feeling in vagina, dinoprostone-induced fever, and fetal distress. Treat dinoprostone-induced fever, which occurs in approximately 50% of patients, with tepid baths and increased fluids. Fever is not to be treated with aspirin. Assess vaginal discharge frequently during use.

FHR, Fetal heart rate; *h,* hour; *min,* minute; *PB,* protein-binding; $t\frac{1}{2}$, half-life; *UK,* unknown.

Nursing Process
Patient-Centered Collaborative Care

Enhancement of Uterine Contractility: Oxytocins

Assessment

- Obtain patient informed consent before inducing or augmenting labor.
- Confirm term gestation before inducing or augmenting labor.
- Collect accurate baseline data before beginning infusion, including maternal pulse and BP, uterine history, uterine activity, and FHR pattern.
- Interview patient and review history to ascertain that there are no contraindications.

Nursing Diagnosis

- Deficient knowledge related to drugs used to promote uterine contractility

PROTOTYPE DRUG CHART 54-1

Oxytocin

Drug Class	Dosage
Oxytocic agent: Oxytocin Trade Names: Pitocin Pregnancy Category: X	For induction or augmentation of labor A: IV: 10 units (1 amp) diluted in 1000 mL lactated Ringer's solution to 10 milliunits/mL. (Resulting concentration is 10 milliunits oxytocin per 1 mL of IV fluid.) Connect to primary IV line close to needle site as a piggyback line. Low-dose oxytocin regimen: start oxytocin at 0.5-1.5 or 2 milliunits/min with an incremental dose of 1-2 milliunits/min or incremental increase of 4 milliunits/min; *max:* 20 milliunits/min unless consult with provider. High-dose oxytocin regimen: begin oxytocin at 4 or 4.5 or 6 milliunits/min IV with an increase in dose by 4 milliunits/min every 15 min or 4.5 milliunits/min every 15-30 min or 6 milliunits/min every 20-40 minutes; *max:* 40 milliunits/min. unless consult with provider. Postdelivery: A: IV: 10-20 units added to 1000 mL electrolyte or dextrose solution; infuse at rate to prevent uterine atony. IM: 10 units after delivery of the placenta Nasal spray: 1 spray into one or both nostrils 2-3 min before nursing or pumping; not for use during pregnancy
Contraindications	**Drug-Lab-Food Interactions**
Contraindicated in vaginal delivery, proven cephalopelvic disproportion, fetal intolerance of labor, hypersensitivity, anticipated nonvaginal delivery, pregnancy (intranasal spray)	Drug: Hypertension with vasopressors, hypotension and/or bradycardia with cyclopropane anesthetics
Pharmacokinetics	**Pharmacodynamics**
Absorption: PO: Not well absorbed; intranasal and IM very rapidly Distribution: PB: Low; widely distributed in extracellular fluid; minute amounts in fetal circulation Metabolism: $t\frac{1}{2}$: 1-9 min; rapidly metabolized in liver Excretion: In urine	IM: Onset: 3-5 min Peak: 40 min Duration: 2-3 h IV: Onset: Within 1 min Peak: UK Duration: 1 h Intranasal: Onset: Few minutes Peak: UK Duration: UK
Therapeutic Effects/Uses	
To induce or augment labor contractions; to treat uterine atony; to stimulate milk letdown (intranasal spray) Mechanism of Action: Promotes uterine contractions by increasing intracellular concentrations of calcium in uterine myometrial tissue, thereby increasing the activity of the calcium-dependent phosphorylating enzyme myosin light-chain kinase. The nasal spray works by forcing milk into larger ducts and sinuses. This occurs because oxytocin promotes milk ejection by causing contraction of the smooth-muscle fibers surrounding the breast alveoli and lactiferous ducts.	
Side Effects	**Adverse Reactions**
Maternal effects with undiluted IV use only: hypertension, dysrhythmias, tachysystole, and uterine hyperstimulation. Tachysystole is 6 or more uterine contractions in a 20-min window. (Hyperstimulation is defined as uterine contractions lasting at least 2 min or 5 or more contractions in a 10-min window.)	Seizures, water intoxication if given in electrolyte-free solution or at a rate greater than 20 milliunits/min. (Water intoxication is manifested by nausea, vomiting, hypotension, tachycardia, and cardiac arrhythmias.) Life-threatening: Patient: Intracranial hemorrhage, cardiac dysrhythmias, asphyxia; fetus: jaundice, hypoxia

A, Adult; *amp,* ampule; *h,* hour; *IM,* intramuscular; *IV,* intravenous; *min,* minute; *PB,* protein-binding; *PO,* by mouth; $t\frac{1}{2}$, half-life; *UK,* unknown.

Planning

- Oxytocin will enhance uterine contractions without adverse maternal or fetal effects.
- Patient's vital signs will be within acceptable ranges throughout labor, delivery, and postpartum period.
- FHR will demonstrate normal rate, pattern, and variability throughout labor and delivery.

Nursing Interventions

- Have tocolytic agents and oxygen readily available.
- Monitor intake and output.

- Monitor maternal pulse and BP, uterine activity, and FHR during oxytocin infusion.
- Maintain patient in sitting or lateral recumbent position to promote placental infusion.
- Monitor for signs of uterine rupture, which include FHR decelerations, sudden increased pain, loss of uterine contractions, hemorrhage, and rapidly developing hypovolemic shock.
- Use an IV pump when administering.

Patient Teaching
- Inform patient that drug is given IV and dosage adjusted in response to uterine contraction pattern.
- For milk letdown, teach patient timing and method of nasal administration.

Evaluation
- Evaluate for effective labor progress.
- Monitor maternal vital signs every 30 to 60 minutes and with every increment in dose, and FHR every 15 minutes and with every increment in dose during first stage of labor and every 5 minutes in second stage of labor. Report changes in vital signs and FHR, specifically late decelerations and any vaginal bleeding.

Ergot Alkaloids

The **ergot alkaloids** (one of a large group of alkaloids derived from a fungus) act by direct smooth-muscle-cell receptor stimulation. These drugs are not used during labor, because they can cause sustained uterine contractions (tetanic contractions), which would result in fetal hypoxia and possibly rupture of the uterus. The uterus becomes more sensitive to these drugs too. After delivery, however, sustained contractions are effective in the prevention or control of postpartum hemorrhage and the promotion of uterine involution.

The most commonly used ergot derivative is methylergonovine maleate (Methergine). Methylergonovine maleate can be given by mouth but is most frequently administered by the IM route. IV administration is not recommended and is given only in emergency situations. If methylergonovine maleate is given IV, administer 0.2 mg over 1 minute. Transient significant elevations in BP can occur, particularly after IV infusion. Patients with gestational hypertension, hypertension, or peripheral vascular diseases should not receive ergot derivatives. Table 54-6 lists commonly used uterotonic drugs and their dosages, uses, and considerations.

Side Effects and Adverse Reactions

Side effects of ergot alkaloids include uterine cramping, nausea and vomiting, dizziness, hypertension with IV administration, sweating, tinnitus, chest pain, dyspnea, itching, and sudden severe headache. Signs of ergot toxicity (**ergotism**) include pain in arms, legs, and lower back; numbness; cold hands and feet; muscular weakness; diarrhea; hallucinations; seizures; and blood hypercoagulability.

Nursing Process
Patient-Centered Collaborative Care

Other Oxytocics: Ergonovine and Methylergonovine

Assessment
- Assess lochia and uterine tone before giving ergonovine or methylergonovine.
- Assess effectiveness of uterine massage and oxytocin administration on local flow and uterine tone.
- Recognize that these two drugs have a vasoconstrictive effect, which may cause hypertension. Ergonovine is more vasoconstrictive than methylergonovine.
- Obtain baseline BP before administration.

Nursing Interventions
- Monitor patient's BP per agency protocol.
- Protect drugs from exposure to light.
- Monitor for side effects or symptoms of ergot toxicity (ergotism). Notify health care provider if systolic BP increases by 25 mm Hg or diastolic BP by 20 mm Hg over baseline.

Patient Teaching
- Advise patient that she will feel more intense uterine cramps after receiving drug but may receive analgesics for pain.
- Encourage patient to avoid smoking. Nicotine increases vasoconstrictive properties of these drugs.

Side Effects
- If patient is breastfeeding, explain that drug lowers serum prolactin levels with potential to inhibit postpartum lactation. Ergonovine has greater potential to inhibit lactation than methylergonovine.

Cultural Considerations
- Recognize cultural influence on patient's expression or lack of expression of discomfort and/or pain.
- Provide an interpreter as appropriate.

Evaluation
- Evaluate effectiveness of drug by assessment of lochia and uterine tone. Count and weigh perineal pads as appropriate.
- Continue monitoring maternal vital signs, specifically pulse and BP. Report changes in maternal vital signs, continued excessive vaginal bleeding, or uterine atony.

SURFACTANT THERAPY IN PRETERM BIRTH

Synthetic Surfactant

One approach to respiratory difficulties in the preterm infant is surfactant replacement therapy. This is used to prevent the

TABLE 54-6 UTEROTONIC DRUGS COMMONLY USED TO ENHANCE UTERINE CONTRACTILITY

GENERIC (BRAND)	ROUTE AND DOSAGE	USES AND CONSIDERATIONS
oxytocin (Pitocin)	See Prototype Drug Chart 54-1.	
15 methyl prostaglandin F_2-alpha or carboprost tromethamine (Hemabate)	0.25 mg as IM with repeat injections every 15-90 min as needed; 4 doses can be given if hypertension is present	Prostaglandin. Direct stimulation of uterine smooth muscle. Treatment of postpartum hemorrhage secondary to uterine atony. IM: Onset: Unknown; Peak: 15-60 min; Duration 24 h. Maximum total dose: 2 mg. Give deep IM with tuberculin syringe. Contraindicated before delivery of placenta. Use with caution in patients with acute renal disease, cardiac disease, hypertension, inflammatory disease of female pelvic organs, and asthma. Adverse reactions: Diarrhea, nausea, vomiting, fever, abdominal pain with cramps. Pregnancy category: C; t½: UK.
methylergonovine maleate (Methergine)	PO: 0.2-0.4 mg, q6-12h; *max:* 1 wk IM: 0.2 mg after delivery of anterior shoulder (if full obstetric supervision), after delivery of placenta, or postpartum; repeat q2-4h; oral doses may follow parenteral IV: Same as for IM; but slowly over 1 min with careful monitoring of BP (IV route for acute emergencies only [e.g., bleeding])	Prevention and treatment of postpartum hemorrhage, subinvolution, and postabortion hemorrhage. Exhibits similar smooth-muscle action to ergotamine, but primarily affects smooth muscle, producing sustained contractions and shortening third stage of labor. IV: Onset: immediate; Duration: 45 min. IM: Onset: 2-5 min; Duration: 3 h. PO: Onset: 5-25 min; Duration: 3 h. Metabolized in liver; eliminated in urine. Not routinely administered IV because of possible sudden hypertensive and cerebrovascular accidents; limit use in patients with hypertension (especially IV). Contraindicated with maternal sepsis, labor induction, threatened spontaneous abortion; do not use with vasodepressors, other ergot alkaloids, or vasoconstrictors. Appears in breast milk, but interference with breastfeeding is less than with ergonovine. Adverse reactions: transient hypertension, diaphoresis, palpitations, dizziness, headache, nausea, vomiting, tinnitus, transient chest pain, dyspnea. Pregnancy category: C; PB: UK; t½: biphasic: initial: 1-5 min; terminal: 30 min-2 h

BP, Blood pressure; *h,* hour; *IM,* intramuscular; *IV,* intravenous; *max,* maximum; *min,* minute; *PB,* protein-binding; *PO,* by mouth; *t½,* half-life; *tab,* tablet; *UK,* unknown; *wk,* week.

development of **respiratory distress syndrome** (RDS) (respiratory disease of the newborn with absence, deficiency, or alteration in surfactant production). **Surfactant** (a lipoprotein in the alveoli that reduces surface tension of pulmonary fluids and keeps alveoli open during expiration) replacement therapy is also used to decrease the severity of RDS after diagnosis. Supplementing the amount of endogenous surfactant available to maintain distention of the alveolar sacs is the focus of this therapy.

The FDA has approved the use of beractant (Survanta), calfactant (Infasurf), and poractant alfa (Curosurf). Beractant lowers alveolar surface tension during respiration and stabilizes alveoli. Beractant intratracheal suspension, a natural bovine-lung extract, contains phospholipids, neutral lipids, fatty acids, and surfactant-associated proteins to which colfosceril palmitate (DPPC), palmitic acid, and tripalmitin are added. Beractant does not require reconstitution. Calfactant is a calf-lung surfactant that can be used preventilatory for prevention of RDS or postventilatory for treatment. Poractantalfa is porcine-lung surfactant and is indicated for rescue treatment. Each of these products defines prophylactic and rescue use differently and has different dosing and administration requirements. Table 54-7 lists the surfactant drugs used for prevention and treatment of RDS and their dosages, uses, and considerations.

All products require a patent endotracheal (ET) tube for administration and specified alterations in positioning the infant throughout the procedure to ensure even drug dispersion. These precise position changes allow gravity to assist in the distribution of the product in the lungs, particularly at the alveolar surface.

Rales and moist breath sounds may be a transient finding after administration of these products, particularly with beractant. Additionally, transient oxygen desaturation has occurred with poractant alfa, and airway obstruction has occurred in 39% of infants in clinical studies with calfactant. Unless obvious signs of airway obstruction are noted, suctioning should not be performed for 2 hours after administration.

Surfactant replacement therapy has been found effective in reducing the severity of RDS; rapid improvements in lung compliance and oxygenation may require immediate decreases in ventilator settings to prevent lung overdistention and pulmonary air leak.

TABLE 54-7 POSTNATAL SURFACTANT THERAPY FOR PREVENTION AND TREATMENT OF RESPIRATORY DISTRESS SYNDROME

GENERIC (BRAND)	ROUTE AND DOSAGE	USES AND CONSIDERATIONS
beractant (Survanta) intratracheal suspension	4 mL/kg per dose ET (divide into 4 quarter doses and give each quarter dose with infant in different position) in one of two modes: Prophylaxis: 1 dose within 15 min of birth if possible; repeat in 6 h if respiratory distress continues; maximum 4 doses in 48 h (6 h apart). Rescue: 4 mL/kg intratracheally (also divide into 4 quarter doses and give each quarter dose with different infant positioning). Give dose as soon as RDS is diagnosed, preferably within 8 h of birth. Repeat in 6 h, giving a maximum of 4 doses in 48 h	Contains phospholipids, neutral lipids, fatty acids, and surfactant-associated proteins to which colfosceril palmitate (DPPC), palmitic acid, and tripalmitin are added. Each 1 mL contains 2.5 mg phospholipids. Must be given by health care personnel experienced with ventilators as prevention or rescue in treatment of RDS. Administered through a 5 French end-hole catheter as a dosing catheter inserted into ET tube. Following administration of each quarter dose, remove catheter from ET tube and ventilate infant for 30 sec until stable. Prophylaxis defined as use in infants less than 1250 g at high risk for RDS or larger infants with evidence of pulmonary immaturity. Rescue defined as treatment of infants with moderate to severe RDS. Biophysical effects occur at the alveolar surface; lowers surface tension on alveolar surfaces during respiration and stabilizes alveoli against collapse at resting pressures. Monitor infant's arterial or transcutaneous measurement of systemic oxygen or carbon dioxide. Drug should appear off-white to light brown. Swirl vial gently; DO NOT SHAKE. Some foaming is normal. Store at 36° to 46° F (2°-8° C); warm 20 min at room temperature or in hand for at least 8 min. Do not artificially warm. For prevention dose, begin preparation before infant's birth. Do not warm or return drug to refrigerator more than once. Adverse reactions: transient bradycardia, oxygen desaturation (associated with dosing procedure); ET tube reflux; ET blockage; pallor; vasoconstriction; hypotension; hypocarbia; hypercarbia; and apnea. All reactions resolve with symptomatic treatment See content below.*
calfactant (Infasurf)	3 mL/kg of birth weight as soon as possible after birth. Give as 2 doses of 1.5 mL/kg each every 12 h for total of 3 doses	Must be given by health care personnel experienced with ventilators and RDS. Stabilization of the premature infant with hypoxemia should occur before administration of calfactant therapy. Give preferably within 30 min after birth. Give through an ET tube. Draw dose with 20-gauge needle; avoid foaming. Gently agitate for dispersion of drug. Does not have to be warmed before administration. Refrigerate at 36°-46° F (2°-8° C). Adverse reactions: bradycardia, airway obstruction, apnea, hypoventilation, cyanosis, ET tube reflux, ET blockage. See content below.*
poractant alfa (Curosurf)	2.5 mL/kg of birth weight. Up to 2 additional doses of 1.25 mL/kg birth weight can be every 12 h; maximum dose 5 mL/kg	Administered via 5 French catheter inserted into ET tube. With infant positioned either right or left side dependent, administer one half dose into each main bronchus. Must be given by health care personnel experienced with ventilators and RDS. Do not suction airways for 1 h after surfactant instillation unless airway obstruction occurs. Multiple-dose regimen has evidenced efficacy. Reduce ventilator inspiratory pressures immediately if chest expansion improves substantially after dosing. Contraindications are previous hypersensitivity to any component of poractant alfa formulations. Adverse reactions: increased incidence of patent ductus arteriosus, hypotension, transient oxygen desaturation, apnea, and flushing
*beractant (Survanta) intratracheal suspension and calfactant (Infasurf)		Does not require reconstitution. Do not dilute or shake. Protect from light. No known contraindications.

ET, Endotracheal; *h*, hour; *min*, minute; *RDS*, respiratory distress syndrome; *sec*, second.

SAFETY: Preventing Medication Errors

Do not confuse ...

- **fentanyl citrate** (Sublimaze) used as an adjunct to general or regional anesthesia, or for postoperative, persistent, moderate to severe pain, with **sufentanil** (Sufenta), used to induce anesthesia in combination with other drugs or as the sole anesthetic agent.

Adverse Reactions

Side effects during administration have included incidents of reflux of product up the ET tube with decreases in oxygenation. Dosing is slowed or halted if the infant (1) becomes dusky colored, (2) becomes agitated, (3) experiences transient bradycardia, (4) has oxygen saturation increases of more than 95%, (5) experiences improved chest expansion, or (6) has arterial or transcutaneous CO_2 levels <30 mm Hg. Pulmonary hemorrhage has been seen in infants treated with Exosurf. Suctioning before dosing decreases the chance for ET tube blockage during dosing. No long-term complications or sequela of synthetic surfactant therapy have been reported.

Nursing Process

Patient-Centered Collaborative Care

Beractant, Calfactant, and Poractant Alfa

Assessment

- Assess for informed consent. Separate consents are needed for multifetal birth.
- Assess infant's vital signs.

Nursing Diagnosis

- Impaired gas exchange related to inadequate lung surfactant secondary to fetal immaturity

Planning

- Infant's oxygen requirement and respiratory effort will decrease.
- Infant's need for mechanical ventilation will be quickly reduced.
- Infant will experience no respiratory distress within 1 hour of surfactant administration.

Nursing Interventions

Beractant Intratracheal Suspension

- Prepare drug with adequate time for drug to warm to room temperature for 20 minutes or in hand for at least 8 minutes. Do not artificially warm drug.
- Do not shake drug.
- Provide only off-white to light-brown product for use in procedure.
- Assist with positioning of infant after each quarter dose as detailed in protocol.

Calfactant

- Avoid excessive foaming.
- Draw up dose using 20-gauge or larger needle.
- Administer through side port of ET tube.
- Administer medication with infant on one-for-one dose, and turn to opposite side for subsequent dose.
- Administer while ventilation is continued over 20 to 30 breaths for each dose, with small bursts during inspiratory cycles.

Beractant Intratracheal Suspension and Calfactant

- Monitor infant carefully for chest expansion, color, arterial blood gases, oxygen saturation, heart rate, facial expression, ET tube patency, BP, and electrocardiogram.
- Monitor ventilator pressure readings and breath sounds.
- Expect infant's lungs to sound wet after administration; do not suction through endotracheal tube for 2 hours.

Poractant Alfa

- Draw up doses using 20-gauge or larger needle.
- Suction before dosing.
- Mucous plugging of ET tube can occur during or after dosing.
- Do not suction airways for 1 hour after surfactant instillation unless signs of airway obstruction present.
- Monitor ventilator inspiratory pressures, which should be reduced immediately if chest expansion improves after dosing administration.

Patient Teaching

General

- Explain to parents what respiratory distress syndrome is and how surfactant helps neonate.
- Explain to parents the purpose of multiple monitoring devices to reduce unrealistic fears about the neonate's condition.
- Ensure informed consent for usage.

Side Effects

- Encourage parents to verbalize understanding about risks associated with use of drug.

Evaluation

- Evaluate preadministration breath sounds and ventilator pressure readings to compare with postadministration findings.

KEY WEBSITES

National Center for Alternative and Complementary Medicine: *nccam.nih.gov*

Clinical Trials: Pregnancy Complications: *clinicaltrials.gov/ct/*

CRITICAL THINKING CASE STUDY

TA (gravida 3, para 0) is at 42 weeks' gestation. At her prenatal visit, her health care provider notes signs and symptoms of pregnancy-induced hypertension and advises TA about a plan to induce labor after administration of prostaglandin gel. TA asks the nurse, "Can you help me understand all of this?"

1. What objective tool (scoring system) can be used to predict the extent to which TA's cervix is "ripe" and therefore favorable for successful induction?

   TA's health care provider orders dinoprostone cervical gel for use in the cervix.
2. What will be accomplished with use of the gel?
3. Who will administer the gel?
4. How often can the gel be administered?
5. How long after the last dose of gel can the IV oxytocic medication be started to induce labor?
6. Why is there a waiting period before starting the oxytocin?
7. Further questioning reveals that TA has been ingesting a pregnancy tonic that includes herbal supplements since she was 36 weeks' gestation. List three concerns specific to pregnancy.

   It is 16 hours since TA first had the gel inserted. Responding to TA's call light, the nurse finds TA in the bathroom, upset because she feels nauseous and is occasionally vomiting a little stomach fluid, and complaining that her stool is watery. "Is something wrong?" TA asks.
8. Analysis of the data about TA's symptoms supports what conclusion?
9. What nursing actions might be taken to support TA?
10. When TA returns to bed and the external fetal monitor is reapplied, what data should the nurse collect, record, and report to the obstetric provider?

It is 24 hours since TA had the first gel instillation and 6 hours since her last insertion. A vaginal examination reveals that TA's cervix is soft, 50% effaced, and 3 cm dilated, and that the presenting part is at 2 station. Contractions are 5 minutes apart and mild. The health care provider elects to begin an oxytocin infusion.

11. TA asks how "a medicine running into my arm is able to make my uterus contract." How should the nurse explain the mode of action of oxytocin to TA?
12. Why is the oxytocin infusion run through a secondary line attached as a "piggyback" to the primary line? At which port along the primary line is the piggyback inserted, and why?
13. Why is oxytocin administered via infusion pump? What is the measurement for dosing?
14. What actions in regard to IV equipment setup should be taken as safety measures before starting the oxytocin?
15. What drugs should be nearby in the event of an emergency with the oxytocin?
16. What information should be recorded during the infusion?
17. While setting up the oxytocin infusion, a new nurse being precepted to labor and delivery asks what criteria is used to know when to slow the rate or stop the infusion. The nurse correctly responds that contractions would be _____ minutes apart with _____ intensity, and the cervix would be dilated at least _____ cm.
18. If uterine hyperstimulation occurs, explain how to handle the situation. Address the following:

    Position TA; rationale: ____________________

    IV fluids; rationale: ____________________

    Oxygen; rationale: ____________________
19. TA asks what side effects can occur if she receives a continuous lumbar epidural. What is the appropriate response?

NCLEX STUDY QUESTIONS

1. A patient, gravida 3, para 2, and 40.6 weeks' gestation, asks, "Is there anything we can do to start labor besides medication? I'm so ready to have this baby." What is the nurse's best response?
   a. "No, there is nothing we can do until you go into labor."
   b. "Amniocentesis should be done to be sure the lungs are mature before we start labor."
   c. "Some women have sex or ride in a car on a bumpy road to start labor."
   d. "Some health care providers may place a balloon catheter or strip the membranes if the cervix is ripe."
2. A patient is to receive 10 mg nalbuphine slow IV push for pain relief during labor. When will the nurse plan to administer nalbuphine?
   a. During the uterine contraction
   b. At the end of the uterine contraction
   c. Between uterine contractions
   d. At any time during the contractions

3. A patient received butorphanol 2 mg IV 10 minutes immediately before delivery. Which of these is important nursing care for this patient?
   a. Subcutaneous administration
   b. Having naloxone (Narcan) available
   c. Fluid bolus IV to the mother
   d. Oxygen 10 L by nasal cannula to the mother
4. A patient is to have lumbar epidural anesthesia. Based on this health care provider order, what would the nurse prepare to administer?
   a. citric acid/sodium citrate (Bicitra)
   b. promethazine (Phenergan)
   c. A bolus of 500 to 1000 mL of a crystalloid IV solution
   d. Rh_O(D) immune globulin (RhoGAM) injection
5. A 33-year-old patient in active labor is experiencing "back labor" with intense pain in her lower back. What is the most effective nursing intervention?
   a. Counterpressure against the sacrum
   b. Pant-blow breathing techniques
   c. Effleurage
   d. Conscious relaxation or guided imagery
6. A patient has an epidural for pain control during labor. During the assessment, the nurse notes a drop in the patient's BP. What is the priority nursing intervention?
   a. Administer low-flow oxygen.
   b. Turn her on her left side.
   c. Assess her urinary output.
   d. Monitor her vaginal bleeding.
7. A patient is to have a stat cesarean section due to late fetal decelerations. Before surgery, the nurse administers citric acid/sodium citrate (Bicitra). What patient response would indicate effective patient teaching regarding citric acid/sodium citrate?
   a. "Citric acid/sodium citrate will prevent infection after the cesarean section."
   b. "The medication will neutralize the contents in my stomach."
   c. "The citric acid/sodium citrate will reduce the need to use pain medication after the cesarean section."
   d. "This medication is administered to prevent vomiting after the cesarean section."
8. Spinal anesthesia with morphine (Duramorph) is administered to a patient for pain relief during cesarean section. The patient complains of itching. The nurse prepares to administer which medication?
   a. diphenhydramine
   b. ephedrine sulfate
   c. butorphanol tartrate
   d. lidocaine (Xylocaine)
9. A nurse administered beractant (Survanta) to a premature infant to prevent respiratory distress syndrome. In assessing the infant's lungs, the nurse auscultated rales and moist breath sounds. What is the priority nursing intervention?
   a. Notify the health care provider.
   b. Suction immediately to remove the beractant.
   c. Turn the infant "back to sleep."
   d. Document the finding; this is a normal transient finding.
10. A patient is gravida 2, para 1 and is admitted to labor and delivery at 39.6 weeks' gestation in active labor. The health care provider performs an amniotomy. What is the nurse's priority intervention?
    a. Monitor uterine contraction frequency and intensity
    b. Check fetal heart rate
    c. Assess for cervical dilation and effacement
    d. Check for umbilical cord compression
11. A patient in labor is to have an epidural administered. Which nursing interventions should the nurse perform before the epidural is administered? (Select all that apply.)
    a. Infuse 500 to 1000 mL of the ordered IV.
    b. Check maternal blood pressure.
    c. Assess fetal heart rate.
    d. Have patient empty her bladder.
    e. Position patient in lithotomy position.
    f. Administer 2 L/min of oxygen via nasal cannula.

Answers: 1, d; 2, a; 3, b; 4, c; 5, a; 6, b; 7, b; 8, a; 9, d; 10, b; 11, a, b, c, d.

CHAPTER 55

Postpartum and Newborn Drugs

Robin Webb Corbett and Laura K. Williford Owens

evolve WEBSITE

http://evolve.elsevier.com/KeeHayes/pharmacology/

- Animations
- Content Updates
- Key Points
- Review Questions for the NCLEX® Examination
- References from the Textbook
- Unfolding Case Studies

OBJECTIVES

- Discuss the purpose, action, side effects, and nursing implications of the drugs commonly administered during the postpartum period.
- Discuss the purpose, action, side effects, and nursing implications of the drugs administered to the newborn.
- Describe the nursing process, including patient teaching, related to drugs used during the postpartum period and drugs administered to the newborn immediately after delivery.

OUTLINE

KEY TERMS

antiflatulents, p. 831
congenital rubella syndrome, p. 836
episiotomy, p. 828
flatus, p. 831
folliculitis, p. 828
lactation, p. 827
necrosis, p. 828
occlusive, p. 828
ophthalmia neonatorum, p. 838
puerperium, p. 827
Rh sensitization, p. 835
$Rh_O(D)$ immune globulin, p. 836
urticaria, p. 837

This chapter focuses on pharmacologic considerations for mothers and infants after delivery. Nonpharmacologic measures and pharmacologic agents related to the relief of common maternal discomforts during the postpartum period are also described. In addition, drugs commonly administered to newborns immediately after delivery are discussed.

DRUGS USED DURING THE POSTPARTUM PERIOD

During the **puerperium** (the period from delivery until 6 weeks postpartum), the maternal body physically recovers from antepartal and intrapartal stressors and returns to its prepregnant state.

Pharmacologic and nonpharmacologic measures commonly used during the postpartum period have five primary purposes: (1) to prevent uterine atony and postpartum hemorrhage; (2) to relieve pain from uterine contractions, perineal wounds, and hemorrhoids; (3) to enhance or suppress **lactation** (production and release of milk by mammary glands); (4) to promote bowel function; and (5) to enhance immunity (Box 55-1).

Whenever possible, nonpharmacologic measures are preferred to the use of drugs or are used in conjunction with drugs (Herbal Alert 55-1). Postpartum nursing care ideally occurs as a partnership between the nurse and the new family. To enhance health and wellness, the nurse collaborates with the mother and family to strengthen the new mother's self-confidence and ability to handle her own health challenges. The nurse's role in this system is threefold:

- To assess and discuss postpartal physical changes and pain management with the patient and determine both healing progress within a standard and effectiveness of medications
- To teach the patient and administer postpartal medications
- To teach the patient and administer narcotic analgesics (as prescribed) when pain control by nonnarcotic products is ineffective.

HERBAL ALERT 55-1

Use of Herbs during Lactation

Because little is known about the safety of herbal supplements, they are not generally recommended during lactation. Breastfeeding patients should be advised to check with their health care provider before taking any herbal supplements; those contraindicated for breastfeeding patients include aloe, belladonna, black tea, bromelain, buckthorn bark, burdock, cat's claw, chondroitin, comfrey, echinachea, ephedra/ma-huang, eucalyptus, flaxseed, kava kava, lavender, licorice, milk thistle, pennyroyal, and saw palmetto. This list is not exhaustive; for more information, refer to Chapter 6.

Pain Relief for Uterine Contractions

"Afterbirth pains" may occur during the first few days postpartum when uterine tissue experiences ischemia during contractions, particularly in multiparous patients and when breastfeeding. Nonsteroidal agents may be used to control postpartal discomfort and pain, with narcotic agents reserved for more severe pain such as that experienced by the patient after cesarean delivery, tubal ligation, or extensive perineal laceration. Box 55-2 lists systemic analgesics commonly used during the postpartum period.

Because some systemic analgesics (e.g., codeine, meperidine) can cause decreased alertness, it is important for the nurse to observe the patient as she cares for her newborn to ensure safety. Patients who receive opioids, such as morphine sulfate or codeine sulfate, should be assessed for bowel function and respirations. With continued opioid use, patient assessment of bowel history is necessary, because these drugs

BOX 55-1 ROUTINE POSTPARTUM MEDICATION ORDERS

Vaginal Delivery Postpartum Medications

Standing Orders

oxytocin (Pitocin) 20 units in 1 L D_5LR or 10 units IM
ferrous sulfate ($FeSO_4$) 325 mg PO b.i.d/t.i.d.
Prenatal vitamin 1 tab PO daily
Motrin 800 mg t.i.d

PRN Orders

docusate sodium (Colace) 100 mg PO b.i.d. PRN for constipation OR
Dulcolax suppository PR PRN for constipation
Lanolin PRN if breastfeeding
Measles-mumps-rubella vaccine if not immunized

Cesarean Birth Postpartum Medications

Standing Orders

cefazolin (Ancef) 1 gram IVPB × 1 dose at time of cesarean section
oxytocin (Pitocin) 20 units in 1 L D_5LR or 10 units IM
POD 1
ferrous sulfate ($FeSO_4$) 325 mg PO b.i.d./t.i.d.
Prenatal vitamin 1 tab PO daily
Motrin 800 mg t.i.d

PRN Orders

POD 1
- nalbuphine 5-10 mg subQ or IV q2-3h OR
- meperidine (Demerol) 50-75 mg IM q3-4h PRN for pain
- acetaminophen/codeine (Tylenol No. 3) 1-2 tab PO q3-4h PRN for pain OR
- oxycodone/acetaminophen (Percocet) 1 tab PO q6h PRN for pain
- hydroxyzine (Vistaril) 25-50 mg IM q3-4h PRN for nausea
- prochlorperazine (Compazine) 10 mg IV q4-6h PRN for nausea OR
- promethazine (Phenergan) 25-50 mg IV q3-4 h PRN for nausea
- A & D cream or Lanolin PRN if breastfeeding

POD 2
- bisacodyl (Dulcolax) suppository PR PRN for constipation OR
- magnesium hydroxide (milk of magnesia) 30 mL PO q6h PRN
- simethicone (Gas-X) 80 mg PO q.i.d. PRN for bloating and/or gas
- Rubella vaccine (Meruvax II) subQ if not immunized

b.i.d., Twice a day; *h,* hour; *IM,* intramuscular; *IVPB,* intravenous piggyback; *PO,* by mouth; *PRN,* as needed; *q.i.d.,* four times a day; *subQ,* subcutaneous; *tab,* tablet; *t.i.d.,* three times a day.

BOX 55-2 COMMONLY USED POSTPARTUM SYSTEMIC ANALGESICS

acetaminophen (Tylenol)
acetaminophen/codeine (Tylenol No. 3)
acetaminophen and propoxyphene
ibuprofen (Motrin)
codeine sulfate
ketorolac tromethamine (Toradol)
acetaminophen and hydrocodone (Lortab)
meperidine (Demerol)
morphine sulfate
nalbuphine oxycodone acetaminophen (Percocet)

can exacerbate the constipation of pregnancy. During the intrapartum period, women are NPO (nothing by mouth) or ingest limited liquids and are not ambulatory, all factors that contribute to decreased bowel activity. In addition, respiratory assessment is important for patients receiving opioids, because respiratory depression may occur. Frequently nonsteroidal agents like ibuprofen and ketorolac tromethamine are used to control postpartum discomfort and pain. Nonsteroidal antiinflammatory drugs (NSAIDs) inhibit the enzyme cyclooxygenase (COX), of which there are two isoenzymes, COX-1 or COX-2; both decrease prostaglandin synthesis. These drugs are effective in relieving mild to moderate pain caused by postpartum uterine contractions, episiotomy, hemorrhoids, and perineal wounds. NSAIDs commonly cause gastrointestinal (GI) irritation, and it is recommended that patients take them with a full glass of water or with food to minimize GI distress. With administration of NSAIDs, a lower narcotic dosage may control pain as a result of the additive analgesic effect. The use of NSAIDs requires ongoing assessment for GI bleeding. These drugs inhibit platelet synthesis and may prolong bleeding time. Patient teaching with this category of drugs is important, because some NSAIDs may be purchased over the counter (OTC). Patient teaching includes avoidance of these drugs while pregnant if symptoms of GI bleeding occur (dark, tarry stools; blood in urine; coffee-ground emesis) and avoidance of the concurrent use of alcohol, aspirin, and corticosteroids, which may increase the risk for GI toxicity.

Pain Relief for Perineal Wounds and Hemorrhoids

Pregnancy and the delivery process increase the pressure on perineal soft tissue. The tissue may become ecchymotic or edematous. Increased edema, ecchymosis, and pain may occur if an **episiotomy** (incision made to enlarge the vaginal opening to facilitate newborn delivery) or perineal laceration is present. The perineum is assessed for *R*edness, *E*cchymosis, *E*dema, *D*ischarge, and *A*pproximation (REEDA). In addition, hemorrhoids that developed during pregnancy may be exacerbated by the pushing during labor. Comfort measures (ice packs immediately after birth, tightening of the buttocks before sitting, use of peribottles and cool or warm sitz baths) and selected topical agents (witch hazel and dibucaine ointment) may relieve pain and minimize discomfort (Table 55-1). Note that rectal suppositories should not be used by women with fourth-degree perineal lacerations.

Side Effects and Adverse Reactions

The most commonly reported side effects of topical or local agents include burning, stinging, tenderness, edema, rash, tissue irritation, sloughing, and tissue **necrosis** (death of tissue caused by disease or injury). The most commonly reported side effects of hydrocortisone local or topical drugs include burning, pruritus, irritation, dryness, **folliculitis** (skin inflammation resulting from contact with an irritating substance or allergen), allergic contact dermatitis, and secondary infection. These side effects are more likely to occur when **occlusive** (i.e., obstructive) dressings are used.

Nursing Process
Patient-Centered Collaborative Care

Pain Relief for Perineal Wounds and Hemorrhoids

Assessment
- Assess patient's cultural framework for health.
- Assess patient's pain using agency pain scale. Assess perineal area for wounds and hemorrhoids (size, color, location, pain scale, REEDA).
- Check expiration dates on topical spray cans, bottles, and ointment tubes.
- Assess for presence of infection at perineal site; avoid use of benzocaine on infected perineal tissue.

Nursing Diagnoses
- Deficient knowledge of causes of pain and discomfort; inexperience with treatment measures, nonpharmacologic and pharmacologic
- Acute pain related to episiotomy, perineal laceration, or hemorrhoids

Planning
- Patient's perineal discomfort will be alleviated by use of topical sprays, compresses, sitz baths, and ointment.

Nursing Interventions
- Teach patient about use of peribottle. Use warm water and direct water on perineum from front to back (clean to dirty).
- Do not use benzocaine spray when perineal infection is present.
- Shake benzocaine spray can. Administer 6 to 12 inches from perineum with patient lying on her side with top leg up and forward to provide maximum exposure. This can also be done with one foot on the toilet seat.

TABLE 55-1 DRUGS USED TO RELIEVE PAIN FROM PERINEAL WOUNDS AND HEMORRHOIDS

GENERIC (BRAND)	ROUTE AND DOSAGE	USES AND CONSIDERATIONS
Perineal Wounds (Episiotomy or Laceration)		
benzocaine (Americaine, Dermoplast)	Spray liberally t.i.d./q.i.d. 6-12 inches from perineum following perineal cleansing Supplied as aerosol benzocaine 20%	Local anesthetic; inhibits impulses from sensory nerves by decreasing permeability of cell membrane to sodium ions. Apply 6-12 inches from affected area. Peak: 1 min; duration: 30-60 min. Hydrolyzed in plasma and liver (to lesser extent) by cholinesterase; eliminated as metabolites in urine. Well absorbed from mucous membranes and traumatized skin. Contraindicated in patients with secondary bacterial infection of tissue and known hypersensitivity
witch hazel pads (Tucks [50% witch hazel with glycerin, water, and methylparaben]) (may also be used for hemorrhoids)	Apply premoistened pads t.i.d./q.i.d. to wound site	Precipitates protein, causing tissue to contract. May be chilled/refrigerated in original container for additional comfort. If liquid, pour over ice and dip absorbent pads into solution; change when diluted. Medical intervention should be sought if rectal bleeding is present. Side effect: local irritation (discontinue use)
Hemorrhoids		
hydrocortisone acetate 10 mg (Anusol-HC, Tucks Ointment [pramoxine HCl 1%, mineral oil 46.7%, zinc oxide 12.5%])	1 suppository b.i.d. for 3-6 d	Relieves pain and itching from irritated anorectal tissue. Anusol-HC contains hydrocortisone acetate, acts as an antiinflammatory agent. Available without hydrocortisone. Wear gloves. Onset: UK; Peak: UK; Duration: UK. Contraindicated in patients with known hypersensitivity. Discontinue if second infection in tissue. If anorectal symptoms do not improve in 7 days or if bleeding, protrusion, or seepage occurs, inform health care provider. Do not use if fourth-degree perineal laceration present. Not known if excreted in breast milk; use cautiously. Pregnancy category: C
hydrocortisone acetate 1% and pramoxine HCl 1% topical aerosol (Proctofoam-HC)	1 applicator transferred to 2-by-2–inch pad and placed against rectum inside peri-pad b.i.d./t.i.d. and after bowel movements	Topical corticosteroid aerosol foam with same action and considerations as above. Also available in nonsteroidal preparation. Shake foam aerosol before use. Onset: UK; Peak: UK; Duration: UK. Extent of percutaneous absorption of topical corticosteroids determined by vehicle integrity, epidermal barrier, and use of occlusive dressings. Not known if any quantity detectable in breast milk. Side effects: burning, itching, irritation; dryness, infrequent folliculitis reactions
dibucaine ointment, USP 1% (Nupercaine)	Apply as above t.i.d./q.i.d., using no more than 1 tube in 24 h	Local anesthetic ointment containing dibucaine 1%. Action same as benzocaine. Onset: within 15 min; Peak: UK; Duration: 2-4 hours. Do not use if rectal bleeding present. Do not use near eyes or over denuded surfaces or blistered areas. Do not use if known hypersensitivity to amide-type anesthetics. Side effects: burning, tenderness, irritation, inflammation, contact dermatitis, urticaria, cutaneous lesions, edema. Pregnancy category: C

b.i.d., Two times a day; *d,* day; *h,* hour; *min,* minute; *q.i.d.,* four times a day; *t.i.d.,* three times a day; *UK,* unknown.

- Use witch hazel compresses (glycerin and witch hazel [Tucks] or witch hazel solution) with an ice pack and a peri-pad to apply cold to the affected area in addition to the active agent.
- Store pramoxine and zinc oxide topical (Anusol) or hydrocortisone acetate (Anusol-HC) suppositories below 86° F (30° C), but protect them from freezing. Use gloves for administration. If patient is breastfeeding, assess to determine whether patient is ready to switch to preparation without hydrocortisone (goal is to discontinue use of suppositories as quickly as possible).
- Check lot numbers and expiration dates.
- Use of pramoxine HCl (Proctofoam-HC) must be explained carefully, because directions instruct patient to place agent inside the anus, which is not generally done with obstetric patients (they may have perineal wounds that extend into the anus). Rectal suppositories should not be used by patients with fourth-degree perineal laceration.

Patient Teaching

General

- Describe the process of perineal wound healing.
- Explain expected action and side effects. With witch hazel a cooling, soothing sensation will provide relief.

Ointment and suppositories will soothe, lubricate, and coat mucous membranes. Pramoxine HCl is not chemically related to "-caine"-type local anesthetics, and there is a decreased chance of cross-sensitivity reactions in patients who are allergic to other local anesthetics.

- Advise patient that drug is not for prolonged use (no more than 7 days) or for application to a large area.
- Explain that topical analgesia lasts for several hours after use.
- Advise patient to store suppositories below 86°F (30°C) so suppositories do not melt but do not freeze. Counsel patient with bleeding hemorrhoids to use drug carefully and to keep health care provider informed if condition exacerbates or does not improve within 7 days.

Self-Administration: Perineal Wounds: Topical Spray Containing Benzocaine

- Apply three to four times daily or as directed.
- Apply without touching sensitive area.
- Hold can 6 to 12 inches from affected area. Administer spray by either lying on side in bed while spraying from behind or by standing with one foot on chair or toilet seat.
- Assess use of complementary and alternative medicines, including herbal supplements.
- Avoid contact of medication with eyes.
- Teach patient not to use perineal heat lamp after application, because this could cause tissue burns.
- If condition exacerbates or symptoms recur within a few days, notify health care provider and discontinue use until directed.
- Keep medication out of children's reach in postpartum unit and later at home. If ingested, contact poison control center immediately.
- Store below 120°F (49°C). Dispose of empty can without puncturing or incinerating.

Self-Administration: Hemorrhoids and Perineal Wounds: Witch Hazel Compresses

- Pour liquid witch hazel over chipped ice; place soft, clean, absorbent squares in solution; squeeze square to eliminate excess moisture; fold and place moist square against episiotomy site or hemorrhoids.
- If using commercial medicated pads, entire container may be placed in refrigerator.
- Avoid touching surface of pad placed next to perineal wound.
- Teach patient when to change compress and how to place ice bag and peri-pad over compress.
- Do not insert medicated pads into rectum.
- Keep product out of children's reach.
- Do not use if rectal bleeding present.
- Discontinue use if local irritation occurs.

Self-Administration: Hemorrhoids: Tucks Ointment and Tucks Suppositories

- Apply ointment externally in postpartum period.
- Place suppository in lower portion of anal canal. Caution: products usually are not inserted rectally if fourth-degree lacerations are present.
- Apply small quantity of ointment onto 2-by-2–inch gauze pad; place inside peri-pad against swollen anorectal tissue approximately 5 times per day.
- If suppository is ordered, tell patient to keep refrigerated but not frozen. Remove wrapper before inserting in rectum (hold suppository upright, and peel evenly down sides). Do not hold suppository for prolonged period, because it will melt. If suppository softens before use, hold in foil wrapper under cold water for 2 to 3 minutes.
- Ascertain patient hypersensitivity to any components of ointment (e.g., pramoxine HCl 1%, mineral oil 46.7%, zinc oxide 12.5%).
- Avoid contact of medication with eyes.
- Ointment may occasionally cause burning sensation in some patients, especially if anal tissue is not intact.
- If erythema, irritation, edema, or pain develops or increases, discontinue use and consult health care provider.
- Notify health care provider if bleeding occurs.

Self-Administration: Hydrocortisone and Pramoxine and Pramoxine HCl

- Advise patient that product is for anal or perianal use only and is not to be inserted into rectum.
- Shake can vigorously before use.
- Fully extend applicator plunger; hold can upright to fill applicator.
- Express contents of applicator onto a 2-by-2–inch gauze pad, and place inside peri-pad against rectum.
- Use two to three times daily and after bowel movements.
- Take applicator apart after each use, and wash with warm water.
- Keep aerosol container out of children's reach in postpartum unit and later at home.
- Store below 120°F (49°C).
- Dispose of aerosol container without puncturing or incinerating.
- Avoid contact of medication with eyes.
- Advise patient that it is not known if topical administration of corticosteroids results in sufficient systemic absorption to produce detectable quantities in breast milk. Burning, itching, irritation, dryness, and folliculitis may occur, especially if occlusive dressings are used.

Self-Administration: Dibucaine Ointment 1%

- Express ointment from applicator on a tissue or 2-by-2–inch gauze pad, and place against the anus. Do not insert applicator into rectum. Effects should be

within 15 minutes and last for 2 to 4 hours. Ointment is poorly absorbed through intact skin, but it is well absorbed through mucous membranes and excoriated skin.
- Do not use product near eyes, over denuded surface or blistered areas, or if there is rectal bleeding.
- Do not use more than one tube (30-g size) in 24 hours.
- Keep medication out of children's reach.
- Ask patient if there is any known hypersensitivity to amide-type anesthetics; if so, product is contraindicated.
- Local effects may include burning, tenderness, irritation, inflammation, and contact dermatitis; inform health care provider if these occur.
- Other side effects may include edema, cutaneous lesions, and urticaria.

Cultural Considerations
- Provide an interpreter with same ethnic background and gender if possible, especially with sensitive topics.

Evaluation
- Reevaluate patient's perception of pain after use of nonpharmacologic and pharmacologic measures. Identify need for additional patient teaching.
- Reassess perineal and anal tissues for integrity, healing, and any side effects.

Lactation Suppression

In the past, lactation was commonly controlled through drug therapy with one of three agents: chlorotrianisene (Tace), Deladumone OB (combination of estrogen plus androgen in the form of estradiol valerate and testosterone enanthate), or bromocriptine mesylate (Parlodel). Estrogenic substances are much less popular than in the past because of the increased incidence of thrombophlebitis associated with the high dosage needed to suppress lactation and concerns about potential carcinogenic effects. Although these drugs are not used now, your patients and their families may ask about these medications, which were given in the past for lactation suppression. Presently nonpharmacologic measures are recommended for lactation suppression, such as wearing a supportive bra 24 hours a day for 10 to 14 days or using axillary ice packs) (Table 55-2). Other strategies include taking 200 mg of pyrioxidine (vitamin B_6) for 5 days, ingesting sage tea approximately every 6 hours, using 3 to 4 mL of alcohol tincture every 6 hours via the mucous membranes, and applying pounded cold cabbage leaves to breasts and aerola, changing every 30 minutes as cabbage leaves wilt.

Promotion of Bowel Function

Constipation is common during the postpartum period. The residual effects of progesterone on smooth muscle decrease peristalsis. This decreased paristalsis, added to decreased liquid intake during labor, decreased activity, and relaxation of the abdominal muscles, amplifies the problem. Patients who deliver by cesarean section are even more likely to experience constipation and **flatus** (intestinal gas). Nonpharmacologic measures (e.g., high-fiber foods, early ambulation, drinking at least 64 ounces of fluids per day, promptly responding to the defecation urge) are generally instituted after delivery.

Pharmacologic measures include the use of stool softeners, laxative stimulants, and for the postcesarean patient, **antiflatulents** (used to treat excessive gas in the stomach and intestines) (Table 55-3).

Side Effects and Adverse Reactions

The following side effects have been reported:
- Docusate sodium (Colace): Bitter taste, throat irritation, rash
- Sennosides and docusate sodium (Peri-Colace): Nausea, abdominal cramping, diarrhea, rash
- Bisacodyl suppositories (Dulcolax): Proctitis and inflammation
- Magnesium hydroxide (milk of magnesia): Abdominal cramps, nausea
- Senna (Senokot): Nausea, vomiting, diarrhea, abdominal cramps; can also cause diarrhea in breastfed infants
- Mineral oil: Nausea, vomiting, diarrhea, abdominal cramps; if aspirated, lipid pneumonitis may occur

Nursing Process
Patient-Centered Collaborative Care

Laxatives

Assessment
- Note time of delivery, predelivery food and fluid intake, ambulation and activity, and predelivery bowel habits. Obtain history of bowel problems.
- Assess patient's bowel sounds in all four quadrants (particularly post–cesarean delivery), and note abdominal distention.
- Assess perineal area for wounds, hemorrhoids, and episiotomy (REEDA).

Nursing Diagnoses
- Risk for constipation related to perineal discomfort, decreased peristalsis, and use of opioids
- Fear of acute pain related to first postdelivery bowel movement secondary to episiotomy, hemorrhoids, or perineal wounds

Planning
- Patient will have bowel movement by 2 to 4 days postpartum.
- Patient will resume normal prepregnancy bowel elimination pattern within 4 to 6 weeks.

TABLE 55-2 NONPHARMACOLOGIC MEASURES FOR COMMON POSTPARTUM NEEDS

INDICATION	INTERVENTION
Uterine contractions	Patient positioned on abdomen with pillow under abdomen for 20-30 min for 3-4 d
	Distraction, breathing techniques, therapeutic touch, relaxation, guided imagery, ambulation
	No heat to abdomen because of risk of uterine relaxation and increased bleeding
Perineal wound resulting from episiotomy or laceration	Ice packs/glove (covered in thin, absorbent material to protect tissue) for 6-8 hours after delivery
	Patient positioned on side as much as possible with pillow between legs
	Early and frequent ambulation
	Perineal exercises (Kegel exercises)
	Cool sitz bath 2-3 h after delivery
	Warm sitz bath 12-24 h after delivery t.i.d./q.i.d.
	Area cleansed front to back using perispray squeeze bottle, cleansing shower, or Surgi-Gator
	Patient tightens buttocks or squeezes buttocks together before sitting and sits tall and flat, not rolled back onto coccyx
	No tampons, douche, or feminine hygiene sprays
	No intercourse until after lochia has ceased or as advised by health care provider
Hemorrhoids	As above but particularly:
	Ice
	Sims position to help increase venous return
	Warm, moist heat; sitz bath
	Witch hazel pads (e.g., Tucks)
Lactation suppression	Tight bra worn continuously for 10-14 days
	Normal fluid intake
	No manipulation or stimulation of breasts
	Pyrioxidine (B_6) 200 mg for 5 days
	Sage tea every 6 hours
	Alcohol tincture 3-4 mL every 6 hours
Engorgement	As above, plus ice to axillary area of breasts if bottle feeding, or apply warm compresses if breastfeeding
	Express small amount of colostrum or milk (if breastfeeding) by hand expression before putting infant to breast to facilitate latching on
Sore or cracked nipples	Wear absorbent breast pads to keep moisture away from nipples
	Do not use soap on nipples
	Air-dry nipples after nursing
	Express small amount of breast milk on nipples to use as a protective lubricant
	Apply hypoallergenic purified lanolin (Lansinoh, PureLan) to nipples as protective lubricant to promote healing
	For cracked nipples, use comfort gel pads (Hydrogel pads)
	Do not use nipple shields because they can promote chafing
	Do not limit infant's nursing time at breast; otherwise milk ducts will not be emptied, and increased pressure may occur
	Ensure proper positioning for feeding; nursing initiated on less sore nipple
	Break suction with little finger after feeding to prevent pulling on nipple

b.i.d., Twice a day; *d,* day; *h,* hour; *min,* minute; *NA,* not applicable; *PB,* protein-binding; *p.c.,* after meals; *PO,* by mouth; *q.i.d.,* four times a day; *t½,* half-life; *t.i.d.,* three times a day; *UK,* unknown; >, greater than.

Nursing Interventions

- *Docusate Sodium and Sennosides with Docusate Sodium*
- Store at room temperature.
- If liquid preparation is ordered, give with milk or fruit juice to mask bitter taste.
- Take with full glass of water.
- Assess patient for history of laxative dependence.
- Drug interaction may occur with mineral oil, phenolphthalein, or aspirin.

Bisacodyl USP

- Store tablets and suppositories below 77° F (25° C), and avoid excess humidity.
- Do not crush tablets.
- Do not administer within 1 to 2 hours of milk or antacid, because enteric coating may dissolve, resulting in abdominal cramping and vomiting.
- Take with full glass of water.

Mineral Oil

- Do not give with or immediately after meals.
- Give with fruit juice or carbonated drink to disguise taste.

Magnesium Hydroxide

- Shake container well.
- Do not give 1 to 2 hours before or after oral drugs because of effects on absorption.
- Take with full glass of water.

TABLE 55-3 DRUGS USED TO PROMOTE POSTPARTUM BOWEL FUNCTION

GENERIC (BRAND)	ROUTE AND DOSAGE	USES AND CONSIDERATIONS
docusate sodium (Colace) 550 mg with 3 mg sodium, 100-mg cap with 5 mg sodium (Dulcolax Stool Softener) 100 mg with 5 mg sodium docusate calcium (Surfak) 240-mg cap	100 mg PO b.i.d. 50-400 mg PO daily in 1-4 divided doses; usual dosage is 50-360 mg daily	Reduces surface tension of the oil-water interface of the stool, resulting in enhanced incorporation of water and fat and subsequent stool softening. Onset: 12-72 h. Docusate salts are interchangeable (amount of Na, Ca, or K per dosage is clinically insignificant). Do not use concomitantly with mineral oil. Contraindicated in patients with intestinal obstruction, acute abdominal pain, nausea, or vomiting. Do not use >1 wk. Prolonged, frequent, or excessive use may cause bowel dependence or electrolyte imbalance. Compatible with breastfeeding. Side effects: rash. Pregnancy category: C; PB: NA; $t\frac{1}{2}$: NA
sennosides with docusate sodium (Peri-Colace, Senokot); docusate sodium 50 mg; sennosides, 8.6 mg	1-2 tabs PO, usually h.s.	Mild stimulant laxative. Take with full glass of water. Onset: 8-12 h, but may require up to 24 h. Contraindicated in patients with abdominal pain, nausea, or vomiting. Compatible with breastfeeding. Adverse reactions: rash, abdominal cramping, diarrhea, nausea. Pregnancy category: C; PB: NA; $t\frac{1}{2}$: NA
bisacodyl USP (Dulcolax) (suppository 10 mg or tab 5 mg)	2-3 tabs PO or 1 supp, 5-15 mg/d given as single dose	Stimulant laxative. Irritates smooth muscle of intestine, possibly colon and intramural plexus; alters water and electrolyte secretion, increasing intestinal fluid and producing laxative effect. Onset PO: 6-10 h; rectally: 15 min-1 h. Absorption: 5% absorbed systemically following oral or rectal form. Metabolized in the liver to conjugated metabolites; excreted in breast milk, bile, and urine. Do not crush tabs (enteric coated). Do not administer within 1 h of milk or antacid, because enteric coating may dissolve, resulting in abdominal cramping and vomiting. Side effects: abdominal cramps, nausea, vomiting, rectal burning, electrolyte and fluid acidosis or alkalosis, hypocalcemia. Pregnancy category: C
magnesium hydroxide (milk of magnesia)	30 mL PO PRN daily or in divided doses	Laxative. Acts by increasing and retaining water in intestinal lumen, causing distention that stimulates peristalsis and bowel elimination. Onset: 4-8 h. Excreted in kidneys (absorbed portion); unabsorbed portion excreted in feces. Poses risk to patient with renal failure, because 15%-30% of magnesium is systemically absorbed. Use with caution in patients with impaired renal function, because hypermagnesemia and toxicity may occur as a result of decreased renal clearance of absorbed magnesium. Contraindicated in patients with colostomy, ileostomy, abdominal pain, nausea, vomiting, fecal impaction, and renal failure. Drug interactions may occur with tetracyclines, digoxin, indomethacin, iron salts, or isoniazid. Milk of magnesia concentrate is three times as potent as regular-strength product. Side effects: abdominal cramps, nausea. Adverse reactions: hypotension, hypermagnesemia, muscle weakness, and respiratory depression. Pregnancy category: B
magnesium hydroxide with mineral oil (Phillips MO)	30-60 mL PO daily	Mild saline laxative. Acts by drawing water into gut, increasing intraluminal pressure and intestinal motility. Onset: 0.5-6 hours. Pregnancy category: B. Equivalent to magnesium hydroxide
mineral oil	15-45 mL PO daily or in divided doses	Lubricant laxative eases passage of stool by decreasing water absorption and lubricating the intestine. Onset: 6-8 hours; Peak: UK; Duration: UK. May impair absorption of fat-soluble vitamins (A, D, E, K), oral contraceptives, coumarin, and sulfonamides. Avoid bedtime doses because of risk of aspiration (lipid pneumonitis). Do not give with food or meals because of risk of aspiration and decreased fat-soluble vitamin absorption. Contraindicated in patients with ileostomy, colostomy, appendicitis, ulcerative colitis, and diverticulitis. Best administered on an empty stomach. Side effects: nausea, vomiting, diarrhea, and abdominal cramps. Pregnancy category: C; PB: NA; $t\frac{1}{2}$: NA

Continued

TABLE 55-3 DRUGS USED TO PROMOTE POSTPARTUM BOWEL FUNCTION—cont'd

GENERIC (BRAND)	ROUTE AND DOSAGE	USES AND CONSIDERATIONS
senna (Senokot)	10-15 mL syrup h.s.; 2-4 tabs PO b.i.d	Stimulant laxative. Acts by local irritant effect on colon to promote peristalsis and bowel evacuation. Also increases moisture content of stool by accumulating fluids in intestine. Onset: 6-24 hours. Metabolized in liver; eliminated in feces (viable) and urine. Drug interactions may occur with (MAOIs, disulfiram, metronidazole, and procarbazine. May discolor urine or feces. Liquid syrup contains 7% alcohol. May create laxative dependence and loss of bowel function with prolonged use. Contraindicated in patients with fluid and electrolyte disturbances, abdominal pain, and nausea and vomiting. Excreted in breast milk. Pregnancy category: C; t½: NA
simethicone (Gas-X chewable tabs, 80 mg; Extra Strength Gas-X chewable tab, 125 mg; Gas-X Extra Strength softgel, 125 mg, Phazyme tab, 90 mg, cap, 125 mg, 180 mg; Mylanta Gas Relief chewable tab, 80 mg; Mylanta Gas Relief Maximum Strength chewable tab, 125 mg)	1 tab or softgel q.i.d. p.c. and h.s; *max:* 6 tabs or 4 softgels/24 h	Antiflatulent. Acts by dispersing and preventing formation of mucus-surrounded gas pockets in GI tract; changes surface tension of gas bubbles and allows them to coalesce, making them easier to eliminate as belching and rectal flatus. Must be chewed thoroughly before swallowing; suggest patient drink a full glass of water after tablets are chewed. Onset: UK. Excreted unchanged in feces. May interfere with results of guaiac tests of gastric aspirates. Do not take double doses to make up for missed doses. Store below 104° F (40° C) in well-closed container. No known side effects. Pregnancy category: C; t½: UK

b.i.d., Twice a day; cap, capsule; *d,* day; *h,* hour; *h.s.,* at bedtime; *MAOI,* monoamine oxidase inhibitor; *min,* minute; *NA,* not applicable; *PB,* protein-binding; *p.c.,* after meals; *PO,* by mouth; *q.i.d.,* four times a day; *supp,* suppository; *tab,* tablet; *t.i.d.,* three times a day.

- Note that milk of magnesia concentrate is three times as potent as regular-strength product.
- Give laxative 1 hour before or 1 hour after any oral antibiotic.

Senna
- Protect from light and heat.

Simethicone
- Administer after meals and at bedtime.
- If chewable tablets are ordered, instruct patient to chew tablets thoroughly before swallowing and follow with full glass of water.

Patient Teaching

General
- Advise patient that stool softeners are given to enable bowel movement without straining.
- Advise patient that measures to prevent and treat constipation include drinking 6 to 8 glasses of fluid per day, ingesting foods high in fiber (bran, fruits, vegetables), and increasing daily ambulation and activity. Instruct patients to avoid/minimize ingestion of gas-forming foods (beans, cabbage, onions) and to increase ambulation/activity.
- Advise patient regarding temperature and storage requirements for particular drugs.
- Caution patient that prolonged, frequent, or excessive use may result in dependence on drug or electrolyte imbalance.
- Advise patient that many laxatives contain sodium. Instruct patient to check with health care provider or pharmacist before using laxative if on low-sodium diet.

Docusate Sodium and Sennosides with Docusate Sodium
- Advise patient to drink at least six 8-oz glasses of liquid daily and to drink one glass of fluid with each dose. Patient should not take drug if already taking mineral oil or having acute abdominal pain, nausea, vomiting, or signs of intestinal obstruction. Patient should not use products for longer than 1 week and should report skin rash or if stomach or intestinal cramping occurs and does not diminish.
- Senna: Instruct patient that drug may discolor urine and feces to yellow-green; to discontinue drug if abdominal pain, nausea, or vomiting occurs; and that syrup form is 7% alcohol.
- Mineral oil: Instruct patient not to take other laxatives (e.g., docusate products) if she is already taking mineral oil; to take on an empty stomach; not to take with food or meals because of risk of aspiration and decreased fat-soluble vitamin absorption; to avoid bedtime doses because of risk of aspiration; and to report nausea, vomiting, diarrhea, or abdominal cramping.

Magnesium Hydroxide
- Advise patient that laxative action generally occurs in 4 to 8 hours and to take with full glass of water.

- Caution patient to note whether drug is regular or concentrated form (concentrate is three times more potent than regular strength).
- Advise patient that drug may interact with tetracyclines, digoxin (Lanoxin), indomethacin (Indocin), iron salts, and isoniazid and to notify health care provider if any of these drugs are used.
- Instruct patient to report any muscular weakness, diarrhea, or abdominal cramps.

Simethicone

- Advise patient that drug will help relieve flatus and associated pain and that it should be taken after meals; if chewable tablets are ordered, instruct patient to chew tablets thoroughly and drink full glass of water. If a dose is missed, patient should take it as soon as possible but should not take double doses.

Cultural Considerations

- In some cultures, pregnancy is considered a "cold" state, so warm foods and activities are encouraged to balance the body. Failure to do so, it is believed, may contribute to later poor health. For example, women of Mexican-American ethnicity may wish to avoid chilling and exposure to drafts and may not accept perineal cold compresses.
- Provide an interpreter with same ethnic background and gender if possible, especially with sensitive topics.
- Be culturally cognizant that different cultures discuss elimination in different ways. Be aware of cultural beliefs and practices.

Evaluation

- Evaluate for return of prepregnancy regular bowel function.

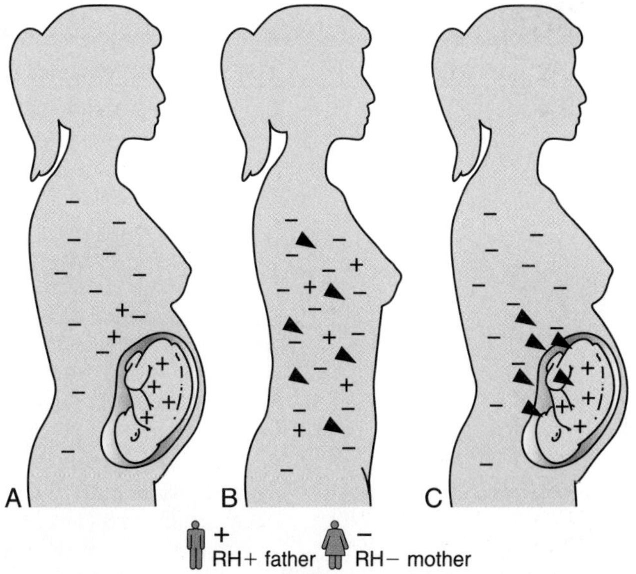

FIGURE 55–1 Understanding Rh isoimmunization. **A**, During pregnancy or delivery, a small amount of fetal blood may enter the mother's circulation. **B**, When the mother is Rh-negative and is pregnant with an Rh-positive fetus, the mother's immune system responds by producing anti-Rh_O(D) antibodies. **C**, In subsequent pregnancies, these antibodies cross the placenta and enter the fetal circulation; when the fetus is Rh-positive, the anti-Rh_O(D) antibodies will attack the fetal red blood cells and cause hemolysis.

IMMUNIZATIONS

Rh_O(D) Immune Globulin

An Rh-negative patient who lacks the Rh factor in her own blood may carry a fetus who is either Rh-negative or Rh-positive. During pregnancy, minimal amounts of fetal blood may cross the placenta. Also, an abortion (spontaneous, therapeutic, or induced), amniocentesis, ectopic pregnancy, previa, and abruption result in some mixing of maternal and fetal blood. Subsequently, anti-D antibodies develop in an Rh-negative mother with an Rh-positive fetus; with the development of these antibodies, the mother becomes sensitized (Figure 55-1). If mother and fetus are both Rh-negative, no incompatibility exists to trigger the maternal antibody response, but if the fetus is Rh-positive, the Rh-negative mother is at risk for **Rh sensitization** (i.e., the development of protective antibodies against incompatible Rh-positive blood). The immune globulin IgM is formed and cannot cross the placenta. Later, IgD antibodies develop, which may cross the placenta with isoimmunization to the D antigen and subsequent hemolysis of fetal red blood cells. Prenatal D isoimmunization occurs in approximately 1% to 2% of Rh-negative women. In later exposure, as with subsequent pregnancies, there is a more rapid IgG (secondary) immune response and increased potential for fetal hemolysis in an Rh-positive fetus. The protective antibodies, once formed, remain throughout life and may result in hemolytic difficulties for fetuses in subsequent pregnancies. Maternal blood is assessed for the D antibody at the initial prenatal laboratory evaluation and at 26 to 28 gestational weeks. Human D immune globulin (RhoGAM, Rh_O[D] immune globulin) is routinely administered to women with maternal/fetal blood mixing, such as after abortion or with threatened abortion at any stage of gestation with continuation of the pregnancy, obstetrical trauma, obstetrical manipulation, or ectopic pregnancy. If abortion occurs up to and including 12 weeks' gestation, the microdose is administered if less than 2.5 mL of Rh incompatible red blood cells were administered. During the postpartum period, Rh_O(D) immune globulin should be administered within 72 hours. Therefore, one full dose (300 mcg) is given postpartum if the newborn is Rh positive, antepartum prophylaxis at 26 to 28 weeks' gestation, after amniocentesis, chorionic villus sampling, and percutaneous umbilical blood sampling. For women with abruption, previa, cesarean births, or manual placental removal, a Kleihauer-Betke analysis (serum test) should be done, because

TABLE 55-4 RH_O(D) IMMUNE GLOBULIN

ROUTE AND DOSAGE	USES AND CONSIDERATIONS
IM in deltoid	Sterile concentrated solution of gamma globulin prepared from human serum containing antibodies to Rh factor (D antigen), also expressed as anti-Rh_0(D). Administered to unsensitized Rh-negative patients. Suppresses active antibody response and formation of anti-Rh_0(D) in Rh-negative patients exposed to fetal Rh-positive blood. Promotes destruction of Rh-positive fetal cells in maternal serum before mother can make antibodies that would cause hemolysis of fetal RBCs in Rh-positive fetuses and newborns in subsequent pregnancies. Use with caution in patients with thrombocytopenia, bleeding disorders, and IgA deficiency. Contraindicated in patients with known hypersensitivity to immune globulins or thimerosal, transfusion of Rh_0(D)-positive blood in previous 3 mo, or previous sensitization to Rh_0(D). 1 vial (300 mcg) prevents maternal sensitization if fetal RBC volume that entered maternal circulation is <15 mL. If the estimated fetal blood and maternal mixing is >15mL, then an additional 300 mcg is administered. When >15 mL maternal-fetal blood mixing has occurred, a fetal RBC is performed to determine appropriate dose. Appears in breast milk (not absorbed by infant). Adverse reactions: lethargy, splenomegaly, elevated bilirubin, myalgia, temperature elevation; most commonly fever (still rare) and pain at injection site. Pregnancy category: C; $t\frac{1}{2}$: 23-26 d
300 mcg (1 vial) (standard dose)	Given at 26-28 wk gestation as prophylaxis and again after normal delivery (within 72 hours) with negative direct and indirect Coombs test. Also 300 mcg (standard dose) given after amniocentesis, chorionic villus sampling, percutaneous umbilical blood sampling, abdominal trauma, obstetrical manipulation, ectopic pregnancy, abortion, or threatened abortion at any stage of gestation with continuation of pregnancy. Larger than standard dose may be given if Kleihauer-Betke analysis shows that large fetal-maternal blood transfusion (>15 mL Rh positive RBCs) has occurred
50 mcg (1 vial) (microdose)	Given after abortion before 12 gestational wk if less than 2.5 mL of Rh incompatible RBCs were administered

d, Day; *IgA,* immunoglobulin A; *IM,* intramuscular; *mo,* month; *RBC,* red blood cell; $t\frac{1}{2}$, half-life; *wk,* week; >, greater than; <, less than.

TABLE 55-5 RUBELLA VIRUS VACCINE, LIVE, MSD

ROUTE AND DOSAGE	USES AND CONSIDERATIONS
Given subQ: 0.5 mL into outer upper arm	Live virus vaccine for immunization against rubella (German measles). Dose is same for all persons, using either single-dose or multidose vials. Do not give immune serum globulin (ISG) concurrent with vaccine. Contraindicated in pregnant women and patients with anaphylactoid reactions to neomycin and/or gelatin, febrile respiratory illness or other febrile infection, active untreated tuberculosis, or immune deficiency conditions. Vaccinated persons can shed but not transmit virus. Defer vaccination for 3 months after blood or plasma transfusions and also after human serum immune globulin. Postpartum patients who received blood products may be vaccinated if repeat titer is drawn 6-8 wk later to ensure that seroconversion has occurred. Excreted in breast milk; use caution. Important for patient to use contraceptive method for 4 weeks following administration, because rubella is teratogenic. Rubella titer may be reassessed 3 mo after administration. Side effects: burning, stinging at injection site; malaise; fever; headache; slight rash 2-4 wk after injection; joint pain 1-3 d within 1-10 wk of injection. Pregnancy category: C

d, Day; *mo,* month; *subQ,* subcutaneous; *wk,* week.

more than 15 mL of fetal-maternal hemorrhage of Rh-positive red blood cells may have occurred, necessitating an increased dose of Rh_O(D) immune globulin. When 15 mL or more of Rh positive red blood cells is suspected, a fetal red blood cell count should be performed to determine the appropriate dose.

The Rh sensitization process can be prevented through the administration of **Rh_O(D) immune globulin** (RhoGAM) to unsensitized Rh-negative patients after each actual or potential exposure to Rh-positive blood (Table 55-4).

Adverse Reactions

Adverse reactions include hypotension, chills, dizziness, fever, headache, pruritus, rash, abdominal pain, diarrhea, and injection site reactions (discomfort, mild pain, redness, swelling).

Rubella Vaccine

Maternal rubella, also called German measles, is a potentially devastating infection for the fetus, depending on gestational age. If an unimmunized woman (rubella titer <1 : 10 or negative titer) contracts the virus during the first trimester, a high rate of abortion and neurologic and developmental sequela associated with **congenital rubella syndrome** (transmission of the rubella virus to the fetus via the placenta) may result. Cataracts, glaucoma, deafness, heart defects, and mental retardation are seen with this syndrome. When infection occurs after the first trimester, there is less risk of fetal damage because of the developmental stage of the fetus. There is no treatment for maternal or congenital rubella infection. The goals are immunization and prevention of rubella in patients of childbearing age (Table 55-5).

Adverse Reactions

Side effects are generally mild and temporary. Burning or stinging at the injection site is caused by the acidic pH of the vaccine. Regional lymphadenopathy, **urticaria** (skin rash caused by an allergic reaction), rash, malaise, sore throat, fever, headache, polyneuritis, arthralgia, and moderate fever are occasionally seen.

Nursing Process
Patient-Centered Collaborative Care
RhO(D) Immune Globulin

Assessment
- Determine blood type and Rh status of all prenatal patients.
- Assess patient for understanding of both her own and her partner's Rh status.
- Ask patient about previous pregnancies and their outcome; ask whether she has ever received $Rh_O(D)$ immune globulin.
- Follow agency policy for Rh blood testing for patient and infant at time of delivery.
- Postpartum, assess data about neonate's Rh type. If infant is Rh negative, drug is not needed. If infant is Rh positive and Rh-negative mother is not sensitized (negative indirect Coombs test) and infant has a negative direct Coombs test, mother is a candidate to receive the injection to prevent antibody production or "sensitization."
- Obtain patient's written consent before administration. Some agencies require a refusal form if the drug is declined.
- Assess for history of allergy to immune globulin products.

Nursing Diagnoses
- Deficient knowledge related to maternal/fetal Rh incompatibility and sensitization
- Deficient knowledge related to $Rh_O(D)$ immune globulin purpose, action, and side effects

Planning
- Patient will receive $Rh_O(D)$ immune globulin as indicated within 72 hours after delivery or abortion.
- Patient will be able to discuss Rh sensitization and actions indicated during subsequent pregnancies.

Nursing Interventions
- Document Rh workup and eligibility of patient to receive drug. Convey information in verbal report and in patient record using agency policy.
- Check lot numbers on vial and laboratory slip for agreement before administration; check expiration date. Check identification band and laboratory slip for matching number. Return required slips to laboratory or blood bank.
- Administer $Rh_O(D)$ immune globulin: dose (microdose/standard dose) according to gestational weeks and exposure and route, according to provider orders and agency. Administer intramuscularly (IM). Normally administered in deltoid muscle within 72 hours after delivery, but if more than 72 hours has passed, administer as soon as possible up to 28 days; a lesser degree of protection may result.
- Intravenous (IV) administration of $Rh_O(D)$ immune globulin is possible, though infrequent. Check provider orders and dose. For IV administration, reconstitute with normal saline. Store at 36° F to 46° F (2° C to 8° C).
- Have epinephrine available to treat anaphylaxis.

Patient Teaching
General
- Explain action, purpose, and side effects of drug.
- Advise patient to avoid live virus vaccines for 3 months after administration.
- Provide written documentation of date of administration for patient's personal health record.

Cultural Considerations
- Provide an interpreter with same ethnic background and gender if possible, especially with sensitive topics.
- Assess patient's religious beliefs. Some patients may refuse $Rh_O(D)$ immune globulin, considering it to be a blood product.

Evaluation
- Evaluate patient's understanding of need for $Rh_O(D)$ immune globulin.

DRUGS ADMINISTERED TO THE NEWBORN IMMEDIATELY AFTER DELIVERY

Drugs administered to the newborn in the immediate period after birth are (1) erythromycin ophthalmic ointment to provide prophylaxis against eye infections (required by U.S. public health law and all states) and (2) vitamin K (Phytonadione, Mephyton) to prevent hemorrhagic disease of the newborn (Table 55-6). Antiinfective agents may be applied to the cord stump (e.g., alcohol, brilliant green/proflavine hemisulfate/gentian violet) during the first few hours after birth; however, literature supports "dry cord care" with no agents applied.

Side Effects and Adverse Reactions

Erythromycin Ophthalmic Ointment. Side effects include chemical conjunctivitis in about 20% of neonates, manifesting as edema and inflammation lasting about 24 to 48 hours.

TABLE 55-6 DRUGS ADMINISTERED TO THE NEWBORN IMMEDIATELY AFTER DELIVERY

GENERIC (BRAND)	ROUTE AND DOSAGE	USES AND CONSIDERATIONS
erythromycin ophthalmic ointment (Ilotycin Ophthalmic)	½-inch ribbon of ointment placed in lower conjunctival sac of each eye (beginning at inner canthus) within 1 h of delivery	Prevention of gonococcal conjunctivitis and chlamydial conjunctivitis **(ophthalmia neonatorum)**, which can cause blindness. Source of infection is birth canal. Contains antibiotic (erythromycin) in sterile base of mineral oil and white petrolatum. Has bactericidal or bacteriostatic action based on concentration per gram and target organisms present. Mandatory administration in U.S. Side effects: Chemical conjunctivitis (swelling, inflammation 24-48 h)
phytonadione, Vitamin K_1 (Mephyton, Aqua-MEPHYTON)	0.5-1 mg IM in vastus lateralis (preferably) or rectus femoris within 1 h after birth (check health care provider or agency standing orders for dosage)	Prevention of hemorrhagic disease of the newborn. Anticoagulant antagonist. Aqueous colloidal solution of vitamin K_1. Newborn does not receive adequate vitamin K transplacentally and unable to synthesize vitamin initially because of limited intestinal flora; therefore production of clotting factors in liver is hindered and low prothrombin levels are evidenced. Phytonadione facilitates production of clotting factors equal to natural vitamin K. Newborns of mothers who received oral anticoagulants, anticonvulsants, antituberculosis drugs, or recent antibiotics during pregnancy may need a higher dosage 6-8 h after first injection. Side effects: Pain and edema at injection site; possible allergic reactions include urticaria and rash; those who receive larger doses may exhibit hyperbilirubinemia and jaundice.

h, Hour; *IM,* intramuscular.

It may interfere slightly with eye-to-eye contact between parents and the neonate.

Vitamin K. Side effects include pain and edema at the injection site. Some allergic reactions, manifested by urticaria and rash, have been reported. Neonates who receive larger doses may exhibit hyperbilirubinemia and jaundice resulting from competition for binding sites.

Immunization during the Newborn Period before Discharge

The American Academy of Pediatrics and the Centers for Disease Control and Prevention (CDC) have recommended that immunization against hepatitis B virus (HBV) begin in the newborn period. HBV infection may result in serious long-term liver disease, cancer, and death in adulthood. The goal of immunization is to reduce the number of chronic carriers of the virus in the population, thus preventing HBV infection.

In pregnancy, HBV transmission occurs vertically, primarily at the time of delivery. Recombinant hepatitis B (Engerix-B, Recombivax HB) provides passive immunization for the newborn (Table 55-7). The current recommendation is that newborns receive recombinant hepatitis B (Engerix-B Pediatric, Recombivax HB) and, if appropriate, hepatitis B immune globulin (HBIG) injections IM in the anterolateral thigh (vastus lateralis [preferred] or rectus femoris muscles) following a protocol based on the mother's HBsAg-positive or -negative status. These injections require signed maternal consent before administration. Infants born to HBsAg-negative mothers will receive only recombinant hepatitis B. Infants born to HBsAg-positive mothers will receive concurrent injections of both hepatitis B immune globulin and hepatitis B vaccine in separate sites within 12 hours of birth, because it is believed that infection can be prevented in 90% of newborns. Determine the mother's HBsAg status as soon as possible. If the mother's HBsAg status is unknown, administer the HepB immunization within 12 hours of delivery. Hepatitis B immune globulin can be given to infants no later than 1 week of age if the mother is HBsAG-positive, but should be given within 12 hours of birth.

Nursing Process
Patient-Centered Collaborative Care

Measles-Mumps-Rubella Vaccine

Assessment

- Review history and laboratory results to determine need for measles-mumps-rubella (MMR) vaccine.
- A rubella titer of less than 1:8/1:10 (agency laboratory), negative, or not immunized indicates the need for MMR vaccine administration.
- MMR vaccine is contraindicated if patient verbalizes (or if medical record review indicates) any of the following. Document the presence of any of these factors:
  Pregnancy
  Receipt of whole blood transfusions, plasma transfusion, or human immune serum globulin within the past 3 months
  History of anaphylactic or anaphylactoid reactions to neomycin (dose contains 25 mcg of neomycin), gelatin, or gelatin-containing products

TABLE 55-7 HEPATITIS B IMMUNIZATION IN THE NEWBORN PERIOD

GENERIC (BRAND)	ROUTE AND DOSAGE	USES AND CONSIDERATIONS
hepatitis B vaccine (Engerix-B, Recombivax HB)	For newborns of mothers who have HBsAg-negative, HBsAg-positive, or unknown HBsAg status: Engerix-B: 0.5 mL (10 mcg) IM within 12 h after birth (first dose); second dose at 1-2 mo, and final dose at >24 weeks (6 mo). Recombivax HB: 0.5 mL (5 mcg) IM within 12 h after birth (first dose), repeated at 1 mo and 6 mo.	A recombinant vaccine that provides passive immunization against all subtypes of HBV. Given to all infants regardless of HBsAg status of mother. Unvaccinated infants <12 mo with mother or primary caregiver with acute hepatitis B are given HBIG because of risk for becoming HBV carrier following infection (also start HBV vaccine series). Iinject IM into vastus lateralis (preferably) or rectus femoris; never inject IV. Following three doses, >90% of infants and children will seroconvert 95%-99%. Protection in those who seroconvert will last 3-7 y with single booster. Contraindicated in patients with hypersensitivity to any component of vaccine or yeast. Neonatal side effects: soreness at injection site with edema, warmth, erythema, and induration. Pregnancy category: C Newborns of HBsAg-positive mothers should also receive HBIG 0.5 mL IM within 12 h of birth. May be given concurrently with first dose of hepatitis B vaccine in separate site (opposite thigh). Newborns of mothers with HBsAg-unknown status whose maternal results are positive within 7 days of birth should receive HBIG (0.5 mL) IM in thigh not used for vaccine.

h, Hour; *HBIG,* hepatitis B immune globulin; *HBsAg,* hepatitis B surface antigen; *HBV,* hepatitis B virus; *IM,* intramuscular; *IV,* intravenous; *mo,* month; *y,* year; >, greater than.

Receipt of other virus vaccines within 1 month (Do not give less than 1 month before or after other virus vaccines.)

Immunosuppressed, radiation therapy, untreated active tuberculosis (TB), AIDS, or symptomatic HIV

Blood dyscrasias, leukemia, lymphomas of any type, or other malignant neoplasms affecting bone marrow or lymphatic system

Any febrile or respiratory illness or other acute illness

- Determine whether patient is also a candidate to receive Rh_O(D) immune globulin. Administration of both drugs may result in suppression of rubella antibodies with need to recheck rubella titer in approximately 3 months.

Nursing Diagnoses
- Deficient knowledge related to risk for rubella infection and benefit of prevention in patients of childbearing age
- Risk for fetal injury related to rubella infection in subsequent pregnancy secondary to lack of immunity

Planning
- Patient will receive MMR vaccine to protect against rubella.
- Patient will plan to prevent pregnancy for 4 weeks after subQ injection.

Nursing Interventions
- Protect vaccine from light, and store at 35.6° F to 46.4° F (2° C to 8° C) before reconstitution.
- Reconstitute with diluent provided, and administer within 8 hours. Administer 0.5-mL vaccine subQ in upper outer arm. Do not administer IV.
- If tuberculin skin test is to be done, administer it before or simultaneously with rubella vaccine (may have temporary depression in tuberculin skin sensitivity). If MMR has been given before tuberculin skin test, postpone tuberculin skin test until 4 to 6 weeks after MMR administration. If giving both simultaneously, use the Mantoux test.

Skill: Reconstitution
- Single-dose vial: withdraw entire amount of diluent into syringe.
- Inject total volume into vial of lyophilized vaccine, and agitate to mix thoroughly.
- Withdraw entire contents into syringe, and inject total volume of restored vaccine.
- Have epinephrine readily available in case of anaphylactic reaction.
- Clearly convey in verbal report and documentation that vaccination has occurred.
- Record date of administration, lot number, manufacturer, name, and title to comply with agency policy.

Patient Teaching
General
- Discuss with patient the importance of immunity to rubella, and help her understand the need to obtain titers to determine immune status.

- Discuss the importance for use of effective contraception for 4 weeks after vaccine injection. Identify contraceptive method of choice, and document instruction.
- Reassure patient that there is no risk to her from being near small children who received the injection, even if she is pregnant and not immune.
- Advise patient regarding drug action, purpose, and side effects.
- Recommend that patient have titer rechecked in 3 months if she also received $Rh_O(D)$ immune globulin.

Side Effects
- The most common side effect is burning or stinging at injection site; some also experience malaise, fever, headache, and slight rash about 2 to 4 weeks after injection. About 1 to 10 weeks after injection, some may experience joint pain that lasts 1 to 3 days.

Cultural Considerations
- Some cultures are opposed to vaccinations. Clarify with the family their desires regarding vaccinations. Explore the legal requirements for vaccinations in your state.

Evaluation
- Evaluate the need for MMR vaccine and administration to patients with titer less than 1:8/1:10 (agency laboratory), not immunized, or negative titer.

Nursing Process
Patient-Centered Collaborative Care

Drugs Administered to the Newborn after Delivery

Assessment

Erythromycin Ophthalmic Ointment (Ilotycin Ophthalmic)
- Assess newborn for signs of hypersensitivity.

Phytonadione, Vitamin K
- Assess newborn for bleeding from umbilical cord, circumcision site, nose, and gastrointestinal tract, and for generalized ecchymoses.

Nursing Diagnoses
- Risk for neonatal injury related to infectious process (congenital) or transient low prothrombin levels in newborn

Planning
- Neonate will experience minimal or no side effects from drugs routinely administered after delivery.

Nursing Interventions

Erythromycin Ophthalmic Ointment
- Refer to Chapter 13 for procedure for administration of eye ointment.
- Promote bonding by facilitating eye contact between parents and infant during this period, but delay instillation no longer than 1 hour after delivery.
- Wear gloves for administration of eye ointment. Do not place tube of ointment under radiant warmer with infant before administration.
- Administer erythromycin ophthalmic ointment before administration of phytonadione and hepatitis B (with maternal consent only) injections. Infant may cry after injections, making administration of ophthalmic ointment more difficult.
- Administer erythromycin ophthalmic ointment (ribbon of ointment about 1 cm long) from inner canthus to outer canthus in lower conjunctival sac of each eye. Do not touch eye with applicator.
- Following administration, close eyes to more evenly distribute ointment. After 1 minute, may blot eye with gauze to remove excess ointment. Do not irrigate eyes after instillation.

Phytonadione, Vitamin K
- Protect drug from light because of photosensitivity of the preparation.
- Cleanse anterolateral site before injecting drug; if alcohol is used, allow to dry before drug administration.
- Wear gloves when administering.
- If phytonadione is in a glass vial, withdraw medication with filter needle. Change needles and use a 25-gauge, ⅝-inch needle to administer into the vastus lateralis muscle.
- Stabilize infant's leg before administration.
- Observe injection site for edema and inflammation (Figure 55-2). Refer to Chapter 13 for a complete discussion of safe pediatric drug injection sites.
- Administer before circumcision.

Patient Teaching

Erythromycin Ophthalmic Ointment
- Instruct parents regarding drug action, purpose, and side effects. Advise parents that drug administration is mandatory in the United States.
- Tell parents that any edema around eyes usually disappears within 24 to 48 hours.
- Explain that administration of eye prophylaxis is federally and state mandated and that there is no risk to vision from the ointment.

Phytonadione
- Instruct parents regarding drug action, purpose, and side effects.

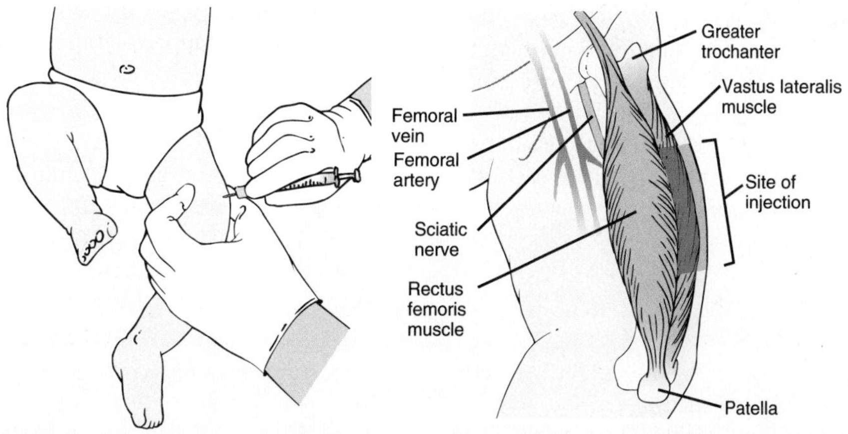

FIGURE 55–2 Site for giving an intramuscular injection to a newborn shortly after birth.

Evaluation

- Evaluate for newborn bleeding, specifically on days 2 and 3 after administration of phytonadione.
- Evaluate for drug hypersensitivity or side effects.
- Evaluate parents' understanding about medications administered to their newborn.

Nursing Process
Patient-Centered Collaborative Care

Hepatitis B Vaccine

Assessment

- Review prenatal record laboratory data for maternal HBsAg status. Validate whether infant is to receive hepatitis B vaccine singly or in concert with HBIG.
- Assess parental knowledge of immunizations, purpose, and childhood immunization schedule.
- Assess for hypersensitivity to yeast (recombinant HB).
- Assess for written maternal consent for newborn vaccine before administration.

Nursing Diagnoses

- Deficient knowledge related to hepatitis B, maternal prophylaxis, and pediatric immunization schedule
- Risk for neonatal injury related to maternal hepatitis B infection

Planning

- Newborn will receive correct dosage of hepatitis B vaccine before discharge. HBIG 0.5 mL is best given within 12 hours of birth if mother is HBsAG-positive.
- Newborn's caregiver will keep scheduled appointments with primary health care provider and verbalizes plans to continue childhood immunizations as recommended by current immunization schedule.

Nursing Interventions

- Shake vial well before withdrawal of medication.
- Discard if other than slightly opaque white suspension.
- Cleanse anterolateral site before injecting drug. If alcohol is used, allow to dry before drug administration.
- Inject complete contents of vial; do not dilute.
- Have epinephrine available for allergic reaction.
- If mother refuses hepatitis B vaccine or HBIG, note in maternal and newborn chart. Assess agency policy; most agencies document medication refusal and also notify local community health department. Monitor newborn's postinjection temperature per agency policy.
- Give IM in vastus lateralis.
- Document administration and site in chart.
- Record lot number, expiration date, name, and title in chart.
- Store product at 35.6° F to 46.4° F (2° C to 8° C).
- Do not freeze (freezing destroys potency).
- Do not confuse hepatitis B vaccine with HBIG or Haemophilus B (Hib, ActHIB) vaccine, because these drugs have different dosages.

Patient Teaching

- Inform patient of implications of her HBsAg-positive or HBsAg-negative status for her newborn, and recommend interventions.
- Have patient read literature and sign consent form for vaccine administration. Place original/copy in newborn's chart per agency policy. Instruct parents regarding childhood immunizations as recommended by current immunization schedule, and inform them when repeat doses should be given. Give parents written information regarding immunization schedule and infant immunization record. Document administration of hepatitis B vaccine on infant immunization record.

Cultural Considerations

- Japanese women may prefer to take their postpartal medications with warm water rather than with cold water.
- Cultural values influence infant care. It is important for nurses to be culturally sensitive to the pregnant patient's cultural belief framework and to try to include this framework, as appropriate, in provision of care and establishing rapport with the patient.

Evaluation

- Evaluate parents' understanding of need for hepatitis B vaccine for newborn.

KEY WEBSITES

Centers for Disease Control and Prevention: Birth defects: *www.cdc.gov/ncbddd/birthdefects/index.html*

National Institutes of Health: National Institute of Child Health and Human Development: *www.nichd.nih.gov/womenshealth/*

Postpartum: *www.babycenter.com/postpartum-health*

CRITICAL THINKING CASE STUDY

TA, an older adolescent, was admitted to the hospital for labor induction/augmentation with signs and symptoms of gestational hypertension at 42 weeks' pregnant (gravida 4, para 1). TA's mother arrived at the hospital when TA was 8 cm dilated, in time for the late stages of TA's labor. Her mother remained as TA's support person throughout the delivery, which occurred at 6:00 AM by vacuum extraction. TA had a continuous epidural for her labor and delivery. An episiotomy was performed at the time of delivery, and a fourth-degree laceration occurred. A cluster of hemorrhoids was evident. Baby JA, weighing 8 lb 7 oz, had Apgar scores of 7 and 9. The infant is alert and active.

TA lives with her parents and has been going to high school while working part time in an automotive parts store. TA wants to keep her infant and to breastfeed "for at least 3 months." She plans to finish school and return to work in 6 weeks.

Immediately after the delivery, the nurse conducts an assessment of TA, analyzes the data, and determines and prioritizes TA's nursing care needs. The same is done for the newborn.

1. Based on the data supplied about her delivery, what is the priority nursing diagnosis for TA?
2. What is a goal for the diagnosis given?
3. How should the nurse intervene in regard to the episiotomy during the early postpartum period, integrating both pharmacologic and nonpharmacologic measures? Orders include benzocaine spray, witch hazel pads, pramoxine hydrochloride, and ibuprofen (Advil, Motrin) tablets (200 mg) at the bedside.
4. TA says that her grandmother wants her to eat warm soup that she will bring to the hospital. The grandmother has also told TA not to take a shower for 4 weeks. What further assessment is necessary?

   Baby JA's newborn medications must be administered within the first hour after delivery. Bonding for TA and JA should also be promoted at this time.
5. Within the standard, how should bonding be promoted, including eye contact between mother and infant, while eye prophylaxis is also administered?
6. What steps should the nurse follow to instill ointment into the infant's eyes, including safety for the nurse administering the ointment?
7. What should TA be taught about the side effects of eye prophylaxis?
8. How should the nurse explain the reason for the vitamin K_1 injection for the infant in terms TA can understand?
9. What steps should the nurse follow to prepare and give the vitamin K_1 injection, including safety for the nurse administering the injection?

   TA is Rh negative. The blood type of the infant's father is unknown. Cord blood was drawn on the infant at the time of delivery. Based on TA's historical data, what is a concern in terms of defining TA as a likely or unlikely $Rh_O(D)$ immune globulin candidate? What information about the mother and the infant is needed to aid in the decision?
10. Assuming TA is a $Rh_O(D)$ immune globulin candidate, what is a nursing diagnosis for TA?
11. What is an outcome-based goal for the diagnosis given?
12. What is the timeframe in which $Rh_O(D)$ immune globulin should be administered? Explain your answer.
13. What is appropriate verbal and written documentation in regard to $Rh_O(D)$ immune globulin administration, both before and after administration?
14. TA's chart reveals that her rubella titer is 1:6. What orders should be expected in regard to rubella vaccine?
15. Neomycin is listed as a known allergy in TA's medication administration record. Considering TA's titer, the standing health care provider's order, and knowledge about this vaccine, how should this situation be handled?
16. In a situation in which a newborn's mother is both a rubella and a $Rh_O(D)$ immune globulin candidate, with

both products being administered, what is the focus of patient teaching for TA in regard to the rubella titer?

Because of her episiotomy, TA is concerned about her first postdelivery bowel movement. It is explained to her that the docusate with sennosides product in her self-administered medication packet will help.

17. TA says that she does not want to take the docusate because she plans to breastfeed. What is the appropriate nursing diagnosis based on TA's communication?
18. How should the nurse address TA's concerns, based on knowledge of the product and breastfeeding?

TA asks what can be done about her hemorrhoids. The mode of action of the ordered pharmacologic products is explained to her. She then states, "So I just have to insert this syringe-type applicator into my rectum once I fill it from the big can?"

19. Analyze TA's statement. What is correct and incorrect concerning the knowledge?
20. What nursing diagnosis is appropriate for TA based on the information supplied?
21. What patient teaching is needed for TA?

Baby JA is ordered to receive hepatitis B vaccine before discharge. TA is HBsAg-negative.

22. Which newborns are eligible to receive hepatitis B vaccine?
23. How many doses constitute the total series, and what is the duration for these?
24. Why is this vaccine given to newborns? Why is it important?
25. TA asks how long the infant's immunity should last. What is the nurse's best response?
26. Where would one expect to find the vaccine stored?
27. What is the written documentation required with administration of this vaccine?

NCLEX STUDY QUESTIONS

1. A patient asks the nurse why her baby is receiving a vitamin K injection. The nurse's best response is based on what knowledge?
   a. Vitamin K causes an increase in newborn platelets.
   b. A newborn's liver is too immature to produce vitamin K.
   c. A newborn cannot synthesize vitamin K without intestinal flora.
   d. Vitamin K is not produced in bone marrow until an infant is 8 days old.
2. In assessing a postpartum patient, the nurse notes saturation of two peri-pads in less than 1½ hours. What is the priority intervention?
   a. Palpate the fundus, and massage if boggy.
   b. Prepare to administer pitocin IV.
   c. Prepare to administer methylergonovine.
   d. Assess maternal blood pressure and pulse for hypovolemic shock.
3. Two hours after delivery, a patient is complaining of pain from her episiotomy. What is the most effective nursing intervention?
   a. Sitz bath for 20 minutes
   b. Application of cold compresses to the perineum
   c. Application of a hydrocortisone acetate suppository
   d. Teaching patient how to use Hydrogel pads to the area
4. A postpartum patient is being discharged from the hospital. The nurse notes that she is Rubella-negative and administers the MMR vaccine. The nurse's teaching includes which instruction?
   a. Avoid people who are immunocompromised for 1 week
   b. Continue to take prenatal vitamins for at least 3 months postpartum
   c. Use a reliable contraceptive for 1 month postpartum
   d. Take ibuprofen 800 mg three times a day for up to 2 weeks
5. It is mandatory to have maternal signed consent before administering which newborn medication?
   a. Erythromycin ophthalmic ointment
   b. Phytonadione
   c. Hepatitis B vaccine
   d. Betamethasone
6. Before administering MMR vaccine to a postpartum patient at discharge, the nurse is reviewing the patient's history for allergies. The nurse plans to withhold the vaccine and notify the health care provider after noting a patient allergy to which item?
   a. Baker's yeast
   b. Eggs
   c. Duck meat or duck feathers
   d. Neomycin
7. The nurse is mentoring a new graduate who is preparing to administer the phytonadione injection to a newborn. Which muscle sites selected by the new graduate would indicate the need for further teaching? (Select all that apply.)
   a. Anterolateral thigh
   b. Vastus lateralis
   c. Rectus femoris
   d. Gluteus maximus
   e. Vastus medialis
8. The nurse is preparing to administer an ophthalmic medication to a newborn. Education for the parents includes which fact about the medication?
   a. Infants of mothers who test positive for syphilis receive this medication.
   b. Eye ointments are administered in the bottom of the eye from the inner to the outer eye.
   c. This medication will prevent congenital cataracts.
   d. Infants with a negative direct Coombs test receive this medication.

9. In assessing a postpartum patient, the nurse notes saturation of one peri-pad in less than 15 minutes and a boggy uterus. The patient is 15 minutes postpartum with vital signs of T 99.7, P 92, R 18, and BP 142/86. The nurse performs fundal massage. Based on the patient's assessment data, the most appropriate nursing action is to withhold which medication?
   a. Carboprost (Hemabate) 0.25 ampule IM
   b. Methylergonovine (Methergine) 0.2 mg IM
   c. Oxytocin (Pitocin) 20 units in 1000 mL of lactated Ringer's solution IV
   d. Bolus of lactated Ringer's solution
10. A newborn is admitted to the nursery. The nurse reviews the maternal history. It is important that the nurse assess the mother's status specific to which infectious process(es)? (Select all that apply.)
   a. Rubeola
   b. Hepatitis A
   c. Hepatitis B
   d. HIV/AIDS
   e. Group B streptococcus
11. A newborn, whose mother is HBsAg positive, is admitted to the nursery. Which immunizations are appropriate for this newborn? (Select all that apply.)
   a. Hepatitis B immune globulin
   b. HepB
   c. *Haemophilus influenzae* type b
   d. Hepatitis A
   e. Phytonadione

Answers: 1, c; 2, a; 3, b; 4, c; 5, c; 6, d; 7, a, c, d, e; 8, b; 9, b; 10, c, d, e; 11, a, b, e.

CHAPTER

56

Drugs for Women's Reproductive Health and Menopause

evolve WEBSITE

http://evolve.elsevier.com/KeeHayes/pharmacology/

- Animations
- Content Updates
- Key Points
- Review Questions for the NCLEX® Examination
- References from the Textbook
- Unfolding Case Studies

OBJECTIVES

- Recognize that successful contraception is essential to the health and well-being of women.
- Describe methods of contraception commonly prescribed, patient selection, mechanisms of action, and possible side effects.
- Identify specific nursing actions that will enhance successful contraception for women and their partners.
- Describe the nursing process, including teaching and risk-benefit–alternative education associated with medications used for contraception and family planning.
- Provide information for nonpharmacologic and pharmacologic interventions for women experiencing menopausal symptoms.
- Differentiate between types of medications used for osteoporosis.
- Describe the nursing process, including teaching and risk-benefit–alternative education associated with medications used for menopausal symptoms

OUTLINE

The authors gratefully acknowledge the work of Marcia Welsh, who updated this chapter for the eighth edition.

KEY TERMS

amenorrhea, p. 847
anovulation, p. 853
breakthrough bleeding, p. 847
chloasma, p. 847
dysmenorrhea, p. 847
dyspareunia, p. 856
ethinyl estradiol, p. 846
hormone therapy, p. 862
menarche, p. 846
menopause, p. 846
menorrhagia, p. 847
mestranol, p. 846
metrorrhagia, p. 851
mittelschmerz, p. 847
oligomenorrhea, p. 856
osteopenia, p. 868
osteoporosis, p. 851
pelvic inflammatory disease, p. 859
progestin, p. 846
withdrawal bleeding, p. 848

Women have specific health care needs throughout their reproductive and postreproductive life cycle. Women's reproductive life cycle begins with **menarche,** the start of spontaneous menstruation, and continues through **menopause,** the permanent cessation of menstruation. Successful contraception is essential to the health and well-being of sexually active women of reproductive age. Successful adaptation to menopause, control of menopausal symptoms, and continued sexual wellness is essential to the health and well-being of older women. This chapter reviews pharmacologic products that may be used throughout the reproductive and menopausal life cycle of women.

In 2011, the Department of Health and Human Services classified contraception as a preventative service under the Affordable Care Act. For many women, this law will reduce the cost of contraception methods and improve access to health care providers.

ESTROGEN-PROGESTIN COMBINATION PRODUCTS

All estrogen-progestin combination products (also known as **combined hormone contraception** [CHC] products) contain a synthetic version of *estrogen* and a compound known as *progestin.* **Ethinyl estradiol** (EE) is the most commonly used synthetic estrogen found in CHC products. An older form of estrogen, **mestranol,** is found in higher-dose (≥50 mcg) oral combination products. Mestranol is converted into ethinyl estradiol in the body. Contraception products with high levels of ethinyl estradiol or mestranol are prescribed only in certain circumstances. Newer CHC products, including low-dose contraception pills, contain only EE as the estrogen component. **Progestins** are natural or synthetic hormones that have *progesterone-like* effects. **Progesterone** is the naturally occurring sex hormone produced in the ovaries of women. **Progestogen** refers to any synthetically produced progesterone compound. Almost all progestins are derivatives of testosterone, a steroid hormone classified under the androgen group. The term *progestin* will be used to describe the compound used in CHC products. Not only do progestins have contraceptive properties, they serve to balance out the effects of estrogen.

One of eight different types of progestins is used in CHC products. Norethindrone, norethindrone acetate, and ethynodiol diacetate are first-generation progestin compounds that were the earliest progestin formulations to be used in contraception pills. Second-generation progestins include norethisterone and levonorgestrel (LNG). LNG is the most commonly used progestin worldwide. Third-generation progestins, also referred to as *new generation* progestins, include desogestrel (etonogestrel), gestodene, and norgestimate. The new generation progestins have a higher efficacy rating and fewer effects on lipid and carbohydrate metabolism when compared to their earlier counterparts. They also have fewer androgenic side effects, which are described later in this chapter.

Drospirenone (DSRP) is a new-generation progestin derived from spironolactone. Because spironolactone is a potassium-sparing diuretic hormone, it can increase serum potassium levels in women taking CHC pills with DSRP, altering water and electrolyte balance. A progestin that comes in an injectable form is medroxyprogesterone acetate (MPA).

Amount of estrogen and type of progestin determine bioactivity and possible side effects of CHC products. The combination of estrogen and progestin causes the products to have estrogen-like activity or *estrogenic activity,* progesterone-like activity or *progestational activity,* and androgen-like activity or *androgenic activity.* The combination of estrogen and the selected progestin also has an effect on the uterine endometrium. The lowest effective dose that successfully prevents conception should be used.

Mechanism of Action

The estrogen component of combined hormone contraceptive products inhibits ovulation by preventing the formation of a dominant follicle. When a dominant follicle does not mature, estrogen remains at a consistent level and is unable to reach the peak level needed to stimulate the luteinizing hormone (LH) surge. The progestin component also suppresses the LH surge. When the LH surge is suppressed, ovulation is prevented and pregnancy does not occur. Any cycle, whether induced by drugs or naturally occurring, in which ovulation does not occur is called an *anovulatory* cycle.

Therefore, CHCs produce drug-induced anovulatory cycles. The estrogen component of CHC products also stabilizes the uterine endometrium, inhibiting proliferation and secretory changes and decreasing occurrence of irregular and/or heavy bleeding. The progestational effects of progestin change the endometrium to make it less favorable for implantation of a fertilized ovum. In addition, progestins have an effect on the quantity and viscosity of the cervical mucus, making it thick and hostile to sperm penetration. Progestins alter the motility of both the muscles of the fallopian tube and the cilia within the tube, impeding the movement of the ovum through the tube.

Route of Delivery

There are several routes of administration for combined hormone contraception products. Most women are familiar with oral contraception, in which a pill is ingested daily, absorbed by the gastrointestinal tract, and metabolized by the liver. CHC products can also be administered through a transvaginal and transdermal route, under the trade names of NuvaRing and the Ortho-Evra transdermal contraceptive patch, respectively. The advantage of these alternative sites for administration is avoiding gastrointestinal absorption and the initial metabolism by the liver, or the "first-pass" effect. Theoretically, side effects such as nausea and vomiting, heart and circulatory risks, and noncompliance with a daily dosage regime may be avoided. Intramuscular and subcutaneous routes of administration for combined hormone contraception are not available in the United States.

Combined Oral Contraception Products

Combined oral contraception (COC) products are one of the most commonly used methods of reversible contraception in the world because of their ease of use, high degree of effectiveness, and relative safety. The theoretical effective rate (absolute correct use) for COC is 99.3%, while typical use effective rate (accounting for patient error) is around 92%. This means that the COC is 92% to 99.3% effective for contraception. When the pill was approved for use by the U.S. Food and Drug Administration (FDA) in 1960, little was known about the best combination of estrogen and progestin or their optimum effective doses. In the 1970s, research provided evidence that the adverse side effects, particularly heart and circulatory effects, were directly related to the dose of estrogen in the oral contraception product. The higher dose of estrogen increased risk for venous thromboembolism (VTE), myocardial infarction (MI), and stroke. Subsequently, "low-dose" oral contraception pills and, more recently, "very low-dose" contraception pills have been introduced. Low-dose COC pills greatly reduce the risk for dangerous side effects. A low-dose COC product contains ≤35 mcg of ethinyl estradiol or ≤50 mcg or less of mestranol and a progestin. Very low-dose CHC pills contain ≤20 mcg of EE and a progestin. Research continues to focus on actual and potential short- and long-term benefits and risks associated with use of low-dose oral contraceptives, particularly in the areas of heart and circulatory risks as well as carcinogenesis. Clinical studies also continue to investigate the venous circulatory effects of new-generation progestins.

COC formulations are differentiated based on the strength of the estrogen component, type of progestin used, and whether estrogen or progesterone (and androgen) activity predominate. Increased estrogenic activity may include side effects such as cyclic breast changes, **dysmenorrhea** (painful periods), **menorrhagia** (heavy periods), **chloasma** (hyperpigmentation of the skin), and VTE, while decreased estrogenic activity may cause **amenorrhea** (absence of periods) or spotting at certain points in the cycle. Increased progestational activity may cause weight gain, depression, fatigue, and decreased libido, while lack of progestational activity may cause **breakthrough bleeding** (BTB) and headaches. BTB is an episode of bleeding that occurs during the active pill cycle of COC products. It is more common at the start of COC use, when a woman changes her COC type of pill, and with progestin-only preparations of contraception. There is no evidence that an episode of BTB is associated with a decrease in the COC's effectiveness as long as the patient continues to take the pill on daily basis and as prescribed. Increased androgenic activity may cause acne, hirsutism, edema, and cholestatic jaundice. The estrogens and progestins in oral contraception pills also have an effect on the uterine endometrium, which may cause changes in the patient's periods, such as irregular bleeding, heavy or light periods, or spotting between periods. The undesirable side effects of hormonal contraception products are discussed later in this chapter.

Most women on COC products experience shorter, lighter periods. Other advantages with COC are decreased blood loss and uterine cramps, elimination of **mittelschmerz** (mid-cycle pain usually associated with ovulation), reduction of symptoms in many forms of benign breast disorders, and prevention of physiologic ovarian cysts. COC products also reduce the incidence of pelvic inflammatory disease (PID) and ectopic pregnancy, reduce endometrial and ovarian cancer risk, and reduce deaths from colorectal cancer. COC products do not reduce the incidence of sexually transmitted infections (STIs).

The goal of therapy is to identify the product that offers the best contraceptive protection while producing the fewest unwanted side effects as a result of either the estrogen or the progestin component. Note: the effectiveness of oral contraceptives can also be compromised by concurrent use of some medications (e.g., antibiotics) or herbal products (Herbal Alert 56-1).

Types of Combined Oral Contraception Products

There are three types of combined oral contraception pill products: monophasic, biphasic, and triphasic. These types of COC pills have also been categorized as "phasic" and "nonphasic" pills. The monophasics, or nonphasic pills, provide a fixed ratio of estrogen to progestin throughout the menstrual cycle. In biphasics, a phasic pill, the amount of estrogen is fixed throughout the cycle, but the amount of progestin varies; reduced in the first half to provide for some

HERBAL ALERT 56-1

St. John's Wort

- St. John's wort may decrease the level of contraceptive hormones in the bloodstream, reducing the effectiveness of CHC products. This may result in breakthrough bleeding and/or a spontaneous ovulation.
- Chasteberry extract is taken by women as an herbal supplement for premenstrual syndrome and menopausal symptoms. Chasteberry extract may alter contraceptive hormone levels in the body making them less effective. Chasteberry extract should be used with caution with CHC or hormone therapy.
- Other herbal remedies that may alter the effectiveness of contraceptive hormones include dong quai, black cohosh, and red clover.

proliferation of the endometrium and increased in the second half to promote secretory development of the endometrium. This simulates the normal physiologic process of menstruation while still inhibiting ovulation. Ortho-Novum 10/11 is an example of a biphasic pill (10 days of norethindrone 0.5 mg and EE 35 mcg followed by 11 days of norethindrone 1.0 mg and EE 35 mcg). The triphasics are the newest form of phasic COC products delivering low doses of both hormones with minimal side effects, including breakthrough bleeding. With triphasics, the amount of either estrogen or progesterone varies throughout the cycle in different ratios during three phases. Ortho Tri-Cyclen is an example of a triphasic pill that varies the dosage of progestin (7 days of norgestimate 0.180 mg and EE 35 mcg; 7 days norgestimate 0.215 mg and EE 35 mcg; 7 days of norgestimate 0.250 and EE 35 mcg). In Ortho Tri-CyclenLo, the progestin change is the same through the three phases as in Ortho Tri-Cyclen, but the dose of EE is lowered to 25 mcg, making this a low-dose pill option for women. Estrostep is an example of a triphasic pill that varies the dosage of estrogen (7 days of EE 20 mcg and norethindrone acetate 1.0 mg; 7 days of EE 30 mcg and norethindrone acetate 1.0 mg; and 7 days of EE 35 mcg and norethindrone acetate 1.0 mg). Ortho Tri-Cyclen, Ortho Tri-CyclenLo, and Estrostep have low androgenic activity and are FDA approved for the treatment of acne. Table 56-1 shows brand-name forms of COC, amounts of EE and type of progestin, and generic equivalents.

A new-generation progestin, Yasmin is a monophasic combination pill with 30 mcg of ethinyl estradiol and 3 mg of drospirenone (DSRP). While the progestin found in other combination oral contraceptives is structurally similar to androgens, drospirenone is the only progestin derived from spironolactone, which is structurally similar to progesterone. As noted, use of drospirenone may increase serum potassium, which can alter water and electrolyte balances in women using this product. Consequently, Yasmin is contraindicated in women with kidney, liver, or adrenal insufficiency and in women who require daily long-term treatment with any of the following medications: NSAIDs (e.g., ibuprofen) taken long-term and daily for arthritis or other diseases or conditions, potassium-sparing diuretics (e.g., spironolactone), potassium supplementation, ACE inhibitors (e.g., Accupril, Lotensin), angiotensin-II receptor antagonists (e.g., Cozaar, Diovan), and heparin.

Femcon Fe (norethindrone 0.4 mg and EE 35 mcg) and Generess Fe (norethindrone 0.8 mg and EE 25 mcg) are mint-flavored, chewable birth control pills for women who have difficulty swallowing pills. They can also be swallowed whole.

Withdrawal Bleeding

Most of the monophasic, biphasic, and triphasic combined oral contraception products are packaged in both 21-day tablet packs and 28-day tablet packs. In the 21-day tablet packs there are 21 days of active pills (pills that contain estrogen and progestin) followed by a 7-day "pill-free" period. A new pack of pills is started after the 7 day pill-free period. In the 28-day tablet pack, there are 21 days of active pills followed by 7 days of inert pills, called counters. The patient takes one pill daily and begins a new pack the day after the last counter pill is taken. During the hormone-free period (counters) or the 7-day pill-free period, the level of estrogen and progestin decreases allowing for a breakdown of the endometrial lining. This causes a pseudomenstruation known as **withdrawal bleeding** or withdrawal menses. The withdrawal bleeding is not a true menstrual period and the bleeding experienced by a woman can vary in amount and duration.

There are 28-day oral contraception pills that do provide medication during the 7-day hormone-free period. Estrostep Fe, Loestrin Fe 1.5/30, Loestrin Fe 1/20, Loestrin 24 Fe, and Generess Fe contain ferrous fumarate, an iron compound, to provide iron supplementation during the phase of withdrawal bleeding. This promotes healthy iron stores in women and protection against menstrual-associated iron-deficiency anemia. Another formulation is Mircette (desogestrel 0.15 mg and EE 20 mcg), which supplies 2 inert pills and 5 pills with 10 mcg of ethinyl estradiol during the counter phase. The use of low-dose estrogen during the "inert" phase of the pill cycle provides a greater degree of ovarian suppression. Another benefit may be the decrease in headaches associated with estrogen withdrawal. Patients who experience headaches associated with the menstrual cycle may benefit from Mircette.

Withdrawal bleeding periods are scheduled monthly to mimic a normal 28-day menstrual cycle; however, researchers have established that a monthly episode of withdrawal bleeding is not necessary to maintain a healthy uterus. There are now FDA-approved formulations of estrogen-progestin combination pills that do one of the following: (1) shorten the period of withdrawal bleeding by extending the number of active pills and decreasing the number of inert pills in the 28-day pill cycle, (2) decrease the number of withdrawal menses per year by having 81 to 84 continuous days of active pills and 7 days of less active pills, resulting in four withdrawal menses per year, or (3) eliminate withdrawal bleeding altogether by continuous oral administration of active pills.

TABLE 56-1 ORAL CONTRACEPTION COMBINATION PRODUCTS: LISTED BY TYPE OF PROGESTIN

PRODUCT TYPE	ESTROGEN (mcg)	PROGESTIN (mg)
Combination Monophasic Products Containing Norethindrone and EE		
Balziva	35 EE	0.4
Brevicon	35 EE	0.5
Femcon Fe	35 EE	0.4
Generess Fe	25 EE	0.8
Junel 21 1/20	20 EE	1.0
Junel Fe 1/20	20 EE	1.0
Junel 21 1.5/30	30 EE	1.5
Junel Fe 1.5/30	30 EE	1.5
Loestrin 1/20	20 EE	1.0
Loestrin Fe 1/20	20 EE	1.0
Loestrin 24 Fe	20 EE	1.0
Loestrin 1.5/30	30 EE	1.5
Loestrin Fe 1.5/30	30 EE	1.5
Microgestin 1/20	20 EE	1.0
Microgestin Fe 1/20	20 EE	1.0
Microgestin 1.5/30	30 EE	1.5
Microgestin Fe 1.5/30	30 EE	1.5
Necon 0.5/35	35 EE	0.5
Necon 1/35	35 EE	1.0
Norinyl 1+35	35 EE	1.0
Ortho-Novum 1/35	35 EE	1.0
Ovcon 35 Fe	35 EE	0.4
Ovcon 50	50 EE	1.0
Combination Monophasic Products Containing LNG and EE		
Altavera	30 EE	0.15
Alesse	20 EE	0.1
Aviane	20 EE	0.1
Lessina	20 EE	0.1
Levlen	30 EE	0.15
Levlite	20 EE	0.1
Levora	30 EE	0.15
Lutera	20 EE	0.1
Nordette	30 EE	0.15
Portia	30 EE	0.15
Quasense	30 EE	0.15
Combination Monophasic Products Containing Norgestrel and EE		
Lo/Ovral	30 EE	0.3
Cryselle	30 EE	0.3
Lo-Ogestrel	30 EE	0.3
Ogestrel 0.5/50	50 EE	0.5
Combination Monophasic Products Containing Ethynodiol Diacetate and EE		
Kelnor 1/35	35 EE	1.0
Zovia 1/35	35 EE	1.0
Zovia 1/50	50 EE	1.0
Combination Monophasic Products Containing Norethindrone and Mestranol		
Necon	50 mestranol	1.0
Norinyl 1+50	50 mestranol	1.0
Ortho-Novum 1/50	50 mestranol	1.0
Combination Monophasic Products Containing Desogestrel and EE		
Apri	30 EE	0.15
Desogen	30 EE	0.15
Ortho-Cept	30 EE	0.15
Reclipsen	30 EE	0.15
Combination Monophasic Products Containing Drospirenone and EE		
Loryna	20 EE	3.0
Ocella	30EE	3.0
Syeda	30 EE	3.0
Yasmin	30 EE	3.0
Yaz	20 EE	3.0
Combination Monophasic Products Containing Norgestimate and EE		
Mononessa	35 EE	0.25
Ortho-Cyclen	35 EE	0.25
Previfem	35 EE	0.25
Sprintec	35 EE	0.25
Combination Extended-Cycle Products Containing LNG and EE		
Camrese	30 EE	0.15
	10 EE	—
Camrese Lo	20 EE	0.1
	10 EE	—
Introvale	30 EE	0.15
Jolessa	30 EE	0.15
LoSeasonique	20/10	0.1
Lybrel	20 EE	0.09
Seasonale	30 EE	0.15
Seasonique	30 EE	0.15
	10 EE	—
Combination Monophasic with Folate in Form of EE/Drospirenone/levomefolate Calcium 451 mcg		
Beyaz	20 EE	3.0
Safyral	30 EE	3.0
Combination Biphasic Products Containing Norethindrone and EE		
Necon 10/11	35 EE	0.5
	35 EE	1.0
Ortho-Novum 10/11	35 EE	0.5
	35 EE	1.0

Continued

TABLE 56-1 ORAL CONTRACEPTION COMBINATION PRODUCTS: LISTED BY TYPE OF PROGESTIN—cont'd

PRODUCT TYPE	ESTROGEN (mcg)	PROGESTIN (mg)
Combination Biphasic Products Containing Desogestrel and EE		
Kariva	20 EE	0.15
	10 EE	—
Mircette	20 EE	0.15
	10 EE	—
Combination Triphasic Products Containing Desogestrel and EE		
Cyclessa	25 EE	0.1
	25 EE	0.125
	25 EE	0.15
Velivet	25 EE	0.1
	25 EE	0.125
	25 EE	0.15
Combination Triphasic Products Containing Norethindrone and EE		
Aranelle	35 EE	0.5
	35 EE	1.0
	35 EE	0.5
Leena	35 EE	0.5
	35 EE	1.0
	35 EE	0.5
Necon 7/7/7	35 EE	0.5
	35 EE	0.75
	35 EE	1.0
Nortrel 7/7/7	35 EE	0.5
	35 EE	0.75
	35 EE	1.0
Ortho-Novum 7/7/7	35 EE	0.5
	35 EE	0.75
	35 EE	1.0
Tri-Norinyl	35 EE	0.5
	35 EE	1.0
	35 EE	0.5
Estrostep Fe	20 EE	1.0
	30 EE	1.0
	35 EE	1.0
Tilia Fe	20 EE	1.0
	30 EE	1.0
	35 EE	1.0
Tri-Legest Fe	20 EE	1.0
	30 EE	1.0
	35 EE	1.0
Combination Triphasic Products Containing Norgestimate and EE		
Ortho Tri-Cyclen	35 EE	0.18
	35 EE	0.215
	35 EE	0.25
Ortho Tri-Cyclen Lo	25 EE	0.18
	25 EE	0.215
	25 EE	0.25
Trinessa	35 EE	0.18
	35 EE	0.215
	35 EE	0.25
Tri-Previfem	35 EE	0.18
	35 EE	0.215
	35 EE	0.25
Tri-Sprintec	35 EE	0.18
	35 EE	0.215
	35 EE	0.25
Combination Triphasic Products Containing Levonorgestrel and EE		
Enpresse	30 EE	0.05
	40 EE	0.075
	30 EE	0.125
Tri-Levlen	30 EE	0.05
	40 EE	0.075
	30 EE	0.125
Trivora	30 EE	0.05
	40 EE	0.075
	30 EE	0.125

EE, Ethinyl estradiol; *LNG*, levonorgestrel; *mcg*, microgram; *mg*, milligram.
CHCs, Pregnancy category X; *progestin-only products*, pregnancy category X.

Extended-Cycle COC Products

Loestrin 24 Fe is a 24-day monophasic hormonal regimen of 20 mcg of ethinyl estradiol tablets and 1 mg of norethindrone acetate, plus 4 ferrous fumarate tablets. It provides 24 days of active hormonal therapy and 4 days of hormone-free pills containing an iron supplement. The active pill days are extended, while the number of inert pill days are reduced, which shortens the period of withdrawal bleeding that the patient will experience. The shorter period of hormone-free tablets increases the contraceptive's efficacy.

Like Yasmin, Yaz (drospirenone 3 mg and EE 20 mcg), another extended-cycle combined hormone pill, contains the progestin drospirenone (DRSP), a spironolactone analogue with antimineralocorticoid properties. The 24-day active hormone pill regimen of Yaz combined with the 30-hour half-life of drospirenone results in less hormonal fluctuation between cycles, compared with traditional oral contraceptives with 21 days of active pills and 7 days of placebos. Preclinical studies indicate that drospirenone also provides an antiandrogenic effect, which means that it counteracts the effects of male hormones in the body. Yaz is FDA approved for the treatment of premenstrual dysphoric disorder (PMDD) as well as acne. It has the same serum potassium precautions as Yasmin. As with Loestrin 24 Fe, women experience a shorter and lighter withdrawal bleeding period with increased ovarian suppression.

Beyaz, with 24 pills containing 3 mg DSRP, 20 mcg of EE, *and* 0.451 mg of levomefolate calcium (a folic acid supplement), and with 4 pills of 0.451 mg of levomefolate calcium in the inert phase, is also available in the United States. Produced by the same pharmaceutical company as Yasmin and Yaz, Beyaz contains DSRP and has the same precautions as Yasmin and Yaz; however, it also contains a form of folic acid throughout the pill cycle promoting healthy folic acid levels for reproductive-age patients. Therefore, Beyaz may help prevent open neural tube defects, should the patient plan to become pregnant. Beyaz is also approved for use in the treatment of PMDD. In April 2012, the FDA issued an updated warning that women taking combined oral contraception products containing drospirenone may have a twofold increased risk for venous blood clot formation compared with women taking CHC products that do not contain DSRP. Women considering a contraceptive product containing DSRP should be made aware of this risk.

Continuous Dosing COC Products

Seasonale (Jolessa) is a continuous dosing combined hormone contraception pill. The 91-day regimen includes 84 days of active pills and 7 days of inert pills. Seasonale (Jolessa) causes withdrawal bleeding to occur just four times per year. The active hormone pills in Seasonale (Jolessa) contain 30 mcg of ethinyl estradiol (EE) and 0.15 mg of levonorgestrel (LNG). Seasonale (Jolessa) is the drug predecessor of Seasonique.

Seasonique is a continuous dosing contraception pill that causes withdrawal bleeding four times per year. It cycles 84 days of tablets that contain 30 mcg of EE and 0.15 mg of LNG, followed by 7 days of tablets that contain 10 mcg EE. During the 7 days of low-dose estrogen pills, women usually experience withdrawal menses. However, by adding very low levels of estrogen in the 7-day "break" period, instead of inert pills, Seasonique provides additional benefits such as a reduction in breakthrough bleeding. LoSeasonique contains 20 mcg of EE and 0.1 mg of LNG, followed by 7 days of 10 mcg of EE, offering a very low-dose continuous CHC product option. Users of extended-cycle birth control pills are more likely to experience bleeding or spotting between periods. The continued progestin dose causes extreme atrophy of the endometrial lining. The atrophic endometrium subsequently breaks down, and the patient experiences uterine bleeding in an irregular pattern.

Lybrel is the first continuous dose combined oral contraception pill to be FDA approved. Lybrel comes in a 28-day pack and contains 20 mcg of EE and 90 mcg of LNG. Lybrel is taken daily and continuously without interruption for withdrawal menses.

Although these products are more commonly known for their contraceptive value, women with menstrual disorders such as menorrhagia (heavy periods), **metrorrhagia** (irregular bleeding between periods, usually heavy), endometriosis, dysmenorrhea, premenstrual syndrome (PMS), and physiologic ovarian cyst formation may benefit from continuous-cycle COC products because of their ability to suppress ovarian function and limit uterine bleeding.

Ortho-Evra Transdermal Patch

The Ortho-Evra patch is a weekly form of combined hormone contraception, consisting of 750 mcg of ethinyl estradiol and 6 mg of the progestin norelgestromin (NGMN) delivered through a transdermal system. It is a thin plastic patch placed on the skin of the buttocks, stomach, upper outer arm, or upper torso. The patch is placed once a week for 3 weeks in a row. The fourth week is patch-free to allow for withdrawal bleeding. It should be placed on clean, dry skin; placement on or near the breasts should be avoided because of the estrogen component. Site of patch placement should be rotated to avoid skin irritation. If the patch partially or completely detaches from the skin, a new patch should be placed. When used correctly, the patch protects against pregnancy on a monthly basis. The theoretical and typical use effective rate for the patch is 99.3% and 92%, respectively, making it 92% to 99.3% effective at preventing pregnancy.

The patch works in a similar manner to COC pills by inhibiting ovulation, thickening cervical mucus to prevent sperm penetration, and preventing a fertilized egg from implanting in the uterus. The patch avoids the first-pass through the liver effect. Advantages include not having to remember to take a pill daily. As with combined oral contraception products, the ability to become pregnant returns quickly when its use is discontinued. There is less menstrual flow and cramping, acne, iron-deficiency anemia, excess body hair, premenstrual symptoms, and vaginal dryness with the patch. As with COC pills, the patch reduces the risk for ovarian and endometrial cancers, PID, breast cysts, ovarian cysts, and **osteoporosis** (loss of bone mass predisposing the patient to fractures). With the patch, there are fewer occurrences of ectopic pregnancy.

Disadvantages of the patch include skin reaction at the site of application, menstrual cramps, and a change in vision or the inability to wear contact lenses; it is not as effective for women who weigh more than 198 lb. In 2005, the FDA approved an addition to the labeling of the Ortho Evra transdermal patch stating that it exposes patients to higher levels of estrogen. In theory, this indicated that women using the patch for contraception may be at an increased risk for venous thromboembolism (VTE). With CHC pills, peak serum estrogen levels are reached rapidly after ingestion and then steadily decline. With the patch, peak serum estrogen levels when reached are 25% less than in women taking the pill, however, these peak levels remain throughout the patch placement week, and then decline, exposing women to 60% more estrogen than with the CHC pill. Ongoing research is necessary to demonstrate exact risk for VTE as well as other cardiovascular complications (particularly heart attack and stroke) in women using the Ortho Evra transdermal patch. Women being prescribed the transdermal route of CHC should be notified of potential risks, and the patch should be used with extreme caution in any patient with increased risk for VTE. Women who are older than 35 years and smoke should not use the Ortho Evra transdermal patch. Other side effects include temporary irregular bleeding, weight gain or loss, breast tenderness, and nausea.

NuvaRing Transvaginal Contraception

NuvaRing is a 2-inch–diameter flexible indwelling ring inserted into the vagina. It is nonbiodegradable, transparent, and colorless to almost colorless. NuvaRing releases 15 mcg of EE and 120 mcg of the progestin *etonogestrel* per day, similar to the quantities of estrogen and progestin found in lower-dose COC products. Etonogestrel is a biologically active metabolite of desogestrel and a new-generation progestin, which may be associated with an increased risk for VTE. Also, NuvaRing has an extended placement schedule, which may mean that the estrogen peak rate, although lower than that of CHC pills, remains sustained longer because of the 3-week ring placement. As with the Ortho Evra transdermal patch, this may expose the patient to higher levels of estrogen. Studies have been inconclusive, and the FDA has placed no additional warning on NuvaRing.

Theoretical effectiveness and typical effectiveness rates are 98% and 92%, respectively, reflecting a rate similar to other leading CHC contraceptive methods. The patient inserts the ring during the first 5 days of the menstrual cycle. She then removes the ring after 3 weeks, remains "ring-free" for 1 week (for withdrawal menses), and then inserts a new ring. Backup contraception is recommended during the first 7 days after the first ring is placed. During this time, the hormones reach an appropriate protective level. After this, contraceptive effects are expected to be continuous provided the ring is correctly inserted. Correct insertion involves placing the ring into the middle or upper third of the vagina. Unlike the diaphragm, it does not need to be placed near or over the cervix. It is the close proximity of the ring to the vaginal mucosa that causes absorption of steroid hormones to occur. The ring remains in place during intercourse, tampon use, or the administration of intravaginal medications. If the ring slips out, it can be rinsed with lukewarm water and reinserted into the vagina. It should be reinserted within 3 hours after becoming dislodged. If the ring remains out for more than 3 hours, additional contraception is required until the ring has been in place for 7 days. Possible side effects include vaginal discharge, irritation, or infection. Other associated risks are the same as for low-dose COC products and are increased in patients who smoke.

PROGESTIN-ONLY CONTRACEPTION PRODUCTS

Progestin-only contraception products do not contain estrogen. The estrogen component of contraceptives increases the risk of circulatory disorders; therefore, these products allow contraception to be available for women who cannot take estrogen-progestin combination products. Advantages of progestin-only contraception products include relative safety, ease of use, spontaneity of sexual intercourse, and reversibility. However, because the estrogen component is missing, these products have a higher incidence of irregular bleeding and spotting, as well as the possibility of depression, mood changes, decreased libido, fatigue, and weight gain. Progestin-only contraception products do not protect women against STIs. Women who cannot take estrogen but may be candidates for progestin-only contraception products include patients with personal or strong family history of VTE or heart disease, breastfeeding patients, smokers older than 35 years of age, and women with uncontrolled hypertension. Women who have an untoward response to estrogenic effects such as chloasma, migraine headaches, or changes in lipid profiles may also be candidates for progestin-only products. Progestin-only contraceptive methods are available in oral, intramuscular, subcutaneous, and implantable routes of delivery.

Progestin-Only Oral Contraception Pill

The progestin-only oral contraception pill (POP), called the *minipill,* has four mechanisms of action: (1) alteration in cervical mucus, making it thick and viscous, which blocks sperm penetration; (2) interference with the endometrial lining, which makes implantation difficult; (3) decreased peristalsis in the fallopian tubes, slowing the transport of ovum; and (4) in approximately 50% of cycles, interference with the LH surge inhibiting ovulation. POPs that contain 0.35 mg of norethindrone as the progestin include Micronor, Nor-QD, Aygestin and their generic equivalents, Errin, Jolivette, Nora-BE and Camila. Ovrette is a POP that contains 0.075 mg of norgestrel. The minipill is taken continuously, without a break for withdrawal bleeding. Patients should be instructed to take the minipill daily, within a 3-hour window.

The theoretical effective and typical use effective rates for the first year of use are similar to that of COC products even though patient adherence to dosage schedule with POPs is more specific. It takes 4 to 6 hours for the progestin to thicken the cervical mucus to prevent sperm penetration, and the duration of the effect of the progestin on cervical mucus lasts just over 24 hours. Risk for pregnancy will increase if a patient misses a pill because POPs do not suppress the release of follicle-stimulating hormone (FSH) and LH to the same degree as COC products. If the minipill is taken more than 3 hours late, a backup contraceptive method should be used for 48 hours. There are no placebo pills in a pack of progestin-only pills. All 28 pills contain active hormones, so the patient continuously takes one active pill daily. Because the endometrial lining is altered, an increase in the amount of irregular bleeding is noted.

Depo-Provera

Depo-Provera is a highly effective, long-acting injectable progestin in the form of depot-medroxyprogesterone acetate (DMPA or MPA), with a theoretical and typical use efficacy rate of 99% and 97%, respectively. This makes Depo-Provera, the brand name for DMPA, one of the most effective hormonal methods of contraception at 97% to 99%. It appeals to women because of its confidentiality of use and convenient dosing schedule. DMPA is popular for adolescents for these reasons. Depo-Provera is administered in a flexible dosing schedule, every 11 to 13 weeks. The mechanism of action of Depo-Provera relies on the progestational activities: thickening of the cervical mucus, thinning of the uterine endometrium, and decrease in fallopian tube motility. Because the progestin in Depo-Provera reaches a higher circulating level than with POPs, DMPA inhibits both FSH and LH secretion from the anterior pituitary gland. This results in both **anovulation** (lack of ovulation) and amenorrhea. Because FSH and LH secretion is inhibited, any formation of a dominant follicle is prohibited and the production of estrogen in the body is greatly decreased. The patient experiences a hypoestrogen state, which can affect bone mineral density (BMD).

The depot-medroxyprogesterone vial or prefilled syringe should be vigorously shaken just prior to administration to ensure a uniform medication suspension. Depo-Provera, 150 mg, is given by deep IM injection into the gluteal, ventrogluteal, or deltoid muscle. Depo-Provera is more effective if given in the ventrogluteus muscle, although research has not supported this. The site should not be massaged after injection. The injection site is documented so that sites can be rotated. The patient is given a personalized calendar for subsequent doses and should return for another injection within 13 weeks. If the patient is late for her injection (13 weeks and 1 day), pregnancy should be ruled out before she receives another injection.

As with oral contraceptives, there is no protection against STIs. There is concern that MPA may cause a loss of bone mineral density, and results of research studies are still controversial. Most recent evidence suggests that at least partial or full recovery occurs in BMD of the spine, with partial recovery occurring in BMD of the hip after the patient discontinues Depo-Provera use. Until ongoing research is conclusive, the FDA recommends that Depo-Provera be discontinued after 2 years of continuous use unless other methods of contraception are inadequate. Many professional provider organizations agree that the concerns of the 2-consecutive-year limit given by the FDA and the BMD effects of DMPA should not prevent the practitioner from considering the benefit-risk ratio for each individual patient. The American College of Obstetricians and Gynecologists (ACOG) states in a committee opinion that "the possible adverse effects of DMPA must be carefully balanced against the significant personal and public health impact of unintended pregnancy." The benefits, risks, and alternatives, as well as the prevention of bone mineral density loss while on Depo-Provera, must be discussed with the patient before administration of the product.

Women taking Depo-Provera should be instructed to increase calcium and vitamin D intake to the daily recommended allowance for their age, as well as to participate in regular weight-bearing exercises. Depo-Provera is safe to receive immediately postpartum. Women can breastfeed while using this contraceptive without affecting milk supply. The most common side effects include initially irregular uterine bleeding or spotting. Menstruation may cease about 1 year after starting Depo-Provera. In addition, Depo-Provera has been shown to cause progressive weight gain in some women. Other side effects include breast tenderness and an increase in depression. The drug is contraindicated in cases of undiagnosed vaginal bleeding and known or suspected pregnancy. Caution should be used in giving DMPA postpartum in women who are at risk for or have a history of postpartum depression.

Depo-subQ Provera 104 is available as an injectable suspension. It contains the same progestin in Depo-Provera, MPA, but it is administered in a subcutaneous injection. The dose is 104 mg/0.65 mL, and it is given to women every 11 to 13 weeks. Depo-subQ Provera 104 has the same mechanism of action, benefits, and risks as Depo-Provera, and women should be counseled about the potential loss of bone mineral density. Depo-Provera and Depo-subQ Provera 104 have a slower return to fertility than other hormonal methods of contraception.

Implantable Progestins

Nexplanon is a single-rod device containing 68 mg of the progestin etonogestrel; it is placed in the same location as Implanon. It is bioequivalent to Implanon, lasting for up to 3 years and removed in the same manner. Training is also provided for practitioners for the insertion and removal of Nexplanon. The difference is that Nexplanon contains barium, a radio-opaque substance that can help locate the device on two-dimensional x-ray, ultrasound, magnetic resonance imaging (MRI) and computed tomography (CT) scanning if necessary. Also, the device comes in a new, preloaded application system that will reduce insertion errors. Nexplanon may not be as effective in women who have a BMI greater than 30 (obese) or are on medications that induce liver enzymes. Patient education will be the same as that for Implanon.

Theoretical and typical effectiveness rates for implantable progestins are the same, at 99.6%.

Pharmacokinetics: Estrogen-Progestin Combination Products EE is rapidly absorbed orally. It undergoes significant first-pass metabolism and elimination via the liver. Mestranol is converted in the liver to EE, which is 97% to 98% bound to plasma proteins. The half-life varies from 6 to 20 hours. Excretion is via bile and urine in a conjugated form. Some enterohepatic recirculation occurs. The steroid hormones in NuvaRing are absorbed through the vaginal mucosa into veins that flow directly into the inferior vena cava. The steroid hormones pass through the circulatory system and directly to the uterus, causing a "first-uterine" pass. The etonogestrel in NuvaRing has a bioavailability of 100% when administered vaginally, compared with EE bioavailability of 55%. With the Ortho-Evra patch, absorption is through the skin into venous circulation, also bypassing the hepatic portal system. Avoiding the liver first-pass effect decreases adverse enterohepatic reactions. The norelgestromin in the patch binds to albumin. Levels of serum steroid hormones in the patch reach constant levels of contraceptive efficacy within 48 hours. It is suggested that the alternative routing may increase the incidence of venous thromboembolitic events because peak levels of serum EE, although lower than that of oral ingestion, remain in the body for a longer duration. Alternative routing may decrease the incidence of irregular bleeding and nausea (NuvaRing only). Also, the avoidance of first-pass through the liver has the potential to decrease adverse drug interactions. Serum hormone levels are rapidly reached and blood levels do not fluctuate as much as is seen with oral contraception products.

Pharmacokinetics: Progestin-Only Products Progestins are also well absorbed orally. Peak plasma levels occur from 0.5 to 4 hours after ingestion, depending on the particular compound. Norethynodrel and ethynodiol diacetate are converted to norethindrone. Levonorgestrel is bioavailable and does not undergo first-pass liver metabolism; norethindrone undergoes first-pass metabolism and is 65% available. The progestins are bound to plasma proteins and to sex-hormone–binding globulin. The half-life of norethindrone varies from 5 to 14 hours; the half-life of levonorgestrel is 11 to 45 hours. MPA is without androgenic and estrogenic activity. Depot-MPA is crystalline suspension. DMPA is not soluble in lipid or water. The crystalline deposits in body tissues and then is reabsorbed. Depo-Provera provides higher peak levels of progestin than POPs and Implanon. Once injected, the levels of MPA increase for 3 weeks, and then remain stable. MPA is not detected in the blood between 120 and 200 days after injection. Nexplanon is a sustained-release system that releases progestin at a level of 60 to 70 mcg/day during the first six weeks after insertion and 35 to 45 mcg/day during the first year. This decreases to 30 to 40 mcg/day after 2 years of implantation and 25 to 30 mcg/day by the end of the third year. Once the rod is inserted, effective contraceptive levels are reached within 8 hours.

Start Date and Dosing Schedule

There are three ways to implement the start of hormonal contraception products unless otherwise indicated by the pharmaceutical company manufacturing the product.

With the *first-day start method,* the contraception product is initiated on the first day of menstruation, or the first day a women experiences bleeding. The first day of bleeding is day 1 of the menstrual cycle. Days are then counted 2, 3, 4, 5, 6, and so on, until the first-day bleeding begins again, usually around day 28. Most methods of contraception can be safely started on day 1 through day 5 of the menstrual cycle, when it is less likely that the patient has an early undiagnosed pregnancy. No backup method of contraception is needed when the product is started on the first through fifth day of menstruation. (A backup method is a second method of contraception that is used until the primary method reaches its peak level of contraceptive effectiveness.) Usually this is a barrier method, such as a condom or diaphragm.

Many products require a *Sunday start* (patient starts the tablets or patch on the Sunday after the first day of menstruation). If menstruation actually starts on Sunday, the patient starts her tablet or patch on that day. The Sunday start aids a woman in remembering the first day of her contraception cycle. If a patient starts her method of contraception later than day 5 of her menstrual cycle, a backup form of contraception should be used for 7 days.

The *quick-start method* of initiating contraception starts the method on the day the patient receives the prescription regardless of where she might be in her menstrual cycle. This method increases patient compliance and resolves the risk for becoming pregnant while waiting for a menstrual period to begin to start the method. Pregnancy should be ruled out prior to the quick-start method, but there is a risk that the patient could have an early pregnancy undetectable by screening. A backup method of contraception must be used for 7 days if the quick-start method is employed after the first 5 days of the menstrual cycle. Both estrogen-progestin and progestin-only contraception methods are contraindicated in pregnancy (Category X). *Nonetheless, there is no evidence of fetal risks associated with these medications when inadvertently used in pregnancy.* If the patient does not get a withdrawal menses when planned, a pregnancy test is administered.

Special Considerations

Depo-Provera and NuvaRing should be started within the first 5 days of the menstrual cycle. (Sunday start and quick-start methods are off-label.) Seasonale (Jolessa) and Seasonique use a Sunday start only. Lybrel uses a first-day start. If the patient is on a 21-day combined oral contraception regimen, she restarts her next pack following the 7-day break whether or not her bleeding has stopped. With 28-day packs, a pill is taken daily without stopping regardless of bleeding pattern. Usually, withdrawal menses occur in a cyclic fashion. In biphasic and triphasic preparations, the day 1 pill is clearly marked and the tablets are taken in the order noted. A difference in the color of the tablets delineates the change in dose of estrogen or progestin through the phases. With the POP, a pill is taken daily without a break. To increase effectiveness, all oral contraception pills should be taken at the same time daily. With the POP, women should strictly adhere to this instruction.

Missed Doses

Table 56-2 presents guidelines for missed doses of oral contraceptives. All patients who are prescribed oral methods of contraception should also be instructed in the use of emergency contraception.

Contraindications

Not every patient is a candidate for use of CHCs. Box 56-1 lists contraindications to CHC use.

TABLE 56-2 GUIDELINES FOR MISSED DOSES OF ORAL CONTRACEPTIVES

MISSED DOSE	RECOMMENDATIONS
Combination Products	
One tablet	Take tablet as soon as realized. Take next tablet as scheduled.
Two tablets	Take 2 tablets as soon as realized and 2 tablets the next day Use backup method of contraception for rest of cycle.
Three tablets	Discontinue present pack, and allow for withdrawal bleeding. Start new package of tablets 7 days after last tablet taken. Use another form of contraception until tablets have been taken for 7 consecutive days.
Progestin-Only Products	
One or more tablets	Take tablet as soon as realized, and follow with next tablet at regular time, PLUS use backup method of contraception for 48 h

h, Hour.

BOX 56-1 CONTRAINDICATIONS FOR CHC PRODUCTS

Absolute Contraindications

Pregnancy (known or suspected)
Venous thrombosis history or risk factors
Vascular disease, including coronary artery disease and CVA and past or current history of DVT or pulmonary embolism
Liver disease; including cirrhosis, viral hepatitis, and benign or malignant liver tumors
Undiagnosed vaginal bleeding or known or suspected endometrial cancer
Breast cancer
Tobacco use of >15 cigarettes per day in patient older than 35 years of age

Cautious Use

Hypertension with associated vascular disease
Hypertension with blood pressure >160/100
Hyperlipidemia
Diabetes mellitus complicated by neuropathy, retinopathy, nephropathy, or vascular disease
Diabetes mellitus >20 year duration
Postpartum <3 weeks
Lactation <6 weeks
Older than 35 years of age and smokes <15 cigarettes/day
Hypercoagulation disorders
Prolonged immobility
Use of drugs that affect liver enzymes (e.g., anticonvulsants, rifampin)

CVA, Cerebrovascular accident; *>,* greater than; *<,* less than.

Drug Interactions

The effectiveness of some drugs is impaired by CHC products; other drugs impair the effectiveness of CHC and progestin-only products. Box 56-2 shows drugs that may have interactive effects with CHC products. Patients receiving low-dose formulations of oral contraceptives need to be particularly cautious about potential interactions. If a patient is on a medication that affects estrogen absorption or metabolism, an estrogen-progestin oral contraception product with a higher dose of EE or mestranol may be prescribed.

Potential Side Effects and Adverse Reactions

It is accepted by health care providers that the risks associated with CHC products and all other methods of hormonal contraception are much less than the risks associated with pregnancy. This is especially true if the patient does not exhibit the contraindications listed in Box 56-1. In most cases, the benefits of any contraceptive method usually outweigh the risks when using a benefit-risk ratio to determine patient eligibility.

Benefit-risk ratio is partially determined by the risk related to the particular contraceptive method as compared to the risk pregnancy poses for the patient. Also included in the benefit-risk ratio is consideration of age, smoking status, allergies and medications, health histories and physical assessments, as well as lifestyle patterns and changes of the patient. These considerations determine patient selection or nonselection for the method as well as continuing or discontinuing a method of contraception.

Most of the untoward side effects are related to differences in the estrogen-progestin ratio of the products and the patient's response to these differences. Side effects primarily caused by an excess of estrogen include nausea, vomiting, dizziness, fluid retention, edema, bloating, breast enlargement, breast tenderness, chloasma (slightly more in dark-skinned patients on higher-dose tablets who are exposed to sunlight), leg cramps, decreased tearing, corneal curvature

BOX 56-2 DRUGS THAT INTERACT WITH CHC PRODUCTS

Drugs That Decrease the Effectiveness of CHC

Use a higher-dose pill or an alternative form of contraception (if the medication is continuous.) Use a backup method for the duration of treatment plus 7 days (if medication is short-term).

Anticonvulsant Medications

carbamazepine (Tegretol)
Hydantoins: ethotoin, mephenyltoin, phenyltoin
succinimide

Antituberculin Medications

rifampin (Rifadin)

Antifungal Medications

griseofulvin (Gris-PEG)

Antibiotics

amoxicillin
ampicillin (Amoxil)
doxycycline (Vibramycin)
metronidazole (Flagyl)
minocycline (Minocin)
neomycin (Neo-Fradin)
nitrofurantoin (Macrobid)
penicillin
tetracycline (Sumycin)

Barbiturates

phenobarbital (Luminal)
primidone (Mysoline)

Hypnotics and Sedatives

Benzodiazepines

Migraine Drugs

topiramate (Topamax)

Drugs That May Increase CHC Activity

acetaminophen (Tylenol)
ascorbic acid (vitamin C)
fluconazole (Diflucan)

Other Drug Interactions

An alternative method of contraception is necessary.
Anticoagulants: CHC products increase clotting factors and decrease the effectiveness of anticoagulants.
Anticonvulsants: CHC products may increase risk for seizure.

alteration, visual changes, vascular headache, and hypertension (in about 1% to 5% of previously normotensive patients within the first few months).

Side effects primarily caused by estrogen deficiency include vaginal bleeding (breakthrough bleeding, especially in the first few cycles after starting therapy) that lasts several days (usually during days 1 to 14); **oligomenorrhea** (very scant periods), especially after long-term use; nervousness; and **dyspareunia** (painful sexual intercourse) secondary to atrophic vaginitis.

Side effects primarily caused by an excess of progestin include increased appetite, weight gain, oily skin and scalp, acne, depression, vulvovaginal candidiasis (vaginitis from the yeast microbe candida, excess hair growth, decreased breast size, and amenorrhea after cessation of use (1% to 2% of patients).

Side effects primarily caused by progestin deficiency include dysmenorrhea, bleeding late in the cycle (days 15 to 21), heavy menstrual flow with clots, or amenorrhea. There may also be changes in laboratory values, including thyroid and liver function, blood glucose, and triglycerides.

The CHC pill may increase the vascularity of the cervical epithelium, extend the area of cervical ectopy, and alter certain immune parameters. Advise pill users to use male or female latex or polyurethane condoms unless they are confident that both partners are free of HIV and other STIs.

Adverse reactions of a more severe nature include cardiovascular and carcinogenetic risks.

Cardiovascular. There is an increased risk for hypertension (usually seen within 3 months after initiating the CHC method in women with preexisting risk) and arterial blood clot complications such as myocardial infarction, pulmonary embolus, and cerebrovascular accident in women using CHC methods as compared to women who are not on CHC methods of contraception. However, in terms of absolute risk for adolescents and women, the rate of dangerous complications from hormonal methods of contraception is extremely low because women younger than 50 years rarely experience heart attack or stroke. The risk for hypertension in women younger than 35 years is also low. Hormonal methods of contraception that contain drospirenone or etonogestrel may double a woman's risk for blood clots in the veins in the form of venous thromboembolitic events. Cardiovascular risks are increased in women older than 35 years who smoke, women older than 45 years, and women with hypertension that is undiagnosed or uncontrolled by medication.

Carcinogenesis. Long-term use of CHC products may increase the risk for breast cancer in younger women, but the risk is minimal. Breast cancer risk returns to normal 10 years or more after discontinuing CHC products. There is an increased risk for benign liver tumors. Risk for cervical cancer is slightly increased, thought to be because CHC methods change cervical epithelium, making it more susceptible to the high-risk human papillomavirus (HPV) pathogen and because condoms may be used less frequently in prevention of STIs. Women who use hormonal methods of contraception have a greatly reduced risk for ovarian and endometrial cancer, and the protective effect is directly related the duration of time the method is used.

Nursing Process
Patient-Centered Collaborative Care
Hormonal Methods of Contraception

Assessment

- Obtain a record of the patient's drug, supplement, and complementary and alternative medicine (CAM) use.
- Obtain baseline vital signs including temperature, pulse, respirations (TPR), BP, weight, and height. Calculate body mass index (BMI). Report abnormal findings.
- Obtain a complete menstrual history including age at menarche, menstrual pattern, cycle length, duration, and amount of bleeding and the first day of the last menstrual period (LMP). A detailed history of the menstrual cycle in reproductive-age and climacteric women should be considered as another vital sign.
- Determine pregnancy status.
- Obtain a family medical history specific to contraindications for CHC and progestin-only product use.
- Obtain family history of premenopausal breast cancer.
- Assess for domestic violence, intimate partner violence, and past or recent sexual abuse/assault.
- Obtain a medical history, assessing for history of allergies to medications, smoking, hypertension, and contraindications to CHC products listed in Box 56-1.
- Obtain a complete obstetrical and gynecologic history including gravida, parity, pregnancy termination and pregnancy loss, age of first and last pregnancy, time frame between pregnancies, complications during pregnancy birth and postpartum, genetic anomalies and health of children, time frame since last Papanicolaou (Pap test), history of abnormal Pap testing, history of gynecologic and/or sexual infections, gynecologic problems and/or surgeries, and gynecologic anomalies.
- Obtain a complete sexual history including sexual expression practices, sexual risk practices, history of STIs and treatment, and past or present sexual abuse and/or assault.
- Recognize need for periodic reassessment of baseline data and side effects. Most patients should be seen in 1 to 3 months after beginning contraceptive regimen.

Nursing Diagnoses

- Deficient knowledge regarding reproduction, reproductive health, and self-care
- Decisional conflicts related to contraception methods
- Decisional conflicts with partner and contraceptive method choice and/or family planning
- Deficient knowledge regarding contraceptive method(s) and appropriate use of method

- Fear related to contraceptive method side effects
- Risk for infections related to unprotected intercourse
- Ineffective expression of sexuality related to fear of pregnancy (and/or method failure)
- Decisional conflicts related to discrepancy between cultural and/or religious beliefs and contraceptive method choice

Planning

- Patients with contraindications to hormonal contraception will be risked out through patient selection and determination of benefit-risk ratio.
- Patient will understand the difference between estrogen-progestin combination products and progestin-only contraception products and their various routes of administration.
- Patient will verbalize understanding the bleeding patterns associated with both types of products by reporting menstrual changes that occur.
- Patient will choose a contraceptive method suitable for her lifestyle and health status.
- Patient will understand the benefits, risks, and alternatives to the method chosen through the BRAIDED method (see below).
- Starting method, dosing schedule, and use of contraceptive method chosen will be explained at patient's level of understanding.
- Explain ACHES and provide contact information (see Side Effects section further on in this section).
- Patient will take oral contraceptives as prescribed and report side effects that occur.
- Patient will place Ortho-Evra patch as prescribed and will report adverse side effects that occur.
- Patient will demonstrate and report comfort with vaginal placement of NuvaRing and report adverse side effects that occur.
- Patient will be aware of specific scheduling needed for progestin-only pills.
- Patient will understand initiation and calendaring of Depo-Provera injection, scheduling, need for weight-bearing exercises, and calcium supplementation.
- Patient will be given time to ask questions related to reproductive health, method choice, benefits, risks and alternatives, and method use.
- Follow-up appointment will be scheduled as needed.

Nursing Interventions

- Separate personal views from those of the patient regarding contraception and use of specific products.
- Address patient's misconceptions, and provide factual, evidence-based information.
- Encourage informed consent for contraceptive method through BRAIDED method: discuss *Benefits* (advantages, positive aspects, and both theoretic and actual effective rates of method), *Risks* (dangers, complications, disadvantages, and failure rates), *Alternatives* (other contraception options available to patient), *Inquiries* (opportunity for patient to ask questions about options proposed), *Decision* (deciding on a method with opportunity to change decision as needed), *Explanation* (health care teaching specific to method chosen), and *Documentation.*
- Use health teaching to encourage effective use of contraceptive method chosen.
- Ensure that patient understands start date, continuation of medication, and appropriate follow-up.
- Recognize that a percentage of patients on hormonal contraceptives will abandon method within 1 year; plan to provide the patient with alternatives and to seek care with a qualified health care provider prior to discontinuing any method of contraception.
- Non-nursing mothers can begin combination hormone contraception 4 to 6 weeks postpartum, regardless of whether or not menstruation has spontaneously occurred. Some sources indicate that a CHC method can be initiated as early as 3 weeks postpartum.
- Non-nursing and nursing mothers can begin Depo-Provera immediately postpartum if there is no increased risk for postpartum depression. POPs can be started at 4 to 6 weeks postpartum.
- Recognize that combined hormonal methods of contraception may decrease breast milk in patients who are currently breastfeeding. (CHC products can be used by breastfeeding mothers; however, CHC methods should be initiated after breastfeeding is well established. This is usually 2 to 3 months after the birth, with some sources stating that 6 weeks is sufficient.)

Patient Teaching

General

- Remind patient that these drugs should be used only under direction of a qualified health care provider.
- Advise patient that concurrent use of some drugs and herbal products decreases effectiveness of hormonal contraceptives. Patient should use a second form of contraception during use of these medications and herbal supplementations and possibly as long as 7 days after discontinuing counteracting medication.
- Patient will understand that hormonal methods of contraception do not prevent transmission of STIs or the pathogen that causes HIV infection and AIDS. If patient is at risk for STI or HIV infections, condoms should be used concurrently with CHC method, and safe-sex practices should be discussed. Inform patient of proper condom use.

Safety

- Counsel patient not to smoke tobacco because of increased cardiovascular risks.
- Advise patient to use barrier method of contraception as needed during first 7 days of contraception use if method is started 5 days or more after first day of

menstrual period. Instruct how to use barrier method properly.

- Teach patient about how to manage missed pills (see Table 56-2). Provide instruction for missed POPs, patch, ring, and injection methods. Review instructions for emergency contraception.
- Advise patient to report any effects from hormonal contraception to provider so therapy can be adjusted to suit her needs. Encourage her not to discontinue use of the method until an adequate trial time frame has been completed, which should be at least 3 to 6 months.
- Counsel patient that health care professionals should be advised of CHC use before surgery in which immobilization for an extended period may be needed.
- Encourage patient to report any irregular bleeding or BTB. A change in dose or type of hormonal contraceptive method may be advised.
- Advise patient to always report that she takes hormonal contraceptives when seeing a health care provider because of possible synergistic or antagonistic responses to other medications and therapies.
- Advise nursing mothers that the use of CHC products may decrease quantity and quality of breast milk.

Side Effects

- Advise patient that rare but serious side effects can occur, including VTE, myocardial infarction, cerebrovascular accident, and retinal vein thrombosis
- Teach patient the acronym ACHES for reporting symptoms of dangerous cardiovascular side effects to health care provider: *A*bdominal pain (severe); *C*hest pain or shortness of breath; *H*eadaches (severe), dizziness, weakness, numbness, speech difficulties; *E*ye disorders including blurring or loss of vision; *S*evere leg pain or swelling in calf or thigh.
- Encourage patient to notify health care provider immediately if she experiences any of these symptoms.
- Advise patient that her menstrual flow may be less in amount and duration because of thinning of endometrial lining with CHC and progestin-only products.
- Advise patient of menstrual changes that can occur at start of combined estrogen-progestin contraception products, when changing types of hormonal contraception products, and with progestin-only products.
- Determine whether or not patient wears contact lenses, and discuss how to handle dry eyes caused by decreased tearing and alterations in the shape of the cornea.
- Counsel patient who experiences post-CHC amenorrhea that 95% of women have regular periods within 12 to 18 months. Advise her that those who participate in endurance fitness activities may have increased post-CHC amenorrhea.
- Advise patient of a possible decrease in libido caused by an alteration in vaginal secretions and decreased levels of testosterone.
- Ensure that patient understands ability to return to fertility after discontinuing a hormonal contraception product and time frame in which pregnancy can be expected.
- Ensure a safe transition between contraceptive methods if a change in method is desired.

Skill

- Teach patient breast health awareness and self-examination.
- Teach patient how to inspect genitalia for abnormalities and note changes in vaginal secretions.
- Show patient the packet of contraception pills, and discuss how to recognize start dates and follow the sequential pill dosing. Demonstrate how to remove pill from pill packet if available.
- Teach patient how to place and remove Ortho-Evra patch.
- Teach patient how to place and remove NuvaRing.
- Teach patient how to use a calendar to record placement and removal of NuvaRing or Ortho-Evra patch.
- Advise patient to return for a Depo-Provera injection within the 13-week time frame.

Diet

- Counsel patient to moderate caffeine intake because elimination of caffeine may be decreased as a result of prescribed CHC products.
- Tell patient to take oral contraception products with a snack or after meals to help eliminate nausea.
- Advise patients using Depo-Provera to increase calcium and vitamin D intake and to do 15 to 30 minutes of weight bearing exercises 3 to 4 times per week.
- Discuss foods that increase iron and iron absorption.

Cultural Considerations

- Be aware of different cultures' contraception practices. For example, in some cultures, methods that involve touching the vagina may be difficult for a woman to use.
- Consider religious and spiritual beliefs with regard to contraceptive choices. Be accepting and supportive of beliefs or practices that are not consistent with personal beliefs.

Evaluation

- Encourage patient in planning follow-up evaluations.
- Evaluate patient's adherence with hormonal contraceptive regimen; assess for changes in sexual partners and/or health status that may compromise the method.

OTHER METHODS OF CONTRACEPTION

Spermicides

Spermicides are chemical agents that inactivate sperm before they can travel through the cervix and into the upper genital tract. The most common form of spermicide is nonoxynol-9.

Nonoxynol-9 is infused into a carrying agent such as jellies and creams, foams, suppositories, and films and is also impregnated into the Today Sponge. Some of the carrying agents contain a short-acting spermicide, while others adhere to the vaginal mucosa to provide extended spermicidal action. When combined with barrier methods such as the condom or diaphragm, spermicides increase protection against pregnancy. Nonoxynol-9–based spermicide products are no longer advised to prevent STIs. Spermicide can cause vulvovaginal abrasions and altered vaginal flora, which can increase susceptibility to pathogens.

The Today Sponge is a polyurethane disc containing nonoxynol-9. It is moistened with water, and the excess is squeezed out. It then should be placed snugly against the cervix. It can be inserted up to 24 hours before intercourse but must remain inserted for 6 hours after. This contraceptive product was discontinued in 1995 because of manufacturing problems, but it is again available over-the-counter in stores.

Barrier Methods

Both male and female condoms are available over-the-counter without a prescription. The female condom is a polyurethane (plastic) pouch with flexible rings at each end. It is inserted deep into the vagina like a diaphragm. The ring at the closed end holds the pouch in the vagina. The ring at the open end stays outside the vulva. Male condoms are available in latex, lambskin, and polyurethane. Latex condoms offer very good protection against STIs and HIV. Other barrier methods include the FemCap, cervical cap, and diaphragm, which require a medical visit for proper fitting. Barrier methods are more effective at preventing pregnancy when paired with a spermicide. Appropriate health care teaching for the use of these methods is essential to enhance pregnancy prevention. Patient with latex allergies need to avoid products containing latex.

Intrauterine Contraception

Intrauterine devices (IUDs) and intrauterine systems (IUSs) are safe methods of contraception with high patient satisfaction rates. Although intrauterine contraception methods are used more widely outside the United States, IUDs and IUSs have the highest effectiveness rates of reversible forms of contraception. Both the expected and typical efficacy rate is 99.9%. Patient selection for IUD and IUS use should consider menstrual factors, known or suspected uterine anomalies and fibroids, risk factors for STIs, and history of **pelvic inflammatory disease** (PID). PID is an infection of the upper genital tract, usually the uterine endometrium, the fallopian tubes, or ovaries. After insertion, the device's filamentous strings protrude through the cervix and into the vagina. The strings ensure that the device remains in place and aid in removal when needed. It was previously thought that the strings can act as a "wick," or a mechanism in which microbes can ascend into the endometrial cavity. However, studies show that risk of upper genital tract infections is related to insertion. Thus, PID incidence is minimal after 20 days of insertion.

If a woman contracts an STI while the device is inserted, in most cases the STI can be treated without removing the device. If the patient contracts PID during IUD/IUS insertion, health care providers will remove the IUD/IUS. Age and parity are not significant factors in patient selection for IUD or IUS use. IUDs and IUSs do not increase the risk for ectopic pregnancy. Currently two IUDs are on the market in the United States.

The ParaGard T 380A releases copper, which primarily interferes with the contractions within the uterus impeding sperm migration. A secondary effect is an inflammation of the endometrium, which also obstructs sperm motility and prevents implantation in the rare case that conception should occur. The ParaGard IUD can increase blood loss during menstruation by 35%, and may also increase uterine cramping and blood clots in menstrual flow. The use of NSAIDs helps to decrease both menorrhagia and dysmenorrhea caused by ParaGard. The ParaGard should be inserted up to day 7 of the menstrual cycle, and can remain in place for up to 10 years.

The Mirena levonorgestrel-releasing intrauterine system (LNG-IUS) causes cervical mucus to become thicker so sperm cannot enter the upper reproductive tract or reach the ovum. Changes in uterotubal fluid also impair sperm migration. Alterations in the endometrium prevent implantation in the rare case that conception occurs with the device in place. The LNG-IUS may also suppress ovulation. Unlike the ParaGard IUD, menorrhagia is improved by 90% with the LNG-IUS. This makes the LNG-IUS an effective treatment for heavy menstrual bleeding caused by hormonal dysfunction, uterine fibroids (as long as the fibroid is not located in the uterine cavity), or endometriosis. The LNG-IUS can also be used to decrease perimenopausal bleeding. Dysmenorrhea is also improved. There is a 20% chance of amenorrhea by 1 year of use, which increases to 60% within 5 years. The LNG-IUS is as effective as female sterilization, decreases a woman's risk of PID by 60%, and may also decrease the risk for ectopic pregnancy. The LNG-IUS should be inserted within 7 days of the start of menstruation. During this time the cervical canal is slightly open, making the insertion of the device easier for the provider. The LNG-IUS is effective for 5 years.

Both the ParaGard and the LNG-IUS can be inserted as early as 6 weeks postpartum. There are no contraindications with breastfeeding women and intrauterine contraception. Contraindications to the LNG-IUS are known or suspected pregnancy, uterine anomalies, and risk for acquiring an STI. The LNG-IUS may be effective at preventing endometrial cancer and invasive cervical cancer. The ParaGard should not be placed in women with a small intrauterine cavity (less than 6 cm) or a large intrauterine cavity (greater than 9 cm). Expulsion risk is 5%. There is a slightly higher expulsion rate in women younger than 20 years of age and when the device is inserted immediately postpartum. Perforation of the uterus is a rare complication of insertion.

Women who choose the IUD or IUS for contraception should be taught how to feel for strings of the device, which extend beyond the cervix. The string check is done monthly after the menstrual cycle and ensures that the device has remained in place. Removal of the device is done at the end of the prescribed time frame, when pregnancy is desired, or at the patient's request. The patient should also be advised that she can become pregnant immediately after removal of the device. The device is also removed in the rare event that a pregnancy has occurred with the device intact. The patient should be advised that removal of the device with an intrauterine pregnancy could possibly end in miscarriage. Both types of IUDs can be located on pelvic and transvaginal ultrasound should a question of proper placement or with the occurrence of full or partial expulsion of the device. The patient should be instructed to use a backup method of contraception until the device is found to be in correct placement. The device should be removed by the provider if it found to be incorrectly placed or partial expulsion has occurred. Reinsertion of a new device or an alternative method of contraception should be prescribed if the patient does not want to become pregnant. Fertility returns immediately after removing the device.

Emergency Contraception

Emergency contraception (EC) can prevent pregnancy after unprotected intercourse. It may be prescribed in three ways: (1) using combined hormonal contraceptive pills in a documented effective regimen; (2) using Plan B, which is a progestin-only EC; or (3) inserting a copper-releasing IUD (ParaGard). It is intended to be used one time in the event that a condom breaks, a diaphragm or a cervical cap is displaced, or doses of a hormonal contraception method are missed. EC is indicated in the event of sexual assault. The only documented contraindication to EC is an established pregnancy. Women should be instructed that EC is most effective when taken within 24 hours after unprotected intercourse.

> **SAFETY: Preventing Medication Errors**
>
> **Do not confuse ...**
>
> - **Mifepristone** (RU486) with **misoprostol** (Cytotec) or **methotrexate.** Mifepristone is used for early pregnancy termination by blocking progesterone. Lack of progesterone causes the uterine lining to shed and ends the pregnancy. Misoprostol causes the uterus to contract and is used for early pregnancy termination or for cervical ripening at any gestational age. It can also be used to control postpartum hemorrhage. Methotrexate is a folate antagonist used to manage ectopic pregnancy.

Combined Hormone Contraceptive Pills. Combined oral contraception pills prevent fertilization after an incidence of unprotected vaginal intercourse or failure of contraceptive method. The method includes using estrogen-progestin contraception pills in multiple dosing. This raises both estrogen and progestin levels to delay or prevent ovulation; interfere with tubal transport of the embryo, egg, or sperm; and change the hormones necessary for the preparation of the uterine lining. Using this method decreases the risk for pregnancy by 75% for each act of sexual intercourse. The major side effect is nausea. To prevent this side effect, an OTC antinausea medicine should be taken 1 hour before administration. Antihistamines are the most commonly used OTC medication used for nausea, and some are marketed specifically for this purpose. Antihistamines include diphenhydramine (Benadryl), dimenhydranate (Dramamine), and meclizine (Antivert). Irregular menstrual bleeding is another side effect. If a woman does not begin menstruation within a few days of the expected time, a pregnancy test should be performed. Patients who are unable to take estrogen should not take the usual EC pill dosage.

The original Yuzpe method involved taking two Ovral tablets (norgestrel 0.5 mg and EE 50 mcg) followed by two more tablets 12 hours later. This method was later expanded to include other types of oral contraception pills. Family planning agencies and women's health organizations provide a full list of CHC pills, as well as the dosage and administration regime for these products when used for EC. Treatment should be initiated within 72 hours of intercourse. The sooner a plan is initiated, the more effective it will be at preventing pregnancy.

The first progestin-only emergency contraceptive pill available in the United States is known as Plan B. In 2006, the FDA approved Plan B without a prescription for women age 18 years or older. In 2009, the FDA stated that both men and women can obtain Plan B One-Step without a prescription if they are older than 17 years. Those younger than 17 years need a prescription.

Plan B should be taken within 72 hours after intercourse, but it is still effective 120 hours afterward. If taken within 24 hours of intercourse, EC reduces the risk of pregnancy by 95%. Just 12 hours after the initial 24-hour postcoital period, the effectiveness rate of EC decreases to approximately 60%. With Plan B, two tablets containing 0.75 mg of LNG are dispensed in one package. One tablet is taken in the initial dose, followed by a second tablet 12 hours later. In an alternative dosing schedule, the two tablets can be taken in one PO dose. Plan B One-Step is a newer preparation of emergency contraception that supplies 1 pill containing 1.5 mg of LNG. Instead of taking two 0.75-mg LNG tablets, the patient takes one 1.5-mg LNG tablet. This single dose improves patient compliance and has an increased efficacy rate. Less nausea is associated with Plan B than with estrogen-containing emergency contraceptive methods. The generic form of the original Plan B is available as Next Choice.

Ella is an emergency contraception product that is FDA approved for up to 120 hours after unprotected intercourse. Patients of all ages need a prescription to obtain ella. Ella contains 30 mg of ulipristal acetate, which is a selective progesterone receptor modulator. This drug inhibits ovulation and is also embryotoxic by its progesterone agonist/antagonist activity. Pregnancy must be excluded before taking ella. Ella is pregnancy category X and is considered to be teratogenic and fetotoxic. It is reported that the manufacturers of ella want to maintain its use as an emergency contraceptive option and not promote off-label use as a product for medical abortion.

Hormonal methods of EC are not considered a method of contraception and should not be promoted as such. CHC products, barrier methods, and IUD/IUS devices are more reliable and effective at preventing pregnancy. Women should be instructed that their next menstrual period could be delayed after a dose of EC. If pregnancy is already established or if implantation occurred since the episode of sexual intercourse, the pregnancy is not disrupted and studies indicate that there are no untoward effects on the fetus.

With ella, if pregnancy has been established when the method is administered, the pregnancy can be disrupted and teratogenic fetal effects may occur. Side effects of ella include headaches, nausea, abdominal pain, dysmenorrhea, and dizziness. Breastfeeding mothers should not use ella.

ParaGard. A copper IUD may be inserted within 5 days of unprotected intercourse as a method of postcoital contraception. The device can be removed after the woman's next menstrual period, or it may remain in place as a method of contraception for up to 10 years. The mechanism of action is interruption of sperm migration and penetration of the ovum.

MEDICAL ABORTION

Medical abortion ends a pregnancy that is less than 63 days from the first day of the LMP, or less than 9 weeks' gestation. Medical abortion uses drugs to disrupt an established pregnancy. (Surgical abortion refers to procedures used to remove the products of conception from the uterus.) *Methotrexate* is a medication that stops the pregnancy in the uterus. It may also be used to treat an *early* ectopic pregnancy that is encapsulated and less than 3 cm in size. *Mifepristone*, first marketed as RU486, is an anti-progestin that blocks the hormone progesterone. Without progesterone, the lining of the uterus breaks down, ending support for the embryo. The hormone human chorionic gonadotropin (hCG) is decreased. hCG is produced by the placenta and is the hormone tested to confirm pregnancy; decreasing levels of hCG signify that the pregnancy has been disrupted. *Misoprostol* is then given to cause the uterus to contract and expel the products of conception.

MENOPAUSE

The transitional process experienced by women as they move from the reproductive years into the nonreproductive stage of life is called **menopause.** Menopause is a naturally occurring event and part of the normal life cycle of women. It occurs for most women between their mid-forties and mid-fifties but may start as early as the late thirties. The climacteric has three stages: perimenopause or premenopause, menopause, and postmenopause, during which certain physiologic events occur. As women go through menopause, providers do not treat the cessation of menses, but address the symptoms that may occur with the menopausal passage.

Perimenopause

The perimenopausal period includes the years before the natural cessation of spontaneous menstruation. During this period, menstrual variations become evident. Women may experience short cycles (less than every 25 days), long cycles (more than every 35 days), heavy bleeding, light bleeding, or periods of longer or shorter duration. Women may start to skip periods or abruptly stop menstruating altogether. Oligomenorrhea (very scant periods) or menorrhagia is common. Symptoms experienced during perimenopause are similar to those during menopause, with the exception that perimenopausal women continue to have some type of cyclic bleeding. The most common symptoms are hot flashes (caused by a surge in LH levels) and vaginal dryness (caused by estrogen withdrawal). Other symptoms include insomnia, headaches, irritability, anxiety or other variations in mood, cognitive difficulties, memory lapses, joint aches, and decreased libido. These unpredictable changes may last a short period of time or for several years.

There are a set number of follicles in the ovaries at birth. They are dormant throughout childhood and become active with puberty. Ovarian follicles are high in number during puberty and until age 35 years but the number of follicles steadily decline after age 35 years, and more rapidly after age 40 years. During the menstrual cycle, these follicles provide high levels of estrogen in the form of estradiol. The highest level of estradiol production in women occurs from puberty until the early thirties. Follicular growth, and therefore the secretion of estradiol, is under the influence of FSH and, to a lesser degree, LH, both of which are released by the anterior pituitary gland.

During the perimenopausal period, ovarian follicles become depleted, causing estrogen levels to diminish. The decrease in estrogen is gradual and allows for fluctuating levels of FSH and LH. Subsequently, menstrual cycles become anovulatory and therefore irregular. The onset of menstrual irregularity is one of the early indications of perimenopause. Symptoms are thought to be related to hormone fluctuations, particularly estrogen withdrawal, and increased levels of LH and FSH. Serum FSH testing is used as a marker of follicular activity, and an elevated level of FSH can be an indication of decreased ovarian function.

Menopause

Menopause is the permanent end of spontaneous menstruation caused by cessation of ovarian function. This natural event is documented as having occurred once a woman has stopped menstruating for 1 year. The triggering event is not known. Women who experience menopause before 40 years of age are said to have premature ovarian failure. Menopause can also occur abruptly as a secondary effect of oophorectomy (surgical removal of the ovaries), radiologic procedures in which ovarian function is destroyed, severe infection, ovarian tumors, or as a temporarily induced state for treatment of conditions such as endometriosis. During this transitional period, and with any episodes of menstrual changes/

irregularities caused by perimenopause, women should use contraception until menstruation has ceased for 1 year if they do not want to become pregnant.

Postmenopause

Postmenopause is the stage when the body adapts to a new hormonal environment. The production of estrogen and progesterone from the ovaries decreases during the late premenopausal and early postmenopausal periods. The ovary continues to secrete androgens (testosterone) in varying amounts as a result of the influence of increased LH levels. During postmenopause, androstenedione (the main androgen secreted by the ovaries and adrenal cortex, which is present in reduced amounts postmenopause) is converted into *estrone,* a naturally occurring estrogen formed in extraglandular tissue of the brain, liver, kidney, and adipose tissue. This represents the main source of available estrogen once the ovaries lose the ability to produce estradiol. Table 56-3 presents common physical effects associated with the climacteric.

SAFETY: Preventing Medication Errors

Do not confuse ...

- **Premarin** with **Prempro** or **Premphase.** Premarin is estrogen only for hormone replacement therapy. Both Prempro and Premphase have combined estrogen and progesterone for use by women with an intact uterus to prevent uterine hyperplasia when estrogen is used.

Hormone therapy (HT) significantly improves vasomotor symptoms and vaginal dryness (two frequently encountered symptoms of menopause) and decreases the risk for osteoporosis and osteoporotic fractures. Vasomotor symptoms have the potential to disrupt sleep quality and exacerbate irritability, mood swings, depression, and problems with concentration. Vaginal dryness and atrophic vaginitis, caused by decreases in systemic estrogen, causes dyspareunia, sexual dysfunction, and atrophic vaginitis. Decreased estrogen also has an effect on libido, sexual arousal, and the achievement of orgasm. It also has an untoward effect on urinary health. While no HT product presently has FDA approval for the treatment of osteoporosis, HT decreases the risk of osteopenia, osteoporosis, and fractures resulting from postmenopausal bone mineral density loss. There are systemic HT products that do have FDA approval for prevention of osteoporosis. HT reduces the risk for postmenopausal osteoporotic fractures in the hip, spine and all other possible fracture areas, even in women who do not have osteoporosis. HT can prevent further BMD loss and even improve BMD in women with osteopenia or osteoporosis.

The FDA has issued a boxed warning that states that HT should be used only for the treatment of menopausal symptoms, at the lowest dose possible, for the shortest duration possible, usually less than 5 years (Box 56-3). Most health care providers adhere to this practice when prescribing HT. Health teaching must be done with menopausal women to ensure that they are aware of the risks and benefits of hormone replacement therapy.

TABLE 56-3 COMMON PHYSICAL EFFECTS ASSOCIATED WITH THE CLIMACTERIC

HYPOESTROGENIC STATE	EFFECTS
Irregular menstruation	Variable frequency, duration, flow
LH surge: hot flashes	Hot flashes: transient sensations of intense heat with or without sweating; tachycardia; sleep disruption
Peripheral vascular dilation: hot flashes and night sweats	Hot flashes: visible flushing in upper chest, neck, and head; visible sweating and chills Night sweats: vasomotor symptoms that occur at night
Vulvar and vaginal atrophy	Dryness; decreased lubrication during sexual stimulation; thinning. Decreased acidity and increased irritation response to stressors such as intercourse can cause increased vaginitis (itching, burning, and discharge). Increased incidence of prolapse/cystocele
Decreased bone mass (osteoporosis)	Backache, reduced height, and sudden fracture, particularly in thin, fair, small-boned women and those with a family history, no pregnancies, sedentary lifestyle, inadequate diet, smoking, alcohol use, or use of drugs that increase calcium loss (anticonvulsants, corticosteroids). Most rapid decrease in mass (particularly in hips, spine, and torso) occurs in first 3 to 5 years postmenopause and slows after 65 years of age
Additional Effects Caused by Menopause Combined with Natural Aging	
Urethral disorders	Loss of urethral tone, painful urination, frequency, and stress incontinence
Decreased breast size	Decrease in fatty tissue in the breast and breast density, increase of fibroglandular tissue; breasts may sag and become more pendulous
Decreased skin elasticity	Facial, neck, and hand wrinkling; variations in quantity and distribution of body hair
Lower HDL levels	Increased risk (3 times) for cardiovascular disease as LDL levels increase
Abdominal fat development	Greater degree of central android abdominal fat accumulates because of altered peripheral resistance to insulin and increase in type II diabetes as aging progresses (lower incidence in estrogen users)
Hyperinsulinemia	Signs and symptoms of low blood sugar
Reduced cognitive function	Normal with aging. Loosely associated with estrogen withdrawal. May be related to sleep disorders and increased stress.

HDL, High-density lipoproteins; *LDL,* low-density lipoproteins; *y,* year.

BOX 56-3 FDA BOXED WARNINGS FOR CHC PRODUCTS AND HT PRODUCTS

CHC pill products: "Cigarette smoking increases the risk of serious cardiovascular side effects from oral contraceptive use. This risk increases with age and with heavy smoking (15 or more cigarettes per day) and is quite marked in women over 35 years of age. Women who use oral contraceptives should be strongly advised not to smoke."

Ortho Evra transdermal patch: "Do not use ORTHO EVRA if you smoke cigarettes and are over 35 years old. Smoking increases your risk of serious cardiovascular side effects (heart and blood vessel problems) from hormonal contraceptives, including death from heart attack, blood clots or stroke. The risk increases with age and the number of cigarettes you smoke."

NuvaRing: "Cigarette smoking increases the risk of serious cardiovascular side effects from combination oral contraceptive use. This risk increases with age and with heavy smoking (15 or more cigarettes per day) and is quite marked in women over 35 years of age. Women who use combination hormonal contraceptives, including NuvaRing, should be strongly advised not to smoke."

Hormone replacement therapies with estrogen and estrogen plus progesterone: "Warning: Cardiovascular disorders, breast cancer, endometrial cancer and probable dementia. ... Estrogens, with or without progestins, should be prescribed at the lowest effective doses and for the shortest duration consistent with treatment goals and risks for the individual woman."

PHARMACOLOGIC AND COMPLEMENTARY AND ALTERNATIVE THERAPY FOR PERIMENOPAUSAL AND MENOPAUSAL SYMPTOMS

Therapies that are presently being used for the treatment of perimenopausal and menopausal symptoms include complementary and alternative medicine (CAM), bioidentical hormone preparations, and HT.

Complementary and Alternative Medicine

Many women have turned to CAM for the relief of menopausal symptoms. While anecdotally women may find them helpful, randomized controlled trials show that most CAM relief measures and supplemental therapy are not more effective than placebos.

The most commonly used products for hot flashes are natural soy and soy derivatives. Natural soy contains phytoestrogens, called *isoflavones,* which have estrogenic effects. Soy has been made available in many over-the-counter nutritional supplements; however, natural soy products are considered more effective at treating hot flashes. Red clover extract is also used to treat hot flashes, although research studies using red clover extract are inconclusive. The herb *Actaea racemosa,* or black cohosh, is used in the over-the-counter preparations of Remifemin and Estroven. Limited studies show that black cohosh may decrease hot flashes. Caution with this herbal product should be used in patients with breast cancer and liver disease. Vitamin E in oral doses of 400 to 800 IU/day or evening primrose oil in oral doses of 1000 IU/day are used with success by some patients experiencing hot flashes; research does not support the effectiveness of either supplement. St. John's wort may be helpful for menopausal women experiencing mild depression or mood alterations. Ginseng may improve sleep, mood changes, and sense of well-being, while valerian is thought to help with insomnia. Melatonin may also be helpful as a sleep aid. Patients should be aware that these products can have side effects, may interfere with other medications, and are not regulated by the FDA. Women should be encouraged to report the use of herbal supplements, CAM, vitamins and minerals, and over-the-counter medications to their health care provider.

Bioidentical Hormone Therapy

Bioidentical hormone therapy includes estrogen-like compounds that have been derived from plants. These compounds are biochemically similar or identical to those produced by the ovaries. They are custom-made for the patient under the direction of the health care provider.

The most common plants to use for bioidentical hormone products are soy and wild Mexican yam root. Bioidentical hormones are more closely formulated after a woman's naturally occurring hormones, whereas natural hormones are those that originate in animal, mineral, or plant form. Women who ask for "natural" estrogen products may actually be requesting the bioidentical formulation. However, the plant components must undergo a chemical process to change them into the necessary estrogen-like structures that are components of the bioidentical hormone product. Although these compounds may be more estrogen-like than their synthesized counterparts, the term *natural* may be confusing.

The most common commercially available compounds are *estrone, estradiol, estriol, testosterone,* and *micronized progesterone.* The route of administration can be oral, sublingual, implantable, injectable, or in vaginal suppository form. Pellet therapy is a form of bioidentical hormones, usually estradiol and estriol, as well as progesterone and testosterone, implanted subcutaneously, in unnoticeable areas. The pellets are about the size of rice and are specifically compounded for each individual according to age, weight, risk factors, symptomology, and serum blood testing of hormonal and metabolic characteristics. Usually one pellet is placed and has a duration of 4 to 6 months. A new pellet is then inserted.

Theoretically, compared with HT, bioidentical hormones have limited side effects, a reduced risk of exacerbating the growth of breast cancer cells, equal osteoporosis prevention benefits, and a decrease in cardiovascular effects. However, clinical research providing evidence of the benefits and risks of bioidentical hormones is limited. Since the FDA has not approved the use of a combined estrogen-progestin bioidentical product in the United States, combination therapy must be compounded and dispensed by a compounding pharmacy. Also, many bioidentical hormones once compounded are not regulated by the FDA, so purity and quality is a concern. The bioidentical hormones have the same benefits and risks as HT.

Tri-est and *Bi-est* are two commonly prescribed bioidentical estrogen products. Bi-est contains 2 mg estriol and 0.5 mg estradiol in an 80/20 ratio, respectively. Tri-est contains 2 mg estriol, 0.25 mg estrone, and 0.25 mg estradiol in an 80/10/10 ratio, respectively. Many bioidentical estrogens or progestins are presently being used in HT products.

Hormone Therapy

Hormone therapy (HT) (Table 56-4) is used only for the relief of symptoms related to menopause, most commonly hot flashes, vaginal dryness, and associated sleep disorders. HT includes estrogen-progestin therapy (EPT) for use with women who have an intact uterus, and estrogen therapy (ET) for use with women who have had a **hysterectomy** (surgical removal of the uterus). Hysterectomy is performed for a variety of gynecologic problems including cancer, fibroids (benign uterine tumors), uterine prolapse, chronic pelvic pain, and heavy/abnormal uterine bleeding. The nurse should determine if the patient has had a hysterectomy in the past prior to administration of HT. It is the estrogen component in HT that relieves the symptoms of menopause. The progestin is added to protect the uterine endometrium from hyperplasia (an abnormal proliferation or overgrowth of tissue.) When the uterus is exposed to unopposed estrogen (estrogen without concurrent progestins), the endometrium becomes hyperplastic, potentiating the development of endometrial cancer. Estrogen alone can be used with women who have had a hysterectomy. With women who still have their uterus, estrogen, most commonly in the form of conjugated equine estrogens (CEE), is taken together with the synthetic progestin. The progestin, however, has the potential to cause unpredictable uterine bleeding.

> **SAFETY: Preventing Medication Errors**
>
> **Do not confuse ...**
>
> - **CHC products** with **HT products.** Oral, transdermal, and vaginal ring preparations for contraception and HT are dispensed in packages and boxes that are very similar. Once opened, CHC products and HT products may have the same disc-dispensing systems and splintered packaging, and similar-appearing skin patches and vaginal rings. Names can also be confused because of similarity, such as Femcon and Femtrace.

HT is available in oral preparations, transdermal applications, and vaginal preparations. Vaginal preparations are creams, suppositories, or rings. All vaginal preparations contain estrogen only and are very effective in treating vaginal dryness. Three types of estrogens are used in HT products: (1) natural or biological estrogens (including bioidentical estrogens), (2) CEE, and (3) synthetic estrogens.

Natural or biologic estrogens are derived from plants, minerals, or animals and are composed of *estrones* (esterified estrogens, CEEs, and piperazine estrone sulfate) and *estradiols* (micronized estradiol, estradiol valerate, and 17-β estradiol).

CEEs are mixtures of natural estrogens isolated from the urine of pregnant mares. Although CEEs are derived from nonhuman sources, they are naturally occurring estrogens. They are generally classified independently of natural or biological estrogens because they are the longest-used and most commonly prescribed form of estrogen in HT. Premarin, the most frequently used conjugated estrogen product, is presented in Prototype Drug Chart 56-1.

Synthetic estrogens include ethinyl estradiol and mestranol, which are both the same estrogens found in CHC products.

Dosage Forms

The oral route is most commonly used because it is well tolerated by most patients and relatively easy to administer. It requires daily dosing. Some patients experience GI upsets, particularly nausea and vomiting. A patient with GI disorders such as colitis, irritable bowel syndrome, peptic ulcer, or a malabsorption disorder may receive inconsistent doses with oral administration, necessitating the use of another route. Oral estrogens have a particularly beneficial effect on lipids by increasing high-density lipoproteins. Although the oral route does result in complete absorption from the GI tract, there is greater impact on liver proteins. In women with an intact uterus, oral estrogen is combined with a progesterone or progestin, completing the combined therapy. This can be given in a separate estrogen tablet combined with a separate progestin tablet (two oral pills taken daily) or in a combined estrogen-progestin tablet (one oral pill taken daily). Oral estrogens are typically used continuously. Common ET products include Premarin (CEE), Estrace (17 β-estradiol), Cenestin (synthetic conjugated estrogen), and Menest (esterified estrogen).

The transdermal skin patch is a convenient method to deliver ET because it does not require daily dosing. The patch is applied to intact skin in the prescribed dosage. Generally the lower abdomen is used, but other sites may be used. As with the Ortho-Evra transdermal patch used for contraception, the HT patch should not be placed on or near the breasts. The transdermal patch allows for absorption of the estrogen directly into the bloodstream through a membrane that limits the absorption rate. All types of transdermal patches, both estrogen only and estrogen-progestin combination patches, contain 17-β estradiol, which is a plant derivative. The advantage is the same as the first-pass avoidance in CHC products using the transdermal route. The GI tract and liver are bypassed initially, which results in less nausea and vomiting and less impact on the hepatic system. Some women prefer to take an estrogen derived from a plant source. Transdermal patches are changed twice a week or weekly, depending on the product. They are used continuously. Examples of transdermal estrogen systems are Climera, Estraderm, Vivelle, and Vivelle-Dot. A progestin should be taken concurrently with the estrogen patch in women with an intact uterus.

TABLE 56-4 ESTROGENS AND PROGESTINS USED IN HORMONE THERAPY

PRODUCT NAME	TYPE OF ESTROGEN OR ESTROGEN/PROGESTIN	ROUTE OF DELIVERY	DOSE
Conjugated Estrogens			
Premarin	See Prototype Drug Chart 56-1.		
Estrogen Products (ET) Oral Administration			
Cenestin	synthetic conjugated estrogen	Tablet	0.3 mg, 0.45 mg, 0.625 mg, 0.9 mg, 1.25 mg daily PO
Enjuvia	synthetic conjugated estrogen	Tablet	0.3 mg, 0.45 mg, 0.625 mg, 0.9 mg, 1.25 mg daily PO
Estrace	micronized estradiol	Tablet	0.5 mg, 1.0 mg, 2.0 mg daily PO
Femtrace	Estradiol	Tablet	0.45 mg, 0.9 mg, 1.8 mg daily PO
Menest	esterified estrogens	Tablet	0.3 mg, 0.625 mg, 1.25 mg, 2.5 mg daily PO
Ogen	Estropipate	Tablet	0.625 mg, 1.25 mg, 2.5 mg daily PO
Ortho-Est	Estropipate	Tablet	0.625 mg, 1.25 mg daily PO
Premarin	CEE	Tablet	0.3 mg, 0.45 mg, 0.625 mg, 0.9 mg, 1.25 mg, 2.5 mg daily PO
Estrogen Products (ET) Transdermal Administration			
Alora	Estradiol	Matrix patch	0.025, 0.05, 0.075, 0.1 mg/d applied to skin 2 times/wk
Climera	Estradiol	Matrix patch	0.025, 0.0375, 0.05, 0.06, 0.075, 0.1 mg/d applied to skin q wk
Divigel	Estradiol	Topical gel	0.25, 0.5, 1.0 mg/packet applied to the skin once daily
Elestrin	Estradiol	Topical gel	0.87 g/pump applied to the skin once daily
Estraderm	Estradiol	Reservoir patch	0.05, 0.1 mg/d applied to skin 2 times/wk
Estrasorb	Estradiol	Topical emulsion	1.74 g/pouch; 2 pouches applied to skin daily
Estrogel	Estradiol	Topical gel	1.25 g/pump; 1 pump applied to skin daily
Evamist	estradiol	Topical spray	1.53 mg/spray; 1 spray/d, may increase to 2-3 times/d PRN
Menostar	Estradiol	Matrix patch	0.014 mg/d applied to skin q wk
Minivelle	Estradiol	Patch	0.0375, 0.05, 0.075, 0.1 mg/d applied to the skin 2 times/wk
Vivelle	Estradiol	Matrix pouch	0.05, 0.1 mg applied to skin 2 times/wk
Vivelle-Dot	Estradiol	Matrix pouch	0.025, 0.0375, 0.05, 0.075, 0.1 mg/d applied to skin 2 times/wk
Vaginal Estrogen Products			
Estrace	Estradiol	Vaginal cream	0.01% (0.1mg/g) daily for 2 wk, then 1- 3 times/wk intravaginal
Estring	Estradiol	Vaginal ring	7.5 mcg/24 h; 1 ring intravaginal q90d
Femring	Estradiol	Vaginal ring	0.05 mg/d, 0.1 mg/d; 1 ring intravaginal q3mo
Premarin	CEE	Vaginal cream	0.625 mg/d intravaginal daily
Vagifem	Estradiol	Vaginal tablet	25 mcg; 1 tab intravaginal daily for 2 wk, then 2 times/wk
Estrogen and Progestin/Progesterone Combination Products (EPT) Oral Administration			
Activella	estradiol and norethindrone acetate	Tablet	0.5 mg and 0.1 mg; 1 mg and 0.5 mg PO daily
Angeliq	estradiol and drospirenone	Tablet	0.5 mg and 0.25 mg; 1 mg and 0.5 mg PO daily
FemHRT	EE and norethindrone acetate	Tablet	2.5 mcg and 0.5 mg; 5 mcg and 1 mg PO daily
Prefest	EE, then EE and norgestimate	Tablet	1.0 mg, then 1.0 mg and 0.09 mg PO daily
Premphase	CEE (14 tabs), then CEE and MPA (14 tabs)	Tablet	0.625 mg (first 14 days), then 0.625 mg and 5 mg PO daily sequentially
Prempro	CEE and MPA (28 tabs)	Tablet	0.3 mg and 1.5 mg; 0.45 mg and 1.5 mg; 0.625 mg and 2.5 mg PO daily
Estrogen and Progestin/Progesterone (EPT) Transdermal Administration			
Climara Pro	estradiol and LNG	Matrix patch	0.045 mg and 0.015 mg/d applied to skin q wk
Combipatch	estradiol and norethindrone acetate	Matrix patch	0.05 mg and 0.14 mg; 0.5 mg and 0.25 mg/d applied to skin 2 times/wk

Continued

TABLE 56-4 ESTROGENS AND PROGESTINS USED IN HORMONE THERAPY—cont'd

PRODUCT NAME	TYPE OF ESTROGEN OR ESTROGEN/PROGESTIN	ROUTE OF DELIVERY	DOSE
Progestins and Progesterone Products			
Used for HT (to prevent endometrial hyperplasia in women with an intact uterus who are on estrogen), to promote withdrawal bleeding in women with amenorrhea, and monthly or bimonthly to cycle withdrawal bleeding as endometrial hyperplasia prophylaxis in women with amenorrhea			
Aygestin	norethindrone acetate	Tablet	HT: 5 mg PO daily (not used for endometrial hyperplasia prevention or amenorrhea) Endometriosis: 5 mg PO daily for 2 wk; increase by 2.5 mg daily for 2 wk. *Max:* 15/mg daily for 6-9 mo
Prometrium	micronized progesterone	Capsule	HT: 100 mg; 200 mg PO daily h.s. Endometrial hyperplasia prevention: 200 mg PO daily h.s. for 12 consecutive days q mo Amenorrhea: 400 mg PO daily for 10 days h.s.
Provera	MPA	Tablet	HT: 2.5 mg; 5 mg; 10 mg PO daily Endometrial hyperplasia prevention: 5-10 mg PO daily for 12-14 d q mo starting on day 1 or day 16 Amenorrhea: 5-10 mg for 5-10 d

CEE, Conjugated equine estrogen; *d,* day; *g,* gram; *h.s.,* at bedtime; *LNG,* levonorgestrel; *max,* maximum; *mcg,* microgram; *mg,* milligram; *mo,* month; *MPA,* medroxyprogesterone acetate; *PO,* by mouth; *PRN,* as needed; *q,* every; *transvag,* transvaginally; *wk,* week
ET, pregnancy category X; *EPT,* pregnancy category X; *Aygestin,* pregnancy category X; *Provera and Prometrium,* exposure in first trimester may cause genital abnormalities in the fetus. HT in nursing mothers is not recommended.

PROTOTYPE DRUG CHART 56-1

Conjugated Estrogens

Drug Class Estrogen replacement Trade Name: Premarin Pregnancy Category: X	**Dosage** A: PO: 0.3, 0.45, 0.625, 0.9, and 1.25 mg daily or cyclically (with or without progestins)
Contraindications Undiagnosed vaginal bleeding, pregnancy, lactation, severe liver disease, venous thrombosis and personal history of breast cancer Caution: Cardiovascular disease, severe renal disease, diabetes mellitus	**Drug-Lab-Food Interactions** Drug: Increase effects with corticosteroids; decrease effects of anticoagulants, oral hypoglycemics; decrease effects with rifampin, anticonvulsants, barbiturates; toxicity with tricyclic antidepressants
Pharmacokinetics Absorption: PO: Well absorbed Distribution: PB: Widely distributed; crosses placenta and enters breast milk Metabolism: $t\frac{1}{2}$: UK Excretion: In urine and bile	**Pharmacodynamics** PO/IV: Onset: Rapid, Peak: UK, Duration: UK IM: Onset: Delayed
Therapeutic Effects/Uses Moderate to severe vasomotor symptoms of menopause and vaginal dryness/atrophy Mode of Action: Develops and maintains female genital system, breast, and secondary sex characteristics; increased synthesis of protein	
Side Effects Nausea, vomiting, fluid retention, breast tenderness, leg cramps, breakthrough bleeding, chloasma	**Adverse Reactions** Jaundice, thromboembolic disorders, depression, hypercalcemia, gallbladder disease Life-threatening: Thromboembolism, cerebrovascular accident, pulmonary embolism, myocardial infarction, endometrial cancer

A, Adult; *d,* day; *IM,* intramuscular; *IV,* intravenous; *PB,* protein-binding; *PO,* by mouth; $t\frac{1}{2}$, half-life; *UK,* unknown.

HT is also available in topical gels, emulsions, and sprays. EstroGel, Divigel and Elestrinare synthetic plant-based transdermal estradiol gels applied once daily for the treatment of moderate to severe vasomotor symptoms. A thin film is applied to one arm from the shoulder to wrist. The gel dries in 2 to 5 minutes. EstroGel and Elestrin are packaged in a non-aerosol, metered-dose pump, while Divigel comes in single-dose packets. The dosage regime is designed to deliver a specific amount of estradiol with each application.

Estrasorb is the first prescription topical emulsion for estrogen therapy. Estrasorb delivers consistent levels of estradiol into the bloodstream in a lotion-like emulsion, applied daily to the skin on the legs for the relief of moderate to severe vasomotor symptoms. Estrasorb should be applied in a comfortable sitting position to clean, dry skin on both legs each morning.

Evamist is delivered in one spray daily to the skin of the inside of the forearm between the elbow and wrist.

With the topical ET products listed above, a progestin should be taken concurrently in women who have an intact uterus.

Medroxyprogesterone acetate or MPA (Provera) is an oral progestin most often administered in combination with estrogen. Other available products are norethindrone acetate (Aygestin) and micronized progesterone (Prometrium).

Combination products contain both estrogen and a progestin, which offers the added convenience of not having to take two pills daily. Combination products have the same adverse effects as estrogen-only and progestin-only HT. Samples of combination oral HT products include Activella (estradiol and norethindrone acetate), FemHRT (EE and norethindrone acetate), and Prempro (CEE and MPA). The newest form HT is Angeliq (0.5 mg drospirenone and 1 mg estradiol). It is the only HT with the unique progestin drospirenone, and it carries the same precautions as those drugs.

Two combination estrogen-progestin transdermal products are available: ClimaraPro is a thin translucent patch containing estradiol and levonorgestrel, and Combipatch contains estradiol and norethindrone acetate. ClimaraPro is the first once-a-week combined HT approved to treat menopausal symptoms such as hot flashes. Combipatch is placed twice a week. The transdermal patch allows for continuous delivery of hormones at much lower doses than in oral HT. This route avoids the first-pass of the liver and may be better tolerated by women.

Vaginal cream preparations are used in the treatment of vaginal atrophy, which causes painful intercourse and urinary difficulties. Estrace contains estradiol cream, while Premarin contains CEE cream. Both preparations are rapidly absorbed into the bloodstream via the mucous membranes that line the vagina. Vaginal creams may be used in conjunction with another method, such as tablets or the transdermal patch. However, vaginal creams do not need a progestin counter because they do not affect the uterine endometrium to the extent that oral and transdermal products will. Vaginal creams are usually delivered in the dose of 0.5 to 2 g intravaginally daily for 2 weeks; then the dosing is decreased to twice weekly.

Estring is an elastomer ring containing 2 mg of 17-β estradiol, a bioidentical estrogen. The Estring ring is inserted into the upper portion of the vagina, where it releases 50% to 60% of estradiol, providing a consistent low dose of estrogen for 3 months. Estring is used to treat local symptoms of urogenital atrophy, which affects 20% to 40% of postmenopausal women.

FemRing is the first vaginal ERT used to treat moderate to severe hot flashes, night sweats, and vaginal dryness in menopause. FemRing contains estradiol acetate, an estrogen, in a soft, flexible silicone ring. It is inserted into the upper vagina for 3 months. It may be left in place during intercourse and during treatment for vaginal infections. The FemRing attains higher levels of serum estrogen than the Estring, so a progestin counterpart must be prescribed for women with an intact uterus.

Vagifem is a vaginal estrogen tablet that contains estradiol. One 25-mcg tablet is inserted intravaginally once daily for 2 weeks, and then the dose is decreased to one 25-mcg tablet twice weekly. Vagifem tablets have lower circulating estrogen levels than vaginal creams.

Contraindications

Contraindications to HT include pregnancy, history of endometrial cancer (when treatment for early endometrial cancer has been completed, it is no longer a contraindication to HT), personal history of breast cancer, history of thromboembolic disorders, acute liver disease or chronic impaired liver function, active gallbladder or pancreatic disease, coronary artery disease (CAD), undiagnosed vaginal bleeding, and endometriosis. Lifestyle factors such as smoking, known to enhance the risk of thromboembolism, should be considered in the treatment decision. The patient with a history of fibroid tumors is not started on HT for a full year after the last menstruation, because estrogen would likely result in tumor growth. The hypoestrogenic state associated with natural menopause usually causes existing fibroids to shrink. The presence of fibrocystic breast disease or diabetes may require extra caution.

Pharmacokinetics Natural estrogens are completely and rapidly absorbed from the GI tract and rapidly metabolized by the liver, necessitating daily doses when oral products that are nonesterified (a process that delays metabolism and lengthens action) are used. About 80% of estradiol is bound to sex-hormone–binding globulin, with 2% unbound and the rest bound to albumin. Estradiol is converted to estrone in the enterohepatic circulation and is conjugated and excreted via the urine. Conjugated estrogens have a longer half-life than natural estradiols. However, it is difficult to measure blood levels of estrogen with conjugated estrogens. Progestin (Provera) is rapidly absorbed and metabolized primarily in the liver with excretion via the kidney; distribution of the agent is not well described. With vaginal creams, there is a systemic absorption of estrogen. The levels are much lower than those found in oral and transdermal preparations. There is a first-pass bypass of the hepatic system with both vaginal and transdermal preparations. On the first day of vaginal ring use, estrogen levels are elevated and then fall quickly to preinsertion levels.

Other Drugs for Menopausal Symptoms

Women who are not candidates for HT (more specifically, women with contraindications and breast cancer survivors) can be prescribed other medications.

SSRIs. Selective serotonin reuptake inhibitors (SSRIs) reduce the number and severity of vasomotor symptoms in women. SSRIs also have the added benefit of reducing depression, which may relieve irritability and mood changes associated with menopause.

Clonidine. Clonidine (Catapres, Kapvay), a medication used for hypertension, also reduces the number and severity of vasomotor symptoms in women. It is currently being used for this purpose for women in whom HT is contraindicated. Blood pressure must be monitored at regular intervals and the medication discontinued if hypotension occurs.

Gabapentin. Gabapentin (Neurontin) is an antiseizure medication that reduces the number and severity of vasomotor symptoms in menopausal women. Gabapentin should be limited to those women who cannot take HT medications and have vasomotor symptoms that are affecting quality of life. Gabapentin can cause drowsiness and should not be used concurrently with other medications with similar precautions, or if the patient's activities of daily living include those that would be affected or even dangerous if sleepiness, dizziness, or syncope occur.

Osteoporosis

Osteoporosis is a progressive, debilitating skeletal disease that affects older men and women. Women older than 50 years are at greatest risk since the loss of estrogen during menopause is directly related to loss in bone mineral density. Bone mass is at its highest density at age 30 years and then steadily declines. Osteoporosis occurs through an imbalance of osteoblasts (bone-building cells) and osteoclasts (cells that break down bone), which causes bone reabsorption to be excelled. This imbalance causes both deterioration of the microstructure within the bone and a decrease bone density. The loss of bone structure and "porous bone" fragility lead to the risk for fractures. Osteoporosis has significant morbidity and mortality in the United States. The most serious fracture site is the hip. Hip fracture is the second most common reason for older women being placed in nursing homes, exceeded only by Alzheimer's disease. Women who experience hip or vertebral fracture may have long-term, progressive, and debilitating health problems that can eventually lead to death. More than half of U.S. women older than 50 years have some degree of **osteopenia** (low BMD) or osteoporosis (severe decline in BMD).

Diagnosis of osteopenia and osteoporosis is made by axial skeletal measurements of bone density in the lumbar spine and hip through dual energy X-ray absorptiometry or DXA scan. The World Health Organization (WHO) defines osteopenia and osteoporosis by transferring the results of the DXA scan into a T-score. Normal BMD is a T-score of –1 or greater. Osteopenia is defined by a T-score of –1 to –2.5 and, osteoporosis is defined by a T-score of –2.5 or less.

HT is no longer recommended for the *treatment* of osteoporosis but should be considered as a *preventive* measure in postmenopausal women who are at risk. Women who have used HT for 5 years or more have been shown to have a reduction in hip and vertebral fractures by 35%. Other medications can manage osteoporosis and prevent fractures without the concerns that are raised by HT. These include bisphosphonates, which can reduce the breakdown of bone microstructure, and selective estrogen receptor modulators (SERMs). SERMs are a new class of synthetic estrogens. SERMs act like estrogens in certain parts of the body (such as the bones) while leaving other parts unaffected. Evista is an example of a SERM used to treat osteoporosis. Contraindications to SERM therapy include past history or risk for VTE and pregnancy. Caution is used in women with heart disease, risk of MI or stroke, and hepatic or renal insufficiency.

The side effects of oral bisphosphonates include nausea, abdominal/stomach pain, difficulty swallowing, esophageal inflammation, reflux, and ulcers. Injectable bisphosphonates do not have the gastrointestinal side effects, and it can be easier for the patient to schedule a quarterly or yearly injection than to remember to take a daily or weekly pill. A rare complication of bisphosphonates is full or partial spontaneous femur fractures. Oral bisphosphonates should not be taken with aspirin, nonsteroidal antiinflammatory drugs (NSIADs), or antacids. Contraindications to bisphosphonates include esophageal abnormalities or delayed emptying of the esophagus, inability to sit or stand for 30 minutes after oral ingestion, and hypocalcemia.

Nursing Interventions

Prevention of osteoporosis includes sufficient intake of calcium and vitamin D throughout the lifespan by either dietary intake or supplementation. The recommended daily requirement of calcium for women age 25 to 50 years is 1000 to 1200 mg/day, while women older than 50 years need 1200 to 1500 mg/day. Calcium should be taken in divided doses and with adequate vitamin D to enhance absorption. The recommended daily allowance of vitamin D is 400 to 800 IU/day for women age 25 to 50 years and 1000 to 2000 IU/day for women older than 50 years. All calcium preparations, with the exception of calcium citrate, should be taken with food. Smoking cessation should be encouraged because smoking interferes with vitamin D absorption. Alcohol consumption should limited to one alcohol drink per day, since alcohol reduces gastrointestinal absorption of calcium. Weight-bearing exercise strengthens the bones, increases muscle strength, and enhances balance. Weight-bearing exercises include walking, jogging, low-impact aerobics, weight training, and yoga. Caution should be used in patients who are prescribed medications that cause hypotension or dizziness. The patient should be assessed for fall risk, and the prevention of falls should be part of the nurse's health care teaching.

Medications

Estrogen is no longer recommended for the treatment of osteoporosis but may be of benefit in the prevention of osteoporosis. The benefit-risk–alternative ratio should be considered in patients who are candidates for HT. Most preparations of HT (oral and transdermal EPT or ET) can be used for prevention of osteoporosis. Vaginal preparations are not effective.

Menostar (estradiol transdermal system) is 14 mcg of 17-β estradiol in a transdermal, once-a-week patch used for prevention of postmenopausal osteoporosis. This estrogen patch is the lowest transdermal dose available. It is available for women who are unable to tolerate alternative therapies. For women with an intact uterus, a progestin is only recommended every 6 to 12 months.

Alendronate (Fosamax) is a bisphosphonate used to treat osteopenia and osteoporosis. It is available in a daily or weekly dose. For prevention, the oral daily dose is 5 mg/day and the oral weekly dose is 35 mg/week. For treatment, the oral daily dose is 10 mg/day, and the oral weekly dose is 75 mg/week. Fosamax must be taken with 8 ounces of water 30 minutes before ingesting any food, liquids, or medication, and the patient must remain upright for 30 minutes. Once-a-week dosing has made this a first-line therapy. Common side effects include abdominal pain and acid reflux. Fosamax Plus D (vitamin D is added) is also available for enhanced absorption of calcium.

Ibandronate sodium (Boniva) is a once-a-month bisphosphonate indicated for the treatment and prevention of osteoporosis in postmenopausal women. It comes in oral dosing and intravenous dosing. The oral dose has the same directions for use and side effects as the other bisphosphonates. Boniva can be administered in 2.5-mg once-daily tablets, 150-mg once-monthly tablets, or 3-mg every 3 months administered IV over 15 to 30 seconds.

Risedronate (Actonel) is also available in a daily or weekly dose. It has similar directions for use and side effects as the bisphosphonates. The dosing schedule is a 5-mg tablet once daily or 35-mg tablet once weekly. Actonel is also available in Actonel with Calcium. The risedronate tablet is taken once weekly followed by a 500-mg tablet taken once daily on days 2 through 7. Atelvia is the only drug used for osteoporosis that has a delayed-release formulation. Atelvia contains 35 mg of risedronate and is taken once a week, immediately following breakfast and with at least 4 ounces of water.

Reclast is a bisphosphonate that is administered IV in a 5-mg dose yearly. The IV dose should be administered over 15 minutes. Kidney failure is a rare but serious condition that may be associated with the use of Reclast in patients with underlying renal disease or renal impairment. Reclast can be given in a 5-mg dose every 2 years for prevention of osteoporosis.

Nurses should teach patients to advise their health care provider of any increased thigh or groin pain, which can be symptoms of rare, atypical femur fractures.

Studies suggest that some patients may be able to discontinue the use of these medications after 3 to 5 years and still benefit from using bisphosphonates. Health care providers should reassess patients on an individual basis every 5 years to determine whether continued therapy is beneficial. It has been determined is that bisphosphonates do work to improve osteoporosis; however the time frame for safe use of these medications needs to be investigated. There is ongoing research to determine whether the use of bisphosphonates increases the risk for esophageal cancer, which is extremely rare in women.

Raloxifene (Evista) is a SERM that increases bone mineral density, decreases bone turnover, and reduces vertebral fractures. A secondary analysis of osteoporotic women treated with raloxifene showed a decrease in the risk for breast cancer. Side effects include hot flashes and increased risk for DVT. Evista is taken orally once a day in 60-mg tablet.

Teriparatide (Fortéo) is a parathyroid hormone used for treatment of postmenopausal osteoporosis. It is administered 20 mcg subQ on a daily basis. It can be used by both men and women who have had a fracture related to osteoporosis or who have multiple risk factors for fracture and cannot use other osteoporosis treatments. The patient can be taught self-administration.

Salmon calcitonin (e.g., Fortical, Miacalcin) is composed of calcitonin, a naturally occurring hormone that regulates calcium in the body and promotes bone metabolism. It is delivered via intranasal spray in a 200-IU dose administered daily.

Denosumab (Prolia) is an osteoclast inhibitor used in women who are at a high risk for osteoporotic fracture, have had a fracture, or have not had improvement in T-score after using the bisphosphonates for osteoporosis. A 60-mg dose is given subcutaneously every 6 months.

Nursing Process
Patient-Centered Collaborative Care

Management of Symptomatic Menopausal Women

Assessment

- Obtain a record of patient's drug, supplement, and CAM use.
- Obtain baseline vital signs including TPR and BP, weight, and height. Report abnormal findings.
- Obtain family history assessing for risk factors regarding osteoporosis, osteoporotic fractures; cardiovascular risks including CAD, ischemic and hemorrhagic stroke, VTE, cognitive disorders, and cancers that affect women.
- Obtain a history of allergies to medications, foods, and supplements.
- Obtain a medical-surgical history, asking about present or past hypertension; falls and fractures; cardiovascular disease; cerebral vascular disorders; hepatic, renal, and urinary tract disorders and infections; gastrointestinal problems; neurologic disorders; and past systemic infections. Assess for past and present history of cancer. Ask about previous surgeries, in particular gynecologic or pelvic surgery. Assess for smoking, alcohol, and illicit drug use. Assess risk for falls, fractures, self-care concerns, and ability to take medications.
- Obtain a complete menstrual history including age at menarche and age at menopause. If the patient is perimenopausal, assess menstrual pattern; cycle length, duration, and amount of bleeding; and first day of LMP

and method used for contraception. If patient is in menopause, assess past and present menopausal symptoms along with effect on quality of life. Assess for any incidence of postmenopausal bleeding.
- Obtain a full gynecologic history, including last Pap testing, results, history of abnormal Pap testing and colposcopy, and gynecologic problems, disorders, and surgeries.
- Obtain a complete sexual history, including sexual expression practices, sexual risk practices, menopausal symptoms and effects on sexual expression, and past or present sexual abuse and/or assault.
- Assess patient's perception of menopause and knowledge of nonpharmacologic and pharmacologic hormone therapies.

Nursing Diagnoses
- Deficient knowledge of perimenopause and menopause
- Decisional conflicts related to starting/continuing HR
- Deficient knowledge related to HR method(s) and appropriate use of method
- Fear related to HR potential side effects
- Risk for infections related to unprotected intercourse
- Risk for alterations in bone mineral density related to systemic decreases in estrogen
- Risk for falls and/or osteoporotic fracture
- Disturbed body image related to changes in body related to menopause
- Ineffective sleep patterns and sleep-wake health related to perimenopause (or menopause)
- Health-seeking behaviors related to seeking relief of symptoms

Planning
- Patients with contraindications to HT will be risked out.
- Patient will verbalize menopausal symptoms and understand nonpharmacologic and pharmacologic measures that may aid in alleviating symptoms.
- If patient elects HT, she will choose the route of administration that is best suited for her lifestyle and will increase safety and effective use of the product.
- Patient will understand difference between EPT and ET.
- Patient will report side effects that occur.
- Patient will self-administer oral, transdermal, topical, or vaginal medications as prescribed.
- Patient will place patch as directed and will report adverse side effects that occur.
- Patient will be comfortable with vaginal placement of medications.
- Patient will report abnormal uterine bleeding and other side effects associated with HT.
- Explain dosing schedule, risks, benefits, and alternatives to patient.
- Patient will schedule follow-up appointment as needed.

Nursing Interventions
- Teach patient about nature of climacteric, its potential effects, and benefits, risks and alternatives of both nonpharmacologic as well as pharmacologic treatment modalities.
- Determine patient's misconceptions about HT, and provide factual, research-based information.
- Use BRAIDED method in assisting patient in choosing a HT method.
- Use health teaching to encourage effective use of HT.
- Place current educational materials in health and community sites.

Patient Teaching

General
- Review risks, benefits, and alternatives for use of HT.
- Review contraindications to HT.
- Advise patient to have a breast examination, pelvic examination, and Pap test before starting HT.
- Tell patient that warm weather and stress exacerbate hot flashes.
- Advise patient to use a fan, drink cool liquids, and decrease intake of caffeine and spicy foods.
- Advise individuals with diabetes, hypertension, or rheumatic heart disease to use vitamin E in low doses with health care provider's approval.
- Encourage patient on HT to have medical follow-up every 6 to 12 months, including blood pressure check, clinical breast examination, and pelvic examination.
- Stress need to use a method of contraception until 1 year after cessation of spontaneous menstruation.
- Suggest to patient that she use a water-soluble vaginal lubricant to reduce painful intercourse (dyspareunia) and prevent trauma.
- Advise patient to decrease use of antihistamines and decongestants if she experiences vaginal dryness.
- Advise patient to wear cotton underwear and pantyhose with a cotton liner and to avoid douches and feminine hygiene products.
- Suggest that patient take HT oral medications after meals to avoid nausea and vomiting.
- Advise patient that she may experience some vaginal bleeding that should stop 3 to 6 months after starting HT.
- Suggest that patient carry sanitary pads or tampons for breakthrough bleeding or irregular menstruation.
- Advise patient to report any heavy bleeding or irregular bleeding patterns and to have hematocrit and hemoglobin evaluated.
- Advise patient that after HT is discontinued, there may be a recurrence of menopausal signs and symptoms such as hot flashes.
- Tell patient that if she wants to stop HT, she should do so with guidance of her health care provider.

Self-Administration

- Teach patient about breast health and to perform regular breast self-examination.
- Teach patient to perform regular genital inspections.
- Advise patient of when she is due for Pap screening.
- If patient uses vaginal cream, review application procedure and suggest that she wear mini-pads.
- If patient uses the transdermal patch, teach her to open the package and apply it immediately and to hold it in place for about 10 seconds; check edges to ensure adequate contact; use the abdomen (except the waistline) for patch; rotate sites with at least 1 week before reuse of a site; do not use breast as a site; do not put patch on an irritated or oily area; do not reapply patch if it loosens, or apply a new one; and follow same cycle schedule.
- Advise patient about appropriate use of gels, sprays, and mists.

Balanced Diet and Exercise

- Teach patient about osteoporosis prevention: (1) weight-bearing exercise; (2) well-balanced diet (high in fiber, vegetables, fruits, whole grains, and plant proteins; low in animal proteins and sugar); (3) supplement of 1000 mg/d calcium (if premenopausal) or 1200 to 1500 mg/d (if menopausal) and vitamin D 1000 to 2000 IU/d; (4) smoking cessation and reduced alcohol consumption.

Evaluation

- Evaluate effectiveness of nonpharmacologic or pharmacologic measures for premenopausal symptoms.
- Determine whether side effects occur. Plan with patient alternative measures to control menopausal symptoms.
- Plan follow-up appointments and health care screenings.

KEY WEBSITES

Planned Parenthood: *www.plannedparenthood.org*
Emergency contraception: *ec.princeton.edu*
North American Menopause Society: *www.menopause.org*
National Osteoporosis Society: *www.nof.org*

CRITICAL THINKING CASE STUDY

TA (gravida 3, para 1) is ready to leave the hospital after delivery of a healthy baby. TA had developed gestational hypertension during her pregnancy, but she had no prior history of hypertension. She plans to breastfeed for 3 months. She desires contraception and asks about hormonal contraceptive methods.

1. TA asks whether she can take combination birth control pills while breastfeeding. What are the nursing diagnoses for TA based on her communication? Are other CHC methods available for TA besides the pill? What CHC start method is best for TA?
2. The nurse tells TA that she may breastfeed and can start using combination pills in about 6 weeks when her milk flow is established. Is this information correct or incorrect? Why? What further information will TA need?
3. What other methods of oral contraception are available for TA that would not affect quantity and quality of breast milk? What nursing health teaching should be stressed with the initiation of these products?
4. TA asks if there are any advantages to using oral contraceptives rather than a Mirena LNG-US. What are four advantages and four disadvantages the nurse could include in the discussion? What health teaching would the nurse provide for TA to ensure that she will use COC pills correctly?

NCLEX STUDY QUESTIONS

1. The nurse is preparing a teaching plan for combined oral contraceptive use. Which information should the nurse include in the teaching plan? (Select all that apply.)
   a. The patient should report abdominal pain, chest pain, headaches, blurred vision and visual disturbances, and severe leg pain.
   b. COCs are safe for smokers older than 35 years who smoke less than 20 cigarettes per day.
   c. COC use will not protect from STIs.
   d. The pills can be missed, but not for more than 12 hours.
   e. Vaginal spotting after starting CHC pills is a sign that the method is not effective in preventing pregnancy.
2. A 54-year-old menopausal patient comes into the gynecology office and is interested in hormone therapy. Which are indications for prescribing hormone therapy? (Select all that apply.)
   a. Relief of hot flashes
   b. Prevention of breast cancer
   c. Prevention of cardiovascular disease
   d. Prevention of osteoporosis in a high-risk patient
   e. Relief of vaginal dryness

3. A 24-year-old patient tells the nurse that she would like to use the minipill for contraception. Nursing evaluation of this patient as a candidate for the progestin-only pill includes what?
   a. Obtaining an obstetrical history to make sure that the patient has given birth in the past.
   b. Obtaining a gynecologic history to assure that the patient has regular periods.
   c. Assessing patient reliability in taking an oral pill daily.
   d. Interviewing the patient about past smoking habits.
4. A 39-year-old patient who smokes one pack per day asks about a contraception method that is best for her. She is normotensive and has used CHC pills in the past. She is in a monogamous relationship and has had two children with no complications during pregnancy. She is not planning any more pregnancies. The nurse determines that which method would be best for this patient?
   a. Combined hormone contraception pills
   b. The Mirena LNG/IUS
   c. Progestin-only pills
   d. Plan B
5. An 18-year-old woman calls the clinic office and tells the triage nurse that she had sex last night and the condom broke. She is concerned about unintended pregnancy. Which statement made by the triage nurse is the best advice for this patient?
   a. "Plan B One-Step is available over the counter."
   b. "You should make an appointment with the provider for a prescription of ulipristal acetate (Ella)."
   c. "You have time to wait a few days to make a decision."
   d. "The provider can insert an intrauterine device. I will make an appointment for you."
6. The nurse is instructing a patient on the use of medroxyprogesterone acetate (Depo-Provera). Which statements are correct? (Select all that apply.)
   a. "Patients using Depo-Provera usually do not have any changes in their periods."
   b. "You should increase your intake of calcium."
   c. "You can expect some irregular bleeding at first."
   d. "You can use Depo-Provera if you are breastfeeding."
   e. "Depo-Provera also helps with postpartum depression."
7. The nurse is counseling a 62-year-old patient with a T-score on her Dexa Scan of –2.0. What is the best advice for this patient?
   a. The patient's diet should be supplemented with daily calcium, 1200 to 1500 mg orally in the morning.
   b. The patient should increase weight-bearing exercises like swimming and cycling.
   c. The patient most likely will be prescribed a drug of the bisphosphonate classification by the health care provider.
   d. The patient should supplement her diet with 1200 to 1500 mg of calcium with vitamin D orally twice daily.
8. A 48-year-old patient arrives at the clinic to discuss her perimenopausal symptoms. She states that her last menstrual period was 8 months ago, and before that they had been irregular. What is the most important nursing advice to give this patient?
   a. Hormone therapy is only used for hot flashes and vaginal dryness.
   b. The patient should be using some form of contraception to avoid pregnancy.
   c. The patient should have a Dexa Scan to test for osteopenia.
   d. At this time, herbal supplementation is probably best to relieve her perimenopausal symptoms.

Answers: 1, a, c; 2, a, d, e; 3, c; 4, b; 5, a; 6, b, c, d; 7, d; 8, b.

CHAPTER

57

Drugs for Men's Health and Reproductive Disorders

evolve WEBSITE

http://evolve.elsevier.com/KeeHayes/pharmacology/

- Animations
- Content Updates
- Key Points
- Review Questions for the NCLEX® Examination
- References from the Textbook
- Unfolding Case Studies

OBJECTIVES

- Describe the effects of gonadal hormone supplementation on the hypothalamic anterior pituitary feedback loop.
- Describe the role of testosterone therapy in managing developmental problems related to primary and secondary male sex characteristics and in spermatogenesis.
- Differentiate common conditions for which androgen therapy and antiandrogen therapy are indicated.
- Describe patients for whom androgen therapy is particularly risky.
- Assess patients for therapeutic and adverse effects of androgen therapy.
- Categorize commonly prescribed medications that can impair male sexual function.
- Explain the nursing process, including patient teaching, related to drugs used to treat male reproductive disorders.

OUTLINE

KEY TERMS

Addison's disease, p. 880
anabolism, p. 877
androgens, p. 874
antiandrogens, p. 878
cryptorchidism, p. 876
delayed puberty, p. 879
ejaculatory dysfunction, p. 880
erectile dysfunction, p. 880
gynecomastia, p. 876
hirsutism, p. 877
hypogonadism, p. 875
hypothyroidism, p. 880
inhibited sexual desire, p. 880
oligospermia, p. 876
priapism, p. 876
spermatogenesis, p. 876
testosterone, p. 874
virilization, p. 877

Reproductive health requires the production of adequate quantities of various hypothalamic, pituitary, and gonadal hormones as well as the appropriate hormone receptors. It requires normal development and patency of the reproductive tract. In addition, reproductive health implies that men and women at developmentally appropriate life stages are fertile (i.e., able to produce gametes [sperm or eggs]). Finally, reproductive health entails the ability to engage in sexual intercourse with ejaculation by the male.

The authors gratefully acknowledge the work of Karen Carmody, who updated this chapter for the eighth edition.

Alterations in male reproductive health reflect a wide range of developmental, endocrine, infectious, inflammatory, hypertrophic, malignant, and psycho-emotional processes. Review the introduction to this unit to gain a better understanding of ways in which reproductive health is affected, including anatomy and physiology, sperm production, regulation of male sexual functioning, and sexual intercourse.

The drug family most clearly associated with male reproductive processes is the androgens. Because synthetic anabolic steroids and antiandrogens affect male reproduction, they are also discussed.

SUBSTANCES RELATED TO MALE REPRODUCTIVE DISORDERS

Androgens

Androgens, or male sex hormones, control the development and maintenance of sexual processes, accessory sexual organs, cellular metabolism, and bone and muscle growth. **Testosterone** is the principal male sex hormone and is an anabolic steroid. It is the prototype of the androgen hormones, synthesized primarily in the testes and, to a lesser extent, in the adrenal cortex. In women, the ovaries synthesize small amounts of testosterone. In men, normal plasma concentrations of testosterone are 250 to 1000 ng/dL, with circadian fluctuations. Prototype Drug Chart 57-1 lists the natural and synthetic androgens and their dosages, uses, and considerations.

Pharmacokinetics Testosterone secretion is greater in men than in women in most stages of life. About 98% of circulating testosterone is bound to both sex hormone–binding globulin (SHBG) and albumin protein, leaving about 2% unbound, or circulating free in the plasma. It is this unbound portion that is biologically active. Estrogen elevates the production of sex hormone–binding globulin, resulting in more protein-bound testosterone in women than in men. The half-life of endogenous (naturally occurring) free testosterone in the blood is 10 to 20 minutes.

Exogenous (supplemental) testosterone is absorbed when taken orally, but because as much as 50% is metabolized on its first pass through hepatic circulation, high doses are needed to achieve effective plasma levels. Synthetic androgens have longer half-lives, so only synthetic androgens are available in oral formulations in the United States. Testosterone can be combined with esters to form esterified testosterone, in an oil base for intramuscular (IM) injection.

PROTOTYPE DRUG CHART 57-1

Testosterone

Drug Class Androgen Trade Names: Depo-Testosterone, First-Testosterone MC, Delatestryl Pregnancy Category: X CSS III	**Dosage** Androgen replacement: IM: 50-400 mg q2-4wk Higher doses used to treat metastatic breast cancer
Contraindications Pregnancy, nephrosis, hypercalcemia, pituitary insufficiency, hepatic dysfunction, benign prostatic hypertrophy, prostatic cancer, history of myocardial infarction, prepubertal status, non–estrogen-dependent breast cancer Caution: Hypertension, hypercholesterolemia, coronary artery disease, gynecomastia, renal disease, seizure disorders; prepubescent patients, older adults	**Drug-Lab-Food Interactions** Drug: Increases effects of anticoagulants; decreases effect with barbiturates, phenytoin, phenylbutazone; antagonizes calcitonin, parathyroid; corticosteroids exacerbate edema Lab: Decreases blood glucose in diabetics; increases serum cholesterol, thyroid, liver function, hematocrit
Pharmacokinetics Absorption: IM: Well absorbed Distribution: PB: 98% Metabolism: $t\frac{1}{2}$: 10-100 min Excretion: In urine and bile	**Pharmacodynamics** IM: Onset: UK Peak: UK Duration: cypionate/enanthate: 2-4 wk
Therapeutic Effects/Uses To achieve normal androgen levels; to slow progress of estrogen-dependent breast cancers Mode of Action: Develops and maintains male sex organs and secondary sex characteristics	
Side Effects Abdominal pain, nausea, diarrhea, constipation, hives, irritation at injection site, increased salivation, mouth soreness, increased or decreased libido, insomnia, aggressive behavior, weakness, dizziness, pruritus FDA boxed warning for children exposed to gel: inappropriate enlargement of the genitalia (penis or clitoris), premature development of pubic hair, advanced bone aging, increased libido, and aggressive behavior	**Adverse Reactions** Acne, masculinization, irregular menses, urinary urgency, gynecomastia, priapism, red skin, jaundice, sodium and water retention, allergic reaction, depression, habituation Life-threatening: Hepatic necrosis, hepatitis, hepatic tumors, respiratory distress

CSS, Controlled Substances Schedule; *d,* day; *IM,* intramuscular; *min,* minute; *mo,* month; *PB,* protein-binding; *PO,* by mouth; *subQ,* subcutaneous; *t* $\frac{1}{2}$, half-life; *UK,* unknown; *wk,* week.

Testosterone is excreted mainly in the urine as the metabolites androsterone and etiocholanolone. About 6% of the hormone is excreted unaltered in the feces. Synthetic androgens may be excreted as unaltered hormone or as metabolites. In some tissues the action of testosterone depends on its reduction to 5-alpha-dihydrotestosterone (DHT), whereas in other tissues testosterone itself is the active hormone. In the central nervous system, the metabolite estradiol affects hormonal action.

Pharmacodynamics Testosterone is responsible for the development of male sex characteristics. The biologic effects of testosterone may be mediated directly by testosterone or by its metabolites. Testosterone and dihydrotestosterone act as androgens by way of a single androgen receptor officially designated NR3A. The hormones bind to sites on certain responsive genes, causing a change to take place in the target cell. The effects of the testosterone depend on which receptor it activates and the tissues in which these effects occur. The manufacture of protein within the target cells results in the buildup of cellular tissue (anabolism), especially in muscles. This leads to development of secondary sex characteristics such as pubic hair growth, beard and body hair growth, baldness, deepening of the male voice, thickening of the skin, sebaceous gland activity, increased musculature, bone development, and red blood cell formation.

Fetal testes begin to produce testosterone during the first 3 months in utero. After birth until just before puberty, production is negligible. During puberty, production increases rapidly and continues until later adulthood. As men age, the number of Leydig cells decreases, sperm production declines, and luteinizing hormone (LH) and follicle-stimulating hormone (FSH) levels rise. Levels of unbound testosterone are reduced in older men to one-third to one-fifth the peak value. If men experience osteoporosis and anemia, and if their testosterone levels are ≤300 ng/dL, testosterone replacement therapy should be considered.

Indications for Androgen Therapy

Table 57-1 lists the natural and synthetic androgens with their dosages, uses, and considerations. The most common clinical use is for androgen deficiency in males, specifically hypogonadism, replacement therapy for testicular failure in adult males, and delayed puberty in adolescents. Occasionally it is used to slow the decline of patients with certain muscle wasting diseases such as COPD and AIDS.

Hypogonadism. The clearest indication for exogenous androgen therapy is **hypogonadism.** Male hypogonadism is a defect of the reproductive system that results in failure of

TABLE 57-1 ANDROGENS (CSS-III)

GENERIC (BRAND)	ROUTE AND DOSAGE	USES AND CONSIDERATIONS
Natural Androgens		
testosterone		
Testoderm scrotal patch	Discontinued in the U.S. Generic versions may still be available.	Androgen replacement, delayed puberty, carcinoma of the breast.
Androderm, Testoderm TTS	Transdermal patch: 5 mg/24 h; apply to nongenital skin; avoid bony areas	Started at full dose and adjusted according to tolerance and therapeutic response.
AndroGel/Testim 1 & 1.62%	1% Gel: 50-100 mg once daily	Less skin irritation with gel than patch. Pregnancy category: X; PB: 98%; t½: 10-100 min
Fortesta 2%	2% Gel: 40-70 mg once daily	
Axiron	Axillary Solution: 60-180 mg/day	
Striant	Buccal: 30 mg twice daily	
Testopel 75 mg/pellet	SubQ implantable pellets: 150-450 mg q3-6mo	
testosterone cypionate (Depo-Testosterone)	IM: 200-400 mg q3-4wk	Androgen replacement, delayed puberty. Therapy generally lasts 3-4 y. Pregnancy category: X; PB: 98%; t½: 8 days
testosterone enanthate (Delatestryl)	IM: 50-400 mg q2-4wk	Androgen replacement, delayed puberty. Pregnancy category: X; PB: 98%; t½: 10-100 min
Synthetic Androgens		
danazol	PO: 100-800 mg/d in 2 divided doses initially	Endometriosis, fibrocystic breast disease, hereditary angioedema. Initial doses are gradually reduced on an individual basis. Pregnancy category: X; PB: UK; t½: 4.5 h
fluoxymesterone (Androxy)	PO: 5 mg 1-4 times/day	Androgen deficiency, carcinoma of the breast. Pregnancy category: X; PB: 98%; t½: 29.2 h
methyltestosterone (Android, Methitest, Testred)	PO: 10-50 mg/d in divided doses initially, reduced for maintenance	Androgen deficiency, carcinoma of the breast. Pregnancy category: X; PB: UK; t½: 2.5-3.5 h
Anabolic Steroids		
oxandrolone (Oxandrin)	A: PO: 2.5-20 mg/d, divided C: PO: <0.1 mg/kg/d	Cachexia, delayed growth/puberty, osteoporotic pain, short stature, Turner's syndrome, alcoholic hepatitis. Pregnancy category: X; PB: 94%-97%; t½: 9.4 h

C, Child; *d,* day; *h,* hour; *IM,* intramuscular; *min,* minute; *mo,* month; *PB,* protein-binding; *PO,* by mouth; *RBC,* red blood cell; *subQ,* subcutaneous; *t½,* half-life; *UK,* unknown; *wk,* week; *y,* year.

the testes to produce testosterone, sperm, or both. Deficiency of sex hormones can result in defective primary or secondary sexual development. Defective sperm development can result in infertility. Hypogonadism is either primary, reflecting testicular abnormality, or secondary, reflecting hypothalamic or pituitary failure. A combination of disorders can also occur. Inadequate pituitary function will severely affect young boys and results in lack of secondary sex characteristics and infertility. Adult men may experience lack of libido, testicular atrophy, impotence, decreased bone density, loss of muscle tone, increased hair growth, or the onset of vasomotor flushing may occur.

The timing and extent of treatment depend on the clinical manifestations. Because accelerated bone maturation can lead to premature closure of bone epiphyses and short stature, androgen therapy should be used cautiously in children and only by specialists aware of the adverse effects on bone maturation. Skeletal maturation must be monitored every 6 months by x-ray of the hand and wrist. Artificial induction of puberty is undertaken only after boys reach age 15 to 17 years and hypothalamic and pituitary function has been assessed. A 4- to 6-month trial of androgen therapy is implemented, followed by a like period of rest for reevaluation. If prolonged therapy is required, testosterone cypionate or testosterone enanthate is used, 50 to 400 mg IM every 2 to 4 weeks. It should be given deep in the gluteal muscle. Inspect vials visually for particulate matter and discoloration before administration. Warm and shake the vial to dissolve any crystals that may have formed during storage. It takes 3 or 4 years for sexual development to occur. Plasma testosterone levels should be monitored and dosages adjusted as needed to maintain normal levels. If the serum testosterone level is below the normal range, the provider will adjust the dose upward. Therapy may be lifelong.

Some young, hypogonadal men are able to resolve erectile dysfunction with testosterone replacement therapy by way of oral, parenteral, or direct injection of drugs into the penis. These therapies may be associated with hypotension, dizziness, pain, and priapism; some of these drugs can cause hepatotoxicity. Given the success and high efficacy of oral erectile dysfunction therapy, discussed later, the use of these medications for adult hypogonadism has decreased markedly.

Testosterone may be administered buccally, orally, transdermally, or parenterally. The selection of an androgen or anabolic steroid depends on the balance of growth and sexual maturation desired and on the preferred route of administration. A buccal muco-adhesive system (Striant) is available at a 30-mg dose every 12 hours. Advise the patient to place the rounded side surface of the system against the gum above an incisor tooth and hold firmly in place with finger over lip and against product for 30 seconds. To remove, slide gently downwards toward tooth to avoid scratching gums. Sites must be rotated with each application. If the product falls off within the 12-hour dosing interval or falls out of position within 4 hours before next dose, remove and apply a new system. The patient should not chew or swallow the tablet. Advise the patient to regularly inspect gums where the system has been applied. With the exception of the buccal system, androgens are considered controlled substances Schedule III.

Many brands of testosterone transdermal patches are available. Testoderm patches are applied to the scrotum; scrotal skin is about five times more permeable than normal skin, and Testoderm will not achieve desired serum concentrations if applied to other skin sites. Serum concentrations of testosterone maximize after 2 to 4 hours, returning to baseline 2 hours after patch removal. Serum concentrations of testosterone approach those of normal males and reach a plateau after 3 to 4 weeks. Testoderm TTS patches achieve adequate serum concentrations when applied to the arm, back, or upper buttocks. Androderm patches can be applied to any healthy skin site other than the scrotum or bony areas. Daily application of two Androderm 2.5-mg skin patches at 10 PM results in serum testosterone concentrations approaching those of healthy young men. The first day of dosing results in morning serum testosterone concentrations within the normal range. There is no testosterone accumulation with continued use. After removal of Androderm, hypogonadal status returns within 24 hours. Keep testosterone gel out of reach of children.

An underarm solution (Axiron) is applied to one or both axillary areas at the same time each day. The patient should not apply Axiron to the genitals. These skin application products can be transferred to others through personal contact with skin or clothing. The treatment eliminates the need for injections and provides circadian fluctuations in dosage.

Other Uses. Other uses of androgens include treatment of refractory anemia in men and women, hereditary angioedema, tissue wasting associated with severe or chronic illness, advanced carcinoma of the breast in women, and endometriosis. The effectiveness of androgens for treatment of **cryptorchidism** (undescended testis) and impotence has not been established. Androgens may be used in combination with estrogens for management of severe menopausal symptoms in women.

Side Effects. Hypogonadal men on androgen therapy may experience frequent erections or **priapism** (painful, continuous erection), **gynecomastia** (mammary gland enlargement in men), or urinary urgency. Continued use of androgens by normal men can halt **spermatogenesis** (formation of spermatozoa). The sperm count may be low (**oligospermia**) for 3 or more months after therapy is stopped.

Other side effects of androgen therapy include abdominal pain, nausea, insomnia, diarrhea or constipation, hives or redness at the injection site, increased salivation, mouth soreness, and increased or decreased sexual desire. Advise the patient to notify the health care provider if side effects persist, worsen, or are bothersome.

Adverse Reactions. Androgen therapy may cause hypercalcemia by stimulating bone resorption in patients with breast cancer or immobilized patients. The drug should be discontinued and appropriate measures instituted if signs of hypercalcemia occur including: nausea and vomiting, lethargy, decreased muscle tone, polyuria, and increased urine and serum calcium.

Virilization refers to the development of male secondary sex characteristics in women or hypogonadal males. Such characteristics include growth of facial hair, acne and skin oiliness, and vocal huskiness. Menstrual irregularities or amenorrhea, suppressed ovulation or lactation, baldness or increased hair growth (**hirsutism**), and hypertrophy of the clitoris may develop in women undergoing androgen therapy. Although most adverse effects slowly reverse themselves after short-term therapy is completed, vocal changes may be permanent. With long-term therapy, as in the treatment of breast cancer, adverse effects may be irreversible.

Children may experience profound virilization as well as impaired bone growth. During pregnancy, androgens can cross the placenta and cause masculinization of the fetus. Virilization can occur in those secondarily exposed to testosterone gel and may cause teratogenic effects in fetuses. Women and children should not handle the gel and should avoid contact with application sites in men using testosterone gel.

Less frequent adverse effects include dizziness, weakness, changes in skin color, frequent headaches, confusion, respiratory distress, depression, pruritus, allergic skin rash, edema of the lower extremities, jaundice, bleeding, paresthesias, chills, polycythemia, muscle cramps, and sodium and water retention. Hepatic carcinoma can occur in patients who have received selected androgens for long-term therapy.

Serum cholesterol may become elevated during androgen therapy. Other alterations in laboratory tests include increased hematocrit, altered thyroid and liver function tests, and elevated urine 17-ketosteroids (a by-product of the breakdown of androgens). Rare complications of long-term therapy include hepatic necrosis, hepatic peliosis (blood-filled cysts), hepatic tumors, and leukopenia.

Contraindications. Androgen therapy is contraindicated during pregnancy and in individuals with nephrosis or the nephrotic phase of nephritis, hypercalcemia, pituitary insufficiency, hepatic dysfunction, benign prostatic hypertrophy, prostate cancer, or history of myocardial infarction. Men with breast cancer are not treated with androgens, nor are women whose breast cancer is not estrogen-dependent.

Caution must be exercised when using androgen therapy in individuals with hypertension, hypercholesterolemia, coronary artery disease, renal disease, or seizure disorder. It is used with caution in infants and prepubertal children because of the potential for growth disturbances and in older men because of their increased risk for benign prostatic hypertrophy and prostate cancer.

Drug Interactions. Androgens potentiate the effects of oral anticoagulants, necessitating a decrease in anticoagulant dosage. Androgens antagonize calcitonin and parathyroid hormones. Because androgens can decrease blood glucose in patients with diabetes, dosages of insulin or other antidiabetic agents may need to be reduced. Concurrent use of corticosteroids exacerbates the edema that can occur with androgen therapy. Barbiturates, phenytoin, and phenylbutazone decrease the effects of androgens.

Anabolic Steroids

Anabolic steroids, or anabolic-androgenic steroids (AAS), are a class of steroid hormones related to the hormone testosterone. They increase protein synthesis within cells, which results in the buildup of cellular tissue (**anabolism**), especially in muscles. Anabolic steroids also have androgenic and virilizing properties, including the development and maintenance of masculine characteristics such as the growth of the vocal cords and body hair. The American College of Sports Medicine notes that AAS, combined with sufficient diet, can contribute to increased body weight, often as lean mass, and that the gain in muscular strength achieved through high-intensity exercise and proper diet can be additionally enhanced by the use of AAS in some individuals.

Testosterone precursors available as nutritional supplements include androstenediol, androstenedione, and dehydroepiandrosterone (DHEA). Older teens are the heaviest users, but more than one-half million junior high school students use them. Marketed as "sport supplements" or "teen formulas," they can be purchased without a prescription in stores and on the Internet. A sudden dramatic increase in weight and body size, increased acne, and changes in mood and behavior can be signs of exogenous anabolic steroid use. Individuals using anabolic steroids may become more aggressive and physical. Health risks can result from long-term use or excessive intake of anabolic steroids; these effects include increased low-density lipoprotein (bad) cholesterol and decreased high-density lipoprotein (good) cholesterol, acne, high blood pressure, liver damage, and dangerous changes in the structure of the left ventricle of the heart. Adverse effects may not be recognized until years later.

Two other steroids that have gained popularity, especially with athletes, are human chorionic gonadotropin (hCG, Pregnyl, Novarel, Ovidrel) and tetrahydrogestrinone (THG). HCG is a hormone used to treat infertility and stimulate testosterone production. THG is a potent androgen developed to escape urine detection. It is not approved by the U.S. Food and Drug Administration (FDA) and is not legally marketed. All major athletic organizations prohibit the use of anabolic steroids, but their continued use despite bans has led to "anti-doping" investigations and punitive action.

Nursing Process
Patient-Centered Collaborative Care

Androgens

Assessment

- Assess the reason for androgen therapy and patient's perception of it. If delayed puberty is the indication, assess patient and family attitudes about the condition.
- Monitor patient's weight, blood pressure, liver and thyroid function, hemoglobin and hematocrit, creatinine, clotting factors, glucose tolerance, serum lipids

and electrolytes, and blood count before and throughout treatment. Note the presence of liver or endocrine dysfunction, or elevation in blood pressure.
- Note concomitant anticoagulant therapy.
- When a prepubertal child is treated, obtain hand and wrist x-rays before, every 6 months during, and after treatment to monitor growth.
- Appraise patient's expressive affect during therapy, particularly aggressiveness in patients taking large doses. Self-concept is an important consideration in the patient on androgen therapy, particularly in children with delayed puberty and in women.

Nursing Diagnoses
- Disturbed body image related to growth delay
- Delayed growth and development related to androgen deficiency
- Situational low self-esteem related to growth delay and/or virilizing effects of androgen therapy
- Sexual dysfunction related to androgen deficiency
- Ineffective sexuality pattern related to antiandrogen therapy and or delayed puberty
- Readiness for enhanced knowledge related to therapeutic regimen management

Planning
- Through collaboration, patient agrees to adhere to prescribed regimen for taking medication and for monitoring; use medication appropriately; report adverse effects immediately; and maintain positive self-concept during long-term treatment.

Patient Teaching
General
- Collaborate with patient and family on proper administration of medications, their reasons for use, and potential undesired effects. Review which effects warrant prompt medical attention (e.g., urinary problems, priapism, respiratory distress).
- Advise patient that an intermittent approach to treatment allows for monitoring of endocrine status between courses of androgen therapy. Explain need to return to health care facility for monitoring, and determine patient's ability to do so. Arrange social service referrals if necessary.
- Counsel family pursuing treatment for a child with delayed puberty about range of normal development.
- Advise patients being treated for tissue wasting to reduce environmental stressors and promote rest and relaxation, because stress hormones are catabolic.
- Encourage patient to monitor muscle strength during treatment.

Self-Administration
- Instruct patient to take oral androgens with food to decrease gastric distress.

Side Effects
- Coach patient about good skin hygiene to decrease severity of acne.
- Urge men undergoing androgen therapy to report priapism promptly so drug dosage can be reduced to avoid subsequent erectile dysfunction.
- Instruct men to report decreased urinary stream promptly so they can be evaluated for prostatic hypertrophy.

Diet
- Assess and review, as needed, nutritional intake of individuals with anemia, osteoporosis, or tissue wasting to ensure adequate intake of essential nutrients.
- Council patient to record body weight several times per week. Restrict sodium if edema develops.
- Advise patients with elevated serum calcium of the need to drink 2 L/day or more of fluid to prevent kidney stones. Individuals on bed rest need range-of-motion exercises, whereas ambulatory patients need to engage in active weight bearing. Hypercalcemia needs prompt medical attention, because it can lead to cardiac arrest.

Cultural Considerations
- Assess how patient's cultural group regards expression of sexuality.
- Ascertain any culturally defined expectations about male-female or male-male relationships, including health care relationship.
- Ask if patient has restrictions related to sexuality, exposure of body parts, or discussion of sexual functioning.

Evaluation
- Monitor patient's ability to adhere to treatment regimen and response to prescribed drugs. Ability to adhere to treatment plan and discuss treatment and effects knowledgeably suggests that teaching has been effective and that patient accepts treatment.
- Ask patient about therapeutic and adverse drug effects on follow-up visits. Monitoring of weight, blood pressure, and laboratory tests will continue throughout therapy, with alterations in the plan of care as needed.
- Periodically assess children and women who experience virilizing effects or acne for ability to cope with these changes and maintain a positive self-concept.
- Assess sexual function when appropriate.

Antiandrogens
Antiandrogens, or androgen antagonists, block the synthesis or action of androgens (Table 57-2). These drugs are used in the treatment of benign prostatic hypertrophy, advanced prostatic cancer, and as hormonal therapy in the treatment of endometriosis. They may also be used to treat male-pattern baldness, acne, hirsutism, virilization syndrome in women,

TABLE 57-2 ANTIANDROGENS

MECHANISM	DRUGS
Elevation of Gn-RH level	goserelin acetate (Zoladex) nafarelin acetate (Synarel) leuprolide acetate (Lupron, Viadur, Eligard)
Inhibition of testosterone synthesis	ketoconazole (Nizoral)
Blocks conversion of testosterone to dihydrotestosterone	finasteride (Proscar)
Receptor inhibitors	flutamide (Eulexin) bicalutamide (Casodex) spironolactone (Aldactone)

Gn-RH, Gonadotropin-releasing hormone.

and precocious puberty in boys, although their effectiveness is not well established. The effectiveness of these drugs to inhibit the sex drive of men who are sex offenders is controversial and not well documented.

Gonadotropin-releasing hormone (Gn-RH), or a synthetic analogue such as leuprolide, is the most effective inhibitor of testosterone synthesis. When such agents are given over time, LH and testosterone levels fall. Normally, Gn-RH is released in a pulsatile fashion, but the sustained activity of leuprolide leads to decreased production of FSH and LH. In the male, this activity stops testosterone production in the testis. In the female, it stops estrogen production in the ovaries. This drug should not be used in combination with herbal or dietary supplements, like black cohosh, DHEA, or chasteberry.

Ketoconazole, an antifungal drug, has testosterone-suppressing effects similar to those of Gn-RH analogues when given at doses higher than those required for antifungal activity. The mechanism of action of this non–Gn-RH drug is unclear. Gn-RH analogues act directly through their impact on testosterone production for the treatment of prostate cancer.

Flutamide is an oral nonsteroidal antiandrogen drug used as an antihormonal agent in the treatment of metastatic prostate cancer. It is most effective when used simultaneously with LHRH agonists such as leuprolide acetate. When used alone, the best response is seen in untreated patients. Flutamide is not effective in treating other hormonally dependent diseases such as breast cancer or benign prostatic hypertrophy. Flutamide competes with androgens at androgen receptor sites in the prostate gland, blocking the conversion of testosterone to dihydrotestosterone. By doing so, it prevents the androgens from stimulating the prostate cancer cells to grow. Men receiving flutamide show elevations in plasma LH and testosterone levels. Bicalutamide (Casodex) is structurally related to flutamide but has a long plasma half-life that allows once-daily dosing, compared with three times daily for flutamide. In addition, bicalutamide is more selective for the peripheral androgen receptor and has less activity at the central androgen receptor on the hypothalamic-pituitary axis.

Spironolactone (Aldactone) is a weak potassium-sparing diuretic used primarily to treat high blood pressure, heart failure, and ascites in patients with liver disease. While not FDA-approved indications, spironolactone has been used to treat acne vulgaris, polycystic ovary syndrome, and female hirsutism. Dosage ranges from 25 to 200 mg/day in divided doses with a maximum adult dose of 400 mg/day. It is a common component in hormone therapy for male-to-female transsexual and transgender surgical patients. It is also used for treating acne in women and can be used as a topical medication for treatment of male pattern baldness.

Finasteride (Propecia/Proscar), a synthetic compound, inhibits conversion of testosterone to 5-alpha-dihydrotestosterone (DHT). This orally active agent decreases the concentration of dihydrotestosterone in plasma and in the prostate without elevated plasma concentrations of LH or testosterone. Finasteride is used to treat benign prostatic hypertrophy (BPH) and male pattern baldness (MPB). The recommended 5-mg daily dose of Proscar for BPH needs to be reevaluated at 6 months and periodically thereafter. The 1-mg dose of Propecia for MPB is taken once a day for 12 months. Continued treatment is recommended for sustained results. Following discontinuation of therapy, reversal of effect is typically seen within 1 year. Adverse reactions include impotence, decreased libido, and decreased ejaculate. Women of childbearing age must not use finasteride and should not handle crushed or broken tablets because the active ingredient may cause abnormalities of a male fetus's sex organs.

Drugs Used in Other Male Reproductive Disorders

Delayed Puberty

A height of two or more standard deviations below the mean for age and sex occurs in 2.5% of normal children. Delay in growth may be a normal part of the maturation process. However, the cause could be androgen deficiency or a deficiency of growth hormone. Secretion of Gn-RH, LH, or FSH is insufficient in up to 5% of cases of **delayed puberty.** Treatment is not initiated before 14 years of age and after a full evaluation. Therapy for 3 to 6 months or less before epiphyseal closure may result in linear growth without adverse permanent effects on hypothalamic, pituitary, or gonadal maturation.

Pituitary, Thyroid, and Adrenal Disorders

Inadequate pituitary function can be another cause of hypogonadism. Menotropins (Menopur, Pergonal, Repronex) are purified combination preparations of the human pituitary gonadotropins, FSH and LH. These drugs are indicated when both LH and FSH levels are low. They encourage spermatogenesis in males with primary or secondary hypogonadism and induce ovulation in anovulatory females. To induce ovulation, Menotropins is given concomitantly with hCG 5,000 to 10,000 IU IM twice a week for at least 3 months. The drug will stimulate testosterone production in men to encourage spermatogenesis when injected three times a week for 4 to 9 months to ensure adequate spermatozoa production. One ampule of Menotropins contains 75 international units (IU) each of LH and FSH. The initial dose is 150 IU SQ/IM once daily for 5 days. Adjust subsequent dose to individual response at intervals no less than every 2 days and not exceeding 75 to 150 IU/adjustment; maximum dose is 450 IU/day. Use lower abdomen (alternating sides) for SQ administration. It must be used immediately after reconstitution and protected from light. Advise patients to discard unused medication. Adverse effects include nausea, vomiting, diarrhea, gynecomastia, and fever.

Inadequate thyroid and adrenal gland function can also affect sexuality. **Hypothyroidism,** a deficiency in thyroid hormone, can be the result of insufficient thyroid hormone production or resistance to its effects at the target organs. The problem can be congenital or acquired. It can cause **inhibited sexual desire** (decreased or lack of interest in sexual activity) and erectile dysfunction. In **Addison's disease**, there is a deficit of both cortisol and the mineralocorticoid aldosterone. Men with Addison disease may experience inhibited sexual desire, erectile dysfunction, or diminished fertility. Both hypothyroidism and Addison's disease are conditions highly responsive to replacement therapy with the appropriate hormones. (Refer to Chapter 51 for discussion of Addison's disease.)

Sexual Dysfunction

Sexual dysfunction is the inability to experience sexual desire, erection, ejaculation, and/or detumescence—the phases of the sexual response cycle. Inhibited sexual desire can result from androgen deficiency, an affective disorder, or discord in the sexual relationship. Many drugs can cause sexual dysfunction (Table 57-3).

Ejaculatory dysfunction (impaired ejection of seminal fluid from the male urethra) can be psychogenic or a result of drug therapy, androgen deficiency, or sympathetic degeneration. Failure of detumescence (reduction of penile engorgement) is most commonly caused by penile disease, systemic disease, trauma, or adverse effects of drugs. Individuals who experience premature ejaculation related to excessive anxiety about sexual intercourse may be helped by treatment with one of the many antidepressants alone or in conjunction with psychotherapy.

Erectile dysfunction (ED) is the inability to achieve or maintain an erection satisfactory for sexual performance. ED happens when not enough blood flows to the penis during sexual stimulation. This may be caused by psychoemotional problems, diabetes, hypertension, lower urinary tract symptoms, a history of pelvic surgery, vascular insufficiency, neurologic disorders, androgen deficiency or resistance, or diseases of the penis. Erectile dysfunction caused by vascular insufficiency is occasionally treated on a short-term basis by local vasoactive drugs, including papaverine, phentolamine, prostaglandin E, and nitroglycerin. Other medication options for the treatment of ED include oral medications, drugs injected into the penis, intraurethral alprostadil, or the male hormone testosterone.

TABLE 57-3 DRUGS THAT CAUSE SEXUAL DYSFUNCTION IN MALES

DRUG CATEGORY	DRUGS OR DRUG FAMILIES
Anticholinergics	atropine scopolamine benztropine trihexyphenidyl
Antidepressants	tricyclic antidepressants monoamine oxidase inhibitors selective serotonin reuptake inhibitors
Antihistamines	diphenhydramine hydroxyzine
Antihypertensives	centrally acting alpha$_2$ agonists alpha- and beta-receptor blockers diuretics angiotensin-converting enzyme inhibitors
Antipsychotics	phenothiazines thioxanthenes butyrophenone
Antiulcer drugs	cimetidine ranitidine famotidine
Sedatives and recreational drugs	alcohol barbiturates diazepam chlordiazepoxide cannabis cocaine opiates methadone
Others	aminocaproic acid baclofen steroids ethionamide digoxin chemotherapeutic agents lithium

A class of drugs called phosphodiesterase (PDE) inhibitors facilitates erections by enhancing blood flow to the penis. PDE-5 inhibitors are currently the most commonly used medical treatment for ED. These medications have a high success rate, are easy to use, and often result in erection when sexually stimulated. The PDE-5 inhibitors currently approved by the FDA are sildenafil (Viagra/Revatio), tadalafil (Cialis), vardenafil (Levitra/Staxyn) and avanafil (Stendra). PDE inhibitors are taken before sexual activity with variations in effective start time and duration of benefit (Table 57-4).

Nitroglycerin and other nitrate medications used to treat heart disease can cause a significant decrease in blood pressure when taken with PDE-5 inhibitors. Therefore, this class of drugs is contraindicated for use by any patient using organic nitrates in any form. Patients with a prescription for PRN sublingual nitroglycerin can take PDE inhibitors, but should still be cautioned about taking them concomitantly. Organic nitrates include nitroglycerin, isosorbide

TABLE 57-4 PDE-5 INHIBITORS FOR ERECTILE DYSFUNCTION

GENERIC (BRAND)	ONSET/ DURATION	SIDE EFFECTS	DRUG INTERACTIONS
sildenafil 20 mg (Viagra, Revatio); works best on an empty stomach	Onset: 30-60 min Duration: 4 h	• Abdominal symptoms, such as diarrhea, heartburn, and upset stomach • Abnormal vision, such as blurring, sensitivity to light and blue-green color tint • Dizziness • Flushing • Headache • Nasal congestion	• Nitrates: isosorbide, nitroglycerin, amyl nitrate, butyl nitrate • Alpha blockers: alfuzosin, doxazosin, prazosin, tamsulosin, terazosin, amiodarone • Antiinfective agents: fluconazole, itraconazole, ketoconazole, clarithromycin, moxifloxacin, erythromycin • Cardiac medications: disopyramide, procainamide, quinidine, sotalol, thioridazine, verapamil • HIV protease inhibitors: atazanavir, indinavir, ritonavir, saquinavir • Other medications: methadone, pimozide, haloperidol
tadalafil 5 mg (Cialis), avanafil 50-200 mg; not affected by food	Onset: 15-60 min Duration: 24-36 h		
vardenafil 5 mg (Levitra, Staxyn); less effective with a high-fat meal	Onset: 25-30 min Duration: 4-5 hours Use once in 24 h		

h, Hour; *min,* minute.

mononitrate, isosorbide nitrate, pentaerythritol tetranitrate, erythrityl tetranitrate, isosorbide dinitrate/phenobarbital, and illicit substances (amyl nitrate/nitrite, butyl nitrate). Sildenafil is contraindicated in patients with significant cardiovascular disease or individuals who have anatomic deformities or conditions predisposing them to priapism.

Studies have shown that vardenafil (Levitra) and tadalafil (Cialis) are safer for patients with heart failure or a history of myocardial infarctions. Like sildenafil, they are contraindicated if the patient is taking nitrate-containing medications. Common side effects of these drugs are headache (most common), dyspepsia, nasal congestion, and nasopharyngitis. Other rare side effects can also occur, and the patient should be taught about them. These effects include blurred vision, photosensitivity, changes in color perception (especially blue and green), and urinary tract symptoms such as frequency or painful urination, and cloudy or bloody urine. Patients are instructed to notify their health care provider of any side effects they experience.

The PDE-5 inhibitors interact with grapefruit juice and grapefruit products by increasing the amount of the PDE-5 inhibitor absorbed, thereby increasing the risk of side effects. Many medications may interact with PDE-5 inhibitors, so be sure to obtain a complete list of medications taken by the patient.

Certain drugs are often abused by individuals seeking a heightened sexual experience. Amyl nitrate is commonly believed to be an aphrodisiac. Sudden death, myocardial infarction, and methemoglobinemia have been reported with its use. Cantharides (Spanish fly) causes bladder and urethral irritation, accounting for its use as a sexual stimulant. Permanent penile damage has been reported with its use.

SAFETY: Preventing Medication Errors

Do not confuse ...

- **Lupron Depot-3 Month** with **Lupron Depot-Ped**
- **Testoderm** with **Testoderm TTS**
- **anabolic steroids** with **corticosteroids**

Natural Products. To self-treat sexual problems or to enhance their sexual performance, consumers use a wide variety of herbs and plant-derived compounds (phytochemicals). Despite new science-based therapies, men are attracted to phytochemicals because they are easy to obtain and may be cheaper than prescription medications, therapies, procedures, or surgeries not covered by insurance. Consumers may perceive natural products as providing health benefits beyond sexual performance because they can be purchased at nutrition centers or health food stores. Common herbs used for sexual health and performance include yohimbine, ginseng, damiana, ginkgo biloba, saw palmetto, muira puama, and Tribulus terrestris. With the exception of yohimbine, which has been scientifically studied, the other compounds do not have benefits proven by research. Their benefits appear to reflect popular or cultural beliefs. Reports in health magazines and advertising are anecdotal and based on a small number of users or health care professionals.

Yohimbine, which is obtained from the bark of the African yohimbe tree, is an alpha-adrenergic antagonist that affects both the central and peripheral nervous system. Studies have shown that men experience a positive effect or improvement in erection. The side effects are headache, hypertension, sweating, anxiety, and sleeplessness. Men who have cardiovascular, neurologic, or psychological problems should not take yohimbine.

Saw palmetto is a popular herbal remedy used to treat symptoms related to BPH and can help shrink enlarged prostate glands. Although effective in the treatment of prostate enlargement, it has not been shown to exert a positive effect on sexual response in men unless erections are inhibited by an enlarged prostate gland. In fact, saw palmetto may reduce androgen action and have a negative effect on sexual response.

Ginkgo biloba leaves have been shown to treat peripheral vascular disease and enhance cerebral blood flow. Research suggests that ginkgo biloba may reduce antidepressant–induced sexual dysfunction caused by selective serotonin reuptake inhibitors. It is not known how it achieves these effects, and further research is needed to substantiate its use. Similarly, ginseng has been shown to improve sexual functioning in animals, but research in humans is contradictory, and further human research is warranted.

Non–Sexually Transmitted Infections

Drugs used to treat acute or chronic prostatitis, orchitis, or epididymitis are the same as those used to treat urinary tract infections (see Chapter 34).

Benign Prostate Hyperplasia

As a man ages, the glandular units in the prostate gland begin to undergo tissue hyperplasia (abnormal increase in the number of cells), resulting in prostatic hypertrophy (enlargement of the gland). The exact cause of BPH is unknown, but its development is almost universal in older men. The enlarged prostate gland contributes to overall lower urinary tract symptoms either through direct bladder outlet obstruction or from resistance within the enlarged gland itself. The man experiences storage and/or voiding disturbances, such as a sensation of bladder fullness, frequency, nocturia, hesitation when trying to begin urinating, dribbling of urine, and erectile dysfunction. Although BPH is not a life-threatening condition, the impact of symptoms on quality of life can be significant. Because these are the same symptoms that prostate cancer may cause, the patient should have a prostate-specific antigen (PSA) blood test and may undergo a prostate biopsy to make sure no cancer is present. Traditionally, the primary goal of treatment has been to alleviate bothersome symptoms. More recently, treatment has also been focused on the alteration of disease progression and prevention of complications. A variety of pharmacologic classes are employed, including alpha-adrenergic antagonists (alpha-blockers), 5-alpha-reductase inhibitors (5-ARIs), anticholinergics, phytotherapeutics, and (most recently) the PDE-5 inhibitor tadalafil. Choosing the correct medical treatment for BPH is complex (Table 57-5). The American Urological Association 2010 Guidelines are a useful reference on the effective evidence-based management of lower urinary tract symptoms caused by BPH. The guidelines advise a discussion of benefits and risks of each recommended treatment alternative (e.g., watchful waiting, medical, surgical, or minimally invasive surgical treatments). The choice of treatment is reached in a shared decision-making process between provider and patient.

With initiation of drug therapy, the patient should be followed every 1 to 3 months, depending on the class of medication chosen, to assess success and inquire about side effects. The patient with an enlarged prostate should avoid medications that can cause urinary retention, such as anticholinergics, antihistamines, and decongestants.

Malignant Tumors

Prostatic cancer accounts for about 10% of all cancer deaths among American men. Most prostatic cancers are adenocarcinomas. Metastasis to lymph nodes, bone, lungs, liver, and

TABLE 57-5 MEDICATIONS USED FOR TREATMENT OF BPH

GENERIC (BRAND)	ROUTE AND DOSAGE	SIDE EFFECTS
5-Alpha-Reductase Inhibitors		
finasteride (Proscar)	PO: 5 mg	Decreased libido, erectile dysfunction
duastride (Avodart)	PO: 0.5 mg	
Safety in Administration		
Caution patients that women of childbearing age must not handle crushed or broken tablets due to possible absorption and potential risk to male fetus; immediately wash contact area with soap and water if contact occurs. Inform patients of increase in high-grade prostate cancer in men treated with 5α-reductase inhibitors indicated for BPH treatment. Inform patients that volume of ejaculate may be decreased and impotence/decreased libido may occur. Instruct to promptly report to physician any changes in breasts (lumps, pain, or nipple discharge).		
Alpha-Adrenergic Blocking Agents		
tamsulosin (Flomax)	PO: 0.4 mg/d 30 min after a meal; titrate up to 0.8 mg/d	Postural hypotension, dizziness, fatigue
doxazosin (Cardura)	PO: Start 1 mg/d h.s.; titrate up to 8 mg/d h.s.	
terazosin (Hytrin)	A: PO: Start 1 mg/d h.s.; titrate up to 10 mg/d *max:* 20 mg/d	
alfuzosin (Uroxatral)	PO: 10 mg/d after a meal	
silodosin (Rapaflo)	PO: 8 mg/d with a meal	
Safety in Administration		
Alpha-adrenergic blocking agents are also used to control blood pressure. To avoid hypotensive episode, advise using at bedtime and reconcile all medications taken before adding another antihypertensive drug. Instruct patient to take medication with food. Counsel about possible symptoms of postural hypotension (dizziness); caution about driving, operating machinery, or performing hazardous tasks. Inform patient that orgasm with reduced or no semen does not pose a safety concern and is reversible when drug is stopped. Advise patient to notify ophthalmologist about use before cataract surgery or other eye procedures.		
PDE-5 Inhibitors		
tadalafil (Cialis)	PO: 5 mg	See Table 57-4
Safety in Administration		
Should not be used by patients taking nitrates such as nitroglycerin because the combination may trigger an unsafe drop in blood pressure. Also tadalafil should not be used with alpha-blockers for the treatment of BPH because the combo therapy has not been adequately studied and may increase the risk of lowering blood pressure.		

d, Day; *h.s.,* at bedtime; *min,* minute.

adrenal glands is common. Prostatic cancer is often asymptomatic, but urinary obstruction is commonly the first sign. Treatment may include a combination of surgical resection, cryotherapy, antiandrogen administration, radiation therapy, chemotherapy, and pain management.

Testicular tumors peak in early adulthood. They include malignant germinal cell tumors and benign Leydig or Sertoli cell tumors. Treatment depends on the type and stage of tumor. Surgical excision, radiation therapy, and chemotherapy are used alone or in combination.

Approximately 1% of breast cancer cases occur in men, most commonly after age 60 years. Treatment, which is similar for men and women, entails surgery, radiation therapy, chemotherapy, and endocrine therapy. Carcinoma of the penis represents less than 1% of all malignancies among men. In situ, treatment entails local excision, radiation therapy, and local application of 5-fluorouracil cream or solution. Invasive carcinoma is treated by surgical resection of the penis and involved nodes. Radiation and chemotherapy follow as needed.

KEY WEBSITES

Harvard Men's Health Watch: *www.health.harvard.edu*

Sexuality Information and Education Council of the United States: *www.siecus.org*

CRITICAL THINKING CASE STUDY

MT, age 16 years, is a high school junior who is 59.3 inches tall and weighs 126 lb. He is having increased feelings of discomfort about not fitting in with the other students at school because he has not yet begun sexual maturation. He is a good student and an accomplished violinist in the school orchestra. His father states that he also was a "late bloomer," but both parents are concerned about MT's increasing social withdrawal and seem determined to seek medical intervention for him. The nurse at the clinic assesses the needs and status of MT and his parents.

1. What is the patient's primary complaint?
2. What is concerning his parents?
3. What information must be included in the history and physical examination?
4. What education should the nurse prepare before the parents decide whether to start their son on androgen therapy?

   The decision is made to prescribe methyltestosterone (Striant) 30 mg twice daily by buccal tablet (held inside the cheek until it dissolves). MT will be on this regimen for 4 months, during which time he is to come to the clinic at monthly intervals.
5. MT asks why he will be treated for 4 months. What will the nurse reply?
6. About what adverse effects do MT and his parents need to be educated?
7. What physical and psychosocial parameters will be assessed at MT's monthly visits?
8. What special hygiene needs does MT have while on this regimen?
9. When should MT have x-rays taken? Explain your answer.
10. During a clinical visit, MT mentions that he heard that the use of anabolic steroids might improve his chances of making the wrestling team. What should he be told about the safety and efficacy of anabolic steroid use?

NCLEX STUDY QUESTIONS

1. A young male patient is referred to the nurse for initiation of intramuscular androgen therapy for hypogonadism. What information should the nurse give this patient? (Select all that apply.)
   a. A 4- to 6-month trial of androgen therapy will be followed by a period of rest for reevaluation.
   b. Sexual development will begin to occur immediately.
   c. Dosages may be adjusted based on periodic plasma testosterone levels.
   d. His growth will be monitored periodically by x-ray.
   e. The patient should not consume alcohol.
2. A married man with two daughters is taking finasteride (Proscar) to treat BPH. Which nursing assessment data are most critical in developing a care plan? (Select all that apply.)
   a. His spouse and children should not handle the drug.
   b. The drug may cause decreased libido and urinary retention.
   c. The dose needs to be reevaluated periodically.
   d. This drug may also cause his hair to grow.
   e. Using finasteride will not increase his risk for developing prostate cancer.
3. The nurse is discussing androgen therapy with a patient. Which statements will the nurse include in the patient education? (Select all that apply.)
   a. "Lower extremity edema associated with androgen therapy can be increased by corticosteroids."
   b. "Only men are prescribed androgen replacement therapy."

c. "Androgen therapy is safe in pregnancy."
d. "Androgen therapy can affect your glucose levels, cholesterol, and thyroid and liver functioning."
e. "Androgen therapy may cause seizures."

4. A man is taking androgen therapy for angioneurotic edema. He is complaining of nausea, increased urination, and loss of muscle tone. Which nursing advice has the highest priority?
   a. "Make an appointment to see the prescribing clinician within 5 to 7 days."
   b. "Follow a clear liquid diet for 24 hours."
   c. "Call 911 for immediate transport to the emergency department."
   d. "Sign up for an exercise group at the local health club."
5. During his annual physical examination, a patient tells the nurse he is in a new relationship and having some problems with erectile dysfunction. He is interested in nutrition and natural therapies. Which are the most appropriate responses by the nurse? (Select all that apply.)
   a. "Herbal therapies are commonly used by men to enhance sexual performance."
   b. "Side effects from using some herbal therapies include increased anxiety, frequent headaches, and trouble sleeping."
   c. "Phytochemicals have been widely researched and are safe to use."
   d. "Men who have cardiovascular, neurologic, or psychological problems should not use some of the herbal products."
   e. "It's a good idea to increase your intake of dietary vitamins."
6. The nurse is interviewing a man with erectile dysfunction who is interested in one of the phosphodiesterase inhibitors. Which response by the nurse is best for this patient?
   a. "The onset of action varies among the different drugs in this class."
   b. "These medications should not be used if you take nitroglycerine for angina."
   c. "Common side effects include headache, blurred vision, photosensitivity, changes in color perception, and urinary tract symptoms."
   d. "There are many causes of sexual dysfunction in men, so a complete history and physical is the first step in treatment."
7. A 17-year-old patient is brought to the health care provider by his father because he has been taking nutritional supplements sold at the gym. Which assessment data are most critical in developing a care plan for this patient? (Select all that apply.)
   a. His blood pressure is low.
   b. His acne is worsening.
   c. He has been in several fist fights with other teenagers.
   d. He has gained 60 pounds.
   e. His liver function tests are abnormal.
8. A patient with AIDS has been started on testosterone for tissue wasting and loss of muscle tone. Which report from the patient is the nurse's highest priority concern?
   a. He reports that his muscle strength is about the same.
   b. He reports that he has morning erections lasting 30 minutes.
   c. He reports that he was out dancing last weekend.
   d. He reports that he has decided to become a vegetarian.
9. A male patient presents with complaints of lower urinary tract symptoms, getting up three times at night to urinate, dribbling after urination, and feeling pressure throughout the day. Recent screening laboratory tests are normal. The provider starts him on doxazosin (Cardura) 1 mg at bedtime. What advice can the nurse give this patient? (Select all that apply.)
   a. Advise the patient about signs and symptoms of low blood pressure.
   b. Tell the patient to notify his ophthalmologist about the doxazosin use before cataract surgery.
   c. Caution the patient that he should not allow his wife to handle the medicine.
   d. Advise the patient to immediately report problems of prolonged erection.
   e. Instruct the patient to take the medication on an empty stomach.

Answers: 1, a, c, d; 2, a, b, c, d; 3, a, d; 4, c; 5, a, b, d; 6, d; 7, b, c, d, e; 8, b; 9, a, b, d.

CHAPTER

58

Drugs for Disorders in Women's Health, Infertility, and Sexually Transmitted Infections

evolve WEBSITE

http://evolve.elsevier.com/KeeHayes/pharmacology/

- Animations
- Content Updates
- Key Points
- Review Questions for the NCLEX® Examination
- References from the Textbook
- Unfolding Case Studies

OBJECTIVES

- Explain the pathophysiology of conditions in women's health, pharmacologic therapies, and expected outcomes of pharmacologic therapies.
- Describe pharmacologic interventions targeting common pathogens causing vulvovaginal infections.
- Understand pharmacologic interventions used in the treatment of infertility in the male and female patient individually and as a couple attempting pregnancy.
- Describe the mechanism of action for ovulatory stimulation therapy.
- Identify drug therapies used for common gynecologic conditions such as dysfunctional uterine bleeding, endometriosis, dysmenorrhea, and premenstrual syndrome.
- Describe the pharmacologic intervention for sexually transmitted infections (STIs) caused by bacterial agents, viral agents, parasites, and other pathogens.
- Describe the nursing process, including teaching, related to drugs used in women's health, infertility, and the treatment of STIs.

OUTLINE

The authors gratefully acknowledge the work of Marcia Welsh, who updated this chapter for the eighth edition.

KEY TERMS

amenorrhea, p. 886
anovulatory cycles, p. 887
dysfunctional uterine bleeding, p. 886
dysmenorrhea, p. 888
endometriosis, p. 889
infertility, p. 893
menometrorrhagia, p. 887
menorrhagia, p. 887
metrorrhagia, p. 887
oligospermia, p. 898
pelvic inflammatory disease, p. 888
polycystic ovarian syndrome, p. 887
premenstrual syndrome, p. 890
sexually transmitted infections, p. 886
vaginitis, p. 891
vaginosis, p. 891
varicocele, p. 898

This chapter discusses the pathophysiology and typical drug regimens for disorders in women's health, including **sexually transmitted infections** (STIs). These gynecologic conditions interfere with a woman's overall health and well-being and may impede a woman's ability to become pregnant. Many of the medications discussed in Chapter 56 may also be used for relief of menstrual disorders and other gynecologic problems. Drugs for female and male infertility are also addressed, with an emphasis on medications that stimulate ovulation.

Sexually transmitted diseases are a threat to reproductive tract integrity and functioning, and to neonatal health. Not only do STIs affect the short-term and long-term health of a woman and her partner(s), they also are detrimental to the health of a community. Some STIs, such as human immunodeficiency virus (HIV), are life-threatening. Drug therapies that are recommended by the Centers for Disease Control and Prevention (CDC) for the treatment of specific STIs are reviewed.

MEDICATIONS USED TO TREAT DISORDERS IN WOMEN'S HEALTH

Common reasons women seek gynecologic health care include alterations in menstrual cycle, menstrual or pelvic pain, and changes in vaginal secretions. Included within these broad categories are irregular uterine bleeding, dysmenorrhea, premenstrual syndrome, and vulvovaginal infections. This section describes common disorders in women's health and presents current pharmacologic approaches to management.

Irregular or Abnormal Uterine Bleeding

Irregular uterine bleeding is a term that describes many different medical conditions or pathologies related to the menstrual cycle. Irregular uterine bleeding, also known as *abnormal uterine bleeding* (AUB), is a common reason women seek gynecologic care. AUB encompasses a wide range of variable bleeding patterns in women, such as amenorrhea, menorrhagia, metrorrhagia, menometrorrhagia, intramenstrual bleeding, and **dysfunctional uterine bleeding** (DUB).

Amenorrhea

Amenorrhea is the absence of menses. *Primary amenorrhea* is defined as no menses by age 14 years of age *without* secondary sex characteristics, or no menses by age 16 years *with* secondary sex characteristics. Primary amenorrhea may be caused by abnormalities in the structures of the female reproductive tract, chromosomal alterations, or endocrine disorders. Many times the cause is just a physiologic delay in the onset of menstruation. *Secondary amenorrhea* is the absence of a spontaneous menstrual period for 6 consecutive months in women who have experienced menstrual cycles in the past. Pregnancy is the most common reason a patient may experience amenorrhea, and breastfeeding or menopausal patients also may not menstruate; therefore, secondary amenorrhea is a *symptom* of these normal physiologic processes. Other causes of secondary amenorrhea include anovulatory cycles (cycles without ovulation), hypothyroidism or hyperthyroidism, and hyperprolactinemia (high levels of the hormone prolactin, which stimulates lactation). Extreme weight loss and anorexia can also cause amenorrhea.

After assessment of the patient's health history, a physical examination, and after pregnancy has been ruled out, a *progestational challenge test* may be administered to determine the underlying cause of amenorrhea. This test uses an oral progestin administered for a limited time to confirm that the hypothalamus-pituitary-ovarian (HPO) responses (the hormonal system mediating the menstrual cycle) are intact.

With the progestational challenge test, a patient is given either micronized progesterone (Prometrium) 400 mg by mouth (PO) at bedtime for 10 days or medroxyprogesterone acetate (Provera) 5 to 10 mg PO for 5 to 10 days. The progestational activity thickens the endometrial lining and increases secretory activity. When the medication is discontinued, progesterone levels decrease, resulting in a breakdown of the endometrial lining and withdrawal bleeding. Withdrawal bleeding should occur within 7 to 10 days after completing the medication and indicates that the HPO axis (the menstrual cycle) is functioning in providing the hormones necessary to regulate the menstrual cycle. Even the smallest amount of bleeding (one incidence of scant spotting) is considered a positive test. However, if there is no withdrawal bleeding, other pathophysiologic problems may exist and further evaluation and diagnostic testing by the health care provider are needed. Micronized progesterone contains peanut oil and thus is contraindicated in those with peanut allergies. The test can also be administered using a combined hormone contraception (CHC) product if the patient desires a form of contraception. The patient starts the CHC method as directed and should have withdrawal menses during the hormone-free phase.

Metabolic Syndrome

Another common cause of secondary amenorrhea is **polycystic ovarian syndrome** (PCOS). PCOS is a form of metabolic syndrome caused by the oversecretion of luteinizing hormone (LH). LH is the hormone responsible for stimulating ovulation, or mid-cycle release of an ovum from the dominant follicle in the ovary. Oversecretion of LH causes the formation of several follicular cysts in the ovaries instead of one dominant follicle. The presence of several follicles increases estrogen levels; however, ovulation does not occur. The cycle then becomes **anovulatory** (the absence of ovulation), and the luteal phase, or the second half of the menstrual cycle in which progesterone is dominant, is inhibited. The endometrium of the uterus is exposed to "unopposed" estrogen from the anovulatory cycles. *Unopposed estrogen* refers to levels of estrogen that are not balanced by a progestational (progesterone) effect. Unopposed estrogen can cause abnormal thickening of the endometrial lining, increasing the patient's risk for endometrial hyperplasia and uterine cancer. In women experiencing secondary amenorrhea, the incidence of PCOS may approach 30% as the cause of sequentially missed or irregular periods. These patients will complain of skipped menstrual cycles, long menstrual cycles (35 days or greater) or no menstruation for several months.

Insulin resistance is a hallmark of PCOS. Insulin resistance is the body's inability to respond to elevated glucose levels. Although insulin is secreted when glucose levels are high, "resistance" to the insulin results in altered glucose metabolism and hyperinsulinemia. Hyperinsulinemia causes higher levels of circulating androgens and predisposes the patient to alterations in lipid metabolism, cardiac disease, and type 2 diabetes mellitus. Women present with one or more of these symptoms: amenorrhea, hirsutism, acne, acanthosis nigricans (increased pigmentation and thickening of the skin, particularly in skinfold areas), or excessive fat along the midsection of the body. PCOS is a common cause of infertility because of the anovulatory cycles.

Pharmacologic treatment of PCOS depends on whether the patient desires pregnancy. If the patient wants to prevent pregnancy, estrogen-progestin combination contraception products are prescribed if the patient is a candidate. CHC products suppress LH and follicle-stimulating hormone (FSH) secretion, limit androgen symptoms, and regulate menstruation by providing a withdrawal bleeding period. With the addition of the progestin in the CHC product and a cycling of a monthly (or 4 times per year, depending on product) withdrawal menses, the risks of unopposed estrogen on the endometrium are significantly reduced.

For women who are attempting to conceive, two drugs, metformin and clomiphene citrate, are used. Metformin (Glucophage) inhibits the production of glucose in the liver and increases peripheral cell sensitivity to insulin, effectively treating insulin resistance and decreasing androgen levels. Metformin administration independently regulates the menstrual period and increases the possibility of ovulation. Metformin is initially prescribed as 500 mg, 1 tablet taken PO twice daily (b.i.d.), and may be increased to 850 mg b.i.d. Because metformin may decrease absorption of vitamin B_{12}, women should be assessed for vitamin B_{12} deficiency. Metformin also has gastrointestinal (GI) side effects (see Chapter 52).

Clomiphene citrate (Clomid or Serophene) is used in conjunction with metformin, or alone to promote a dominant follicle and induce ovulation; it is described in "Medications Used to Promote Fertility."

Abnormal Uterine Bleeding Patterns

The normal menstrual cycle occurs every 25 to 35 days and lasts 2 to 7 days, with an estimated blood loss of no more than 80 mL. **Menorrhagia** is *regular* uterine bleeding greater than 80 mL or lasting more than 7 days. Women with menorrhagia may describe their periods as very heavy or state the need to change a tampon or sanitary pad frequently. **Metrorrhagia** is *irregular* uterine bleeding greater than 80 mL or lasting more than 7 days. Women with menorrhagia describe their periods as irregular and heavy. They may state that they have no idea when bleeding will occur, and that when it does happen it will soak through sanitary products or clothing. **Menometrorrhagia** is a combination of these two. Intramenstrual bleeding is an episode of bleeding, usually light, that occurs between menstrual periods.

A common complaint that brings a woman into the gynecologic health care setting is that she is having menstrual cycles that are suddenly different from the pattern she usually experiences. In women of reproductive age, pregnancy should always be considered first as the possible cause of AUB. However, AUB can result from physiologic processes such as stress, severe dieting and weight loss, eating disorders, or excessive exercise. Irregular bleeding patterns are a sign of decreasing ovarian function or approach of menopause in older women. AUB can also be caused by pathologic processes such as endocrine disorders, thyroid disease, leiomyomata (benign tumors in the uterus), ovarian cysts, infections of the genital tract, or cancer. If a woman is pregnant, uterine bleeding may indicate ectopic pregnancy or impending miscarriage. Some pharmacologic medications, substances, and herbal preparations can also cause irregular bleeding, including anticoagulants, antipsychotics, benzodiazepines, hormone therapy, ginkgo, ginseng, and soy products. Once physiologic, pathologic, and pharmaceutic causes have been ruled out, the patient may be diagnosed with DUB.

Dysfunctional Uterine Bleeding

DUB is the most common classification of irregular bleeding. Diagnosis of DUB is made when no organic pathology can be determined to cause the irregular bleeding. Pharmacologic treatment of DUB primarily involves normalizing the bleeding pattern and correcting anemia that may have resulted from chronic or acute blood loss. In the normal physiologic menstrual cycle, estrogen and progesterone levels are low during menstruation. Once estrogen levels start to rise with the formation of a dominant follicle, uterine bleeding is effectively stopped, ending menstruation. Increasing levels of estrogen by administration of an extraneous estrogen drug product is usually effective in stopping prolonged DUB.

Since estrogen is never used alone in treatment (because of the detrimental effects of unopposed estrogen on the uterine endometrium and the risk for endometrial cancer), estrogen-progestin combination products are used. Progestins alone are not as effective as estrogen in reducing an episode of acute bleeding; however, because *prolonged* progestin administration causes atrophy of the endometrial lining, they can be very effective if long-term control is needed. Depot-medroxyprogesterone acetate (Depo-Provera) intramuscular (IM) injection or IUS/LNG (Mirena) inserted into the uterus are the products used for extended progestin therapy.

Pharmacologic Management of Irregular Bleeding

Nonsteroidal antiinflammatory drugs (NSAIDs) can be used for the treatment of menorrhagia. The mechanism of action for the management of uterine bleeding is not well understood. NSAIDs block the production of prostaglandin, which decreases both excessive bleeding and uterine cramps. Common NSAIDs used for menorrhagia are mefanamic acid (Ponstel), ibuprofen, and naproxen sodium. Only mefanamic acid has U.S. Food and Drug Administration (FDA) approval for menorrhagia. Ibuprofen and naproxen sodium are used by providers as an "off-label" option. The correct dosage of mefanamic acid is 500 mg PO once, followed by 250 mg PO every 6 hours for 2 to 3 days. Mefanamic acid should be taken with food.

CHC products can be used to decrease and regulate DUB. Monophasic products and products that have a dosage schedule of 21/7, 24/4, or 84/7 (see Chapter 56) are first-line drug therapy if the patient is a candidate for CHC products. The increase in estrogen stops uterine bleeding and maintains the endometrial lining. Withdrawal bleeding is cycled in to regulate periods of bleeding. If bleeding does not respond, the CHC can be increased to a schedule of 1 pill PO twice daily for 5 to 7 days, or until the bleeding stops, then 1 pill PO daily for 21 days. Reduction in flow should be seen within 24 hours. If a heavy flow continues for more than 48 hours, the patient should be reevaluated. Benefits, risks, and patient instructions are the same as if the product were being used for contraception. Women who are not a candidate for estrogen therapy or CHC products should excluded. Women using a CHC product for DUB should see their periods normalize within the first 3 months of use. The patient can continue the method for contraception or discontinue use in 6 to 9 months, depending on the effectiveness in controlling bleeding.

Progestins are not as effective as estrogens at reducing episodes of irregular bleeding. However, progestins are effective in the long-term treatment of AUB and may be the method of choice in women who have contraindications to estrogen use. Progestins can be given cyclically (e.g., norethindrone acetate 5 mg PO daily for 10 to 14 days) to produce a monthly withdrawal bleed, or in a continuous dose (e.g., medroxyprogesterone acetate 5 to 10 mg PO daily). Medroxyprogesterone acetate, norethindrone, and micronized progesterone are used in this manner. Depot-medroxyprogesterone acetate and the LNG-IUS are also be used for treatment of DUB. Long-term use of progesterone has an atrophic effect on the uterine endometrium, consequently decreasing incidences of irregular bleeding. Women using depot-medroxyprogesterone acetate or the LNG-IUS for DUB should see heavy bleeding patterns decrease within 3 to 6 months.

Dysmenorrhea

Dysmenorrhea is pelvic pain associated with the menstrual cycle. It is also called cyclic pelvic pain (CPP). Other symptoms that may occur are uterine cramping, lower back pain, abdominal cramps, changes in bowel patterns, increased bowel movements, and nausea and vomiting. Dysmenorrhea is experienced by approximately 80% of women in their late teens and early twenties, when it is more prevalent. It is the most common reason young women miss school or work. Dysmenorrhea is classified as either primary dysmenorrhea or secondary dysmenorrhea, depending on whether there is a known etiology for the menstrual pain. Primary dysmenorrhea is diagnosed when there is no apparent underlying pathology. It is caused by larger-than-normal amounts of prostaglandins at the start of the menstrual period. Prostaglandins cause arterioles in the uterus to contract, decreasing blood flow to the endometrium. All of these mechanisms are necessary for breakdown of the endometrial lining and for menstruation to occur. However, this process causes increased pain in some women.

In secondary dysmenorrhea, there is an underlying cause for the pelvic pain. Conditions that may cause secondary dysmenorrhea are urinary tract infections (UTIs), **pelvic inflammatory disease** (PID), irritable bowel syndrome (IBS), uterine leiomyomata (fibroids), and endometriosis.

Pharmacologic Management of Dysmenorrhea

Herbal, Botanical, and Vitamin/Mineral Therapy. The following vitamin therapy may provide pain relief in patients with mild dysmenorrhea: vitamin E (400 to 800 units/day), magnesium (dose ranges varied in clinical trials), thiamine (vitamin B_1, 100 mg/day), and zinc (1 to 3 mg/day a few days before menstruation). Omega-3 fatty acids (1 to 2 g/day) decreased the use of ibuprofen in women with dysmenorrhea in small clinical trials. Omega-3 fatty acids must be used with caution in individuals on anticoagulant therapy.

NSAIDs. NSAIDs block pain by preventing synthesis of prostaglandins. The mechanism of drug action is the inhibition of cyclooxygenase (COX). The COX enzyme converts arachidonic acid into prostaglandins, which cause constriction of the uterine arterioles, necrosis of the endometrial lining, uterine contractions, and menstrual pain. Usually nonselective and COX-2 inhibitors are used. The most commonly used NSAIDs for relief of pain associated with dysmenorrhea include naproxen sodium (Anaprox), diclofenac potassium (Cataflam), ibuprofen (Motrin), naproxen (Naprosyn), celecoxib (Celebrex), and mefenamic acid (Ponstel). Many NSAIDs can be purchased over the counter, so the nurse should include health information about the benefits, risks, and alternatives as well as specific dosage amounts, other drug interactions, and how to take the medication. Some (diclofenac potassium, celecoxib, and mefenamic acid) are by prescription only. Patients must understand the differences in these medications and avoid them if they have allergies to and/or side effects from any of the ingredients. They should avoid taking two different NSAID medications at the same time. GI upset is a common side effect of NSAIDs, so most drugs in this category should be taken with food and water. NSAIDs can also be taken with an antacid or calcium supplement to prevent GI upset. NSAIDs should not be taken for more than 10 days.

Hormonal Contraception. CHC products are effective in the treatment of dysmenorrhea. Extended-cycle CHC products such as 24/4 day products or 87/7 day products may be more effective. CHC products limit the thickness of the uterine endometrium. The 24/4 day CHC products shorten withdrawal bleeding periods, and the extended-cycle CHC products decrease the number of withdrawal menses per year or eliminate them altogether. Depo-Provera, Implanon, and the LNG-IUS decrease dysmenorrhea in patients who are candidates for these methods. Long-term progestin-only products cause atrophy of the uterine lining, limiting the occurrence of dysmenorrhea and the amount of bleeding during menstruation.

Endometriosis

Endometriosis is the abnormal location of endometrial tissue outside the uterus. The tissue is known as *ectopic endometrial implants.* It is a common cause of dysmenorrhea, chronic pelvic pain, and infertility. The ectopic endometrial implants can be found affixed to the ovaries, the posterior surface of the uterus, the uterosacral ligaments, the broad ligaments, or the bowel. They also can be found on other organs within the pelvic or thoracic cavity. The ectopic endometrial implants respond to hormonal control, particularly estrogen, in the same way as the normal endometrial tissue located inside the uterus. Thus, when menstruation occurs, the ectopic endometrial implants proliferate and then bleed. As the number of menstrual cycles increases, inflammation of surrounding organ tissue, scar tissue formation, and adhesions result, causing pelvic pain.

Diagnosis of endometriosis is based on laparoscopic evidence of endometrial tissue, or implants, outside the uterus. The most common symptoms of endometriosis are dysmenorrhea and pelvic pain, sometimes including chronic pelvic pain, which lasts more than 6 months and is not associated specifically with menstruation. The patient may experience back pain; painful, sometimes bloody, bowel movements; and dyspareunia (painful sexual intercourse). An increased number of women with endometriosis experience primary or secondary infertility; although a specific cause linking the two has not been established. It is theorized that the ectopic endometrial implants, or the resultant scar tissue and adhesions, obstruct or affect the motility of the fallopian tubes or other reproductive organs. Affected women have an increased risk for ectopic pregnancy.

Pharmacologic Management of Endometriosis

Pharmaceutic treatment strategies for endometriosis include drugs that decrease the amounts of circulating estrogen and limit or eliminate menstruation. This interrupts internal bleeding and irritation associated with the ectopic endometrial implants and may even cause them to recede.

CHC Products. These drugs suppress gonadotropin-releasing hormone (Gn-RH) release, prevent ovulation, and cause atrophy of the uterine lining, actions thought to relieve pelvic pain by causing a regression of the endometrial implants. CHCs relieve the pain of endometriosis in approximately 75% of women. Extended-cycle CHC products can also manage endometriosis by causing fewer cycles per year or eliminating withdrawal menses altogether.

Progestational Products. These drugs suppress ovulation and cause long-term endometrial atrophy. They also inhibit Gn-RH release, similar to CHCs. Over time, progestins can shrink or eliminate endometrial implants. The most commonly used progestin is depot-medroxyprogesterone acetate (DMPA) in the form of Depo-Provera and Depo-subQ 104 Provera. With DMPA, 70% to 90% of patients experience relief of symptoms associated with endometriosis. This effect may last months after discontinuing the medication. Benefits and risks are the same as if using DMPA for contraception, so concerns for bone mineral density (BMD) loss and prevention, irregular bleeding or amenorrhea, possible weight gain, and mood changes should be discussed with the patient (see Chapter 56). The injection is given every 11 to 13 weeks.

A progestin that can be taken in an oral form is norethindrone acetate (Aygestin), 5 mg PO daily for 2 weeks, then increasing the dose by 2.5 mg every 2 weeks until a dose of 15 mg per day is reached. This is continued for 6 to 9 months.

Gn-RH Agonists. Gn-RH agonists are potent drugs that inhibit Gn-RH release and create a hypoestrogenic environment. The side effects are also menopause-like, with hot flashes, atrophic vaginitis, vaginal dryness, decreased sex drive, and potential for bone loss. Leuprolide (Lupron Depot 3.75 mg) is given in a 3.75-mg dose IM monthly for up to 6 months. Leuprolide is also available in a 3-month dosage schedule (Lupron Depot-3 Month 11.25 mg) given via IM injection once every 3 months for up to 6 months. Leuprolide should be initiated in the first 3 days of the menstrual cycle as it is pregnancy category X. Women may be able to become pregnant on leuprolide, so a barrier method of contraception should be used. Progestins or CHC products can also be prescribed to prevent pregnancy and reduce bone loss.

Nafarelin (Synarel Nasal Spray) is administered in a 400-mcg/day dose; with 1 spray (200 mcg) into one nostril in morning and 1 spray (200 mcg) into the other nostril in evening for up to 6 months. Goserelin (Zoladex) is administered in a 3.6-mg dose in a subcutaneous implant placed in the abdominal wall every 28 days for 6 months. The Gn-RH agonists should be used for only 6 months. Use of these medications past 6 months, as well as retreatment, can cause irreversible adverse changes in BMD. Approximately 90% of women experience relief of symptoms with gonadotropin inhibitors and Gn-RH agonists.

Studies investigating DMPA preparations compared with Gn-RH inhibitors/agonists report that Depo-SubQ 104 Provera is as effective as leuprolide in reducing symptoms of endometriosis and shrinking or eliminating endometrial implants. DMPA preparations are much less expensive for the patient than leuprolide. Leuprolide causes a higher hypoestrogen state than DMPA; therefore, menopause-like symptoms are much more severe. DMPA, in studies, caused irregular bleeding including menorrhagia, weight gain, and prolonged time returning to menstruation after the treatment was discontinued. DMPA also causes BMD changes, and preventive measures must be reviewed with the patient before initiating treatment.

Aromatase inhibitors (nastrozole, letrozole) suppress the conversion of androgens into estrogens and are prescribed for up to 6 months.

Premenstrual Syndrome

Premenstrual syndrome (PMS) comprises a collection of cyclic physical symptoms and perimenopausal mood alterations. Symptoms increase in the 2 weeks before menstruation and subside after menses begins. These physical, emotional, and behavioral symptoms interfere to varying degrees with a woman's ability to function. PMS falls under the classification of cyclic perimenstrual pain and discomfort.

PMS can result in decreased work effectiveness and distressing mood variations. PMS affects 40% of all adult women, with about 5% exhibiting debilitating symptoms. These debilitating symptoms may be classified as premenstrual dysphoric disorder (PMDD) if severe mood swings are exhibited. PMDD is recognized by the American Psychiatric Association as a "depressive disorder not otherwise specified." The hallmark of PMS and PMDD is that symptoms occur in a repetitive pattern during the luteal phase (days 15 to 28) of the menstrual cycle and decrease significantly in the early follicular phase (days 1 to 14).

There is no universal agreement about the definition, etiology, symptoms, or treatment of PMS. Researchers theorize that the etiology of PMS could be hormonal excess or deficits, fluid or sodium retention, or nutritional deficiencies. It is also proposed that an imbalance in the HPO axis function exists. Other hypotheses center on the neuroregulatory effects of estrogen and progesterone on the release or uptake of serotonin.

A patient can help with the diagnosis of PMS by recording three variables on a perimenstrual assessment calendar: (1) group of symptoms (Box 58-1), (2) severity of symptoms, and (3) impact on function (degree of distress). Diagnosis of PMS can be made when the patient's symptoms consistently occur in a cyclic pattern at least 1 week before the menstruation cycle and decrease significantly after menses begins. Symptoms usually have a negative impact on the ability to function effectively. Other endocrine abnormalities must be ruled out. Also, it should be noted that not every symptom associated with the menstrual cycle is indicative of PMS.

BOX 58-1 GROUPING OF SYMPTOMS OF PREMENSTRUAL SYNDROME

Physical

Weight gain	Acne flare-ups
Edema	Joint pain
Bloating in lower abdomen	Constipation
Breast soreness	Headache
Fatigue	Insomnias, alterations in sleep patterns, lack of healthy sleep hours
Backaches	

Emotional

Anger	Difficulty with concentration
Anxiety	Irritability
Agitation	Tearfulness
Feelings of being out of control	Depression
Labile emotions and rapid mood alterations	Suicidal thoughts
Tension	

Behavioral

Increased or decreased sexual desire	Cravings for foods high in sugar or salt
Impulsive behavior	Sudden increase or decrease in activity
Increased appetite	
Acting out aggression or emotional alterations	

Pharmacologic and Complementary and Alternative Treatment of PMS

Pharmacologic treatment of PMS should consider evidence-based recommendations that are appropriate in treating the patient's specific symptoms. The following treatments have been identified.

Nonpharmacologic Treatment. Nonpharmacologic treatment modalities are very important in treating women with PMS. They include expression of empathy, support from family and friends, correction of knowledge deficits about PMS, exercise, and dietary changes. Aerobic exercise improves general health, heightens endorphin levels, and may facilitate an overall sense of well-being. Dietary changes include limiting salty foods, alcohol, caffeine, and concentrated sweets. Eating four to six small, high-carbohydrate, low-fat meals may also help relieve some symptoms. Stress-reduction exercises are also helpful. These measures may help the patient feel proactive regarding her diagnosis of PMS.

Herbal, Botanical, and Vitamin/Mineral Therapy. Some patients experience improvement with selected symptoms through use of vitamin B_6 (pyridoxine), which is popular but not found superior to placebo. Increased calcium intake through diet, not via supplementation, has also been suggested for symptom relief of PMS. Studies indicate that calcium has an inverse relationship with PMS: the higher the intake of calcium, the lower the PMS risk. Since calcium and B_6 are relatively benign when taken in the recommended allowances, both can be used by women to treat PMS symptoms.

Studies on evening primrose oil have had mixed results, although supporters say that it lessens premenstrual mood alterations, helps alleviate breast tenderness, and decreases fluid retention. Chasteberry may help with some PMS symptoms as well as breast pain. Chasteberry prevents progesterone overproduction and inhibits prolactin release (prolactin may be elevated in women with breast tenderness).

St. John's wort has demonstrated efficacy for mild depression that may accompany PMS and PMDD. The mechanism of action is unclear. St. John's wort should not be used if the patient is taking monoamine oxidase inhibiters or has been prescribed selective serotonin reuptake inhibitors (SSRIs). Many herbal or botanical supplements have variations in active ingredient dosing and purity because they may not be approved by the FDA for a specific use.

Antidepressant and Antianxiety Medications. Severe PMS is improved with SSRIs or SSRI medications. The American College of Obstetricians and Gynecologists suggests that SSRIs be taken either continuously or cyclically on days 15 to 28 of the menstrual cycle. Symptom relief includes a decrease in irritability, mood swings, fatigue, tension, and breast tenderness. SSRIs block the reuptake of serotonin into nerve terminals in the CNS, regulating serotonin use by the brain. The most commonly used SSRIs are fluoxetine hydrochloride (Prozac) and sertraline hydrochloride (Zoloft), although paroxetine hydrochloride (Paxil) and citalopram (Celexa) have also demonstrated relief in patients with severe PMS symptoms. Fluoxetine has been repackaged and remarketed to women as Sarafem.

For the management of severe PMS or PMDD, antianxiety medications may be prescribed to reduce or eliminate anxiety and control panic disorders. Antianxiety medications may also help with depression and headaches associated with PMS. The most commonly used medications include alprazolam (Xanax), diazepam (Valium), lorazepam (Ativan), and buspirone (BuSpar). These medications should be used in the short term because of their potential for tolerance or addiction. Patients should be warned that they also may cause sedation. Antianxiety medications are not recommended as first-line of treatment for severe PMS. Treatment for longer than 8 weeks warrants continued medical or psychiatric surveillance.

Hormonal Therapy. Long-term suppression of ovulation has been shown to decrease cyclic physical discomforts and normalize mood variations in some women. Monophasic CHC products such as oral contraception pills, Ortho-Evra, and Nuva Ring can be used in this manner. Caution should be used with progestin-only products because they may exacerbate symptoms of depression. Oral contraceptives such as Yaz, Beyaz, and Lybrel are approved by the FDA for treatment of PMDD.

Common Vulvovaginal Infections

Another common reason women seek out gynecologic care is changes in vaginal secretions or vulvar and vaginal pruritus, irritation, or pain. Vaginal secretions are normal, may change throughout a women's menstrual cycle, lubricate the vaginal and external genitalia, and maintain a healthy vaginal microecosystem. Normal vaginal secretions are clear to white, may be slightly slippery or sticky, and have a mild odor; the secretions may turn yellow on underwear or panty liners. Three vaginal infections change normal vaginal secretions into abnormal vaginal discharge and cause different vulvar or vaginal symptoms: vulvovaginal candidiasis (VVC), bacterial **vaginosis** (BV), and trichomoniasis. **Vaginitis** is the term used to describe inflammation in the vaginal area.

Vulvovaginal Candidiasis. VVC is a yeast infection of the vulva or vaginal area. It causes inflammation, irritation, pruritus, excoriations, and burning on urination or intercourse, and it usually presents with a thick, white, curdlike discharge. The causative agent is most often an overgrowth of *Candida albicans,* normal flora in the vagina; other *Candida* species can also cause VVC. Uncomplicated VVC is treated with topical drugs from the azole category. There are 1-day antifungal agents, as well as 3- and 7-day vaginal treatments. Some antifungal medications can be purchased over the counter; others need a prescription. Table 58-1 lists common medications used to treat VVC.

Bacterial Vaginosis. BV causes larger amounts of homogenous, thin, white vaginal discharge with a strong fishy odor. Normal, healthy bacteria in the vagina—lactobacilli—are replaced with anaerobic bacteria, most commonly *Gardnerella vaginalis* or *Mobiluncus.* BV can be transmitted via sexual contact but is not considered an STI. BV is treated with metronidazole (Flagyl) 250 mg PO three times a day for 7 days, 500 mg PO twice a day for 7 days, or 750 mg extended-release tablet (Flagyl ER) once daily for 7 days. Metronidazole can also be taken in a one-time 2-g dose by taking four 500-mg tablets PO. Since metronidazole can cause stomach upset, it should be taken with food or a full glass of water or milk. Alcohol causes severe nausea and vomiting when ingested with metronidazole, so the patient should be instructed not to drink alcoholic beverages or use products that contain alcohol (such as mouthwash) for the duration of drug therapy and for 48 hours after treatment. These vaginal preparations are also effective in treating BV: metronidazole gel 0.75%, one full applicator intravaginally at bedtime for 5 nights; or clindamycin cream 2%, one full applicator intravaginally at bedtime for 5 days.

Tinidazole (Tindamax) is also used to treat BV. It is prescribed in two 500-mg tablets that are taken in 1 dose PO for 5 days or four 500-mg tablets taken in 1 dose daily PO for 2 consecutive days. Tinidazole has the same precautions with alcohol as metronidazole and should be taken with food. Tinidazole causes slightly less GI upset than metronidazole.

TABLE 58-1 COMMON VAGINAL INFECTIONS AND PHARMACOLOGIC TREATMENT

INFECTION	CDC-RECOMMENDED REGIMENS	NOTES
Vulvovaginal Candidiasis		
Recurrent vulvovaginal candidiasis may be indicative of other disease, such as diabetes or HIV infection.		
Vaginal Preparations with Butoconazole		
Femstat-3 (OTC)	Butoconazole 2% cream 5 g intravag for 3 d or	Pregnancy category: C Number following brand name indicates number of days product is to be used.
Gynezole-1 (Rx only)	Butoconazole 2% cream 5 g (Butaconazole-1) single intravag application	All suppositories and creams listed are inserted intravaginally.
Vaginal Preparations with Clotrimazole		
Gyne-Lotrimin 7 Cream (OTC)	Clotrimazole 1% cream 5 g intravag for 7-14 d or	Pregnancy category: B
Gyne-Lotrimin 7 Combination Pack (OTC)	Clotrimazole 100-mg vag tab for 7 d or	
Gyne-Lotrimin 3 Cream (OTC)	Clotrimazole 100-mg vag tab, 2 tab for 3 d	
Vaginal Preparations with Miconazole		
Monistat-7 Cream (OTC)	Miconazole 2% cream 5 g intravag for 7 d or	Monistat comes in a variety of products, cream only, vaginal suppository only, and combination packs with both vaginal suppositories and cream.
Monistat-7 Suppositories (OTC)	Miconazole 100-mg vag supp, 1 supp for 7 d or	Pregnancy category: C; use is not recommended in first trimester.
Monistat-3 Suppositories (OTC)	Miconazole 200-mg vag supp, 1 supp for 3 d or	Number following brand name indicates number of days product is to be used.
Monistat-1 Combination Pack (OTC)	Miconazole 1,200-mg vag supp, 1 supp for 1 d	
Vaginal Preparations with Nystatin		
Nystatin (Rx only)	Nystatin 100,000-unit vag tab, 1 tab for 14 d	Pregnancy category: A
Vaginal Preparations with Terconazole		
Terazol 7 Cream (Rx only)	Terconazole 0.4% cream 5 g intravag for 7 d or	Pregnancy category: C
Terazol 3 Cream	Terconazole 0.8% cream 5 g intravag for 3 d or	
Terazol 3 Suppositories	Terconazole 80-mg vag supp, 1 supp for 3 d	
Vaginal Preparations with Tioconazole		
1-Day (OTC)	Tioconazole 6.5% ointment 1 applicatorful in a single dose	Pregnancy category: C
Vagistat-1 Ointment (OTC)	Tioconazole 6.5% ointment 1 applicatorful in a single dose	Complete relief may take up to 7 days.
Oral Preparations		
Diflucan (Rx only)	Fluconazole 150-mg oral tablet, one tab PO in a single dose	Pregnancy category: D
Bacterial Vaginosis		
Clindamycin		
Cleocin Vaginal Cream (Rx only)	Clindamycin cream 2% 1 full applicator (5 g) intravag h.s. for 3-7 d or	Pregnancy category: B
Cleocin Vaginal Ovules (Rx only)	Clindamycin ovules 100 mg intravag h.s. for 3 d or	
Clindesse (Rx only)	Clindamycin cream 2% 1 full applicator intravag in a single dose or	
Oral Clindamycin	Clindamycin 300 mg PO b.i.d. for 7 d	

TABLE 58-1 COMMON VAGINAL INFECTIONS AND PHARMACOLOGIC TREATMENT—cont'd

INFECTION	CDC-RECOMMENDED REGIMENS	NOTES
Metronidazole		
Flagyl ER Oral Tablets (Rx only)	Metronidazole 750-mg tab PO for 7 d or	Pregnancy category: B All ETOH products should be avoided when taking oral metronidazole during treatment and for 3 days after use.
Flagyl (Rx only)	Metronidazole 500 mg PO b.i.d. for 7 d or	Should be taken with food.
Flagyl (Rx only)	Metronidazole 2 g PO in a single dose or	Oral metronidazole should not be used in first trimester of pregnancy.
MetroGel Vaginal (Rx only) or Vandazole (Rx only)	Metronidazole vaginal 0.75% gel 1 full applicator 1-2 times/d for 5 d	Second and third trimester: Pregnancy category: B
Tinidazole		
Tindamax (Rx only)	250-mg or 500-mg tabs 2 grams daily PO for 2 d or 1 gram daily PO for 5 d Tinidazole 2 g/d for 2 d or 1 g/d for 5 d	When taking oral tinidazole, avoid all ETOH products during treatment and for 3 days after use. Take with food. Do not use oral tinidazole in the first trimester of pregnancy. Second and third trimester: Pregnancy category: B Fewer GI side effects than metronidazole

b.i.d., Twice a day; *d*, day; *ER*, extended-release; *g*, gram; *GI*, gastrointestinal; *h.s.*, at bedtime; *intravag*, intravaginally; *mg*, milligram; *OTC*, over-the-counter; *PO*, by mouth; *q*, every; *Rx*, prescription; *supp*, suppository; *tab*, tablet; *vag*, vaginally.

Both medications should not be taken in the first trimester of pregnancy.

Trichomoniasis. Trichomoniasis is sometimes grouped with other vulvovaginal infections because of the changes *T. vaginalis* causes in vaginal secretions and associated vaginal irritation. However, trichomoniasis is an STI and is discussed in the section on STIs later in this chapter.

MEDICATIONS USED TO PROMOTE FERTILITY

Infertility is defined as the inability to conceive a child after 12 months of unprotected sexual intercourse. Women older than 35 years may be considered infertile after 6 months of attempting pregnancy. Infertility is considered primary infertility if a couple has never conceived or has never carried a pregnancy to term. Secondary infertility describes a couple who has conceived and brought a pregnancy to term but is unable to conceive afterward. Approximately 15% to 20% of couples in the United States experience infertility. Fertility rates decrease in both men and women as they get older; however, the risk for infertility increases more abruptly in women than in men as women reach the end of the reproductive life cycle. The monthly chance of achieving pregnancy decreases to 5% after age 40 years.

Assessing the Infertile Couple

Causes of infertility are numerous (Table 58-2). Infertility can be attributed to a female factor, a male factor, and many times, a combination of both. In the female partner, the most common causes for infertility are alterations in ovarian function and anatomic disorders. Alterations in ovarian function are categorized as *ovulatory dysfunction disorders*. Any process, whether a disease state or the normal biologic process of aging, that causes anovulation (lack of ovulation) or a decrease in ovulation cycles will affect the process of conception. Many of these women present with irregular menstrual periods. Causes of ovulatory dysfunction include alterations in the HPO axis, such as metabolic disorders (most commonly PCOS), and age approaching the end of the reproductive spectrum. Fertility declines sharply in women after age 35 years, and infertility becomes a factor from age 38 to 40 years. Endocrine disorders such as hyperprolactinemia (increase in circulating prolactin, the hormone that promotes breastfeeding) or thyroid disorders (hypothyroidism or hyperthyroidism) also can cause anovulatory cycles. Ovulation can be disrupted by eating disorders (anorexia and bulimia) and by stress.

The most common anatomic disorder is blocked fallopian tubes. Blocked tubes can be the result of a history of STI or PID. STIs, treated or undiagnosed, and PID can lead to scarring within the tubes, impeding sperm or ovum transport. A previous ectopic pregnancy or other tubal surgery can also result in infertility. Other causes include endometriosis, uterine leiomyomata (fibroids), or scarring within the uterine endometrium.

Male causes of infertility include any disease process that prevents sperm production or blocks sperm transport. Undescended testicles, surgical removal of the testes, STIs or other

TABLE 58-2 CAUSES OF INFERTILITY

Female Factors	
Genetic	Chromosomal abnormalities, enzyme defects
Tubal or peritoneal	Infection, occlusion, fimbriae damage, pelvic adhesions, endometriosis
Ovarian	Anovulation, oligoovulation, inadequate luteal phase, polycystic ovarian syndrome (PCOS)
Cervical	Cervicitis, poor-quality cervical mucus, diethylstilbestrol exposure (daughter and granddaughter of DES exposure)
Uterine	Uterine fibromas, congenital malformations, adhesions, endometrial abnormalities
Endocrine	Panhypopituitarism, hypothyroidism, adrenal insufficiency, congenital adrenal hyperplasia, Cushing's disease, cirrhosis, hyperprolactinemia, hormone receptor defects
Other	Age, drugs, malnutrition, excess alcohol intake, tobacco use
Male Factors	
Genetic	Chromosomal genetic abnormalities
Seminal	Failure of semen to liquefy, inadequate volume, low sperm count, decreased or erratic sperm motility, sperm dysmorphology, varicocele
Transport	Hypospadias, micropenis, retrograde ejaculation, epididymitis, impotence, ductal occlusion, ductal adhesions
Testicular	Oligospermia/azoospermia, cryptorchidism, testicular agenesis, history of high fever, postpubertal orchitis, testicular injury/surgery, varicocele
Endocrine	Panhypopituitarism, hypothyroidism, adrenal insufficiency, congenital adrenal hyperplasia, Cushing's disease, cirrhosis, hormone receptor abnormalities
Other	Age, drugs, excess alcohol intake, tobacco use, pollution, malnutrition, scrotal heat exposure, autoimmunity to sperm, infectious processes, allergies
Couple Factors	Sexual technique, frequency or timing of intercourse, immune response to sperm

infections of the internal genitalia, hypospadias, environmental factors, and sexual dysfunction can also contribute to infertility. Some medications affect sperm quality and migration.

Treatment of infertility depends on the cause. General health assessment of the infertile couple includes (1) complete health history, including nutritional, reproductive, and social histories; medications; herbal and illicit drug use; and gynecologic, menstrual, obstetric, and sexual histories as they pertain to each partner; (2) complete physical examinations with breast and pelvic examinations of the female partner and examination of male genitalia and function; (3) Pap testing, HPV testing, collections of cultures for STI testing;

TABLE 58-3 COMMON TESTS FOR INFERTILITY

TEST	PURPOSE
Physical examination	Assess secondary sex characteristics, reproductive tract function, and patency by gross examination Assess for hyperandrogen symptoms
Hematology, liver and renal function	Rule out disease processes
Hysterosalpingogram, tubal insufflation	Evaluate fallopian tube patency
Cervical mucus test	Assess viscosity of mucus and its effect on sperm motility
Plasma progesterone	Assess function of corpus luteum
Endometrial biopsy	Assess ovulatory status or adequacy of corpus luteum
Semen analysis	Check number, structure, movement of sperm
Basal body temperature	Determine whether ovulation occurs; document temperatures daily in chart
Sperm penetration assay	Determine ability of sperm to penetrate and fertilize ovum
Laparoscopy	Visualize female pelvic organs
Hysteroscopy	Visualize uterus
Echohysteroscopy	Assess structure of woman's internal reproductive organs
Hormone assays	Assess Gn-RH, FSH, LH, progesterone, estrogen, prolactin, testosterone, and thyroid hormone levels
Immunologic testing	Assess cervical immunity against sperm, seminal fluid immunity against sperm, and serum antisperm antibodies in either partner
Imaging	Pituitary integrity

FSH, Follicle-stimulating hormone; *Gn-RH,* gonadotropin-releasing hormone; *LH,* luteinizing hormone.

and (4) laboratory tests and other diagnostic tests. Semen evaluation is also necessary. Common tests to determine the specific causes of infertility are listed in Table 58-3.

One of the leading causes of infertility in women is ovulatory dysfunction disorders, usually in the form of PCOS or other metabolic syndromes. The first line of pharmacologic treatment for ovulatory dysfunction disorders is usually induction of ovulation by oral drug therapy.

Induction of Ovulation

Clomiphene citrate (CC) is an estrogen antagonist that binds with estrogen receptors within the hypothalamus. By binding to the estrogen receptors, the hypothalamus is led to believe that circulating estrogen levels are low. This sets the hypothalamus in motion to secrete more Gn-RH, stimulating the HPO axis. The Gn-RH instructs the anterior pituitary gland to release FSH and LH to initiate a response from the ovarian follicles. Estrogen levels increase in response to FSH and LH,

PROTOTYPE DRUG CHART 58-1

Clomiphene Citrate

Drug Class Ovulation stimulant Trade Names: Clomid, Serophene Pregnancy Category: X	**Dosage** A: PO: 50-150 mg/d for days 5-9 of cycle If ovulation does not occur with 50 mg/d, increase next course to 100 mg/d. Maximum dose is 150 mg/d; maximum sequential cycles is three. Under strict supervision by physicians specializing in infertility, as much as 250 mg/d may be used.
Contraindications Pregnancy, undiagnosed vaginal bleeding, depression, fibroids, hepatic dysfunction, thrombophlebitis, primary pituitary or ovarian failure	**Drug-Lab-Food Interactions** Drug: None are significant; danazol may inhibit response; decrease effects of ethinyl estradiol Lab: Increase in serum thyroxine
Pharmacokinetics Absorption: Readily absorbed from GI tract Distribution: PB: UK Metabolism: t½: 5-8 d Excretion: In feces	**Pharmacodynamics** PO: Onset: 5-14 d Peak: UK Duration: UK
Therapeutic Effects/Uses To stimulate ovarian follicle growth Mode of Action: Stimulates release of follicle-stimulating hormone and luteinizing hormone	
Side Effects Breast discomfort, fatigue, dizziness, depression, anxiety, nausea, vomiting, constipation, increased appetite, headache, flatulence, multiple gestation, hot flashes, fluid retention	**Adverse Reactions** Visual disturbances, abdominal pain, weight gain, hair loss, ovarian hyperstimulation, anxiety, ovarian cysts, ectopic pregnancy

A, Adult; *d*, day; *GI*, gastrointestinal; *PB*, protein-binding; *PO*, by mouth; *t ½*, half-life; *UK*, unknown.

and a follicle becomes dominant, producing the level of estrogen needed for the LH surge. The LH surge causes ovulation of an ovum from the dominant follicle. It is important that LH reach a level high enough to produce an ovulatory cycle and that the timing of the LH surge be at the height of follicle formation, which is mid-cycle.

CC is the most commonly used ovulation stimulant (Prototype Drug Chart 58-1). Women with PCOS may need concurrent treatment for hyperinsulinemia with metformin. Metformin alone will help regulate the menstrual cycle and promote ovulation; however, when it is paired with CC, the success rate is increased.

CC is given in a 50-mg oral dose on days 5 through 9 of the menstrual cycle. If ovulation does not occur, the dose can be increased by 50-mg increments to 100 mg, then 150 mg, up to 250 mg orally on days 5 through 9, in sequential cycles, until ovulation is achieved. Usually, no more than three cycles of CC are used. Women are at an increased risk for multiple gestation; usually no more than a twin gestation is experienced.

Recombinant FSH, LH, and human chorionic gonadotropin (hCG) promote normal hormone levels with minimal adverse effects (Table 58-4). Recombinant FSH (Bravelle, Follistim, Gonal F) and recombinant LH (Luveris) work directly on ovarian function to stimulate follicle maturation and promote ovulation. These therapies supply women with exogenous hormones to enhance the normal physiologic process of the menstrual cycle, promoting ovulation and increasing the probability of conception. HCG (A.P.L., Pregnil, Novarel, Ovidrel) ensures development of the corpus luteum *after* ovulation. The corpus luteum provides for adequate levels of both estrogen and, more importantly, progesterone, to maintain the uterine endometrium and a pregnancy, should one occur. These drugs are more potent than CC and have an increased risk for multiple births. HCG further enhances ovulation in women who have been pretreated with gonadotropins, FSH, or LH.

Pharmacokinetics Data on the pharmacokinetics of CC are limited, but clomiphene is readily absorbed from the GI tract. It is partially metabolized in the liver and excreted in the feces via biliary elimination. CC has a half-life of about 5 days.

Pharmacodynamics The mechanism of action of CC is unknown, but it is hypothesized that it competes with estrogen at receptor sites. The perception of decreased circulating estrogen by the hypothalamus and pituitary gland triggers the negative feedback response that increases secretion of FSH and LH. The results are ovarian stimulation, maturation of the ovarian follicle, ovulation, and development of the corpus luteum.

Side Effects. Side effects of CC include breast discomfort, fatigue, dizziness, depression, nausea, increased appetite, dermatitis, urticaria, anxiety, weakness, heavier menses, vasomotor flushing, and abdominal bloating or pain. Antiestrogenic effects include interference with endometrial maturation and cervical mucus production. Paradoxically, this may interfere with fertilization or implantation.

TABLE 58-4 OVULATORY STIMULANTS AND OVULATION CONTROL

GENERIC (BRAND)	ROUTE AND DOSAGE	USE AND CONSIDERATIONS
bromocriptine mesylate (Parlodel)	1.25-2.5 mg/d; may increase by 2.5 mg every 2-7 d; *max:* 2.5-15 mg/d	Normalizes prolactin levels. Possibly teratogenic. Pregnancy category: C; PB: 92%; $t_{1/2}$: 50 h
clomiphene citrate (Clomid, Serophene)	See Prototype Drug Chart 58-1.	
Gn-RH analogues Agonists: Synarel Antagonists: Cetrotide, Ganirelix	Synarel: Spray up to 800 mcg/d (200 mcg per nostril b.i.d.) Cetrotide: 0.25 mg in a single dose subQ daily on stimulation day 5 or day 7, or 3 mg subQ in a single dose on stimulation day 7 (to control day of LH surge) Ganirelix: 250 mcg subQ once daily after initiating FSH, during mid to late follicular stage.	Enhances ovulation stimulation for IVF cycles by suppression of a spontaneous LH surge. (Controls fertility cycle, improving pregnancy outcomes.) PB: UK; $t_{1/2}$: 11-23 h
human menotropic gonadotropins (Humegon, Pergonal, Serono, Repronex)	IM injection: Humegon, Pergonal, Serono subQ: Repronex Dosage determined by patient 75:75 units of FSH:LH or 150:150 units of FSH:LH once daily for 5 or more days	Possesses same activities as FSH and LH therefore will induce ovulation in women with hypothalamic amenorrhea. Ovarian hyperstimulation is a risk. Multiple gestation is a risk. Pregnancy category: X
recombinant FSH (Gonal-F, Follistim) human menopausal gonadotropin or hMG (similar to FSH) (Repronex, Menopur) recombinant LH (Luveris, Novarel, A.P.L., Pregnyl); recombinant human chorionic gonadotropin or hCG (Ovidrel)	Recombinant FSH: subQ or IM injection; dosage individualized for each patient, usually 75-150 units daily, early follicular phase continuing for 10-14 d Recombinant LH: subQ 75 units given subQ along with an FSH or recombinant FSH Recombinant hCG 250 mcg prefilled syringe subQ injection given 1 d after last dose of gonadotropin (FSH and/or LH) 5000-10,000 units IM 1 d after last dose of gonadotropin (FSH and/or LH)	Recombinant FSH possesses same hormonal activities as FSH. Ovarian hyperstimulation remains a risk, though minimal, with recombinant products. Multiple gestation is a risk, which is reduced by careful monitoring. PB: UK; $t_{1/2}$: 23-77 h IM, 13-35 h subQ Pregnancy category: X Avoid herbal supplements containing black or blue cohosh

d, Day; *FSH,* follicle-stimulating hormone; *Gn-RH,* gonadotropin-releasing hormone; *h,* hour; *hCG,* human chorionic gonadotropin; *IM,* intramuscular; *LH,* luteinizing hormone; *min,* minute; *PB,* protein-binding; *subQ,* subcutaneously; $t_{1/2}$, half-life; *UK,* unknown.

Adverse Reactions. Adverse reactions include photophobia, mastalgia, diplopia, and decreased visual acuity. Ovarian hyperstimulation may result in ovarian enlargement, mid-cycle ovarian pain, and cysts. Reversible hair loss has been noted. The effect of CC on fetal development is unclear. Neural tube defects have been reported but have not been confirmed by controlled studies. Adverse reactions of other ovulatory stimulants are listed in Table 58-4.

Contraindications. Contraindications for treatment with CC include undiagnosed vaginal bleeding, pregnancy, uterine fibroids, clinical depression, history of hepatic dysfunction or thromboembolic disease, and primary pituitary or ovarian failure. CC may cause existing ovarian cysts to enlarge. Contraindications to the use of other ovulatory stimulants are listed in Table 58-4.

Drug Interactions. There are no known significant drug interactions with CC. Danazol may inhibit patient response to CC, and CC may suppress response to ethinyl estradiol. There are no known drug interactions with human menopausal gonadotropin or hCG.

Luteal Phase Defects

Another leading cause of infertility is related to decreased progesterone levels in the luteal phase of the menstrual cycle (the phase after ovulation). With the decrease in circulating progesterone, the luteal phase is shortened and the progesterone-mediated endometrial changes vital to implantation do not occur. This condition is identified by low serum progesterone levels, taken through serum blood testing on days 21 through 25 of the menstrual cycle.

Women with inadequate luteal-phase progesterone output, called *luteal phase deficiency* (LPD), are treated with progesterone in vaginal, oral, or IM dosing (called luteal phase support). Progesterone supports the luteal phase that occurs immediately after ovulation. The extraneous progesterone is continued until 10 to 12 weeks' gestation, well after the placenta is functioning independently to support the pregnancy.

Progesterone cream or gel (Crinone 8%, Prochieve 8%) contains 90 mg of progesterone in a prolonged-release vaginal gel. It is administered intravaginally once or twice daily. Micronized progesterone (Endometrin 100 mg) is a vaginal suppository containing 100 mg of progesterone that is inserted twice or three times daily. Progesterone for injection comes in a 50 mg/mL vial; the usual dose is 50 mg daily (or 1 mL/day) given by deep IM injection. The progesterone comes in sesame oil, which makes it viscous and difficult to inject. An allergy to sesame seeds or oils should be determined by the nurse. Prometrium is micronized progesterone taken in an oral dose of 200 mg twice a day or 100 mg three times a day. It is used by practitioners treating women with infertility conditions caused by lack of progesterone output; however, this is an off-label use. Clinical trials are producing evidence that progestins and micronized progesterone are not teratogenic and cause no ill effects to a fetus. Nevertheless, these drugs carry a category X pregnancy warning. The use of progesterone after ovulation enhances successful conception and implantation in women with LPD.

For some women, the cause of LPD is the result of a premature LH surge. With an early LH surge, the follicle has not been given the time needed to mature and the cycle becomes anovulatory. A Gn-RH antagonist is used and can be given subcutaneously or by IM injection. Drugs that stimulate ovulation and their side effects are listed in Table 58-4.

Other Drug Treatments

Endocrine disorders include hyperprolactinemia and thyroid disorders. In women with hyperprolactinemia, an elevated level of prolactin is the causative factor of infertility. Prolactin is a hormone secreted by the anterior pituitary gland and elevated during pregnancy and postpartum to support milk production. Breastfeeding causes a natural rise in prolactin, and hyperprolactinemia can be seen in women who are breastfeeding or have recently discontinued breastfeeding.

Drug therapies, such as haloperidol (Haldol), metoclopramide (Reglan), methyldopa, reserpine, and long-term CHC use have been known to cause hyperprolactinemia. The most common cause of pathologic hyperprolactinemia is a small benign pituitary tumor called a *pituitary adenoma.* Most women, regardless of the cause of hyperprolactinemia, can be treated with the ergot derivative bromocriptine (Parlodel). Bromocriptine binds to dopamine receptors in the pituitary gland and inhibits prolactin secretion. Treatment continues until pregnancy is confirmed. Clomiphene can be introduced if needed after 2 months.

In addition, hypothyroidism or hyperthyroidism and adrenal dysfunction must be assessed and managed to attain euthyroid levels. Endometriosis can be treated with a course of danazol, leuprolide, or DMPA to suppress gonadotropin output.

Nursing Process
Patient-Centered Collaborative Care

Infertility

Assessment

- Assess general health history, including drug and herbal product use. Physical examination, including speculum and bimanual exam, are required. Assess patients' reproductive and sexual histories, with attention to history of abnormal Pap testing and treatment, history of vaginal infections and STIs and treatment, past use of contraception methods, pelvic surgery and past and present gynecologic abnormalities, and pregnancy and birth history and complications.
- Complete menstrual history including menarche; last menstrual period; length, duration, and flow of bleeding; and any signs or symptoms related to the menstrual cycle.
- Complete assessment of sexual practices including use of lubricants and timing and technique of intercourse.
- Assess couple's mental health status, with a referral to support group or counseling as needed. Infertility can be isolating, because many couples may have several peers who are pregnant or already have children.
- The couple will undergo an exhaustive battery of diagnostic tests to evaluate the cause of infertility. Once this is determined, conditions that contraindicate the treatment of choice are ruled out.
- It is particularly important that the couple's interpretation of their infertility be explored, along with its impact on their relationship. The nurse should help the couple discuss their feelings in a safe, supportive environment.

Nursing Diagnoses

- Deficient knowledge related to menstrual cycle, ovulation, conception, causes of infertility, prognosis, and assisted reproductive technologies
- Deficient knowledge related to treatment regimen and outcomes
- Ineffective sexuality pattern related to infertility
- Risk for sexual dysfunction related to assisted reproduction strategies
- Disturbed body image related to inability to conceive
- Situational low self-esteem related to infertility
- Anxiety related to infertility and treatment medication and procedures
- Powerlessness related to infertility diagnosis
- Decisional conflicts related to discrepancy between cultural and/or religious beliefs and assisted reproductive therapies
- Grieving related to loss of the plan to have a biologic child

Planning

- Patient will understand normal physiologic process of conception.
- Patient will identify basic concepts that increase fertility.
- Patient will adhere to medical regimen with minimal adverse effects physically, psychologically, emotionally, and spiritually.
- Patient will report adverse effects of treatment or pharmacologic therapy.
- Long-term goal is a successful pregnancy. If pregnancy cannot be achieved, patient will be able to consider alternatives and make the transition with confidence, relationship, and sense of self-worth intact.
- Patient will recognize that many treatment regimens for infertility must be repeated before successful conception is attained.

Nursing Interventions

General

- Initiate teaching to assist the patient (and her partner) in understanding the menstrual cycle, patterns and symptoms of ovulation, temperature changes with ovulation, specific physiologic signs of ovulation, use of ovulation predictor kits, and timing of sexual intercourse.
- Help the patient to understand the interrelationships among the menstrual cycle, ovulation, and coitus as they relate to conception.
- Advise the patient on the sexual techniques that enhance fertilization: placement of a pillow under the woman's hips during coitus, placement of the woman in a supine position with the hips elevated for about 30 minutes after her partner ejaculates.
- Initiate drug treatment regimens as prescribed by the provider. The patient and partner(s) will understand the treatment regimen and the expected outcomes of the treatment regimen.
- Provide the patient and her partner psychological counseling and support.

Specific

- Counsel the patient to report adverse effects such as abdominal pain or visual disturbances to her infertility specialist at once and to be cautious with tasks that require alertness. If she misses a dose of her medication, she should call her infertility specialist.
- Advise the patient that treatment increases the chance of multiple births.
- Ensure that patient understands the risks, benefits, and alternatives to pharmacologic therapy.

Patient Teaching

- Teach couples how to evaluate and record on a chart the woman's basal body temperature and changes in the cervical mucus. The first day of menses is day 1 of the cycle. Ovulation is predicted by a 0.5° F drop in basal body temperature followed by a 1° F rise. Over-the-counter diagnostic kits for assessing ovulatory status can also be used to time coitus. The couple is advised to engage in coitus frequently from 4 days before to 3 days after ovulation, but if the semen analysis reports a lowered sperm count, intercourse should occur every other day to maximize the man's sperm count.
- Advise male partner to wear boxer shorts during infertility treatment. Briefs hold the scrotum close to the body, and the heat reduces sperm count. For the same reason, if he is seated all day in his work, he is counseled to take a walk every hour or so.
- Advise male partner to avoid use of certain herbs that affect sperm production (Herbal Alert 58-1).
- Advise female partner to take medication at same time each day to maintain steady blood levels.

HERBAL ALERT 58-1

Herbs and Male Infertility

- *Saw palmetto* may cause metabolic changes in the sperm.
- *St. John's wort* affects sperm cells and causes decreased sperm motility and decreased viability.

- Encourage patient and partner to verbalize concerns and express feelings about treatment successes and failures.

Cultural Considerations

- A number of churches and religions do not support the use of reproductive technologies. Some couples may opt for adoption instead of reproductive assistance. Some may suffer additional anxiety if they go against their religious or cultural traditions and use reproductive technology.
- Some women may prefer to be examined only by a female health care provider. These women should remain covered as much as is possible and appropriate. Some patients combine traditional practices with conventional medicine; therefore, a complete history of nonpharmacologic therapy is needed.
- Use of a certified medical interpreter is necessary for individuals who have limited English skills; one of the same gender and culture is preferred for sensitive topics.
- In male-dominated cultures, the male partner may be unwilling to undergo an infertility evaluation, because infertility is viewed as a female problem.

Evaluation

- Successful outcomes of fertility treatment include avoidance of ovarian hyperstimulation and other untoward effects. Pregnancy that results in the birth of a live infant fulfills the objectives of treatment. If pregnancy is not achieved, intervention is aimed at helping the couple consider alternatives to childbearing without adverse impact on their self-esteem or harm to their relationship.

Drug Therapy for Male Infertility

For most infertile men, no specific causal factor can be identified. These patients are identified as having idiopathic **oligospermia** (semen with a low concentration of sperm) and **asthenospermia** (low sperm motility). There is no documented cost-effective treatment for this large group of men. Most drug regimens used have shown little promise in controlled studies, with the exception of using testosterone (or other hormonal) therapy to attain physiologic levels. Assisted reproductive techniques appear to hold more promise than drug therapy. Some surgical techniques, such as removal of a **varicocele** (an enlarged vein in the scrotal sac), can sometimes improve male infertility. Some herbal products contribute to male infertility problems (see Herbal Alert 58-1).

MEDICATIONS USED IN THE TREATMENT OF SEXUALLY TRANSMITTED INFECTIONS

Healthy sexual relationships are important to patients' health and well-being. The reproductive process, including pregnancy and birth, and the healthy expression of sexual intimacy between partners should be free from the threat of STIs. STIs are infections that are primarily transmitted through sexual contact. Pathogens implicated in STIs include bacteria, viruses, protozoal microbes, and certain parasites (Table 58-5).

Depending on the causative organism, STIs may be localized lesions affecting the skin or mucosa, or they may spread upward through the reproductive tract, increasing the risk for pelvic infection and infertility. Many are life-threatening and can be transmitted through pregnancy and birth to a fetus or neonate. Approximately one in four Americans will experience an STI in their lifetime. The incidence increases in communities with lower socioeconomic status and/or limited access to health care, in socially disparate communities, and in developing nations. Prevention and control of STIs are essential not only for the health of individuals, but also for the health of the community.

Transmission and Risk

Sexual transmission of pathogens can occur through breaks in the vaginal or cervical mucosa or the skin covering the shaft or glans of the penis. Each act of coitus results in tiny, friction-induced fissures on these surfaces. The problem is exacerbated by inadequate vaginal lubrication, which may occur after menopause, postpartum, just after menses, or when the woman is not sufficiently aroused before penetration.

Semen, sperm cells themselves, vaginal secretions, blood, and other body fluids can carry pathogens. Skin and mucosal lesions can be penetrated by microorganisms, and they can also shed them. Sexual contact can involve skin-to-skin, mouth-to-mouth, oral-genital, oral-anal, or hand-anal transmission of pathogens through breaks in the skin or mucosal surfaces or from inoculation by infectious body fluids. Anal penetration is particularly risky because of the likelihood of tissue trauma that results in the partner's exposure to enteric microorganisms. The risk for contracting an STI increases with substance abuse, imprisonment, sexual activity with a partner who has been imprisoned, sexual activity with individuals being paid for sex acts, and rape or sexual assault.

Patients engaging in sexual activity with multiple partners are at high risk for transmission of STIs, particularly HIV. Investigators at the National Institutes of Health suggest that the risk for acquiring STIs is markedly increased among individuals who have more than one sexual partner per year versus those who have fewer partners. Other high-risk practices are anal or vaginal intercourse without a condom, hand-anal contact and contact with menstrual blood during sexual activity, use of an enema before anal intercourse, and urination on broken skin or inside the body. Women have an increased incidence of acquiring an STI than men do. Risk-reducing behaviors for avoidance of STIs are listed in Box 58-2.

STIs are often manifested as multiple infections. Individuals undergoing treatment for one STI should be assessed for others, including HIV. This is especially true if genital or perianal ulcerations are present.

Vertical transmission, or perinatal infection, occurs when a fetus or neonate is infected by its mother. Microbes can travel up the reproductive tract from the vagina or cervix and

TABLE 58-5 PATHOGENS THAT CAUSE SEXUALLY TRANSMITTED INFECTIONS

	MODE OF TRANSMISSION		
PATHOGEN	**PREDOMINANTLY SEXUALLY TRANSMITTED**	**CAN BE TRANSMITTED BY SEXUAL CONTACT**	**SEXUAL CONTACT WITH ORAL-FECAL EXPOSURE**
Bacteria	*Calymmatobacterium granulomatis* *Chlamydia trachomatis* *Haemophilus ducreyi* *Neisseria gonorrhoeae* *Treponema pallidum* *Ureaplasma urealyticum*	*Escherichia coli** *Gardnerella vaginalis** *Haemophilus vaginalis* *Mobiluncus curtisii, Mobiluncus mulieris,** *Peptostreptococcus* *Group B streptococcus** *Mycoplasma hominis**	*Shigella Campylobacter*
Viruses	Cytomegalovirus Hepatitis B Herpes simplex virus type 2 Human papillomavirus Molluscum contagiosum virus	Human T-lymphotrophic virus-1 Herpes simplex virus type 1 Epstein-Barr virus	HIV-1, HIV-2 Hepatitis C, D Hepatitis A
Protozoa, fungi, ectoparasites	*Trichomonas vaginalis* *Phthirus pubis* *Sarcoptes scabiei*	*Candida albicans** *Candida glabrada** *Candida tropicalus**	*Giardia lamblia* *Entamoeba histolytica*

*These microbial infections are frequently caused by alterations in the vaginal microecosystem or from an intestinal-to-vaginal route exposure but can be transmitted through certain sexual practices.
HIV, Human immunodeficiency virus.

BOX 58-2 RISK-REDUCING BEHAVIORS FOR AVOIDANCE OF STIS

- Patient screening for STIs at all gynecologic encounters
- Sexual abstinence or sexual contact with one partner who also is monogamous and tested for STIs before sexual intimacy
- Consistent and correct use of male or female condom
- Washing and urinating before and after intercourse
- Avoiding sex with someone who has genital or anal lesions
- Reducing use of alcohol or drugs, both of which impair judgment about sexual risk and may decrease immune response
- Avoiding sexual contact with HIV-infected persons, IV drug users, individuals who have present or past imprisonment, or sexual partners of all such individuals
- Never sharing hypodermic needles, razors, or any item that may be exposed to blood or body fluids
- Reporting, testing, and treating any exposure

STI, Sexually transmitted infection.

enter the intrauterine environment. Organisms that are of little consequence to healthy adults can be devastating to a fetus. Transmission can occur through contact with the mother's blood at birth or through breast milk, as in the case of HIV and hepatitis B virus. Many STIs, such as syphilis, are transmitted through the placenta and membranes. Others, the herpes simplex virus type 2 (HSV-2) for example, require actual contact by the infant with microorganisms in the birth canal. Because of the risk for blindness caused by *Chlamydia trachomatis* and *Neisseria gonorrhoeae,* erythromycin ointment is routinely administered in the eyes of neonates as prophylaxis. This is usually done in within the first hour after birth.

CDC guidelines for the primary treatment of various STIs are listed in Table 58-6. All sexual contacts of an infected individual should be informed of the exposure so they can be treated. Partners should refrain from sexual activity until each is clear of infection on follow-up evaluation or, at the very least, should use condoms.

STI Pathogens

Bacterial Pathogens

Sexually transmitted bacterial pathogens can be effectively treated with antibiotic therapy. These infections are found in the cervix, urethra, oropharynx, Bartholin's glands, and Skene's glands. They can cause a friable cervix and mucopurulent discharge. Many times they go undetected. Some women will complain of vaginal bleeding or spotting, increased discharge, and pelvic pain. Bacterial pathogens are a common cause of PID. Common bacterial pathogens are *Neisseria gonorrhoeae* and *Chlamydia trachomatis. Treponema pallidum* is a spirochete that causes syphilis. Syphilis, if not treated early in the infection process, is a systemic disease that has stages of active disease process and periods of dormancy. Left untreated, it can be fatal. The drug of choice for syphilis is Benzathine penicillin G, 2.4 million units given IM once in the early stage of syphilis, or, if the infective process is known to be greater than 1 year, Benzathine PCN G 2.4 million units IM once weekly for 3 weeks.

Viral Pathogens

Viral pathogens are not curable. Medication therapy is palliative. These include herpes simplex virus I (with cross-contamination from oral to genital) and herpes simplex virus II (HSV-1 or HSV-2), human papilloma virus (HPV), and HIV.

Human Papillomavirus. There are more than 80 different strands of HPV, about 30 of which are sexually transmitted. There are approximately 12 types, called "low-risk," that cause external lesions, and approximately 15 types, called "high-risk," that cause cervical lesions. It is now recognized that it is the high-risk types of HPV that cause cervical cancer in women, and up to 60% of sexually active women in their late teens or early twenties harbor the virus. For most young women, the virus is effectively suppressed by the immune system before causing cervical changes. However, if the HPV persists, it can cause the cervical cells to grow abnormally. The Pap test detects cervical dysplasia, which can be a precursor to cervical cancer if left untreated. While the Pap test can determine whether the cervical cells are abnormal, a digene test can detect the presence of 13 high-risk HPV types.

Gardasil is a vaccine indicated in male and female patients' age 9 to 26 years for the prevention of cervical cancer caused by HPV. Gardasil protects against HPV types 6 and 11, which cause genital lesions and have a lower risk for carcinoma, and HPV types 16 and 18, which are highly invasive and have the potential to cause cervical dysplasia. Gardasil should be administered in three separate IM injections in the upper arm over a 6-month period with the first dose at an elected date, the second dose 2 months after the first dose, and the third dose 6 months after the first dose. Gardasil does not substitute for routine cancer screening, and women who receive Gardasil should continue to undergo screening per standard of care.

Herpes Simplex Virus. HSV-2 is a recurrent viral infection that causes small, painful vesicles over the genital area, anus, thighs, and buttocks. Associated symptoms may be fever, pelvic pain, malaise, and other flulike symptoms. HSV-1 causes oral lesions ("cold sores") that can be transmitted to male or female genitalia during oral sexual practices. It is reported that 80% of adult individuals have oral herpes lesions. The length of time of viral eruption is shortened with antiviral medications; however, HSV remains recurrent and painful, and treatment is mostly palliative.

HIV. See Chapter 35 for drugs used to treat HIV.

Other Pathogens

Pediculosis refers to parasitic infections. *Pediculosis humanus capitus* are head lice, *pediculosis humanus corporus* are body lice, and *Phthirus pubis* are pubic lice. These infestations present with extreme pruritus of the body part or area where the lice are moving and laying egg cases. An infection that causes increased pruritus in the vaginal area with copious

Text continued on p. 905

TABLE 58-6 **CURRENT GUIDELINES FOR PRIMARY THERAPIES FOR COMMON SEXUALLY TRANSMITTED INFECTIONS***

INFECTION	PRIMARY THERAPY	NOTES
Nongonococcal urethritis	Recommended: azithromycin 1 g PO in a single dose or doxycycline 100 mg PO b.i.d. for 7 d Alternative regimens: erythromycin base 500 mg PO q.i.d. for 7 d or erythromycin ethylsuccinate 800 mg PO q.i.d. for 7 d or levofloxacin 500 mg PO daily for 7 d or ciprofloxacin 300 mg PO b.i.d. for 7 d	Use of fluoroquinolones and tetracyclines is not recommended during pregnancy.
Chancroid	azithromycin 1 g PO in a single dose or ceftriaxone 250 mg IM in a single dose or ciprofloxacin 500 mg PO b.i.d. for 3 d or erythromycin base 500 mg PO t.i.d. for 7 d	Use compresses to remove necrotic material; clean ulcerative lesions t.i.d.
Chlamydia	Recommended: azithromycin 1 g PO for 1 d or doxycycline 100 mg PO b.i.d. for 7 d Alternative regimen: erythromycin base 500 mg PO q.i.d. for 7 d or erythromycin ethylsuccinate 800 mg PO q.i.d. for 7 d or ofloxacin 300 mg PO b.i.d. for 7 d or levofloxacin 500 mg PO daily for 7 d Pregnancy recommended: azithromycin 1 g PO for 1 dose or amoxicillin 500 mg PO t.i.d. for 7 d Pregnancy alternative: erythromycin base 500 mg PO q.i.d. for 7 d or erythromycin base 250 mg PO q.i.d. for 14 d or erythromycin ethylsuccinate 800 mg PO q.i.d. for 7 d or erythromycin ethylsuccinate 400 mg PO q.i.d. for 14 d Infants (ophthalmia neonatorum): erythromycin base or ethylsuccinate 50 mg/kg/d PO divided into 4 doses for 14 d	TOC needed 3-4 mo after initial treatment. Second course of therapy may be required.
Epididymitis	If likely cause GC or CT: ceftriaxone 250 mg IM for 1 d and doxycycline 100 mg PO b.i.d. for 10 d If likely cause enteric bacteria or allergy to above medications: ofloxacin 300 mg PO b.i.d. for 10 d or levofloxacin 500 mg PO daily for 10 d	Treat for gonorrhea; follow with treatment for nongonococcal urethritis.
Genital warts	Provider applied: cryotherapy or cryoprobe; repeat application q1-2wk or podophyllin 10%-25% in compound tincture of benzoin once/wk for 6 wk; wash off 4-6 hours after application. or trichloroacetic acid (TCA) or dichloroacetic acid (BCA) 80%-90% applied to visible warts and allowed to dry. Application is once/wk	Nothing eradicates HPV. Podophyllin contraindicated during pregnancy. Safety during pregnancy has not been established. Pregnancy category: C Pregnancy category: C Pregnancy category: C

Continued

TABLE 58-6 CURRENT GUIDELINES FOR PRIMARY THERAPIES FOR COMMON SEXUALLY TRANSMITTED INFECTIONS—cont'd

INFECTION	PRIMARY THERAPY	NOTES
	Patient applied: imiquimod 5% cream, applied h.s., 3 times/wk for up to 16 wk. Wash treatment area with soap and water 6-10 h after application. or sinecatechins 15% ointment applied to each wart t.i.d. for up to 16 weeks. or podofilox 0.5% solution or gel applied to warts with cotton swab b.i.d. for 3 d then discontinued for 4 d. Repeat cycle for 4 wk.	
Gonorrhea	Recommended: ceftriaxone 250 mg IM in a single dose *plus* either azithromycin 1 G PO in a single dose or doxycycline 100 mg PO b.i.d. for 7 d or Alternative if ceftriaxone not available: cefixime 400 mg PO in a single dose *plus* azithromycin 1 G PO in a single dose or doxycycline 100 mg PO b.i.d. for 7 d plus Test of cure in 1 week If cephalosporin allergy: azithromycin 2 G PO in a single dose *plus* Test of cure in 1 wk Pregnancy recommended: CDC suggests that cephalosporins be used for treatment of gonorrhea in pregnancy. ceftriaxone 250 mg IM in a single dose *plus* azithromycin 1 G PO in a single dose would be the treatment of choice Ophthalmia neonatorum: ceftriaxone 25-50 mg/kg IM/IV in a single dose; *max:* 125 mg Ophthalmia neonatorum prophylaxis: erythromycin (0.5%) ophthalmic ointment; 1 application each eye in a single dose	Patient should be concurrently treated for chlamydia. Fluoroquinolones are not recommended for treatment of GC infection due to high prevalence of fluoroquinolone resistance in these populations. Oral cephalosporins should not be given if parenteral cephalosporins are available. If it is given, a 1-wk follow-up for a test of cure is required. Use of fluoroquinolones and tetracyclines is not recommended during pregnancy.
Granuloma inguinale	azithromycin 1 g PO in a single dose or ceftriaxone 250 mg IM in a single dose or ciprofloxacin 500 mg PO b.i.d. for 3 d or erythromycin base 500 mg PO t.i.d. for 7 d	
Hepatitis A	No specific therapy exists.	Vaccine available as HAVRIX or VAQTA. Available in 2- and 3-dose series for eligible children 1-18 y. Available for patients older than 18 y with risk for obtaining HAV (men who have sex with men, drug users, sex workers, patients with HBV or HCV).
Hepatitis B	HAV and HBV are two STIs for which a vaccine exists.	CDC recommends vaccination of all infants and adolescents. ACIP recommends vaccination of all persons with recent STI and those with more than one partner in last 6 mo. Combined hepatitis A and B vaccine has been developed for adults.
Hepatitis C	Alpha interferon and oral agent ribavirin may be used to treat HCV chronic liver disease	No vaccine available.

TABLE 58-6 CURRENT GUIDELINES FOR PRIMARY THERAPIES FOR COMMON SEXUALLY TRANSMITTED INFECTIONS—cont'd

INFECTION	PRIMARY THERAPY	NOTES
Genital herpes simplex	First episode: acyclovir 400 mg PO t.i.d. for 7-10 d or acyclovir 200 mg PO five times/d for 7-10 d or famciclovir 250 mg PO t.i.d. for 7-10 d or valacyclovir 1 g PO b.i.d. for 10 d Recurrent episode: acyclovir 400 mg PO t.i.d. for 5 d or acyclovir 800 mg PO b.i.d. for 5 d or acyclovir 800 mg PO t.i.d. for 2 d or famciclovir 125 mg PO b.i.d. for 5 d or famciclovir 1,000 mg PO b.i.d. for 1 d or famciclovir 500 mg PO once followed by 250 mg PO b.i.d. for 2 d or valacyclovir 500 mg PO b.i.d. for 3 d or valacyclovir 1 g PO daily for 5 d Suppressive therapy: acyclovir 400 mg PO b.i.d. or famciclovir 250 mg PO b.i.d. or valacyclovir 500 mg PO daily or valacyclovir 1 g PO daily Neonatal: acyclovir 20 mg/kg IV q8h for 21 d	Types 1 and 2 cannot be distinguished clinically. No cure is known. Systemic disease is life-threatening to neonates; neurologic damage may result. Viral shedding is most prevalent when symptomatic; patient should avoid sexual relations at this time. Acyclovir, famciclovir, and valacyclovir may be used in pregnancy for HSV suppression therapy from gestational week 36 until delivery. Acyclovir and valacyclovir must be used with caution in first trimester of pregnancy. Visit the CDC website for information on treatment of HSV in immunosuppressed patients, including those with HIV/AIDS. For severe HSV disease, in-hospital parenteral (IV) therapy may be needed.
Lymphogranuloma venereum	doxycycline 100 mg PO b.i.d. for 21 d or erythromycin 0.5 g PO q.i.d. for 21 d	
Molluscum contagiosum	cryoanesthesia and curettage or caustic chemicals (podophyllin, trichloroacetic acid, silver nitrate) and cryotherapy	If all lesions not eradicated, may recur.
Mucopurulent cervicitis	azithromycin 1 g PO in a single dose or doxycycline 100 mg PO b.i.d. for 7-10 d	
Pelvic inflammatory disease (PID)	Inpatient regimen A: cefotetan 2 g IV q12h or cefoxitin 2 g IV q6h plus doxycycline 100 mg PO or IV q12h Inpatient regimen B: clindamycin 900 mg IV q8h plus gentamicin (loading dose) 2 mg/kg IM/IV followed by maint 1.5 mg/kg q8h Ambulatory care: ceftriaxone 250 mg IM in a single dose *plus* doxycycline 100 mg PO b.i.d. for 14 d	Often polymicrobial. This regimen may not treat anaerobes, pelvic mass, or IUD-associated PID.

Continued

TABLE 58-6 CURRENT GUIDELINES FOR PRIMARY THERAPIES FOR COMMON SEXUALLY TRANSMITTED INFECTIONS—cont'd

INFECTION	PRIMARY THERAPY	NOTES
	with or without metronidazole 500 mg PO b.i.d. for 14 d or cefoxitin 2 g IM in a single dose *plus* doxycycline 100 mg PO b.i.d. for 14 d with or without metronidazole 500 mg PO b.i.d. for 14 d or other parenteral third-generation cephalosporin (e.g., ceftizoxime or cefotaxime) *plus* doxycycline 100 mg PO b.i.d. for 14 d with or without metronidazole 500 mg PO b.i.d. for 14 d	
Proctitis	ceftriaxone 250 mg IM in a single dose, and doxycycline 100 mg PO b.i.d. for 7 d	
Pubic lice	permethrin 1% cream rinse: Apply to affected area, and wash off after 10 min or pyrethrins with piperonyl butoxide: Apply to affected area, and wash off after 10 min	Use lindane only if other therapy fails. Decontaminate clothes and bedding. Second treatment 7-10 d after first to kill newly hatched lice. Treat partner also.
Scabies	Recommended: permethrin cream 5% applied to all affected areas from neck down and washed off after 8-14 h or ivermectin 200 micrograms/kg PO, repeat in 2 wk. Alternative regimen: lindane 1% applied to all affected areas from neck down and thoroughly washed off after 8 h	
Sexual assault	ceftriaxone 250 mg IM in a single dose or cefixime 400 mg PO in a single dose *plus* metronidazole 2 g PO in a single dose plus azithromycin 1 g PO in a single dose or doxycycline 100 mg PO b.i.d. for 7 d	Tetanus booster and gamma globulin, as well as baseline HIV testing and follow-up, are recommended.
Syphilis	Primary, secondary, or <1 y duration (early latent syphilis): benzathine penicillin G, 2.4 million units IM in a single dose Unknown duration or >1 y (late latent syphilis): benzathine penicillin G, 7.2 million units divided in 2.4 million IM weekly in three doses Allergic to penicillin: see infectious disease specialist Infants and children: benzathine penicillin G 50,000 units/kg IM in a single dose, up to 2.4 million units.	Pregnant patients who are allergic to penicillin should be desensitized. Administration of Benzathine penicillin G in patient with syphilis may cause the Jarisch-Herxheimer reaction from the breakdown of the *T. pallidum* spirochete. This acute febrile reaction is often accompanied by headache, myalgia, and fever. In pregnant patients, this can cause preterm labor or fetal distress.
Trichomoniasis	Recommended: metronidazole 2 g PO in a single dose or tinidazole 2 g PO in a single dose Alternative regimen: metronidazole 500 mg PO b.i.d. for 7 d STIs have potentially serious sequela; partners of infected patients should be treated simultaneously to prevent reinfection.	Pregnant women can be treated after the first trimester. Metronidazole vaginal gel should not be given for trichomoniasis Tindamax is contraindicated during the first trimester of pregnancy.

*The most recent guidelines and alternative treatments are available from *www.cdc.gov/STD/treatment.*

A, Adult; *ACIP*, Advisory Committee on Immunization Practices; *b.i.d.*, twice a day; *C*, child; *CDC*, Centers for Disease Control and Prevention; *d*, day; *GI*, gastrointestinal; *h*, hour; *HAV*, hepatitis A virus; *HBV*, hepatitis B virus; *HCV*, hepatitis C virus; *HIV*, human immunodeficiency virus; *HPV*, human papillomavirus; *h.s.*, at bedtime; *IM*, intramuscular; *IUD*, intrauterine device; *IV*, intravenous; *maint*, maintenance; *max*, maximum; *min*, minute; *mo*, month; *PO*, by mouth; *q.i.d.*, four times a day; *STI*, sexually transmitted infection; *t.i.d.*, three times a day; *wk*, week; *y*, year; >, greater than; <, less than.

green-yellow, malodorous vaginal discharge is *Trichomonas vaginalis.* This microbe can be visualized under a microscope as one-celled protozoa with flagella. All pathogens that are sexually transmitted are shown in Table 58-5.

Because STIs can threaten reproductive health, neonatal health, fertility, and even life, early diagnosis and treatment are crucial but are less effective than prevention. For some, drug therapies may offer relief.

Nursing Process

Patient-Centered Collaborative Care

Sexually Transmitted Infections

Assessment

- Assess a medical history before gathering physical data. Address less-sensitive issues before more personal issues so trust can be established. Use the term *partner* when discussing sexual activity rather than value-laden terms such as *wife* or *boyfriend.* Include the following questions for all patients, regardless of gender or sexual orientation: "Do you have sex with women?" and "Do you have sex with men?"
- Assess patient history including chief complaint, description of course of illness, review of systems and general health history, gynecologic history including reproductive history and sexual history, review of lifestyle and social habits, and identification of allergies.
- Physical examination includes inspection and palpation of mouth, oropharynx, throat and lymph nodes, abdomen, and inguinal lymph systems. Also perform a physical examination of the genitalia and other points of inoculation. Allow men to swab themselves for cultures if preferred. Gonorrhea and chlamydia may also be obtained from a urine specimen.
- Laboratory tests include wet slide with microbe-specific setting agents, urinalysis, culture, Pap smear, complete blood count, syphilis serology, and HSV-2 and HSV-2 antibodies.

Nursing Diagnoses

- Deficient knowledge related to transmission and prevention of STIs
- Deficient knowledge related to pharmacologic treatment of STIs
- Noncompliance related to known prevention strategies
- Impaired tissue integrity related to lesions, ulcerations, and excoriations
- Pain related to inflammation and infection
- Situational low self-esteem related to potential stigma of diagnosis
- Ineffective sexuality patterns related to unsafe sex practices
- Risk for infection related to unsafe sex practices
- Medical diagnosis of HIV disease may bring these additional nursing diagnoses: (1) fatigue related to diagnosis, (2) anxiety related to potential outcome of disease, (3) anticipatory grieving related to fear of death, (4) risk for loneliness related to possible stigma of diagnosis, and (5) ineffective therapeutic regimen management/health maintenance related to focus on daily concerns with diagnosis

Planning

- Short-term goals include patient's adherence to treatment regimen and avoidance of adverse effects.
- Long-term goals include patient's return for follow-up evaluation and adoption of risk-reducing sexual behaviors.

Nursing Interventions

- Counsel patient about procedures performed during evaluation and how to administer prescribed medications and treatments. Review side effects and adverse reactions that require immediate intervention.
- Provide needed support as patient deals with the fact that infection is sexually transmitted.
- Advise patient to notify sexual partners so they can be evaluated and treated.
- Counsel patient to avoid sexual contact during treatment. At the least, patient should use condoms until both partners are shown to be clear of infection.
- Schedule follow-up visits from 4 days to 4 weeks later, depending on type of infection and treatment.
- Counsel patient about being tested for HIV.

Patient Teaching

- Review mode of transmission of STIs, relationship of all STIs to HIV infection, and how HIV risk is avoided.
- Counsel patient on effective use of both male and female condoms.
- Discuss condom use negotiation.
- Advise patient to plan periodic reproductive health checkups.

Cultural Considerations

- Some women prefer to be examined only by a female health care provider.
- Use a certified medical interpreter of same gender and culture, especially for sensitive topics.
- In male-dominated cultures, male patient may be unwilling to undergo testing or treatment.

Evaluation

- Intervention has been successful if the individual's infection is clear on reevaluation or, in the case of viral infections, the individual experiences quiescence of the virus.
- The infection is not transmitted to other individuals.
- The patient is able to avoid sexual practices that carry risk for acquiring STIs, including intercourse without the use of a condom.

KEY WEBSITES

Centers for Disease Control and Prevention: STI treatment guidelines: *www.cdc.gov/STD/treatment*

InterNational Council on Infertility Information Dissemination: *www.inciid.org*

MedlinePlus: *www.nlm.nih.gov/medlineplus/sexuallytransmitteddiseases.html*

CRITICAL THINKING CASE STUDY

DD is 32 years old and has never been pregnant. She has been diagnosed with infertility for 3 years. For the last year, she and her male partner TD have been trying to conceive without success. DD's nurse practitioner learns that DD has had three previous sexual partners and was treated for chlamydia at age 23 years; DD's partner TD was treated in the past for HSV. DD's menstrual history reveals an erratic pattern of unpredictable periods, occurring about every 3 to 4 months. DD and TD are referred to an infertility specialist by the nurse practitioner.

1. What is the relevance of DD's past sexual history to the current complaint?
2. Why would the infertility specialist consider cultures for *Chlamydia trachomatis* and *Neisseria gonorrhoeae* years after exposure?
3. What other tests would reveal damage resulting from STIs?
4. What is abnormal about DD's menstrual history? What about her menstrual pattern makes conception difficult? What are the possible diagnoses and pharmacologic treatments for the patient to help with conception? For what would the nurse want to observe when she examines the patient?
5. How can TD prevent DD from getting HSV? How can DD be tested for HSV?

   After a complete evaluation of both DD and TD, metformin is prescribed for DD along with a course of clomiphene citrate.
6. What side effects can DD expect from these medications?
7. When should DD take the medications? What patient instructions are needed when clomiphene citrate is prescribed?
8. When should DD and TD have sexual intercourse to enhance the possibility of conception?
9. What other possible disease conditions can cause infertility?
10. DD becomes pregnant after four cycles on clomiphene citrate. What is one potential risk factor with this pregnancy?

    DD gives birth to a boy after an uneventful pregnancy. She decides to breastfeed for 12 months. After discontinuing breastfeeding, her menstrual cycles return to a normal monthly pattern. However, she experiences fatigue, breast tenderness, and mood swings for a few days before her periods. She states that she cries and gets frustrated with her partner and child. She also has very painful periods and has missed work on several occasions because of her symptoms. She wants to wait 3 years before having another child.
11. What are the possible conditions that DD is experiencing? What nursing diagnoses accompany these conditions?
12. What type of complementary and alternative and/or drug therapies can be used to help DD with these conditions?
13. What method of contraception would be best for DD?
14. List the complete health teaching for DD.

NCLEX STUDY QUESTIONS

1. A patient with infertility asks the nurse what is causing her to have irregular cycles leading to her diagnosis of PCOS. What is the nurse's best response?
   a. "PCOS is caused by damage to the female reproductive tract by pathogens."
   b. "Increased levels of progesterone with PCOS cause the sperm to be unable to penetrate cervical mucus."
   c. "PCOS causes your body to have menstrual cycles in which ovulation does not occur."
   d. "PCOS is a state in which there is a lack of estrogen that interferes with the menstrual cycle."
2. A patient has been prescribed clomiphene citrate therapy by her doctor. The patient asks the nurse, "How does my new medicine work?" What is the nurse's best response to convey the mechanism of action of clomiphene citrate therapy to this patient?
   a. "This medication works by stimulating the ovaries, increasing the chance of ovulation."
   b. "This medication increases circulating progesterone levels."
   c. "This medication usually does not work on the first cycle."
   d. "This medication helps the ovaries form multiple follicles."
3. A patient at the STI clinic asks why he is not prescribed antibiotics. He has been diagnosed with HSV-2. The nurse's best response is based on what knowledge? (Select all that apply.)

a. Antibiotics will not lessen the symptoms of HSV.
b. HSV can be cured with antiviral medications only.
c. Antibiotics are used to successfully treat viral infections.
d. HSV symptoms may be relieved with palliative antiviral medications.
e. Antibiotics combined with antiviral medications are the best treatment for HSV-2 infections.

4. The nurse is reviewing risk factors for STIs with a patient. Which behavior has the least risk for acquiring an STI?
a. Abstinence
b. Use of a male condom
c. Sexual relations within a mutually monogamous relationship
d. Sexual relations with a previous IV substance user

5. The nurse prepares a class for high school students. What best describes why ulcerative STIs increase an individual's risk for HIV infection?
a. Ulcerative STIs decrease the amount of lubrication.
b. STIs are commonly associated with other high-risk behaviors.
c. STIs are only found in individuals with multiple sexual partners.
d. A break in the skin increases the transmission of pathogens.

6. The nurse is reviewing a patient's medications with her. The nurse knows that effective pharmacologic treatment for vulvovaginal candidiasis includes which drug?
a. metronidazole
b. fluconazole
c. metformin
d. ibuprofen

7. The nurse is meeting with a couple during the early phase of treatment for primary infertility. Which content would be appropriate to include in a generic teaching plan to be personalized for this couple? (Select all that apply.)
a. Ways to alleviate feelings of low self-esteem related to infertility
b. Sexual techniques that enhance fertilization
c. Recommended avoidance of guaifenesin
d. Necessity of repetitive treatment regimens before successful conception
e. Infertility is 100% curable.

Answers: 1, c; 2, a; 3, a, d; 4, a; 5, d; 6, b; 7, a, b, d.

UNIT XIX

Emergency Agents

This final unit focuses on adult and pediatric emergency drugs. Chapter 59 considers oxygen as an emergency drug and discusses pharmacologic treatment for five categories of emergency situations: (1) cardiac disorders, (2) intracranial hypertension, (3) poisoning, (4) shock, and (5) hypertensive crises and pulmonary edema. Specific drug protocols and dosages for the pediatric patient are included.

CHAPTER

59

Adult and Pediatric Emergency Drugs

Linda Laskowski-Jones

evolve WEBSITE

http://evolve.elsevier.com/KeeHayes/pharmacology/

- Animations
- Content Updates
- Key Points
- Review Questions for the NCLEX® Examination
- References from the Textbook
- Unfolding Case Studies

OBJECTIVES

- Describe indications for the emergency drugs listed in this chapter.
- Define the basic mechanism of action for each emergency drug.
- Discuss pertinent nursing considerations and actions specific for each agent.
- Explain how to administer the drugs properly.
- Describe significant adverse effects of each drug.

OUTLINE

KEY TERMS

anaphylactic shock, p. 921
angina pectoris, p. 911
asthma, p. 921
asystole, p. 912
bradycardia, p. 912
cathartic, p. 919
dysrhythmias, p. 913
extravasation, p. 920
fraction of inspired oxygen, p. 910
glycogenolysis, p. 922
heart block, p. 912
hypertensive crisis, p. 922

hypomagnesemia, p. 914
hypovolemic shock, p. 919
hypoxemia, p. 910
myocardial infarction, p. 911
paroxysmal supraventricular tachycardia, p. 912
preload, p. 924
pulse oximetry, p. 910
tachycardia, p. 911
torsades de pointes, p. 914

The drugs described in this chapter are first-line agents used to treat various medical emergencies. Nurses must have knowledge of the indications and actions of these agents, because medical and surgical emergencies can occur in virtually any area of nursing practice. Learning key nursing implications *before* a crisis situation enables the nurse to function at the highest possible level when the patient requires lifesaving intervention.

At the end of each discussion of a group of emergency drugs is a summary prototype drug chart that contains dosages and indications. Common adult doses are listed in the drug charts; pediatric dosages may vary widely depending on the child's age and weight. For the purpose of drug dosing, advanced cardiac life support guidelines consider adults to be older than 8 years and children to be 8 years or younger; infants are younger than 1 year. The drug charts list only the most common indications and dosages for the emergency drugs discussed; they *do not* describe all possible uses and dosing regimens for the agents.

OXYGEN AS AN EMERGENCY DRUG

Oxygen can be classified as a drug, because it can have both beneficial and adverse effects on the body based on the amount and manner in which it is administered. Oxygen is essential to life—without it brain death begins within 6 minutes. Inadequate oxygenation produces **hypoxemia** (inadequate oxygen in the blood) and significant physiologic sequela to all body systems; therefore oxygen is a first-line drug for all emergency situations. Depending on the circumstances, adequate oxygenation may be all that is necessary to effectively treat physiologic disturbances such as chest pain, bradycardia, and cardiac dysrhythmias. Oxygen also acts as a potent pulmonary vasodilator and is beneficial for patients in heart failure.

Before the other pharmacologic agents discussed in this chapter are administered, ensure that the patient's airway and breathing are addressed to promote optimal oxygenation and ventilation. Giving a drug to treat a disorder brought on by hypoxemia without effectively correcting the cause of the hypoxemia is ineffective and ultimately does not produce the desired outcome. **Pulse oximetry**, which provides a digital display of oxygen saturation, is an essential monitoring tool that should be used in emergency situations to assess the adequacy of oxygenation and guide further interventions. Ideally oxygen saturation should be kept at or above 94%. It is important to recognize, however, that certain pathophysiologic states can make pulse oximetry readings inaccurate. These conditions include vasoconstriction, severe anemia, hypothermia, carbon monoxide poisoning, and shock.

The ambient room air contains approximately 21% oxygen. When patients breathe room air, the oxygen they inspire constitutes 21% of the total volume of gas they take in with each breath. This measure is termed the **fraction of inspired oxygen** (FiO_2). As a general rule, patients suffering from severe physiologic stress such as shock states, traumatic injury, acute myocardial infarction (AMI) with hemodynamic instability, and cardiac arrest initially require supplemental oxygen in high concentrations (i.e., an FiO_2 close to 100%). The initial emergency oxygen delivery devices of choice for these conditions include a nonrebreather mask with an oxygen reservoir (oxygen flow rate set at 10 to 15 L/min) for spontaneously breathing patients, and a bag-valve-mask device attached to an oxygen source at a flow rate of 15 L/min for patients who require assisted ventilation until definitive airway management and a mechanical ventilator are available.

Although caution must be exercised for patients with chronic obstructive pulmonary disease (COPD), who may lose their hypoxic respiratory drive when given oxygen in high concentration, oxygen should never be denied to a patient who needs it. In the case of COPD, the nurse should be prepared to ventilate the patient manually with a bag-valve-mask if respiratory depression or arrest occurs. Some patients in respiratory distress as a result of obstructive pulmonary disease or acute cardiogenic pulmonary edema may also benefit from oxygen therapy delivered through noninvasive mask ventilation via a CPAP or BiPAP circuit; these devices deliver oxygen via a positive-pressure mechanism.

Whatever the underlying injury or disease process, as the patient's condition stabilizes, the oxygen concentration should be decreased to achieve an arterial oxygen saturation of ≥94%. An FiO_2 above 50% for a prolonged period can lead to oxygen toxicity and other detrimental effects to the pulmonary system in both adults and children.

For emergency situations that do not involve severe physiologic stress (e.g., angina, dysrhythmias, pulmonary disease), supplemental oxygen delivered by nasal cannula at 1 to 6 L/min or by simple face mask at 6 to 10 L/min may have significant physiologic benefit. Young children may better tolerate a face tent with a high oxygen flow of 10 to 15 L than a face mask.

EMERGENCY DRUGS FOR CARDIAC DISORDERS

Drugs described in this section are indicated for cardiac emergencies such as angina, MI, disturbances of cardiac rate or rhythm, and cardiac arrest. In a resuscitation situation, the foundation of patient therapy is based upon proper oxygenation and ventilation, performance of optimal CPR, and application of electrical therapy (cardioversion and defibrillation) according to established treatment algorithms and standards. Pharmacologic agents are used as adjuncts in synchrony with these efforts when indicated to enhance the likelihood of a successful outcome. These drugs often must be prepared and administered rapidly. A sound knowledge base as well as easy access to the drugs and necessary equipment is essential for the best patient response in a cardiac emergency. Usually in an emergency, detailed personal, medical, drug, and herbal histories are unavailable (Herbal Alert 59-1). Treatment is based on patient presentation.

HERBAL ALERT 59-1

Herbs and Emergency Medications

In emergency situations, a detailed personal health history is often not available; therefore, treatment is based on patient presentation. Herbal products with anticoagulation properties or those that interact with catecholamines (which may cause hypertensive crisis) could adversely influence the effectiveness of medications used to treat emergency conditions.

Aspirin

Aspirin is a first-line emergency drug used to decrease platelet aggregation in the management of acute coronary syndromes and myocardial infarction. It is best administered at the onset of chest pain in doses of 160 to 325 mg orally. The patient should be asked to chew the tablet to speed absorption of the drug instead of swallowing the tablet whole. For patients experiencing nausea and vomiting, an aspirin rectal suppository in a dose of 300 mg can be given as an alternative. Aspirin is also indicated in the initial treatment algorithm for patients suffering from acute ischemic stroke who are not candidates for fibrinolytic therapy. Contraindications to aspirin administration include a true drug allergy, presence of cerebral hemorrhage on CT scan, and recent GI bleeding.

Nitroglycerin

Nitroglycerin dilates coronary arteries and improves blood flow to an ischemic myocardium. It is therefore the treatment of choice for **angina pectoris** (chest pain) and **myocardial infarction** (heart attack). Nitroglycerin is also considered a first-line drug in the management of patients with acute cardiogenic pulmonary edema due to its ability to decrease both preload and afterload. A focused medication history is essential prior to administration, even in emergency situations, because nitroglycerin in combination with drugs for erectile dysfunction (i.e., sildenafil [Viagra], vardenafil [Levitra], tadalafil [Cialis]) causes profound hypotension that may be refractory to treatment when taken within a 24- to 48-hour period. This combination is contraindicated. Nitroglycerin is available in sublingual, translingual aerosol spray, oral, topical, and intravenous (IV) forms. Only the sublingual, translingual aerosol spray, and intravenous preparations are discussed.

Sublingual nitroglycerin (0.3 to 0.4 mg) and the translingual aerosol spray (0.4-mg metered dose) preparations are indicated for patients experiencing an acute anginal attack who have a systolic blood pressure >90 mm Hg. The patient is taught to sit or lie down and moisten 1 sublingual nitroglycerin tablet with saliva and then place it under the tongue to allow it to dissolve slowly. If the chest pain is not relieved, sublingual nitroglycerin may be repeated at 3- to 5-minute intervals as long as the patient's systolic blood pressure remains >90 mm Hg until a total of 3 tablets has been taken. Patients prescribed the translingual aerosol preparation should be reminded that the spray should not be inhaled. Instead, it should be sprayed onto or under the tongue. The patient should be instructed not to swallow for approximately 10 seconds to allow absorption of the drug. As with sublingual nitroglycerin, up to 3 doses may be taken within 15 minutes. If pain persists despite 3 doses of the sublingual or aerosol forms, further interventions are necessary in an emergency or critical care setting. An ambulance should be called if the patient is outside the hospital. Blood pressure and heart rate must be monitored closely. Hypotension is a common adverse effect, especially the first time a patient takes nitroglycerin. **Tachycardia** (abnormally high heart rate in adults; >100 beats/min) or, uncommonly, bradycardia also may occur. Patients who take sublingual or translingual aerosol spray nitroglycerin while wearing a nitroglycerin patch may be at higher risk for hypotension. This situation warrants caution. Though tolerance to nitrates can develop in individuals who take nitroglycerin preparations daily and can offer some protection against hypotension, the nitroglycerin patch may need to be removed if blood pressure instability occurs. To prevent arcing and the potential for skin burns, the nitroglycerin patch must also be removed prior to cardioversion or defibrillation.

IV nitroglycerin is reserved for patients with unstable angina or an AMI. A continuous infusion is usually initiated at a rate of 10 to 20 mcg/min and increased by 5 to 10 mcg/min every 5 to 10 minutes, based on chest pain and blood pressure response. Continuous blood pressure and heart monitoring are required, because hypotension is a common adverse effect. Hypotension usually is treated by reducing or discontinuing the nitroglycerin infusion (see Chapter 42) and by placing the patient in a supine position with legs elevated if tolerated.

Morphine Sulfate

Morphine sulfate, a narcotic analgesic, is used to treat the chest pain associated with AMI. It also is indicated for acute cardiogenic pulmonary edema. Morphine relieves pain, dilates venous vessels, and reduces the workload on the heart. The standard dosage of morphine sulfate is 1 to 4 mg IV over 1 to 5 minutes, repeated every 5 to 30 minutes until chest pain is relieved. Because respiratory depression and hypotension are common adverse effects, the drug must be administered slowly and carefully titrated to achieve the desired therapeutic effects. Close patient monitoring is essential. It is important to realize that although morphine can produce respiratory depression, this agent can relieve the dyspnea caused by pulmonary edema. In this situation, respiratory distress is not a contraindication to morphine administration. The narcotic antagonist naloxone (Narcan) may be ordered to reverse the action of morphine if adverse effects pose a significant risk to the patient. The dose is 0.4 to 2 mg every 2 minutes as indicated (see Chapter 26).

Atropine Sulfate

Atropine sulfate is the primary agent indicated for the treatment of hemodynamically significant **bradycardia** (slow heart rate) and some types of **heart block** (e.g., atrioventricular block at the nodal level). Atropine acts to increase heart rate by inhibiting the action of the vagus nerve (parasympatholytic effect). Atropine sulfate is also used as an emergency drug to reverse the toxic effects of organophosphate pesticide and nerve agent exposure, which include bradycardia and excessive secretions.

In symptomatic bradycardia, atropine is administered IV in 0.5-mg doses at 3- to 5-minute intervals until the desired heart rate is achieved or until 0.04 mg/kg (not more than 3 mg) is given. Dosing in this manner may be repeated every 3 to 5 minutes up to a limit of 0.04 mg/kg (usually not more than 3 mg IV).

The adult IV atropine dose should never be less than 0.5 mg. Doses below 0.5 mg can produce a paradoxical bradycardia; at doses of 0.04 mg/kg or greater, vagal activity is considered completely blocked, and further atropine administration may have no benefit. However, in the case of organophosphate insecticide or nerve agent poisoning, *very high* doses of atropine may be necessary to counteract the pathophysiologic effects of these toxins. Therefore, the typical dosing range and limits do not apply under these circumstances.

If venous access is not available in an emergency situation, atropine sulfate should be administered through the intraosseous (IO) route. As a last resort, atropine may be given via the endotracheal tube (ETT) route if venous or intraosseous access cannot be achieved. The dose for endotracheal administration is 2 to 2.5 times the venous dose, diluted with normal saline or sterile water. Accordingly, 2 to 3 mg of atropine would be diluted in 10 mL of normal saline or sterile water and instilled deep into the ETT via a feeding tube attached to a syringe. After endotracheal administration, the patient should be ventilated vigorously with a bag-valve device to enhance absorption of the drug.

Continuous cardiac and blood pressure monitoring is essential for the patient who receives atropine sulfate. Significant adverse effects include cardiac dysrhythmias, tachycardia, myocardial ischemia, restlessness, anxiety, mydriasis, thirst, and urinary retention. See Chapter 19 for more information on atropine and other anticholinergics.

Pediatric Implications

The definition of bradycardia is variable and age-specific for the pediatric population. Knowledge of normal ranges is essential. Because cardiac output is dependent on heart rate in infants younger than 6 months, bradycardia (heart rate <100 beats/min for infants) must be treated. In fact, a heart rate <60 beats/min in an infant requires performance of CPR. Before administration of drugs, efforts always should be targeted first toward restoring adequate ventilation and oxygenation. For the neonate with a spontaneous heart rate of less than 80 beats/min, epinephrine 0.01 mg/kg IV or IO every 3 to 5 minutes as indicated should be given prior to atropine to elevate the heart rate, because stressed neonates quickly deplete their own stores of catecholamines. If these interventions do not produce the desired clinical response, then atropine is indicated in the presence of increased vagal tone or atrioventricular (AV) block. Other pediatric indications for atropine include management of organophosphate toxicity and as pretreatment to prevent bradycardia after succinylcholine administration during rapid-sequence intubation.

The pediatric dose of atropine is 0.02 mg/kg IV or IO. It is important to be cognizant that in the pediatric population, the minimum single dose is 0.1 mg and the maximum single dose is 0.5 mg IV. The maximum total pediatric dose is 1 mg in a child and 3 mg in an adolescent (defined as an individual who has reached puberty). Note: When referring to general age groupings of patients, *infants* are considered to be younger than 1 year; a *child* is considered to be age 1 year to adolescence (puberty), and an *adult* is considered to be an adolescent or older. See Chapters 7 and 11 for more information on pediatric medication dosing and monitoring.

Adenosine

Adenosine is the first-line drug of choice to treat **paroxysmal supraventricular tachycardia** (PSVT), a sudden, uncontrolled, rapid rhythm (exceeding 150 beats/min in adults) that originates above the ventricles. The goal is to convert PSVT to sinus rhythm. A natural substance found in all body cells, adenosine slows impulse conduction through the heart's AV node, interrupts dysrhythmia-producing reentry pathways, and restores a normal rhythm in patients with PSVT. Because the half-life is less than 5 seconds, adenosine is best administered rapidly via a peripheral IV site in the port most proximal to the patient as a 6-mg IV bolus over 1 to 3 seconds followed by a 20-mL saline flush. A 12-mg bolus may be given 1 to 2 minutes after the initial dose if PSVT persists. Higher doses are not recommended.

Nursing considerations include continuous cardiac monitoring and frequent assessment of vital signs. Adenosine is inhibited by methylxanthines such as caffeine and theophylline, so higher doses may be needed. Though usually transient, ventricular ectopy, bradycardia, flushing, chest pain, and dyspnea may occur. In addition, a short period of **asystole** may follow injection of adenosine (up to 15 seconds). Spontaneous cardiac activity typically resumes. Adenosine is contraindicated in patients with poison- or drug-related tachycardia, second- and third-degree heart block, and in patients with sick sinus syndrome, except those with functioning pacemakers. If the tachycardia originated in the ventricles, the patient could deteriorate and become hypotensive after adenosine administration. See Chapter 42 for more information on antidysrhythmic drugs.

Diltiazem

Diltiazem is a calcium channel blocker and is administered as an IV bolus to treat PSVT and to slow the ventricular response rate in atrial fibrillation or flutter. It is considered a second-line agent after adenosine. Diltiazem has less of a negative inotropic effect than other similar calcium channel blockers, but it has strong negative chronotropic actions. Therefore, IV diltiazem is less likely to cause cardiac depression, but is very effective in controlling heart rate.

The usual initial bolus dose of IV diltiazem is 0.25 mg/kg given over 2 minutes. If the supraventricular tachycardia does not convert to a normal sinus rhythm in 15 minutes, a second IV bolus of 0.35 mg/kg over 2 minutes may be necessary. For ongoing control of the ventricular rate in patients with atrial fibrillation or flutter, a continuous infusion of diltiazem is indicated at a dose range of 5 to 15 mg/hour, titrated according to the desired heart rate.

The nurse must carefully monitor blood pressure and heart rate and rhythm after administering IV diltiazem. Arrhythmias, bradycardia, heart block, and hypotension may develop. Diltiazem can elevate serum digoxin levels, predisposing the patient to digitalis toxicity. Simultaneous use of calcium channel blockers and beta blockers is contraindicated, because their negative inotropic and negative chronotropic effects are synergistic, causing myocardial depression and bradycardia. Other contraindications include preexisting heart block or sick sinus syndrome in the patient without a pacemaker, Wolff-Parkinson-White syndrome, and heart failure.

Amiodarone

The IV form of amiodarone is considered a first-line agent in the advanced cardiac life support algorithms for the treatment of life-threatening ventricular dysrhythmias and cardiac arrest. It has alpha- and beta-adrenergic blocking effects and acts on sodium, potassium, and calcium channels. Indications for use include pulseless ventricular tachycardia and ventricular fibrillation (after defibrillation and epinephrine), hemodynamically stable ventricular tachycardia, PSVT refractory to adenosine, ventricular rate control in atrial fibrillation, and pharmacologic treatment of atrial fibrillation.

Amiodarone is especially good for patients with impaired heart function who have atrial and ventricular dysrhythmias. It has been found to be more effective and to have fewer proarrhythmic properties than other agents with similar actions.

For patients who have a pulse (i.e., not in cardiac arrest), amiodarone 150 mg IV is given over 10 minutes, followed by a continuous infusion of 1 mg/min for 6 hours, then 0.5 mg/min over 18 hours as a maintenance infusion. For patients in cardiac arrest because of pulseless ventricular tachycardia or ventricular fibrillation, a dose of 300 mg diluted in 20 to 30 mL D_5W is given as a rapid infusion followed by a continuous infusion as described earlier. Additional doses of 150 mg may be given by rapid infusion if ventricular fibrillation or ventricular tachycardia recurs. The maximum daily dose is 2.2 g per 24-hour period.

Significant adverse effects include hypotension and bradycardia. The nurse should slow the infusion rate to prevent or treat these effects and be prepared to administer IV fluids, vasopressors, and agents to increase heart rate. A temporary pacemaker may be needed. Amiodarone has a very long half-life. It should not be given concurrently with pharmacologic agents that prolong Q-T interval on ECG (e.g., procainamide).

Pediatric Implications

Amiodarone is given for pulseless ventricular tachycardia and ventricular fibrillation as a 5 mg/kg rapid IV/IO bolus, which can be repeated up to a maximum dose of 15 mg/kg per 24 hours. For responsive children who have supraventricular (junctional and atrial) tachycardia and ventricular dysrhythmias with pulses present, amiodarone is given as a 5 mg/kg IV/IO loading dose (300 mg maximum) over 20 to 60 minutes and repeated to a maximum daily IV dose of 15 mg/kg per 24-hour period.

Lidocaine

Lidocaine may be used to treat significant ventricular **dysrhythmias** (irregular heartbeats) such as frequent premature ventricular contractions (PVCs), ventricular tachycardia, and ventricular fibrillation as an alternative agent to amiodarone. Lidocaine exerts a local anesthetic effect on the heart, thus decreasing myocardial irritability. Typically a patient with ventricular dysrhythmias is given a 1- to 1.5-mg/kg bolus of lidocaine, followed by 0.5 mg/kg to 0.75 mg/kg every 5 to 10 minutes until the dysrhythmia is controlled or a total dose of 3 mg/kg has been administered via the IV or intraosseous (IO) route. A continuous lidocaine infusion is initiated at a rate of 1 to 4 mg/min to maintain a therapeutic serum level. Lidocaine may also be administered via the endotracheal route in doses of 2 to 4 mg/kg.

Important nursing considerations for the patient receiving lidocaine include continuous cardiac monitoring and assessment for signs and symptoms of lidocaine toxicity (e.g., confusion, drowsiness, hearing impairment, cardiac conduction defects, myocardial depression, muscle twitching, and seizures). Because lidocaine is metabolized by the liver, patients with hepatic impairment, heart failure, shock, and advanced age (older than 70 years) are at higher risk for toxicity. In these patients, the lidocaine dose may need to be reduced by as much as 50% (see Chapter 42). Lidocaine is contraindicated as a *prophylactic* agent to prevent ventricular dysrhythmias following acute myocardial infarction.

Pediatric Implications

Ventricular ectopy is uncommon in children. Metabolic causes should be suspected if ventricular dysrhythmias occur. The pediatric dose of lidocaine is 1 mg/kg IV or via the IO route. The endotracheal tube (ETT) dose is 2 to 3 mg/kg. A maintenance infusion of 20 to 50 mcg/kg/min is

PROTOTYPE DRUG CHART 59-1

Lidocaine HCl

Drug Class	Dosage
Antidysrhythmic, class IB Trade Name: Xylocaine Pregnancy Category: C	A: IV/ IO: 1-1.5 mg/kg; may repeat 0.5 mg/kg q5-10min up to 3 mg/kg *(max)* ETT*: 2-4 mg/kg Drip: 1-4 mg/min C: IV/IO: Initially: 1 mg/kg; maint: 20-50 mcg/kg/min is recommended after bolus ETT*: 2-3 mg/kg Therapeutic range: 1.5-5 mcg/mL
Contraindications	**Drug-Lab-Food Interactions**
Hypersensitivity, advanced atrioventricular block Caution: Liver disease, heart failure, older adults	Drug: Increase effects with phenytoin, quinidine, procainamide, propranolol; increase risk for toxicity with cimetidine, beta-adrenergic blockers
Pharmacokinetics	**Pharmacodynamics**
Absorption: IV Distribution: PB: 60%-80%; concentrates in adipose tissue Metabolism: $t\frac{1}{2}$: Initial: 7-30 min; terminal: 9-120 min Excretion: Through the liver	PO: Onset: 45-60 sec Peak: 45-60 sec Duration: 10-20 min
Therapeutic Effects/Uses	
Antiarrhythmic drug to treat ventricular dysrhythmias such as premature ventricular contractions (PVCs), ventricular tachycardia, and ventricular fibrillation Mode of Action: Decreases automaticity; increases electrical threshold of ventricle	
Side Effects	**Adverse Reactions**
Drowsiness, confusion, dyspnea, lethargy, hypotension, nausea, vomiting	Life-threatening: Seizures, cardiac arrest

*Note: For endotracheal drug administration, dose should be 2 to 4 mg/kg in adults.

A, Adult; *C,* child; *ETT,* endotracheal tube; *IO,* intraosseous; *IV,* intravenous; *PB,* protein-binding; *maint,* maintenance; *max,* maximum; *min,* minute; *sec,* seconds; $t\frac{1}{2}$, half-life.

recommended following the bolus dose. Prototype Drug Chart 59-1 lists the pharmacologic data for lidocaine.

Procainamide

Procainamide is an antidysrhythmic agent prescribed for ventricular tachycardia, PVCs, and rapid supraventricular dysrhythmias unresponsive to adenosine. The typical IV loading dose of procainamide is 20 to 50 mg/min until the dysrhythmia is successfully treated. Other endpoints to procainamide administration include a total administration of 17 mg/kg of the drug, the development of hypotension, and specific changes on the ECG (e.g., widening of the QRS complex by 50% or more). A continuous maintenance infusion of 1 to 4 mg/min may be ordered following the loading dose.

The nurse must monitor vital signs and the ECG with particular attention to heart rate and rhythm, as well as blood pressure and the width of the QRS complex. Procainamide administration can cause severe hypotension. Heart block, rhythm disturbances, and cardiac arrest can occur. Procainamide is contraindicated in patients with **torsades de pointes,** an unusual polymorphic ventricular tachycardia often associated with a prolonged Q-T interval. The drug is eliminated via the kidneys; therefore patients with renal failure are at higher risk of adverse effects and often require a lower dosage.

Pediatric Implications

Procainamide is given to children for ventricular tachycardia that is recurrent or refractory to other measures and for supraventricular tachycardia. The loading dose is 15 mg/kg/ IV or IO given over 30 to 60 minutes. The same monitoring guidelines, adverse effects, and contraindications described for adults are relevant in the pediatric population.

Magnesium Sulfate

Magnesium is an essential element in multiple enzymatic reactions in the body, including function of the sodium-potassium adenosine triphosphatase (ATPase) pump. Its physiologic effects can be likened to a calcium channel blocker with neuromuscular blocking properties. Hypomagnesemia is associated with the development of atrial and ventricular dysrhythmias.

The primary indications for emergency administration of magnesium sulfate are refractory ventricular tachycardia, refractory ventricular fibrillation, cardiac arrest associated with **hypomagnesemia** (low serum magnesium level), and life-threatening ventricular dysrhythmias from digitalis toxicity. It is also the drug of choice for the treatment of torsades de pointes.

Magnesium is administered by diluting 1 to 2 g (2 to 4 mL of a 50% solution) in 10 mL of D_5W. For cardiac arrest caused by hypomagnesemia or torsades de pointes, magnesium is given by direct IV push or via the IO route over 5 to 20 minutes. For patients experiencing torsades de pointes who are not in cardiac arrest, a magnesium infusion of 1 to 2 g diluted in 50 to 100 mL of D_5W can be given IV/IO over 5 to 60 minutes followed by a continuous infusion of 0.5 to 1g/h.

Although magnesium toxicity is rare, the nurse should monitor the patient's response to magnesium administration. Hypotension is the most common adverse effect when magnesium is given by rapid IV push. Other effects include mild bradycardia, flush, and sweating. True hypermagnesemia can cause diarrhea, respiratory depression, deep tendon reflex impairment, flaccid paralysis, and circulatory collapse. Because magnesium is eliminated via the kidneys, it should be administered with caution in patients with renal impairment.

Pediatric Implications

Indications for magnesium sulfate in pediatric patients include torsades de pointes, hypomagnesemia, and status asthmaticus that is unresponsive to beta-adrenergic agents. The magnesium sulfate dose is 25 to 50 mg/kg IV/IO (maximum dose of 2 g) given as a bolus for pulseless ventricular tachycardia, slowly over 10 to 20 minutes for ventricular tachycardia with pulses, and over 15 to 30 minutes for status asthmaticus.

Epinephrine

Epinephrine is a catecholamine with alpha- and beta-adrenergic effects. It has multiple uses. Emergency cardiac indications for administration of IV/IO epinephrine include profound bradycardia and hypotension, asystole, pulseless ventricular tachycardia, and ventricular fibrillation. Epinephrine is thought to improve perfusion of the heart and brain in cardiac arrest states by constricting peripheral blood vessels. In addition, epinephrine increases the chances for successful electrical countershock (defibrillation) in ventricular fibrillation. It is important to be aware that epinephrine is available in two primary concentrations: 1:1000 and 1:10,000. The 1:10,000 concentration is used when administering a single IV/IO dose of epinephrine. The 1:1000 form is used when preparing a continuous epinephrine infusion or when giving epinephrine via the IM or subQ route. The IM route has a more predictable absorption and is, therefore, preferred over the subQ route.

For profound bradycardia or hypotension, an epinephrine infusion may be ordered at 2 to 10 mcg/min. For asystole, pulseless ventricular tachycardia, and ventricular fibrillation, epinephrine is administered in 1-mg doses (1:10,000 solution) IV/IO every 3 to 5 minutes until the desired clinical response is achieved (usually return of effective cardiac activity). Epinephrine also may be given via the ETT route in doses of 2 to 2.5 mg diluted in 10 mL of normal saline.

Nursing implications for patients receiving epinephrine include constant cardiac and hemodynamic monitoring. Epinephrine can cause myocardial ischemia and cardiac dysrhythmias. Epinephrine should neve r be administered in the same site as an alkaline solution such as sodium bicarbonate, because alkaline solutions inactivate epinephrine. In addition, the presence of metabolic or respiratory acidosis decreases the effectiveness of epinephrine. All efforts should be made to correct acid-base imbalances in the patient. More drug information about epinephrine and other adrenergic drugs can be found in Chapter 18.

PREVENTING MEDICATION ERRORS

Epinephrine

- Ensure that the correct concentration (1:1000 vs. 1:10,000) is administered. The 1:10,000 preparation is meant to be given intravenously.

Pediatric Implications

The pediatric dose of epinephrine is 0.01 mg/kg (1:10,000 solution) given every 3 to 5 minutes IV or via the intraosseous (IO) route for cardiac arrest. The ETT dose of 0.1 mg/kg should be given using the 1:1000 solution.

Vasopressin

Vasopressin is indicated for the treatment of ventricular fibrillation that is refractory to defibrillation. It is found in the human body as endogenous antidiuretic hormone. The therapeutic dose is significantly higher than the amount normally present in humans. The effects of vasopressin as a cardiac emergency drug include nonadrenergic peripheral vasoconstriction. When used as an emergency agent, it appears to increase coronary artery perfusion during cardiopulmonary resuscitation (CPR) and to exhibit vasopressor effects. It is given to patients in cardiac arrest before or after epinephrine administration as a single 40 units IV or intraosseous dose. Although vasopressin can be given via the ETT route, a specific effective dose has not yet been established through research. Vasopressin is considered an adjunct to epinephrine and can replace either the first or second epinephrine dose in the cardiac arrest algorithm. Because vasopressin can induce myocardial ischemia and angina, it is contraindicated in responsive patients who have coronary artery disease (CAD), that is, patients with CAD who are not in cardiac arrest.

Pediatric Implications

Vasopressin is indicated for pediatric patients in cardiac arrest as well as those with catecholamine-resistant hypotension. The dosage for vasopressin in pediatric cardiac arrest is 0.4 to 1 unit/kg given as a bolus to a maximum dose of 40 units. A vasopressin infusion of 0.2 to 2 milliunits/kg/min can be initiated for catecholamine-resistant hypotension.

Sodium Bicarbonate

Sodium bicarbonate is prescribed to treat the metabolic acidosis that may accompany cardiac arrest and the hyperkalemia and acidotic states related to specific drug overdose situations. The current standard in resuscitation is to give sodium bicarbonate only *after* adequate ventilation, chest compressions, IV fluids, and drug therapy fail to correct the acidotic state. Sodium bicarbonate is not considered a first-line drug for the treatment of cardiac arrest; it is preferentially given based on results of arterial blood gas analysis when acidosis is severe. If a patient has been in arrest for a prolonged period and blood gas analysis is not available, sodium bicarbonate may be ordered as part of the ongoing resuscitation attempt. The standard initial IV dose of sodium bicarbonate is 1 mEq/kg. Subsequent dosing depends on arterial blood gas analysis.

Important nursing considerations relevant to sodium bicarbonate include careful monitoring of arterial blood gas analysis results. Sodium bicarbonate administration can lead to metabolic alkalosis, which may be very difficult to reverse and have deleterious physiologic effects. Catecholamines such as epinephrine, norepinephrine, and dopamine should not be infused in the same site as sodium bicarbonate, because they are inactivated by solutions containing sodium bicarbonate.

Table 59-1 lists emergency cardiac drugs and their dosages, uses, and considerations.

Pediatric Implications

If severe metabolic acidosis persists after attention has been directed at maintaining optimal ventilation and oxygenation, sodium bicarbonate may be given to the pediatric patient in a 1-mEq/kg dose via the IV or intraosseous route. It may also

TABLE 59-1 EMERGENCY CARDIAC DRUGS

GENERIC (BRAND)	ROUTE AND DOSAGE	USES AND CONSIDERATIONS
adenosine	A: IV: Initially: 6 mg; then 12 mg in 1-to 2 min if needed	For paroxysmal supraventricular tachycardia. Pregnancy category: C; PB: UK; $t\frac{1}{2}$: <10 sec
amiodarone IV	A: IV: with pulse: 150 mg over 10 min; then continuous infusion 1 mg/min, for 6 h; then 0.5 mg/min over 18 h. Cardiac arrest: 300 mg diluted in 20-30 mL D_5W rapidly; second dose 150 mg, followed by continuous infusion as above; *max:* 2.2 g/d. C: IV: without pulse: 5 mg/kg administered as rapid IV/IO bolus. With pulse: 5 mg/kg IV/IO loading dose over 20-60 min; repeated to max daily dose of 15 mg/kg	Part of ACLS algorithm for treatment of both atrial and ventricular dysrhythmias. Pregnancy category: C: PB: UK; $t\frac{1}{2}$: 26-107 d
atropine sulfate	IV/IO: 0.5-1 mg; can repeat up to 0.04 mg/kg or 3 mg (max) ETT: 2-3 mg diluted in 10 mL normal saline	For symptomatic bradycardia; asystole. Pregnancy category: C; PB: 60%-80%; $t\frac{1}{2}$: 2-3 h
diltiazem	IV: 0.25 mg/kg; repeat in 15 min at 0.35 mg/kg IV: drip: 5-15 mg/h	For supraventricular tachycardia and atrial fibrillation and flutter. Pregnancy category: C; PB: 80%; $t\frac{1}{2}$: 2-5 h
epinephrine	IV/IO: 0.5-1 mg; may be repeated q3-5min ETT: 2.0-2.5 mg diluted in 10 mL normal saline	For cardiac arrest. Pregnancy category: C; PB: UK; $t\frac{1}{2}$: UK
lidocaine	See Prototype Drug Chart 59-1.	
magnesium sulfate	Dilute 1-2 g (2-4 mL of 50% solution) in 10 mL of D_5W. Give IV/IO in cardiac arrest over 5-20 min. Torsades de pointes: 1-2 g diluted in 50-100 mL of D_5W given IV over 5-60 min, followed by continuous infusion of 0.5-1 g/h	For hypomagnesemia, ventricular tachycardia, and ventricular fibrillation. Drug of choice for torsades de pointes. Rapid infusion can cause hypotension. Pregnancy category: D; PB: 25%-35%; $t\frac{1}{2}$: 30 min
morphine sulfate	IV: 1-4 mg q5-30min	For chest pain, unstable angina, pulmonary edema. Pregnancy category: C; PB: 35%; $t\frac{1}{2}$: 2-2.5 h
nitroglycerin	SL: 0.3-0.4 mg; Translingual aerosol spray: 0.4-mg metered dose, up to 3 sprays in 15 min onto or under tongue IV: drip: 10-20 mcg/min, increased 5-10 mcg/min q5-10 min (titrated)	For chest pain, angina, unstable angina, MI. Hypotension can occur; contraindicated in patients taking drugs for erectile dysfunction (e.g., Viagra). Pregnancy category: C; PB: 60%; $t\frac{1}{2}$: 1-4 min
procainamide HCl	IV: 20-50 mg/min; *max:* 17 mg/kg Recognize endpoints: Hypotension QRS widens >50% Total dose of 17 mg/kg given Drip: 1-4 mg/min	For PVCs, ventricular tachycardia, ventricular fibrillation, atrial dysrhythmias. Pregnancy category: C; PB: 20%; $t\frac{1}{2}$: 3-4 h
sodium bicarbonate	IV: Initially: 1 mEq/kg; then dose based on ABG results	For metabolic acidosis. Pregnancy category: C; PB: UK; $t\frac{1}{2}$: UK
vasopressin	A: IV/IO/ETT: single 40-unit dose before or after epinephrine administration	For ventricular fibrillation refractory to defibrillation. Contraindicated in responsive patients with CAD. Pregnancy category: C; PB: UK; $t\frac{1}{2}$: 10-20 min

A, Adult; *ACLS,* Advanced Cardiac Life Support; *C,* child; *CAD,* coronary artery disease; *d,* day; *ETT,* endotracheal tube; *h,* hour; *IO,* intraosseous; *IV,* intravenous; *max,* maximum; *MI,* myocardial infarction; *min,* minute; *PB,* protein-binding; *PVC,* premature ventricular contraction; *sec,* second; *SL,* sublingual; *t,* half-life; *UK,* unknown; >, greater than; <, less than.

be given as treatment for a tricyclic antidepressant overdose. Sodium bicarbonate is hyperosmolar and should be diluted from an 8.4% solution (1 mEq/mL) to a 4.2% solution (0.5 mEq/mL) for infants.

EMERGENCY DRUG FOR INTRACRANIAL HYPERTENSION

Mannitol

Mannitol is an osmotic diuretic used in emergency, trauma, critical care, and neurosurgical settings to treat cerebral edema and to reduce increased intracranial pressure (intracranial hypertension), which may occur following head trauma, neurosurgery, malignancy, and other types of intracranial pathology. Mannitol may be given as an IV bolus or via a continuous drip. The usual initial bolus dose of mannitol is 1g/kg IV of a 20% to 25% solution. Subsequent dosing is highly variable and is influenced by serum osmolality. In general, mannitol is held when serum osmolality exceeds 310 to 320. Mannitol is highly irritating to veins. The nurse must use a filter needle when administering mannitol, because crystals may form in the solution and syringe and be inadvertently injected. When a filter needle is used to draw up the mannitol, a *new* filter needle *must* be used to administer the mannitol IV. In addition, the nurse should carefully assess the patient's neurologic status; monitor laboratory studies, including electrolytes and serum osmolality; and keep accurate intake and output records to assess fluid volume status, because diuresis may be substantial. Prototype Drug Chart 59-2 lists the pharmacologic data for mannitol.

EMERGENCY DRUGS FOR POISONING

Although there are numerous antidotes for specific types of poisoning, the drugs presented in this section are the most commonly prescribed agents in cases of drug overdose and ingestion of toxic substances, with pertinent exceptions noted. Particular attention must be given to administration guidelines to achieve the best possible clinical outcome for the patient. These drugs are cross-referenced to their specialty chapters.

Naloxone

Naloxone is classified as an opiate antagonist. It reverses the effects of all opiate drugs (e.g., morphine, meperidine, codeine, propoxyphene, heroin) by competitively binding to opiate receptor sites in the body. Naloxone is indicated for individuals who have taken an overdose of opiate drugs, those experiencing respiratory or cardiovascular depression from therapeutic doses of opiates given in a health care setting, and those brought to the emergency department in a coma of unknown etiology (which may be drug induced).

PROTOTYPE DRUG CHART 59-2

Mannitol

Drug Class Osmotic diuretic Trade Name: Osmitrol Pregnancy Category: C	**Dosage** A: IV: Initially 1g/kg of 20%-25% sol as a bolus Highly individualized dosing
Contraindications Hypersensitivity, severe dehydration Caution: Pregnancy, breastfeeding, current intracranial bleeding	**Drug-Lab-Food Interactions** Drug: May decrease effectiveness with lithium
Pharmacokinetics Absorption: IV Distribution: PB: Confined to extracellular space Metabolism: t½: 100 min Excretion: In urine	**Pharmacodynamics** Decrease in intracranial pressure: IV: Onset: 30-60 min Peak: 1 h Duration: 6-8 h Diuresis: IV: Onset: 1-3 h Peak: 1 h Duration: 6-8 h
Therapeutic Effects/Uses To treat increased intracranial pressure, cerebral edema Mode of Action: Inhibits reabsorption of electrolytes and water by affecting pressure of glomerular filtrate	
Side Effects Temporary volume expansion, hyponatremia/hypernatremia, hypokalemia/hyperkalemia, dehydration, blurred vision, dry mouth	**Adverse Reactions** Pulmonary congestion, fluid/electrolyte imbalances Life-threatening: Convulsions

A, Adult; *h*, hour; *IV*, intravenous; *min*, minute; *PB*, protein-binding; *sol*, solution; *t ½*, half-life.

The typical dose of naloxone for actual or suspected opiate overdose in adults is 0.4 to 2 mg IV administered every 2 minutes until the patient's condition improves to an acceptable level. If there is no improvement within 10 minutes after 10 mg of the drug has been injected, nonopiate drugs or disease must be suspected. Although naloxone should be administered IV in emergency situations, it also may be given via the intramuscular (IM), intraosseous (IO), or subcutaneous (subQ) routes if IV access is not readily obtainable. In addition, naloxone appears to have efficacy when given via the intranasal route in doses of 1 mg per nostril, which reduces the risk of needlestick injuries to health care personnel.

Because most opiate drugs have a longer duration of action than naloxone, the nurse must monitor the patient closely for signs and symptoms of recurrent opiate effects such as respiratory depression and hypotension. In this situation, naloxone administration may need to be repeated several times or a continuous IV infusion ordered. Naloxone has no major adverse effects, but can precipitate withdrawal symptoms in patients addicted to opiate drugs and rarely cause anaphylaxis. In addition, pulmonary edema has been reported following naloxone administration in patients who have had an overdose of morphine (see Chapter 26). Nurses also must be on guard for combative or violent behavior following naloxone administration, especially in patients who have overdosed on an illicit drug; having security personnel available to stand by is prudent. Prototype Drug Chart 59-3 lists the pharmacologic data for naloxone.

Pediatric Implications

For narcotic reversal in children, give 0.01 to 0.1 mg/kg, repeating the drug as necessary based upon desired therapeutic effects up to 2 mg. Naloxone can be administered as an IV bolus or continuous infusion, as well as IO, IM, or subQ in children.

Flumazenil

Flumazenil is the reversal agent for the respiratory depressant and sedative effects of benzodiazepine medications (e.g., diazepam [Valium], midazolam [Versed], chlordiazepoxide [Librium]). It is administered to counteract the effects of benzodiazepines given as sedative or anesthetic agents, as well as to treat accidental or intentional benzodiazepine overdose. Flumazenil does not reverse the central nervous system (CNS) depressant effects of nonbenzodiazepine agents such as alcohol, opiates, and barbiturates and may not reverse amnesia induced by benzodiazepines.

PROTOTYPE DRUG CHART 59-3

Naloxone HCl

Drug Class Narcotic antagonist Trade Name: Narcan Pregnancy Category: B	**Dosage** IV/IM/IO/subQ: 0.4-2 mg; repeat every 2-3 min as indicated
Contraindications Hypersensitivity, respiratory depression Caution: Opiate-dependent patients, cardiac disease, breastfeeding neonates of opiate-dependent mothers	**Drug-Lab-Food Interactions** Drug: Naloxone can precipitate withdrawal in a patient dependent on narcotic analgesics Lab: Urine vanillylmandelic acid (VMA), 5-hydroxyheptadecatrienoic acid (5-HIAA), urine glucose
Pharmacokinetics Absorption: IM/subQ: Well absorbed Distribution: PB: UK Metabolism: t½: Adults: 1-4 h; neonates: 1-3 h Excretion: In urine metabolites	**Pharmacodynamics** subQ/IM: Onset: 2-5 min Peak: UK Duration: 1-4 h IV/IO: Onset: 1-2 min Peak: UK Duration: 1-4 h
Therapeutic Effects/Uses To treat respiratory depression caused by narcotics; to treat narcotic-induced depressant effects and narcotic overdose Mode of Action: Blocks effects of narcotics by competing for receptor sites	
Side Effects Negligible pharmacologic effect without narcotics in body	**Adverse Reactions** Nausea, vomiting, tremulousness, sweating, tachycardia, elevated blood pressure Life-threatening: Atrioventricular fibrillation, pulmonary edema (with overdose of morphine)

h, Hour; *IV,* intravenous; *IM,* intramuscular; *min,* minute; *PB,* protein-binding; *subQ,* subcutaneous; *t½,* half-life; *UK,* unknown.

TABLE 59-2 EMERGENCY DRUGS FOR POISONING

GENERIC (BRAND)	ROUTE AND DOSAGE	USES AND CONSIDERATIONS
Flumazenil	IV: Initial dose 0.2 mg over 15 sec. Additional doses of 0.3-0.5 mg over 30 sec every 1 min as indicated. For resedation, may repeat at 20-min intervals to total dose of no more than 3 mg.	Reversal agent for benzodiazepine overdose; may precipitate seizures in patients with long-term use or abuse of benzodiazepines and those with seizure disorders; may precipitate emergent reactions. Pregnancy category: C; PB: 50%; t½: Variable (40-80 min)
naloxone (Narcan)	See Prototype Drug Chart 59-3.	
activated charcoal	A/C: 1-2 g/kg PO	For poisoning. Onset: <1 min. Pregnancy category: C; PB: NA; t½: NA

A, Adult; *C*, child; *IV*, intravenous; *min*, minute; *NA*, not applicable; *PB*, protein-binding; *PO*, by mouth; *sec*, second; *t½*, half-life; <, less than.

For suspected benzodiazepine overdose, flumazenil is given IV in an initial dose of 0.2 mg over 15 seconds. A second dose of 0.3 mg may be given over 30 seconds. A third dose and subsequent doses of 0.5 mg IV may be given every minute until the desired clinical response is achieved or until a total dose of 3 mg is given within any given hour. If sedation occurs again, doses of flumazenil may be repeated at 20-minute intervals (not to exceed 1 mg at a time) to a total hourly dose of no more than 3 mg IV.

Nursing considerations include careful assessment of respiratory rate and effort, blood pressure, and mental status. If the benzodiazepine is reversed too rapidly, patients may have emergence reactions in which they become agitated and confused and experience perceptual distortions. Because seizures are precipitated by benzodiazepine withdrawal, seizure precautions must be implemented for patients at risk (those with long-standing benzodiazepine use or abuse) or for those who have a known seizure disorder.

Activated Charcoal

Activated charcoal may be prescribed for poisoning as a means to prevent absorption of toxins into the body if the ingested substance is known to be affected by charcoal in the gastrointestinal (GI) tract. A poison control center should be contacted as soon as possible to help guide medical therapy. In cases of known or suspected poisoning, activated charcoal is prepared as a slurry and given to the patient orally or via a gastric tube, ideally within 30 minutes to 1 hour of ingestion, sometimes following gastric lavage. The dose is dependent on the amount of poison ingested; the typical adult and pediatric dose is 1 to 2 g/kg, up to 25 to 60 g per dose. Activated charcoal dosing may need to be repeated for certain types of poisoning, particularly from agents such as salicylates, slow-release drug preparations, and *Amanita phalloides* (death cap mushrooms), to name a few.

Since vomiting is a common adverse reaction, patients with an impaired gag reflex and/or an impaired mental status are at high risk for aspiration after ingesting activated charcoal. Aspiration pneumonia and death can occur. To promote safety, these patients may need intubation for airway protection followed by installation of the activated charcoal via a gastric tube. Activated charcoal should not be administered with milk products, because they decrease its adsorptive properties. Activated charcoal is ineffective and should not be given to patients who have ingested some forms of pesticides, hydrocarbons, alcohol, acids or alkalis, lithium, solvents, and iron supplements. A **cathartic** (a purgative resulting in bowel movements) may be ordered following administration of activated charcoal to speed elimination of the charcoal-toxin complex from the body. The patient should be told that charcoal produces black stools.

Table 59-2 lists the emergency drugs for poisoning and their dosages, uses, and considerations.

EMERGENCY DRUGS FOR SHOCK

Drugs may be required to elevate blood pressure and to improve cardiac performance in various types of shock states. Therapeutic agents described in this section are primarily indicated in conditions such as cardiogenic shock, neurogenic shock, septic shock, anaphylactic shock, and insulin shock. A noteworthy exception to the list is **hypovolemic shock** (shock resulting from loss of blood or fluid volume); drugs should never be used as the primary therapy to correct the hypotension associated with this condition. Administration of fluids or blood products or both is the only acceptable initial means to treat hypovolemic shock. However, if hypotension persists after appropriate volume resuscitation, vasoactive drugs may be necessary to elevate and sustain blood pressure. The drugs that follow are cross-referenced to their specialty chapters.

Dopamine

Dopamine is a sympathomimetic agent often used to treat hypotension in shock states. Dopamine may also be used to increase heart rate (beta1 effect) in bradycardic rhythms when atropine has not been effective. The dose range is 2 to 20 mcg/kg/min. Dopamine enhances cardiac output by increasing myocardial contractility and increasing heart rate (beta$_1$ effect) and elevates blood pressure through vasoconstriction (alpha-adrenergic effect). Alpha effects predominate at higher doses—vasoconstriction of renal, mesenteric, and peripheral blood vessels occurs. Such vasoconstriction, although sometimes necessary to maintain adequate blood pressure in severe shock, can lead to poor organ and tissue perfusion, decreased cardiac performance, and reduction of urine output. The lowest effective dose of dopamine should be used. Patients must be weaned gradually from dopamine; abrupt discontinuation of the infusion can cause severe hypotension.

Dopamine is typically mixed as a concentration of 400 to 800 mg in 250 mL D_5W or normal saline solution and administered IV by an electronic infusion pump for precision, preferably in a central vein. Sodium bicarbonate will inactivate dopamine; it should not be infused in the same IV line. Continuous heart and blood pressure monitoring is essential. The nurse must carefully document vital signs, the cardiac rhythm and intake and output as prescribed. Significant adverse effects include tachycardia, dysrhythmias, myocardial ischemia, nausea, and vomiting. The IV site must be assessed hourly for signs of drug infiltration; **extravasation** (escape into tissues) of dopamine can produce tissue necrosis that may necessitate surgical debridement and skin grafting. If extravasation occurs, the site should be injected in multiple areas with phentolamine (Regitine), 5 to 10 mg diluted in 10 to 15 mL of normal saline, to reduce or prevent tissue damage. Prototype Drug Chart 59-4 lists the pharmacologic data for dopamine.

PREVENTING MEDICATION ERRORS

Do not confuse...
- **dopamine** with **dobutamine**

Dobutamine

Dobutamine is a sympathomimetic drug with beta adrenergic activities. The $beta_1$ effects include enhancing the force of myocardial contraction (positive inotropic effect) and increasing heart rate (positive chronotropic effect). The $beta_2$ effects produce mild vasodilation. Dobutamine is indicated in shock states when improvement in cardiac output and overall cardiac performance is desired. Blood pressure is elevated only through the increase in cardiac output. The usual IV dose range of dobutamine is 2 to 20 mcg/kg/min administered via an electronic infusion pump for precision. A typical concentration of dobutamine is 250 mg to 1000 mg mixed in 250 mL of D_5W or normal saline. Like dopamine, dobutamine administration should be tapered gradually as the patient's condition warrants; abrupt discontinuation can precipitate clinical deterioration.

Continuous cardiac and blood pressure monitoring are required for patients receiving dobutamine infusions. Adverse effects are dose-related and include myocardial ischemia, tachycardia, dysrhythmias, headache, nausea, and tremors. The nurse must carefully monitor intake and output and assess for any signs or symptoms of myocardial ischemia such as chest pain or development of dysrhythmias.

Norepinephrine

Norepinephrine is a catecholamine with extremely potent vasoconstrictor actions (alpha-adrenergic effect). It is used in

PROTOTYPE DRUG CHART 59-4

Dopamine HCl

Drug Class Adrenergic Trade Name: Dopamine Pregnancy Category: C	**Dosage** A: IV: Drip: 2-20 mcg/kg/min (>10 mcg/kg/min may be ordered if lower doses are ineffective)
Contraindications Hypersensitivity, tachydysrhythmias, ventricular fibrillation, pheochromocytomas Caution: Safety in children is not known.	**Drug-Lab-Food Interactions** Drug: May result in hypertensive crisis when used within 2 wk of MAOIs; concurrent IV administration of phenytoin may result in hypotension and bradycardia; sodium bicarbonate solutions inactivate dopamine—do not administer through same IV line
Pharmacokinetics Absorption: IV Distribution: PB: UK Metabolism: t½: 2 min Excretion: In urine	**Pharmacodynamics** IV: Onset: 1-2 min Peak: <5 min Duration: <10 min
Therapeutic Effects/Uses To treat hypotension in shock states after adequate fluid and/or blood product resuscitation; to increase heart rate in atropine-refractory bradycardia. Mode of Action: Stimulates receptors to cause cardiac stimulation; increases systemic vascular resistance	
Side Effects Palpitations, tachycardia, hypertension, ectopic beats, angina, IV line site irritation, piloerection, nausea, vomiting	**Adverse Reactions** Cardiac dysrhythmias, azotemia, tissue sloughing (from extravasation) Life-threatening: MI, gangrene in extremities (from vasoconstriction)

A, Adult; *IV*, intravenous; *MAOIs*, monoamine oxidase inhibitors; *MI*, myocardial infarction; *min*, minute; *PB*, protein-binding; *t ½*, half-life; *UK*, unknown; *wk*, week; >, greater than; <, less than.

shock states, often when drugs such as dopamine and dobutamine have failed to produce adequate blood pressure, or as an alternative to dopamine. Like high-dose dopamine, the peripheral vasoconstriction that results has the potential to impair cardiac performance and decrease organ and tissue perfusion. In general, 4 to 8 mg of norepinephrine are added to 250 mL D_5W or normal saline solution and infused at 0.5 to 35 mcg/min (titrated) for adults. Continuous cardiac monitoring and precise blood pressure monitoring are required. The drug must be tapered slowly; abrupt discontinuation can result in severe hypotension.

Nursing actions and considerations are the same as those for dopamine. Norepinephrine should not be used as an initial therapy to treat hypotension in hypovolemic patients; fluid, blood, or both must be administered to restore adequate volume first. Adverse effects of norepinephrine include myocardial ischemia, dysrhythmias, and impaired organ perfusion. Extravasation of norepinephrine causes tissue necrosis, so attention to the IV site is essential. If extravasation occurs, the area should be infiltrated with phentolamine, as described for dopamine.

Epinephrine

Epinephrine is the drug of choice in the treatment of **anaphylactic shock,** an allergic response of the most serious type, brought about by an antibody-antigen reaction. Anaphylactic shock can be fatal if prompt treatment is not initiated. Severe bronchoconstriction and hypotension resulting from cardiovascular collapse are its hallmarks. Epinephrine is also indicated for an acute, severe asthmatic attack.

Administration of epinephrine causes bronchodilation, enhanced cardiac performance, and vasoconstriction to increase blood pressure. In severe asthma and anaphylactic shock, epinephrine is given in a dose range of 0.2 to 0.5 mg IM or subQ for adults via a tuberculin syringe for accuracy (1 : 1000 solution). IM administration is preferable to subQ administration, because the IM route has a more predictable pattern of absorption. As an alternative, epinephrine can be given in a dose of 0.1 to 0.25 mg IV over 5 to 10 minutes (1 : 10,000 solution). Epinephrine administration can be repeated every 5 to 15 minutes if necessary.

The patient who receives epinephrine must be closely monitored for tachycardia, cardiac dysrhythmias, hypertension, and angina. Patients who are given IV epinephrine must be on a cardiac monitor, with resuscitation equipment immediately available. Other adverse effects include excitability, fear, anxiety, and restlessness. In addition, the nurse should be alert to the possibility that the anaphylactic response may recur and necessitate repeated treatment. For this reason, steroids are commonly ordered and are slowly tapered over days to weeks to prevent recurrence. Examples of steroids are hydrocortisone sodium succinate, prednisone, and methylprednisolone. Patient education should include strict avoidance of the agents responsible for the anaphylactic reaction and follow-up care with a physician. For some patients, such as those with severe allergic responses to bee stings, the physician may prescribe an epinephrine kit or pen to be carried with the patient for self-medication in the event of contact with the antigen. Proper patient education regarding the use of the kit or pen is essential. See Chapters 18 and 41 for more information.

Albuterol

Albuterol is a beta-adrenergic bronchodilator used to reverse bronchoconstriction in anaphylactic shock, **asthma** (inflammation and narrowing of the airways caused by enhanced responsiveness of the tracheobronchial system to a variety of stimuli), and COPD. In emergency situations, it is typically administered via nebulizer (adults: 0.5 mL of 0.5% inhalation solution in 2.5 mL saline). Albuterol is also supplied as a metered-dose inhaler, which the patient can carry to self-administer a "rescue" dose of the drug during an acute episode of bronchospasm. The nurse should assess breath sounds before and after administration; effectiveness is evidenced by relief of bronchospasm. In severe bronchospasm, wheezing may not be audible. As the bronchospasm is relieved, wheezing may become more pronounced, indicating that the drug is producing the desired therapeutic effect. Assessment of the patient's subjective feelings of respiratory distress before and after administration is especially important. Adverse effects of albuterol include tachycardia, tremor, nervousness, cardiac dysrhythmias, and hypertension.

Diphenhydramine Hydrochloride

Diphenhydramine, an antihistamine, is often administered with epinephrine to treat anaphylactic shock. This agent is effective for treating the histamine-induced tissue swelling and pruritus common to severe allergic reactions. The standard adult dose is 25 to 50 mg administered IV or deep IM. Oral pill and liquid forms of the drug exist, but the parenteral form is preferred in emergencies. However, the patient may be instructed to keep an oral formulation on hand in the home setting for emergency self-administration during an allergic reaction prior to receiving medical assistance. An important tip for patient teaching is that the liquid diphenhydramine is easier to swallow than a pill, especially in the presence of tissue edema in the mouth or throat. Adverse effects include drowsiness, sedation, confusion, vertigo, excitability, hypotension, tachycardia, GI disturbances, and dry mouth (see Chapter 40).

Dextrose 50%

Dextrose 50% is a concentrated, high-carbohydrate solution given to treat insulin-induced hypoglycemia or insulin shock. When insulin shock is known or suspected and the patient's state of consciousness is impaired such that oral administration of sugar solutions is contraindicated, 50 mL of dextrose 50% is commonly ordered and given as an IV bolus. Dextrose 50% is highly irritating to veins and should be administered in a large peripheral or central vein whenever possible. Phlebitis can occur. Extravasation of the solution can cause tissue sloughing and necrosis. The nurse must monitor the patient's blood sugar carefully; hyperglycemia is common, especially after rapid injection. Urine output should be accurately

TABLE 59-3 AGENTS FOR EMERGENCY TREATMENT OF SHOCK

GENERIC	ROUTE AND DOSAGE	USES AND CONSIDERATIONS
albuterol	A: nebulizer: 0.5 mL of 0.5% inhalation solution in 2.5 mL saline	For bronchoconstriction secondary to anaphylactic shock, asthma, and COPD. Adverse effects include tachycardia, tremor, nervousness, cardiac dysrhythmias, and hypertension. Pregnancy category: C; PB: UK; t½: 3.7-5 h
dextrose 50%	A: IV: 50 mL C: 0.5-1.0 g/kg IV of dextrose 25% sol	For insulin shock; severe hypoglycemia. Pregnancy category: C; PB: UK; t½: UK
diphenhydramine	IM/IV: 25-50 mg	For anaphylactic shock; acute allergic reaction. Pregnancy category: C; PB: 98%-99%; t½: 3-8 h
dobutamine	IV: drip: 2-20 mcg/kg/min	For low cardiac output. Effects antagonized by beta blockers. Pregnancy category: C; PB: UK; t½: 2 min
dopamine HCl	See Prototype Drug Chart 59-4.	
epinephrine	IM/subQ: 0.2-0.5 mg (1 : 1000 sol) IV/IO: 0.1-0.25 mg (1 : 10,000 sol) ETT: 2-2.5 mg diluted in 10 mL normal saline	For anaphylactic shock; severe acute asthmatic attack. May cause hypertensive crisis with MAOIs, increased dysrhythmias with cardiac glycosides. Pregnancy category: C; PB: UK; t½: UK
glucagon	subQ/IM/IV: 0.5-1 mg; may repeat once	Insulin shock; severe hypoglycemia; beta blocker overdose (reverses effects of beta blockers). Pregnancy category: B; PB: UK; t½: 3-10 min
norepinephrine	IV: drip: 0.5-30 mcg/min (titrated)	Hypotension not responsive to other therapies. Pregnancy category: D; PB: UK; t½: UK

A, Adult; *C*, child; *COPD*, chronic obstructive pulmonary disease; *ETT*, endotracheal tube; *h*, hour; *IM*, intramuscular; *IV*, intravenous; *MAOIs*, monoamine oxidase inhibitors; *min*, minute; *PB*, protein-binding; *sol*, solution; *subQ*, subcutaneous; *t½*, half-life; *UK*, unknown.

recorded, because osmotic diuresis can occur when blood sugar is elevated, and a hyperosmolar state can result. Patient education must be centered on teaching about diabetes, nutrition, physical activity, and insulin administration.

Pediatric Implications

Glycogen stores in infants and children may be quickly depleted in stress states produced by severe illness. Because adequate amounts of glucose are essential to strong myocardial function, hypoglycemia must be corrected to provide the greatest chance for successful resuscitation. After determining that hypoglycemia is present by the fingerstick or heelstick method of rapid blood glucose testing, dextrose 25% or less may be administered per physician order. Because glucose is supplied in a 50% concentration, it must be diluted 1:1 in sterile water before administration to reduce its osmolarity and prevent sclerosis of peripheral veins. The standard dose is 0.5 to 1g/kg IV or IO.

Glucagon

Glucagon is a pancreas-produced hormone that elevates blood sugar by stimulating glycogen breakdown (**glycogenolysis**). Glucagon, like dextrose 50%, is indicated in the treatment of severe insulin-induced hypoglycemia or insulin shock. In an emergency when dextrose 50% is unavailable or cannot be administered IV, glucagon is an effective agent. Glucagon may be given subQ, IM, or IV. The standard dose for adults and children is 0.5 to 1 mg, which can be repeated in 15 minutes for persistent coma. If the coma has not resolved after two doses, dextrose 50% must be administered. Adverse effects from glucagon are uncommon, but can include nausea, vomiting, and a hypersensitivity reaction that may produce bronchospasm and respiratory distress. Glucagon can also be used as an agent to reverse the effects of calcium channel blocker and beta-blocker overdose; in this situation, 5 to 10 mg IV of glucagon is administered initially, followed by an IV infusion of 3 to 5 mg/hr.

Table 59-3 lists the emergency drugs for shock and their dosages, uses, and considerations.

EMERGENCY DRUGS FOR HYPERTENSIVE CRISES AND PULMONARY EDEMA

A variety of pharmacologic agents may be prescribed to treat **hypertensive crisis,** generally defined as a diastolic blood pressure that exceeds 110 to 120 mm Hg, and pulmonary edema. Three of the most commonly prescribed drugs are discussed in this section. The drugs are cross-referenced to their specialty chapter.

Labetalol

Labetalol is an alpha- and beta-adrenergic blocker that acts by inhibiting the effects of the sympathetic nervous system. Its pharmacologic actions include lowering heart rate, blood pressure, myocardial contractility, and myocardial oxygen consumption, and reducing the vasoconstriction that results from sympathetic nervous system stimulation. This agent is indicated for the acute management of clinically significant hypertension in the presence of ischemic and hemorrhagic stroke, as well as for hypertensive crisis.

Initially 10 to 20 mg of labetalol is administered IV push over 2 minutes. This starting dose can be repeated or doubled every 10 minutes until the desired clinical response is achieved, to a maximum dose of 300 mg. As an alternative approach, a continuous infusion of labetalol mixed with D_5W can be prepared to deliver 2 mg/min until the target therapeutic response is attained; the maximum dose with this approach is also 300 mg.

Important nursing considerations during the administration of labetalol include the use of an electronic infusion pump for accurate continuous infusion medication delivery, cardiac monitoring, and frequent blood pressure measurement. Documentation of blood pressure may need to be as often as every 5 minutes during IV push dosing or at the initiation of the continuous infusion. Serious adverse effects include hypotension, bradycardia, ventricular dysrhythmias, and bronchospasm. Dizziness is also a frequently reported adverse reaction. Labetalol is contraindicated in patients with bronchial asthma or COPD because of the risk of bronchospasm and in patients with severe bradycardia or apparent heart failure.

Nitroprusside Sodium

Nitroprusside sodium is an IV agent used to reduce arterial blood pressure in hypertensive emergencies. The mechanism of action is immediate direct arterial and venous vasodilation. Antihypertensive effects end when nitroprusside sodium is discontinued; blood pressure increases as soon as drug administration is stopped. Continuous and accurate blood pressure measurement is required. In general, 50 mg of nitroprusside sodium is mixed in 250 mL D_5W. The typical dose range for adults is 0.25 to 5 mcg/kg/min, titrated to the desired clinical response. The maximum dose is 10 mcg/kg/min.

There are several important nursing considerations:

- Nitroprusside sodium is rapidly inactivated by light; the IV bottle or bag must be wrapped with aluminum foil or another opaque material to protect the solution from degradation.
- Although a faint brown tint is typical, blue or brown discoloration of the solution indicates degradation and necessitates that the solution be discarded.
- When nitroprusside sodium therapy is prolonged, or infused at the maximum dose of 10 mcg/kg/min for more than 10 minutes, patients are at risk for toxicity resulting from elevated serum thiocyanate or cyanide levels (by-products of drug metabolism). Signs and symptoms include metabolic acidosis, profound hypotension, dyspnea, dizziness, and vomiting. Serum thiocyanate levels should be monitored every 24 to 72 hours for patients receiving prolonged infusions of more than 2 mcg/kg/min. Patients with renal insufficiency or failure are at a higher risk, because the metabolites are excreted in the urine.
- Patients should be placed on an oral antihypertensive agent as soon as possible so that nitroprusside sodium can be tapered slowly. Drug data for nitroprusside sodium are presented in Prototype Drug Chart 59-5.

PROTOTYPE DRUG CHART 59-5

Nitroprusside Sodium

Drug Class Vasodilator Trade Name: Nipride Pregnancy Category: C	**Dosage** A: IV: Drip: 0.25-5 mcg/kg/min; begin at 0.25 mcg/kg/min, and titrate to desired effect
Contraindications Hypersensitivity, hypertension (compensatory), decreased cerebral perfusion, coarctation of the aorta Caution: Increased intracranial pressure	**Drug-Lab-Food Interactions** Drug: Antihypertensives, general anesthetics Note: Do not mix with any other drug in syringe or solution. Lab: Decrease in PCO_2, Ph
Pharmacokinetics Absorption: IV only Distribution: PB: UK Metabolism: $t\frac{1}{2}$: <10 mi Excretion: In urine	**Pharmacodynamics** IV: Onset: 1-2 min Peak: Rapid Duration: 1-10 min
Therapeutic Effects/Uses To treat hypertensive crisis and to decrease systemic vascular resistance to improve cardiac performance Mode of Action: Stimulates smooth muscle of veins and arteries; produces peripheral vasodilation	
Side Effects Dizziness, headache, nausea, abdominal pain, sweating, palpitations, weakness, vomiting	**Adverse Reactions** Thiocyanate toxicity: hypotension, tinnitus, dyspnea, blurred vision, metabolic acidosis Life-threatening: Severe hypotension, loss of consciousness, profound cardiovascular depression

A, Adult; *IV*, intravenous; *min*, minute; *PB*, protein-binding; *PCO2*, partial pressure of carbon dioxide; $t\frac{1}{2}$, half-life; *UK*, unknown; <, less than.

TABLE 59-4 EMERGENCY DRUGS FOR HYPERTENSIVE CRISES AND PULMONARY EDEMA

GENERIC (BRAND)	ROUTE AND DOSAGE	USES AND CONSIDERATIONS
nitroprusside sodium	See Prototype Drug Chart 59-5.	
furosemide (Lasix)	IV: Initial bolus of 0.5-1.0 mg/kg over 1-2 min, up to 2 mg/kg	For acute pulmonary edema from left ventricular dysfunction; hypertensive crisis. Adverse effects: hypovolemia, dehydration, electrolyte disturbances
morphine	IV: 1-4 mg q5-30min	For pulmonary edema, chest pain, unstable angina, MI
labetalol hydrochloride	IV: Initial push 10-20 mg over 2 min, repeated or doubled q10min up to a max of 300 mg; continuous infusion 2 mg/min	For hypertension in CVA and for hypertensive crisis. Adverse effects: ventricular dysrhythmias, hypotension, bronchospasm. Contraindications: bronchial asthma, COPD, severe bradycardia, heart failure

COPD, Chronic obstructive pulmonary disease; *CVA,* cerebrovascular accident; *IV,* intravenous; *max,* maximum; *MI,* myocardial infarction; *min,* minute.

Furosemide

Furosemide (Herbal Alert 59-2) is classified as a *loop diuretic* that acts by inhibiting sodium and chloride reabsorption from the ascending loop of Henle and the proximal and distal tubules. It promotes the renal excretion of water, sodium, chloride, magnesium, hydrogen, and calcium, and it depletes potassium. Furosemide also has peripheral and renal vasodilating effects that can lower blood pressure. The main indications for use of furosemide as an emergency drug are acute pulmonary edema from left ventricular dysfunction and hypertensive crisis.

HERBAL ALERT 59-2

Furosemide

Ginseng can inhibit its efficacy. Licorice can promote potassium loss, enhancing the potential for severe hypokalemia. These herbs should not be taken concurrently with furosemide.

Furosemide is given as an initial bolus of 0.5 to 1 mg/kg IV over 1 to 2 minutes. For patients who take furosemide on a regular basis, the effective dose may be much higher (up to 2 mg/kg). The vasodilatory effects occur *before* diuresis begins and act to lower blood pressure. Central venous pressure is reduced through a decrease in venous return to the heart once vasodilation is achieved. Diuresis should start within 10 minutes of drug administration and may continue for approximately 6 hours.

The most significant adverse effects are severe hypovolemia, dehydration, and electrolyte disturbances (hypokalemia, hypomagnesemia, hyponatremia, and hypochloremia). Patients on digitalis preparations are at an increased risk of digitalis toxicity from hypokalemia. The patient's fluid and electrolyte status, BUN, and creatinine must be carefully assessed before and after furosemide administration, including auscultation of breath sounds for rales, strict surveillance of intake and output, and review of laboratory data when available. An indwelling urinary catheter might be necessary. Electrolyte and careful fluid replacement may be required during furosemide therapy to prevent physiologic consequences. The nurse must also exercise caution when giving nephrotoxic agents when furosemide is prescribed and in administering the drug to patients with sulfonamide sensitivity, because furosemide is a sulfonamide derivative and can produce an allergic reaction.

Morphine Sulfate

Like furosemide, morphine sulfate is also indicated for acute pulmonary edema, because it produces venous vasodilation that decreases cardiac **preload** (the amount of blood returning to the right ventricle). The net effect is a decrease in pulmonary venous congestion. Morphine has been discussed previously in this chapter.

Table 59-4 lists emergency drugs used for hypertensive crises and pulmonary edema and their dosages, uses, and considerations.

KEY WEBSITES

American Association of Critical-Care Nurses: *www.aacn.org*

American Heart Association: *www.americanheart.org*

Emergency Nurses Association: *www.ena.org*

CRITICAL THINKING CASE STUDY

DW, age 19 years, suffered a gunshot wound to the head and a spinal cord injury from a stab wound over the thoracic spine 1 hour ago. He was transported immediately from the injury scene to the trauma center by paramedics. Upon hospital arrival, DW was awake and following simple commands, but his neurologic status has subsequently deteriorated. At this point, he has undergone initial resuscitation and a rapid diagnostic workup. He is now orally intubated, has two functional IV catheters (one peripheral line in the right forearm and one triple-lumen central line in the left subclavian vein), an oral gastric tube, and an indwelling urinary catheter. His current vital signs are BP 88/56, HR 56, temperature 96.8° F (36° C), and RR 16 on a mechanical ventilator. His mother reported that DW is addicted to opioids, including heroin. He also abuses oral diazepam (Valium) and other street drugs.

DW's diagnoses include a penetrating head injury with intracerebral hemorrhage diagnosed by computed tomography (CT) scan, a penetrating spinal cord injury at the T4 level, and drug abuse. DW opens his eyes spontaneously, does not follow commands, and withdraws to pain with only his upper extremities; his lower extremities do not move.

1. On arrival to the trauma center, should DW have received supplemental oxygen based on his mechanism of injury? What type of oxygen delivery device would be appropriate for DW on his initial presentation when he was breathing spontaneously?
2. The physician orders 50 g of mannitol to be given now, IV push. On hand are several 50-mL vials of "mannitol, 25%" solution. How many milliliters of mannitol from this vial need to be drawn up into the syringe to administer 50 g?
3. Describe the type of needle that must be used when administering mannitol. Explain your answer. What size syringe should be used? Which IV line should be used to administer the mannitol?
4. What are the indications for mannitol administration? List at least three nursing considerations when giving mannitol.
5. DW has a history of heroin and diazepam abuse. List the reversal agents that could be used if the trauma team believes recent illicit drug use may be a contributing factor to his altered mental state.
6. Because of DW's spinal cord injury, he is exhibiting signs of neurogenic shock: bradycardia, warm skin, and hypotension. What is the drug of choice that the nurse should keep at the bedside in case DW requires emergency treatment for symptomatic bradycardia? Name the drug, its mechanism of action, and dosing considerations.
7. The physician orders a dopamine infusion, 800 mg/250 mL D_5W, to be titrated to maintain systolic BP>110 mm Hg. Which IV site would be the best choice for a continuous dopamine infusion in DW?
8. What is the consequence of dopamine extravasation?
9. Describe the treatment for dopamine extravasation.
10. What vital sign parameters must be monitored while DW receives dopamine? Name at least four adverse effects of dopamine.

Antibiotics are initiated as prophylaxis for infection due to the nature of DW's penetrating injuries. Upon infusion of the antibiotic, a bodywide rash, swelling of the lips and tongue, and hypotension develop.

11. After antibiotic administration, what condition has developed in DW?
12. What are the drugs of choice to treat DW's condition now?
13. How can the nurse evaluate the effectiveness of these drugs?

NCLEX STUDY QUESTIONS

1. The nurse is administering atropine 0.3 mg IV to a 75-year-old patient with a heart rate of 45, and his heart rate decreases to 38. What is the most likely explanation?
   a. Atropine exerts its effects by stimulating the vagus nerve.
   b. The ordered dose was too low.
   c. Adenosine was indicated, not atropine.
   d. Atropine typically slows heart rate first and then increases it.
2. An 80-year-old woman with a hip fracture received morphine 3 mg IV 20 minutes ago. The patient's son runs to the nurses' station and says that his mother is no longer responding to him. What actions should the nurse take?
   a. Assess the patient; call for additional assistance; support breathing with a bag-valve-mask device as indicated, and prepare to administer flumazenil.
   b. Call the physician and report that the patient most likely suffered a stroke and now has elevated intracranial pressure; prepare to administer mannitol.
   c. Assess the patient; call for additional assistance; support breathing with a bag-valve-mask device as indicated, and prepare to administer naloxone.
   d. Explain to the patient's son that the morphine is taking effect and that unresponsiveness is the desired outcome to best manage her pain.
3. The nurse is caring for a 21-year-old woman with a closed head injury. Her intracranial pressure is 35 (normal <20). Her serum osmolality is 330. The nurse should anticipate which action?
   a. Administer mannitol.
   b. Withhold mannitol at this time, but take other measures to reduce intracranial pressure.
   c. Administer sodium nitroprusside.

d. Take no action at this time because the patient has a serum osmolality of 330, which will offset the effects of the elevated intracranial pressure.

4. A dopamine infusion was started in a patient's antecubital vein during resuscitation after cardiac arrest. The electronic infusion device is now sounding an alert for an occlusion. What is the most important immediate concern for the nurse?
   a. Infiltration with phentolamine will be necessary if there is extravasation.
   b. An interruption in the infusion can produce hypotension in the patient.
   c. The device will need to be reported to the hospital's clinical engineering department for service.
   d. The patient could develop hypertension as a result of the alarm.
5. Adenosine is ordered for a patient in the emergency department. Immediately after intravenous administration, the nurse observes a short period of asystole on the cardiac monitor that resolves spontaneously. What is the most appropriate initial action for the nurse?
   a. Call for the doctor.
   b. Prepare epinephrine and atropine for intravenous administration.
   c. Initiate CPR.
   d. Closely observe the patient and the cardiac monitor.
6. A patient on the medical-surgical unit has suffered an acute anaphylactic reaction during infusion of an IV antibiotic with hives and bronchospasm. The nurse practitioner has written a number of stat medication orders. What is the priority medication to administer first?
   a. steroid dose pack
   b. dopamine
   c. epinephrine
   d. diphenhydramine
7. The nurse receives a stat order to administer 50% dextrose solution intravenously to a 1-year-old child with hypoglycemia. How should this medication best be prepared for safe administration to the child?
   a. Use a filter needle.
   b. Draw the medication into a tuberculin syringe.
   c. Dilute 1 : 1 with sterile water to produce dextrose 25%.
   d. Shake the solution vigorously before injection.
8. A 51-year-old woman has been reportedly taking Xanax for a severe anxiety disorder following her mother's death. She was brought into the emergency department because she became unresponsive while at work in an insurance office. Knowing her history, what should the nurse anticipate administering?
   a. mannitol
   b. naloxone
   c. activated charcoal
   d. flumazenil
9. A 25-year-old woman was admitted to the emergency department after a successful prehospital resuscitation from cardiac arrest owing to an asthma attack. On arrival, her pulse oximeter reading is 85%. Given her condition, what is the most important initial medication to administer as ordered?
   a. epinephrine
   b. sodium bicarbonate
   c. albuterol
   d. oxygen
10. The nurse practitioner orders epinephrine 0.3 mg IM for a severe allergic reaction to a bee sting in an adult patient. Which concentration of epinephrine should the nurse select to administer this particular dose?
    a. 1 : 10,000
    b. 1 : 1000
    c. 1 : 100
    d. 1 : 10
11. The emergency physician orders activated charcoal for a teenage girl who took an intentional overdose of aspirin and several unknown drugs from her parent's medicine cabinet. Upon preparing to administer the activated charcoal by mouth, the nurse notes that the patient has become very somnolent and opens her eyes only to a noxious stimulus. Which action by the nurse is most appropriate at this point?
    a. Immediately discuss the change in the patient's mental status with the physician so that the plan of care can be reevaluated.
    b. Immediately insert a nasogastric tube, and administer the activated charcoal.
    c. Immediately elevate the head of the patient's stretcher, and coax her to drink the activated charcoal while applying noxious stimuli as necessary to keep her awake.
    d. Give only half the dose now, and wait until her mental status improves before giving the remainder of the dose.
12. While getting dressed to go home after minor outpatient surgery on his leg for removal of a mole, a 62-year-old patient notifies the nurse that he has severe chest pain. He is also diaphoretic and complains of shortness of breath. The surgeon is notified and orders administration of aspirin 325 mg PO while quickly making arrangements to transfer the patient to the emergency department. Which is the best course of action by the nurse?
    a. Question the aspirin order because the patient just had a surgical procedure and might have bleeding complications.
    b. After checking for drug allergies, first instruct the patient to chew the aspirin tablet and then administer the aspirin.
    c. After checking for drug allergies, instruct the patient to swallow the aspirin tablet whole.
    d. Suggest to the surgeon that the enteric-coated form of aspirin might be better tolerated by the patient to avoid GI distress.

Answers: 1, b; 2, c; 3, b; 4, b; 5, d; 6, c; 7, c; 8, d; 9, d; 10, b; 11, a; 12, b.

APPENDIX A

Therapeutic Drug Monitoring*

Selected drugs are monitored by serum and urine to achieve and maintain therapeutic drug effect and to prevent drug toxicity. Drugs with a wide therapeutic range (window), the difference between effective dose and toxic dose, are not usually monitored. Drug monitoring is important in maintaining a drug concentration–response relationship, especially when the serum drug range (window) is narrow, such as with digoxin and lithium. Therapeutic drug monitoring (TDM) is the process of following drug levels and adjusting them to maintain a therapeutic level. Not all drugs can be dosed and/or monitored by their blood levels alone.

Drug levels are obtained at peak time and trough time after a steady state of the drug has been achieved in the patient. Steady state is reached after four to five half-lives of a drug and can be reached sooner if the drug has a short half-life. Once steady state is achieved, the serum drug level is checked at the peak level (maximum drug concentration) and/or at trough/residual level (minimum drug concentration). If the trough or residual level is at the high therapeutic point, toxicity might occur. Careful assessment is needed by both physical and laboratory means.

TDM is required for the following:

- Drugs with a narrow therapeutic index or range (window)
- When other methods for monitoring drugs are not effective, such as blood pressure (BP) monitoring
- To determine when adequate blood concentrations are reached
- To evaluate a patient's compliance to drug therapy
- To determine whether other drugs have altered serum drug levels (increased or decreased) that could result in drug toxicity or lack of therapeutic effect
- To establish a new serum drug level when the dosage is changed

Drug groups for TDM include analgesics, antibiotics, anticonvulsants, antineoplastics, bronchodilators, cardiac drugs, hypoglycemics, sedatives, and tranquilizers. To effectively conduct TDM, the laboratory must be provided with the following information: drug name and daily dosage, time and amount of last dose, time blood was drawn, route of administration, and patient's age. Without complete information, serum drug reporting might be incorrect.

HIV drugs are primarily dosed based on the patient's viral load or CD4 counts. Many of these drugs have dosage adjustments for renal and/or hepatic impairment.

*Revised by Ronald J. Lefever, RPh, Lead Pharmacist, VCU Medical Center, Richmond, Virginia.

DRUG	THERAPEUTIC RANGE	PEAK TIME	TOXIC LEVEL
acetaminophen (Tylenol)	10-20 mcg/mL	1-2.5 h	>50 mcg/mL Hepatotoxicity: >200 mcg/mL
acetohexamide (Dymelor)	20-70 mcg/mL (dosed according to blood glucose levels)	2-4 h	>75 mcg/mL
alcohol	Negative		Mild toxic: 150 mg/dL Marked toxic: >250 mg/dL
alprazolam (Xanax)	10-50 ng/mL	1-2 h	>75 ng/mL
amikacin (Amikin)	Peak: 20-30 mcg/mL Trough: <10 mcg/mL	Intravenously: 0.5 h Intramuscular: 0.5-1.5 h	Peak: >35 mcg/mL Trough: >10 mcg/mL
aminocaproic acid (Amicar)	100-400 mcg/mL	1 h	>400 mcg/mL
aminophylline (see theophylline)			
amiodarone (Cordarone)	0.5-2.5 mcg/mL	2-10 h	>2.5 mcg/mL
amitriptyline (Elavil) + nortriptyline (parent and active metabolite)	110-225 ng/mL	2-4 h (and up to 12 h)	>500 ng/mL
amobarbital (Amytal)	1-5 mcg/mL	2 h	>15 mcg/mL Severe toxicity: >30 mcg/mL
amoxapine	20-100 ng/mL	2.5 h; steady state 2-7 d	>100 ng/mL
amphetamine: serum: urine	20-30 ng/mL	Detectable in urine after 3 h; positive for 24-48 h	0.2 mcg/mL >30 mcg/mL (urine)
aspirin (see salicylates)			
atenolol (Tenormin)	200-500 ng/mL	2-4 h	>500 ng/mL
beta carotene	48-200 mcg/dL	Several weeks	>300 mcg/dL
bromide	20-80 mg/dL		>100 mg/dL
butabarbital (Butisol)	1-2 mcg/mL	3-4 h	>10 mcg/mL
butalbital	10-20 mcg/mL		>40 mcg/mL
caffeine	Adult: 3-15 mcg/mL Infant: 8-20 mcg/mL	0.5-1 h	>50 mcg/mL
carbamazepine (Tegretol)	4-12 mcg/mL	6 h (range 2-24 h)	>9-15 mcg/mL
chloral hydrate	2-12 mcg/mL	1-2 h	>20 mcg/mL
chloramphenicol (Chloromycetin)	10-20 mg/L		>25 mg/L
chlordiazepoxide (Librium)	1-5 mcg/mL	2-3 h	>5 mcg/mL
chlorpromazine (Thorazine)	50-300 ng/mL	2-4 h	>750 ng/mL
chlorpropamide (Diabinese)	75-250 mcg/mL (Diabinese)	3-6 h	>250-750 mcg/mL
clonidine (Catapres)	0.2-2 ng/mL (hypotensive effect)	2-5 h	>2 ng/mL
clorazepate (Tranxene)	0.12-1 mcg/mL	1-2 h	>1 mcg/mL
cimetidine (Tagamet)	Trough: 0.5-1.2 mcg/mL	1-1.5 h	Trough: >1.5 mcg/mL
clonazepam (Klonopin)	10-60 ng/mL	2 h	>80 ng/mL
codeine	10-100 ng/mL	1-2 h	>200 ng/mL
cyclosporine	100-300 ng/mL	3-4 h	>400 ng/mL
dantrolene (Dantrium)	1-3 mcg/mL	5 h	>5 mcg/mL
desipramine (Norpramin)	125-300 ng/mL	4-6 h	>500 ng/mL
diazepam (Valium)	0.5-2 mg/L 400-600 ng/mL therapeutic	1-2 h	>3 mg/L >3,000 ng/mL
digitoxin (rarely administered)	10-25 ng/mL	Noticeable: 2-4 h Peak: 12-24 h	>30 ng/mL
digoxin	0.5-2 ng/mL	PO: 6-8 h IV: 1.5-2 h	2-3 ng/mL
Dilantin (see phenytoin)			
diltiazem (Cardizem)	50-200 ng/mL	2-3 h	>200 ng/mL
disopyramide (Norpace)	2-4 mcg/mL	2 h	>4 mcg/mL
doxepin (Sinequan)	150-300 ng/mL	2-4 h	>500 ng/mL
ethosuximide (Zarontin)	40-100 mcg/mL	2-4 h	>150 mcg/mL
flecainide (Tambocor)	0.2-1 mcg/mL	3 h	>1 mcg/mL
5-flucytosine	Peak: 100 mcg/mL Trough: 50 mcg/mL		Peak: >125 mcg/mL Trough: >125 mcg/mL
fluoride			>15 µmol/L
fluoxetine	90-300 ng/mL	2-4 h	>500 ng/mL

DRUG	THERAPEUTIC RANGE	PEAK TIME	TOXIC LEVEL
flurazepam (Dalmane)	20-110 ng/mL	0.5-1 h	>1500 ng/mL
folate	>3.5 mcg/mL	1 h	
gentamicin (Garamycin)	Peak: 6-12 mcg/mL Trough: <2 mcg/mL	IV: 15-30 min	Peak: >12 mcg/mL Trough: >2 mcg/mL
haloperidol (Haldol)	5-15 ng/mL	2-6 h	>50 ng/mL
hydrocortisone	135-637 nmol/L at 8 AM	1-2 h (PO)	>700 nmol/L at 8 AM
hydromorphone (Dilaudid)	1-30 ng/mL	0.5-1.5 h	>100 ng/mL
ibuprofen (e.g., Motrin)	10-50 mcg/mL	1-2 h	>100 mcg/mL
imipramine (Tofranil) + desipramine (parent and active metabolite)	200-350 ng/mL	PO: 1-2 h IM: 30 min	>500 ng/mL
isoniazid (INH, Nydrazid)	1-7 mcg/mL (dose usually adjusted based on liver function tests)	1-2 h	>20 mcg/mL
kanamycin (Kantrex)	Peak: 15-30 mcg/mL	PO: 1-2 h IM: 0.5-1 h	Peak: >35 mcg/mL Trough: >10 mcg/mL
lead	<20 mcg/dL Urine: <80 mcg/24 h		>80 mcg/dL Urine: >125 mcg/24 h
lidocaine (Xylocaine)	1.5-5 mcg/mL	IV: 10 min	>6 mcg/mL
lithium	0.8-1.2 mEq/L	0.5-4 h	>1.5 mEq/L
lorazepam (Ativan)	50-240 ng/mL	1-3 h	>300 ng/mL
meperidine (Demerol)	0.4-0.7 mcg/mL	2-4 h	>1 mcg/mL
meprobamate (Equanil, Miltown)	15-25 mcg/mL	2 h	>50 mcg/mL
methadone (Dolophine)	100-400 ng/mL	0.5-1 h	>2000 ng/mL or >0.2 mcg/mL
methaqualone	1-5 mcg/mL		>10 mcg/mL
methotrexate	<0.1 mmol/L after 48 h	1-2 h	1×10^6 at 48 h
methsuximide	<1 mcg/mL	1-4 h	>40 mcg/mL
methyldopa (Aldomet)	1-5 mcg/mL	3-6 h	>7 mcg/mL
methylprednisolone (Depo-Medol)	135-637 nmol/L at 8 AM	PO: 1-2 h IM: 4-8 d	>700 nmol/L at 8 AM
methyprylon (Noludar)	8-10 mcg/mL	1-2 h	>50 mcg/mL
metoprolol (Lopressor)	75-200 ng/mL	2-4 h	>225 ng/mL
mexiletine (Mexitil)	<0.5-2 mcg/mL	2-3 h	>2 mcg/mL
morphine	10-80 ng/mL	IV: Immediately IM: 0.5-1 h subQ: 1-1.5 h	>200 ng/mL
netilmicin (Netromycin)	Peak: 0.5-10 mcg/mL Trough: <4 mcg/mL	IV: 30 min	Peak: >16 mcg/mL Trough: >4 mcg/mL
nifedipine (Procardia)	50-100 ng/mL	0.5-2 h	>100 ng/mL
nortriptyline (Aventyl)	50-150 ng/mL	8 h	>200 ng/mL
oxazepam (Serax)	0.2-1.4 mcg/mL	1-2 h	
oxycodone (Percodan)	10-100 ng/mL	0.5-1 h	>200 ng/mL
pentazocine (Talwin)	0.05-0.2 mcg/mL	1-2 h	>1 mcg/mL Urine: >3 mcg/mL
pentobarbital (Nembutal)	1-5 mcg/mL	0.5-1 h	>10 mcg/mL Severe toxicity: >30 mcg/mL
phenmetrazine (Preludin)	5-30 mcg/mL (urine)	2 h	>50 mcg/mL (urine)
phenobarbital (Luminal)	15-40 mcg/mL	6-18 h	>40 mcg/mL Severe toxicity: >80 mcg/mL
phenytoin (Dilantin)	10-20 mcg/mL	4-8 h	>20-30 mcg/mL Severe toxicity: >40 mcg/mL
pindolol (Visken)	0.5-6 ng/mL	2-4 h	>10 ng/mL
primidone (Mysoline)	5-12 mcg/mL	2-4 h	>12-15 mcg/mL
procainamide (Pronestyl)	4-10 mcg/mL	1 h	>10 mcg/mL
procaine (Novocain)	<11 mcg/mL	10-30 min	>20 mcg/mL

Continued

DRUG	THERAPEUTIC RANGE	PEAK TIME	TOXIC LEVEL
prochlorperazine (Compazine)	50-300 ng/mL	2-4 h	>1,000 ng/mL
propoxyphene (Darvon)	0.1-0.4 mcg/mL	2-3 h	>0.5 mcg/mL
propranolol (Inderal)	>100 ng/mL	1-2 h	>150 ng/mL
protriptyline (Vivactil)	50-150 ng/mL	8-12 h	>200 ng/mL
quinidine	2-5 mcg/mL	1-3 h	>6 mcg/mL
ranitidine (Zantac)	100 ng/mL	2-3 h	>100 ng/mL
reserpine (Serpasil)	20 ng/mL	2-4 h	>20 ng/mL
salicylates (aspirin)	10-30 mg/dL	1-2 h	Tinnitus: 20-40 mg/mL Hyperventilation: >35 mg/dL Severe toxicity: >50 mg/dL
secobarbital (Seconal)	2-5 mcg/mL	1 h	>15 mcg/mL Severe toxicity: >30 mcg/mL
streptomycin	Peak: 5-20 mcg/mL Trough: <5 mcg/mL		Peak: >40 mcg/mL Trough: >40 mcg/mL
sulfadiazine	100-120 mcg/mL		>300 mcg/mL
sulfamethoxazole	90-100 mcg/mL		>300 mcg/mL
sulfapyridine	75-90 mcg/mL		>300 mcg/mL
sulfisoxazole	90-100 mcg/mL		>300 mcg/mL
theophylline (Theo-Dur)	10-20 mcg/mL	PO: 2-3 h IV: 15 min (depends on smoking or nonsmoking)	>20 mcg/mL
thiocyanate	4-20 mcg/mL		>60 mcg/mL
thioridazine (Mellaril)	100-600 ng/mL 1-1.5 mcg/mL	2-4 h	>2000 ng/mL >10 mcg/mL
timolol (Blocadren)	3-55 ng/mL	1-2 h	>60 ng/mL
tobramycin (Nebcin)	Peak: 5-10 mcg/mL Trough: 1-1.5 mcg/mL	IV: 15-30 min IM: 0.5-1.5 h	Peak: >12 mcg/mL Trough: >2 mcg/mL
tocainide (Tonocard)	4-10 mcg/mL	0.5-3 h	>12 mcg/mL
tolbutamide (Orinase)	80-240 mcg/mL	3-5 h	>640 mcg/mL
trazodone (Desyrel)	500-2,500 ng/mL	1-2 wk	>4,000 ng/mL
triamcinolone (Aristocort, Kenalog)	135-637 nmol/L at 8 AM	1-2 h (PO/IM)	>700 nmol/L at 8 AM
trifluoperazine (Stelazine)	50-300 ng/mL	2-4 h	>1,000 ng/mL
trimethoprim/sulfamethoxazole (TMP/SMX)	Peak: trimethoprim: >5 mcg/mL Peak: sulfamethoxazole: >100 mcg/mL		
valproic acid (Depakene)	50-100 mcg/mL	0.5-1.5 h	>100 mcg/mL Severe toxicity: >150 mcg/mL
vancomycin (Vancocin)	Peak: 20-40 mcg/mL Trough: 5-10 mcg/mL	IV: Peak: 5 min IV: Trough: 12 h	Peak: >80 mcg/mL
verapamil (Calan)	100-300 ng/mL	PO: 1-2 h IV: 5 min	>500 ng/mL
warfarin (Coumadin)	1-10 mcg/mL (dose usually adjusted by PT 1-2.5 control) or INR: 2-3	1.5-3 d	>10 mcg/mL INR: >4

d, Day; *h*, hour; *min*, minute; *wk*, week; >, greater than; <, less than.

HIV DRUGS

DRUG	PEAK TIME (TMAX)	ELIMINATION HALF-LIFE	NEW TO TDM	SPECIAL CONSIDERATIONS
Nucleoside/Nucleotide Reverse Transcriptase Inhibitors (NRTIs)				
abacavir (Ziagen)	0.7-1.7 h	1.5 h		Dose adjustment for hepatic impairment
abacavir + lamivudine + zidovudine (Trizivir)	See individual agents	See individual agents		
didanosine (Videx)	0.25-1.5 h	1.5 h		
emtricitabine (Emtriva)	1-2 h	10 h	Y	
emtricitabine + Tenofovir (Truvada)	1-2 h	10-17 h	Y	
lamivudine (Epivir)	0.9-3.2 h	5-7 h		Dose adjustment for renal impairment suggested
lamivudine + abacavir (Epzicom)	See individual agents	1.5-7 h	Y	Abacavir: $t_{1/2}$: 1.5 h; lamivudine: $t_{1/2}$: 5-7 h Dose adjustment for renal impairment required
lamivudine + zidovudine (Combivir)	See individual agents		Y	
stavudine (Zerit)	1-1.5 h	1.5 h (8 h with renal impairment)		
tenofovir (Viread)	1 h	17 h	Y	Dose adjustment for renal impairment required
zidovudine (Retrovir)	0.5-1.5 h	1 h (1.4-2.9 h with renal impairment)		
Non-Nucleoside Reverse Transcriptase Inhibitors (NNRTIs)				
delavirdine (Rescriptor)	1 h	2-11 h	Y	
etravirine (Intelence)	2.5-4 h	41 h	Y	NRTI and first-line NNRTI (delavirdine, efavirenz, or nevirapine) experienced or contraindicated, with either detectable viral load or intolerance to current regimen
efavirenz (Sustiva)	3-5 h	40-55 h		
nevirapine (Viramune)	4 h	25-30 h		
Multiclass Combination Agents				
efavirenz + emtricitabine + tenofovir (Atripla)	See individual agents	See individual agents	Y	
Protease Inhibitors (PIs)				
atazanavir (Reyataz)	2.5 h	7 h	Y	
darunavir (Prezista)	2.5-4 h	15 h	Y	Elimination half-life when co-administered with ritonavir.
fosamprenavir (Lexiva)	1.5-4 h	7.7 h	Y	
indinavir (Crixivan)	0.8 h	2 h (3 h with hepatic impairment)		
lopinavir + ritonavir (Kaletra)	4 h	5-6 h		
ritonavir (Norvir)	2-4 h	3-5 h		
tipranavir (Aptivus)	2.9-3 h	5.5-6 h	Y	Female and male, respectively
maraviroc (Selzentry)	0.5-4 h	14-18 h	Y	NRTI and NNRTI experienced or contraindicated and prior experience with one or more PIs, or raltegravir, or intolerance to current regimen
Integrase Inhibitor				
raltegravir (Isentress)	3 h	9 h	Y	

h, Hour; $t_{1/2}$, half-life.

APPENDIX B

Selected Potential Weapons of Bioterrorism

Refer to the following online resources for updates to this information:

- Centers for Disease Control and Prevention (CDC): *www.bt.cdc.gov/agent/agentlist.asp*
- Journal of the American Medical Association (JAMA): *www.jama.ama-assn.org/cgi/collection/bioterrorism*
- U.S. Food and Drug Administration (FDA): *www.fda.gov/oc/opacom/hottopics/bioterrorism.html*

AGENT/ETIOLOGY	TRANSMISSION/CLINICAL MANIFESTATIONS	DRUG TREATMENT/CONSIDERATIONS
Bacteria and Viruses		
Anthrax, pulmonary/*Bacillus anthracis*	Inhalation of spores; incubation up to 60 d Initially ILS: fever, malaise, fatigue, nonproductive cough, chest discomfort. Later, (2 to 3 d) severe respiratory distress, stridor, cyanosis, septicemia, increased fever, and hemorrhagic meningitis	Early treatment with antibiotics IMPORTANT; IV route preferred; ciprofloxacin and doxycycline drugs of choice; PLUS use of additional antibiotics to avoid drug resistance in both adults and children; duration for IV and PO 60 d. Low morbidity when treated early; with onset of respiratory distress, morbidity near 100%. Recombinant vaccine in development
Anthrax, cutaneous/*Bacillus anthracis*	Spores enter through nonintact skin; incubation up to 60 d; papule becomes fluid-filled vesicle that dries and forms dark eschar	Ciprofloxacin or doxycycline PO for 7 to 10 d; with systemic symptoms or risk of inhalation, treat as above. Morbidity up to 24% if untreated; treated <1%. Goal: prevention of systemic complications
Smallpox/variola virus	Respiratory droplets and pustule drainage; incubation 12 to 14 d; prodrome 2 to 4 d of ILS; papular rash that becomes deep vesicles, then scabs; mostly face and extremities; does involve palms and soles	Supportive; research continues on new antivirals (e.g., cidofovir); proven treatment unknown. Treat corneal lesions with idoxuridine; vaccinate patient, all contacts, and health care workers in facility. Antibiotics for secondary infections. Morbidity: 30% likely; in rare hemorrhagic form: up to 90%. *For terrorist attack:* Follow with vaccination prophylaxis.
Plague, pneumonic/*Yersinia pestis*	Inhaled droplets; incubation: 2 to 3 d; begins as ILS; rapid 24-h progression to severe pneumonia, hemoptysis, and then respiratory distress and failure. Can be transmitted by coughing	Antibiotics of choice are streptomycin and gentamicin. In mass casualty environment, PO administration is more usual with doxycycline or ciprofloxacin. No vaccine available. Morbidity 100% if untreated
Tularemia/*Francisella tularensis*/"rabbit fever"	Inhaled or through skin; incubation 2 to 5 d (up to 14 d); begins as ILS; progresses over days to pneumonia with dyspnea and hilar adenopathy. Not transmitted person to person	Antibiotics of choice: IV streptomycin or gentamicin; po doxycycline or ciprofloxacin in mass breakout. Morbidity <5%
Viral hemorrhagic fevers; Ebola	Blood or secretions; incubation 2 to 10 d; prodrome of ILS; bleeding day 3; desquamation day 5; progresses rapidly to multisystem organ failure and delirium	Supportive care; transfusions and fresh frozen plasma; dialysis
Biotoxins		
Botulinum/*Clostridium botulinum*	Inhaled; incubation of 24 to 72 h; symmetric descending flaccid paralysis; eyes, bulbar muscles, then respiratory and skeletal effects	Supportive; antitoxin (from Centers for Disease Control and Prevention or Public Health) may decrease progress; BabyBIG for children <1 year. No antibiotics. Morbidity uncertain; long recovery

AGENT/ETIOLOGY	TRANSMISSION/CLINICAL MANIFESTATIONS	DRUG TREATMENT/CONSIDERATIONS
Ricin/*Ricinus communis*	Inhalation: onset within hours; coughing, chest tightness, dyspnea, nausea, and muscle ache. Later, edematous airway; cyanosis and death may follow Ingested: GI hemorrhage, vomiting, and diarrhea. Later, liver and kidney failure; may die within 10 to 12 d Injection: severe symptoms and death; route unlikely to terrorists	Supportive; no antidote for ricin. Vaccine in development
Chemical Weapons		
Nerve agents (e.g., Sarin, VX, GA, GB)	Absorbed through skin and mucous membranes and inhaled; onset rapid when inhaled; skin or mucous membrane onset 30 min to 18 h. Early signs: eye pain, rhinorrhea, and local sweating if droplet. Classic toxidrome: diarrhea, urination, miosis, bronchospasm, bronchorrhea, bradycardia, emesis, lacrimation, and salivation	Mechanical ventilation support with oxygen. Atropine IV or IM in high doses: 2 mg q3-5min; pralidoxime chloride (2-PAM) 1 to 2 g IV over 30 to 60 min; may need drip of 500 mg over 24 h; valium or Versed PRN for seizures; homatropine for ciliary spasm. Morbidity potentially high, depending on concentration and duration of exposure
Chlorine or phosgene	Inhaled, mucous membranes, and eyes; rapid irritant effects; pulmonary effects (distress and edema) may be seen in 6 to 24 h	Humidified oxygen; bronchodilators; ventilatory support with PEEP for ARDS; monitor for 24 h if suspected significant exposure. Morbidity depends on exposure level; phosgene higher than chlorine
Sulfur mustard (Mustard gas)	Mainly absorbed through skin; can affect airway, eyes, GI tract, and bone marrow. Delayed onset of >6 h with few warning symptoms of contact; blistering of affected areas. Later, seizures and dysrhythmias	Requires rapid decontamination. Intubation if severe airway damage. Wash with dilute sodium thiosulfate (2.5% solution); prednisone may have antidote effects; Neupogen for later leukopenia. Morbidity under 5% to 10%
Cyanide	Absorbed in GI tract via contaminated products; inhaled vapors or via skin; generally rapid onset of symptoms; delayed if low concentration; sudden loss of consciousness with high concentration; cyanosis and severe respiratory distress	Inhaled amyl nitrite, sodium nitrite IV, sodium thiosulfate. Morbidity varies by exposure level
Radiologic Agents		
Nuclear bombs	Immediate threat: blast Delayed threat: radioactive fallout	Potassium iodide blocks uptake by thyroid of radioactive iodine, thus reducing risk of cancer; tablets for this purpose are released by public health after determining the presence of iodine-131. FDA recommended doses: Birth to 1 mo: 16 mg; >1 mo to 3 y: 32 mg; >3 y to 18 y: 65 mg; >18 y or lactating: 130 mg

ARDS, Adult respiratory distress syndrome; *d,* day; *FDA,* Food and Drug Administration; *GI,* gastrointestinal; *h,* hour; *ILS,* influenza-like syndrome; *IM,* intramuscular; *IV,* intravenous; *min,* minute; *mo,* month; *PEEP,* positive end-expiratory pressure; *PO,* by mouth; *PRN,* as needed; *y,* year; *>,* greater than; *<,* less than.

REFERENCES

Agency for Healthcare Research and Quality. (2012). *Evidence-based practice center systemic review protocol: Otitis media with effusion: comparative effectiveness of treatments.* Retrieved from *www.effectivehealthcare.ahrq.gov/ehc/products/387/1013/OME_AmendedProtocol_20120807.pdf.*

American Academy of Ophthalmology. (2010). *Preferred practice pattern: Primary angle closure.* Retrieved from *http://one.aao.org/CE/PracticeGuidelines/PPP_Content.aspx?cid=92bea8f6-5459-49a6-9233-4528343dc4c3.*

American Academy of Ophthalmology. (2010). *Preferred practice pattern: Primary open-angle glaucoma.* Retrieved from *one.aao.org/CE/PracticeGuidelines/PPP_Content.aspx?cid=93019a87-4649-4130-8f94-b6a9b19144d2.*

American Academy of Pediatrics. (2012). Active and passive immunization. In L. K. Pickering, C. J. Baker, D. W. Kimberlin, et al. (Eds.), *Red book: 2012 report of the committee on infectious diseases* (29th ed.). Elk Grove Village, IL: American Academy of Pediatrics.

American Association of Clinical Endocrinologists. *Medical guidelines for clinical practice for the evaluation and treatment of male sexual dysfunction: a couple's problem—2003 update.* Retrieved from *www.aace.com/files/sexdysguid.pdf.*

American Heart Association. (2011). *Advanced cardiovascular life support professional provider manual.* Dallas: American Heart Association.

American Heart Association, American Academy of Pediatrics. (2011). *Pediatric advanced life support professional provider manual.* Dallas: American Heart Association.

Arroyo, J. G. (2012). Age-related macular degeneration: Epidemiology, etiology, and diagnosis. In H. N. Sokol (Ed.), *Up-to-date.* Retrieved from *www.uptodateonline.com.*

Arroyo, J. G. (2012). Age-related macular degeneration: Treatment and prevention. In H. N. Sokol (Ed.), *Up-to-date.* Retrieved from *www.uptodateonline.com.*

AWHONN, Mattson, S., & Smith, J. E. (Eds.). (2011). *Core curriculum for maternal newborn nursing* (4th ed.). Philadelphia: Elsevier.

Bartlett, J. G., & Gallant, J. E. (2009). *Medical management of HIV infection* (2009-2010 ed., pp. 29–32). Durham, NC: Knowledge Source Solutions.

Birnbach, D., & Brown, I. (2010). Anesthesia for obstetrics. In R. Miller, L. Eriksson, L. Fleisher, et al. (Eds.), *Miller's anesthesia for obstetrics.* (pp. 2203–2240). Philadelphia: Elsevier.

Birt, C. M., Buys, Y. M., Ahmed, I. I. K., et al. (2010). Toronto Area Glaucoma Society: Prostaglandin efficacy and safety study undertaken by race (The PRESSURE study). *Glaucoma, 19*(7), 460–467.

Bloski, T., & Pierson, R. (2008). Endometriosis and chronic pelvic pain: unraveling the mystery behind the complex condition. *Nurs Women's Health, 12,* 382.

Bo, S., Menato, G., Villois, P., et al. (2009). Iron supplementation and gestational diabetes in midpregnancy. *Am J Obstet Gynecol, 200,* 158e1–158e6.

Bonanno, C., & Wapner, R. (2009). Antenatal corticosteroid treatment: what's happened since Drs Liggins and Howie? *Am J Obstet Gynecol, 200,* 448–457.

Bonvillain, N. (2010). *Cultural anthropology* (2nd ed.). Upper Saddle River, NJ: Pearson.

Bosarge, P. M., & Freeman, S. (2009). Bioidentical hormones and compounding. *J Nurse Pract, 5*(6).

Breathnach, F., & Geary, M. (2009). Uterine atony: definition, prevention, nonsurgical management, and uterine tamponade. *Semin Perinatol, 33*(2), 82.

Brown, C. G. (2010). *A guide to oncology symptom management.* Oncology Nursing Society, ONS Publishing Division.

Brunton, L., Lazo, J., & Parker, K. (2010). *Goodman and Gilman's the pharmacological basis of therapeutics* (12th ed.). New York: McGraw-Hill.

Campinha-Bacote, J. (2008). African-Americans: In L. Purnell & B. Paulanka (Eds.), *Transcultural health care: a culturally competent approach* (3rd ed.). Philadelphia: FA Davis.

Centers for Disease Control and Prevention. (2012). Recommended immunization schedules for persons aged 0 through 18 years—United States. *MMWR, 61*(5), 1–4.

Centers for Disease Control and Prevention. (2012). Recommended adult immunization schedule–United States. *MMWR, 61*(4), 1–7.

Centers for Disease Control and Prevention. (2011). General recommendations on immunization. *MMWR, 60*(2), 1–61.

Centers for Disease Control and Prevention. (2010). National, state and local area vaccination coverage among children aged 19-35 months—United States, 2009. *MMWR, 59*(33), 1171–1177.

Centers for Disease Control and Prevention. (2006). *HIV/AIDS facts.* Retrieved from *CDCinfo@CDC.gov.*

Center for Substance Abuse Treatment. (2009). *Buprenorphine: a guide for nurses.* DHHS Pub. No. (SMA) 09-4376. Rockville, MD: Substance Abuse and Mental Health Services Administration.

Chan, P. D., & Johnson, S. M. (2011). *Gynecology and obstetrics* (2011 ed.). Blue Jay, CA: Current Clinical Strategies.

Chavez, J. (2009). Preventing and treating osteoporosis: pharmacological and nonpharmacological approaches. *J Nurse Pract, 5,* 6S1.

Cheng, J. W. (2009). A meta-analysis of topical prostaglandin analogs in the treatment of chronic angle-closure glaucoma. *J Glaucoma, 18*(9), 652–657. doi: 10.1097/IJG.0b013e31819c49d4.

Clayton, B. D., Stock, Y. N., & Harroun, R. D. (2007). *Basic pharmacology for nursing* (14th ed.). St Louis: Elsevier.

Cooper, M., Grywalski, M., Lamp, J., et al. (2007). Enhancing cultural competence: a model for nurses. *Nurs Womens Health, 11*(2), 148–159.

Cunningham, F. G., Gant, N. F., Leveno, K. J., et al. (2010). *Williams obstetrics* (23rd. ed.). New York: McGraw-Hill.

Curtis, C. (2009). Factors affecting compliance with eye drop therapy for glaucoma in a multicultural outpatient setting. *Contemp Nurse, 31*(2), 121–128.

Davidson, M., London, M., & Ladewig, P. (2008). *Olds maternal-newborn nursing and women's health across the lifespan* (8th ed.). Upper Saddle River, New Jersey: Pearson Prentice Hall.

Davis, R., Cook, D., & Cohen, L. (2013). A community reliance approach to reducing ethnic and racial disparities in health. *Am J Public Health, 95*(12), 2168.

De Backer, D., Aldecoa, C., Njimi, H., et al. (2012). Dopamine versus norepinephrine in the treatment of septic shock: A meta-analysis. *Crit Care Med, 40*(3), 725–730.

De Backer, D., Biston, P., Devriendt, J., et al. (2010). Comparison of dopamine and norepinephrine in the treatment of shock. *NEJM, 362*(9), 779–789.

Department of Health and Human Services. *Adult and Adolescent Treatment Guidelines*. Retrieved from *hyyp://aidsinfo.nih.gov*.

Devine, P. (2009). Obstetric hemorrhage. *Semin Perionatol, 33*(2), 76.

Dickey, R. P. (2010). *Managing contraceptive pill patients* (14th ed.). Dallas: EMIS Medical.

Diclegis. (2013). Retrieved from *http://diclegis.com/pdf/Diclegis_Full_Prescribing_Information.pdf.*

DiPiro, J., Talbert, R., Yee, G., et al. (2008). *Pharmacotherapy: a pathophysiologic approach* (7th ed.). New York: McGraw-Hill.

Dlugosz, C. K., Chater, R. W., & Engle, J. P. (2006). Appropriate use of non-prescription analgesics in pediatric patients. *J Pediatr Health Care, 20*(5), 316.

Duley, L. (2009). The global impact of pre-eclampsia and eclampsia. *Semin Perionatol, 33*(2), 130.

Emergency Nurses Association. (2009). *Sheehy's emergency nursing principles and practice* (6th ed.). St Louis: Elsevier.

Ezekial, M. R. (2007). *Handbook of anesthesiology* (2008 ed.). Laguna Hills, CA: Current Clinical Strategies.

Faridi, U. A. (2010). Comparative study of three prostaglandin analogues in the treatment of newly diagnosed cases of ocular hypertension, open-angle and normal tension glaucoma. *Clin Experiment Ophthalmol, 38*(7), 678–682. doi: 10.1111/j.1442-9071.2010.02305.x.

Flockhart, D. A. (2007). *Drug interactions: Cytochrome P450 drug interaction table.* Indiana University School of Medicine. Retrieved from *www.medicine.iupui.edu/clinpharm/ddis/table/aspx.*

Fowler, G. C. (2011). Corneal abrasions and removal of corneal and conjunctival foreign bodies. In J. L. Pfenninger & G. C. Fowler (Eds.), *Pfenninger and Fowler's procedures for primary care* (3rd ed., pp. 433–439). Philadelphia: Elsevier.

Gahart, B., & Nazareno, A. R. (2012). *Intravenous medications* (28th ed.). Philadelphia: Elsevier.

Giger, J., & Davidhizar, R. (2013). *Transcultural nursing: assessment and intervention* (6th ed.). St Louis: Elsevier.

Gleason, K. M., Brake, H., Agramonte, V., et al. (2011). *Medications at Transitions and Clinical Handoffs (MATCH) Toolkit for medication reconciliation*. Prepared by the Island Peer Review Organization, Inc., under Contract No. HHSA2902009000 13C. AHRQ Publication No. 11(12)-0059. Rockville, MD: Agency for Healthcare Research and Quality.

Guyton, A. C., & Hall, J. E. (2010). *Book of medical physiology*. Philadelphia: Elsevier.

Haddad, B., & Sibai, B. (2009). Expectant management in pregnancies with severe pre-eclampsia. *Semin Perionatol, 33*(3), 143.

Hammer, S. M., Eron, J. J., Reiss, P., et al. (2008). Anti-retroviral treatment of adult HIV infection: 2008 recommendations of the International AIDS Society—USA Panel. *JAMA, 300*(5), 555–570.

Harrington, B. (2013). Complications specific to neuraxis block: meningeal puncture headache. In J. Neal & J. Rathmell (Eds.), *Complications in regional anesthesia and pain medicine* (2nd ed., pp. 96–114). Philadelphia: Lippincott.

Hatcher, R. A., Trussell, J., Nelson, A., et al. (2008). *Contraceptive technology* (19th ed.). New York: Irvington.

Heitmann, K., Nordeng, H., & Longe, H. (2013). Safety of ginger use in pregnancy: Results from a large population-based cohort study. *Eur J Clin Pharmacol, 69*, 269–277. doi 10.1007/s00228-012-1331-5.

Hemmings, H., & Hopkins, P. (2006). *Foundations of anesthesia: basic sciences for clinical practice* (2nd ed.). Philadelphia: Elsevier.

HIV. (2009). *Sourcebook for the primary care provider*. Mountain Plains AIDS Education and Training Center. Retrieved from *www.mpaetc.org.*

Hockenberry, M. J., & Wilson, D. (2007). *Wong's nursing care of infants and children* (8th ed.). St Louis: Elsevier.

Hodgson, B., & Kizior, R. (Eds.), (2012). *Saunders nursing drug handbook 2012*. Philadelphia: Elsevier.

Holst, L., Wright, D., Haavik, S., et al. (2011). Safety and efficacy of herbal remedies in obstetrics—review and clinical implications. *Midwifery, 27*(1), 80–86. doi: 10.1016/j.midw.2009.05.010.

Horowitz, B. Z. *Emergent management of calcium channel blocker toxicity, Medscape reference: drugs, diseases & procedures.* Retrieved from *http://emedicine.medscape.com/article/813485-overview.*

Human Genome Project. *Information*. Retrieved from *www.oml.gov/sci/techresources/Human_Genome/medicine/pharma.*

Indian Health Service. (2012). Retrieved from *www.ihs.gov/PublicInfo/PublicAffairs/Welcome Info/IHSintro.asp/.*

James, J. J., & Lyznicki, J. M. (2010). Biologic agents reference chart: symptoms, tests, and treatment. In E. T. Bope & R. D. Kellerman (Eds.), *Conn's current therapy 2012*. Philadelphia: Elsevier.

Johnson, J. M. (2009). Management of acute cardiogenic pulmonary edema: a literature review. *Adv Emerg Nurs J, 31*(1), 36–43.

Kampman, K. M. (2008). The search for medications to treat stimulant dependence. *Addict Sci Clin Pract, 4*(2), 28–35.

Kee, J. L. (2010). *Laboratory and diagnostic tests with nursing implications* (9th ed.). Upper Saddle River, NJ: Prentice Hall.

Kee, J. L., Marshall, S. M. (2013). *Clinical calculations* (7th ed.). Philadelphia: Elsevier.

Kee, J. L., Paulanka, B., & Polek, C. (2009). *Fluids and electrolytes with clinical applications* (8th ed.). New York: Delmar.

Kinsey, B. M., Jackson, D. C., & Orson, F. M. (2009). Anti-drug vaccines to treat substance abuse. *Immunol Cell Biol, 87*, 309–314.

Knudtson, M. (2009). Osteoporosis: background and overview. *J Nurse Pract, 5*(6, Suppl 1).

Kriebs, J. M., & Gegor, C. L. (2009). *Varney's pocket midwife* (2nd ed.). Boston: Jones & Bartlett.

Kudzma, E., & Carey, E. (2009). Pharmacogenomics: personalizing drug therapy. *Am J Nurs, 109*(10), 50–57.

Languages spoken at home. Retrieved from *www.census.gov/population/cen2000/phc-t20/tab06.xls.*

Laskowski-Jones, L. (2010). Trauma and shock. In J. L. Kee, B. J. Paulanka, & C. Polek (Eds.), *Fluids and electrolytes with clinical applications: a programmed approach* (8th ed.). Clifton Park, NY: Delmar Cengage Learning.

Laskowski-Jones, L. (2013). Care of patients with common environmental emergencies. In D. Ignatavicius & L. Workman

(Eds.), *Medical-surgical nursing: patient-centered collaborative care* (7th ed., pp. 136–154). St. Louis: Elsevier.

Laskowski-Jones, L., & Toulson, K. L. (2013). Concepts of emergency and trauma nursing. In D. Ignatavicius & L. Workman (Eds.), *Medical-surgical nursing: patient-centered collaborative care* (7th ed., pp. 121–135). St. Louis: Elsevier.

Lee, N. M., & Saha, S. (2011). Nausea and vomiting in pregnancy. *Gastroenterol Clin North Am, 40*(2), 309–334. doi: 10.1016/j.gtc.2011.03.009.

Lefever, R. J. (2010). Therapeutic drug monitoring (TDM). In J. L. Kee (Ed.), *Laboratory and diagnostic tests with nursing implications* (9th ed.). Upper Saddle River, NJ: Prentice Hall.

Levine, A. J., & Oren, M. (2009). The first 30 years of p53: growing ever more complex. *Nat Rev Cancer, 9*, 749–758.

Lewis, S. L., Dirksen, S. R., Heitkemper, M. M., et al. (2010). *Medical-surgical nursing: assessment and management of clinical problems* (8th ed.). St Louis: Elsevier.

Lindsay, M., & Burnett, E. (2013). The use of narcotics and street drugs during pregnancy. *Clin Obstetr Gynecol, 56*(1), 133–141.

Liquori, G. (2013). Hemodynamic complications. In J. Neal & J. Rathmell (Eds.), *Complications in regional anesthesia and pain medicine* (2nd ed., pp. 59–71). Philadelphia: Lippincott.

Lowdermilk, D. L., & Perry, S. E. (2011). *Maternity nursing* (8th ed.). St Louis: Elsevier.

Magee, L., & von Dadelsze, P. (2009). The management of severe hypertension. *Semin Perinatol, 33*(3), 138.

March of Dimes. *Caffeine in pregnancy*, March of Dimes Fact Sheet. Retrieved from *www.marchofdimes.com/professionals/14332_1148.asp.*

March of Dimes. *Folic acid*, March of Dimes Fact Sheet. Retrieved from *www.marchofdimes.com/.*

Matthews, A., Dowswell, T., Hassa, D. M., et al. (2010). Interventions for nausea and vomiting in early pregnancy. *Cochrane Database Syst Rev, 9*, CD007575. doi: 10.1002/14651858.CD007575.pub2.

Merlin, M. A., Saybolt, M., Kapitanyan, R., et al. (2010). Intranasal naloxone delivery is an alternative to intravenous naloxone for opioid overdoses. *Am J Emerg Med, 28*, 296–303.

Minkin, M. J., & Gibli, K. (2004). *Manual of management counseling for the preimenopausal and menopausal patient: a clinician's guide.* London: Informa Healthcare.

Mirza, F., & Gaddipati, S. (2009). Obstetric emergencies. *Semin Perionatol, 33*(2), 97.

Mosby's nursing drug reference. (2012). St Louis: Elsevier.

National Academies Press. *Improving birth outcomes: meeting the challenge in the developing world.* Retrieved from *www.nap.ecu/openbook/0309086140/html/243.html.*

National Institute on Drug Abuse. (2007). *Drugs, brains, and behavior—the science of addiction.* Retrieved from *www.drugabuse.gov/science of addiction/brain.html.*

National Research Council. (2013). *Implementing guidelines on weight gain and pregnancy.* Washington, DC: National Academies Press.

Nebivolol (Bystolic) for hypertension. (2008). *Med Lett, 50*(1281), 17–19.

North American Nursing Diagnosis Association. (2009). *Nursing diagnoses: definitions and classifications 2009-2011.* Oxford, UK: Wiley-Blackwell.

Olson, K. R. (2010). Activated charcoal for acute poisoning: one toxicologist's journey. *J Med Toxicol, 6*, 190–198.

Peacock, W. F., Varon, J., Baumann, B. M., et al. (2011). CLUE: a randomized comparative effectiveness trial of IV nicardipine versus labetalol use in the emergency department. *Critical Care, 15*, R157. Retrieved from *www.ccforum.com/content/15/3/R157.*

Polovich, M., Whitford, J., & Olsen, M. (2012). *Chemotherapy and biotherapy guidelines and recommendations for practice* (3rd ed.). Oncology Nursing Society, ONS Publishing Division.

Powers, M. (2010). Performance-enhancing drugs. In J. Houglum, G. Harrelson, & D. Leaver-Dunn (Eds.), *Principles of pharmacology for athletic trainers* (2nd ed.). Thorofare, NJ: Slack.

Powers, M. (2005). Performance-enhancing drugs. In J. Houglum, G. Harrelson, & D. Leaver-Dunn (Eds.), *Principles of pharmacology for athletic trainers.* New York: Thomson Delmar Learning.

Purnell, L., & Paulanka, B. (2008). *Transcultural health care: a culturally competent approach* (3rd ed.). Philadelphia: FA Davis.

Rausch, A. V., Gross, A., Droz, S., et al. (2009). Group B streptococcus colonization in pregnancy: prevalence and prevention strategies of neonatal sepsis. *J Perinat Med, 37*(2), 124.

Rhee, D. J., & Roy, H. (2012). *Medscape reference: Drug-induced glaucoma.* Retrieved from *www.emedicine.medscape.com/article/1205298-overview.*

Sadelain, M., Papapetrou, E., & Bushman, F. (2012). Safe harbours for the integration of new DNA in the human genome. *Nat Rev Cancer, 12*, 51–58, doi:10.1038/nrc3179.

Satia, J. A., Littman, A., Slatore, C. G., et al. (2009). Associations of herbal and specialty supplements with lung and colorectal cancer risk in the Vitamins and Lifestyle Study. *Cancer Epidemiol Biomarkers Prev, 18*, 1419–1428.

Satia, J. A., Littman, A., Slatore, C. G., et al. (2009). Long-term use of beta-carotene, retinol, lycopene, and lutein supplements and lung cancer risk: results from the VITamins and Lifestyle (VITAL) Study. *Am J Epidemiol, 7*, 815–828.

Scott, S. (2011). Personalizing medicine with clinical pharmacogenetics. *Genet Med, 12*, 987–995.

Seo, W. S., & Oh, H. S. (2010). Alterations in Serum Osmolality, Sodium, and Potassium Levels After Repeated Mannitol Administration. *J Neurosci Nurs, 42*(4), 201–207.

Skidmore-Roth, L. (2010). *Mosby's handbook of herbs & natural supplements* (4th ed.). St. Louis: Elsevier.

Soto, E., & Bahado-Singh, R. (2013). Fetal abnormal growth associated with substance abuse. *Clin Obstetr Gynecol, 56*(1), 142–153.

Stargrove, M., Treasure, J., & McKee, D. (2008). *Herb, nutrient and drug interactions: clinical implications and therapeutic strategies.* St. Louis: Elsevier.

Tatro, D. (2009). *Drug interaction facts: The authority on drug interactions.* St Louis: Wolters-Kluwer.

Tehranifar, P., Neugut, A. I., Phelan, J. C., et al. (2009). Medical advances and racial/ethnic disparities in cancer survival. *Cancer Epidemiol Biomarkers Prev, 18*, 2701–2708.

Therapeutic Research Center. (2011). Drugs that cause or exacerbate glaucoma. *Prescriber's Letter.* Retrieved from *prescribersletter.therapeuticresearch.com.*

Therapeutic Research Center. (2009). Drugs treatments for swimmer's ear: an update. *Prescriber's Letter.* Retrieved from *prescribersletter.therapeuticresearch.com.*

Thorpe, B. M. (2009). Integrating osteoporosis prevention and treatment into clinical practice. *J Nurse Pract, 5*(6, Suppl 1), S21–S33.

Tita, A., Rouse, D. (2009). Progesterone for preterm birth prevention: an evolving intervention. *Am J Obstet Gynecol, 200*(3), 219–224.

Tsen, L. (2012). Anesthesia for obstetric care and gynecologic surgery. In D. Longnecker, D. Brown, M. Newman, et al. (Eds.), *Anesthesiology* (2nd ed., pp. 1148–1162). New York: McGraw Hill.

Tsen, L. (2011). Anesthesia for cesarean delivery. In C. Vacont, P. Sikka, R. Urman, et al. (Eds.), *Essential clinical anesthesia* (pp. 751–756). New York: Cambridge University Press.

Tuuri, R. E., Wright, J. L., He, J., et al. (2011). Does Prearrival communication from a poison center to an emergency department decrease time to activated charcoal for pediatric poisoning? *Pediatric Emergency Care, 27*(11), 1045–1051.

U.S. Department of Health and Human Services. (2009). *Guidelines for prevention and treatment of opportunistic infections in HIV-infected adults and adolescents.* Retrieved from *www.cdc.gov/mmwr/preview/mmwrhtml/rr5804a1.htm.*

U.S. Department of Health and Human Services. (2008). *Guidelines for the use of antiretroviral agents in HIV-1 infected adults and adolescents.* Retrieved from *www.cdc.gov/mmwr/preview/mmwrhtml/00054080.htm.*

U.S. Department of Health and Human Services, Centers for Disease Control and Prevention. (2009). *Guide to vaccine contraindications and precautions.* Retrieved from *www.cdc.gov/vaccines/recs/vac-admin/downloads/contraindications_guide.pdf.*

U.S. Food and Drug Administration. (2007). *Carbamazepine prescribing information to include recommendation of genetic test for patients with Asian ancestry.* Retrieved from *www.fda.gov/NewsEvents/Newsroom/PressAnnouncements.*

U.S. Food and Drug Administration. (2011). *FDA drug safety communication: new warnings against use of terbutaline to treat preterm labor.* Retrieved from *www.fda.gov/Drugs/DrugSafety/ucm243539.htm.*

U.S. Food and Drug Administration. (2012). *Approved drug products with therapeutic equivalence evaluations* (32nd ed.). Retrieved from *www.fda.gov/downloads/Drugs/DevelopmentApprovalProcess/UCM071436.pdf.*

U.S. Food and Drug Administration. (2013). *FDA approves Diclegis for pregnant women experiencing nausea and vomiting.* Retrieved from *www.fda.gov/NewsEvents/Newsroom/PressAnnouncements/ucm347087.htm.*

Vance, M. L. (2014). Hypopituitarism. In R. E. Rakel (Ed.), *Conn's current therapy 2014.* Philadelphia: Elsevier.

Von Dadelszen, P., Menzies, J., Payne, B., et al. (2009). Predicting adverse outcomes in women with severe pre-eclampsia. *Semin Perionatol, 33*(3), 152.

Wang, S., Peyrollier, K., & Bourguignon, L. (2007). The influence of hyaluronan-CD44 interaction on topoisomerase II activity and etoposide cytotoxicity in head and neck cancer. *Arch Otolaryngol Head Neck Surg, 133*, 281.

Wells, S., Director of The Genographic Project. (2009). *The human family tree* (television broadcast). New York: National Geographic.

WHO, UNAIDS. (2010). *AIDS epidemic update.* Retrieved from *www.unaids.gov.*

Yarbro, C., Wujcik, D., & Gobel, B., (2010). *Cancer Nursing: Principles and Practice* (7th ed.). Boston: Jones & Bartlett.

Young, R. P., Hopkins, R. J., & Hay, B. A. (2009). A gene-based risk score for lung cancer susceptibility in smokers and ex-smokers. *Post Graduate Med J, 85*, 515–524.

Younkers, K., Wisner, K., Stewart, D., et al. (2009). The management of depression during pregnancy: a report from the American Psychiatric Association and the American College of Obstetricians and Gynecologists. *Gen Hosp Psychiatry, 31*, 403–413.

INDEX

Page numbers followed by *f*, *t*, and *b* indicate figures, tables, and boxes, respectively.

LIST OF FEATURES

Prototype Drug Charts

Nursing Process